Inflammation and Diseases of Connective Tissue

A Hahnemann Symposium

Edited by

LEWIS C. MILLS, M.D.

HEAD, SECTION OF ENDOCRINOLOGY AND METABOLISM,
HAHNEMANN MEDICAL COLLEGE AND HOSPITAL

And

JOHN H. MOYER, M.D.

PROFESSOR AND CHAIRMAN OF
THE DEPARTMENT OF MEDICINE,
HAHNEMANN MEDICAL COLLEGE AND HOSPITAL

W. B. SAUNDERS COMPANY

Philadelphia and London   1961

To

the memory of

JOHN G. BILL

whose devotion to the
health of mankind
nurtured this symposium

*"The measure of a man is not solely what
he contributes to the world, but what
he inspires others to contribute."*

————ROBERTSON

CONTRIBUTORS

HANNA ABU-NASSAR, M.D. Research Fellow in Infectious Diseases, Department of Medicine, Baylor University College of Medicine, Houston, Texas.

KENNETH S. ALLEN. Research Assistant, Department of Medicine, University of Southern California School of Medicine, Los Angeles, California.

D. MURRAY ANGEVINE, M.D. Professor of Pathology and Chairman of Department, University of Wisconsin Medical School, Madison, Wisconsin.

RITSU N. ARISON, Ph.D. Research Associate, Merck Institute for Therapeutic Research, Rahway, New Jersey.

S. HOWARD ARMSTRONG, JR., M.D. Director of Biological Sciences and Medical Education, Cook County Hospital; Professor of Medicine, University of Illinois College of Medicine, Chicago, Illinois.

GLEN E. ARTH, Ph.D. Research Associate, Fundamental Research, Merck Sharp and Dohme Research Laboratories, Rahway, New Jersey.

GUSTAV ASBOE-HANSEN, M.D. Director, Connective Tissue Research Laboratory, University Institute of Medical Anatomy, Copenhagen, Denmark.

PETER BARLAND, M.D. Postgraduate Fellow, National Foundation; Staff, Albert Einstein College of Medicine, Yeshiva University, New York City.

ROBERT J. BARNET, M.D. Research Fellow in Pediatrics, Harvard Medical School; Research Fellow, House of the Good Samaritan (Children's Hospital Medical Center), Boston, Massachusetts.

RAYMOND B. BAYER. Department of Endocrinology, The Upjohn Company, Kalamazoo, Michigan.

J. CLAUDE BENNETT, M.D. Resident in Medicine, University Hospital, Birmingham, Alabama; Fellow in Rheumatic Diseases, Massachusetts General Hospital, Boston, Massachusetts.

DONALD BERKOWITZ, M.D.   Associate, Department of Medicine, Hahnemann Medical College and Hospital, Philadelphia, Pennsylvania.

DAVID L. BERLINER, M.D.   Assistant Research Professor, Department of Anatomy, University of Utah College of Medicine, Salt Lake City, Utah.

ARNOLD BLACK, M.D.   Assistant Professor of Medicine, Chicago Medical School; Chief, Arthritis Clinic, Mount Sinai Hospital, Chicago, Illinois.

ROGER L. BLACK, M.D.   Senior Investigator, National Institute of Arthritis and Metabolic Diseases, Bethesda, Maryland; Clinical Assistant Professor of Medicine, Georgetown University School of Medicine, Washington, D. C.

EDWARD W. BOLAND, M.D.   Clinical Professor of Medicine, University of Southern California School of Medicine; Director of Medicine, St. Vincent's Hospital, Los Angeles, California.

ALFRED J. BOLLET, M.D.   Associate Professor of Internal Medicine and Preventive Medicine, University of Virginia School of Medicine, Charlottesville, Virginia; Markle Scholar in Medical Sciences.

AMEDEO BONDI, Ph.D.   Professor and Chairman, Department of Microbiology, Hahnemann Medical College and Hospital, Philadelphia, Pennsylvania.

BARBARA J. BOWMAN, A.B.   Department of Endocrinology, The Upjohn Company, Kalamazoo, Michigan.

ALBERT N. BREST, M.D.   Associate, Department of Medicine; Director, Hypertension Unit, Hahnemann Medical College and Hospital, Philadelphia, Pennsylvania.

SELWYN BRODY, M.D.   Chief Psychiatrist, Children's Village, Dobbs Ferry, New York.

ERNEST M. BROWN, M.D.   Assistant Professor of Medicine, School of Medicine and Graduate School of Medicine, University of Pennsylvania, Philadelphia, Pennsylvania.

JAMES G. BULGRIN, M.D.   Assistant Professor of Radiology, University of Southern California School of Medicine, Los Angeles, California.

JOSEPH J. BUNIM, M.D., Sc.D.   Clinical Director, National Institute of Arthritis and Metabolic Diseases, National Institutes of Health, Bethesda, Maryland.

GEORGE F. CAHILL, JR., M.D.   Director, Endocrine-Metabolic Unit, Peter Bent Brigham Hospital, Boston, Massachusetts.

BENJAMIN CASTLEMAN, M.D.   Clinical Professor of Pathology, Harvard Medical School; Chief, Department of Pathology, Massachusetts General Hospital, Boston, Massachusetts.

ZEV W. CHAYES, M.D.   Fellow in Endocrinology and Metabolism, Hahnemann Medical College and Hospital, Philadelphia, Pennsylvania.

IRWIN CLARK, Ph.D.   Associate Professor of Biochemistry, Department of Orthopaedic Surgery, Columbia University College of Physicians and Surgeons, New York City.

PHILLIP COMENS, M.D.   Instructor in Medicine, Washington University School of Medicine, St. Louis, Missouri.

GABOR CZONICZER, M.D.   Research Associate in Pediatrics, Harvard Medical School; Associate Research Director, House of the Good Samaritan (Children's Hospital Medical Center), Boston, Massachusetts.

C. WILLIAM DAESCHNER, JR., M.D.   Professor and Chairman, Department of Pediatrics, University of Texas Medical Branch, Galveston, Texas.

WINTHROP N. DAVEY, M.D.   Professor of Internal Medicine, University of Michigan Medical Center, Ann Arbor, Michigan.

BERNARD DEITCH, M.D.   Instructor, Department of Medicine, Hahnemann Medical College and Hospital, Philadelphia, Pennsylvania.

HUGH DEMPSEY, M.D.   Research Fellow, University of Alabama Medical Center; Resident in Medicine, University Hospital, Birmingham, Alabama.

JOSEPH F. DINGMAN, M.D.   Associate Professor of Medicine, Tulane University School of Medicine, New Orleans, Louisiana.

VINCENT D. DI RAIMONDO, M.D.   Assistant Professor of Medicine, University of California Medical Center, San Francisco, California.

WARREN F. DODGE, M.D.   Assistant Professor of Pediatrics, University of Texas Medical Branch, Galveston, Texas.

THOMAS F. DOUGHERTY, Ph.D.   Professor of Anatomy, University of Utah College of Medicine, Salt Lake City, Utah.

ALVIN DUBIN, M.S.   Director of Biochemistry, Cook County Hospital; Assistant Professor of Biochemistry, University of Illinois College of Medicine, Chicago, Illinois.

EDMUND L. DUBOIS, M.D.   Assistant Clinical Professor of Medicine, University of Southern California School of Medicine; Director, Collagen Disease Clinic, Los Angeles County General Hospital, Los Angeles, California.

THOMAS M. DURANT, M.D.   Professor and Chairman, Department of Medicine, Temple University School of Medicine, Philadelphia, Pennsylvania.

GEORGINA FALUDI, M.D.   Research Instructor in Medicine, Hahnemann Medical College and Hospital, Philadelphia, Pennsylvania.

CUTTING B. FAVOUR, M.D.   Professor and Chairman, Department of Preventive Medicine, and Associate Professor of Medicine, Georgetown University School of Medicine; Chief, Georgetown Medical Service, District of Columbia General Hospital, Washington, D. C.

CHARLOTTE I. FERENCZ, M.D.   Assistant Professor of Pediatrics, University of Buffalo School of Medicine; Pediatric Cardiologist, Meyer Memorial Hospital, Buffalo, New York.

EDWARD E. FISCHEL, M.D.   Director, Department of Medicine, The Bronx Hospital; Associate Clinical Professor of Medicine, Albert Einstein College of Medicine, Yeshiva University, New York City.

MAURICE FOX, M.D.   Instructor in Medicine, Vanderbilt University School of Medicine, Nashville, Tennessee.

THOMAS F. FRAWLEY, M.D.   Professor of Medicine and Head of Subdepartment of Endocrinology and Metabolism, Albany Medical College of Union University, Albany, New York.

JOSEF FRIED, Ph.D.   Director, Section of Organic Chemistry, Squibb Institute for Medical Research, New Brunswick, New Jersey.

MORTON FUCHS, M.D.   Assistant Professor of Medicine, Hahnemann Medical College and Hospital, Philadelphia, Pennsylvania.

LEONARD D. GARREN, M.D.   Research Assistant, Department of Medicine, Harvard Medical School, Peter Bent Brigham Hospital, Baker Research Clinic Laboratory, Boston, Massachusetts.

E. MYLES GLENN, Ph.D.   Research Associate, Department of Endocrinology, The Upjohn Company, Kalamazoo, Michigan.

MICHAEL GLYNN, M.D.   Teaching Fellow, Stritch School of Medicine of Loyola University; Resident in Internal Medicine and Research Fellow (Nephritis), Cook County Hospital, Chicago, Illinois.

THOMAS A. GOOD, M.D.   Assistant Professor of Pediatrics, University of Maryland School of Medicine, Baltimore, Maryland.

DAN M. GORDON, M.D.   Assistant Professor (Clinical) of Surgery (Ophthalmology), Cornell University Medical College; Assistant Attending in Surgery, New York Hospital, New York City.

SEYMOUR J. GRAY, M.D., Ph.D.   Associate Professor of Medicine, Harvard Medical School, Boston, Massachusetts.

DAVID HAMERMAN, M.D.   Assistant Professor of Medicine, Albert Einstein College of Medicine, Yeshiva University, New York City.

A. McGEHEE HARVEY, M.D.   Director, Department of Medicine, The Johns Hopkins University School of Medicine and The Johns Hopkins Hospital, Baltimore, Maryland.

S. RICHARDSON HILL, JR., M.D.   Associate Professor of Medicine and Director, Division of Endocrinology and Metabolism, University of Alabama Medical Center, Birmingham, Alabama.

JOSEPH L. HOLLANDER, M.D.   Associate Professor of Medicine, School of Medicine and Graduate School of Medicine, University of Pennsylvania; Chief, Arthritis Section, Hospital of the University of Pennsylvania, Philadelphia, Pennsylvania.

HOWARD L. HOLLEY, M.D.   Professor of Medicine and Chief of Division of Rheumatic Diseases, Medical College of Alabama, Birmingham, Alabama.

HALSTED HOLMAN, M.D.   Professor of Medicine, Stanford University Medical Center, Palo Alto, California. Formerly, Assistant Professor of Medicine, The Rockefeller Institute, New York City.

JOHN M. HOWARD, M.D.   Professor and Chairman, Department of Surgery, Hahnemann Medical College and Hospital, Philadelphia, Pennsylvania.

HARRY J. HURLEY, M.D.   Professor of Dermatology, Hahnemann Medical College and Hospital, Philadelphia, Pennsylvania.

JOSEPH E. IMBRIGLIA, M.D.   Professor and Chairman, Department of Pathology, Hahnemann Medical College and Hospital, Philadelphia, Pennsylvania.

DAVID S. JACKSON, Ph.D.   Assistant Professor of Biochemistry, University of Oregon Medical School, Portland, Oregon; Helen Hay Whitney Research Fellow.

SYLVIA FITTON JACKSON, Ph.D.   Medical Research Council External Staff, Strangeways Research Laboratory, Cambridge, England.

GEORGE JACOBSON, M.D.   Professor of Radiology and Head of Department, University of Southern California School of Medicine; Chief, Department of Radiology, Los Angeles County Hospital, Los Angeles, California.

PIERRE JEAN, M.D.   Research Assistant, Institut de Médicine et de Chirurgie Expérimentales, Université de Montréal, Montréal, Québec, Canada.

DALTON JENKINS, M.D.   Associate Professor of Medicine and Head of Section of Endocrinology, University of Colorado Medical Center, Denver, Colorado.

J. SHEKAR JHAVERI, M.D.   Research Fellow in Pediatrics, Harvard Medical School; Research Fellow, House of the Good Samaritan (Children's Hospital Medical Center), Boston, Massachusetts.

NORMAN B. KANOF, M.D., Med.Sc.D.   Associate Clinical Professor of Dermatology and Syphilology, New York University Post Graduate Medical School, New York University-Bellevue Medical Center, New York City.

MELVIN H. KAPLAN, M.D.   Assistant Professor of Medicine, Western Reserve University School of Medicine; Associate Physician, Cleveland Metropolitan General Hospital, Cleveland, Ohio. Established Investigator, American Heart Association.

VINCENT C. KELLEY, M.D.   Professor of Pediatrics, University of Washington School of Medicine; Director of Research, Children's Orthopaedic Hospital, Seattle, Washington.

MARGARET A. KELSALL, Ph.D.   Director, Laboratory of Tissue Culture, Cleveland Psychiatric Institute and Hospital, Cleveland, Ohio. Formerly, Research Staff (Biology), University of Colorado, Boulder, Colorado.

E. KARL KOIWAI, M.D.   Associate Professor of Pathology, Hahnemann Medical College and Hospital, Philadelphia, Pennsylvania.

DANIEL S. KUSHNER, M.D.   Associate Director of Biological Sciences and Medical Education, Cook County Hospital; Assistant Professor of Medicine, Northwestern University Medical School, Chicago, Illinois.

DANIEL L. LARSON, M.D.   Assistant Professor of Medicine, Columbia University College of Physicians and Surgeons, New York City.

JAMES H. LEATHEM, Ph.D.   Professor of Zoology and Assistant Director, Bureau of Biological Research, Rutgers University, New Brunswick, New Jersey.

STANLEY L. LEE, M.D.   Associate Professor of Medicine, State University of New York Downstate Medical Center; Director, Hematology Division, Maimonides Hospital of Brooklyn, Brooklyn, New York.

GRANT W. LIDDLE, M.D.   Associate Professor of Medicine and Director of Endocrine Service, Vanderbilt University School of Medicine, Nashville, Tennessee.

WILLIAM LIKOFF, M.D. Director, Cardiovascular Section, Department of Medicine, Hahnemann Medical College and Hospital, Philadelphia, Pennsylvania.

L. MAXWELL LOCKIE, M.D. Professor and Head of Department of Therapeutics, University of Buffalo School of Medicine, Buffalo, New York.

BENNET P. LUSTGARTEN, M.D. Visiting Physician, Veterans Administration Hospital, Bronx, New York City.

ABRAHAM MARKOWITZ, Ph.D. Director of Immunochemistry, Hektoen Institute for Medical Research of the Cook County Hospital; Assistant Professor of Biochemistry, University of Illinois College of Medicine, Chicago, Illinois.

DANIEL MASON, M.D. Assistant Professor of Medicine, Hahnemann Medical College and Hospital, Philadelphia, Pennsylvania.

BENEDICT F. MASSELL, M.D. Research Director, House of the Good Samaritan, Children's Hospital Medical Center; Assistant Clinical Professor of Pediatrics, Harvard Medical School, Boston, Massachusetts.

DANIEL J. McCARTY, M.D. Assistant Professor of Medicine, Hahnemann Medical College and Hospital, Philadelphia, Pennsylvania.

ROBERT P. McCOMBS, M.D. Professor of Graduate Medicine, Tufts University School of Medicine; Senior Physician, Pratt Diagnostic Clinic, New England Center Hospital, Boston, Massachusetts.

RAYMOND C. MELLINGER, M.D. Associate Physician, Division of Endocrinology, Henry Ford Hospital, Detroit, Michigan.

*VALY MENKIN, M.D. Professor of Pathology and Chairman of the Department, University of Kansas City School of Dentistry, Kansas City, Missouri.

JOHN P. MERRILL, M.D. Director, Cardiorenal Section, Peter Bent Brigham Hospital; Assistant Professor of Medicine, Harvard Medical School, Boston, Massachusetts.

LEWIS C. MILLS, M.D. Associate Professor of Medicine and Chief, Section of Endocrinology and Metabolism, Hahnemann Medical College and Hospital, Philadelphia, Pennsylvania.

RAYMOND W. MONTO, M.D. Physician-in-Charge, Division of Clinical Hematology, Henry Ford Hospital, Detroit, Michigan.

EVAN R. MORGAN, B.S. Research Assistant, Merck Institute for Therapeutic Research, Rahway, New Jersey.

JOHN H. MOYER, M.D. Professor and Chairman, Department of Medicine, Hahnemann Medical College and Hospital, Philadelphia, Pennsylvania.

HELEN M. MUIR, Ph.D. Medical Unit, St. Mary's Hospital; Research Fellow, Pearl Assurance Company, London, England.

ARNOLD L. NAGLER, Ph.D. Research Fellow in Pathology, New York University Medical Center, New York City.

DAVID H. NEUSTADT, M.D. Instructor in Medicine, University of Louisville School of Medicine, Louisville, Kentucky.

* Deceased.

BENJAMIN NEWMAN, M.D. Resident in Medicine, Hahnemann Hospital, Philadelphia, Pennsylvania.

CHARLES A. NICHOL, Ph.D. Director, Department of Experimental Therapeutics, Roswell Park Memorial Institute; Research Professor of Pharmacology, University of Buffalo Graduate School, Buffalo, New York.

EDWIN M. ORY, M.D. Assistant Professor of Medicine, Baylor University College of Medicine, Houston, Texas.

LAMAR S. OSMENT, M.D. Associate Professor of Dermatology, The Medical College of Alabama, Birmingham, Alabama.

CARL M. PEARSON, M.D. Associate Professor of Medicine, University of California Medical Center, Los Angeles, California.

MAURICE M. PECHET, M.D., Ph.D. Research Associate, Harvard Medical School; Tutor in Biochemical Sciences, Harvard University; Assistant, Massachusetts General Hospital, Boston, Massachusetts.

BURTON J. POLANSKY, M.D. Instructor in Medicine, Boston University School of Medicine; Clinical Associate in Medicine, Boston City Hospital, Boston, Massachusetts.

ABOU D. POLLACK, M.D. Pathologist-in-Chief, Baltimore City Hospitals; Associate Professor of Pathology, The Johns Hopkins University School of Medicine, Baltimore, Maryland.

VICTOR E. POLLAK, M.D. Research Assistant Professor of Medicine, University of Illinois College of Medicine; Research Associate, Hektoen Institute for Medical Research of Cook County Hospital, Chicago, Illinois. Established Investigator, American Heart Association and Illinois Heart Association.

ROBERT E. PRIEST, M.D. Research Assistant Professor of Pathology, University of Washington School of Medicine, Seattle, Washington.

JOHN W. REBUCK, M.D., Ph.D. Physician-in-Charge, Division of Laboratory Hematology, Department of Laboratories, Henry Ford Hospital, Detroit, Michigan.

HOBART A. REIMANN, M.D. Professor of Medicine, Professor and Chairman of Department of Public Health, Hahnemann Medical College and Hospital, Philadelphia, Pennsylvania.

RAFAEL A. RIZEK, M.D. Research Fellow in Hematology, Henry Ford Hospital, Detroit, Michigan.

GERALD P. RODNAN, M.D. Assistant Professor of Medicine and Chief of Section of Rheumatic Diseases, University of Pittsburgh School of Medicine, Pittsburgh, Pennsylvania.

MONROE J. ROMANSKY, M.D. Professor of Medicine, George Washington University School of Medicine; Chief, George Washington Medical Division, District of Columbia General Hospital, Washington, D. C.

GEOFFREY A. ROSE, D.M. Senior Registrar to Medical Unit, St. Mary's Hospital, London, England.

MARILYN L. ROTH, B.A. Department of Orthopaedic Surgery, Columbia University College of Physicians and Surgeons, New York City.

CLARENCE E. RUPE, M.D. Physician-in-Charge, Fourth Medical Division, Henry Ford Hospital, Detroit, Michigan.

DAVID D. RUTSTEIN, M.D. Professor and Head of Department of Preventive Medicine, Harvard Medical School, Boston, Massachusetts.

MARVIN SACKNER, M.D. Resident in Medicine, Philadelphia General Hospital, Philadelphia, Pennsylvania.

ARTHUR L. SCHERBEL, M.D. Head, Rheumatic Disease Department, Cleveland Clinic and Cleveland Clinic Hospital, Cleveland, Ohio.

WILLARD C. SCHMIDT, M.D. Assistant Professor of Pediatrics, Preventive Medicine and Microbiology; Established Investigator of the Helen Hay Whitney Foundation, Western Reserve University School of Medicine, Cleveland, Ohio.

EUGENE SCHUPAK, M.D. Assistant Clinical Instructor in Medicine, Chicago Medical School; Resident in Internal Medicine and Research Fellow (Nephritis), Cook County Hospital, Chicago, Illinois.

BEATRICE CARRIER SEEGAL, M.D. Professor of Microbiology, Columbia University College of Physicians and Surgeons, New York City.

THOMAS F. SHELLEY, M.D. Research Fellow in Medicine, Department of Endocrinology and Metabolism, Albany Medical College of Union University, Albany New York.

WILLIAM B. SHERMAN, M.D. Associate Clinical Professor of Medicine, Columbia University College of Physicians and Surgeons, New York City.

RICHMOND W. SMITH, JR., M.D. Physician-in-Charge, Division of Endocrinology, Henry Ford Hospital, Detroit, Michigan.

WILLIAM A. SODEMAN, M.D. Dean, The Jefferson Medical College and Medical Center, Philadelphia, Pennsylvania.

LOUIS J. SOFFER, M.D. Clinical Professor of Medicine, State University of New York Downstate Medical Center, Brooklyn; Attending Physician and Head of Endocrinology, Mount Sinai Hospital, New York City.

LEON SOKOLOFF, M.D. Chief, Section of Rheumatic Diseases, Laboratory of Pathology and Histochemistry, National Institute of Arthritis and Metabolic Diseases, Bethesda, Maryland.

DAVID M. SPAIN, M.D. Clinical Professor of Pathology, State University of New York Downstate Medical Center; Director of Pathology, Beth El Hospital, Brooklyn, New York.

RAYMOND W. STEBLAY, M.D. Research Associate, Department of Obstetrics and Gynecology, University of Chicago School of Medicine, Chicago, Illinois.

SANFORD L. STEELMAN, Ph.D. Director of Endocrinology, Merck Institute for Therapeutic Research, Rahway, New Jersey.

MALLORY STEPHENS, M.D. Visiting Investigator, Rockefeller Institute; Staff, Albert Einstein College of Medicine, Yeshiva University, New York City. Formerly, Trainee, National Institute of Arthritis and Metabolic Diseases.

HERBERT C. STOERK, M.D. Director of Experimental Pathology, Merck Institute for Therapeutic Research, Rahway, New Jersey.

PAUL B. SZANTO, M.D. Director of Pathology, Cook County Hospital; Professor of Pathology, Chicago Medical School, Chicago, Illinois.

JOHN H. TALBOTT, M.D. Editor, Journal of the American Medical Association, Chicago, Illinois.

CHARLES M. THOMPSON, M.D. Professor of Medicine and Head, Section of Gastro-enterology, Department of Medicine, Hahnemann Medical College and Hospital; Chairman, Department of Medicine B, Philadelphia General Hospital, Philadelphia, Pennsylvania.

WAYNE THORNBURG, Ph.D. Associate Professor of Cytology, Dartmouth Medical School, Hanover, New Hampshire.

SIBYLLE TOLKSDORF, Ph.D. Director, Endocrinology Department, Biological Research Division, Schering Corporation, Bloomfield, New Jersey.

DEMETRIOS TZIROS, M.D. Chief Surgical Resident, Department of Surgery, Hahnemann Medical College and Hospital, Philadelphia, Pennsylvania.

JOHN H. VAUGHAN, M.D. Associate Professor of Medicine and Assistant Professor of Bacteriology (Immunology), University of Rochester School of Medicine and Dentistry and Strong Memorial Hospital, Rochester, New York.

ALFRED VOGL, M.D. Professor of Clinical Medicine, New York University College of Medicine, New York City.

BERNARD M. WAGNER, M.D. Professor and Chairman, Department of Pathology, New York Medical College, New York City.

MAX H. WEIL, M.D., Ph.D. Assistant Professor of Medicine, University of Southern California School of Medicine, Los Angeles, California.

ROBERT I. WISE, M.D. Magee Professor of Medicine and Head of Department, Jefferson Medical College, Philadelphia, Pennsylvania.

ELLARD YOW, M.D. Professor of Medicine, Baylor University College of Medicine, Houston, Texas.

CHRIS J. ZARAFONETIS, M.D. Professor of Clinical and Research Medicine, Temple University Medical Center, Philadelphia, Pennsylvania.

SALVADOR B. ZINGALE, M.D. Fellow, National Council for Technical and Scientific Investigations of the Argentine Republic.

BENJAMIN W. ZWEIFACH, Ph.D. Professor of Pathology, New York University School of Medicine, New York City.

PREFACE

In the not too distant past, the connective tissues of the body received little more than passing interest from investigators in the basic sciences and from clinicians alike; they were regarded merely as supportive tissues of the body and of little relative importance to the function of other apparently more important structures and organs. However, in recent years the recognition and study of the so-called "collagen" diseases has stimulated interest in these tissues, and indeed it has been shown that these tissues are of major importance in the normal body physiology. In addition, the isolation of cortisone and the subsequent synthesis of this compound as well as other chemical substances having a closely related structure have led to intensive investigation of the biochemical alterations in diseases of connective tissues and have provided effective pharmacologic agents for their therapy. However, because the understanding of these processes is still in its infancy, it seemed particularly appropriate to arrange a symposium devoted to a discussion of current aspects of the biochemistry and functions of connective tissues and to the pathogenesis and therapy of the diseases of these tissues. Investigators from the United States and abroad, whose interests ranged from basic biochemistry to clinical management of patients, from immunology and bacteriology to pathology and pharmacology, were invited to contribute to the symposium, which was held in Philadelphia in December 1960. Each investigator presented one or more papers and participated in the panel discussions which followed each series of papers on a given subject. The discussions were transcribed from tape recordings and were edited by the editors of this volume. It was hoped that through this type of program the clinicians might obtain a better understanding of the fundamental abnormalities of these diseases and the basic scientists a greater appreciation of their clinical implications. The biochemical, pathological and immunological abnormalities were discussed at the beginning of the symposium, and it is apparent that much has been learned about these mechanisms. It is also apparent that these mechanisms are extremely complex and that further intensive investigation will be necessary to clarify them. In addition, it appears that many of the immunological phenomena observed in the collagen diseases are not causative factors but rather results of the diseases. It is yet to be determined whether certain of these diseases are actually due to antigen-antibody reactions, although at the present time this is the favored theory.

Subsequently, the participants discussed the pharmacology and metabolic actions of anti-inflammatory steroids. An exciting development was the report that in addition to separation of the sodium and water retaining effects from the anti-inflammatory effect, it may be possible to abolish certain other undesirable properties of the synthetic anti-inflammatory steroids. Of course we must await further confirmatory trials in humans, but the reported data suggest that indeed it may be possible to synthesize an anti-inflammatory steroid which will have minimal effects on other biochemical processes. The development of such a compound would have extremely widespread basic and clinical implications and applications.

In the last two days of the symposium, the use of various anti-inflammatory agents in the therapy of the collagen diseases was discussed. Anti-inflammatory steroids are usually effective in abolishing the acute manifestations in many of these disease processes, but it was disappointing to hear reports of unrelenting progression of joint damage in patients with rheumatoid arthritis and of valvular disease in patients with rheumatic fever. Such reports were counterbalanced at least to some extent by others of the effectiveness of these agents in the treatment of lupus nephropathy, a process thought until recently to be unaffected by steroid therapy. Although there was not complete agreement among the participants about the effectiveness of the steroids, the favorable studies were well controlled and apparently valid. In these studies, the principal determinants of positive response were the high dosage and long duration of steroid therapy; this observation offers hope that more satisfactory results can be obtained in patients with rheumatoid arthritis and rheumatic fever, since in these two diseases therapy usually has been given at minimal dose levels or for only relatively short periods of time.

In addition, the so-called antimalarial compounds appear to offer considerable promise as effective therapeutic agents for certain connective tissue diseases, and the reports on such compounds should stimulate research into the as yet unstudied biochemical abnormalities underlying these conditions. These data also suggest that it may be possible to synthesize other nonsteroidal compounds which may in the end prove to be the agents of choice in the therapy of the collagen diseases.

Finally, some of the undesirable effects of steroid therapy were discussed. Infection, activation of peptic ulcer disease and the development of mental aberrations, as well as many other effects, must always be kept in mind, but it is also apparent that with careful and intelligent use of these compounds and institution of appropriate prophylactic therapy as indicated, the frequency and seriousness of these effects will be greatly reduced.

Even from this brief résumé of a few of the major areas discussed by the participants, it must be apparent that there is still much to be learned. In fact, in many areas only the outward manifestations of a process are presently known; in others we are beginning to understand some of the internal mechanisms, and the excellent presentations of the participants in this symposium are powerful aids to our understanding.

Many other investigators and clinicians are concerned with the problems represented here. We hope that the papers and discussions in this volume will be of interest to them and will serve to stimulate further investigation. We hope that this symposium will also be of value, because of its large number of references to related areas, as a summarizing source of information about connective tissues and their diseases.

LEWIS C. MILLS, M.D. and JOHN H. MOYER, M.D.

CONTENTS

Part I. CURRENT CONCEPTS OF CONNECTIVE TISSUE

Part II.   GENERAL CHARACTERISTICS OF INFLAMMATION

Part III.   IMMUNOLOGY OF INFLAMMATION AND
CONNECTIVE TISSUE DISEASES

Part IV.   ETIOLOGY AND PATHOGENESIS OF COLLAGEN DISEASES

Part V. BIOCHEMISTRY AND PHARMACOLOGY OF
ANTI-INFLAMMATORY STEROIDS

Part VI. EFFECTS OF ANTI-INFLAMMATORY AGENTS ON
THE GENERAL INFLAMMATORY PROCESS

Part VII. THERAPEUTIC USE OF STEROIDS AND OTHER DRUGS IN SPECIFIC INFLAMMATORY STATES

Part VIII. TREATMENT OF OTHER DISEASES

Part IX. EFFECTS OF STEROIDS ON SPECIFIC NEPHROPATHIES

Part X. STEROIDS AND INFECTION

Part XI. UNDESIRABLE EFFECTS OF STEROIDS

Part I | CURRENT CONCEPTS OF
CONNECTIVE TISSUE

Cytological Organization
of Connective Tissues

WAYNE THORNBURG

Dartmouth Medical School

In an earlier day the connective tissues of the body were described in terms of the shape, distribution and staining properties of a few basic elements—the cells, fibers and ground substance. With the hundredfold increase in resolving power that has become available through the use of the electron microscope, the structural picture of these elements has been considerably refined. The resulting progress, however, is more than a matter of descriptive morphology. Many correlations can now be made with biochemical studies, and these are discussed in subsequent papers in this volume. My comments will deal in rather general terms with the various classes of cellular membranes and with their probable role in the cytological organization of connective tissue.

The fibroblast has a plasma membrane, a double nuclear membrane, mitochondria with an outer membrane and an inner convoluted membrane, cytoplasmic membranes which after suitable fixation show attached ribonucleoprotein particles, smooth membranes which probably account for the reticular apparatus seen in classical Golgi preparations, and one or more types of membrane-bound vesicles. All of these membranes appear as black lines in electron micrographs, all of them are about 100 Å thick, and all of them are occasionally resolved as paired black lines. In undamaged sections they are probably always closed curves. Not only do the several membranes of fibroblasts look very much alike, but they also look very much like the corresponding membranes seen in chondrocytes, osteoblasts and almost all other cells of both plants and animals.

These generalities stand in sharp contrast to the vast differences in behavior and function even among those cells which appear to be structurally identical. The dilemma is reinforced by the fact that cells of apparently identical function exhibit, under normal biological conditions, a variety of configurational states. Some of these are the result of external physical and biochemical stimuli which are referred to collectively as biological control systems. Others are undoubtedly a consequence of intrinsic functional cycles. The dilemma also has a practical aspect in that it has probably led to two common mistakes in cytology—the over-classification of cells and the dismissal of significant differences in membrane configuration as mere "biological variability."

With present techniques the structural correlatives of functional specialization can be established in three general ways. The first is through the cytochemical identification of characteristic storage products or secretory products in the cytoplasm. Membrane-bound vesicles have been seen which probably contain the fibrous proteins and polysaccharides destined to form the extracellular components of connective tissue, but beyond this point the cytochemistry of connective tissue cells has not been particularly informative.

3

Secondly, it is possible to make some statistical generalities about the quantity and distribution of cellular membranes. The plasma membrane of fibroblasts, for instance, is thrown into elaborate folds and pseudopod-like processes. Endoplasmic reticulum, which accounts for the cytoplasmic basophilia of most cells, is relatively sparse. Finally, in a growing number of cases, individual macromolecules can be identified directly in electron micrographs of tissue sections. Identification of the collagen molecule from periodic striations in native protofibrils has already contributed importantly to the study of fibrogenesis.

Although there are still many arguments over details, a tentative interpretation of the events in fibrogenesis can be given as follows: The collagen molecule, like many other proteins, is synthesized on the surface of a class of cytoplasmic membranes which is often referred to in the cytological literature as endoplasmic reticulum and in the biochemical literature as the microsomal fraction. These membranes contain the ribonucleoprotein particles which are produced by the nucleus. They provide the genetically determined template on which protein synthesis is ordered. The membranes themselves are probably elaborations of the outermost of the two membranes which enclose the nucleus. After synthesis, the collagen molecules and, by inference at least, all other macromolecules which contribute to the extracellular elements of connective tissue are accumulated into membrane-bound vesicles and transported to the cell surface. Here they are released and either lie directly on the outer surface of the plasma membrane where, under its influence, they become organized into fibrous bundles, or they diffuse into extracellular spaces where, by accretion, they contribute to the maturation of pre-existing structure.

The remarkable motility of the fibroblast, its plasma membrane and all of its organelles has been amply demonstrated by time-lapse photography in both intact tissues and in culture. The gross aspects of connective tissue organization clearly depend upon the movements of these cells and the obscure biological stimuli by which they are controlled. The importance of motility in membranes and organelles can only be presumed. The wavelike activity of the plasma membrane which Lewis[7] described as pinocytosis is of interest in several other respects. There is good evidence that an analogous process (also called pinocytosis) is responsible for the transport of particulate materials[1] through the formation of membrane-bound vesicles which are ten to one hundred times smaller than those originally observed. Various experiments demonstrate that the mechanism may be applicable quite generally to the transport of proteins,[4] small molecules,[2] and even water.[6] Wavelike activity of the plasma membrane may be responsible for the aggregation of precursors on the plasma membrane which Porter and Pappas[10] have observed. Polarization of such waves may account for the very regular patterns of collagen fibers found in some tissues.[12]

The importance of membrane systems leads to a consideration of the structure of membranes themselves. There is little doubt that they contain layers of protein and oriented lipid molecules. These are the relatively stable components which are recovered in biochemical preparations and are preserved by the fixatives used in electron microscopy. Except for differences in the lipid analysis of certain organelles, however, this membrane fraction has so far proved to be rather uninteresting. At least it has not yet provided a structural basis for explaining the numerous different and highly specialized activities of membranes.

The necessary complexity appears to depend, instead, on the more labile elements of membrane structure, elements which are attached through a spectrum of binding energies and are often lost during fixation, centrifugal separation or other preparative procedures. Two pertinent examples are provided by studies on the structured enzyme systems of mitochondria[5] and the nucleoproteins associated with cytoplasmic membranes.[11] In each case a complex function is performed by a specialized molecular structure which in turn appears to be sensitive to configurational changes in the membrane of which it is a part. It also appears that the external surface of the plasma membrane of all cells is associated with some form of structural sugar—in plant cells the celluloses, in yeast and bacteria the zymosans and type-specific polysaccharides, in invertebrates the chitins, in vertebrate epithelial cells the basement membranes, cement substances, mucins, surface antigens, and so on. Under limiting conditions these may be the sugars associated with the cerebroside fraction. The hyaluronic acids and chondroitin sulfates of connective tissue are consistent with this pattern. An extended model for membrane structure is therefore proposed which includes not only the relatively stable lipoprotein framework that appears as black lines in electron micrographs, but also the nucleoproteins, polysaccharides, mucoproteins and adsorbed enzymes which are generally associated with membranes in living cells. Such a model, of course, destroys any nice anatomical definition of a membrane. But so long as nice anatomical models remain there will be little room for speculation which is appropriate to the functional complexity of a structure which is very much alive.

Although the origin of the characteristic fibers and sheets found in elastic tissues is unknown, a theory based upon an analogy with a quite different structure, the stratum lucidum of human skin, is worthy of mention. It was suggested by the fact that the stratum lucidum and the internal elastic lamina of a blood vessel happened to look very much alike in electron micrographs prepared independently by Odland[8] and by Parker.[9] In each case a rather dense and homogenous matrix was seen which seemed to contain some delicate fibrils. There are some other similarities between these structures which might be of interest. The analogy proposed here, however, is restricted to the mechanism of morphogenesis.

The stratum lucidum is a stage in the differentiation of the epithelial cells. In normal subjects it is a coherent, glassy layer about two microns thick which is believed to be the definitive diffusion barrier of the skin.[3] On one side are the normal cells of the malpighian layer; on the other, cornified epithelium. Were it not for the continuity of this membrane in the face of the continual sloughing of epithelial cells it might not have been recognized as a stage in cellular differentiation. Because of the relative rarity of transition stages seen in sections between cells with a full complement of normal organelles and the homogenous band which gives no evidence of its cellular origin, the transition must be comparatively rapid.

There is some evidence that the elusive "elastoblast" is actually a fibroblast which, in addition to its other functions, has been induced to synthesize, store and perhaps secrete the characteristic proteins of elastic tissue. If such cells have as a terminal stage in their morphogenesis prompt transformation into a homogenous material, the cellular origin of the resulting sheets and fibers might well pass undetected. Encouraged by the absence of another satisfactory interpretation, I cautiously propose such a process as the source of elastic fibers and lamellae.

REFERENCES

1. Alksne, J. F.: The passage of colloidal particles through dermal capillary wall under the influence of histamine. Quart. J. Exper. Physiol., 44:51, 1959.
2. Bennett, H. S.: The concepts of membrane flow and membrane vesiculation as mechanisms for active transport and ion pumping. J. Biophys. & Biochem. Cytol., 2(suppl.): 99, 1956.
3. Buettner, K. and Odland, G. F.: Physical factors of the skin barrier layer and water diffusion into human skin. Fed Proc., 16:No. 75, 1957.
4. Chapman-Andresen, C. and Holtzer, H.: The uptake of fluorescent albumin by pinocytosis in Amoeba proteus. J. Biophys. & Biochem. Cytol., 8:288, 1960.
5. Green, D. E.: Electron transport and oxidative phosphorylation. Adv. Enzymol., 21: 73, 1959.
6. Holter, H.: Pinocytosis. Internat. Rev. Cytol., 8:481, 1959.
7. Lewis, W. H.: Pinocytosis. Bull. Johns Hopkins Hosp., 49:17, 1931.
8. Odland, G. F.: The fine structure of the interrelationships of cells in human epidermis. J. Biophys. & Biochem. Cytol., 4:529, 1958.
9. Parker, F.: An electron microscope study of coronary arteries. Am. J. Anat., 103: 247, 1958.
10. Porter, K. R. and Pappas, G. D.: Collagen formation by fibroblasts of the chick embryo dermis. J. Biophys. & Biochem. Cytol., 5:153, 1959.
11. Siekevitz, P. and Palade, G. E.: A cytochemical study of the pancreas of the guinea pig. IV. Chemical and metabolic investigation of the ribonucleoprotein particles. J. Biophys. & Biochem. Cytol., 5:1, 1959.
12. Weiss, P. and Ferris, W.: The basement lamella of amphibian skin. Proc. Nat. Acad. Sc., 40:528, 1954.

Some Biochemical Characteristics

of Connective Tissues

SYLVIA FITTON JACKSON

Medical Research Council Strangeways Research Laboratory, Cambridge, England

The connective and skeletal tissues are concerned throughout the body with the formation and maintenance of structure. They have as a common origin the embryonic mesenchymal cell, which in the course of differentiation forms the connective tissue proper, cartilage and bone. The texture of these tissues depends upon the orientation of the cells, their physical and chemical properties, the spatial organisation of the various constituents with respect to each other and the relative amount of each substance present. The connective tissue cells are required to produce a wide variety of extracellular materials, and according to present knowledge the fundamental assumption has to be made that the same cell is capable of synthesising the various specialised products, either simultaneously or in alternating phases. It is convenient to classify the extracellular moiety into the following phases: (1) the fibrous proteins, collagen and elastin; (2) the acid mucopolysaccharides, usually found as complexes with noncollagenous protein; (3) the neutral or heteropolysaccharides; (4) the interstitial fluids with their content of plasma proteins; and (5) lipid constituents. The composition of these phases will be outlined in the first part of the paper, and the second part will detail certain biochemical characteristics and their resultant structural order in four representative tissues, skin, aorta, compact bone and hyaline cartilage.

EXTRACELLULAR PHASES

Fibrous Proteins.   Native collagen fibres give a typical x-ray fibre diagram[1] and the protein has a characteristic amino acid composition;[14] one-third of the residues are glycine and the two amino acids, proline and hydroxyproline, together account for about two in every nine residues. Most fibrils demonstrate an axial periodicity of about 640 Å,[2] and the diameter of the fibrils varies from about 100 Å to over 1000 Å depending upon the type of tissue from which they are derived. The collagen fibrils are inextensible and they are readily converted to gelatine.

In contrast, elastin gives a poor x-ray fibre diagram; amino acid analyses[45] show that glycine residues constitute about a third of the total, but the content of hydroxyproline is low and the amount of valine is about seven times that in collagen. Electron microscopy has shown that the elastin fibrils are only about 70 Å in diameter and are grouped into bundles visible with the light microscope; axial periodicity is absent[50] but the fibres are highly elastic. Elastin cannot be converted into gelatine.

Considerable information is available on the molecular structure of collagen, but little on that of elastin. Two helical structures for collagen have been proposed;[8, 49, 51] each model is composed of three polypeptic chains, hydrogen-bonded together and forming a coil or major helix. It is not known, however, whether all three polypeptide chains have the same amino-acid composition with a similar sequence of residues along their length, but it is a stereochemical requirement that every third residue along each of the three component minor helices must be glycine. The monomeric unit, termed "tropocollagen,"[21] is now thought to be 2800 Å in length and acts as a rigid rod.[4] Collagen fibres are soluble and under appropriate conditions may be induced to reaggregate into "quarter-stagger" packing arrangements of parallel arrays with all like features in register;[26, 27, 55] the 2800 Å unit thus gives a repeat pattern of 640 Å. The variations in the rate of precipitation with ionic strength and pH indicate that it is controlled to a significant degree by electrostatic interaction between the soluble collagen particles.[64]

The controlling factors involved in the alignment of the macromolecular units into fibrous structures in tissues are not understood. Seven successive stages, however, which have been shown to be concerned in the production and aggregation of the collagen macromolecules in tissues, have been defined and may be regarded as a skeleton of the fibrogenetic processes.[30] In studies of the synthesis of collagen, proline has been established as a major precursor of hydroxyproline in the intact animal[57] and in tissue culture;[32] the evidence suggests that bound, or "activated," hydroxyproline is not synthesised from proline and incorporated with it into collagen as part of a large molecule,[52] but that proline and activated hydroxyproline enter the precollagen molecule as individuals; the first macromolecules synthesised would thus contain both amino acids.[32] Fractionation studies of collagen-producing cells[29] have indicated that such activated hydroxyproline is found in association with cellular particles the size of which is larger than that of the ribosomal particles usually associated with the synthesis of globular proteins. The problems of how the synthesising mechanisms within the cell obtain or receive information about the state and order of the many macromolecules outside the cell and how such information can regulate both synthesis and breakdown require study in the immediate future.

Acid Mucopolysaccharides and Protein: Polysaccharide Complexes. Several types of acid mucopolysaccharide have been identified in various proportions in different tissues and may be divided into two classes:[44] (1) the non-sulphated hyaluronic acid, a glucuronic acid containing acetylglucosamine and glucuronic acid moieties, and chrondroitin, (2) the sulphated mucopolysaccharides, chondroitin sulphates A, B and C, composed of equimolar concentrations of N-acetylgalactosamine, uronic acid and sulphate ester; heparitin sulphate containing equal proportions of glucosamine, uronic acid and sulphate; and lastly, the uronic-acid-free keratosulphate composed of equimolar amounts of N-acetylglucosamine, galactose and sulphate residues. The properties and distribution of these substances will be discussed in detail in the next paper in this volume.

The sequence of mechanisms involved in the synthesis of mucopolysaccharides is not as yet known, but several stages have been identified. The isolation and characterisation of uridine nucleotides containing various carbohydrate moieties[6, 12] and the demonstration of the role of uridine nucleotides in the activation of monosaccharides, as first described by Cardini et al.[7] in the synthesis of sucrose, suggested that such compounds were involved in a general pattern of polysaccharide synthesis.[41] Studies by Dorfman on the biosynthesis of hyaluronic acid have shown that glucose, without previous scission of the molecule, is a direct precursor of both glucosamine and glucuronic acid moieties of hyaluronic acid;[10] an enzyme has been isolated from a strain of Group A Streptococcus and has been shown[41] to be capable of catalyzing the synthesis of this mucopolysaccharide from uridine diphosphoglucuronic acid, incorporated into the glucuronate moiety, and from uridine diphospho-N-acetylglucosamine and N-acetylglucosamine-1-phosphate incorporated into the acetylglucosamine moiety of hyaluronic acid. These authors propose that a mechanism of synthesis may involve a single enzyme with three active sites, chain formation occurring in five sequential steps; such a mechanism "could be extended to explain the formation of more complex chains which contain more than two different monosaccharide units." An alternative mechanism would involve two enzymes, one for the formation of the disaccharide uridine nucleotide and a second for polymerisation of disaccharide units to polymers. No critical evidence is yet available to enable a choice to be made between these mechanisms.[41] In studies of sulphation of mucopolysaccharides, which may be applicable to connective tissues, Suzuki and Strominger have shown that the sulphation of mono-, tri-, penta- and polysaccharides containing terminal N-acetylgalactosamine may be achieved with an enzyme found in a cellular fraction derived from hen oviduct[60] via phosphoadenosine-phosphosulphate labelled with S^{35} as sulphate donor.[59]

Ample evidence is available that the sulphated mucopolysaccharides exist in the tissues as firmly bound complexes with noncollagenous protein;[46, 56] these complexes can be split only with mild acid or alkali[44] or similar disruptive treatment.[40] On the other hand, the bonding is comparatively weak in tissues where protein is in loose complex with nonsulphated mucopolysaccharide.[44] The amino-acid analysis of the protein fraction of the complex found in bovine nasal septa is quite different from that of collagen and is notable for a high tyrosine content; hydroxyproline is absent and proline and glycine are in low concentrations compared with those in collagen.[47]

Physical chemical studies[3, 42] have indicated that the protein polysaccharide complex is composed of macromolecular units of average MW of 4×10^6. The complex isolated from bovine nasal cartilage consists of 45 per cent of the total dry weight of the cartilage, and on degradation at pH 12.4 yields 38 per cent chondroitin sulphate A.[16] The complex may be separated into two major fractions by ultracentrifugation; both fractions contain protein and polysaccharide. The heavier fraction, not necessarily a single component, sediments completely at $10,000 \times g$ and consists of 13 per cent of the total dry weight of the complex; this fraction is composed of roughly equal proportions of protein and polysaccharide. The lighter fraction sediments in a manner indicating a single component and comprises 75 per cent of the total dry weight, consisting of 15 per cent protein and 85 per cent polysaccharide. Gerber et al.[16] point out that these fractions cannot be characterised as chemical individuals at present since preparative procedures might have caused degradation of a native complex, giving the fractions as end products. These data strongly suggest, however, that the sulphated mucopolysaccharide protein complex, possibly itself in loose combination with collagen, must be considered as a component of structural significance in the tissues.

The mechanisms involved in the formation of the protein polysaccharide complex in cartilage are unknown but must involve the synthesis of both moieties, possibly within the same cell; present knowledge of modes of synthesis indicates the extreme complexity of such processes. A recent study[22] of the rate of the simultaneous metabolism of the protein and mucopolysaccharide moieties by means of their specific labelling in rat costal cartilage has shown that there is no difference in the rate of their turnover; the log rates of turnover, however, were not linear with time, which indicates that the metabolic pool of the complex was not homogeneous. Though the rate of turnover is a function of synthesis as well as of degradation, the data suggest that the complex may be metabolised as a unit within the cell, possibly in the basic molecular form of MW 4×10^6, and thence extruded into the matrix where further aggregation may take place. These studies are of interest since it has been pointed out[27] that alterations in the normal pattern of cellular synthesis in connective tissues could lead to the production of abnormal forms of extracellular substances; employment of similar methods used in these experiments in conjunction with studies of cellular fractions would clearly aid in the elucidation of many problems.

Heteropolysaccharides. Small but significant amounts of heteropolysaccharides,[9] which do not contain hexuronic acid or sulphate residues, are present in the extracellular regions and can be distinguished from the plasma proteins. The functional significance of these substances is not known.

Interstitial Fluid. The large macromolecular components detailed above, which form the two main extracellular phases, are bathed in interstitial fluid. This substance contains matter of low molecular weight such as amino acids, simple sugars, peptides, nucleotides, and precursor and degradation products of the other phases. In addition, free electrolytes and considerable quantities of soluble tyrosine-rich globular proteins, such as those from plasma, are present. It should be mentioned that it is improbable that the interstitial fluid is in a free fluid state, but rather in colloidal suspension.

Lipid Constituents. Small amounts of lipid have been found in association with both collagen and elastin fibres,[54] but since most of the analytical work in the connective tissue field has been based on fat-free material, little information is as yet available.

TISSUE CHARACTERISTICS

Skin. The chief component of the epidermis of skin is formed by the insoluble fibrous protein keratin; the main fibrous component of the dermis, however, is collagenous protein, and the small proportion of about 3 per cent elastin is considered to be responsible for the compliance of the tissue. The content of dermal mucopolysaccharide is less than 10 per cent and three types have been clearly identified in pig skin:[44] chondroitin sulphate B (the L-iduronic acid containing mucopolysaccharide[58] designated dermatin sulphate by Jeanloz and Stoffyn[33]), hyaluronic acid and small amounts of chondroitin sulphate C; some keratosulphate may also be present. In calf skin Bowes et al.[5] have recorded that between 2 and 10 per cent of a noncollagenous protein can be extracted, the amount depending upon age, pH and temperature; the removal of this fraction appears to parallel a decrease in the cohesion of the skin. In view of the spreading factor first noted by Duran-Reynals[11] it should be mentioned that whereas hyaluronic acid is hyaluronidase labile, the main mucopolysaccharide of skin, chondroitin sulphate B, is resistant to this enzyme.[44]

In general, studies of aging have indicated a decrease of total mucopolysaccharide per unit dry weight, chronological age being coincident with an increase in collagen content. Meyer et al.[44] have found that in the skin of embryonic pigs close to term the total content of mucopolysaccharide is much higher than in adults, there being a marked diminution of hyaluronic acid and an increase of chondroitin sulphate B with age; the analyses show that the ratio of these substances in the embryo is 0.20, whereas in the adult it is 1.25. Comparable figures for collagen content are unfortunately not available.

Cold neutral-salt extracts of connective tissue are thought to represent a stage in fibrogenesis that precedes the formation of collagen fibrils. It is of interest, therefore, that such a collagen fraction cannot be extracted from tissues of the normal chick embryo of about 17 days incubation;[39] this result suggests that in rapidly developing connective tissue the transformation of collagen macromolecules into fibrils may occur at such a rate that the "free" macromolecules are not available for extraction or are no longer labile to the ionic environment of neutral salts. On the other hand, studies[19] on the formation of collagen in the dermis of young growing guinea pigs, where collagen formation may occur at a slower rate, have shown that about 10 per cent of the total collagen is extracted by neutral salts, the amount extracted varying directly with growth rate. Other studies on the aging of collagen have demonstrated increased lateral bonding in mature fibrils.[20]

Human Aorta. Vascular tissue, such as human aorta, is composed chiefly of elastic fibres which constitute more than 50 per cent of the dry weight in an adult of 26 years.[62] The elastic fibres are closely associated with collagen fibrils (20 per cent of the unit dry weight) and are disposed in a wickerwork pattern about the circumference of the blood vessels, this arrangement being largely responsible for the physical properties of the tissue. Four mucopolysaccharide fractions have been identified by Kaplan and Meyer,[37] and their total content and galactosamine to glucosamine ratios, expressed as chondroitin sulphate C plus B to hyaluronic acid plus heparitin sulfate were constant throughout all stages studied. At least equal quantities of noncollagenous protein have been found in association with the mucopolysaccharides,[62] and the amount of plasma proteins and neutral sugars is of the order of 10 per cent in the tissue. Two of the mucopolysaccharides isolated, namely, chondroitin sulphate B and heparitin sulphate, have anticoagulant properties[23] equivalent to between 1 and 4 per cent heparin activity.[38, 65]

The familiar histological pattern of aging in the human aorta is striking. In a study[62] of material obtained from patients in an age range of 8 to 86 years, it has been found that the elastin content per unit dry weight remains approximately constant, but that the relative amount of collagen decreases with age; these data, however, do not demonstrate local changes in density of the fibrous components. The mineral that is deposited with age in the aorta has been shown to be associated with the elastic fibres as opposed to the collagen fibres, and the deposition increases from approximately 0.1 per cent at age 21 to 28.2 per cent per unit dry weight at age 86.[63] The mineral has been identified as a hydroxyapatite similar to that which occurs in bone, but a preferred orientation of the crystals in relation to the elastic fibres has not been observed. Quantitative changes in the relative amounts, but not in types, of individual mucopolysaccharides have been reported by Kaplan and Meyer[37] in an examination of seven age groups ranging from 21 to 72 years. Increased amounts of chondroitin sulphate B (8 to 15 per cent) and heparitin sulphate (6 to 21 per cent) were noted, and reductions occurred in the quantities of hyaluronic acid (20 to 12 per cent) and of chondroitin sulphate C (66 to 52 per cent). These alterations were accompanied by an increase in the degree of atherosclerosis. As mentioned previously, the total content of mucopolysaccharide remains constant. The authors have suggested that these complex alterations in pattern not only may be due to age changes *per se,* but also may reflect simultaneous degenerative and reparative processes.

Compact Bone. In compact bone, at least 95 per cent of the organic matter is formed of collagen fibres.[13] Analyses have shown that mucopolysaccharides are present in amounts not much exceeding 0.5 per cent per unit dry weight,[53] and in these, chondroitin sulphate A, hyaluronic acid and keratosulphate have been identified.[43] Small amounts of heteropolysaccharides have been isolated,[9] and a protein moiety with an amino-acid composition altogether different from that of collagen is also present.[13] The mineral phase of bone constitutes about 70 per cent of the total dry weight and is found as a hydroxyapatite. The suggestion has been made that the epsilon amino groups of the lysine component of the collagen fibrils act as initial sites for nucleation of the apatite crystals,[17] and evidence obtained from the examination of sections of embryonic bone viewed in the electron microscope indicates that individual apatite particles are organised precisely within and in relation to the periodic structure of the newly formed collagen fibrils;[28] this precise localization may have a bearing on the subsequent alignment of the apatite crystals in relation to the collagen fibrils[31] as demonstrated by x-ray diffraction.[15] Such an intimate relation between the individual collagen fibrils and the mineral phase, and the varying orientation of the collagen fibres, are means of providing the requisite strength of bone without unnecessary weight.

Hyaline Cartilage. On the other hand, cartilage is a supporting tissue with a firm, resilient matrix combining rigidity with flexibility. These characteristics of cartilage have been attributed to its high concentration of protein-polysaccharide complex mentioned earlier, which may constitute as much as half the dry weight of the tissue.[40] About 35 per cent of it is collagen. The analyses that are available on the gross total of constituents in cartilage show that the amounts of different substances vary considerably from tissue to tissue, from species to species and with age. In further contrast to bone, the quantity of substances of low molecular weight flowing through the matrix may be considerable;[35] the matrix, however, may be impermeable to substances of high molecular weight, since Paulson et al.[48] have provided evidence which suggests that the free pore size in the cartilage of nucleus pulposus is only of the order of 10 to 15 Å.

Kaplan and Meyer[36] have demonstrated that profound changes occur in the mucopolysaccharide fraction of human costal cartilage during aging. The total amount of chondroitin sulphate present decreases linearly with age; in infants this fraction occurs exclusively as chondroitin sulphate A, but in adults it appears predominantly as type C. Keratosulphate is absent in infants, negligible in amount in the very young, but increases linearly with age to a plateau which even in senescence appears to be maintained at about 50 per cent of the total mucopolysaccharide present. These alterations in amount as well as in type of mucopolysaccharide suggest that considerable changes must occur in the structural organisation of the cartilage matrix and that certain other changes, as yet unknown, occur which enable the cells to synthesise different specialised products. Enzymes which degrade chondroitin sulphate, which is often the predominent mucopolysaccharide in cartilage, have not yet been isolated, but a loss in structural integrity in the cartilage of rabbit ears following intravenous injection of papain has been demonstrated by Thomas;[61] the effect is believed to be due to the direct enzymatic action of papain on the protein polysaccharide complex, since the chondroitin sulphate fraction is released from the cartilage.

A study[34] of the protein polysaccharide complex in human costal cartilage has shown that the proportion of protein to mucopolysaccharide varies rather widely in different individuals, but the total complex represents about 35 per cent of the dry weight of the tissue. The complex has been fractionated by ultracentrifugation, and 50 per cent of the complex is separated into one light and one heavy fraction, such as those found in bovine nasal cartilage and discussed earlier in this paper, but the relative proportion of the light fraction is greatly reduced. In costal cartilage the light and heavy fractions contain 21 per cent and 66 per cent of noncollagenous protein, respectively, whereas in the nasal cartilage these fractions contain 15 per cent and 50 per cent, respectively. It is thus apparent that certain distinct differences occur in the relative proportions of two main constituents of the protein polysaccharide complex in these cartilages from different sources. These authors point out that recent improvements in technique in the isolation and fractionation of these complexes should aid in studies of the changes that may occur in total amount and condition of the complex in the cartilage of rheumatic patients.

A review of the biochemical characteristics of the tissues which have been outlined in this paper emphasises the enormous complexity of the connective tissue constituents and their interrelationship with and interdependence on each other. Many abnormalities in connective tissue diseases may be due to intracellular changes occurring secondarily perhaps to extracellular damage. Thus, studies of how damage to extracellular constituents is related to intracellular synthetic sites may help to elucidate some of the problems concerned in the cellular response to inflammation and disease of connective tissue.

REFERENCES

1. Astbury, W. T.: Proc. Roy. Soc. B. Lond., *134*:303, 1947.
2. Bear, R. S.: Adv. Prot. Chem., 7:69, 1952.
3. Bernardi, G.: Nature, Lond., *186*:93, 1957.
4. Boedtker, H. and Doty, P.: J. Am. Chem. Soc., *78*:4267, 1956.
5. Bowes, J. H., Elliot, R. G. and Moss, J. A.: In Connective Tissue. C.I.O.M.S., 1957, p. 264.
6. Cabib, E. L., Leloir, L. F. and Cardini, C. E.: J. Biol. Chem., *203*:1055, 1953.
7. Cardini, C. E., Leloir, L. F. and Chiribogo, J.: J. Biol. Chem., *214*:149, 1955.
8. Cowan, P. M., McGavin, S. and North, A. C. T.: Nature, Lond., *176*:1062, 1955.
9. Dische, Z., Danilezenko, A. and Zelmenis, G.: In Chemistry and Biology of Mucopolysaccharides. Ciba Foundation Symposium, 1958, p. 116.
10. Dorfman. A.: Pharmacol. Rev., 7:1, 1955.
11. Duran-Reynals, F.: Bact. Rev., 6:197, 1942.
12. Dutton, G. J. and Storey, F. D. E.: Biochem. J., *57*:275, 1954.
13. Eastoe, J. E.: In Bourne, G. H. (ed.): The Biochemistry and Physiology of Bone. New York, Academic Press, 1956, p. 81.
14. Eastoe, J. E. and Leach, A. A.: In Stainsby, W. (ed.): Recent Advances of Gelatine and Glue Research. New York, Pergamon Press, 1957, p. 173.
15. Engstrom, A. and Zetterstrom, R.: Exper. Cell Res., 2:268, 1951.
16. Gerber, B. M., Franklin, E. C. and Schubert, M.: J. Biol. Chem., *235*:2870, 1960.
17. Glimcher, M. J.: Rev. Mod. Phys., *31*:359, 1959.
18. Gross, J.: J. Exper. Med., *107*:247, 1958.
19. Gross, J.: J. Exper. Med., *107*:265, 1958.
20. Gross, J.: Nature, *181*:556, 1959.
21. Gross, J., Highberger, J. H. and Schmitt, F. O.: Proc. Nat. Acad. Sc., *40*:679, 1954.
22. Gross, J. I., Mathews, M. B. and Dorfman, A.: J. Biol. Chem., *235*:2889, 1960.
23. Grossman, B. J. and Dorfman, A.: Pediatrics, *20*:506, 1957.
24. Hass, G. M.: Arch. Path., *35*:19, 1943.
25. Harkness, R. D., Marko, A. M., Muir, H. M. and Neuberger, A.: Biochem, J., *56*:558, 1954.
26. Hodge, A. J. and Schmitt, F. O.: Proc. Nat. Acad. Sc., *44*:418, 1958; *46*:186, 1960.
27. Jackson, S. Fitton: Proc. 3rd Internat. Congr. Clin. Path., 1957, p. 697.
28. Jackson, S. Fitton: Proc. Roy. Soc. B. Lond., *146*:270, 1957.
29. Jackson, S. Fitton: In Roberts (ed.): Microsomal Particles and Protein Synthesis. New York, Pergamon Press, 1958, p. 121
30. Jackson, S. Fitton: In Nicholson (ed.): Bone as a Tissue. New York, McGraw-Hill Book Co., 1960, p. 165.
31. Jackson, S. Fitton and Randall, J. T.: Nature, Lond., *178*:798, 1956.
32. Jackson, S. Fitton and Smith, R. H.: J. Biophys. & Biochem. Cytol., 3:897, 1957.
33. Jeanloz, R. W. and Stoffyn, P. J.: Fed. Proc., *17*:249, 1958.
34. Johnson, B. and Schubert, M.: J. Clin. Invest., *39*:1752, 1960.
35. Joseph, N. R., Catchpole, H. R., Laskin, D. M. and Engel, M. B.: Arch. Biochem., *84*:224, 1959.
36. Kaplan, D. and Meyer, K.: Nature, Lond., *183*:1267, 1959.
37. Kaplan, D. and Meyer, K.: Proc. Soc. Exper. Biol. & Med., *105*:78, 1960.
38. Kirk, J. E.: Nature, Lond., *184*:309, 1959.
39. Levene, C. I. and Gross, J.: J. Exper. Med., *110*:771, 1959.
40. Malawista, I. and Schubert, M.: J. Biol. Chem., *230*:535, 1958.
41. Markovitz, A., Cifonelli, A. and Dorfman, A.: J. Biol. Chem., *234*:2343, 1959.
42. Mathews, M. B. and Lozaityte, I.: Arch. Biochem., *74*:158, 1958.
43. Meyer, K.: In Bone Structure and Metabolism, Ciba Foundation Symposium, 1956, p. 65.
44. Meyer, K., Hoffman, P. and Linker, A.: In Connective Tissue. C.I.O.M.S., 1957, p. 86.
45. Partridge, S. M. and Davis, H. F.: Biochem. J., *61*:21, 1955.
46. Partridge, S. M. and Davis, H. F.: In Chemistry and Biology of Mucopolysaccharides, Ciba Foundation Symposium, 1958, p. 93.

47. Partridge, S. M. and Davis, H. F.: Biochem. J., 68:298, 1958.
48. Paulson, S., Sylvan, B., Hirsch, C. and Snellman, O.: Biochim. et biophys. acta, 7: 207, 1951.
49. Ramachandran, J. and Kartha, G.: Nature, Lond., 174:369, 1954.
50. Rhodin, J. and Dalhamn, T.: Exper. Cell Res., 9:371, 1955.
51. Rich, A. and Frick, F. C. H.: Nature, Lond., 176:915, 1955.
52. Robertson, van B., Hewett, J. and Herman, C.: J. Biol. Chem., 234:105, 1959.
53. Rogers, H. J.: Nature, Lond., 164:625, 1949.
54. Saxl, H.: Gerontologia, 1:142, 1957.
55. Schmitt, F. O.: Proc. Nat. Acad. Sc. U. S., 42:806, 1956.
56. Shatton, J. and Schubert, M.: J. Biol. Chem., 211:565, 1954.
57. Stetten, M. R.: J. Biol. Chem., 181:31, 1949.
58. Stoffyn, P. J. and Jeanloz, R. W.: J. Biol. Chem., 235:250, 1960.
59. Suzuki, S. and Strominger, H. L.: J. Biol. Chem., 235:257, 1960.
60. Suzuki, S. and Strominger, H. L.: J. Biol. Chem., 235:267, 1960.
61. Thomas, L.: J. Exper. Med., 104:245, 1956.
62. Weissmann, G.: Unpublished results.
63. Weissmann, G. and Weissmann, S. J.: J. Clin. Med., 39:1657, 1960.
64. Wood, G. C. and Keech, M. K.: Biochem. J., 175:588, 1960.
65. Yu, S. Y. and Blumenthal, H. T.: J. Gerontol., 13:366, 1958.

Sulphated Polysaccharides of Connective Tissue

HELEN MUIR

Medical Unit, St. Mary's Hospital, London, England

The ground substance of connective tissue contains several similar acidic polysaccharides which are, however, chemically quite distinct and are probably synthesised by different enzymes. It seems likely that these polysaccharides have different functions because they are not evenly distributed in connective tissue[47] and their proportions change with age, although they are apparently all linear unbranched polymers containing hexosamine and another sugar, usually uronic acid, arranged alternately. Apart from hyaluronic acid and chondroitin of cornea, the connective tissue polysaccharides are all sulphate esters and are therefore highly charged polyanions, which show considerable interaction with themselves and with proteins and which also bind salts and water to a marked degree. The coiling and extension of such polyanions are greatly influenced by the ionic strength,[41, 43] so that water or salt depletion of a tissue should alter the characteristics of its ground substance. Furthermore, in the native state, the polysaccharides of connective tissue are probably all combined with noncollagenous protein[53, 54] forming very large complex molecules with molecular weights of several million.[44] When one considers their functions, all these properties must be considered, and also the fact that the ground substance contains other soluble proteins with which the polysaccharides can interact. Some of these proteins are probably identical with plasma proteins even though they are not in metabolic equilibrium with them.[20, 29] The importance of these polysaccharides to the physical behaviour of connective tissue, such as its resistance to compression, has been pointed out by Fessler;[15] hence, relatively small changes in structure are likely to lead to appreciable changes in the behaviour of connective tissue. Chondroitin sulphate is the most widely distributed sulphated polysaccharide and its macromolecular structure alone has so far been studied. In the native state it probably all exists as a protein complex with a molecular weight of several million, whose physical properties are not at all like that of the free polysaccharide, whose molecular weight is only about 50,000. Furthermore, these complexes can form large aggregates with molecular weights of fifty million,[44] which must influence considerably the properties of such tissue as cartilage where there is a high concentration of chondroitin sulphate combined with a noncollagenous protein.[40, 65] This protein is attacked by papain both *in vitro*[52, 53, 57] and *in vivo*, and by streptokinase-activated plasminogen.[35]

In vivo papain causes chondroitin sulphate to be leached out of cartilage matrix of rabbits[45, 67, 71, 72] and to appear in the blood and in the urine,[3] which normally contain only very small amounts. Papain also decreases the polysaccharide content of rabbit aorta,[17] and repeated injections of papain into suckling rats produces a chondrodysplasia in which the whole skeleton develops abnormally.[46] It is noteworthy that in hereditary deforming chondrodysplasia, affected individuals in two families that have been studied excreted large quantities of chondroitin sulphate.[39] It therefore seems that integrity of the protein moiety is important in retaining chondroitin sulphate in the tissues and is essential for the high viscosity of the complex, which contains only about 10 per cent protein,[53] and which appears to be metabolised as a single unit, since labelled lysine and sulphate were found to have the same turnover rates.[18] It is possible that natural proteases of the body, such as plasmin, may be involved in pathological processes by causing dissolution of chondroitin sulphate by breakdown of the protein moiety. Cell-free extracts of rheumatoid synovial membranes have been found to decrease the viscosity of chondroitin sulphate complexes, while extracts of uninflamed membranes do not.[74]

The shape of the molecule of the complex of chondroitin sulphate A has been shown by Mathews[44] to be quite unlike that of hyaluronic acid, which behaves as a long, randomly kinked coil, well suited to act as a lubricant.[15] The chondroitin sulphate complex, on the other hand, consists of a protein backbone to which are attached laterally about 60 chondroitin sulphate chains, whose mutual electrical repulsion, due to charged sulphate groups, lends rigidity to the molecule, which behaves as a rigid rod.[44] The chondroitin sulphate chains are not looped but attached at one point only.[57] The protein-carbohydrate link of chondroitin sulphate A complexes from both cartilage and aorta appears to be a weak covalent bond which, like an ester, is irreversibly disrupted by dilute alkali,[53, 54] after which protein-free chondroitin sulphate can be isolated. This bond resists attack by a variety of proteolytic enzymes, because even after prolonged proteolysis a peptide fragment remains attached to chondroitin sulphate which can be removed by dilute alkali in the same way as the protein of the whole complex.[53] Different enzymes could attack these complexes at the peptide, glycoside and protein-carbohydrate bonds.

The protein moiety of the complexes of different connective tissue polysaccharides may not be the same, nor may they have the same shape, so that although the free sulphated polysaccharides are alike in many respects, their protein complexes may be very different, and this may explain why they are not evenly distributed in different tissues and why their proportions change with age and disease. In support of this view it has been found that chondroitin sulphate A and B from aorta after prolonged proteolysis retained peptide fragments which had different amino acid patterns.[55]

The chemical structures of those sulphated polysaccharides that have so far been established have been determined mainly as a result of the work of Meyer and his co-workers. It is only in the last few years that the structural differences between the three chondroitin sulphates have been finally determined, although chondroitin sulphate was first isolated in 1861. Chondroitin sulphates A and C are often found together in cartilage. The rib cartilage of the newborn contains chondroitin sulphate A, but in the adult it is replaced largely by chondroitin sulphate C,[47] although there is a progressive decrease throughout life of chondroitin sulphate in this cartilage.[33] Chondroitin sulphates A and C have identical carbohydrate chains, consisting of alternate galactosamine and glucuronic acid units linked by β-glycosidic bonds, at the same positions on the monosaccharide components.[9, 11, 23, 24, 26, 27] However, the two polysaccharides have different *infra* red spectra at certain frequencies associated with the sulphate group.[24, 56] The differences disappear when the sulphate groups are removed.[24] The *infra* red spectra of chondroitin sulphates A and B do not differ in this region,[42] and as Jeanloz and his co-workers[31] have proved that the sulphate group is situated on C_4 of the galactosamine moiety of chondroitin sulphate B, it is concluded that it is also at this position in chondroitin sulphate A, which leaves C_6 of the galactosamine as the only available alternative for the sulphate group in chondroitin sulphate C. Thus, chondroitin sulphates A and C differ only in the relative positions of their sulphate groups.

Chondroitin sulphate B, however, differs from chondroitin sulphate A in containing iduronic acid in place of glucuronic acid,[6, 22, 30] in which C_5 has the opposite configuration; but there appear to be no other structural differences.[26] However, this makes chondroitin sulphate B resistant to hyaluronidase, which attacks chondroitin sulphates A and C.[47] Chondroitin sulphate B is the chief sulphated polysaccharide of adult skin, replacing chondroitin sulphate C of embryonic skin,[37] but in adult rib cartilage chondroitin sulphate C replaces A,[47] and so a particular chondroitin sulphate cannot be associated with immaturity.

The corneal polysaccharide chondroitin discovered by Meyer[10] is considered to be the same polysaccharide as chondroitin sulphates A or C but lacking the sulphate groups.

Besides these closely related compounds, considerable quantities of keratosulphate are present in cornea,[51, 73] nucleus pulposus,[16] rib cartilage,[49] a small amount in the aorta,[4] and it may also be present in small amounts elsewhere. Keratosulphate is made up of disaccharide units like chondroitin sulphate but contains glucosamine in place of galactosamine and galactose in place of uronic acid.[51] The sulphate groups are situated on C_6 of the hexosamine residues, as they are in chondroitin sulphate C, and the hexosamine amino groups are also similarly acetylated, while the glycosidic bonds likewise have the β-configuration[21, 61] but are not susceptible to the enzymes which break down the chondroitin sulphates. The metabolic behaviour of keratosulphate in the ageing process appears to be different from that of chondroitin sulphate. In intervertebral discs the relative proportion of keratosulphate increases with age[19] while that of chondroitin sulphate decreases. In herniated discs the total polysaccharide is greatly reduced, but the loss of chondroitin sulphate is greater than the loss of keratosulphate.[12] In Marfan's syndrome there is an increased excretion of chondroitin sulphate, and the rib cartilage contains more than the normal amount of keratosulphate.[2]

Heparin is probably not strictly an extracellular component of connective tissue. Although it is reported to be present in appreciable quantities in rat skin,[63] it probably arises from the numerous mast cells that are present. However, sulphated polysaccharides that appear to be structurally related to heparin, containing glucosamine and glucuronic acid,[26, 32, 36] have been found in several tissues.[5, 32, 36, 62] These compounds vary in optical rotation and in acetyl and sulphate content, which is much less than that of heparin.[25] It is not possible to decide yet whether they are distinct compounds or mixtures. They appear also in certain pathological conditions such as liver amyloid[47] and in quantity in the organs and urine of patients with Hurler's syndrome,[13, 38, 48, 50] when they are often accompanied by chondroitin sulphate B. If it is assumed that a single gene is involved in the abnormality, then a very early stage in the biosynthesis of these dissimilar polysaccharides must be affected, since they contain different hexosamines and uronic acids namely, glucosamine and glucuronic acid in the heparin derivative and galactosamine and iduronic acid in chondroitin sulphate B. Furthermore, the monosaccharide residues are probably linked in each case by sterically opposite glycosidic bonds. Since chondroitin sulphate A and C do not appear to be involved in the abnormality, these may be synthesised by a different pathway. This suggestion is supported by a recent finding that enzymes that synthesise glucosamine-6-phosphate from hexose-6-phosphate and glutamine were not found in some tissues (such as cartilage, nucleus pulposus and arterial wall) that are known to synthesise polysaccharides.[58] In these tissues there may be another source of hexosamine.

The uptake of radioactive sulphate has been used extensively to indicate synthesis of sulphated polysaccharides, both *in vivo* and *in vitro*. It has been shown by Schiller and her co-workers,[64] using two labels simultaneously, that the sulphate and carbohydrate chain of chondroitin sulphate B of skin turn over at the same rate, so that the sulphate group, in this instance, does not exchange independently. However, Strominger[68] has recently shown that hen oviduct contains enzymes which can transfer inorganic sulphate to preformed polysaccharides, such as sulphated and desulphated chondroitin sulphates A, B and C. Similar enzymes appear to be present in rabbit skin.[8] Meyer had previously postulated that corneal chondroitin might be a precursor of chondroitin sulphate, but attempts to show this had failed.[1] However, chondroitin may not be an obligatory intermediate since monosaccharides and oligosaccharides can also act as sulphate acceptors, although the velocity of the reaction increases with chain length.[69] These results make it necessary to treat with caution conclusions drawn from experiments in which radioactive sulphate uptake alone is assumed to imply *de novo* polysaccharide synthesis, as exchange reactions could account for much of the incorporated radioactivity. Furthermore, although cartilage slices show a vigorous uptake of radioactive sulphate when incubated in Kreb's buffer, there is an over-all breakdown of chondroitin sulphate.[7] The sulphate transferred by Strominger's enzyme system[70] is not evenly distributed along the carbohydrate chain as some oligosaccharides could be obtained which possessed more than one sulphate group per hexosamine and others less than one, so that analysis of the whole polymer represents a statistical average. Such an uneven distribution of sulphate might explain the variable sulphate content of the polysaccharides related to heparin discussed above.

Mixtures of polysaccharides obtained from connective tissue are difficult to separate quantitatively, but work so far carried out shows that they not only behave differently in the ageing process but are differently influenced by hormones[14] and deficiencies. Ascorbic acid deficiency depresses chondroitin sulphate synthesis but not that of hyaluronic acid.[28, 34, 59, 60, 66] Since the connective tissue polysaccharides have different chemical structures, it would be surprising if their metabolic behaviour were the same, and each may also behave differently in different sites in the body under hormonal and other influences. It is thus clear that further understanding of their function awaits reliable quantitative methods of separating them.

REFERENCES

1. Adams, J. B.: Biochim. et biophys. acta., *32*:559, 1951.
2. Berenson, G. S. and Serra, M. T.: Fed. Proc., *18*:190, 1959.
3. Bryant, J. H., Leder, I. G. and Stetten, D.: Arch. Biochem. Biophys., *76*:122, 1959.
4. Buddecke, E.: (1960). Hoppe-Seyl. Ztschr., *318*:33, 1960.
5. Cifonelli, J. A. and Dorfman, A.: Fed. Proc., *18*:204, 1959.
6. Cifonelli, J. A., Ludoweig, J. and Dorfman, A.: Fed. Proc., *16*:165, 1957.
7. Coelho, R. R. and Chrisman, O. D.: J. Bone & Joint Surg., *42A*:165, 1960.
8. Davidson, E. A.: Fed. Proc., *19*:146, 1960.
9. Davidson, E. A. and Meyer, K.: J. Am. Chem. Soc., *76*:5686, 1954.
10. Davidson, E. A. and Meyer, K.: J. Biol. Chem., *211*:605, 1954.
11. Davidson, E. A. and Meyer, K.: J. Am. Chem. Soc., *77*:4796, 1955.
12. Davidson, E. A. and Woodhall, B.: J. Biol. Chem., *234*:2951, 1959.
13. Dorfman, A. and Lorincz, A. E.: Proc. Nat. Acad. Sci. Wash., *43*:443, 1957.
14. Dorfman, A. and Schiller, S.: Recent Progr. Hormone Res., *14*:427, 1958.
15. Fessler, J. H.: Biochem. J., *76*:124, 1960.
16. Gardell, S.: Acta chem. scandinav., *9*:1035, 1955.
17. Grant, R. A., Hathorn, M. and Gillman, T.: Biochem. J., *76*:412, 1960.
18. Gross, J. I., Mathews, M. B. and Dorfman, A.: Fed. Proc., *18*:239, 1959.
19. Hallen, A.: Acta chem. scandinav., *12*:1869, 1958.
20. Harkness, R. D., Marko, A. M., Muir, H. M. and Neuberger, A.: (1954). Biochem. J., *56*:558, 1954.
21. Hirano, S., Hoffman, P. and Meyer, K.: Fed. Proc., *19*:146, 1960.
22. Hoffman, P., Linker, A. and Meyer, K.: Science, *124*:1252, 1956.
23. Hoffman, P., Linker, A. and Meyer, K.: Arch. Biochem. & Biophys., *69*:435, 1957.
24. Hoffman, P., Linker, A. and Meyer, K.: Biochim. et biophys. acta., *30*:184, 1958.
25. Hoffman, P., Linker, A. and Meyer, K.: Fed. Proc., *17*:1078, 1958.
26. Hoffman, P., Linker, A., Sampson, P., Meyer, K. and Korn, D. E.: Biochim. et biophys. acta., *25*:658, 1957.
27. Hoffman, P., Meyer, K. and Linker, A.: J. Biol. Chem., *219*:653, 1956.
28. Hughes, R. E. and Kodicek, E.: Biochem. J., *77*:3P, 1960.
29. Humphrey, J. H., Neuberger, A. and Perkins, D. J.: Biochem. J., *66*:390, 1957.
30. Jeanloz, R. W. and Stoffyn, P. J.: Fed. Proc., *17*:249, 1958.
31. Jeanloz, R. W., Stoffyn, P. J. and Tremege, M.: Fed. Proc., *16*:201, 1957.
32. Jorpes, J. E. and Gardell, S.: J. Biol. Chem., *176*:267, 1948.
33. Kaplan, D. and Meyer, K.: Nature, Lond., *183*:1268, 1959.
34. Kodicek, E. and Loewi, G.: Proc. Roy. Soc. B., *144*:100, 1955.
35. Lack, C. H. and Rogers, H. J.: Nature, Lond., *182*:948, 1958.
36. Linker, A., Hoffman, P. and Meyer, K.: Fed. Proc., *17*:264, 1958.
37. Loewi, G. and Meyer, K.: Biochim. et biophys. acta., *27*:543, 1958.
38. Lorincz, A. E.: Fed. Proc., *17*:266, 1958.
39. Lorincz, A. E.: Fed. Proc., *19*:148, 1960.
40. Malawista, I. and Schubert, M.: J. Biol. Chem., *230*:535, 1958.
41. Mathews, M. B.: Arch. Biochem. & Biophys., *61*:367, 1953.
42. Mathews, M. B.: Nature, Lond., *181*:421, 1958.
43. Mathews, M. B.: Biochim. & biophys. acta., *35*:9, 1959.

44. Mathews, M. B. and Lozaityte, I.: Arch. Biochem. & Biophys., *74*:158, 1958.
45. McCluskey, R. T. and Thomas, L.: J. Exper. Med., *108*:371, 1958.
46. Merkow, L. P. and Lalich, J. J.: Fed. Proc., *19*:145, 1960.
47. Meyer, K., Davidson, A. E., Linker, A. and Hoffman, P.: Biochim. et biophys. acta., *21*:506, 1956.
48. Meyer, K., Grumbach, M. M., Linker, A. and Hoffman, P.: Proc. Soc. Exper. Biol., N.Y., *97*:275, 1958.
49. Meyer, K., Hoffman, P. and Linker, A.: Science, *128*:896, 1958.
50. Meyer, K., Hoffman, P., Linker, A., Grumbach, M. M. and Sampson, P.: Proc. Soc. Exper. Biol., N.Y., *102*:587, 1959.
51. Meyer, K., Linker, A., Davidson, A. E. and Weissman, B.: J. Biol. Chem., *205*:611, 1953.
52. Muir, H. M.: Biochem. J., *62*:26P, 1956.
53. Muir, H. M.: Biochem. J., *69*:195, 1958.
54. Muir, H. M.: Abstr. Comm. 4th Int. Congr. Biochem., Vienna., No. 18, 1958.
55. Muir, H. M.: Unpublished material, 1959.
56. Orr, S. F. D.: Biochim. et biophys. acta., *14*:173, 1954.
57. Partridge, S. M., Davis, H. F. and Adair, G. S.: Biochem. J., *73*:32P, 1959.
58. Priest, R. E.: Fed. Proc., *19*:148, 1960.
59. Reddi, K. K. and Norström, A.: Nature, Lond., *173*:1232, 1954.
60. Robertson, W. van B. and Hinds, H.: J. Biol. Chem., *221*:791, 1956.
61. Rosen, O., Hoffman, P. and Meyer, K.: Fed. Proc., *19*:147, 1960.
62. Schiller S.: Biochim. et biophys. acta., *32*:315, 1959.
63. Schiller, S. and Dorfman, A.: Nature, Lond., *185*:111, 1960.
64. Schiller, S., Mathews, M. B., Cifonelli, J. A. and Dorfman, A.: J. Biol. Chem., *218*:139, 1956.
65. Shatton, J and Schubert, M.: J. Biol. Chem., *211*:565, 1954.
66. Slack, H. G. B.: Biochem. J., *69*:125, 1958.
67. Spicer, S. S. and Bryant, J. H.: Amer. J. Path., *34*:61, 1958.
68. Suzuki, S. and Strominger, J. L.: J. Biol. Chem., *235*:257, 1960.
69. Suzuki, S. and Strominger, J. L.: J. Biol. Chem., *235*:267, 1960.
70. Suzuki, S. and Strominger, J. L.: J. Biol. Chem., *235*:274, 1960.
71. Thomas, L.: J. Exper. Med., *104*:245, 1956.
72. Tsaltas, T. T.: J. Exper. Med., *108*:507, 1958.
73. Woodin, A. M.: Biochem. J., *51*:319, 1952.
74. Ziff, M., Gribetz, H. M. and Lospalluto, J.: J. Clin. Invest., *39*:405, 1960.

Trephocytic Activity of Lymphocytes, Plasmacytes and Mast Cells in Relation to the Metabolism of Connective Tissue[*]

MARGARET A. KELSALL

Cleveland Psychiatric Institute and Hospital, Cleveland, Ohio

Lymphocytes, plasmacytes and mast cells synthesize and release several substances that are important in the metabolism of connective tissues. Fluctuations in the rate of formation, infiltration and lysis of these cells provide cellular mechanisms for several systems of balances and counterbalances that control activities of interstitial fluids and metabolism of connective tissues.

Lymphocytic infiltration and plasmacytogenesis, such as occur in inflammations, concentrate nucleoproteins in an area of connective tissue. By dialytic exchange, cytoplasmic budding and lysis, lymphocytes release trephones into interstitial fluids. Plasmacytogenesis in connective tissue is a process of synthesizing antibodies, RNA and other proteins, and a means by which these proteins are stored intracellularly between the period of increased capillary permeability and proliferation of connective tissue and other cells. Thus, lymphocytic and plasmacytic infiltrations, which are preceded by mast cell-induced hyperemia and increased capillary and tissue permeability, can increase protein metabolism and proliferation of cells in localized areas of connective tissue.[18, 19]

Eosinophils may also be important in connective tissue metabolism because histamine, hormones, hypersensitivity, inflammation, foreign protein reaction, infestation, necrosis and other conditions affect their numbers in tissues and blood and their infiltration-responses. The function of the eosinophil has not been established but is probably related to its primary component, the peroxidase-bearing granules.[15] Several investigators suggest that eosinophils, or slightly modified peroxidase from their granules,[1] inhibit the action of histamine (Vercauteren's antihistiminicum)[22] and detoxicate bacterial and necrotic toxins.[15]

MAST CELL-HISTAMINE CHAIN

Mast cells synthesize, store and release histamine, which incites hyperemia and induces capillary leakage of proteins. In 1953, Riley and West[30] established the importance of mast cells as a source of endogenous histamine. The experimental methods and tests used to establish the presence and func-

[*] These studies have been sponsored in part by grants from the Thorne Ecological Research Station, Grant A-1272 (C2) from the Institute of Arthritis and Metabolic Diseases of the United States Public Health Service, and various contributions.

tion of histamine have been evaluated and discussed at length.[5, 6, 10, 11, 14, 19, 26, 29, 31, 34, 35] The mast cell is an important source of histamine in most animals, but histamine is also abundant in blood platelets of some species and occurs in physiologic quantities in nearly all mammalian tissues and body fluids.[3, 10, 14, 19, 26, 29, 31] Endogenous and exogenous histamine are potent inductors of hyperemia and of increased capillary and tissue permeability.[4, 5, 10, 19, 26, 35] A close relationship between the mast cell population and the histamine and/or heparin content of tissues has been found in a number of animals and tissues.[5, 6, 13, 19, 26, 29]

Heparin is considered an adjuvant of histamine in increasing capillary and tissue permeability and in increasing other mucopolysaccharides.[2, 19] Heparin is abundant in the granules of mast cells,[13, 29, 34] and practically all histamine-releasing agents release heparin, as well as histamine, from mast cells.[5, 19, 29, 30]

Release of histamine and heparin from mast cells speedily induces dilation of capillaries and increased permeability and reduces the viscosity of hyaluronic acid in interstitial fluid. Usually, these changes result in increased passage of plasma proteins, including the largest molecules, from terminal vascular structures into the interstices, with formation of protein-rich edema.[5, 19]

Edema has been considered a factor in initiating and continuing collagen degeneration. Swelling of collagen fibers is one of the early changes in collagen diseases.[2, 9, 23] In 1933, Klinge noted mucoid swelling in intercellular material in early alteration of connective tissues in rheumatic fever and rheumatoid arthritis.[21] Edema appears in skeletal muscle in dermatomyositis,[28] in degeneration of muscle fibers (Fig. 1) and in walls of vessels in periarteritis nodosa.[12]

MASTOCYTOGENESIS

Variations in the numbers of mast cells in connective tissues have been described in many physiological and pathological conditions.[24, 26, 27, 29] Observations from several experimentally induced conditions that increased formation of mast cells suggested to us that mastocytogenesis is related to increased formation of stem cells and to increased protein in interstitial fluid.

Estrogen. Mastocytogenesis increased in the mammary gland of female hamsters that received estrogen,[17] but the number of mast cells in several nontarget organs (pancreas, stomach, intestine, lymph nodes, spleen, submaxillary glands, thymus) was not increased.[17] In addition, estrogen did not induce formation of mast cells in the stroma of the ovary, brain, adrenal, kidney or hepatic lobules,[17] organs in which mast cells are normally absent or very rare in hamsters. Three to 29 parenteral administrations of aqueous estrogen (1.4 to 29 mg. during 1 to 64 days) to 19 virgin hamsters, 42 to 96 days old, increased mast cells in the mammary glands (see Figs. 14 and 15 in reference 19). This increase of mast cells in the mammary glands was definitely evident in regions of small ducts, but was not as evident in the white fibrous periductal tissue of the larger ducts.[17]

Testosterone. A second relation which presents the possibility that mast cells may be a significant part of the mechanism by which sex hormones act on their target organs is indicated by the mastocytogenesis that occurred in the connective tissue surrounding the lumbodorsal sebaceous glands of

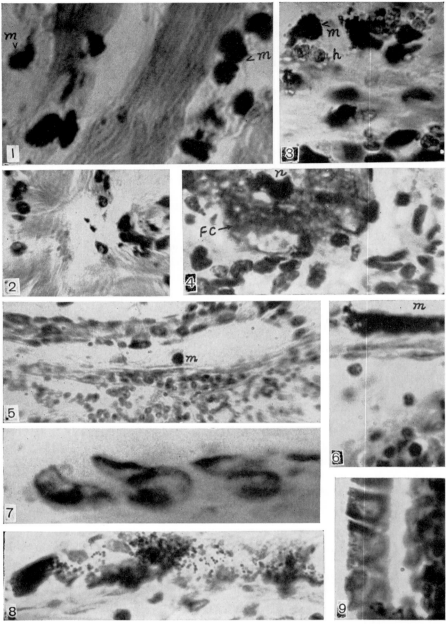

Fig. 1.   Mast cells (m) and edema between muscle fibers degenerating as a result of pressure necrosis (2 μ, hamster).

Fig. 2.   Mast cells in the dartos muscle of the scrotum of a hamster that was killed 10 days after total body irradiation of 995 r (6 μ).

Fig. 3.   Hemosiderin (h) and mast cells (m) in region of scar tissue in a hamster (4 μ).

Fig. 4.   Large foam cells (f c) of a lymph node depleted by cortisone (6 μ, hamster). The dark bodies (n) are nuclei.

Figs. 5-9 are from lymph nodes of hamster that received 14 injections of bovine gamma globulin over 35 days. Tissues were cut at 6 μ and stained with toluidine blue.

male hamsters that received testosterone. Mast cells increased along capillaries and in the connective tissue surrounding these sebaceous glands in adult male hamsters that received 14 to 40 injections of aqueous testosterone (77.5 to 300 mg.) over a period of 65 to 164 days. This pigmented gland, which is a secondary sexual character in male hamsters, hypertrophied up to four times normal size in some adult males of this group.

X-irradiation. During involution following total body x-irradiation (995 r to 1200 r) of 33 female and 22 male hamsters 82 to 101 days old, mast cells increased in 17 to 25 thymi in the inversion stage and in 12 of 23 extremely depleted thymi.[16] This increase in mast cells may be a result of increased extracellular proteins from the lymphocytolysis that occurs during the earlier periods of depletion by x-irradiation.

Necrosis of Muscle. A great increase in mastocytogenesis accompanied the edema that occurred between fibers of skeletal muscle that were degenerating as a result of pressure necrosis (Fig. 1) from the formation of turpentine cysts, or from pressure necrosis of growing transplantable tumors. Mast cells were also abundant in the atrophying dartos muscle layer of the scrotum of hamsters that received 995 r total body irradiation (Fig. 2).

Hemorrhage. Large aggregations of mast cells often occurred near deposits of hemosiderin (Fig. 3) that resulted from extirpation of transplanted tumors, in sites of old hemorrhages in the scrotum and testes of x-irradiated hamsters and in regions of old hemorrhages subsequent to chemical or surgical methods.

Cortisone. Mast cells were very rare along the afferent lymphatics and in other regions of lymph nodes and were decreased in most of the other tissues in 15 males and 3 females that received 20 to 21 injections (1 mg./ 100 g.) of cortisone acetate (Merck) for 1 to 37 days. However, aggregates of foam cells, presumably macrophages that had phagocytized the vehicle of the cortisone, were especially abundant in afferent lymphatics of depleted lymph nodes (Fig. 4).

Bovine Gamma Globulin. Injections of bovine gamma globulins into 6 male and 4 female hamsters (10 to 21 injections of 0.25 ml. each over 15 to 47 days) increased the formation of mast cells along the afferent lymphatics of the lymph nodes regional to the injection sites (Figs. 5-9). This increased formation of mast cells was accompanied primarily by hyperplasia of the germinal centers in the cortex. Some of these proximal nodes hypertrophied from four to eight times their normal size.[20]

SIGNIFICANCE OF THE MAST CELL-HISTAMINE CHAIN

Histamine increases capillary permeability, which in turn increases proteins in interstitial fluid. Increased interstitial proteins stimulate formation of the stem cells of mast cells and their synthesis of histamine and heparin

---

Fig. 5. Mast cells around an afferent lymphatic and a mast cell in the cortical sinus of a lymph node proximal to the sites of injections.

Fig. 6. Large mast cell (m) and two lymphocytes in the cortical sinus.

Figs. 7, 8 and 9. Two stages of developing mast cells (7 and 9) along a vessel in the cortical sinuses of two lymph nodes proximal to injection sites of bovine gamma globulin. Fig. 8 shows lysis of mast cells along a capillary in the cortex of a submaxillary lymph node.

(Fig. 10). This chain of events can be accelerated by an increase in the activity of one or more of the four steps (Fig. 10) if other steps are not inhibited or counterbalanced. A wide variety of factors or agents incite release of histamine from mast cells.[5, 8, 19, 25, 29, 33] Some sources of histamine include the increased formation of mast cells, and cytolysis of mast cells and other cells by foreign proteins, antigen-antibody reaction, x-irradiation, UV, and compound 48/80, a formaldehyde polymere of p-methoxyphenyhel-methylamine. In addition to the release of histamine, activity of the chain

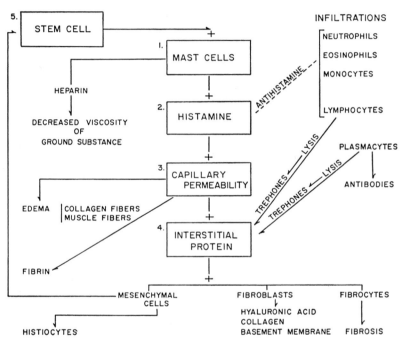

Fig. 10. Concept of the mast cell-histamine chain and relations of some trephocytes to several metabolic processes in connective tissue.

can be accelerated by increased capillary permeability, or fragility, which can result from increased capillary pressure, leukotaxin, acetylcholine, possibly hyaluronidase and other factors or conditions. Furthermore, the mast cell-histamine chain may be activated by the increases in interstitial proteins that result from hemorrhage, erythrocytolysis, capillary fragility, atrophy and necrosis of cells, interstitial fibrin formation and occlusion of lymphatics.

The mast cell-histamine chain can be decelerated by many methods. For example, histamine may be decreased, bound, inhibited or degraded by cortisone, antihistamines, histaminase(s) and possibly Vercauteren's antihistiminicum from eosinophil granules, by decreased stem cell production of mast cells, by decrease of proteins in tissue fluid and by inhibition of histidine decarboxylase. Capillary permeability may be decreased by epinephrine or cortisone or by supplementing bioflavonoids, ascorbic acid or calcium if a deficiency of one of these substances is a cause of increased capillary fragility.

Cortisone is a very effective inhibitor of the mast cell-histamine chain. The earliest and most striking action of cortisone is antiphlogistic, as indicated by amelioration of arthritic and other allergic conditions.[19] This hormone inhibits connective tissue growth and growth processes in general chiefly by progressively inhibiting utilization of available proteins and other substances that are essential in intermediary metabolism.[7, 18, 19] Some of the means by which this hormone decelerates the mast cell-histamine chain and induces conditions unfavorable for proliferative processes are the following: (a) Cortisone causes lymphocytolysis and inhibits formation of lymphocytes and plasmacytes[7, 18, 19] and of mast cells.[2, 19] (b) Cortisone tones histamine-dilated arterioles[19] and decreases permeability of existing capillaries and interstitial substances, probably by inhibiting the action of hyaluronidase(s),[2, 19] of histidine decarboxylase,[32] and of histaminase.[14] (c) Cortisone inhibits edematous swelling and degeneration of collagen fibers.[9, 23, 28] (d) Cortisone inhibits vascularization and decreases proliferation of mast cells and their stem cells.[19]

The mast cell-histamine chain has varied effects on metabolism of connective tissues:

1. A sudden decrease in an activator can revert the chain to the status quo, as in serum sickness.

2. Repetition of acceleration of the mast cell-histamine chain in the same area of a tissue or organ results in subacute or chronic inflammation.

3. Progression of this chain into alveolar, adipose or other connective tissues is effected by growth of capillaries accompanied by formation of stem cells of mast cells in the pericapillary tissue; thereby, as the capillaries grow, they carry with them potential sources of readily available histamine. Examples of this extension of increased vascularity occur in granulation tissue, hypertrophy of mammary glands and resorption of bone. The formation of polyps and synovial villi extends capillary growth into areas that become sites of chronic inflammation (i.e., repetition of the mast cell-histamine chain in the same area).

4. If these steps replace fibrinoid degeneration of collagen, the mast cell-histamine chain may be terminated by fibroblastic production of hyaluronic acid, or by deposition of collagen, fibrosis or other replacement processes.

5. Prolonged repetition of the mast cell-histamine chain at spaced time intervals in the same area is conducive to excessive formation of some cells and may be a factor in formation of tumors, such as plasmacytoma, mastocytoma and several kinds of sarcomas.

6. The failure of fibroblasts to produce basement membranes could be a contributing factor in initiating carcinogenesis by increasing hyperemia and availability of interstitial proteins for epithelial cells. In addition, heparin from the increased number of mast cells might augment the availability of protein by decreasing the viscosity of the ground substance in the basement membranes. For example, we have observed that granules of mast cells often occur within basement membranes underlying stratified squamous epithelium during carcinogenesis induced by 9,10-dimethyl-1,2-benzanthracene applied to the skin of hamsters.

7. Release of histamine from granules of mast cells primes the mast cell-histamine chain (Fig. 10) and possibly indicates a contributing factor in the predilection of the following tissues or organs to lesions in collagen diseases: (a) abundance of mast cells in the pleura—pleurisy of rheumatoid arthritis;

(b) "cuffing" of mast cells around arterioles—periarteritis nodosa; (c) foreign protein release of mast cell-histamine in serum sickness.

8. There are also several correlations between pathological changes in certain collagen diseases and increased formation of mast cells: (a) edema and mastocytogenesis in skeletal muscle—the frequency of occurrence of muscle lesions in many collagen diseases; (b) the presence of mast cells—resorption of bone.

This concept of a mast cell-histamine chain in regulating metabolism of connective tissue and the multiple factors involved in its balancing and counterbalancing systems may account for some of the reasons for individual differences in response to the same agent and for variations in the localization, extent and progression of lesions in collagen diseases.

REFERENCES

1. Agner, K.: Acta physiol. scandinav., *2*(suppl. 8):1, 1941.
2. Asboe-Hansen, G.: Physiol. Rev., *38*:446, 1958.
3. Barron, D. H.: In Fulton, J. F. (ed.): A Textbook of Physiology. Philadelphia, W. B. Saunders Co., 1949, pp. 283-314.
4. Best, C. H. and McHenry, E. W.: Physiol. Rev., *11*:371, 1931.
5. Crabb, E. D.: Univ. Colorado Stud. Ser. Biol., *4*:1, 1958.
6. Crabb, E. D.: Univ. Colorado Stud. Ser. Biol., *4*:36, 1958.
7. Crabb, E. D. and Kelsall, M. A.: J. Nat. Cancer Inst., *12*:91, 1951.
8. Davies, G. E. and Low, J. S.: Brit. J. Exper. Path., *41*:335, 1960.
9. Duff, G. L.: Canad. M. A. J., *58*:317, 1948.
10. Feldberg, W.: In Wolstenholm, G. E. W. and O'Connor, C. M. (eds.): Histamine. Boston, Little, Brown and Co., 1956, pp. 4-13.
11. Haddy, F. J.: Am. J. Physiol., *198*:161, 1960.
12. Hughes, W. F., Jr.: In Traut, E. F. (ed.): Rheumatic Diseases. St. Louis, C. V. Mosby Co., 1952, pp. 626-634.
13. Jorpes, J. E.: Heparin: Its Chemistry, Physiology and Applications in Medicine. Oxford, Oxford University Press, 1939.
14. Kapeller-Adler, R.: In Wolstenholm, G. E. W. and O'Connor, C. M. (eds.): Histamine. Boston, Little, Brown and Co., 1956, pp. 356-380.
15. Kelsall, M. A.: Univ. Colorado Stud. Ser. Biol., *4*:62, 1958.
16. Kelsall, M. A. and Crabb, E. D.: Science, *115*:123, 1952.
17. Kelsall, M. A. and Crabb, E. D.: Anat. Rec., *124*:415, 1956.
18. Kelsall, M. A. and Crabb, E. D.: Ann. N. Y. Acad. Sc., 72:293, 1958.
19. Kelsall, M. A. and Crabb, E. D.: Lymphocytes and Mast Cells. Baltimore, Williams & Wilkins Co., 1959.
20. Kelsall, M. A. and Crabb, E. D.: Anat. Rec., *136*:339, 1960.
21. Klemperer, P.: In Asboe-Hansen, G. (ed.): Connective Tissue in Health and Disease. Copenhagen, Ejnar Munksgaard, 1954.
22. Lindahl, K. M.: Arkiv. Zool., *6*:569, 1954.
23. MacLeod, C. M.: In Lawrence, H. S. (ed.): Cellular and Humoral Aspects of the Hypersensitive States. New York, Paul B. Hoeber, Inc., 1959, pp. 615-627.
24. Michels, N. A.: In Downey, H. (ed.): Handbook of Hematology. New York, Paul B. Hoeber, 1938, vol. I, pp. 231-372.
25. Mongar, J. L.: In Wolstenholm, G. E. W. and O'Connor, C. M. (eds.): Histamine. Boston, Little, Brown and Co., 1956, pp. 74-91.
26. Mota, I., Beraldo, W. T., Ferri, A. G. and Junqueira, L. C. U.: In Wolstenholm, G. E. W. and O'Connor, C. M. (eds.): Histamine. Boston, Little, Brown and Co., 1956, pp. 47-50.
27. Padawer, J.: Tr. N. Y. Acad. Sc., *19*:690, 1957.
28. Percival, G. H., Drennan, A. M. and Dodds, T. C.: Atlas of Histopathology of the Skin. Baltimore, Williams & Wilkins, 1947.
29. Riley, J. F.: The Mast Cells. Baltimore, Williams & Wilkins, 1959.
30. Riley, J. F. and West, G. B.: J. Physiol. (London), *120*:528, 1953.
31. Rocha e Silva, M.: Histamine: Its Role in Anaphylaxis and Allergy. Springfield, Ill., Charles C Thomas, 1955.

32. Schayer, R. W.: In Wolstenholm, G. E. W. and O'Connor, C. M. (eds.): Histamine. Boston, Little, Brown and Co., 1956, pp. 183-188.
33. Sylvén, B.: In Turnbridge, R. E. (ed.): A Symposium. Oxford, Blackwell Scientific Publications, 1957.
34. West, G. B.: In Wolstenholm, G. E. W. and O'Connor, C. M. (eds.): Histamine. Boston, Little, Brown and Co., 1956, pp. 14-19.
35. Whelan, R. F.: In Wolstenholm, G. E. W. and O'Connor, C. M. (eds.): Histamine. Boston, Little, Brown and Co., 1956, pp. 220-234.

Panel Discussion

Gustav Asboe-Hansen, *Moderator*

Dr. Asboe-Hansen: Dr. Menkin, what is the mechanism of repair in inflammation?

Dr. Menkin: A number of years ago we became interested in whether there was a mediator similar to leukotaxine that might explain the mechanism of repair in inflammation. We found that after injections of exudative material into the ears of rabbits for a period of six months to a year, a nodular prominence formed; subsequently, we found that this was due to a growth-promoting factor. We could not obtain this response when blood serum was substituted. We also found that a more convenient and more responsive site to demonstrate the effects of this factor was the breast tissue of nonpregnant rabbits. The response to injections in this area was a very active one, and proliferation of the epithelium in the lining of the ducts and acini and of the stromal connective tissue occurred. After repeated injections, the changes were similar to those found in cystic hyperplasia and chronic cystic mastitis. Likewise, this could not be duplicated with material from the blood serum. The active component was diffusible and could be dialyzed from the exudate; upon concentration of the diffusate the active principle was recovered. This material also affects cartilaginous and osseous tissue and can cause metaplastic transformations in epithelial cells. Regarding the nature of this material, chromatographic studies indicate that in the hydrolysate of the diffusate there is a peptide, and inactivation by chymotrypsin indicates activity in the peptide portion. Additional observations indicate that this factor has a nucleotide structure, since spectrophotometric analysis shows a peak in the nucleotide range, and since in the host the activity is abolished by ribonuclease. Therefore, it seems likely that the activity lies in both the peptide and nucleotide groups, and there is a good possibility that the compound is a nucleopeptide. The presence of this endogenous growth-promoting factor offers a reasonable explanation for the mechanism of repair in inflammation.

Dr. Asboe-Hansen: Dr. Menkin has given one answer to this question, but there may be some other comments on this. Dr. Jackson, would you comment on this mechanism?

Dr. D. Jackson: I think that the mechanism of repair is a far more complicated one. Using the example of the simple wound, there are several phenomena taking place almost simultaneously. There is the inflammatory response, fibroblastic proliferation, epithelization, capillary growth and a whole host of things, all interdependent, all taking place at the same time. I personally think that it is a little too simple to try and look for one single growth factor and say that this is the mechanism by which repair takes place.

Dr. Kelsall: I certainly agree with Dr. Jackson. In presenting our concept of the role of the cells in the metabolism and growth of other cells, I did not point out the significance of the enzymatic relations. I think that even if the cells are as significant as I have considered, they are merely one facet of an advanced problem.

Dr. Menkin: It is perfectly true that the mechanism of repair is much more complex than I presented, but nevertheless, the growth promoting factor is a complete factor that causes proliferation in the medium involved in the mechanism of repair. That there are other factors is perfectly possible, and the presence of the factor which I described does not preclude the possibility that there are other factors, but the point in question is how to isolate them. The factor I described at least is one which we can identify and provides at least an initial building block in the development of our knowledge concerning the mechanism of repair.

Dr. Asboe-Hansen: Dr. Menkin, what do you think of the stimulatory effect of the edema alone in inflammation? There is definite evidence that edema influences connective tissue cells to produce or to release some substances. I have some data regarding the effects of edema on mast cells, and although I have not studied fibroblasts from this viewpoint, I am not in doubt that such studies would show something too. If you increase tissue water or even if you use isotonic fluids and increase the water concentration of tissues, this will provoke the production or release of polysaccharides, for example, mucopolysaccharides, which may have some primary role in the growth or repair process. I think that water is one of the real stimulators for connective tissue repair and regeneration. The water is the primary thing, the mucin the secondary thing, and the collagen deposition the third thing, and by this mechanism the regeneration process is initiated.

Dr. Menkin: When you refer to edema fluid, what does that really mean? Does that mean edema fluid *per se,* or does it mean edema fluid which may contain products of cellular injury? Who knows what products are in this fluid in cellular injury? The growth-promoting factor which I referred to a few minutes ago may be present. Unless you can demonstrate that water by itself will stimulate proliferation without causing injury, and I do not see how that can be done when it is injected *in vivo,* it is difficult to draw any conclusions about the effect of the water itself.

Dr. Asboe-Hansen: You need not inject the water. If you take a connective tissue surface and drop a physiological fluid on it, a drop of water on it, a protein-rich fluid on it, or a polysaccharide-rich fluid on it, the regeneration process can be induced that way.

Dr. Kelsall, what are some of the possible factors that may stimulate the production of mast cells?

Dr. Kelsall: I think, from my work, that an increase in protein, whether produced by increased capillary permeability, by a chemical process in other cells, or by any of the means in which proteins are increased in interstitial fluids, can stimulate production of mast cells. Furthermore, as I mentioned, erythrocytolysis may be a very important stimulating factor for mast cells through the stimulation of the mesenchymal cells in the presence of increased histidine since the mast cell does contain histidine decarboxylase. In addition, in many growth processes, mast cells form where there is growth of capillaries, and in target organs sex hormones also increase the number of mast cells.

Dr. Wagner: Dr. Kelsall, did you say that an increase in interstitial proteins increased the number of mast cells in an area?

Dr. Kelsall: Yes.

Dr. Wagner: In naturally occurring or experimental amyloidosis, there are massive deposits of protein in the connective tissue, but I am not aware that there is any increase in mast cells as a result of this.

Dr. Kelsall: I have not observed the formation of mast cells in organs or areas in tissues in which they do not normally occur, for example, the parenchyma of the kidney or the adrenal gland. So there is a specificity and one does not expect mast cells to form where normally their precursors do not occur.

Dr. Asboe-Hansen: I think the conditions you mentioned, including the protein-rich edema and the hormonal states, all include the growth process. It is well known that there is a mast cell accumulation preceding any growth process, and I was unable to find any specific condition in which growth or regeneration did not take place in the studies we have done.

Dr. Kelsall: During the period of involution of the thymus gland there is very little proliferation.

Dr. Asboe-Hansen: If there is involution of the thymus there is connective tissue proliferation.

Dr. Kelsall: At a period of from three to ten days following total body irradiation, there would be very little proliferation in the thymus.

Dr. Asboe-Hansen: In that situation there is irradiation and the response observed may be due to the irradiation.

Dr. Angevine: Dr. Kelsall, do you have any information on how mast cells divide? The question of mitosis in mast cells has always been an interesting one. Do you feel that their rapid division is a mitotic one, or have you seen mitoses?

Dr. Kelsall: I have not seen mitoses in a cell that I could definitely identify as a mast cell. However, we very frequently find chains or groups of two mast cells with very fine granules in the early stage of differentiation. I have not seen a mitotic figure in a mast cell that has large well developed granules.

Dr. Asboe-Hansen: There is a paper by an American author on degranulation of mast cells and a description of mitoses and mitotic phenomena in these cells. These workers found many mitoses after degranulation. I think this was after 48/80 injection (a formaldehyde polymer of p-methoxyphenylhelmethylamine). In our studies in mice with precancerous papillomas we administered tritiated thymidine. This goes into the premitotic stage of the nuclei and we found, although there were very few, some mast cells which were incorporating thymidine in the premitotic stage.

Dr. Angevine: Dr. Muir, can nonsulfated polysaccharides become sulfated *in vivo,* and if so, would you comment on the mechanism?

Dr. Muir: I think that Meyer suggested that chondroitin is in fact the precursor of chondroitin sulfate. A number of people have tried to prove this by making enzyme extracts from tissues synthesizing polysaccharides actively, but entirely failed to demonstrate sulfate transfer. However, rather recently, an enzyme system has been obtained from the chick oviduct that will transfer sulfate not only to chondroitin but also to artificially desulfated chondroitin sulfate and heparin monosulfate. Interestingly enough, the sulfate is not distributed evenly along the polysaccharides, and some polysaccharides may be without sulfate and others with more than one.

DR. WAGNER: Where is the sulfate removed *in vivo* and where does it come off?

DR. MUIR: An interesting paper has been published concerning a soluble enzyme system derived from rabbit skin which will desulfate chondroitin sulfate B, but will not desulfate chondroitin A.

DR. ASBOE-HANSEN: Dr. Jean, would you comment on the production of connective tissue in glass tubes implanted under the skin of experimental animals?

DR. JEAN: I would like to present a brief résumé of some experiments in which we have obtained what we call an *"in vivo"* culture of connective tissues. We have implanted Pyrex glass tubes under the skin of rats, and one might expect that regeneration would have sealed the tube; but much to our surprise, a thin central cord of connective tissue developed, forming a bridge between the two openings of the tube. This single beam of connective tissue might be a good test object for further biochemical studies.

DR. D. JACKSON: This is very similar to the results of some experiments reported three or four years ago, in which the same thing occurred in implanted tubes of tantalum mesh. In fact, this same investigator has laminated structures which he has recently used to replace sections of the aorta of the dog, apparently quite successfully. Experimental growth of connective tissue is a very odd phenomenon. In some cases, the connective tissue response results in growth on the outside of a foreign body, and in other cases growth occurs on the inside. While the phenomenon of the production of collagen is a common one, it is very difficult to understand why these different reactions take place. When sponges in which there are interstices are implanted, the collagen growth occurs both on the outside and the inside of the sponge, the fibroblast migrating through into the interstices of the sponge. This is another example of growth on the inside. On the other hand, there is another reported experiment in which a balloon was inserted subcutaneously and inflated. In this experiment the cells could not get through and connective tissue grew only on the outside of the balloon. There are obviously some factors involved in this mechanism that we are not aware of and which decide where the connective tissue is going to grow. It is just another very nice example of a model of connective tissue growth which will be very useful for studies of its biochemistry.

DR. ASBOE-HANSEN: Dr. Jackson, Meyer has suggested that the different polysaccharides of connective tissues are synthesized by different sorts of fibroblasts. Is there any evidence for this suggestion from tissue culture studies? What are the different sorts of fibroblasts? Is a mast cell a fibroblast?

DR. S. FITTON JACKSON. I think this a question of semantics. There are in a sense all sorts of different fibroblasts, for example, fibroblasts in different stages of differentiation. There is a differentiation factor which causes gradual development of the mesenchymal cell until it is, in full, a protein-producing cell of a collagen type; alternatively, it is yet to be proved that the fibroblast is in actual fact producing mucopolysaccharide. It is quite possible that there is only one morphologically recognizable cell, a comparable situation to the chondroblast in cartilage. But again one can see variations both at the cytochemical level and at the fine structure level within this one type of cell, and it may be that at one precise moment it is producing mucopolysaccharide exclusively and then at another moment it may be producing the noncollagenous protein which is required for the chondromucoprotein complex. At a third and different time, it may be producing a collagen protein. It is quite obvious that the fibroblast, the chondroblast or the osteoblast theoretically should be in different stages, and therefore, one may say that they are different cells if one considers the end product they are producing.

DR. ASBOE-HANSEN: Dr. Kelsall, one usually concedes that metabolites in transfer between cells are small molecules and that large complex molecules are subsequently synthesized by cells. In what manner are the complex molecules of trephocytes, for example, proteins of lymphocytes, transferred to other cells?

DR. KELSALL: At this time, it is my opinion that those large molecules are free in the interstitial fluid and then subsequently are broken down to various levels of size and depolymerization of the nuclear protein. Some may be at the stage of the mononucleotide or even smaller.

DR. SOKOLOFF: This is an area which requires further investigation, and I think Dr. Kelsall has presented an interesting hypothesis, but I find it a little difficult to understand. For example, how can lymphocytes store proteins, nuclear proteins and other complex proteins for immediate use by the adjacent cells, unless there is some mechanism available for the metabolism of these large molecules which must involve some extracellular mechanism or some other hypothesis to account for the function of the lymphocytes in these areas?

DR. KELSALL: In that respect, I think that lymphocytes by releasing different types of cytoplasm and by disintegrating within a specific area of connective tissue, can release into the interstitial fluid various proteins which can be broken down by enzymes in the interstitial fluids or in other areas. In the case of the small lymphocytes that occur within the columnar epithelial cells, there may be a very direct transfer within the cell.

DR. WAGNER: I think there has to be general agreement that when cells break up, whatever substances they break up into are released into the immediate area. The unanswered problem is how these substances are utilized. One has to consider the detailed analysis of the split products as cells degenerate by enzyme degradation and how these substances might be reincorporated from a metabolic pool. It is on this point that there is insufficient knowledge. A small lymphocyte has many attributes that have been reported in the literature. How many of these are correct, I do not know, but in regard to whether or not it liberates materials into the area of the lymphocytolysis, there is some evidence that the purine bases that are derived from the nuclear protein break down and stimulate oxidative phosphorylation and thereby play a role in synthetic mechanisms. Conceivably then, with lymphocytolysis and break down of nuclear protein materials, a number of substances are liberated into the adjacent metabolic pool that may be utilized by other cells, for example, by an adjacent plasma cell; then these products may be useful in synthesizing proteins.

The Formation and Breakdown of Connective Tissue*

DAVID S. JACKSON

University of Oregon Medical School

The rise of interest in the connective tissue diseases since 1948 has stimulated workers in a wide range of scientific disciplines and focused attention on the structure, formation, metabolism and function of the connective tissues, particularly of the extracellular elements. From this work a fairly clear picture has appeared of the formation of collagen and certain other extracellular elements, such as the mucopolysaccharides, in normal conditions.

What may well prove to be more important to those interested in the connective tissue diseases is the problem of connective tissue resorption. Here information is scanty. What little work has been done serves only to point up our ignorance of this subject. Indeed, despite the vast amount of research by basic scientists on the connective tissues, it would not be an exaggeration to say that this work has thrown very little light as yet on the problem of the connective tissue diseases.

In this communication I will concentrate on the collagen component of the connective tissues and will discuss the question of fibrogenesis in the normal connective tissues. I will indulge in some speculation on the problem of resorption and briefly mention some recent work done in my laboratory on the relationship between inflammation and fibrogenesis which may throw some light on both of the preceding questions.

In view of the nature of this review, readers will be referred mainly to review articles for the bibliography.

FIBROGENESIS IN THE NORMAL GROWING ANIMAL

Few if any detailed biochemical studies of fibrogenesis have been carried out on any normal connective tissues except the dermis and, to a lesser extent, on tendon. It is possible that detailed studies on the other tissues may show greater or lesser divergence from the hypothesis put forward here.

It is generally accepted that collagen is a product of the fibroblast or the analogous cells in the more specialized connective tissues such as bone and cartilage.[1] The collagen part of the connective tissue fibers has been shown by a wide variety of methods to be made up essentially of aggregates of the basic collagen molecule, now called tropocollagen.[6] This basic molecule is an elongated stiff rod 2860 Å long by 13.6 Å in diameter consisting of three helical polypeptide chains whose rigidity is maintained by intramolecular crosslinks which are mainly of the hydrogen bond type[18] but may also include ester-like linkages.[5] Hodge et al.[12] have recently produced evidence that these molecules have short polypeptide extensions by which end-to-end linkage is achieved. Transverse intramolecular bonds maintain the fibrous struc-

* This investigation was supported by PHS grants A-3565 from the Institute of Arthritis and Metabolic Diseases and RG-6483 (C1).

ture, and are visible at both electron microscope and light microscope magnifications.[10]

Synthesis of the Collagen Molecule. Since collagen is a protein, it must be assumed that collagen molecules are synthesized by the same mechanism as obtains for other proteins and that this occurs intracellularly. Since collagen is made up of three separate polypeptide chains, these chains must be somehow synthesized and then put together in a precise steric configuration. The mechanism by which this is carried out is unknown. However, recent studies have demonstrated that there is a protein-containing hydroxyproline closely associated with the microsomal fraction, which can be extracted from these intracellular particles with saline.[15] In solution it behaves very similarly to normal collagen and also has essentially the same amino acid composition. Since it is labeled with C^{14} amino acids more rapidly than any other collagen fraction so far isolated, it must be assumed that this is the earliest form of fully formed collagen molecules so far demonstrated. Orekhovitch[16] has claimed that the two major components of the collagen molecule, the alpha and beta fractions, are synthesized at different rates, but this finding has so far not been substantiated.

The problem of collagen synthesis is further complicated by the fact that neither endogenous hydroxyproline nor hydroxylysine can be incorporated directly into the collagen molecule. In both cases the corresponding non-hydroxylated amino acids, proline and lysine, are the precursors of the hydroxy amino acids.[13] Precisely at what stage this hydroxylation takes place is not known, but an earlier hypothesis that suggested that a nonhydroxylated collagen precursor was first formed and later hydroxylated has been shown to be untenable.[17] A possible hypothesis is that the hydroxy amino acids cannot undergo the activation step necessary before amino acids can be incorporated into protein and that the hydroxylation of proline and lysine takes place after these amino acids have been activated.

The Formation of Collagen Fibers from the Tropocollagen Molecule. The question as to where recognizable collagen fibers with the characteristic 640 Å spacing first occur has been much debated. Earlier evidence indicated that they first appear extracellularly. It was also suggested[14] that the site was at the cell surface, which acted as a template to orient the collagen molecules. More recently, however, evidence has been put forward that the first stage of aggregation takes place in the cell cytoplasm (Wardley, personal communication). These fibers seem to be secreted by the cell, which loses its membrane at the point of secretion. The cell may also simultaneously release other intracellular components such as microsomes and mitochondria during the expulsion of the collagen fibers.[3]

It was suggested long ago by Schwann and Virchow that the fibers were formed extracellularly from a secreted soluble precursor formed by the cell. Two soluble fractions obtained from the connective tissues of young growing animals have been claimed as having identity with this postulated soluble precursor. The evidence for and against these claims has been recently reviewed critically.[13, 14] and the neutral salt-extractable collagens have been shown to be the most likely candidates. Further experiments, however, have shown that none of the extractable collagens can be claimed to be *the* precursor since all are heterogeneous from a biologic point of view.[14] Thus, at a given time in developing connective tissue there exists a continuous spectrum of soluble fractions ranging from those soluble in saline to completely insoluble collagen. These fractions differ only in their state of aggregation in the tissues at the time when they were extracted. The longer the time that has elapsed since the constituent molecules were synthesized, the more strongly aggregated they are and the more difficult to extract. In this work a direct correlation between the dispersing power of the extracting solution and the rate of uptake of C^{14} glycine into the collagen molecules extracted was established.

SCHEME OF FIBROGENESIS

The scheme of fibrogenesis which emerges from the data available is as follows:

The cell synthesizes the collagen molecule, which is found in its completed form closely associated with the microsomal fraction. On leaving the microsome the first fibrils are formed intracellularly by end-to-end aggregation, through a double helix formation of polypeptide appendages on the collagen molecule, and also by transverse intermolecular cross linking. These early fibrils are visible only with the electron microscope and are secreted by the cells into the extracellular space. Here they appear to increase in size by the accretion of more collagen molecules from the extracellular space, and not by side-to-side linking of these early fibrils. Hence, it must also be assumed that nonfibrillating collagen molecules are also secreted by the cell or that some of the fibrils must disaggregate and their constituent molecules are then captured by other fibrils. In young growing connective tissue two things go on simultaneously: (1) formation of new fibrils and the addition of more molecules onto the fibrils formed earlier by the cell; as Porter has suggested, these fibrils probably act as templates to extend the polymerization of collagen; (2) increasing strength of cross linking in the older fibrils. At this point extraction with 0.14 M sodium chloride will remove the new fibers and also the molecules laid down on the older fibers at the same time. The remainder of the fibers will now be extractable only with sodium chloride of higher concentration. Eventually the main process will be the increase in diameter of the fibers by accretion of tropocollagen molecules. The deeper in the fiber the collagen molecule is, the more firmly will it be cross linked, as with time, molecules move into more favorable steric apposition under the influence of thermal agitation. This increasing cross linkage will be largely, if not entirely, intermolecular. Hence, there will be a decrease in the proportion of the collagen fractions extractable with aqueous solvents as the tissue ages. The outer layers will be more loosely aggregated and, hence, the more easily extractable. When synthesis of new collagen ceases and collagen becomes relatively metabolically inert, the only process continuing will be a spreading of the region of maximal cross linkage through the whole of the fiber.

FACTORS AFFECTING FIBROGENESIS

The major factors affecting the formation of collagen, which will be briefly discussed, are protein starvation, ascorbic acid deficiency, and cortisone treatment.[4]

Protein Starvation. When an animal is deprived of protein, wounds fail to heal[4] and collagen is absent in the granulation tissue. Healing and collagen formation can be restored to normal by feeding methionine or cystine. As collagen is completely deficient in cystine, its absence cannot be responsible directly for the failure of collagen formation. Practically nothing is known about the role of methionine, although it has been shown by autoradiography[4] to be taken up rapidly by the fibroblasts.

Gross has shown that the amount of neutral salt-extractable collagen present in the skin of guinea pigs is directly proportional to the growth rate.[7] Starving the animal for two days causes almost complete disappearance of this collagen fraction probably because synthesis has ceased and the collagen which was neutral salt-extractable becomes more insoluble and, hence, is not available to such an extraction. No new collagen replaces this fraction which thus disappears. It takes five days following resumption of a normal diet before newly formed collagen again appears.[7]

Ascorbic Acid Deficiency. Although it has been known since the time of Lind that ascorbic acid deficiency leads to the failure of wound healing, the actual role of ascorbic acid in this situation is still unknown.[2, 4] Several authors have shown that there is less collagen produced in scurvy and others have shown a reduced uptake of C^{14} amino acids into collagen.[17] One theory put forward on several occasions is that ascorbic acid is involved in the hydroxylation of proline and lysine to give the corresponding hydroxy amino acids, but this remains unproved.[17] Furthermore, it has been shown that fibroblasts in tissue culture do not require ascorbic acid to synthesize collagen.[9] It has also been shown that collagen is formed in normal amounts in Ivalon sponges implanted in the anterior chamber of the eye of scorbutic guinea pigs (Geever, personal communication), despite the fact that sponges implanted subcutaneously in the same animal had considerably less than the normal collagen content. Since the anterior chamber of the eye is avascular, this suggests that some factor in the plasma is responsible for the reduction in collagen formation. Gould,[9] however, has suggested that there is ascorbic acid-independent and ascorbic acid-dependent collagen biosynthesis, the former being "growth collagen," the latter being "repair collagen." However, the finding by the same author that collagen in sponges is resorbed if the animal is made scorbutic, and is resorbed more slowly with increase of the time interval between sponge implantation and ascorbic acid depletion, suggests that in scurvy some collagen may be destroyed as it is formed and, hence, is no longer metabolically inert, and that ascorbic acid somehow protects the collagen molecule against this destruction. Preliminary results obtained in this laboratory suggest an increased turnover rate of newly formed collagen in scurvy, although what new collagen remains unaffected becomes more insoluble at the same rate as that found in a normal animal.

Effect of Cortisone. It was early found that wound healing in patients receiving cortisone failed or was delayed. This was confirmed in animal experiments. A reduction in the rate of synthesis of both collagen and mucopolysaccharides has been demonstrated.[4] However, it is also known that cortisone is effective in delaying healing only if given prior to or during the inflammatory phase.[4] Once fibroplasia has begun, cortisone appears to be ineffective in slowing down wound healing. Thus, it would appear that there is some direct relationship between inflammation and subsequent fibrogenesis.[4]

FIBROGENESIS FOLLOWING INFLAMMATION

There is evidence of a direct relationship between the acute inflammatory response and the subsequent reparative process. The studies of Selye[19] demonstrate a specific relationship between the severity and nature of an inflammatory response and the subsequent healing process. Moreover, it is well known that the connective tissue which forms around a foreign body which has provoked inflammation may subsequently be resorbed, provided that the foreign body is removed from the locus of inflammation; the carrageenin granuloma is a typical example of this phenomenon. However, if the foreign body is not removed, as, for example, in the case of the Ivalon sponges, complete collagen resorption does not take place. Boucek et al.[1] have suggested that in this instance synthesis is eventually balanced by resorption, the total amount of collagen present remaining constant.

Recently in this laboratory studies have been made concerning the effect of bacterial endotoxins on collagen formation. The rate of synthesis of collagen in implanted Ivalon sponges is greatly increased by the intraperitoneal injection of a single dose of a few micrograms of bacterial endotoxin. The maximum collagen content is reached by 12 days as compared with 20 days for the control animals. However, in studies with incised and open wounds no effect on either the tensile strength or the amount of collagen in the granulation tissue could be demonstrated. It is possible that in the wounds the optimal inflammatory response is normally evoked, so that the added effect of endotoxin is minimal. On the other hand, in the sponges, in which the inflammatory response is mild, endotoxin brings it up to optimal conditions leading to a higher rate of collagen synthesis. In the extreme case, sponges implanted with practically no local inflammatory response evoke minimal collagen formation.

THE BREAKDOWN OR RESORPTION OF COLLAGEN

Collagen is normally considered to be relatively metabolically inert, so inert that it has so far been impossible to measure the half-life of the constituent collagen molecules of mature collagen fibers. However, several instances have been reported in which collagen was resorbed very rapidly. In the carrageenin granuloma the tissue formed is rapidly resorbed.[21] After reaching its maximum weight by the tenth day, the granuloma rapidly decreases and disappears completely in about thirty days. During this resorption period, there is a large increase in the amount of extractable collagen, collagen which appears to behave in many respects like normal collagen.[14] Thus, it appears that resorption takes place by a disaggregation process, presumably followed by complete breakdown of the collagen molecule. The dermal collagen above the area of the granuloma has also been found to disappear simultaneously, to be replaced by fat.[21] Increasing amounts of extractable collagen have also been demonstrated in the resorbing skin (unpublished data).

Recently it has been shown that there is a similar increase in extractable collagen from the tissues of animals on a lathyrogenic diet. (Several nitriles have been shown to be the responsible agents.) This occurs both in chick embryo and in adult guinea pigs and rats.[8]

As has already been noted, collagen formed in implanted Ivalon sponges also resorbs when the animals are placed on a scorbutogenic diet. In this instance, however, no increase in extractable collagen could be demonstrated. Gould[9] suggests that the collagen is partially degraded, since the younger collagen at least appears susceptible to trypsin in these circumstances.

The most striking example of collagen resorption in a normal physiological situation occurs during the postpartum involution of the uterus.[11] The uterus returns to normal size within about 48 hours, during which time the collagen content returns to normal levels. No reports of increasing amounts of extractable collagen occurring during this resorption have so far been made.

Mechanism of Resorption. Little or nothing is known of the mechanism by which resorption is effected. In the instances quoted, there is no evidence of any change of cell type accompanying resorption to cells analogous to the osteoclast present during bone resorption. Boucek et al.[1] have reported an increase in the proteinases active at pH 3.5 (cathepsins) in the later stages of sponge implantation. Harkness,[11] however, was unable to demonstrate any relationship between proteinase activity and collagen released into the media during incubation of homogenized uteri at various stages of pregnancy. Recently Hodge et al.[12] have demonstrated that trypsin and other proteolytic enzymes affect the aggregating properties of the collagen molecule in solution, probably by hydrolyzing away the peptide appendages (discussed in the previous section), but leaving the rodlike structure unchanged. Proteolytic enzymes have also been shown to affect the mature collagenous tissues in such a way that most of the collagen can be extracted with aqueous solvents. In this instance, too, the collagen molecule appears to remain intact.

Thus, resorption may take place by the local production of proteolytic enzymes by the cells or by activation of a circulating enzyme normally inactive. Such an enzyme has been reported in guinea pig serum by Spector et al.[20] Reinjection of such diluted serum seems also to cause increased capillary permeability.[20]

REFERENCES

1. Boucek, R. J., Noble, N. L. and Woessner, J. F.: In Page, I. H. (ed.): Connective Tissue, Thrombosis and Atherosclerosis. New York, Academic Press, 1959, p. 193.
2. Bourne, G. H. (ed.): Biochemistry and Physiology of Bone. New York, Academic Press, 1959, p. 593.
3. Chapman, J.: J. Biochem. Biophys. Cytol. In press, 1960.
4. Edwards, L. C. and Dunphy, J. E.: New Engl. J. Med., *259*:224, 1958.
5. Gallop, P.: Nature, *183*:1659, 1959.
6. Gross, J.: J. Biophys. Biochem. Cytol., *2*(suppl.):261, 1956.
7. Gross, J.: J. Exper. Med., *107*:265, 1959.
8. Gross, J. and Levere, C. I.: J. Exper. Med., *110*:771, 1959.
9. Gould, B. S.: Conference on Vitamin C. Ann. N. Y. Acad. Sc. In press, 1960.
10. Gustavson, K. H.: The Chemistry and Reactivity of Collagen. New York, Academic Press, 1956.
11. Harkness, R. D. and Moralee, B. E.: J. Physiol., *132*:502, 1956.
12. Hodge, A. J., Highberger, J. H., Deffner, S. W. and Schmitt, F. O.: Proc. Nat. Acad. Sc., *46*:197, 1960.
13. Jackson, D. S.: New Engl. J. Med., *259*:814, 1958.
14. Jackson, D. S. and Bentley, J. P.: J. Biochem. Biophys. Cytol., 7:37, 1960.
15. Lowther, D. A. and Green, N. M.: J. Biochem. Biophys. Cytol. In press.
16. Orekovtich, V. N., Shpikiter, V., Kasakova, O. and Mauzourov, V.: Arch. Biochem. Biophys., *85*:554, 1959.
17. Robertson, W. van B.: Conference on Vitamin C. Ann. N. Y. Acad. Sc. In press, 1960.
18. Schmitt, F. O.: In Page, I. H. (ed.): Connective Tissue, Thrombosis and Atherosclerosis. New York, Academic Press, 1959, p. 43.
19. Selye, H.: In Jasmin, G. and Robert, A. (eds.): Symposium on Mechanism of Inflammation. Montreal, ACTA, Inc., 1953, p. 53.
20. Spector, W. G. and Willoughby, D. A.: J. Path. Bact., *77*:1, 1959.
21. Williams, G.: J. Path. Bact., *73*:557, 1957.

Endocrine Control
of Connective Tissue

G. ASBOE-HANSEN

University of Copenhagen

The chemical structure of the hormones influencing connective-tissue cells determines their actions upon the target. The detailed chemical mediation of the hormone effects, however, is not completely known. A circulating hormone may act by stimulating or depressing certain enzyme systems of the cells. It may influence the synthesis of enzymes, co-enzymes, activators or inhibitors, as well as participate in the enzymic process itself. On their passage from the blood to the connective tissue cells the hormones may influence the permeability of the capillary wall, the connective-tissue ground substance, the membranes of the cells, nuclei, mitochondria, granules, etc. These boundaries separate areas with different enzyme systems, and the constant influence of several hormones of widely different chemistry results in a constant control, allowing for wide variations, of the metabolism of the tissues.

The hormonal control of connective tissue is exerted primarily on the cells of mesenchymal origin, a minute fraction of the total tissue mass. These cells manufacture the much greater amount of extracellular substances, fibrils as well as amorphous ground substance. Hormones influencing connective-tissue cells control the regeneration and growth processes as well as other functions of connective tissues.

Regeneration and repair of connective tissue is initiated by tissue edema, which brings about a release of water-binding mucopolysaccharide from the mast cells and, thereby, a mucinous organization of the water. The presence of mucopolysaccharides stimulates deposition of collagen fibrils and fibrous organization. The process of regeneration, repair and growth may be influenced by hormones. The most sensitive point of attack is the formation of hyaluronic acid, which has a rapid turnover. Its biological half-life is about two days, whereas that of chondroitin sulfate is several times longer. Once deposited, collagen, at least in certain organs, is a practically inert substance with a very slow turnover.

GLUCOCORTICOIDS

In tissues influenced by the adrenal steroids cortisone and cortisol (hydrocortisone), the number and size of the *mast cells* is diminished, their outlines are irregular and bizarre, and the cytoplasm is vacuolated. The cytoplasmic granules form irregular aggregates, and the size of the granules varies. The stainability changes from metachromatic to orthochromatic with toluidine blue.

Cortisone inhibits the uptake of S^{35}-labeled sulfate in skin mast cells. The binding of new histamine to rat skin after depletion is inhibited.

In tissue cultures of embryonic skin and spleen, cortisone (free alcohol) has been shown to inhibit mast cell activity.

38

Several investigators have been able to demonstrate an inhibition of the growth and migration of *fibroblasts* in tissue cultures, and cytoplasmic vacuoles have been observed at an early stage of outgrowth. The number of mitoses has been found unchanged. Some workers could not find any influence on fibroblasts *in vitro*.

Cortisone and cortisol inhibit the production of collagen, and high doses of steroids reduce the number of fibroblasts in induced skin wounds.

In inflammation, the emigration of *polymorphonuclear granulocytes* and *macrophages* and the regeneration of reticuloendothelial cells are restricted by cortisone. The number of *plasma cells* has been found to decrease. In blood the *lymphocyte* count may show a temporary fall as a response to cortisone effect, and the numbers of *eosinophil* and *basophil* granulocytes are decreased.

The connective-tissue ground substance is changed, and the content of acid mucopolysaccharide is reduced. As an immediate response to cortisone the polymerization of the hyaluronic acid of synovial fluid may be increased. New formation, however, is inhibited, as is the synthesis of chondroitin sulfuric acid in regenerating connective tissue. The incorporation of S^{35} is reduced.

Cortisone brings about an increase of *spreading* of injected fluids and corpuscular elements in connective tissues, evidently by changing the ground substance. The activity of hyaluronidase is inhibited for a similar reason. The permeability of blood capillaries is consistently reduced.

THYROTROPHIC HORMONE

The biologic effect of purified thyrotrophic anterior pituitary extract is a stimulation of the thyroid gland and a stimulating effect directly on connective tissues.

In thyroidectomized guinea pigs systemic administration of a thyrotrophic pituitary extract brings about *a mobilization of fat from the normal depots*, hyperlipemia and deposition of lipids in the liver, the kidneys and the skeletal and cardiac muscles. During this transport the blood leukocytes phagocytize fat droplets.

Along with the fat mobilization goes a *stimulation of mucin production*. In the tissues the number and size of mast cells is increased, and acid mucopolysaccharide of the hyaluronic acid type is released from these cells. To a certain extent also chondroitin sulfate production seems to be stimulated. A replacement of retrobulbar fat with water-binding acid mucopolysaccharides due to a stimulation of hyaluronate production in glands, muscles and loose connective tissue results in exophthalmos. The *ophthalmotrophic or exophthalmogenic effect* may well be identical with the fat-mobilizing and mucotrophic principles. If this is true, a connective-tissue stimulating factor is present in the extract together with and closely linked to a thyroid-stimulating factor. These two factors may be separated by chemical means and may be different hormones. However, thyroxine inhibits all the above-mentioned effects.

Thyroidectomy, as well as administration of thyrotrophin, is followed by an increase in the viscosity and in the glucosamine content in the vitreous body of rabbits. An increased uptake of S^{35}-sulfate has been observed in skin, cornea, sclera and retrobulbar tissues.

Thyrotrophin stimulates the mucopolysaccharide production to the fluids of the labyrinth. Disturbances in the vestibular functions have been observed after administration of thyrotrophic hormone to thyroidectomized guinea pigs.

By increasing the hyaluronic acid content in connective tissue, thyrotrophin inhibits spreading in the skin and increases the spreading effect of hyaluronidase that finds an almost ideal substrate to act upon.

THYROID HORMONES

Thyroid hormone inhibits the tissue effects of thyrotrophic hormone. In thyrotoxic subjects the content of acid mucopolysaccharide, sulfated as well as non-sulfated, in connective-tissue ground substance is decreased, and so is the water-binding capacity of the skin. The mast cells appear small and faintly granulated; there are few of them, occurring predominantly around the vessels. The blood count of basophil leukocytes decreases as a response to d,l-thyroxine.

Thyroxine increases spreading of fluids in skin and subcutaneous tissue. This hormone has been found to reduce the incorporation of S^{35}-labeled sulfate into sulfomucopolysaccharides of growing connective tissue.

SOMATOTROPHIC HORMONE

In many respects the tissue effects of this anterior pituitary hormone is similar to that of thyrotrophic hormone. Somatotrophin, however, gives a stronger stimulation of fibroblast activity, and especially of collagen formation and deposition.

SEX HORMONES

In several animals, *estrone* induces an increase in the content of acid mucopolysaccharide, particularly hyaluronic acid, in all connective tissues. This implies a decrease of spreading in the skin and of vascular permeability. The activity of mast cells is increased, especially in the reproductive organs, and the incorporation of radiosulfate into the mucous membranes of the uterus, Fallopian tubes and vaginal wall is stimulated by estrogens. *Progesterone* seems to counteract the tissue effect of estrone. *Relaxin* increases the tissue content of water and mucin, predominantly in the pelvic connective tissues.

Testosterone. During the growth of the cock's comb, which is controlled by testosterone activity, there is an accumulation of hyaluronic acid, whereas only traces of chondroitin sulfate have been demonstrated. Testosterone has been found to increase collagen formation in the skin of capons.

REGENERATION AND REPAIR

Adrenal steroids. As a result of the effect on the formation of ground substance and collagen, the healing of wounds is inhibited by cortisol, cortisone and related steroids in human subjects as well as in other mammalian species. During cortisone treatment the ingrowth of vessels is restricted, the oxygen uptake by wound tissue is reduced, and so is the tensile strength of sutured experimental wounds.

The targets of the hormonal effect are the mesenchymal cells of the wound. In rabbits, the formation of granulation tissue has been found to be delayed for a few weeks; thereafter the granulations develop unrestricted.

Healing of bone fractures is retarded, the absorption of blood, formation of callus and production of collagen being inhibited and delayed.

Intraperitoneal injection of cortisol (hydrocortisone) acetate prevents the development of serosal adhesions after surgical injury, sprinkling with talc and separation of fully developed adhesions.

Thyroxine. Moltke observed that l-thyroxine reduced the tensile strength of healing incised wounds in normal as well as in thyroidectomized guinea pigs. No similar effect was noted under the influence of d-thyroxine. The metabolic effect of this isomer is only moderate, but the thyrotrophin inhibition is considerable. Neither isomer reduced the lowered tensile strength in scorbutic guinea pigs. Administration of thyroxine together with a dehalogenase inhibitor caused an even greater restriction and retardation of wound healing, presumably because of the prevention of a deiodination and inactivation. Thyroxine acts on some target in the wound tissue, interfering with the formation of collagen fibrils.

Thyroxine increases epinephrine-induced vascular lesions to the extent that, in experimental animals, arteriosclerosis—including changes in mucopolysaccharides of the media and intima and calcification—is aggravated and accelerated.

Thyrotrophic hormone, in the above-mentioned experiments, did not convincingly influence the tensile strength of the wounds.

Somatotrophic hormone, because of its stimulation of collagen formation, increases the tensile strength of healing wounds, especially in low doses.

Sex hormones. In the presence of somatotrophin, testosterone and estradiol have been found to stimulate the formation of granulation tissue in inflammatory processes.

INFLAMMATION

Any change in connective tissue influences inflammatory processes. Glucocorticoids inhibit vascular permeability and exudation, fibrin formation, the concourse and phagocytotic activity of leukocytes and macrophages, the blood flow, and the formation of granulation tissue.

In contrast to thyroxine, thyrotrophin and somatotrophin stimulate the inflammatory reactions of connective tissue to injury.

TUMORS

The stroma plays an important role in the integrity, development, growth and spreading of various tumors. By influencing their connective tissue some hormones change the conditions for the tumors.

Adrenal steroids. Systemic administration of cortisone inhibits the development and prolongs the lag period of skin papillomas in mice induced by painting with carcinogenic hydrocarbons such as 9,10-dimethyl-1,2-benzanthracene or benzpyrene. In some experiments with methylcholanthrene, however, an increase of the incidence has been observed.

Fully developed skin papillomas regress in response to local injections of cortisol acetate into the stroma. Carcinomas, on the other hand, after initially showing a similar response, start growing after 8 to 11 weeks despite continued treatment.

The problem of whether mast cells and their mucopolysaccharide products form a barrier against spread of tumors is still unsettled.

Thyroxine. In thyroidectomized mice, thyroxine decreases the number of tumor-takes after one painting of the skin with 9,10-dimethyl-1,2-benzanthracene. On the other hand, thyroidectomy or thyrotrophin treatment increases the number of tumors.

Other hormones such as growth hormone exert a certain influence on the growth of some tumors, but the role of connective tissue changes is still obscure.

INFECTION

Some bacteria produce hyaluronidase, a spreading enzyme that facilitates invasion in the connective tissues. The hyaluronate is changed from a viscous to a watery material, and the bacteria as well as their toxins are allowed to spread. Some break-down products of acid mucopolysaccharides counteract the enzyme, reducing the permeability of the tissues. This process is influenced by hormones.

Adrenal steroids. Long-term treatment with adrenal steroids reduces resistance against infection. Low doses, however, may have a protective effect.

Thyrotrophin, growth hormone and *estrogens* inhibit spreading, but may render the tissues more susceptible to the influence of hyaluronidase.

FERTILITY

The production of hyaluronate in the ovarian follicles is subject to hormonal control, and so is the growth of the follicles to the point of rupture.

Fertilization, i.e., fusion of the spermatozoon with the ovum, takes place only if the hyaluronidase of the sperm is able to break down the hyaluronate of the mucinous mass surrounding the egg after release from the ovary. This is a target of hormonal action.

Thyroidectomy causes polycystic ovaries and an increase in the total amount of acid mucopolysaccharide. Ovulation is restricted.

ENDOCRINE DISEASES

In Cushing's disease the above-mentioned tissue effects of glucocorticoids are responsible for most of the changes represented in the clinical picture.

The effects of growth hormone and thyrotrophin are evident in acromegaly and gigantism, and those of thyrotrophin in malignant exophthalmos, circumscribed pretibial myxedema and hypothyroid myxedema. The importance of the ophthalmotrophic factor is most pronounced in acromegaly and gigantism, even in cases of thyrotoxicosis. In hypothyroid myxedema the mucotrophic and the fat-mobilizing factors are predominantly active. In thyrotoxicosis the thyroid-stimulating factor is immediately recognized.

Premenstrual tension may be due to water-binding by the ground-substance hyaluronate subject to sex-hormonal control.

HORMONE THERAPY

It is evident that hormone drugs are in use not only as substitution therapy in endocrine disorders, but also in diseases of connective tissue.

Systemic mesenchymoses, especially in phases of progression, may respond readily to hormone treatment. Disorders in the mucinous system can be influenced—e.g., by adrenocortical steroids—and a beneficial effect may be reflected within hours or a few days. Severe diseases of the skin, joints, eyes, muscles, bone marrow and other organs may be symptomatically relieved by a profound alteration of the physico-chemical state of the ground substance of the entire mesenchymal system.

Thyroid hormone, sex hormones, etc., are utilized as specific or symptomatic treatment.

Side effects due to overdosage of hormones should be considered on the basis of the above-mentioned knowledge of the properties of the hormones. In treatment of patients it may be a hard task to balance between beneficial effects that normalize pathologic processes and untoward side effects that affect even normal tissues and functions.

REFERENCES

Asboe-Hansen, G. (ed.): Connective Tissue in Health and Disease. Copenhagen, Munksgaard, 1954.

Asboe-Hansen, G.: Connective tissues under hormonal control. In Connective Tissue, Transactions of the 5th Conference. New York, Josiah Macy, Jr. Foundation, 1954.

Asboe-Hansen, G.: Hormonal effects on connective tissue. Physiol. Rev., 38:446, 1958.

Asboe-Hansen, G.: Endocrine control of connective tissue. Am. J. Med., 26:470, 1959.

Boseila, A-W. A.: The Basophil Leucocyte and Its Relationship to the Tissue Mast Cell. Copenhagen, Munksgaard, 1959.

Larsen, G.: Experimental studies on the mesenchymal structures and fluids of the eye. (In press.)

Lorenzen, I.: Epinephrine-induced alterations in connective tissue of aortic wall in rabbits. Proc. Soc. Exper. Biol. & Med., 102:440, 1959.

Moltke, E.: Experimental Investigations into the Influence of Thyroxine on Healing Wounds. Copenhagen, Munksgaard, 1958.

Poulsen, H.: Influence of Myxoedematous Connective-tissue Changes on Labyrinthine Function. Copenhagen, Munksgaard, 1959.

Thorsde, H.: Effect of thyroidectomy on ovarian mucopolysaccharides. Acta endocrinol. (In press.)

Zachariae, F.: Acid Mucopolysaccharides in the Female Genital System and Their Role in the Mechanism of Ovulation. Copenhagen, Periodica, 1959.

Zachariae, L.: Local Effect of Hydrocortisone on Connective Tissue. Copenhagen, Coster, 1956.

Hormonal Control of Acid Mucopolysaccharide Synthesis

ROBERT E. PRIEST

University of Washington School of Medicine

Acid mucopolysaccharides (AMP) are prominent components of the intercellular material in connective tissues. The importance of the AMP in fibrillogenesis, in osteogenesis and in fluid and electrolyte exchange is generally acknowledged, although a precise identification of the role of the AMP in these processes is still lacking. The elaboration of AMP by the connective tissues as well as their destruction or removal, as with other metabolic processes, is not static, but is greatly influenced by the environment of the connective tissues themselves. The hormonal status of the organism controls this metabolic process to a considerable extent.

The accumulation and regression of the intercellular substance in accordance with the hormonal state, as seen in the cock's comb and in the sex skin of certain primates, has intrigued investigators for a long time.[1, 8] The usefulness of radioactive tracers in the elucidation of the metabolism of AMP has been recognized by a number of workers, and hormonal influences on this metabolism have been demonstrated repeatedly by these techniques. Adrenal gluco-steroids have been shown to reduce incorporation of sulfate labelled with S^{35} into the sulfated acid mucopolysaccharides;[2, 5] growth hormone stimulates it,[3, 4] and insulin increases it in the diabetic animal.[7]

Efforts to delineate the mechanism of action of these hormones have been severely hampered because procedures for extraction are not quantitative, methods of separating different AMP from one another are insufficiently refined, and the knowledge of the mechanisms of biosynthesis is still sketchy. Indeed, it seems likely that not all of the kinds of AMP have as yet been identified. Nonetheless, some pertinent information has been gathered about the mechanism of hormonal influences on AMP metabolism.

The influence of estradiol can be taken as an example.[6] When estradiol is given to young adult male rats and is followed by an intraperitoneal injection of sulfate labelled with S^{35}, less radioactivity is incorporated into cartilage and other connective tissues than in animals not given the hormone. Since mammalian tissues appear to lack the capacity to convert this oxidized sulfur to the reduced form found in amino acids, the radioactivity incorporated is in the form of sulfate and except for small amounts found in sulfated nucleotides, cerebroside sulfate, etc., has been incorporated into the sulfated AMP. The reduction of incorporation into the AMP isolated from connective tissues of animals given estradiol parallels the reduction of incorporation into the tissues themselves (Table 1).

The reduction of incorporation of radioactive sulfate into connective tissues following administration of estradiol represents, then, a diminution in incorporation into the sulfated AMP. With injection of the radioactive material into the intact animal, such diminution could as well represent an increased rate of excretion of the isotope as a decrease in metabolic activity

44

TABLE 1. COMPARISON OF INCORPORATION OF S^{35}-LABELLED SULFATE
INTO CARTILAGE AND INTO THE AMP ISOLATED FROM
CARTILAGE WITH ADMINISTRATION OF ESTRADIOL

	TISSUE CPM/mg.	AMP CPM/μg.SO$_4$
Control	27.2	69.7
Estradiol	11.3	31.9
E/C × 100	41.7%	45.8%

of the sulfated AMP. If, however, one administers estradiol to animals, removes the tissues and then incubates them *in vitro* in the presence of radioactive sulfate, diminished incorporation is still evident. This clearly indicates that one is dealing with an alteration in the metabolic activity of the sulfated AMP rather than an alteration in size of the miscible pool of sulfate.

The fact that this effect of estradiol is not demonstrable by these techniques until more than a day following the administration of the hormone suggests that it could be mediated through another endocrine gland. Since hypophysectomized animals respond similarly and since testosterone fails to produce a significant alteration in sulfate incorporation, this possibility seems unlikely. Estradiol does produce a loss of weight in these animals, but differences in consumption of food cannot account for the effect on sulfate incorporation, because animals which are force fed still show the diminution when injected with estradiol and animals treated with estradiol show diminished incorporation of sulfate when compared to untreated animals whose diet has been restricted.

Although one is reasonably secure in regarding the incorporation of sulfate into connective tissues as a measure of metabolic activity of sulfated AMP, it is not so well established that this represents synthesis of these components of connective tissues. It is entirely conceivable that hormonal influences on the metabolism of the sulfated AMP measured by the incorporation of sulfate could represent influences on the mechanism of sulfation without significant effects upon the rate of synthesis of the polysaccharide backbone of the molecule. However, the radioactivity of the AMP isolated from tissues incubated in the presence of glucose labelled with C^{14} can be regarded as a measure of synthesis of the polysaccharide portion of the molecule. The incorporation of glucose-C^{14} and sulfate-S^{35} into AMP can be measured separately. When this is done in tissues from animals which are under the influence of estradiol, the incorporation of each isotope is found to be reduced by about the same degree (Table 2). It can be concluded, then, that the reduction of incorporation of S^{35}-sulfate into connective tissues which follows the administration of estradiol does, indeed, represent reduced synthesis of sulfated AMP.

TABLE 2. SIMULTANEOUS INCORPORATION OF C^{14}-GLUCOSE AND
S^{35}-SULFATE INTO THE AMP OF RAT CARTILAGE MEASURED
IN CPM PER μg. OF SULFATE

	C^{14}	S^{35}
Control	3.16	45.5
Estradiol	1.54	21.1
E/C × 100	48.7%	46.4%

Which step in the series of enzymic reactions in the biosynthesis of AMP is the rate-limiting one has yet to be determined for estradiol or for the other hormones. Whether the hormone affects the quantity of available substrate, certain cofactors or the enzyme itself remains at this point only a provocative question.

REFERENCES

1. Boas, N. F. and Ludwig, A. W.: The mechanism of estrogen inhibition of comb growth in the cockerels, with histologic observations. Endocrinology, 46:299, 1950.
2. Clark, I. and Umbreit, W. W.: Effect of cortisone and other steroids upon *in vitro* synthesis of chondroitin sulfate. Proc. Soc. Exper. Biol. & Med., 86:558, 1954.
3. Denko, C. W. and Bergenstal, D. M.: The effect of hypophysectomy and growth hormone on S^{35} fixation in cartilage. Endocrinology, 57:76, 1955.
4. Ellis, S., Huble, J. and Simpson, M. E.: Influence of hypophysectomy and growth hormone on cartilage sulfate metabolism. Proc. Soc. Exper. Biol & Med., 84:603, 1953.
5. Layton, L. L.: Effect of cortisone upon chondroitin sulfate synthesis by animal tissues. Proc. Soc. Exper. Biol. & Med., 76:596, 1951.
6. Priest, R. E., Koplitz, R. M. and Benditt, E. P.: Estradiol reduces incorporation of radioactive sulfate into cartilage and aortas of rats. J. Exper. Med., 112:225, 1960.
7. Schiller S. and Dorfmann, A.: The metabolism of mucopolysaccharides in animals. IV. The influence of insulin. J. Biol. Chem., 227:625, 1957.
8. Zuckermann, S., Von Wagenen, G. and Gardiner, R. H.: The sexual skin of the Rhesus monkey. Proc. Zool. Soc., London, Series A, 108:385, 1938.

Panel Discussion

Gustav Asboe-Hansen, *Moderator*

Dr. Asboe-Hansen: Dr. Wagner, how do you identify a fibroblast?

Dr. Wagner: This is a matter of definition. Should the parameters of the definition be restricted exclusively to histological criteria or should the functional status be included? This is the real problem, because one defines a fibroblast in terms of "guilt by association." We study the area surrounding the cell and see what is there and then make an assumption that the cell is probably a fibroblast. I am quite sure that I must agree with Dr. Muir's earlier remarks that we must identify these cells in terms of a specific function at a given time. Then I think we might have some interesting answers.

Dr. Asboe-Hansen: I think it will be quite impossible to identify fibroblasts even by chemical methods. There is no doubt that a fibroblast in one place is different from a fibroblast in a neighboring place; even two fibroblasts quite close to each other may have different cytochemical properties. Although this is not definitely proved for fibroblasts, it is proved for mast cells. The mast cell in one animal has a different cytochemistry from a mast cell in a different species, and even two mast cells within the same tissue and the same grade of tissue may have different cytochemistries. We have only very crude histological and chemical methods, and these methods are insufficient and too undeveloped for identification of cells, so at the present time we cannot differentiate between different mesenchymal cells.

Dr. S. Fitton Jackson: I think we may be able to develop adequate chemical methods in the near future; for example, I have been doing some tissue culture work using "plated-out" cell suspensions, in which the presence of hydroxyproline can be detected chemically within 12 hours after the cell has been plated out. By electron microscopy and x-ray diffraction the presence of collagenous protein can not be identified for 45 hours. This indicates that chemically one may be able to pick up the presence of protein prior to morphological evidence of it.

DR. ASBOE-HANSEN: Dr. Jackson, would you also comment about the present methods for identification of a fibroblast, and define what a fibroblast is?

DR. S. FITTON JACKSON: I agree with Dr. Wagner that identification is usually "guilt by association." One says a certain cell is a fibroblast if it is surrounded by recognizable collagenous material. In addition, we know from embryological studies that many of the early undifferentiated cells that we see become fibroblasts; there is a great deal of work supporting this, showing how the mesenchymal cells move into the right areas. Of course, this brings up all the old embryological and genetic problems as well as the exterior situations that convert cells and stimulate them to produce their chemical substances. I think it will take a very long time to define precisely the process which produces these morphological and cytochemical hallmarks.

DR. ANGEVINE: May I make some comments about the identification of fibroblasts and mast cells? Although we must keep an open mind and accept new advances, we are training people in this field as well as doing investigations, and I would not like to leave the impression that this panel of experts would say that they do not know what these cells are. I know what a fibroblast is, and although I may not know all of its functions, I think I know many of them. We must retain our present concepts at this time, in order to make progress and learn more about these cells. In regard to the mast cell, typical examples of it have been shown in many of the slides which have been presented. Cells without granules may not be mast cells and one may be reluctant to call certain cells mast cells if no granules are present; but I think the only way we can work with the problem is to accept the present morphological criteria for identification of these cells.

DR. ASBOE-HANSEN: In living organisms living cells which are partly degranulated can still be identified as mast cells; if they have a cytoplasmic mass you can still identify them. At least that is the criterion we use. Morphological criteria can be used for identification of fixed fibroblasts, certain mast cells and degranulated mast cells. You can even tell the difference between a mast cell and a macrophage which has taken up granules from a disintegrated mast cell; however, I think that within a very short time different criteria for identification of these cells may be available and the names of some of them may have to be changed.

DR. ANGEVINE: The investigators who work with these cells at the molecular level and with the electron microscope have to know what they start with before they can relate the information derived from these advanced techniques to previous morphological data.

DR. ASBOE-HANSEN: I agree. I believe you are referring to the studies of neutral collagen by investigators who have picked out a single cell or two of these cells which they think are fibroblasts; then they isolate them and state that these cells are producing polysaccharides or other chemical substances in the culture media. However, these cells might have been in the embryotic state, and instead of being real fixed fibroblasts, might have been young mast cells.

DR. S. FITTON JACKSON: Surely, Dr. Asboe-Hansen, there is not any question of the fact that a specific type of cell was used, and I am sure that this applies to cells that are defined as fibroblasts. A fibroblast is a fibroblast even if it is in a young stage of differentiation. As this cell becomes more mature, then its function may change a little, but it will still be a fibroblast. However, if it is in a certain area, just for semantic reasons one calls it an osteoblast if it is concerned with laying down bone or another name if it is concerned with production of a different type of connective tissue.

DR. MENKIN: I think that we are dealing with a primitive mesenchymal cell which has a multipotential. In the last analysis, it is the intracellular substance that is formed which defines the cell type. If it forms collagenous material it is a fibroblast, or if it forms chondromucin it is a cartilaginous cell, or if it forms osseous matrix it is an osteoblast.

DR. SOKOLOFF: I would like to ask Dr. Kelsall and Dr. Asboe-Hansen about the mechanisms of degranulation of mast cells that occurs in variety of physiologic and pathologic states.

DR. KELSALL: I do not think that the degranulation of mast cells in the peritoneal cavity reported in most of the studies pertains to the lysis of mast cells in most situations. In sections of tissue not exposed to water or other substances which cause rapid lysis, mast cells may release only a few granules at a time instead of a large number simultaneously. Furthermore, after the granules are released we often see that the granules within the cells increase in size to some extent.

DR. ASBOE-HANSEN: I agree with Dr. Kelsall.

DR. WAGNER: The mast cell granule is supposed to contain histamine, 5-hydroxytryptamine and heparin. Will anyone comment on how these are "packaged" in the granule, how they are released, and what is the mechanism for release?

DR. ASBOE-HANSEN: The exact mechanisms will be difficult to define until we have more information about them. Some investigators think that heparin and mucopolysaccharides are outside the cells or are located in the cytoplasm between or on the surface of the granules, rather than inside the granules. The data are not clear and there is no proof of which theory is correct. What do you think, Dr. Kelsall?

DR. KELSALL: I think recent reports have definitely established by diversified techniques that the mast cell is a very significant source of histamine and heparin. One would expect that whatever was in a mast cell would be primarily located within the granule because that is the major portion of a mast cell. However, if the mast cell does contain histamine, one would have to be most careful in evaluating the significance of the mast cell as the source of hyaluronic acid.

DR. ASBOE-HANSEN: I also think that some of these substances are in the mast cell and must be in the granule, but I do not know where the histamine is located. Perhaps, although we have not proved this, the mucopolysaccharide is also in the granule.

DR. PRIEST: I haven't worked with mast cell granules, but it is my impression, right now, from the data which have been presented using histochemical techniques, that histamine in the living mast cell is located in the granule in association with the metachromasia.

DR. KELSALL: I would like to ask Dr. Asboe-Hansen how one can differentiate between the possibility that mast cells are a direct source of hyaluronic acid and the possibility that histamine from mast cells acting on fibroblasts increases the formation of hyaluronic acid?

DR. ASBOE-HANSEN: This is the same problem again: Is there any difference between a degranulated mast cell and a fibroblast? As far as we can identify mast cells, these cells contain mucopolysaccharides. No one has any method for identifying mucopolysaccharides in a fibroblast. I believe that Dr. Kelsall thinks that histamine is bound, necessarily bound, to the mucopolysaccharide fraction of mast cells and that these two substances are released together, but I think that it may be possible for the mast cell to release the histamine without releasing the mucopolysaccharide.

Dr. Kelsall, is there any evidence that histamine can be released associated with mucopolysaccharides?

DR. KELSALL: Most of the procedures used to release histamine also release heparin concomitantly, and both substances are increased following lysis of mast cell granules. There are several theories about the way in which heparin and histamine are combined, and one of these is that the two substances are linked by a cross-type linkage since release of granules is associated with simultaneous release of histamine and heparin.

DR. PRIEST: It was demonstrated some years ago that concomitant with degranulation of mast cells in breast tissue there was a release of histamine and 5-hydroxytryptamine, which is found in these particular mast cells. Later, *in vitro* studies with isolated mast cells indicated that, with degranulation, there was nearly total release of histamine, 5-hydroxytryptamine, and partial release of chymotryptic activity.

DR. ASBOE-HANSEN: Dr. Kelsall, how do you identify the heparin?

DR. KELSALL: As far as identifying it is concerned, I would call it an acid mucopolysaccharide and let it go at that.

DR. WAGNER: Even the biochemists have trouble telling what heparin is. Many arguments have taken place regarding its chemical identification. It is very difficult to be sure heparin is present and not some related substance.

DR. THORNBURG: In regard to release of these substances, I think that it is worth remembering that the granule in a mast cell appears to have a membrane, and secondly, that the structural site of the effect of histamine appears to be the membrane, the histamine causing gross changes in transport by pinocytosis. Finally, it may be that the release of the material in the granules involves a pinocytotic mechanism in which the membrane of the granules adjoins the plasma membrane of the cell at the time of release.

I would also like to comment on the hormonal control of the synthesis of various cellular products. In the first place, all research which has attempted to identify hormonal control of soluble systems has failed. On the other hand, there are several theses of data that indicate that hormones do influence membranes and transport processes, for instance, in the endothelial cells, and that they also affect other secretory functions which are essentially membrane functions.

Secondly, it appears that the transport process may be pre-eminent here and as a result of the transport, and perhaps the secretion, synthesis is stimulated, so that the mechanisms of hormonal reactions may be mediated through structural changes in membranes. Again, we have many models for this because when there are structural abnormalities in membranes, there are at the same time differences in secretory rates.

The third comment has to do with the problem of identifying cell particulates, either those exerting hormonal control or the synthetic products which we expect to find in these cells. The problem here is one that biochemists generally have not been aware of; that is, in the process of the separation of these cell particulates, the cells are subjected in the ultra-centrifuge to hydrostatic pressures in the range of a thousand pounds or more which are known to cause specific membrane damage and fragmentation of membranes. Thus, it seems quite likely that there is an abnormal system in these cell particulates, particularly those that are dropped down at higher speeds, and as such the system might no longer be subject to hormonal control. The data taken from these studies may have led to incorrect conclusions about hormonal control of synthesis in these elements.

Part II | GENERAL CHARACTERISTICS
OF INFLAMMATION

The Inflammatory State— General Remarks*

VALY MENKIN

University of Kansas City School of Dentistry

There have been many definitions of inflammation, all of which have no doubt been adequate to a person having his particular views in interpreting this basic phenomenon of pathology. I have defined it as the complex vascular, lymphatic and local tissue reaction elicited in higher animals by the presence of viable or of nonviable irritants.[1] It represents a basic or elemental reaction to injury whereby the deleterious agent tends to be localized and ultimately destroyed. When caused by viable irritants, inflammation may be regarded as the physical basis of infectious processes. The inflammatory reaction may be truly viewed as an immunological mechanism of definite significance.

The subject of inflammation has, as far back as Hippocrates (about 460-377 B.C.), played a dominant part in the history of medicine.[2] Hippocrates regarded inflammation as being closely associated with fever. I shall not take time to go over the history of this subject, for, as Boyd appropriately states in his textbook, the history of inflammation is the history of pathology. A few highlights, however, may be pointed out. Celsus (about 25 B.C. to A.D. 45) stated the classic cardinal features. Galen, and later on John Hunter, stressed the loss in function. Hunter regarded inflammation as an adaptive defense mechanism which ultimately restored the injured part to its normal function. In this respect, this investigator (1728-1793) was the first to understand the immunological implication of inflammation.

It was, however, in the 19th century that serious analysis of the phenomenon of inflammation had its start. Cohnheim analyzed the process involved from the standpoint of disturbed local capillary physiology.[3] To Cohnheim the central point of the inflammatory reaction was the increased permeability of the capillary wall. The outward migration of leukocytes was regarded by Cohnheim as being closely associated with this phenomenon. This investigator took the very definite position that the events of inflammation were all referable to alteration in the vessel wall, for he categorically stated, and I quote: "I believe I can prove strictly *that it is only and solely the vessel wall which is responsible for the entire series of events.*"

In the latter part of the 19th century a different theory to explain inflammatory processes was advanced by Metchnikoff.[4] This investigator was primarily a zoölogist, and his views represented the outcome of careful observations in the realm of comparative pathology. He rejected the views of Cohnheim that the inflammatory reaction was essentially referable to alteration in the permeability of the vascular wall. To Metchnikoff the primary function of inflammation involved the phagocytic capacity of leukocytes, which in this way disposed of the irritant; inflammation was an adaptive

* The studies embodied in this communication have been aided by grants from the United States Public Health Service, Bethesda, Maryland.

phagocytic reaction to injurious material that had penetrated into tissues.

In 1940 in a monograph entitled "Dynamics of Inflammation," I pointed out that the early views of Hunter, who conceived inflammation as a defensive reaction; those of Cohnheim, who regarded the reaction as essentially one of vascular alteration; and finally, the phagocytic theory of Metchnikoff should not be considered separately, but rather as major interdependent sequences in the development of the inflammatory reaction.[1] At that time I also indicated that the overwhelming influence of Metchnikoff had disadvantages, for inflammation, even to that day, was still regarded erroneously by numerous pathologists as exclusively a leukocytic response. Cohnheim, on the other hand, failed to consider the immunological implication of inflammation. In my opinion these early views could be shown to have a synthetic relationship to more modern observations that concerned themselves with the various mechanisms involved.[1]

Inflammation is no longer to be considered as a relatively static phenomenon, as its morphological picture often suggests to students or beginners. It is a manifestation of severe cellular injury in the vertebrate kingdom. It represents a constantly changing dynamic state consisting of several interdependent reactions incited in the host by an irritant. Foreign substances, whether viable or nonviable, in contact with otherwise normal tissue will induce an inflammatory reaction, the intensity of which may vary from a barely visible hyperemia to an intense suppurative process. It is only for obvious reasons that the interest of the microbiologist in problems of tissue injury has primarily been focused on bacterial infection.[1]

Inflammation is initiated by a disturbance in local fluid exchange. This is manifested primarily, as Cohnheim first conceived it, by an increase in capillary permeability. Since this reaction is the pivot response on which all subsequent sequences depend, an understanding of the mechanism involved looms as one of definite significance. This phase of inflammation will accordingly be discussed with some detail during the course of this symposium.

The immunological implication of inflammation as a site that limits or "walls off" the irritant is closely linked with the initial increase in capillary permeability. It is with the enhanced passage of plasma protein that fibrinogen accumulates in the area of injury. With the formation of a fibrinous network as well as with the occlusion of draining lymphatics by thrombi, the site of inflammation is to a large extent circumscribed. The rapidity and the intensity with which this process of "walling off" occurs is of importance in envisaging the dissemination of the irritant, especially if this happens to be a pathological microorganism. In this way it has been shown that the staphylococcus as a highly injurious organism in turn induces rapid local fixation. On the other hand, the hemolytic streptococcus is a milder organism, and consequently is more invasive. One can thus arrive at a formulation that dissemination from the site of inflammation bears an inverse ratio to the degree of induced local injury. This can be expressed as $D = \dfrac{Kt}{I}$, where D refers to dissemination, t to time, K being a constant depending on the irritant and its anatomical location, and I to the degree of induced injury. Such studies have led to the interpretation that the role of inflammation in immunity is that of a regulator of bacterial invasiveness.[1] Finally, in pointing to the immunological aspect of inflammation one cannot overlook the abundant studies on allergic and anaphylactic inflammation with all the implications involved in various states of hypersensitiveness.

The early work at the beginning of this century, particularly by Opie, has indicated the significance of intracellular enzymes in the phagocytic cells at the site of inflammation.[5] Even though these studies have been amplified by the finding of other enzymes besides leukoprotease and the lymphoprotease of Opie, nevertheless the conclusions drawn by this distinguished investigator remain essentially true to this day. The studies of Opie have stimulated further probing into the mechanism that regulates the cellular sequence in inflammation consisting of polymorphonuclear leukocytes followed by mononuclear phagocytes. This sequence had been described as early as 1893 by Borrel in France.[6] The studies of Schade in Germany have stressed the developing acidosis in an area of inflammation.[7] In 1934 I interpreted from experimental observations on canine exudate that the hydrogen ion concentration of the exudate conditions this cellular sequence at the site of inflammation.[8] This study demonstrated that in exudates the central problem centered around that of survival of leukocytes. In brief, the polymorphonuclear leukocytes were incapable of surviving in exudates of an acid pH. The inability of polymorphonuclear leukocytic survival with developing acidosis has nothing to do with the actual process of emigration. This study has been confirmed by several investigators.[9, 10] When the pH falls below 6.0, all types of white cells are injured, and pus results. Pus formation in acute inflammation is virtually a function of the hydrogen ion concentration. Further studies have indicated that the mechanism of acidosis was primarily referable to a developing glycolysis.[1] The final conclusion drawn was that the cellular sequence at the site of inflammation is conditioned by the local pH, which in turn is determined by disturbance in the intermediary carbohydrate metabolism.

Studies on phagocytosis have progressed considerably since the days of Metchnikoff. These include the important studies of Mudd and his collaborators in the late 1920's and early 1930's.[11] These investigators pointed out the importance of the opsonins and bacteriotropins as protein films around particles to be ingested. These globulins acted as promoters of phagocytosis. Increased phagocytosis was ascribed to changes in surface tension. The subsequent studies of Barry Wood, Jr., and collaborators pointed out that the physical character of the surface seems to be an important element in the promotion of phagocytosis.[12] The subject is now also being studied from the standpoint of cellular energy as an important element in phagocytosis.[13] Cellular biologists have also considerably interested themselves in demonstrating the close relationship of pinocytosis to phagocytosis.[14]

Active biochemical studies of inflammation were initiated in my laboratory at the Harvard Medical School in the middle 1930's. The early studies indicated that injured cells at the site of inflammation release a permeability and chemotactic factor which was termed *leukotaxine*.[15] This finding initiated the studies on the recovery of mediators from inflammatory exudate. These mediators or common denominators have been shown to explain in a reasonable fashion specific biological manifestations of inflammation.[16] The mechanism for the local increase in capillary permeability, migration of leukocytes, leukocytosis, leukopenia, the pattern of injury in inflammation and the pathogenesis of fever each had an explanation in the recovery of a specific common denominator.[17] Some were shown to be polypeptides; others still require further chemical investigation. None of these mediators have been as yet obtained as complete, pure entities. Each of them, however, is specific. The leukocytosis is ascribed to two factors, the leukocytosis-promoting factor

(LPF) and the thermostable leukocytosis factor.[18-21] Leukocytosis cannot be initiated by any of the other known mediators. The migration of leukocytes is initiated in large part by leukotaxine. The increase in capillary permeability may be referable to several mediators, but leukotaxine and exudin have been found to be important in this mechanism.[22-24] In brief, these mediators are biologically specific, but not as yet fully chemically purified. It is hoped that this fact will induce chemists to probe further into the exact chemical configuration of these important substances.

The finding of polypeptides in inflammatory exudate with the biological properties described has stimulated considerable further work throughout the world.[1, 17] In the United States, England, Germany, South America, Russia, Italy and Japan there have been considerable studies on the mediators at the site of inflammation.[25-31] The presence of a number of the known mediators has already been confirmed; time has been inadequate to substantiate the presence of the others. Some of these mediators no doubt have practical clinical application. I am referring, for instance, to the leukocytosis-promoting factor and possibly to pyrexin, one of the two factors concerned in the pathogenesis of fever.

Another important field in the modern studies of inflammation is the effect of anti-inflammatory agents. This work had its inception in the Harvard Medical School Laboratories in 1936-1940, when it was shown that adrenocortical extract suppresses the increase in capillary permeability caused by leukotaxine.[32] In 1942 the same effect was shown to occur with Compound E, which came to be known as cortisone.[33] These early experiments were the first studies on the anti-inflammatory property of the corticoids. They have received considerable attention by clinicians, biochemists, physiologists and pathologists in the last eleven years following the brilliant discovery by Hench and Kendall of the therapeutic value of cortisone and ACTH in some arthritic conditions.[34] Attempts have been made to elucidate the anti-inflammatory mechanism of cortisone. The mode of action of cortisone is still under study. It is possible that the suppression in cell activity caused by cortisone may be referable to a repression in protein synthesis. This would entail, I believe, an inhibition in the formation of the polypeptides or mediators by the injured cell.[17, 35] By suppressing the formation of the mediators by injured cells at the site of inflammation, the manifestation of the inflammatory reaction would be correspondingly reduced. Suppression of cellular activity seems to be a significant factor in the anti-inflammatory mechanism.

Many studies have been made, and many are still in progress, on the mechanism of repair in inflammation.[17, 36-40] This has been shown to be referable to the liberation of an endogenous growth-promoting factor. A knowledge of the chemistry of this growth-promoting factor is of paramount importance. Its diffusibility, thermostability and ultraviolet spectrophotometric curve as well as its inactivation by trypsin and ribonuclease suggest the possibility that it may be a nucleopeptide. The liberation of this growth-promoting factor at the site of inflammation is probably significant in explaining the mechanism of repair with inflammation. It seems also to be of importance in explaining the role of inflammation in carcinogenesis. Recent studies indicate that this role may be that of a cocarcinogen via the endogenous growth-promoting factor liberated at the site of inflammation by injured cells.

REFERENCES

1. Menkin, V.: Dynamics of Inflammation. New York, The Macmillan Co., 1940 (reprinted 1950).
2. Hippocrates; Translated by W. H. S. Jones. London and New York, Loeb Classical Library, 1923.
3. Cohnheim, J.: Virchow's Arch., *40*:1, 1867; Lectures on General Pathology, London, New Sydenham Society, 1889.
4. Metchnikoff, E.: Leçons sur la Pathologie Comparée de l'Inflammation. Paris, G. Masson, 1892.
5. Opie, E. L.: J. Exper. Med., 7:316, 1905; Arch. Int Med., *5*:541, 1910; Physiol. Rev., 2:552, 1922.
6. Borrel, A.: Ann. Inst. Pasteur, 7:593, 1893.
7. Schade, H.: Die Molekular-pathologie der Ehtzündung. Dresden and Leipzig, Theodor Steinkopff, 1935.
8. Menkin, V.: Am. J. Path., *10*:193, 1934.
9. Rugiero, H. R. and Tanturi, C. A.: Semana Med., *8*:13, 1942.
10. Bennett, I. L., Jr.: J. Exper. Med., *88*:279, 1948.
11. Mudd, S., McCutcheon, M. and Lucké, B.: Physiol. Rev., *14*:210, 1934.
12. Wood, W. B., Jr. and Smith, M. R.: Science, *106*:86, 1947.
13. Gordon, G. B. and King, D. W.: Am. J. Path., *37*:279, 1960.
14. Bennett, H. S.: Report before Xth International Congress on Cell Biology, Paris, Sept. 6, 1960.
15. Menkin, V.: J. Exper. Med., *67*:129, 145, 1938.
16. Menkin, V.: Ann. N. Y. Acad. Sc., *59*:956, 1955.
17. Menkin, V.: Biochemical Mechanisms in Inflammation. Springfield, Illinois, Charles C Thomas, 1956
18. Menkin, V.: Am. J. Path., *16*:13, 1940.
19. Menkin, V.: Arch. Path., *30*:363, 1940.
20. Menkin, V.: Blood. J. Hemat., *4*:1323, 1949.
21. Menkin, V.: Proc. Soc. Exper. Biol. & Med., *75*:738, 1950.
22. Menkin, V.: Am. J. Physiol., *166*:509, 1951.
23. Menkin, V.: Proc. Soc. Exper. Biol. & Med., *77*:592, 1951.
24. Menkin, V.: Am. J. Physiol., *166*:518, 1951.
25. Reifenstein, G. H., Ferguson, J. H. and Weiskotten, H. G.: Am. J. Path., *17*:233, 1941.
26. Cullumbine, H. and Rydon, H. N.: Brit. J. Exper. Path., *27*:23, 1946.
27. Pasquali, L.: Ric. e studi d. Med. Speciment, *18*:209, 1947.
28. Minami, G. and Inugami, K.: Tr. Soc. Path. Jap., *30*:389, 1940.
29. Busse Grawitz, P.: Prensa méd. argent., *32*:1902, 1945.
30. Spector, W. G.: J. Path. & Bact., *63*:93, 1951.
31. Morimoto, M.: Naika No Ryoiki, *1*:401, 1953.
32. Menkin, V.: Am. J. Physiol., *129*:691, 1940.
33. Menkin, V.: Proc. Soc. Exper. Biol. & Med., *51*:39, 1942.
34. Hench, P. S., Kendall, E. C., Slocumb, C. H. and Polley, H. F.: Proc. Staff Meet., Mayo Clin., *24*:181, 1949.
35. Menkin, V.: Science, *120*:1026, 1954.
36. Menkin, V.: Cancer Res., *1*:548, 1941.
37. Menkin, V.: Cancer Res., *19*:544, 1959.
38. Menkin, V.: Brit. M. J., *1*:1585, 1960.
39. Menkin, V.: Proc. Soc. Exper. Biol. & Med., *104*:312, 1960.
40. Menkin, V.: Biologic Cocarcinogens. Extracted from Progress in Experimental Tumor Research. Basel, Switzerland, Karger, *1*:279, 1960.

Inflammatory States Due to Bacterial Infection Having a Histopathological Resemblance to the Dyscollagenoses

E. KARL KOIWAI

Hahnemann Medical College and Hospital, Philadelphia

Biopsies of skin and skeletal muscle are often submitted to pathologists for establishing the diagnosis of a dyscollagenosis. Distinguishing vascular changes, connective tissue alterations, and inflammatory changes are often used to identify the presence of a collagen disease.[7, 8] Demonstration in postmortem material of histopathological changes, such as granulomatous lesions with perivascular or subendocardial fibrinoid changes in the myocardium, often denotes the presence of a collagen disease. Changes described as being consistent with the diagnosis of a dyscollagenosis are acknowledged to be the result of an allergic phenomenon[10] or of production of autoantibodies.[1] However direct action of bacteria and their toxins, for example hemolytic streptococci, on the heart muscle may produce a similar lesion.[3, 6] Both theories have been supported by some experimental evidence. The pathologist is often committed to make a definite diagnosis, and depending upon the clinical picture he acknowledges the presence or absence of a dyscollagenosis.

Recently Ginsburg and associates[4] have produced cardiac lesions in the rabbit by intramyocardial injection of various micro-organisms. They obtained endomyocardial changes at the site of a single intramyocardial injection of living or killed hemolytic streptococci, their cell-free extract, and other micro-organisms: enterococci, lactobacilli, *Bact. coli* and *L. casei.* The lesions consisted of fibroblastic and histiocytic cell proliferation in the endocardium mingled with round cell infiltration. In both the endocardium and the myocardium, granulomatous lesions with giant cells were produced. Although not so described by Ginsburg,[4] they resembled granulomatous lesions of rheumatic fever. However, no lesions were produced by injection of various micro-organisms either intravenously or intracardially without first traumatizing the heart with a sterile needle. Since well developed granulomata were found seven days after one single injection, the role of sensitization in the production of these lesions was questioned. Gross and associates[6] produced similar myocardial changes following intracardiac injection of α-hemolytic streptococci, and regardless of whether single or repeated injections were given, the histological changes were identical. Glaser et al.[5] found myocardial granulomata 48 to 72 hours following intrapharyngeal injection of hemolytic streptococci. Ginsburg and his group[4] felt that these observations made it unlikely that sensitization or allergy played a significant role in the production of myocardial lesions of this type.

To verify the observations above, the following study was done using

Pseudomonas aeruginosa and *Staphylococcus aureus*. These organisms were used because of their resistance to many of the antibiotics; furthermore, in Pseudomonas infections the mechanism of development of the infection and of the tissue reaction is not clear.

MATERIALS AND METHODS

Micro-organisms. *Pseudomonas aeruginosa* (pigmented) and *Staphylococcus aureus* of strain S-1 from stock cultures from the Department of Microbiology were grown on agar slants incubated 24 hours at 37° C. For inoculation two loops of the organisms streaked from the agar slants were suspended in 5 cc. of sterile normal saline and 0.2 cc. was given intramyocardially.

Animals. Seventeen rabbits weighing 2 to 3 kg. were used. They were fed on Staley's Rockland vitamin C fortified rabbit diet and water.

Methods. The rabbits were anesthetized with ether; the heart was traumatized by intracardiac puncture with a 20-gauge needle attached to a sterile syringe and intraventricular blood was removed for initial antibody titers and paper electrophoresis of the rabbit's serum. While still in place, the needle was pulled out slightly and negative pressure was applied on the syringe until there was no evidence of blood coming from the heart chamber. This indicated that the needle was in the myocardium and not in the heart chamber. At this point 0.2 cc. of normal saline containing the micro-organisms was injected into the myocardium.

Eleven rabbits were injected intramyocardially with *Pseudomonas aeruginosa* and six rabbits with *Staphylococcus aureus,* strain S-1. On the seventh day blood was removed from the heart of ten of the rabbits injected with the Pseudomonas suspension. Of those, seven were killed and autopsied, and the remaining three rabbits were given a second dose of 0.2 cc. of Pseudomonas intramyocardially after ventricular blood was removed for antibody studies. These last three rabbits were sacrificed 14 days after the initial injection of the micro-organisms. One of the 11 rabbits injected with the Pseudomonas suspension expired on the day of the first injection.

Six rabbits were injected similarly with Staphylococci, S-1, after cardiac blood was drawn. Only one rabbit survived seven days; the remaining rabbits expired two to four days after injection. All six rabbits had cardiac blood drawn for initial antibody studies, but only the one rabbit which survived seven days had blood removed for the second determination.

Histological Preparations. The animals were autopsied and the organs were fixed in cold neutral 10 per cent formalin solution. Paraffin sections were stained with hematoxylin-eosin, Alcian blue-periodic acid Schiff stain, Brown-Bren stain, McGee-Russell's alizarin-red method for calcium, and Gomori's trichrome stain.

Paper Electrophoresis. Pre- and postinfection blood samples were taken and the serum protein patterns were determined using the Spinco Model R Paper Electrophoresis system and the bromphenol blue stain.

Antibody Determinations. Preparation of the Antigen. The colonies from the agar-slant were picked and streaked on a blood agar plate and incubated at 37° C. for 12 hours. After 12 hours the blood agar plate was flooded with sterile normal saline and the surface of the colony was dissolved by touching it lightly with a warm platinum loop. The antigen mixture was transferred to a test tube and diluted with normal saline until the desired turbidity was obtained The antigen mixtures were thus prepared from Pseudomonas and Staphylococcus colonies.

SLIDE AGGLUTINATION TEST. A drop of serum and a drop of the above prepared antigen were mixed on a slide with a toothpick and after one minute were read for possible agglutination. The result was compared with a control of saline and the prepared antigen. The results were read 0 to 4 plus, depending on the quantity of agglutination.

QUANTITATIVE TITRATION. Tube dilutions for quantitative analysis of the presence of antibodies were done by starting with the first tube containing 0.2 cc. of rabbit serum, 0.8 cc. of normal saline and 0.5 cc. of the prepared antigen of either Pseudomonas or Staphylococcus and then taking 0.5 cc. aliquots to make serial dilutions of 1/5, 1/10, 1/20, 1/40 and 1/50. These were compared with a control containing normal saline and the antigen after incubation for one hour at 37° C. and then overnight at room temperature.

RESULTS

Pseudomonas-Injected Rabbits. Of the 11 rabbits injected intramyocardially, the rabbit that expired on the day of the injection failed to show any myocardial lesions except for the intramyocardial hemorrhage caused by the needle; the remaining 10 rabbits showed both gross and microscopic lesions. On the epicardium at the apparent site of injection there was often a patch of yellowish gray exudate covered with fibrin and sometimes surrounded by focal areas of hemorrhage. Epicardial and pericardial cultures were, however, sterile.

Microscopically, all ten rabbits had both subendocardial and myocardial granulomatous lesions (Fig. 1). These lesions were present in the animals killed on both the seventh and the fourteenth day after the initial injection

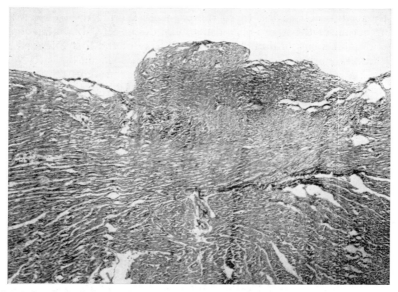

Fig. 1. Subendocardial granulomatous lesion with fibrinoid necrosis formed in a rabbit injected with *Pseudomonas aeruginosa* intracardially. H&E. × 26.

of the micro-organisms. There was a marked fibroblastic proliferation with infiltration of histiocytes, lymphocytes, and mononuclear and giant cells (Figs. 2 and 3).

These giant cells had basophilic or slightly eosinophilic cytoplasm. On Trichrome stain the cytoplasm stained similarly to the muscle and the nuclei

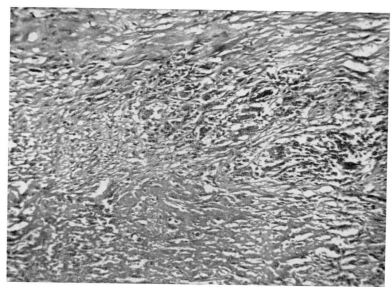

Fig. 2. The granulomatous lesion contains giant cells and is infiltrated with lymphocytes, mononuclear cells and histiocytes. Contiguous with the granuloma there are areas of fibroblastic proliferation and fibrinoid changes. H&E. × 80.

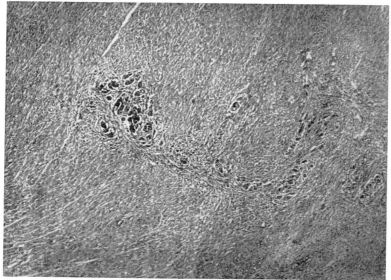

Fig. 3. Within the myocardium, there are multiple granulomatous lesions containing giant cells which resemble Aschoff bodies of rheumatic myocarditis. H&E. × 26.

were vesicular, containing prominent nucleoli (Fig. 4). Histologically, the changes in the giant cells corroborate Murphy's concept that these multinucleated structures are of myogenic origin.[9] The fibroblastic proliferation extended into the adjacent myocardial fibers. With the granulomatous lesion there were areas of fibrinoid changes most frequently found beneath the endocardium. The lesions were not related to the blood vessels. Within the same granulomatous areas there was amorphous material which took a basophilic stain with H&E but was positive with the PAS stain and

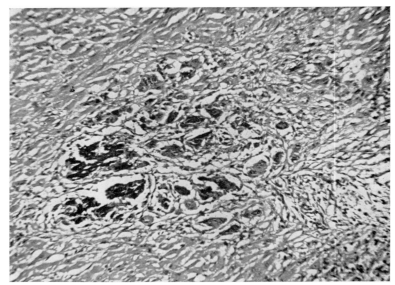

Fig. 4. The intramyocardial granulomatous lesion contains giant cells with prominent vesicular nuclei, while the cytoplasm takes on a basophilic stain and still others take a slightly eosinophilic stain. H&E. × 175.

stained irregularly with the calcium stain. The Brown-Bren stain failed to reveal any bacteria. The exact nature of this material is not certain, although it may be remnants of myocardial fibers.

Staphylococci-Injected Rabbits. Only one of the six rabbits injected intramyocardially survived seven days. Three rabbits which expired one to two days after injection failed to show any granulomatous lesions. The remaining three rabbits surviving three, four and seven days after the initial trauma and injection with staphylococci had a fibroblastic reaction in the myocardium with granulomatous changes similar to those present in the myocardium of the Pseudomonas-injected rabbits. These findings corroborate those of Ginsburg.[4] Lesions of the myocardium were found as early as three days after injection. The animals which expired before the seventh day were found to have hemorrhagic bronchopneumonia. Cultures of the pericardium were negative for staphylococci and the Brown-Bren stain for bacteria in the myocardium was also negative.

Histological examination of the heart in both the Pseudomonas- and staphylococci-injected groups was positive for a granulomatous lesion in all rabbits that survived three days or more. According to this experiment, it is unlikely that sensitization or allergy plays a significant role in the production of these lesions. However, in order to rule out the possible role of

TABLE 1. ANTIBODY STUDIES ON RABBITS INJECTED INTRAMYOCARDIALLY WITH PSEUDOMONAS AERUGINOSA AND STAPHYLOCOCCUS AUREUS*

| RABBIT | DAYS SURVIVED | LESIONS | PRE-INJECTION Ps. Antigen Slide | 7TH DAY POSTINJECTION Ps. Antigen | | Staph. Antigen | 14TH DAY POSTINJECTION Ps. Antigen | |
				Slide	Tube	Tube	Slide	Tube
*PR- 1	0	−	0	0	0	0		
PR- 2	7	+	−	−	0	0		
PR- 3	7	+	−	2+	0	0		
PR- 4	7	+	−	2+	0	0		
PR- 5	7	+	−	3+	0	0		
PR- 6	7	+	−	4+	−	1/30		
PR- 7	7	+	−	4+	0	0		
PR- 8	14	+	−	4+	−	1/20		
PR- 9	7	+	−	4+	1/20	0		
PR-10	14	+	−	4+	1/20	1/20	4+	1/20
PR-11	14	+	1+	4+	1/10	0	3+	
†S-12	7	+	1+	3+	0	1/30		
S-13	2	−	0	0	0	0		
S-14	2	−	0	0	0	0		
S-15	4	++	0	0	0	0		
S-16	3	++	0	0	0	0		
S-17	1	−	0	0	0	0		

* PR = Pseudomonas-injected rabbits.
† S = Staphylococci-injected rabbits.

hypersensitivity, paper electrophoretic patterns were done on the serum before and after intramyocardial injections of the micro-organisms. Slight to marked alterations of the electrophoretic pattern were found after injection, notably in the albumin, α_2, β and γ globulin fractions. These alterations suggested the possibility of formation of antibodies; therefore, antibody studies were initiated. The previously described procedures were done: first, the slide agglutination test and then quantitative titration.

Results of Serum Antibody Studies (Table 1). In one Pseudomonas-injected rabbit, PR-2, no agglutination took place, but all others showed 2 to 4 plus agglutination at seven days as well as 14 days after injection. The only serum collected from the Staphylococci-injected group was from rabbit S-12 since the remaining rabbits expired before the seventh day. By mistake, the serum of S-12 was used against the prepared Pseudomonas antigen, which showed 1 plus agglutination pre-injection and 3 plus agglutination post-injection. This implied that this agglutination was nonspecific. Meanwhile quantitative titrations were done on the available rabbit serums. The rabbits PR-6 and PR-8, although having a 4 plus reaction on slide agglutination, had a negative reaction by the tube dilution method. However, rabbits PR-9, PR-10 and PR-11 had a positive reaction at 1/20, 1/20 and 1/10 dilutions, respectively, thereby indicating the possible presence of a specific antibody. Nevertheless, when the above mistake was discovered, staphylococcal antigen was used in the tube titration and it was discovered that the serum from rabbits PR-6, PR-8 and PR-10 had titers of 1/30, 1/20 and 1/20, respectively. The rabbit S-12, which was injected with Staphylococci, had a titer of 1/30 with the staphylococcal antigen. The results of these tests indicate that these reactions in the slide agglutination and tube titration methods are nonspecific. The true nature of these nonspecific reactions should be further investigated.

DISCUSSION

The intramyocardial lesions resembling a dyscollagenosis were produced by a single trauma of a sterile needle and the injection of saline suspensions of *Pseudomonas aeruginosa* or *Staphylococcus aureus*. Paper electrophoretic and antibody studies indicate that hypersensitivity does not play a role in the production of these lesions. This experiment agrees with the findings of Ginsburg and his associates,[4] who showed that neither trauma to the heart muscle alone nor the intravenous injection of living or heat-killed hemolytic streptococci caused any pathological changes in the heart. On the other hand, well developed granulomatous lesions appeared in the heart when the intravenous injections of these organisms were preceded by puncturing the myocardium with a sterile needle. They suggest that trauma to the heart is of importance in production of myocardial changes; there is also the possibility that products of various organisms—toxins and enzymes—may cause "trauma" to the heart muscle, thereby predisposing it to the effect of the micro-organisms.

The question arises as to whether the routine biopsies of skin and skeletal muscle for determining the presence of collagen disease actually represent examples of the above theory. Such an example is the vasculitis with thrombosis which is often present in a gangrenous leg and is frequently categorized as thromboangiitis obliterans (Figs. 5 and 6). This, however, may represent a case of marked arteriosclerosis with vasculitis caused by trauma and bacteria enzymes and toxins. Therefore the findings appear to be in agreement with those of Wessler and his associates,[11] who state that the entity described as thromboangiitis obliterans does not exist.

The cardiac lesions produced by this experiment also resemble the granulomatous lesions in humans described by Churg and Strauss[2] as "allergic

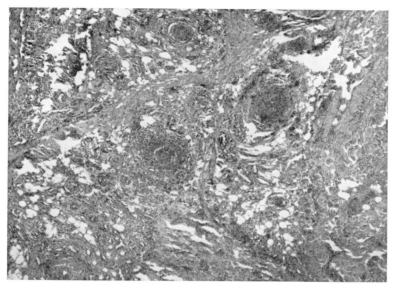

Fig. 5.   The multiple vessels show marked thickening with obliteration of the lumens and marked inflammatory infiltration. The section taken was from a 57-year-old white female whose toes were amputated for gangrene. H&E. × 80.

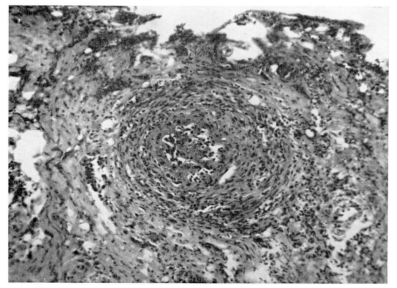

Fig. 6.   The same case as Figure 5 which shows the microscopic features of thromboangiitis obliterans and complete obliteration of the lumen due to a thrombus which contains giant cells. The thickened wall and perivascular tissue are markedly infiltrated with an acute and chronic inflammatory cells. H&E. × 175.

granulomatosis." They have described, in addition to the central eosinophilic core of necrotic cells and altered collagen fibers surrounded by radially arranged macrophages and giant cells, the presence of small dense aggregates of eosinophiles. Eosinophilic infiltration was not evident in these experimental animals. Without this eosinophilic infiltration the differentiation between the two types of lesions would be difficult.

Zeek's critical review of periarteritis nodosa[12] brings out the confusion and the difficulty of classifying "necrotizing angiitis" accurately. "Not only the gross and microscopic morphology of the lesions are important but also their distribution in the body. It is no longer adequate to state the lesions are characteristic of periarteritis nodosa in every respect."

Therefore, it can be added that before a diagnosis of a collagen disease can be definitely established, the possibility that the histological changes present may be the result of trauma and bacterial action should also be considered.

SUMMARY

Granulomatous lesions having a histopathological resemblance to the dyscollagenoses were produced in the endomyocardium of rabbits. They were produced by cardiac trauma and intramyocardial injection of *Pseudomonas aeruginosa* or *Staphylococcus aureus*. It is unlikely that hypersensitivity played a role in their production because well developed granulomata were produced in three days after one single injection of the micro-organism and no specific antigen-antibody reaction was demonstrable.

The diagnosis of dyscollagenosis on the basis of histopathological changes alone is inadequate.

REFERENCES

1. Calvelti, P. A.: Studies on the pathogenesis of rheumatic fever, Part 1 and Part 2. Arch. Path., *44*:1, 13, 1947.
2. Churg, J. and Strauss, L.: Allergic granulomatosis, allergic angiitis and periarteritis nodosa. Am. J. Path., *27*:277, 1951.
3. Clawson, B. J.: Experimental endocarditis with fibrinoid degeneration in the heart valves of rats. Arch. Path., *50*:68, 1950.
4. Ginsburg, I., Laufer, A. and Rosenberg, S. Z.: Cardiac lesions produced in the rabbit by intramyocardial injections of various micro-organisms. Brit. J. Exper. Path., *41*:19, 1960.
5. Glaser, R. J., Thomas, W. A., Morse, S. I. and Darnell, J. E.: The incidence and Pathogenesis of myocarditis in rabbits after group A streptococcal pharyngeal infections. J. Exper. Med., *103*:173, 1956.
6. Gross, P., Cooper, F. B. and Phillips, J. D.: The cytologic response of rats and mice to a strain of Greening streptococci. Am. J. Path., *17*:377, 1941.
7. Klemperer, P.: Concept of collagen diseases. Am. J. Path., *26*:505, 1950.
8. Klemperer, P., Pollack, A. D. and Baehr, G.: Diffuse collagen diseases, J.A.M.A., *119*:331, 1942.
9. Murphy, G. E.: Nature of rheumatic heart disease with special reference to myocardial disease and heart failure. Medicine, *39*:289, 1960.
10. Rich, A. R. and Gregory, J. E.: The experimental demonstration that periarteritis nodosa is a manifestation of hypersensitivity. Bull. John Hopkins Hosp., *72*:65, 1943.
11. Wessler, S., Ming, S., Gurewich, V. and Freiman, D. G.: A critical evaluation of thromboangiitis obliterans. New Engl. J. Med., *262*:1149, 1960.
12. Zeek, P. M.: Periarteritis nodosa: a critical review. Am. J. Clin. Pathol., *22*:777, 1952.

The Inflammatory State—Response to Chemical and Physical Agents*

PIERRE JEAN

Institut de Médecine et de Chirurgie expérimentales, Université de Montréal

The contribution of our Institute in the field of inflammation is closely related to stress research. Investigations were planned to elucidate the role played by hypophyseal and corticoid hormones in the nonspecific response of the body to systemic stress, which affects the whole body, and to topical stress, whose manifestations are limited to a circumscribed region. The response of the body to systemic stress is the "general adaptation syndrome" (G.A.S.), characterized by manifold morphologic and functional changes throughout the organism. Conversely, topical stress elicits a "local adaptation syndrome" (L.A.S.), whose manifestations consist, on the one hand, of degeneration, atrophy and necrosis, and on the other, of inflammation, hypertrophy and hyperplasia.

The purpose of the present communication is to present the interrelationship between the G.A.S. and the L.A.S. and to give two experimental models of inflammation: one, the "granuloma-pouch technique," being the response to chemical agents; the other, the "tissue-scaffolding technique," being the response to physical agents.

RELATIONSHIP BETWEEN THE G.A.S. AND THE L.A.S.

Both the G.A.S. and the L.A.S. can be elicited by a great variety of agents. This nonspecificity of action led to the definition of systemic stress as "the sum of all the nonspecific, systemic biologic phenomena (including damage and defense)."[1] In the same sense, we may say that local stress is "the sum of all nonspecific local biologic phenomena (including damage and defense)."

Inflammation has often been described as "the reaction to topical injury." In addition to this defense reaction, the L.A.S. includes the initial tissue damage itself. In practice, the manifestations of damage are often inseparable from those of defense. The phenomena of cellular degeneration, atrophy and necrosis are predominantly injurious. On the other hand, the subsequent formation of an inflammatory granulomatous barricade is fundamentally a protective phenomenon that shields the adjacent tissues against the irritant.

Like the G.A.S.,[1, 2] the L.A.S. is essentially a triphasic biologic reaction:

1. The local alarm reaction. When a strong irritant is introduced into a circumscribed region of the body, the cells and connective tissue fibers undergo degenerative changes, frequently progressing towards necrosis; the direct effect of injury might be considered the "shock phase." In the surrounding region, mature fibroblasts dedifferentiate into rounded elements of

* The experimental work on which this article is based was supported by grants from the National Science Foundation and the National Cancer Institute of Canada.

a more embryonic type that can give rise to phagocytes or to elements resembling white-cell types of circulating blood. This "counter-shock phase" is essentially what we call acute inflammation.

These first two phases of the local alarm reaction are extremely non-specific, in that their manifestations are essentially the same irrespective of the nature of the eliciting injurious agent.

2. The local stage of resistance. Depending upon the particular irritant used, the dedifferentiated cells are transformed predominantly into fibroblasts, lymphocytic elements, macrophages and foreign body giant-cells. Varying proportions of hematogenous leukocytes or erythrocytes may accumulate within the injured region.

One of the most striking characteristics of this "local stage of resistance" is that the wall of the inflammatory focus becomes highly resistant to further treatment with otherwise necrotizing doses of the irritant originally used to produce it ("specific-resistance"). Indeed, it even exhibits a high degree of tolerance to cognate substances that would normally evoke the formation of a histologically similar type of granuloma ("cross-resistance"). Conversely, resistance to irritants that would normally produce different types of granuloma is significantly diminished ("cross-sensitization"). These facts will be illustrated later by experiments in which the "granuloma-pouch technique" was used.

3. The local stage of exhaustion. Defense against a severe irritant cannot be maintained indefinitely; degeneration and necrosis occur. But if the intensity of the irritant is mild, healing takes place without the "local stage of exhaustion."

Both the L.A.S. and the G.A.S. are singularly sensitive to the so-called "adaptive hormones" (ACTH, STH, corticoids). The effect of these hormones on the general inflammatory process is discussed elsewhere in this volume.

RESPONSE TO CHEMICAL AGENTS

A few years ago, a technique was devised in our Institute in order to produce local inflammation, the so-called "granuloma-pouch technique," a procedure that has been described elsewhere.[3] In principle, it consists in the injection of 25 ml. of air into the loose connective tissue of the rat, under the shaved skin of the back. If a chemical irritant is then injected into the regular ellipsoid air-space thus created, the lining connective tissue is transformed into a granuloma. For instance, a few days after the introduction of a dilute solution of croton oil into the pouch, the air is replaced by an inflammatory exudate, which can be measured by transillumination or by aspiration into a syringe; the walls of the cavity are gradually transformed into a well-delimited granulomatous membrane.

Various chemical irritants have been used for the production of a "granuloma pouch." Croton oil induces a hemorrhagic exudate and an intensely fibrous capsule; formalin, at a low concentration, provokes a fibroblastic reaction, while higher concentrations readily induce necrosis; turpentine facilitates pus formation; fine particulate matter (India ink, kaolin) stimulates macrophage production; and gross particles (mustard powder) result in giant-cell formation.

The "granuloma-pouch technique" has furnished interesting findings that have led us to formulate the concepts of "specific- and cross-resistance." A pouch produced with dilute croton oil becomes resistant to normally necrotizing doses not only of croton oil itself[4] but also of formic acid, hypertonic NaCl, mustard oil, NaOH, HCl, trypsin, ox bile and boiling water.[5]

Conversely, at the same time, the croton-oil pouch is less resistant to formaldehyde,[5] which normally produces a different type of granuloma ("cross-sensitization"). The wall of an inflammatory focus seems to differentiate in such a manner as to afford optimum protection against the evocative agent or cognate irritants. However, at the same time, it loses the ability to adapt itself for other purposes.

Thus, the "granuloma-pouch technique" is a useful tool for studying the response of the tissue to chemical injury.

RESPONSE TO PHYSICAL AGENTS

Recent experiments were planned in our laboratory to elucidate the response of connective tissue to agents that are irritant only by their physical structure. For this purpose, we used the "tissue-scaffolding technique," which furnished us with tools for the systematic analysis of the influence exerted by various mechanical factors upon tissue reactivity.[6] For animal experiments, our standard scaffolding of this kind is a straight Pyrex glass tube 30 mm. long, with a bore of 10 mm., and open at both ends. Usually, we envelop it tightly (leaving the opening free) in nylon muslin, which is readily encapsulated by the connective tissue; the tube is, thereby, rigidly fixed in the desired position (Fig. 1). Soon after such a scaffolding is implanted under the skin of the rat, its two ends are closed by round "basal plates" of the adjacent connective tissue. Two weeks after implantation, the tube is completely or almost completely filled with a citrine fluid and a straight axial cord has developed between the two openings. This cord consists of a broad, central spindle made up of fibrin threads and histiocytes. Within a month or so, the fibrin thread is invaded by a tendon-like, dense connective tissue (Van Gieson-positive and well vascularized), which forms a bridge between the central points of the two basal plates (Figs. 2, 3). It is not yet clear why once such a connection is complete and well vascularized it does not increase in thickness and gradually fill the tube.

It has been possible to demonstrate that if the inner surface of the tube is also lined with a layer of nylon muslin, the entire cavity rapidly becomes filled with loose connective tissue. Here, the arrangement of fibers and blood vessels is quite irregular, presumably owing to the many surfaces for attachment provided by the nylon trellis. By providing simple glass tubes with one or more lateral openings, it was possible, furthermore, to construct filiform beams of tendon-like connective tissue, with lateral anastomoses at predictable points.

The same "tissue-scaffolding technique" permitted us to study the reaction of tissue to another physical agent, pressure.[7] When small chambers having only a single, relatively narrow opening are introduced into the subcutaneous tissue of the rat, a considerable negative pressure develops as a result of the absorption of air introduced at the time of implantation or of subsequently formed exudate. In such cases, the surrounding connective tissue is sucked into the lumen and there gives rise to the formation of pads that are indistinguishable macroscopically and microscopically from normal fat tissue

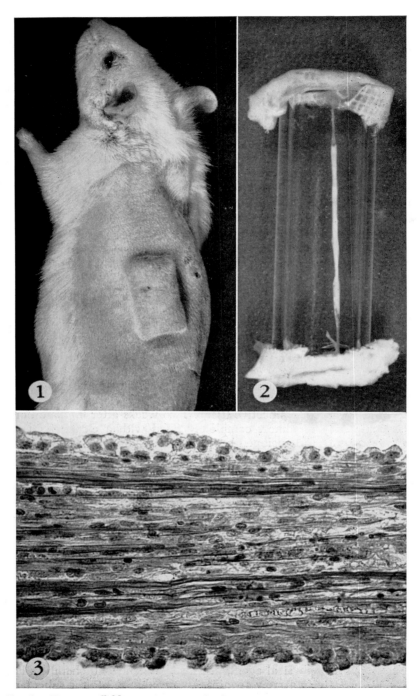

Fig. 1. Tissue-scaffolding as it appears in situ.

Fig. 2. Axial-cord formation within simple glass tube. The disk-like basal plates **at** the opening are intact; here, the nylon-muslin, which envelops the tube in situ, has been removed. Note the invasion of the two extremities of the fibrin thread by connective tissue.

Fig. 3. Longitudinal section of an axial cord. Numerous histiocytes are seen on the surface. Spindle-shaped fibrocytes and capillaries run parallel to the fully developed connective tissue fibers. (Van Gieson stain × 480).

(Figs. 1, 2, 3 after Selye, H.: Medizinische, No. 14, 617, 1959.)

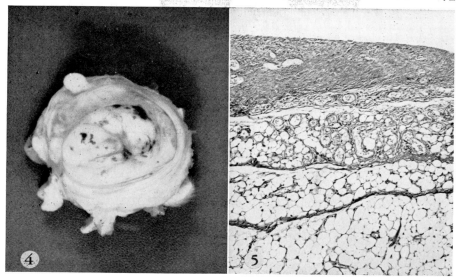

Fig. 4. Basal plate at the opening of a bottle-shaped glass chamber. Note the bulging fat pad, with multiple petechiae underneath the surface and two pedunculated small lipomas near the margin.

Fig. 5. Histologic section through a similar fat pad. Note the typical aspect of the adipose tissue, whose lobules are separated by connective-tissue bands. (Van Gieson stain × 100).

(Figs. 4, 5 after Selye, H., Jean, P. et al.: Plast. and Reconstruct. Surg., 24:250, 1959.)

(Figs. 4, 5). It is assumed that suction itself is chiefly responsible for this phenomenon.

These experiments illustrate the reaction of tissue to agents that are irritant only by virtue of their physical structure or by mechanical factors. It is hoped that such a "tissue-scaffolding technique" may prove useful in the study of inflammation and wound-healing.

SUMMARY

The general adaptation syndrome (G.A.S.) and the local adaptation syndrome (L.A.S.) are closely interrelated. The former represents the sum of all nonspecific systemic biologic phenomena, and the latter includes all nonspecific local biologic phenomena. Both are nonspecific reactions, comprising damage and defense; both are triphasic, with typical signs of "cross-resistance" or, depending upon the stressors used, "cross-sensitization" during the second stage.

Two experimental models of tissue reactivity to injury have been presented. The "granuloma-pouch technique" illustrates the response to chemical irritants, and the "tissue-scaffolding technique" demonstrates the response to physical agents.

REFERENCES

1. Selye, H.: Stress; the Physiology and Pathology of Exposure to Systemic Stress. Montreal, Acta Inc., 1950.
2. Selye, H.: The Story of the Adaptation Syndrome. Montreal, Acta Inc., 1952.

3. Selye, H.: On the mechanism through which hydrocortisone affects the resistance of tissues to injury. J.A.M.A., 152:1207, 1953.
4. Selye, H.: Induction of topical resistance to acute tissue injury. (An experimental study with the "granuloma-pouch technique.") Surg. Clin. North America, 33:1417, 1953.
5. Selye, H.: Induction of local "crossed resistance" to various necrotizing agents. J. Exper. Med. & Surg., 11:81, 1953.
6. Selye, H.: Diaphragms for the analysis of the mechanics of connective-tissue growth. Nature, 184:701, 1959.
7. Selye, H., Jean, P., Cantin, M. and Lemire, Y.: Induction of adipose tissue development by mechanical means. Plast. & Reconstruct. Surg., 24:250, 1959.

Some Studies on Biochemical
Changes in Inflammation*

VALY MENKIN

University of Kansas City School of Dentistry

An inflammatory reaction is initiated by a disturbance in local fluid exchange.[1] There is a preliminary vasoconstriction followed by a vasodilatation, and, most important of all, an increase in capillary permeability.[1] The extent of this increased permeability is evinced by the passage of graphite particles or of bacteria through the endothelial wall (Fig. 1).[2] It is of significance to determine the mechanism of this increased capillary permeability in an inflamed area. More than twenty-four years ago it was observed that an inflammatory exudate *per se* induces an increase in capillary permeability.[3] There seems to exist a permeability factor in the exudate. The exudate, in turn, is considered to represent the products of cell injury admixed with elements from the circulating blood. Untreated blood serum, however, is incapable of inducing such a reaction. The permeability factor present in exudates can be precipitated with 20 per cent sodium sulfate or at half saturation with ammonium sulfate.

By preliminary deproteinization with pyridine or dioxan and acetone, the permeability factor was purified. Subsequently it was treated with butyl alcohol or N acetic acid (cf. Scheme of Extraction and Figure 2).[4, 5] The purified product consisted of doubly refractile granules in an ill-defined matrix.[4, 6] This could at times be brought to the crystalline state as needle-like crystals, although this may entail some difficulty.[4] In addition, this substance induced first the close adherence of polymorphonuclear leukocytes to the endothelial wall, as well as their subsequent migration or diapedesis into the extracapillary spaces (Fig. 3). This migratory activity failed to occur when blood serum was extracted by the same scheme. This substance is diffusible from the whole exudate and it is thermostable.[1, 4, 6] Recent studies

* These studies were aided by grants from the U. S. Public Health Service, Bethesda, Maryland.

indicate that it can be extracted in the very first few hours of inflammation (4 to 5 hours), at a time when the exudative material first appears in measurable amounts at the site of inflammation.[7] It displays two of the important biological properties of inflammation, namely the ability of increasing capillary permeability and of inducing the migration of leukocytes.[1, 6] It has been

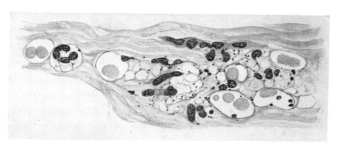

Fig. 1. Camera lucida drawing, showing passage of graphite particles through capillary walls into area of inflammation induced by croton oil (about 6 hours' duration). Magnified approximately × 970. (From Menkin: J. Exper. Med., 53:647, 1931, and Dynamics of Inflammation, New York, The Macmillan Co., 1940.)

LEUKOTAXINE (SCHEME OF EXTRACTION)

50 cc. exudate (usually at an alkaline pH)
↓
Dioxan (1:1)
↓
Stir for 1 hour
↓
Centrifuge
↓
Supernatant
↓
Acetone (1:1)
↓
Centrifuge
↓
Evaporated to dryness *in vacuo* at about 50° C.
↓
25 cc. of N acetic acid
↓
On ice for about 1 day or longer
↓
Centrifuge
↓
Wash precipitate with distilled water by stirring and subsequent centrifugation (repeat procedure twice)
↓
Precipitate contains leukotaxine in amorphous state admixed with leukotaxine crystals
↓
Add 5 cc. distilled water to precipitate
↓
Dialyze 18 hours against 50 cc. distilled water, stirring the dialyzing bag throughout the dialysis
↓
Concentrate diffuse *in vacuo* at 50° C.
↓
Active doubly refractile crystalline leukotaxine

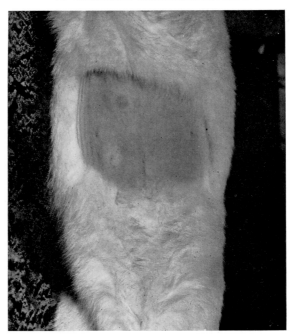

Fig. 2. Effect of leukotaxine by N acetic acid method. Upper area shows accumulation of trypan blue from the circulation in area treated with leukotaxine in saline. Lower area shows complete inactivity with physiological saline.

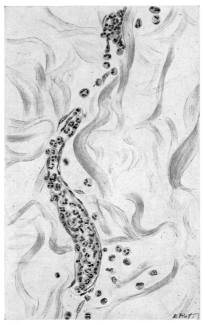

Fig. 3. The effect of leukotaxine on the diapedesis of leukocytes 44 minutes after the introduction of leukotaxine into the cutaneous tissue of a rabbit. The material injected was crystalline-like. It also induced a marked increase in capillary permeability. Note that the capillary lumen is crowded with polymorphonuclears active in migrating into the extracapillary space. About × 700.

termed *leukotaxine*.[4, 8] The chemotactic property elicited by leukotaxine can be demonstrated by *in vitro* studies (Figs. 4 and 5).[1, 6] As controls, neither carbon particles nor reduced iron powder is capable of inducing any such chemotactic response.[1, 6, 9] Recently we have found that an exudate composed primarily of mononuclear phagocytes, as encountered in the later or acid stage of an acute inflammation, when in contact *in vitro* with leukotaxine,

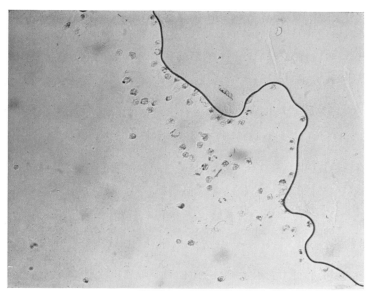

Fig. 4. Chemotactic effect of leukotaxine on polymorphonuclear leukocytes. The polymorphonuclears are derived from an exudate of a dog. The pH of that exudate is 7.2, and the differential count consists of 80 per cent of these cells. The cells are supravitally stained with neutral red, and the chemotaxis is studied *in vitro*. Note the gradual orientation and in many cases the adherence of the leukocytes to a mass of leukotaxine. This photograph is an example of the chemotactic property of leukotaxine. × 255. (From Menkin: Biochemical Mechanisms in Inflammation. Springfield, Illinois, Charles C Thomas, 1956.)

likewise exhibits within a period of hours a peripheral aggregation of these phagocytes (Fig. 5).[6, 9] It is therefore conceivable that leukotaxine is perhaps also chemotactic for the mononuclear phagocytes. These cells, however, as shown by Harris, are slower than the polymorphonuclears in their mobility towards an identical target.[10] It is therefore possible that the peripheral spatial location of these cells in an inflamed area is also referable in part to leukotaxine.[9] Further *in vivo* observations are necessary in order to substantiate this view.

Leukotaxine appears to be a polypeptide.[4, 7] This was demonstrated by inactivation with aminopeptidase.[7] Chromatographic studies further substantiate this view (Fig. 6).[6] Whether there is a prosthetic group attached to leukotaxine remains yet to be determined. In brief, this substance is biologically specific. It has been purified to some extent, but still considerable studies are required in order to obtain complete purity, as well as additional chemical information concerning the precise structure of this significant biological substance. Recent studies by differential centrifugation, in an endeavor to localize the cytologic precursor of leukotaxine, indicate its close association

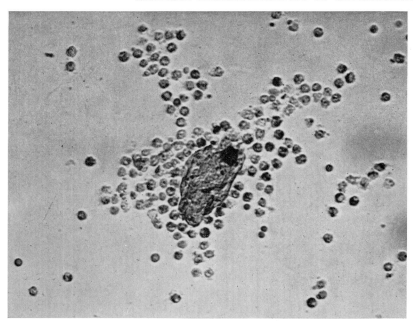

Fig. 5. The gradual aggregation of primarily mononuclear phagocytic cells around a mass of leukotaxine. This response may be seen within 1 day or less after exposure to leukotaxine. These types of cells are derived from an acid exudate, and they are supravitally stained with neutral red. × 255. (From Menkin: Biochemical Mechanisms in Inflammation. Springfield, Illinois, Charles C Thomas, 1956.)

with the "mitochondrial" fraction and often with the "microsomal" fraction of the homogenate of inflamed tissue when the exudate is at an alkaline pH.[11]

Leukotaxine is capable of essentially reproducing the effect of the whole exudate as far as increasing local capillary permeability and inducing the

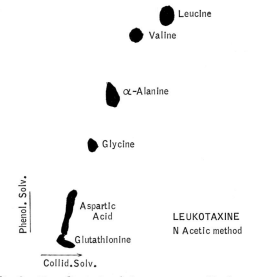

Fig. 6. Two-dimensional chromatogram of leukotaxine.

emigration of polymorphonuclear leukocytes are concerned. This fact, important as it is, does not, however, preclude the possibility that other factors may also contribute to the phenomenon of increased capillary permeability at the incipient stage of the inflammatory reaction (Menkin, 1940; Miles and Wilhelm, 1955; Spector, 1956; Menkin, 1960). The postulated globulin described by Spector (1956) may play a role. Menkin has recently expressed the view that the blood serum permeability factor of Miles may, by seeping into an area of inflammation, reinforce the effectiveness of leukotaxine.[12]

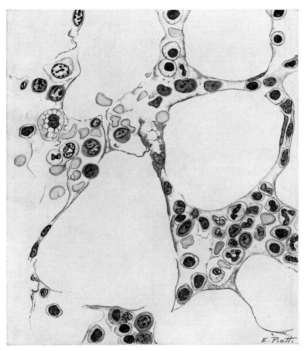

Fig. 7.   Dog 7-50 G. Section of femoral bone marrow injected several days previously with pseudoglobulin fraction from blood serum. Note that the bone marrow is essentially normal. × 1300.

Let us turn now to another common denominator liberated by injured cells at the site of an acute inflammation. Leukocytosis or elevation in the number of circulating leukocytes is frequently associated with some acute inflammatory conditions. The intravascular introduction of an exudate, derived from the site of an inflammation in a dog with leukocytosis, into a recipient dog induces in the latter a state of leukocytosis.[13, 14] Leukotaxine introduced into the circulation fails to induce such an effect.[13] The rise in the number of circulating leukocytes is referable to a discharge of immature granulocytes from the bone marrow.[13, 14] The evidence thus indicates that there is present a leukocytosis-promoting factor (abbreviated as the LPF) in an inflammatory exudate. Its presence reasonably explains in part the mechanism of leukocytosis with inflammation. This specific factor is non-diffusible and it is thermolabile.[6, 15] It can be purified by ammonium sulfate fractionation.[6] It is absent in blood serum unless there is a concomitant acute inflammation.[16] It causes specific hyperplasia of granulocytes and of mega-karyocytes in the bone marrow (Figs. 7 and 8).[17] Chromatographic studies indicate that one is apparently dealing with a polypeptide.[6] Aging the material causes a loss in biological potency and the LPF becomes insoluble.[18] Centrifugation of the suspended aged material in an aqueous medium indicates, however, that the active principle is confined to the supernatant phase.[18] This substance recovered from canine exudate is likewise active in human beings.[6, 19] This may prove to be of clinical significance in various

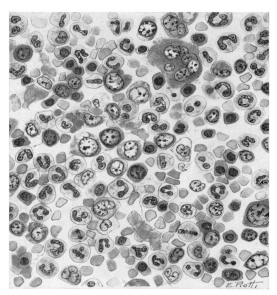

Fig. 8. Femoral bone marrow, Dog 7-64 G, several days after injection of 87 mg. of leukocytosis-promoting factor (LPF) into the circulation. This injection caused a marked leukocytosis and distinct hyperplasia of the bone marrow involving the myelocytic type of cells, as well as the megakaryocytes. Note the mitotic figure.

states of persistent leukopenia that are accompanied with only some degree of aplasia of the hematopoietic tissue in the marrow. Finally, studies by differential centrifugation of the homogenate of inflamed tissue in 0.25 M sucrose indicate that the precursor of the LPF appears to be in the soluble phase or S_2 fraction.[11]

Inflammation is considered to be a manifestation of severe cellular injury in vertebrates. The basic pattern was first described at the beginning of our era by Celsus. This entails the well-known classic signs of redness, swelling, heat and pain. Galen and, later on, John Hunter added another cardinal sign, loss of function. We have pointed out the presence of an additional bio-chemical cardinal sign, namely, proteolysis.[20] Is there a chemical factor concerned in the basic mechanism of the pattern of injury in inflammation? The ultimate character of the injury may be modified by the inherent chemistry of the irritant or by the anatomical location of the lesion. In brief, a number of years ago, it was found that the primary reaction seems to be referable to a toxic euglobulin liberated by injured cells at the site of inflammation, and which I have termed *necrosin* (Fig. 9).[21] The alpha globulins of exudates,

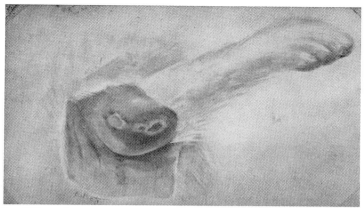

Fig. 9. Effect of necrosin injected into the skin of foreleg of Rabbit 22-25. The acute inflammatory reaction with areas of central necrosis was drawn about 22 hours after the cutaneous injection of 1 ml. of an aqueous suspension of necrosin derived from the exudate of a dog. (From Menkin: Arch. Path. 36:269, 1943.)

containing the leukocytosis-promoting factor (LPF), are inactive in inducing any such characteristic lesion. The euglobulin of blood serum is likewise inactive.[21] The first morphological type of injury induced by necrosin affects the collagenous bundles (Fig. 10).[21] Within ten minutes these may be swollen.[21] Necrosin induces the formation of thrombi in lymphatics (Fig. 11). The significance of lymphatic blockade in inflammation has been described elsewhere.[1] It may therefore well be referable to the liberation of necrosin by the severely injured cells. Thrombi in small blood vessels may likewise be

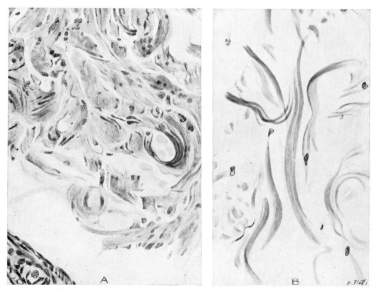

Fig. 10. A. Effect of a suspension of necrosin 10 minutes after its intracutaneous injection in the rabbit. Note that the collagenous bundles are markedly swollen. This seems to be the first evidence of injury following the injection of necrosin. B. It appears that the euglobulin fraction of normal blood serum is solely without effect on the appearance of the collagenous bundles of the skin even after 45 minutes.

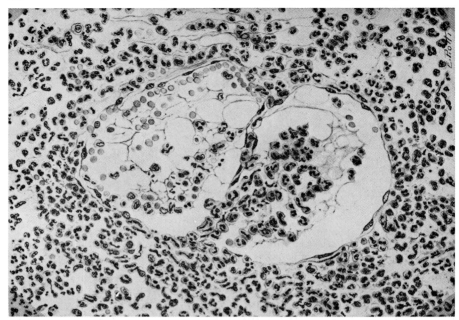

Fig. 11. The drawing of thrombosed lymphatic in a zone of dense leukocytic infiltration of a subcutaneous area into which necrosin had been injected about 23 hours and 30 minutes previously. (From Menkin: Arch. Path., 36:269, 1943.)

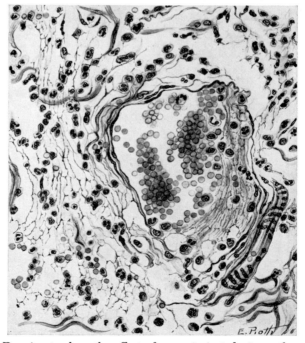

Fig. 12. Drawing to show the effect of necrosin in inducing a thrombus in a small blood vessel. This is taken from the same section as Figure 11. (From Menkin: Arch. Path., 36:269, 1943.)

found at the site of the acute injury (Fig. 12).[21] Intravascular injections of necrosin frequently induce hepatic injury (Fig. 13).[21] Repeated injections of necrosin into dogs in an endeavor to duplicate a prolonged inflammatory process may be followed by a curious denudation of the cytoplasmic contents of liver cells.[19] There is a replacement by glycogen, as evidenced by

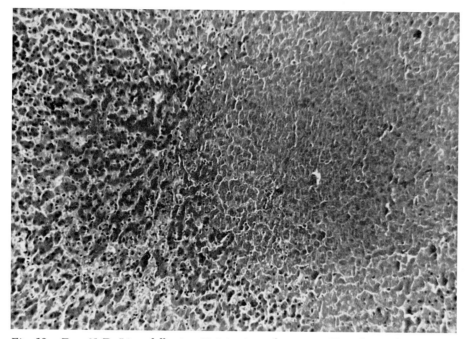

Fig. 13. Dog 61-D. Liver following 22 injections of necrosin. Note the marked necrosis of hepatic tissue in the section. × 202.

appropriate cytochemical staining (Best carmine). This glycogen deposition does not seem to be referable to diet. Starving an animal for one or even sometimes two days yields the same abundance of glycogen in the liver of a dog repeatedly injected with necrosin.[19] The kidney is another organ that may be frequently involved following repeated injections of this substance.[21] This may be in the form of damage to glomeruli and to the lining epithelium of the tubules, and there may be irregular foci of leukocytic infiltration (Fig. 14).

The euglobulin fraction of inflammatory exudates contains four chemical factors or mediators which have definite biological significance in inflammation. It was noted in the early studies of this fraction of exudate that, in addition to the injury induced, leukopenia, leukocytosis and fever were frequent accompaniments following the injection into dogs of this toxic euglobulin. This is particularly true when the euglobulin is derived from acid exudates.[6]

Let us examine, in brief, the primary mechanism of fever with acute inflammation. First, it is noted that the whole euglobulin fraction of exudates fails to enter readily into solution in the presence of electrolytes. However, after precipitating out the euglobulin at one-third saturation with ammonium sulfate prior to the dialyzing out of the sulfate ions, the precipitate is treated with distilled water. Under such circumstances, a true euglobulin is found to enter into solution in the presence of the sulfate ions.[22] This euglobulin is necrosin. The residual insoluble fraction contains the pyrogenic factor.[22] By

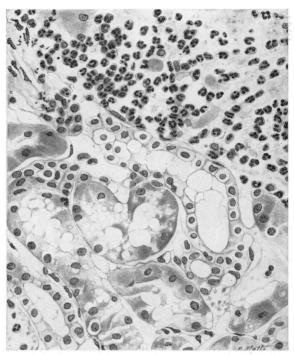

Fig. 14. Section through a kidney of Dog 7-40 about 7 hours after a single intra-vascular injection of 10 ml. of necrosin obtained from another dog's exudate. Note the focus of polymorphonuclear leukocytic infiltration with very few mononuclear cells. The tubules likewise show, in many instances, prominent intracellular vacuolation of the lining epithelial cells with irregular contour of their surface. × 760. (From Menkin: Arch. Path., 36:269, 1943.)

this simple dissociation we have succeeded in separating necrosin from the fever-inducing factor, which has in turn been termed *pyrexin*.[22] At times this dissociation is not readily performed. One can then resort to merely allowing necrosin in the fluid state to stand in the refrigerator; this causes, within a few days to a few weeks, the sedimentation of pyrexin to the bottom of the container.[6] Pyrexin has also been crystallized from a 50 per cent acetic acid mother liquor.[23] The crystals appear to be rhomboid, but on slight dehydration they tend to assume a needle-like appearance. These crystals are active in inducing fever in rabbits, in contrast to the ineffectiveness of the mother liquor.[23] Necrosin contains proteolytic activity, especially when fibrinogen is utilized as a substrate.[24] It is interesting to note that the incubation of necrosin is frequently followed by an end-product which is *per se* pyrogenic.[6, 22] Conceivably, pyrexin in the euglobulin fraction of exudates may perhaps be an end-product of proteolytic activity by necrosin. Recent studies by differential centrifugation of both exudates and homogenates of inflamed tissue indicate the presence of two pyrogenic factors, namely, a thermostable factor identical with pyrexin and a thermolabile factor.[11] This latter thermolabile factor may yet prove to be similar to the factor recently studied by Bennett and Beeson, and Wood, Jr., with his associates.[25, 26] The pathogenesis of fever in inflammation, as I have pointed out, may be referable to a thermolabile and a thermostable factor (pyrexin).[6, 11] The thermolabile factor would account for fever in the earlier stages of inflammation when the exudate is at an alkaline pH and there is an abundance of polymorphonuclear leukocytes.[6, 11] Pyrexin would explain the mechanism of fever in the later phases of an acute inflammation when the pH tends to be on the acid side.[6, 11]

This is a general picture of the inflammatory reaction, illustrating how the liberation by injured cells of various chemical factors or mediators reasonably explains some of the biological manifestations of this important process. It can be viewed as the physical basis of infectious diseases, even though inflammation in itself is a much more inclusive term, and, as pointed out above, it may be caused by nonviable irritants as well. There are other factors, such as the thermostable leukocytosis factor and the leukopenic factors. Some of these mediators are also recovered in the euglobulin fraction of exudates.[6] There is insufficient time, however, to enter into a description of the other already identified factors. These have been adequately described elsewhere.[6, 27] We are already familiar with some of the cytologic precursors of these significant chemical mediators.[11] It may well be that Ungar's view that histamine liberation is referable to the activity of a protease[28] may perhaps also prove to apply to the formation of these various chemical factors which I have identified.[6] These factors are biologically very specific. For instance, pyrexin induces fever, whereas the injection of the leukocytosis-promoting factor is followed by a leukocytosis. These factors, however, are not as yet chemically pure. This looms as an important task for the future.

The mechanism of repair following acute inflammation appears to be referable to the liberation of an endogenous diffusible growth-promoting factor (GPF) at the site of inflammation. Its extraction and properties have been fully described in other recent communications.[29, 30, 31, 32]

As a central idea, I should like to restate a biochemical view of inflammation, namely, that the liberation of chemical mediators by injured cells at the site of an acute inflammation reasonably explains the diverse biological manifestations of this basic immunological process. Finally, inflammation is indeed an admirable system in which to study the biochemistry of injured cells.

REFERENCES

1. Menkin, V.: Dynamics of Inflammation. New York, The Macmillan Co., 1940 (reprinted 1950).
2. Menkin, V.: J. Exper. Med., 53:647, 1931.
3. Menkin, V.: J. Exper. Med., 64:485, 1936.
4. Menkin, V.: J. Exper. Med., 67:129, 1938.
5. Menkin, V.: Arch. Exper. Path. u. Pharmakol., 219:473, 1953.
6. Menkin, V.: Biochemical Mechanisms in Inflammation. Springfield, Illinois, Charles C Thomas, 1956.
7. Menkin, V.: Leucotaxine and Exudin in Relation to Inflammation, extracted from Polypeptides which Affect Smooth Muscles and Blood Vessels. London, Pergamon Press, 1960.

8. Menkin, V.: J. Exper. Med., 67:145, 1938.
9. Menkin, V.: Ann. N. Y. Acad. Sc., 59:956, 1955.
10. Harris, H.: Physiol. Rev., 34:529, 1954.
11. Menkin, V.: Am. J. Path., 34:921, 1958.
12. Menkin, V.: Fed. Proc., 19:March 1960.
13. Menkin, V.: Am. J. Path., 16:13, 1940.
14. Menkin, V.: Arch. Path., 30:363, 1940.
15. Menkin, V.: Proc. Soc. Exper. Biol. & Med., 64:448, 1947.
16. Menkin, V. and Kadish, M. A.: Arch. Path., 33:193, 1942.
17. Menkin, V.: Am. J. Path., 19:1021, 1943.
18. Menkin, V.: Blood. J. Hematol., 3:939, 1948.
19. Menkin, V.: Arch. Path., 41:376, 1946.
20. Menkin, V.: A Mechanism in Bodily Defense, extracted from Medico-Surgical Tributes to Harold Brunn. Berkeley, University of California Press, 1942, p. 275.
21. Menkin, V.: Arch. Path., 36:269, 1943.
22. Menkin, V.: Arch. Path., 39:28, 1945.
23. Menkin, V.: Arch. Internat. Pharmacodyn., 89:229, 1952.
24. Menkin, V.: Am. J. Physiol., 147:379, 1946.
25. Bennett, I. L., Jr. and Beeson, P. B., Jr.: Exper. Med., 98:477, 1953.
26. Wood, B., Jr.: Lancet, July 12, 1958, p. 53; Menkin, V.: Lancet, October 18, 1958, p. 851.
27. Menkin, V.: Brit. M. J.: May 21, 1960, p. 1521.
28. Ungar, G.: Fibrinolytic System and Inflammation, extracted from Jasmin, G. and Robert, A. (eds.): Mechanism of Inflammation. Montreal, ACTA, Inc., 1953, p. 151.
29. Menkin, V.: Cancer Research, 1:548, 1941.
30. Menkin, V.: Cancer Research, 17:963, 1957.
31. Menkin, V.: Cancer Research, 19:544, 1959.
32. Menkin, V.: Biologic Cocarcinogens, extracted from Progr. Exper. Tumor Res. 1:1960, Basel, Switzerland, S. Karger.

Role of Catechol Amines
in the Genesis of Tissue Injury*

BENJAMIN W. ZWEIFACH and
ARNOLD L. NAGLER

New York University Medical Center

Among the many different forms of tissue injury available for experimental study, the hemorrhagic necrosis following administration of bacterial endotoxin first reported by Apitz[1] and Shwartzman,[9] has attracted much attention because of its obvious importance in immunological reactions. Recent evidence[13] dealing with the genesis of the tissue destruction following locally administered bacterial extracts suggests that epinephrine in the presence of products of cellular damage is a central factor in the mediation of the ensuing vascular disruption. The mechanism by which catechol amines accelerate tissue damage is not well understood, and it is the purpose of this paper to clarify this aspect of the injury reaction.

Rather than attempt to review critically the many concepts which have been advanced, it would be more useful to discuss the successive steps in the

* Supported by a grant from the U. S. Public Health Service (H-2267).

evolution of an experimental investigation of a particular model of tissue injury. Such an exercise would then make it possible to attempt to synthesize the facts into an acceptable schema of the injury reaction.

The hemorrhagic necrosis produced in the skin of rabbits by two spaced injections of bacterial products, the local Shwartzman reaction, was selected as the test model for the current studies. This lesion develops slowly and involves almost every aspect of the inflammatory process—hyperemia, edema, endothelial damage, extravasation of blood cells, depolymerization of plasma proteins and thrombosis.[5] It differs from most inflammatory processes in progressing through a phase of hemorrhagic disruption and ultimate necrosis. The latter phase of the reaction thus serves as a useful end point for quantitating the effects of different agents in the production of tissue injury.

Under normal circumstances, local tissue homeostasis is maintained by an interaction between blood-borne vasoactive materials and locally produced mediators.[15] In particular, the catechol amines and adrenal corticosteroids are the important circulating components of these mechanisms. On a local scale, various agents, including acetylcholine,[3] histamine,[8] 5-hydroxytryptamine[10] and various polypeptides[2] and metabolites, serve to modulate the effect of the vasotonic amines on vascular smooth muscle. Under abnormal circumstances, the local milieu is disturbed to the extent that many of the aforementioned mediators accumulate in excessive amounts, or new products are formed as a consequence of the altered physico-chemical environment.

For many years, it has been apparent that some of the systemic and local effects of bacterial endotoxins were similar to those resulting from the elaboration of catechol amines. More recently, Thomas found[13] that he could produce an accelerated form of dermal necrosis by using epinephrine in place of one of the two injections of bacterial endotoxins. Thus, the conventional technique has been to inject intradermally into rabbits a small amount of a gram-negative bacterial extract (50 to 100 μg. of *E. coli* lipopolysaccharide) and after an interval of some 14 to 18 hours to inject the same material intravenously. There follows over a period of four to six hours a slowly developing inflammation and a marked hemorrhage into the affected site. Thomas obtained the same tissue necrotizing effect by combining epinephrine with endotoxin and injecting the mixture into the skin. Hemorrhage and necrosis developed within three to five hours. Others have shown that the typical Arthus reactions which normally progress to inflammation and edema could be converted into a hemorrhagic phenomenon by injecting epinephrine into or near the skin site.[4] A similar potentiating action of epinephrine has been described for other inflammatory phenomena, including antigen-antibody interactions.

In the present study microcirculatory techniques were used to determine the vascular effects of such combinations. Observations were made on both rats and rabbits in which the mesentery was exposed for microscopic examination. It was found that epinephrine injected locally in concentrations from a fraction of a gamma to 50 gamma produced only extensive vasoconstriction with no evidence of capillary damage or disruption. When repeated applications of epinephrine were made, the muscular arterioles and venules became sensitized and shut down completely. As a result, after one to two hours breakdown of capillary vessels occurred, with a swelling of the endothelium and complete closure of the capillary lumen. Such tissue destruction did not involve capillary hemorrhage but progressed directly into necrosis.

In experiments in which combinations of epinephrine and endotoxin were given, the initial phase of intense vasoconstriction was in turn replaced by a period of erythema during which the blood capillaries and especially the collecting venules lost their normal permeability characteristics. Complete stasis developed in many of the small vessels. After a variable phase of stasis, red blood cells began to leak through the vessel walls, especially in the venules; many of the vessels disrupted completely. The hemorrhagic phase of the reaction, once started, progressed rapidly so that within 20 to 30 minutes numerous petechial hemorrhages were present in the capillary bed and large areas showed complete stasis of blood.

Attempts were then made to determine whether the influence of bacterial extracts on vascular behavior was in fact dependent upon particular mediator systems. In this regard, studies were made with histamine and 5-hydroxy-tryptamine, alone and in combination with epinephrine (Table 1). Hista-

TABLE 1. EFFECTS OF MIXTURES OF CATECHOL AMINES AND
VASOTOXIC AGENTS

| TOPICALLY APPLIED | DOSE (μg.) | MICROCIRCULATORY* | | | | DERMAL Hem. necrosis |
		Vaso-genic	Cell adhesion	Endoth. damage	Stasis	
Epinephrine	1-50	VCS	0	0	0	0
Epin. + Endotoxin†	250	VCS	+	++	+	+++
Histamine	1-50	VDIL	+	+	+	0
Epin. + Histamine†	50	VCS	+	++	+	0
5-HT	1-250	0	0	0	0	0
Epin. + 5-HT†	250	VCS	+	++	+	++
Gamma globulin	1-500	0	0	0	0	0
Epin. + Globulin†	500	VCS	+	++	++	+++

* Studied in mesentery of rat and rabbit and in skin of rabbit.
† Concentration of epinephrine in mixtures kept at 50 μg.
VCS = Vasoconstriction.
VDIL = Vasodilatation.

mine, when introduced locally into the mesenteric tissue, produced in low concentrations (below 1 μg.) only a swelling of the endothelial cells and an extensive dilation of the muscular vessels. Increased adhesion of platelets and leukocytes to the vessel walls seemed to occur secondarily after damage to endothelium was evident. This distinction was made by introducing colloidal carbon into the circulation. Under normal circumstances, endothelium does not sequester such colloid from the blood stream. Under the influence of histamine, the inner surface of the affected vessels became coated with carbon; many of the particles were seen to be engulfed or phagocytized by the endothelial cells. Thus, endothelial phagocytosis is stimulated by histamine. The endothelial stimulation occurs before leukocytes and platelets adhere to the vessel wall.

Combinations of epinephrine and histamine were administered locally. Although the endothelial damage was more extensive and progressed to capillary stasis more rapidly under these circumstances, tissue hemorrhage did not develop. Various combinations, of epinephrine and histamine were used without reproducing cardinal manifestations of the Shwartzman phenomenon or of hemorrhagic necrosis.

It has long been known[10] that 5-hydroxytryptamine (5-HT) increases capillary permeability locally. Local injection of this agent in concentrations

TABLE 2.   EFFECT OF INCREASING DOSAGE OF 5-HT
ON RESPONSE TO EPINEPHRINE

MIXTURE APPLIED LOCALLY		RAT MESENTERY		
Epin. (μg./ml.)	5-HT (μg./ml.)	Artles.	Precaps.	Venules
1.0	. .	+	+	none
1.0	0.1	++	+	++
1.0	5.0	+	++	+++
5.0	1.0	+	++	+++
. .	1.0	±	none	none

+ = vasoconstriction

ranging from 0.1 to 10 μg. had no effect on capillary endothelium (Table 2). The amine rendered the arterioles less responsive to the constrictor action of epinephrine. When combinations of 5-HT and epinephrine were administered, an interesting synergism was uncovered. Two separate sets of events could be recognized. First, the muscular venules, which are ordinarily the least responsive constituents of the microcirculation, became inordinately sensitive to the catechol amines. As a result, normally threshold amounts of epinephrine introduced into the circulation caused intense constriction of the venules and engorgement of the capillary vasculature. Second, the simultaneous presence of these two amines had a deleterious effect on vascular endothelium. Colloidal carbon was removed from the blood stream and taken up by the endothelium of the capillaries and small venules. A marked increase in permeability occurred and extensive capillary stasis was present within 10 to 15 minutes after the local application of a mixture containing 1 μg. of epinephrine and from 2 to 3μg. of 5-HT.

These experiments led us to explore the possibility that combinations of 5-HT and epinephrine might be capable of eliciting a dermal hemorrhagic reaction similar to that evoked by combinations of epinephrine and bacterial endotoxins. This was found to be true. Mixtures containing 100 μg. of epinephrine and 50 μg. of 5-HT produced in about 30 to 40 per cent of the rabbits, upon injection into the skin, a diffuse hemorrhagic area which developed within four hours and persisted for several days. Subsequently, it was possible to increase the reproducibility of this reaction by using as test animals rabbits which had been pretreated with a moderate stress, such as sublethal hemorrhage, manipulation of the intestines, or blockade of the reticuloendothelial system with Thorotrast. Under these circumstances the dermal necrotizing reaction developed in almost 90 per cent of the animals.

The fact that tissue responses depend upon the interaction of both blood-borne and locally elaborated agents led us to examine the effects of substances known to deplete tissues of their local stores of biogenic agents. For this purpose we used reserpine and compound 48/80. Although both of these substances effect the release of vasoactive products, such as histamine and 5-HT, they achieve their end result by different mechanisms.[7] With reserpine, the evidence seems to indicate that storage of substances such as 5-HT is suppressed, leading to a lowered tissue content. Compound 48/80, on the other hand, leads to a disruption of mast cells which both form and store these amines.

Reserpine-treated rats and rabbits showed no differences in their susceptibility to tissue damage when treated with combinations of either epinephrine and endotoxin or epinephrine and 5-HT. This was tested in two ways—by the dermal hemorrhagic necrotic reaction and by the response of the microcirculation of the mesentery. On the other hand, animals which were pretreated with 48/80 for several days showed a remarkable resistance to the vasotoxic effects of the two epinephrine-mediated combinations (Table 3). Thus, rats which had received 48/80 (50 μg. i.v.) for four days did not

TABLE 3.   *EFFECT OF DEPLETION WITH 48/80 ON VASCULAR RESPONSE*

| AGENT APPLIED | RAT SKIN | |
LOCALLY	Controls	Treated
Epinephrine	++	+
5-Hydroxytryptamine	00	none
E and 5-HT	+++	+
Histamine	00	00
Acetylcholine	00	0

+ to +++ = vasoconstriction
0 = vasodilation

develop the vascular symptoms of capillary damage—adhesion of colloidal carbon, or leukocyte and platelet thrombi in the mesentery—following the local injection of a mixture of epinephrine and 5-HT. Although hyperemia and a moderate edema did develop, no hemorrhage or necrosis was observed. Interestingly enough, the response to histamine alone or in combination with epinephrine was not affected. In passing, it should be noted that rats pretreated with 48/80[7] for several days also showed an enhanced capacity to withstand traumatic shock and acutely lethal doses of bacterial endotoxin.

In further explorations of the mechanisms involved in this type of tissue damage, attention was given to the possible role of a blood-borne component. Among the many constituents which have been made suspect in this regard are the blood globulins. A number of investigations have shown that the systemic administration of globulin preparations causes animals such as mice and rats to become more susceptible to the systemic and local effects of bacterial endotoxins. It seemed plausible to us that the altered permeability in locally damaged areas might permit the influx of blood globulins and that their presence might affect the subsequent vascular reaction. Indeed, such an explanation has been proposed both by Spector[11] and by Miles and co-workers[6] as a basis of the inflammatory reaction. In both of these instances the mechanism appeared to involve the production of a vasoactive polypeptide which was then responsible for the ensuing altered permeability, edema and local accumulation of leukocytes. We therefore substituted preparations of blood globulins for both epinephrine and endotoxin in the accelerated hemorrhagic reaction which has been described above.

It was found that globulins could not be used in place of epinephrine in combinations of epinephrine and bacterial endotoxin. On the other hand, combinations of epinephrine and globulin (highly purified human gamma globulin, or rabbit or rat globulin*) produced hemorrhagic necrosis in the skin of rabbits with the same regulatory and pattern of development as did combinations of epinephrine and bacterial endotoxins. Lesions produced by both combinations were found to be strikingly similar on gross and microscopic examination. When globulin-epinephrine mixtures were injected into

* Prepared by Dr. George Y. Shinowara, New York University Medical Center.

the mesentery, a pattern of endothelial swelling, sequestration of carbon and capillary disruption was encountered. Interestingly enough, the terminal stage of petechial hemorrhage and capillary stasis occurred without extensive diapedesis of leukocytes or formation of platelet thrombi. There was a marked tendency for the reaction to spread beyond the immediate area of application. Lesions of this kind were produced in the rabbit with mixtures containing 100 μg. of epinephrine and as little as 0.1 to 2.0 μg. (protein content) of purified human globulin. In the rat mesentery it was necessary to use somewhat higher concentrations of globulin—from 200 to 500 μg.—to produce capillary rhexis.

Although the globulin experiments clearly suggested the involvement of antibodies, it seemed equally plausible that these preparations might be effective because of their known content of blood enzymes,[14] proteolytic enzymes in particular. We therefore carried out the same set of experiments in animals which had been pretreated with inhibitors of proteolytic activity. The most useful agents in this class were tosyl arginine methyl ester (TAME) and epsilon aminocaproic acid (EACA).[16] Both of these agents, acting as competitive substrates, inhibit the inactivation of proteolytic enzymes of the trypsinogen or plasminogen type. Rabbits and rats pretreated with 20 to 30 mg. of these inhibitors were protected against the development of the epinephrine-accelerated reactions. In the case of TAME, it was possible to rule out the nonspecific action of this material by using tosyl arginine (TA), a metabolic by-product which is not an effective inhibitor. Such animals developed the usual tissue necrotizing response with various epinephrine mixtures. The fact that two different competitive substrates had an inhibitory action and that a similar effect was obtained with another inhibitor—soybean trypsin inhibitor (SBTI)—would seem to substantiate the conclusion that the protective effect was mediated by suppression of proteolytic enzyme activity.

One other possibility was investigated, namely, the involvement of a change in local redox potential by virtue of changes in tissue acidity or in sulfhydryl groupings. Many investigators have suspected the local shift in pH and the accumulation of lactic acid as an important determinant of the ensuing inflammatory response.[12] We therefore measured the pH of all of our reaction mixtures and, with the exception of the globulin mixtures, found the pH to be below 4; that of the globulin mixture was 6.1. We therefore buffered the active agents to keep them at a pH of 4. This factor by itself greatly increased the severity of the hemorrhagic necrosis and rendered the tissue more sensitive to these mixtures. For example, it was now possible to produce the same type of vascular damage in the rabbit by using from 1 to 10 μg. instead of 100 μg. of epinephrine in combination with 5-HT and/or globulin. The lesions were also much more reproducible. In addition, tissue sites which received acid-buffered epinephrine produced local hemorrhage and necrosis in about 50 to 60 per cent of the animals. Mixtures of cysteine and epinephrine injected into the mesentery resulted in capillary stasis but had to be applied several times before a damaging effect on the endothelium could be elicited. The intravenous administration of cysteine had no observable effect on any of the epinephrine combinations used to produce local tissue injury.

In general, the experimental models which we have discussed require at least two constituents in the genesis of hemorrhagic necrosis and capillary stasis. Epinephrine is common to all these phenomena. In addition, another factor presumably involves activation of some lytic enzyme system. The evidence is not clear as to the precise system which is involved. Although emphasis has been placed on a proteolytic factor, the possibility still remains that some other hydrolytic or cytolytic enzyme may be concerned. The effectiveness of epinephrine in the development of hemorrhagic necrosis is clearly aborted by agents which inhibit such systems. Epinephrine does not seem to be involved in the local inflammatory response *per se,* but rather in the subsequent development of endothelial damage and rhexis. Its effects in this regard are mediated by an action over and above the well known constrictor action on vascular smooth muscle.

REFERENCES

1. Apitz, K.: A study of the generalized Shwartzman phenomenon. J. Immunol., *29*:255, 1935.
2. Bhoola, K. O., Calle, J. D. and Schachter, M.: The effect of bradykinin, serum kallikrein and other endogenous substances on capillary permeability in the guinea pig. J. Physiol., *152*:75, 1960.
3. Florey, H. W.: Inflammation. In Florey, H. W. (ed.): General Pathology. Philadelphia, W. B. Saunders Co., 1958.
4. Gatling, R. R.: Altered reactivity to epinephrine in the hypersensitive rabbit. J. Exper. Med., *108*:441, 1958.
5. Menkin, V.: Biology of inflammation. Science, *123*:527, 1956.
6. Miles, A. A. and Wilhelm, D. L.: Enzyme-like globulins from serum reproducing the vascular phenomenon of inflammation. I. An activable permeability factor and its inhibitor in guinea pig serum. Brit. J. Exper. Path., *36*:71, 1955.
7. Paton, W. D. M.: Histamine release by compounds of simple chemical structure. Pharmacol. Rev., *9*:669, 1957.
8. Rowley, D. A. and Benditt, E. P.: 5-Hydroxytryptamine and histamine as mediators of the vascular injury produced by agents which damage mast cells in rats. J. Exper. Med., *103*:399, 1956.
9. Shwartzman, G.: Phenomenon of local tissue reactivity. New York, Paul B. Hoeber, Inc., 1937.
10. Sparrow, E. M. and Wilhelm, D. L.: Species differences in susceptibility to capillary permeability factors: histamine, 5-hydroxytryptamine and compound 48/80. J. Physiol., *137*:51, 1957.
11. Spector, W. G.: Activation of a globulin system controlling capillary permeability in inflammation. J. Path., *74*:67, 1957.
12. Stetson, C. A., Jr.: Studies on the mechanism of the Shwartzman phenomenon. Certain factors involved in the production of hemorrhagic necrosis. J. Exper. Med., *93*:489, 1951.
13. Thomas, L.: The role of epinephrine in the reactions produced by the endotoxins of gram-negative bacteria. I. Hemorrhagic necrosis produced by epinephrine in the skin of endotoxin-treated rabbits. J. Exper. Med., *104*:865, 1956.
14. Wroblewski, F. and Wroblewski, R.: The clinical significance of lactic dehydrogenase activity of serous effusions. Ann. Int. Med., *48*:813, 1958.
15. Zweifach, B. W.: General principles governing the behavior of the microcirculation. Am. J. Med., *23*:684, 1957.
16. Zweifach, B. W., Nagler, A. L. and Troll, W.: Some effect of proteolytic inhibitors on tissue injury and systemic anaphylaxis. J. Exper. Med., *113*:437, 1961.

Observations on the Inflammatory Process in Diseases of Connective Tissue

D. MURRAY ANGEVINE

University of Wisconsin Medical School

Historically, Morgagni was concerned with diseases of organs and Virchow with alterations of cells. Diseases were next considered by systems, such as syphilis of the nervous system or tuberculosis of the genitourinary tract, and only relatively recently those conditions that involve the connective tissue, or "dyscollagenoses," have been described.

About 20 years ago Klemperer, Pollack and Baehr[4] expressed the opinion that the morphologic alterations in systemic lupus erythematosus (S.L.E.) were the result of extensive damage in the connective tissues, but that the underlying functional disturbances responsible for such alterations were not evident. They also indicated that the same common denominator, namely, degeneration of connective tissue, was present in periarteritis nodosa, rheumatic fever and scleroderma. This led to the concept of a group of diseases involving principally the "collagen" of connective tissue. Almost immediately the structural and supporting components of the body that heretofore had been relatively neglected began to attract wide attention; currently this is a most active field of interest and investigation.

Before discussing the inflammatory reaction in this group of diseases, I shall speculate briefly upon the site and nature of the alterations responsible for the varied inflammatory responses observed in these conditions. One of the most conspicuous and constant alterations associated with injury of connective tissue is the presence of "fibrinoid degeneration." This is a controversial and still unsettled problem, but studies on it have served as a catalyst in arousing interest in the subject. Since fibrinoid is intimately associated with both the injury and associated reactions, it seems essential to record a few comments about some of its special characteristics. The principal current differences of opinion between various workers seem to revolve largely around their definitions of the term, rather than upon the interpretation of their observations.

Our concept of fibrinoid is that of a homogeneous, eosinophilic, relatively acellular refractile substance with some of the tinctorial properties of fibrin.[1] This opinion coincides with that of Pagel,[8] who states that "the ill-defined homogeneous substance (fibrinoid) remains unstained by Weigerts' method for fibrin, phosphotungstic acid, hematoxylin and acid picro-Mallory method." In our studies, especially of early lesions and of those adjacent to the circulation, as in periarteritis nodosa, we frequently observed "a blue fibrillar material, presumably fibrin, in some of the phosphotungstic acid hematoxylin preparations. In serial sections it was noted that the blue material could not be correlated anatomically with the deep eosinophilic substance." The same situation was observed and described for vegetations on

91

the heart valves in rheumatic fever, gastric ulcers, and Nitabuch's membrane of the placenta. On the basis of such studies it was concluded that fibrinoid formed as a co-precipitate of acid mucopolysaccharide of the ground substance with a basic protein. It was also suggested that amyloid formation, hyalinization and sclerosis may be laid down in tissues by a similar mechanism.

The observations of the presence of fibrin in experimentally induced arteritis[7] are not in disagreement with our reported studies.[1] They do not, however, satisfactorily explain the nature of the hyaline material that fails to take the accepted stains for fibrin. We have never at any time excluded the possibility that some altered form of fibrin may play a role in the formation of fibrinoid, but believe that we have ruled out collagen, reticulum, elastin and muscle as possible components. Whether the precise initial site of injury is in the ground substance, as we are strongly inclined to believe, or whether it involves primarily the collagen fibers or perhaps both, is not germane to this discussion. On the basis of experience with other problems, it would seem fair to assume that both sites are probably affected to some extent. I have never been as much impressed by the degeneration of collagen in the very early stages of injury to connective tissue as most observers appear to be, but I do not, of course, question the fact that collagen is eventually altered.

As investigators explore more deeply into cellular function at the molecular level by the use of newer cytochemical techniques, it becomes increasingly evident that when one component or fraction of a cell is altered this is almost immediately reflected, somewhat as a chain reaction, by an alteration in some other component. There is little reason to doubt that some similar relation will hold for alterations that may occur in the structures that occupy the extracellular body spaces. Whatever may be the nature of the injurious agent or wherever it may strike, the resulting injury to the tissues is regularly followed by or associated with some degree of inflammatory reaction.

The resulting cellular reactions vary greatly in the different diseases as well as in different patients with the same disease, being dependent upon or modified by one or more of the following factors:

1. The severity of the illness.
2. The capacity of the patient to react to injury, dependent upon age, nutrition, etc.
3. The resistance of the patient to the injury.
4. The time in the disease at which the tissue is examined.
5. The degree of sensitization (if hypersensitivity is a factor).
6. The nature of the therapy administered.

As a general rule, the pattern of inflammatory reaction to several different though related agents is remarkably constant, this being especially true for many pyogenic microorganisms; the predominant alterations, namely necrosis and formation of pus, depend to a large extent upon the toxins and enzymes elaborated by the causative organism which, of course, must be isolated culturally to be incriminated.

Other organisms, such as *B. typhosus, B. tularensis* and *B. tuberculosis,* elicit responses with special histologic patterns so that one may suspect the etiologic agent with a fair degree of accuracy. This statement is, of course, only relative because the similarity of the characteristic lesions in tuberculosis, histoplasmosis and coccidioidomycosis well illustrate how almost identical reactions can be elicited by very dissimilar organisms. It is not surprising, therefore, to have a somewhat analogous situation in a variety of diseases such as those under consideration in which the cellular reaction is most probably associated with or is the result of the response to an antigen-antibody reaction.

I shall now discuss briefly the principal characteristics of the inflammatory reaction seen in the significant lesions observed in rheumatic fever, rheumatoid arthritis, systemic lupus erythematosus, serum sickness and polyarteritis. It cannot be too strongly emphasized that the significant microscopic criteria by which such diseases are recognized in establishing a diagnosis depend primarily upon the architectural and cytologic aberrations of the particular tissue in conjunction with the location and configuration of the lesion, the cellular characteristics of the inflammatory reaction being less evident. To illustrate, one can usually recognize a typical Aschoff body at a glance with a low power objective, the number and/or type of inflammatory cells attracting little attention. One must, of course, be aware that somewhat comparable lesions are found in the heart in uremic coma, scarlet fever and rheumatoid arthritis. Although difficult to evaluate, the influence of therapy upon different lesions must also be recognized and taken into consideration since cortisone and acetylsalicylic acid undoubtedly modify the microscopic picture.

Let us now turn to the reactions observed in the synovial membranes of patients with rheumatoid arthritis. Initially the injury, whatever the cause, is characterized by many neutrophils and subsequently mononuclear cells with plasma cells playing a predominant role. Several years ago I was intrigued by the plethora of plasma cells, but had no idea of their significance. Somewhat later it was recognized that these cells were concerned with antibody formation, and now on the basis of newer techniques it has been demonstrated that they are apparently concerned with the production of rheumatoid factor.[5] The precise initiating cause of this reaction is still very much a mystery, even though the lesion may be imitated fairly closely in experimental animals sensitized to various microorganisms or to an agent such as horse serum.[2] The histology of the Arthus phenomenon has been studied experimentally by More and Movat[6] in both the joints and skin of rabbits. Their observations indicate that the intense mononuclear (macrophage and plasma cellular) response is out of proportion to that expected in acute inflammation of normergic animals. It is of interest that their illustrations of the synovial membrane reactions are indistinguishable from many of those seen in typical cases of rheumatoid arthritis. Observations such as these suggest that the reaction of the synovial membrane to a variety of injurious agents will elicit a pattern of inflammation with many similarities, so that from histologic examination alone one cannot regularly obtain a definitive answer.

It has not been my intent to belittle the value of microscopic observation, but rather to emphasize the importance of the wide experience necessary for accurate interpretation of reactions such as those that occur in the synovia. I have considerable concern about the cytologist who, with limited experience, restricts himself to the interpretation of tissue reactions of only one disease or group of diseases. I have on more than one occasion been most surprised and occasionally somewhat shocked by the interpretation made of some relatively simple pathologic lesions by observers whose microscopic horizons do not extend beyond the restricted limitations of their specialty.

In S.L.E., a disease in which there is nothing characteristic about the cellular reaction, the presence of L.E. bodies in association with variously distributed lesions in the kidney and spleen is of the greatest help. Teilum[11] has described epithelioid cell granulomas in fatal S.L.E. and has used this as an argument to indicate that the disease is allergic in nature. Pollack,[9] who has had a wide experience, states that the lesion is very rare. I have yet to be convinced that a granulomatous reaction is always indicative of hypersensitivity, although I am fully aware that such lesions are not infrequently observed in hypersensitive states.

Because some diseases of this group have certain features of hypersensitivity, there has been a tendency to consider them all as allergic without an adequate basis, so that there is considerable confusion in the literature on this point which I trust may be somewhat clarified here.

There are two diseases, namely, serum sickness and polyarteritis, that seem clearly to be the result of sensitization. The descriptive histology of serum sickness is minimal because of the few fatal cases observed. Clark and Kaplan[3] have recorded proliferation of cardiac endothelium with aggregations of histiocytes beneath and also focal accumulations of lymphocytes in various organs. Fibrinoid was not a conspicuous feature, but Rich[10] later observed several cases in which fibrinoid was more evident; however, his cases had received sulfonamides in addition to serum.

Because the inflammatory process in polyarteritis will be presented subsequently, I shall merely indicate that initially the inflammatory exudate in the typical case is essentially similar to that observed in experimentally induced serum sickness, namely, damage to vascular endothelium, the appearance of fibrinoid in the subendothelium and media followed by proliferation of histiocytes, lymphocytes and sometimes eosinophilic leukocytes. In some instances of polyarterities, granulomatous inflammation is a conspicuous feature—a finding that has led to the creation of several new disease entities and, although perhaps of some clinical value, has not contributed much to our comprehension of the nature of this disease.

In summary, I wish to stress two principal points. (1) The cellular reactions associated with inflammation are not as helpful in the designation of this group of diseases as the structural alterations in the connective tissue. (2) There is a wide variation in both the extent and character of the cellular reactions in the connective tissue diseases which are for the most part nonspecific.

REFERENCES

1. Altshuler, C. H. and Angevine, D. M.: Histochemical studies on the pathogenesis of fibrinoid. Am. J. Path., 25:1061, 1949.
2. Angevine, D. M., Cecil, R. L. and Rothbard, S.: The influence of various types of immunization on the pathogenesis of experimental hemolytic streptococcus arthritis. A.M.A. Arch. Path., 34:18, 1942.
3. Clark, E. and Kaplan, B. J.: Endocardial, arterial and other mesenchymal alterations associated with serum disease in man. Arch. Path., 24:458, 1937.
4. Klemperer, P., Pollack, A. D. and Baehr, G.: Pathology of disseminated lupus erythematous. Arch. Path., 32:569, 1941.
5. Mellors, R. C., Heimer, R., Corcos, J. and Korngold, L.: Cellular origin of rheumatoid factor. J. Exper. Med., 110:875, 1959.
6. More, R. H. and Movat, H. Z.: Cellular and intercellular changes in the arthus phenomenon. A.M.A. Arch. Path., 67:482, 1959.
7. Movat, H. Z. and More, R. H.: Nature and origin of fibrinoid. Am. J. Clin. Path., 28:331, 1957.

8. Pagel, W.: Polyarteritis nodosa and the "rheumatic" diseases. J. Clin. Path., *4*:137, 1951.
9. Pollack, A. D.: Pathology of systemic lupus erythematosus. In Baehr, G. and Klemperer, P. (eds.): Systemic Lupus Erythematosus. New York, Grune and Stratton, 1959.
10. Rich, A. R.: Role of hypersensitivity in periarteritis nodosa. Bull. Johns Hopkins Hosp., *71*:123, 1942.
11. Teilum, G.: Pathogenetic studies on lupus erythematosus disseminatus and related diseases. Acta med. scandinav., *123*:126, 1946.

Panel Discussion

D. Murray Angevine, *Moderator*

Dr. Angevine: The term "granulomatous inflammation" has been used several times this afternoon, and I am sure some of the other panelists will use it. It is a term very widely employed and very commonly used by people to imply that there is a hypersensitive type of inflammation. I wonder what this term means to some of the panelists?

Dr. Sokoloff: I had occasion to look in several medical dictionaries to see how "granuloma" was defined, and no two dictionaries had definitions that corresponded to one another. One source defined this as an inflammatory reaction with a predominance of lymphocytes, another as inflammation characterized by the formation of granulation tissue but it did not state what granulation tissue was. Still another source stated that the basic inflammatory cell was a mononuclear cell or derivative of it. Finally, one dictionary defined it as a focal lesion leading to nodular areas of scar formation. I would define a "granuloma" as a chronic inflammatory lesion that is apparently nodular and leads to formation of a scar. Quite frequently, but not necessarily, necrosis is present, and I do not think hypersensitivity or another type of allergic reaction is always implicated.

Dr. Pollack: I agree more or less with this. I do not think the type of cells that are seen in granulomatous inflammation have anything to do with the persistence of the granuloma itself. For example, characteristically in brucellosis, the granuloma consists of epithelioid cells, with or without leukocytes. This would fall into the definition of a granuloma, but it is not a persistent lesion. It will resolve for some reason or another in spite of the fact that there are epithelioid cells.

Dr. Wagner: I agree with Dr. Sokoloff's comments, except that I would specify that the cells that compose the granuloma be derived from the mesenchyme. We have seen lesions in muscle composed of multinucleated cells of myogenic origin associated with necrosis and inflammatory cells. This is not a granuloma. I would further restrict the cell population to the characteristic chronic inflammatory cells including those mononuclear cells derived from the mesenchyme.

Dr. Priest: However we define this lesion, the specificity of it must be presented in morphologic terms because of our present lack of knowledge about it.

Dr. Koiwai: In the lesions we produced in the myocardium by injections of Pseudomonas, a nodular pattern was present with a mononuclear type of cell infiltration, including epithelioid cells, fibroblasts in some areas and also "round cells." To me, this is a granuloma.

DR. MENKIN: I would like to comment on the biochemical mechanisms in granuloma formation. In studying the hydrogen ion concentration in the conditioned cellular sequence of the appearance of polymorphonuclear cells followed by mononuclear phagocytes, we found that changes in pH were due to changes in intermediary carbohydrate metabolism. In tubercles the glycolytic index was much higher and more lactic acid was produced in tuberculous lesions. Therefore, further experimental studies of the changes in hydrogen ion concentration and of the biochemical changes in the intermediary carbohydrate metabolism might be useful in distinguishing the various types of inflammation.

DR. ANGEVINE: Someone has to tell a biochemist what a granuloma is before he knows what he is going to work on.

DR. THORNBURG: A common difficulty in establishing biological definitions may be that we are seeking single structural entities or single pathways in the time sequence and causation, when, as a matter of fact, we know that biological systems are systems of very high orders of action and interaction. In many processes there are undoubtedly multiple biochemical reactions taking place at the same time, one influencing another, and possibly different end results occur, depending on which sequence of events initiates the process or takes place first.

DR. ZWEIFACH: In reference to specific mediators in the production of the various characteristics of inflammation, we must analyze the data with respect to a particular effect on the inflammatory process. For example, bacterial endotoxins carried in the blood can produce tissue damage by an effect on the muscular arterioles and venules as a result of vasospasm or increased vascular reactivity. Very frequently the important change is in activity of the venules, the small venules which are normally very unreactive becoming highly reactive to vasotropic materials; the lumen closes and capillary pressure increases, and this increases the tendency toward rupture. We then must consider the mediator with respect to its target in terms of the blood. Very often many of these mediators initiate changes in proteolytic systems. They may induce thrombotic phenomena and diminish the blood supply to the tissue, and thereby destroy the tissue. We also have mediators, presumably such as 5-hydroxytryptamine, which I discussed, which seem to alter the vascular endothelium and increase its capacity to phagocytize material. This may cause this kind of cells to take up materials which they do not normally take up; they may take up antigen-antibody complexes; they may take up denatured proteins, which normally they do not. Finally, one must give consideration to the fact that when an injury persists for some time a hemorrhagic phase may occur. This may occur very suddenly and dramatically over a period of as little as 10 minutes. An area which is merely inflamed can become hemorrhagic. It appears as if some lytic or proteolytic process were being activated by the release of a particular agent. Therefore, when we talk about histamine or any of the so-called mediators of tissue injury we should attempt to relate them in their proper perspective to the tissue involved and to the various constituents of the tissue.

DR. ANGEVINE: This is why I object to the term "inflammatory states" and why I like the term "inflammatory process"; it means that something is going on all the time.

DR. MUIR: Dr. Zweifach, am I right in thinking that you said that the tissue injury is independent of the pressor activity of epinephrine?

DR. ZWEIFACH: The tissue injury that I was referring to was the production of a hemorrhagic endpoint. If one applies adrenalin repeatedly on the same site, one obtains vasoconstriction; if one continues to apply the adrenalin, one ends up with closure of the vessel and a massive white necrotic area. In contrast, the type of injury that occurs with many of the biological agents, such as antigen-antibody combinations, antitoxins and products of their interaction with various blood components, involves not only an inflammatory response but a spreading of the reaction with extensive hemorrhage and later necrosis. This is independent of the vasoconstrictor activity of adrenalin since other vasoconstrictor agents can be used without producing this effect. It is our definite impression that adrenalin has an effect on many cells; we believe it has an effect on the metabolism of endothelial cells, and it is this metabolic effect which is important in terms of its tissue cytotoxic activity. Whether or not some energy-dependent system is affected is not known.

Dr. Pollack: May I ask a question of Dr. Zweifach? When you speak of local injury, such as when you used hemorrhage as the endpoint of injury, how do you differentiate between injuries to the capillary wall and endothelial cells, and injuries to the ground substance and to the basement membrane or a complex of both which is transversed by the capillary which is an endothelial lined tube? For example, one says very glibly that in scurvy there is endothelial damage and therefore hemorrhage, but we know that connective tissue ground substance is altered in scurvy. When one applies various agents locally, where do you think the damage is taking place—in the ground substance or in the capillary wall and endothelium?

Dr. Zweifach: I think this is an excellent point. One should emphasize the fact that the capillary wall does not exist as an entity in itself, but is an integral part of the tissue, and as such it has not only an endothelial component and intercellular forces which keep it together, but it has a basement membrane and is surrounded by the general connective tissue ground substance. Obviously, changes in what we call capillary permeability involve many different factors. You can produce dissolution or shifts in the physiochemistry of the ground substance and produce changes in capillary permeability. In the literature, there are all sorts of references to mediators of capillary permeability. There is no such entity as capillary permeability; this is actually a misnomer. Many of the studies of capillary permeability involve the exudation of a blue dye and the exudation of the dye is dependent on blood flow. If you reduce blood flow there is no exudation of dye. How are you going to measure the extent or severity of capillary injury using a technique of that kind?

However, I would like to emphasize that one can observe changes in the endothelial cells *per se* by administration of agents which seem to be toxic to endothelium, such as histamine. These seem to cause the cell to swell, and if one introduces particulate elements into the blood stream, the endothelial cell may phagocytose them. If high concentrations of histamine are given, other attributes of injury such as adhesion of platelets and deposition of fibrinoid or fibrin-like material on the interface between the blood and the endothelium occur. Therefore, it is difficult to say that substance "A" affects the ground substance and substance "B" affects something else.

You mentioned capillary fragility resulting from vitamin C deficiency in the scorbutic animal. In this condition there is no evidence of a change in the endothelium as evidenced by swelling or adhesion of platelets or uptake of particulate matter, and yet the capillary begins to show signs of weakness and ruptures. One might interpret this as being due to a change in the ground substance or basement membrane.

I do not think that there is any one permeability factor. There are materials which can destroy the integrity of the intercellular forces that hold the endothelium together; there are materials which are cytotoxic to the endothelium; there are materials which cause the endothelial cells to become phagocytic, and degeneration or injury may occur as a result of the uptake of some substance; and there are materials which seem to affect the ground substance. Whether any one material will affect one particular aspect and not another is open to question.

Dr. D. Jackson: I want to comment on the term "ground substance" and its use in the singular. By some it is known simply as mucopolysaccharide, whereas, in fact, the amount of lipids, plasma-type proteins and other components, and even soluble collagen, present in the so-called ground substance is greater than the amount of mucopolysaccharides. I also find it very difficult to understand what is meant by injury to the ground substance.

Dr. Pollack: I think the term "ground substance" is just as permissible as the use of the term "collagen disease." I think everyone realizes that the term "ground substance" refers to a group of materials, some of which have been defined and others which have not been defined. It is merely a term of convenience.

Dr. D. Jackson: I would tend to disagree with you on this because the more I read and the more I see, the more I realize that people do get completely confused about what is meant by the ground substance. Time and time again I have heard people say that the ground substance contained a certain amount of hexosamine and that this meant that there was a certain amount of polysaccharide there. We all know that the mucoproteins contain hexosamine in larger or just as large quantities as the polysaccharides, so determination of hexosamine does not measure the amount of mucopolysaccharides alone. I know that certain people know perfectly well what they are talking about when they talk about ground substance, but I am worried about what other people may think when they hear the term used in the singular as if it were a continuous entity. Quite frequently it is not a continuous entity. Different changes can take place in different components. I think that we ought to be a little more careful in the use of the word.

In addition, as a biochemist, I would like to ask the pathologists on the panel how they define "injury." The term seems to include many things, from the easily observable reactions to injury that Dr. Zweifach has just talked about to the reaction to microinjury in which there is no easily observable damage at all. For example, we have implanted sponges treated with certain materials as a method of producing injury. In this situation, only minimal damage is produced, there is no necrosis, and mast cells do not appear; so where does the histamine come from, if histamine is involved in this reaction? In other words, are there different pathways or different mechanisms involved in each type of inflammation, or is there a common mechanism only a part of which is involved in some types of inflammation?

Dr. Menkin: We do not know what injury really is and we do not know the exact mechanism involved. The whole process is very interesting. We have had the concept for some time that the degree of injury is important in determining whether inflammation, proliferation or neoplasia will occur. Inflammation seems to be a manifestation of more severe injury and proliferation seems to be referable to a very mild degree of injury. We can produce a minimal type of injury by piercing the ears of rabbits with staples. When the staples are left in place for periods of four months to two years, about 25 per cent of the rabbits develop proliferative nodules, and these are found to be chondrofibromas histologically. Why this particular reaction to mild injury occurs in only 25 per cent of the rabbits is unknown, but we believe that the group of rabbits we used had a genetic susceptability to neoplasia. This may be the reason that one finds an inflammatory reaction so often around neoplastic tissue. Perhaps both malignancy and inflammation are basically manifestations of cell injury.

Dr. Wagner: Unfortunately, unlike mathematicians, we are dealing with biological systems, and observational disciplines are involved; consequently, we have to recognize the limits of this technique and begin from there. I think it is better if we say "alteration" rather than injury. For example, if the cristae of mitochondria are bent in half, is this an injury? There are great gaps in our definitions relating to biological systems, but we must begin someplace. The biologist must first know the normal process and its variations. Only then can he begin to observe alterations or deviations from the usual pattern and try to classify them. In biology at this point, there are two groups of people, the "lumpers" and the "splitters." The "lumpers" will place all of the alterations under one big heading, and the "splitters" will place them in many small categories. Year by year we "lump" and "split" until we do find the proper place and sequence of each observation.

Since the discussion has progressed into the area of definitions, I wonder whether we do enhance our concept of connective tissue diseases by introducing new terms. What do these concepts really tell us? To illustrate this, there are two other terms I want to discuss. "Fibrinoid" was originally defined by Neumann in 1880. He was impressed by some observations on inflamed serous membranes. He noted some peculiar looking, eosinophilic, refractile material occurring in clumps or bands when the sections were stained with eosin and said it looked like fibrin; but when he applied a picrocarmine stain to it, he found that it was not fibrin, and he called it "fibrinoid." That initiated the use of this term. Other German pathologists then began to look for the material, and soon fibrinoid was found to be present in normal placentas and in many diseased tissues. Even if you pinch the skin of a rabbit, you can then find fibrinoid. Actually, what I am saying is that there is a very definite limitation in the techniques used in identifying the materials under observation.

Subsequently, Klinge produced fibrinoid in experimental animals in various hypersensitivity experiments; this started the concept that when one sees fibrinoid its pathogenesis is hypersensitivity. Now, this was a tremendous generalization, and Klinge kept it going with some support by other investigators, but obviously this cannot be the whole answer. Connective tissue has a limited capacity to respond, and our techniques limit us in determining exactly what is happening. One of the key problems, as I see it, in connective tissue disease research is the need for a more meticulous definition of "fibrinoid," that is, what it is and how it can be identified by its principal component.

The same thing holds true for amyloid. There are many ways in which one can produce amyloid. For example, one can produce amyloid in certain strains of mice by daily gamma irradiation; there are strain A mice who naturally develop amyloid. In other animals amyloid can be produced by injections of protein products from cells. Are all of these amyloids the same type of amyloid?

Finally there is the term "dyscollagenosis." If we agree with Klinge that fibrinoid in the hypersensitivity experimental model is not degenerated collagen fibers *per se*, but an alteration in the ground substance in which the fibers are embedded, then we are not talking about a collagen disease *per se*, but a disease of the ground substance. I believe Dr. Pollack rejected the sweeping generalization of hypersensitivity in regard to the fibrinoid in scleroderma and lupus and went back to the original idea of Neumann simply to serve as a concept. To stimulate other pathologists to study this, he coined the term "collagen disease" rather than some other term. I do not think the term "dyscollagenosis," which contains the word "collagen," should be used since we know that in many of these diseases the collagen fibers *per se* may not be the site of primary involvement. I prefer to use the term "connective tissue disease."

DR. ANGEVINE: I agree with everything that you said. Dr. Pollack, would you comment on this?

DR. POLLACK: The term "collagen disease" was used as a "telegraphic" term to indicate that the connective tissue was involved. In the original paper, we were talking about the connective tissue as a whole. It became corrupted subsequently by others who used the word "collagen" because of its convenience. It originally did not have the meaning it has acquired since, and I think it would be just as well to use the term "connective tissue disease." However, it is important to remember that all of the diseases which we refer to now as connective tissue diseases are not necessarily the result of primary disorders of this tissue, since there are a number of diseases, some related and some not, in which anatomical symptoms occur in the connective tissue.

DR. D. JACKSON: I would like to emphasize the relation of fibrinoid to connective tissue. We all assume that the fibrinoid has its own identity and that proteolytic enzymes have no effect on it except to coagulate it. Recently it has been obvious that some enzymes will in fact cause rather subtle changes in the fibrous tissue which are not apparent when one looks at it, even through a microscope. This problem can be approached in a slightly different way by putting this tissue into slightly acid solution, and you find that the whole structure spontaneously falls apart. In other words, something is being attacked by proteolytic enzymes; it is not collagen but is very closely associated with it, and once that happens, the collagen is no longer a stable fiber. It is quite clear that it is falling apart. It is the kind of phenomenon one sees in many of these diseases. Therefore, it is quite obvious that in many situations, a minor change in these components will reflect quite strongly on the collagen, but the latter will be purely a secondary phenomenon. Nothing will happen to the collagen fiber molecule as such.

DR. ASBOE-HANSEN: I think it is extremely useful to speak about terminology. Many things we talk about have not been definitely settled, and the terminology used in one hospital is often different from that used in another. Aside from this, there are other factors, and I particularly want to stress the differences resulting from the methods used for fixation of tissues. In one institution mast cells may be fixed with formalin, in another with formalin and water, and in a third only by freeze drying. These different methods give quite different results. For example, when formalin-water fixation is used, the granules of a mast cell may go out into the water, altering the appearance of the cell, and it may be called a fibroblast. Another example is the use of formalin fixation and subsequent staining with P.A.S. The Schiff reagent stains formalin as well as polysaccharides, and how can anyone determine the amount of polysaccharides in tissue slices if the formalin is also stained?

DR. WAGNER: I think that the periodic acid Schiff reaction is a useful reaction, but only if one realizes the limitations in the chemistry of it, as Dr. Asboe-Hansen has pointed out. I would agree completely that it is impossible to relate data from one laboratory to another when you do not know how the tissue has been fixed and prepared, and consequently I would like to reemphasize the point that when we talk about P.A.S.-positive granules and metachromasia we should define the systems used.

Part III | IMMUNOLOGY OF INFLAMMATION AND CONNECTIVE TISSUE DISEASES

Immunity and Inflammation*

BERNARD M. WAGNER

New York Medical College

The immune state and its deviations are currently under intensive study by a variety of methods. The acquisition of immunity to a specific biological agent requires detailed analyses of many variables. The cellular responses associated with the development of immunity may be considered as part of the inflammatory process; as Florey[5] has aptly written, "Inflammation is a process and not a state." Certain patterns of response have emerged and serve as the basis in recognizing unusual variants. The purpose of this paper will be to examine the role of the lymphocyte in chronic inflammation, with special attention to immune phenomena.

CHRONIC INFLAMMATION

Most pathologists agree that lymphocytes, plasma cells and histiocytes, when arranged in a focal manner, suggest chronic inflammation. By utilizing appropriate systems, almost all antigens are capable of eliciting this response in the tissues of the host as a local reaction. What, then, is the function of these cells, especially in the elaboration of antibody? It is beyond the scope of this paper to list the many publications devoted to this question. The reader is referred to recent critical reports.[9] However, certain pertinent observations are necessary.

The cytoplasmic ultrastructure of the lymphocyte and plasma cell has been studied by Bernhard and Granboulan.[2] The lymphocyte is primarily a container of DNA since the cytoplasm is minimal and contains a few mitochondria. The plasma cell demonstrates an ultrastructure comparable to that of pancreatic acinar cells. Such structural similarity strongly suggests functional similarity and serves to support the theory that protein antibodies are produced by plasma cells. The obvious and vexing next question is whether lymphocytes can become plasma cells. There appears to be no proof of a direct transformation of typical lymphocytes into plasma cells. Dixon and his associates[4] reported the presence of plasma cells in tissues into which homologous lymph node cells had been transferred after antigenic stimulation. A possible interpretation of this observation would relate the antibody induction process to a recognizable lymphocyte and antibody synthesis to a cell with the structural configuration of a plasma cell. A major stumbling block continues to be at the cytological level in fixing morphological criteria for purposes of cellular identification. Nevertheless, the overwhelming data implicate the plasma cell as the major source of protein antibody. What, then, may be the status of the lymphocyte in the immune process?

POSSIBLE ROLE OF THE LYMPHOCYTE IN THE IMMUNE PROCESS

There continues to be a substantial body of information relating the lymphocyte to the cellular production of antibodies. Extensive cell transfer

* Supported in part by U. S. Public Health Service Grant H-5822.

studies by Harris and his associates[7] present the most convincing evidence that lymphocytes are intimately involved in the mechanism leading to antibody synthesis. Some years ago, while working in the laboratory of Dr. William Ehrich, we decided to test the hypothesis that lymphocytes might be carriers of essential materials[1, 3] required by the plasma cell for protein synthesis.[11] Several considerations led to this hypothesis; the key ones were (1) the rapid turn-over rate of lymphocytes and (2) their constant presence in areas elaborating antibody. Since lymphocytolysis releases DNA and its subsequent degradation products into the local environment, attention was paid to the possible role of these products in stimulating synthetic mechanisms. The original experiments have been repeated, confirmed and extended. A total of 86 rabbits have been studied.

MATERIALS AND METHODS

A system producing glucose-6-PO_4 at a low rate via oxidative phosphorylation was used. The efficiency of the system was expressed by comparing the quantity of inorganic phosphate esterified with the quantity of oxygen consumed. Figure 1 represents the oxidative phosphorylation system

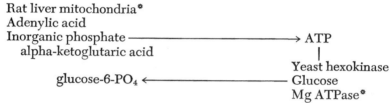

Fig. 1. Scheme of oxidative phosphorylation. Certain preparations* are purposely prepared and utilized to maintain a low efficiency.

used according to Polis et al.[10] Standard biochemical techniques were used and may be found in any standard text. New Zealand male rabbits weighing 1.5 to 2.0 kg. were inoculated in the footpad of the right hind leg with 0.5 ml. of a commercial typhoid vaccine. The regional lymph node, the popliteal, was excised, trimmed of fat and weighed. These nodes were sampled daily by sacrificing pairs of animals from 1 to 15 days after antigen administration. In addition, the contralateral popliteal nodes were also removed and served as controls. At the time of lymph node removal the animal was exsanguinated and the serum used for determining agglutinin titer. The nodes were homogenized at 4° C. and suspended in 0.25 M sucrose solution. Differential centrifugation allowed for the removal of cellular débris. The clear supernate was used for the determination of enzyme activity.

The method of differential enzymatic spectrophotometry designed by

PURINE	REACTION	ENZYME	E	
Xanthine	Oxidation	Xanthine oxidase	$- E_{270}$	$+ E_{290}$
Hypoxanthine	Oxidation	Xanthine oxidase	$- E_{250}$	$+ E_{290}$
Uric acid	Oxidation	Uricase		$- E_{290}$
Adenine compounds	Deamination	Adenosine deaminase	$+ E_{240}$	$- E_{265}$

Fig. 2. The symbol E represents the change in extinction during the reaction.

Kalckar[8] was employed to measure the presence of xanthine oxidase, adenosine deaminase and adenase. The full technical details will be the subject of a future publication.[12] Figure 2 lists the substrate-enzyme reactions and the change in extinction coefficients at specific wavelengths. The rate of change allows for calculation of enzyme concentration. A typical experiment is noted in Figure 3.

TIME (min.)	E_{265}	$- E_{265}/min.$	TIME (min.)	E_{265}	$- E_{265}/min.$
0.5	0.826		6	0.544	
		0.082			0.015
1	0.744		8	0.510	
		0.068			0.010
2	0.676		10	0.500	
		0.058			0.002
3	0.618		15	0.490	
		0.046			0.000
4	0.572		20	0.490	
		0.032			

Fig. 3. Determination of adenosine deaminase in 6-day lymph node. Temp. 22° C., 4×10^{-5} M adenosine in PO_4 buffer, pH 7.40. Volume in cuvette 3.0 ml., 0.03 ml. tissue extract in Cl^-/HCO_3^- buffer. Beckman DU spectrophotometer.

Total nitrogen was determined by a micro-Kjeldahl method. According to the basic procedures of Kalckar[8] as used in this laboratory, enzymatic determinations were made with a Beckman model DU spectrophotometer using 1 cm. cuvettes. The control cuvettes contained all the reactants except the substrate. The alterations of the purine molecule which result in marked spectral changes at appropriate wavelengths after enzyme addition are utilized to calculate the concentration of the particular substrate. Under the conditions of the experiment used, the rate of increase or decrease in extinction was directly proportional to tissue concentration. All determinations were carried out at two tissue concentrations, and the rates of change for a given time interval when the rate was constant were averaged, then calculated as micromoles of substrate used, by use of optical constants.

Adenosine deaminase was determined by measuring the rate of decrease in absorption at 265 mμ. and increase at 240 mμ. The values obtained at 265 were used in the calculations. Under the conditions of the determination only adenosine was deaminated. The deamination of adenine could not be detected. The composition of the reaction mixture was 0.5 ml. of 0.25 M glycylglycine buffer, pH 7.4, a suitable aliquot of the tissue preparation, and distilled water to make a final volume of 3.0 ml. After equilibration at 22.0° C., 0.1 ml. of 4×10^{-5} M adenosine was added and readings were taken at 1-minute intervals for the first 4 minutes and then at 2-minute intervals for a period of 20 minutes. Readings were made at 265 and 240 mμ.

RESULTS

Table 1 expresses the relationships between lymph node weights, predominant cellular response, agglutinin titers and enzyme activity. By the

TABLE 1. POPLITEAL LYMPH NODE RESPONSES AND RELATIONSHIP
TO ANTIBODY TITER AND ENZYME ACTIVITY

DAY	NODE WT. C	NODE WT. R	LYMPH. C	LYMPH. R	PLASMA CELLS C	PLASMA CELLS R	GERM. C. C	GERM. C. R	AGG. TITER	ADENOSINE D. C	ADENOSINE D. R
0	1	1	1	1	0	0	1	1	0	0	0
1	1	2	1	2	0	0	1	1	0	0	0
3	1	2	2	2	0	1	1	1	10	0	1
5	1	3	2	3	1	3	2	3	200	0	3
6	2	3	3	3	2	3	2	3	350	2	3
7	2	3	3	4	3	4	2	3	300	3	4
9	2	4	3	4	3	4	3	4	200	3	4
11	2	4	3	4	3	3	3	4	100	3	4
15	2	4	3	4	2	3	3	4	100	3	4

Note: An arbitrary unit system has been used to allow for ease of comparison.
C = contralateral node, R = regional node.
Node Wt. = Lymph node weight in mg. control value = 1 and 4 is the maximal weight
    observed.
Lymph. = Lymphocytes. Normal distribution and quantity = 1, and 4 is maximal lympho-
    cytosis-lymphocytolysis.
Plasma cells = Normal distribution and quantity of plasma cells = 1, and 4 is maximal
    number observed.
Germ. C. = Germinal centers. Normal cortical centers = 1, and 4 is maximal number
    of active centers.
Agg. Titer = Agglutination titer. Values based on multiples of 10.
Adenosine D. = Adenosine deaminase. Minimal activity = 1, and 4 is maximal activity
    observed.

TABLE 2. STIMULATING EFFECTS OF CERTAIN PURINES
ON OXIDATIVE PHOSPHORYLATION

$$\frac{\text{Esterified Phosphate}}{\text{Oxygen Consumption}} = \text{Efficiency of the System (E)}$$

Compound	E
control	1
xanthine	100
adenine	90
hypoxanthine	60
inosine	40
uric acid	20

techniques employed, adenosine deaminase was the only enzyme that showed
significant changes. Table 2 shows the effects of added purines, including
inosine, on the efficiency of the oxidative phosphorylation system used. These
substances served to stimulate the system and agree with the results of
Polis et al.

DISCUSSION

The exquisite sensitivity of the differential spectrophotometric method
allowed for the study of certain enzymes associated with nucleoprotein
synthesis in antibody-producing lymph nodes. The assumption is made that
the enzyme pattern is directly related to the cellular events in the node. It
would seem from the limited data that enzyme activity is greatest at the

time the node shows its most active increase and destruction of lymphocytes. However, the adenosine deaminase activity was also elevated during the plasma cellular phase.

The purines, nucleotides and nucleosides may function as key intermediates in the rapid synthesis of nucleoprotein. There is evidence supporting inosine as such a compound. The amino groups released by the deaminase may serve as important building blocks in amino acid synthesis. A great deal of additional work is contemplated along these lines. It is most tempting to speculate that lymphocytolysis serves the useful purpose of supplying the needs of the local metabolic pool. The DNA degradation products, in addition to serving as intermediates for nucleoprotein synthesis, may serve other functions as well. Thus, they may function as important co-factors. The *in vitro* demonstration of the ability of adenine, xanthine, hypoxanthine, inosine and adenosine to substantially stimulate oxidative phosphorylation may suggest such a role *in vivo*. Such metabolic rate regulators would be most useful to cells actively engaged in protein synthesis.

THE HISTIOCYTE

These cells are also key figures in areas of chronic inflammation and antibody production. There is some suggestion that they may be transformed into plasma cells. Given an experimental situation in which antigen concentration is increasing locally, the first morphological evidence of immunity will be the perivascular arrangement of mononuclear cells. The origin of these cells is controversial. A variety of possibilities exist, such as local histiocytes, vascular endothelium, lymph nodes and RE cells. Gell[6] refers to the reaction as a perivascular island and suggests that these cells, by virtue of their position, may protect the vessel against the injurious effects of antibody interacting with local antigen. The perivascular island reaction, as produced experimentally with tuberculin, is usually equated with hypersensitivity of the delayed type. For this and other reasons, similar observations in human rheumatic diseases have suggested a relationship to hypersensitivity.

SUMMARY

The development of immunity is intimately related to cellular responses which characterize chronic inflammation. It is accepted that the plasma cell is a major source of antibody. Evidence is briefly presented relating the activity of adenosine deaminase to lymphocytosis-lymphocytolysis in antibody-producing lymph nodes. Certain purine bases and allied compounds significantly stimulate *in vitro* oxidative phosphorylation. The hypothesis is advanced that lymphocytes may supply key intermediates to the local metabolic pool which serve to ultimately influence protein synthesis. The perivascular collection of histiocytic cells is the earliest morphological indication of delayed hypersensitivity. Similar changes in certain connective tissue diseases may indicate a similar process.

REFERENCES

1. Barnes, J. M.: The enzymes of lymphocytes and polymorphonuclear leukocytes, Brit. J. Exper. Path., *21*:264, 1940.
2. Bernhard, W. and Granboulan, N.: Ultrastructure of immunologically competent cells. In Cellular Aspects of Immunity. Boston, Little, Brown and Co., 1960, p. 92.

3. Conway, W. and Cooke, R.: The deaminases of adenosine and adenylic acid in blood and tissues. Biochem. J., 33:479, 1939.
4. Dixon, F. J., Weigle, W. D. and Roberts, J. C.: Comparison of antibody responses associated with the transfer of rabbit lymph node, peritoneal exudate and thymus cells. J. Immunol., 78:56, 1957.
5. Florey, H.: General Pathology. 2nd ed. Philadelphia, W. B. Saunders Co., 1958, p. 21.
6. Gell, P. G. H.: Cytologic events in hypersensitivity reactions. In Lawrence, H. S. (ed.): Cellular and Humoral Aspects of the Hypersensitive States. New York, Paul B. Hoeber, Inc., 1959, p. 43.
7. Harris, T. N. and Harris, S.: Cellular sources of antibody: a review of current literature. Ann. N.Y. Acad. Sc., 86:948, 1960.
8. Kalckar, H. M.: Differential spectrophotometry of purine compounds by means of specific enzymes. III. Studies of the enzymes of purine metabolism. J. Biol. Chem., 167:461, 1947.
9. Lawrence, H. S. (ed.): Cellular and Humoral Aspects of the Hypersensitive States. New York, Paul B. Hoeber, Inc., 1959.
10. Polis, B. D., Polis, E., Jedeikin, L. and Kety, S.: The effect of insulin and ATPase in a reaction coupling oxidation with phosphorylation. Am. J. M. Sc., 218:715, 1949.
11. Wagner, B. M. and Ehrich, W. E.: Adenosinase, adenase and xanthine oxidase of lymphoid tissues. Fed. Proc., 9:347, 1950.
12. Wagner, B. M.: Biochemical activity of antibody-producing lymph nodes. I. Purine metabolism. To be published.

Immunopathologic Studies in Rheumatic Heart Disease; Concept of Autoantibodies to Heart in Rheumatic Fever and Postcommissurotomy Syndrome[*]

MELVIN H. KAPLAN

Western Reserve University School of Medicine

The concept that a hypersensitivity mechanism participates in the pathogenesis of rheumatic fever was initially given strong impetus by the histopathologic and experimental studies of Klinge[14] and Rich and Gregory,[20-22] who emphasized similarities to serum sickness in man and the experimental lesions of serum sickness in animals. However, the relationship of such a postulated hypersensitivity mechanism to the specific cardiac stigmata of rheumatic fever has remained obscure. The current arguments for and against the role of hypersensitivity in rheumatic fever have been reviewed by McCarty[16] and MacLeod,[15] and there seems little point in summarizing them again.

[*] This work was done during the tenure of an Established Investigatorship of the American Heart Association and was supported by grants-in-aid from the National Heart Institute, U. S. Public Health Service and the Cleveland Foundation.

In this paper, I should like to summarize the results obtained in our laboratory by application of fluorescent antibody methods[7] to immunopathologic studies of rheumatic heart tissues and of the tissue-reactive properties of sera from patients with rheumatic fever. These studies were begun in 1954 and were originally undertaken in a search for evidence of bound gamma globulin* in rheumatic heart tissue from biopsied auricular appendages, on the assumption that such deposits might give indirect evidence of participation of immune factors in pathogenesis. It soon became evident that presence of bound gamma globulin could not be accepted as *a priori* evidence of an immunologic reaction. However, the origin and function of gamma globulin deposits in these tissues became of special interest also from other points of view, as will be described.

One hundred auricular appendages were made available for this study in Boston and Cleveland from 1954 to 1959.† Of these 100 specimens, 18 gave unequivocal evidence of bound gamma globulin in a characteristic pattern of distribution.[10] These auricular tissue specimens were from patients considered to be in an inactive stage of their disease by clinical criteria prior to surgery. However, the same distribution of bound gamma globulin was also observed in postmortem heart tissue from an 11-year-old boy who died following a severe attack of acute rheumatic fever, with congestive failure and cardiac arrhythmia. This child also gave serologic evidence of recent streptococcal infection indicated by an antistreptolysin O titer of 2500 Todd units.‡ Bound gamma globulin in the involved rheumatic hearts occurred in patchy distribution in the following histologic sites: (1) within segments of sarcolemma of myofibers, (2) within adjacent subsarcolemmal sarcoplasm and intermyofibrillar loci in the sarcoplasm in apparent continuity with sarcolemma, (3) in interstitial connective tissue between myofibers in deposits frequently confluent with involved sarcolemma and myofiber sarcoplasm, (4) in segments of walls of arterioles and venules, and (5) occasionally in scattered foci in connective tissue of endocardial and epicardial layers. This histologic distribution is illustrated in Figures 1, 2 and 3. Control non-rheumatic pathologic heart tissue specimens obtained at postmortem as well as those available from biopsies at cardiac surgery did not give evidence of such bound gamma globulin deposits.

Other serum proteins, including albumin and fibrin, were not found in the involved sites, thus indicating that gamma globulin was selectively fixed in these hearts. Histopathologic study further demonstrated that the sites of gamma globulin fixation in these tissues also exhibited, in most cases, objective evidence of tissue alteration, as indicated by an enhanced affinity for eosin, shown by a selective fluorochrome staining technique[10] (Fig. 4), an enhanced reaction with the periodic acid-Schiff reagent, and an intense metachromatic stain with toluidine blue. These staining reactions were much more prominent in unfixed frozen sections than in formalin-fixed preparations. Since these histochemical changes are precisely those characteristic of fibri-

*By *bound* gamma globulin is meant gamma globulin that cannot be removed from tissues following repeated washings of unfixed frozen sections, in contrast to the diffusible and completely extractable gamma globulin of normal heart tissue.

† We are grateful to Drs. Dwight E. Harken, Gustave Dammin, Gordon Scannell and Laurence Kunz, of Boston, Mass., and George H. Clowes, of Cleveland, Ohio, for making these tissues available for study.

‡ The collaboration of Dr. Robert Bolande, Institute of Pathology, Western Reserve University, in the study of the tissues of this patient is acknowledged.

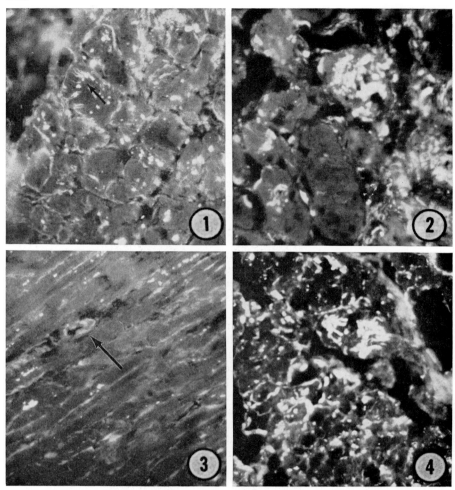

Fig. 1. Auricular appendage, Patient Mey. Bound gamma globulin in sarcolemma, in intermyofibrillar sites extending from sarcolemma (arrow) and within substance of sarcoplasm of some myofibers. Spherical bodies scattered in sarcoplasm are pigment granules. × 312.

Fig. 2. Auricular appendage, Patient For. Bound gamma globulin in amorphous deposits within sarcoplasm of myofibers, in segments of sarcolemma and in interstitial connective tissue sites. × 400.

Fig. 3. Auricular appendage, Patient Mey. Bound gamma globulin in segmental distribution in walls of small vessel (arrow) and in sarcolemma and interstitial connective tissue. × 312.

Fig. 4. Auricular appendage, Patient For. Eosin binding by eosin-fluorochrome technique. Sites with affinity for eosin include sarcolemma, amorphous or rodlike deposits within sarcoplasm and sites in interstitial connective tissue. These same sites in this specimen exhibited intense reaction with periodic acid-Schiff reagent and metachromasia with toluidine blue. × 200.

noid[1, 26] it appeared that the distribution of bound gamma globulin actually reflected the localization of fibrinoid material in these hearts.

These observations in rheumatic hearts were thus analogous to those made in studies of classic lesions of other connective tissue diseases by Mellors and associates[17] and Vazquez and Dixon,[25] with respect to the

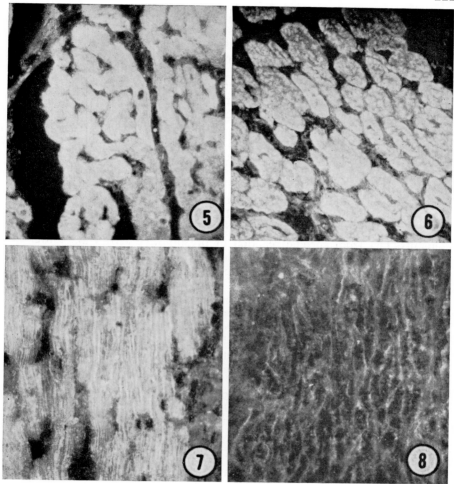

Fig. 5.   Diffuse sarcoplasmic pattern of immunofluorescent reaction with myofibers. × 200.

Fig. 6.   Subsarcolemmal-sarcoplasmic pattern of immunofluorescent reaction. Staining involves particularly subsarcolemmal sites and sites within remaining sarcoplasm which give "mottled" distribution. × 200.

Fig. 7.   Intermyofibrillar pattern of immunofluorescent reaction. Intense reaction with myofiber constituents concentrated between or adjacent to myofibrils. × 200.

Fig. 8.   Sarcolemmal pattern. Staining involves the connective tissue sheaths surrounding myofibers, in this case without reaction with sarcoplasmic constituents. × 200.

presence of gamma globulin in fibrinoid material in the "wire-loop" glomerular lesions and "onion-skin" vascular lesions of disseminated lupus, and in the subcutaneous nodules of rheumatoid arthritis.

In their studies of rheumatic heart tissue, Vazquez and Dixon[25] reported gamma globulin also in Aschoff lesions and in adjacent altered perivascular connective tissue. In our own material, *bound gamma globulin* was not noted in Aschoff bodies, nor was the occurrence of gamma globulin in auricular appendage specimens found to be correlated with either the presence or absence of Aschoff lesions.[10] It is possible that these divergent results represent either a difference in the clinical materials studied or in the immuno-fluorescent techniques employed.[11]

It was of interest that the distribution of gamma globulin and fibrinoid material in rheumatic hearts in this work resembled in many respects the distribution of sites of early fibrinoid change (Fruh-infiltrat) described by Klinge[14] in his illuminating histopathologic studies of the initial stages of "rheumatic inflammation" observed in patients dying early in the course of acute rheumatic fever. The implication which perhaps arises is whether deposits of bound gamma globulin in fibrinoid material in rheumatic auricular appendages hold special significance as an index of subclinical rheumatic activity analogous to the Aschoff lesion.

The more central problem concerns the origin and function of the bound gamma globulin in these rheumatic hearts and the relationship of such deposits to fibrinoid alteration. Several hypothetical possibilities may be considered (cf. references 25 and 11): Deposition of bound gamma globulin may result (1) from nonspecific binding of this protein to altered tissue elements, (2) from specific reaction of presumptive serum autoantibodies with tissue antigen, (3) from a specialized inflammatory process involving either local production or deposition of gamma globulin, or both.

Nonspecific binding of circulating gamma globulin to altered tissue sites was opposed by the following experimental observations. When the distribution of gamma globulin was compared in adjacent sections with the distribution of other plasma proteins and of altered tissue as defined by each of the following staining reactions, eosin-binding, metachromasia and enhanced periodic acid-Schiff reaction, a direct correspondence was frequently not observed, as shown in Table 1. In occasional tissue specimens, intense and

TABLE 1. *COMPARISON OF BOUND GAMMA GLOBULIN WITH OTHER HISTOCHEMICAL OBSERVATIONS AT SITES OF DEPOSITION*

HEART TISSUE SPECIMEN	BOUND GAMMA GLOBULIN	ALBUMIN	FIBRIN	METACHROMASIA	EOSIN BINDING
Gas	++++	0	Traces	+++	++++
San	++++	0	Traces	+++	+++
Cap	+++	0	0	+++	++
Hut	++++	0	0	+++	0
Mey	++++	0	0	++++	0
DeA	+	0	0	+++	++++
Rou	0	0	0	++++	+++

widespread evidence of altered staining by all three histochemical techniques was observed, although bound gamma globulin was sparse or entirely absent.* Other tissue specimens have been observed with extensive deposits of bound gamma globulin, associated with metachromatic and P.A.S.-positive material, which did not exhibit eosin binding by the standard method of test.[10] In none of these sections was either fibrinogen/fibrin or albumin associated with sites of localization of gamma globulin. It would seem that if deposition of gamma globulin resulted simply from nonspecific binding of serum proteins to fibrinoid, a more direct correspondence of gamma globulin and perhaps of other proteins with sites of altered histochemical reaction should have been observed.

---

* This sparseness or absence of bound gamma globulin in sites of fibrinoid alteration in these tissues may have some relevance to the fibrinoid material in subcutaneous nodules in the rheumatoid arthritis of agammaglobulinemic individuals.[3]

The second proposition, derivation of bound gamma globulin from circulating autoantibody, was approached directly by examining the serologic activity of sera of patients with rheumatic fever against heart tissue sections, using the indirect immunofluorescent technique. Serologic reactions of rheumatic sera with heart tissue have been reported in the literature by Brockmann and associates,[4] Cavelti,[6] Osler and associates,[18] Rejholec and Wagner,[19] Butler and Moeschlin,[5] and Steffen,[24] employing such techniques as complement-fixation with aqueous or alcoholic extracts of heart, collodion particle agglutination and antiglobulin consumption tests. These reports have been recently reviewed.[12] Except for Cavelti,[6] these authors have not found such serologic reactions specific for rheumatic fever. Positive tests were reported in rheumatoid arthritis, renal and other parenchymatous diseases, and with sera of some normal individuals.

In the present work, evidence was obtained pointing to the multiple nature of presumptive autoimmune globulins reactive with heart in rheumatic as well as in other pathologic sera.[13] These serologic factors could be differentiated, using the indirect immunofluorescent technique, by the histologic or cytologic distribution of reactive antigens in the tissue section. Reactants were found to include primarily constituents of myofiber sarcoplasm and sarcolemma. In the case of sarcoplasmic-reactive factors, three cytologic patterns of reaction could be distinguished, termed descriptively (1) diffuse sarcoplasmic, (2) subsarcolemmal-sarcoplasmic, and (3) intermyofibrillar. These serologic reactions are illustrated in Figures 5, 6, 7 and 8. Sera giving diffuse sarcoplasmic or subsarcolemmal-sarcoplasmic reactive patterns of staining with myofibers frequently showed complement-fixation reactions with alcoholic extracts of heart as antigen. All three types of sera gave flocculation reactions with alcohol extract of heart, using a latex-particle agglutination technique. In all three cases, the reactant was distinct from the Wassermann antigen, cardiolipin, which was also observed to be a constituent of myofiber sarcoplasm.

It was possible to distinguish between 7S and 19S gamma globulin immunochemically by employing anti-19S gamma globulin labelled with fluorescein in the indirect staining technique. Sarcoplasmic-reactive factors were found associated with 19S gamma globulins infrequently. In one series of tests, only 6 of 50 sera reactive with fluorescent anti-human gamma globulin exhibited a reaction when tested with fluorescent anti-19S gamma globulin. Five of these yielded a subsarcolemmal-sarcoplasmic pattern; one, an intermyofibrillar pattern.

Sera with reactive properties for sarcolemma, with or without reactivity for sarcoplasmic constituents, were observed infrequently in patients with rheumatic fever. These sarcolemmal-reactive factors were also associated in some sera with 19S gamma globulins.

None of the sarcoplasmic and sarcolemmal-reactive factors were specific for rheumatic fever or rheumatic heart disease. The diffuse sarcoplasmic pattern of reaction was particularly nonspecific; it was observed in patients with infectious, neoplastic and parenchymatous diseases, and may possibly represent an immunofluorescent counterpart of such serologic reactions as the universal serologic reaction of Kahn.[9] The subsarcolemmal-sarcoplasmic and intermyofibrillar patterns of reaction were observed infrequently[12] except in diseases of connective tissue, including rheumatic fever, rheumatic heart disease, rheumatoid arthritis and disseminated lupus, and in liver disease.

TABLE 2. DISTRIBUTION OF SARCOPLASMIC REACTIVE FACTORS IN
"CONNECTIVE TISSUE DISEASE"

DIAGNOSTIC CATEGORY	NO. OF PATIENTS	NO. OF POSITIVE REACTIONS WITH REACTIVE PATTERN			PER CENT POSITIVE	PER CENT POSITIVE WITH S AND I PATTERNS
		D*	S	I		
Acute rheumatic fever	40	21	10	0	77.4	25.0
Rheumatic heart disease, inactive	79	33	14	3	63.3	21.5
Rheumatic heart disease, post-cardiotomy	45	9	29	6	97.8	77.8
Rheumatoid arthritis	27	10	5	1	59.3	22.2
Lupus erythematosus	11	6	2	3	100.0	45.4
Liver disease	38	25	7	2	89.5	23.7

* D = Diffuse sarcoplasmic; S = Subsarcolemmal-sarcoplasmic; I = Intermyofibrillar.

The frequency distribution of these serologic factors in these disorders is given in Table 2.

In acute rheumatic fever, 21 of 40 patients, or 52.5 per cent, exhibited serologic reactions of the diffuse-sarcoplasmic type; 10, or 25 per cent, showed subsarcolemmal-sarcoplasmic reactions; and none showed an intermyofibrillar reaction. Positive reactions were noted most frequently during the acute stages of the disease, and in such patients reaction usually persisted for some weeks after C-reactive protein tests had become negative. In a few patients, serologic activity was first detectable in the serum only after the C-reactive protein tests had become negative. Serologic reactions with sarcolemma were usually noted in patients with chronic or cyclical rheumatic activity.

It will be noted in Table 2 that positive serologic tests were observed in some patients with rheumatic heart disease considered clinically inactive, as, for example, those selected for surgical correction of mitral stenosis. Approximately two weeks after mitral surgery, a marked increase in frequency of serologic reactions was noted, particularly with respect to subsarcolemmal-sarcoplasmic and intermyofibrillar-reactive factors. Thus, as shown in the table, serologic reactions of these types increased from a frequency of 21.5 per cent in adult rheumatic patients clinically inactive, to 77.8 per cent after cardiac surgery. Evidence that surgery itself was the event stimulating these serum factors was afforded by simultaneous tests of paired sera from rheumatic patients collected prior to and two weeks after surgery. Serologic activity was tested both against autologous auricular appendage and normal non-rheumatic heart by immunofluorescence and by flocculation tests with alcoholic extract of normal heart. Development of or increase in serologic activity of postsurgical sera by both methods of test was observed in a majority of rheumatic patients subjected to cardiac surgery (Table 3).

The serologic changes observed in a group of 19 patients in whom auricular tissue and pre- and postsurgical sera were available were as follows: Ten of the 19, or 52.6 per cent, showed development of subsarcolemmal-sarcoplasmic reactive factor following surgery. Five patients revealed the presence of such serum factors both before and after cardiotomy; however, of these, two exhibited a marked increase in serologic activity following cardiotomy. The remaining four patients exhibited no serologic activity.

TABLE 3.   *CHANGE IN SEROLOGIC REACTION WITH HOMOLOGOUS HEART FOLLOWING CARDIAC SURGERY IN 7 RHEUMATIC PATIENTS AS INDICATED BY IMMUNOFLUORESCENT AND FLOCCULATION REACTIONS**

PATIENT	SERUM SPECIMEN†	INTENSITY OF IMMUNOFLUORESCENT REACTION	FLOCCULATION REACTION AT SERUM DILUTION					
			1/2	1/4	1/8	1/16	1/32	1/64
Gra	Presurgical	+ (S)	+	+	±	0	0	0
	Postsurgical	+++++ (S)	+++	++	+	+	+	0
Con	Presurgical	++ (D)	+++	+	0	0	0	0
	Postsurgical	+++++ (S)	++++	++++	++++	±	0	0
Nel	Presurgical	0	0	0	0	0	0	0
	Postsurgical	+++ (D)	++	++	+	0	0	0
Wag	Presurgical	+ (I)	0	0	0	0	0	0
	Postsurgical	++ (I)	++++	++++	+++	0	0	0
Clif	Presurgical	++ (D)	++	++	±	0	0	0
	Postsurgical	+++++ (S)	++	+	+	±	0	0
Fla	Presurgical	+ (D)	++	++	0	0	0	0
	Postsurgical	++++ (S)	++	++	+	0	0	0
Sha	Presurgical	++ (D)	++	+++	++	++	0	0
	Postsurgical	+++++ (S)	+++	+++	++	+	±	0

* The same heart was used for tissue sections and for preparation of the alcoholic extract.
† Serum specimens were obtained 0 to 5 days before and 11 to 14 days after surgery.

Thus, in this group of 19 individuals, 12, or 63.2 per cent, either developed or showed increase in serologic activity following cardiotomy.

We may now turn to the question posed previously: Can the deposition of bound gamma globulin at sites of fibrinoid alteration in rheumatic heart tissue be attributed to a reaction of serum autoantibodies with tissue antigen? Attempts to correlate the presence of bound gamma globulin in auricular appendage material with serologic activity present either prior to or at the time of surgery did not support such a relationship. As shown in Table 4,

TABLE 4.   RELATIONSHIP OF BOUND GAMMA GLOBULIN TO PRESENCE IN
SERUM OF SARCOPLASMIC-REACTIVE FACTOR

HEART SPECIMEN	BOUND GAMMA GLOBULIN IN AURICULAR APPENDAGE*	SERUM REACTION† 0-5 DAYS PRIOR TO SURGERY
Gas	++++	+++ (S)
Hut‡	++++	0
San	++++	0
Cap	+++	++ (D)
Lau	+++	+ (D)
Spi	+++	+++ (I)
Sil	++	0
DeA	+	0
Zam	+	+++ (S)
Gog	+	+ (D)
Fav	0	+++ (D)
Ebb	0	0
Geo	0	+ (D)
Eis	0	+++ (S)
Wic	0	0
Gil	0	++ (S)
Tro	0	0
Ara	0	++ (S)

   * Graded by extent of distribution in myocardium within myofibers and interstitium.
   † As determined with autologous heart tissue sections. Intensity of immunofluorescent staining graded from 0 to 5 +.
   ‡ Postmortem heart and serum from patient with acute rheumatic fever.

certain of the patients with bound gamma globulin in auricular appendage tissue gave evidence of serologic activity with heart tissue; others, also with such gamma globulin deposits, did not show serologic activity. Many patients without gamma globulin in auricular tissue exhibited marked serologic reaction. Thus, derivation of bound gamma globulin from the circulating auto-antibodies described in the present work is not supported by the present data.

Do these circulating autoantibodies to heart have any pathologic significance? During the postcardiotomy period, development of or increase in serologic activity was, in most cases, not found associated with appearance of clinical signs or symptoms. However, those patients with the postcommissurotomy syndrome[8, 23] who have been studied in our laboratory have all given evidence of remarkable serologic activity which persisted from several weeks to months concurrent with the duration of this disorder.

Thus, while a direct pathogenetic relationship of these serologic factors to the immunopathologic changes observed in rheumatic hearts and to the pathogenesis of the postcommissurotomy syndrome probably cannot be supported, it is probable that such autoantibodies do reflect a state of immunologic hyper-responsiveness. These heart reactive factors may perhaps be held analogous to the lupus serum factors reactive with nuclear material. Although not directly involved in pathogenesis, such autoantibodies in the serum may possibly point to an underlying immunopathologic state yet to be uncovered.

Association of gamma globulin with a specialized process of rheumatic inflammation was the third hypothesis presented above in interpretation of the association of bound gamma globulin with fibrinoid material. As yet this hypothesis must be considered without supportive evidence. However, of relevance to this concept is the observation of Anderson and McCarty[2] of a close relationship of serum gamma globulin concentration to clinical and laboratory evidences of rheumatic activity. Such gamma globulin fluctuations were not found related necessarily to specific antistreptococcal antibody. The nature, origin and function, if any, of such gamma globulin and its relationship to the rheumatic process present us with an array of "unknowns" which remain to be attacked in further investigation of the association of gamma globulin with fibrinoid material.

REFERENCES

1. Altschuler, C. H. and Angevine, D. M.: Histochemical studies on pathogenesis of fibrinoid. Am. J. Path., 25:1061, 1949.
2. Anderson, H. C. and McCarty, M.: Unpublished data. Cited by McCarty: The immune response in rheumatic fever. In Thomas, L. (ed.): Rheumatic Fever, a Symposium. Minneapolis, University of Minnesota Press, 1952, p. 136.
3. Bridges, R. A. and Good, R. A.: Connective tissue diseases and certain serum protein components in patients with agammaglobulinemia. Ann. N. Y. Acad. Sc., 86:1089, 1960.
4. Brockmann, H., Brill, J. and Frendzell, J.: Komplement Ablenkung mit organ Extrakten von Rheumatiken bei sogenannten gelenk Rheumatismus. Klin. Wochschr., 16:502, 1937.
5. Butler, K. and Moeschlin, S.: Antikorper gegen verschiedene Gewebszellen bei rheumatischen und anderen Erkrankungen. Helv. Med. Acta., 23:592, 1956.
6. Cavelti, P. A.: Autoantibodies in rheumatic fever. Proc. Soc. Exper. Biol. & Med., 60:379, 1945.
7. Coons, A. H. and Kaplan, M. H.: Localization of antigen in tissue cells. II. Improvements in a method for the detection of antigen by means of fluorescent antibody. J. Exper. Med., 91:1, 1950.
8. Elster, S. K., Wood, H. F. and Seely, R.: Clinical and laboratory manifestations of the post-commissurotomy syndrome. Am. J. Med., 17:826, 1954.
9. Kahn, R. L.: An introduction to universal serologic reaction in health and disease. New York, The Commonwealth Fund, 1951.
10. Kaplan, M. H. and Dallenbach, F. D.: Immunologic studies of heart tissue. III. Occurrence of bound gamma globulin in auricular appendages from rheumatic hearts. Relationship to certain histopathologic features of rheumatic heart disease. J. Exper. Med., 113:1, 1961.
11. Kaplan, M. H.:The fluorescent antibody technic as a research tool in the study of connective tissue disease. Arthritis Rheum., 2:568, 1959.
12. Kaplan, M. H.: The concept of autoantibodies in rheumatic fever and in the post-commissurotomy state. Ann. N. Y. Acad. Sc., 86:974, 1960.
13. Kaplan, M. H., Meyeserian, M. and Kushner, I.: Immunologic studies of heart tissue. IV. Serologic reactions with human heart tissue as revealed by immunofluorescent methods: isoimmune, Wassermann, and autoimmune reactions. J. Exper. Med., 113:17, 1961.
14. Klinge, F.: Der Rheumatismus. Ergebn. d. allg. Path. u. path. Anat., 27:32, 1933.
15. MacLeod, C. M.: Hypersensitivity and disease. In Lawrence, H. S. (ed.): Cellular and Humoral Aspects of the Hypersensitive States. New York, Paul B. Hoeber, Inc., 1959, p. 615.
16. McCarty, M.: Nature of rheumatic fever. Circulation, 14:1138, 1956.
17. Mellors, R. C., Ortega, L. G. and Holman, H. R.: Role of gamma globulins in the

pathogenesis of renal lesions in systemic lupus erythematosus and chronic membranous glomerulonephritis, with observations on the L. E. cell reaction. J. Exper. Med., *106*:191, 1957.

18. Osler, A. G., Hardy, P. H. and Sharp, J. T.: Fixation of complement by human sera and alcoholic extracts of human cardiac tissue. Am. J. Syph., *38*:554, 1954.
19. Rejholec, V. and Wagner, V.: Antimyocardial antibodies in rheumatic fever. Experientia (Basel), *11*:278, 1955.
20. Rich, A. R. and Gregory, J. E.: Experimental evidence that lesions with the basic characteristics of rheumatic carditis can result from anaphylactic hypersensitivity. Bull. Johns Hopkins Hosp., *73*:239, 1943.
21. Rich, A. R. and Gregory, J. E.: Further experimental cardiac lesions of the rheumatic type produced by anaphylactic hypersensitivity. Bull. Johns Hopkins Hosp., *75*:115, 1944.
22. Rich, A. R.: Hypersensitivity in disease. The Harvey Lectures, *42*:106, 1946-47.
23. Soloff, L. A., Zatuchin, J., Janton, O. H., O'Neill, T. J. E. and Glover, R. P.: Reactivation of rheumatic fever following mitral commissurotomy. Circulation, *8*:481, 1953.
24. Steffen, C.: Nachweis und wirkung von Gewebs Autoantikorpern bei primarchronischer Polyarthritis im vergleich mit anderweitig auftretenden Gewebs Autoantikorpern. Immunopathologie I. Internationales Symposium, Basel/Seelisberg, p. 376. Basel, Switzerland. Benno Schwabe, 1958.
25. Vazquez, J. J. and Dixon, F. J.: Immunohistochemical study of lesions in rheumatic fever, systemic lupus erythematosus, and rheumatoid arthritis. Lab. Invest., *6*:205, 1957.
26. Wagner, B. M.: Hypersensitivity. The role of the connective tissue. In Mellors, R. C. (ed.): Analytical Pathology. New York, McGraw-Hill Book Co., 1957, p. 429.

Hypersensitivity and Rheumatoid Arthritis

JOHN H. VAUGHAN

University of Rochester School of Medicine and Dentistry

Rheumatoid arthritis is a disease of unknown etiology. Evidence in favor of its being a hypersensitivity disease is only circumstantial and depends upon the drawing of parallelisms.

Taking experimental serum disease as a model for hypersensitivity (Fig. 1), the essential ingredients in the system are: the introduction of an antigen into the body, the development of lymphoid tissue hyperactivity and an antibody response to the antigen, the accumulation of antigen and antibody in the tissues, and the development of tissue lesions characterized by endothelial damage, fibrinoid, cellular infiltration, specific staining reactions indicating the presence of the antigen and the antibody in the tissues, and occasionally granuloma formation. Clinically, the major pathology presents itself as urticaria, arthritis, nephritis, carditis and sometimes neuropathy.

Delayed hypersensitivity differs from the model in Figure 1 by having a cellular rather than a humoral antibody component from the lymphoid tissue. Also there might be emphasis on the granulomatous rather than on the vasculitic features of the tissue lesions. A typical distribution of the major clinical pathology cannot be defined.

When Klinge[4] pointed out that the histological features of rheumatic fever resemble those of experimental serum sickness, he also included rheumatoid arthritis in the parallelism. Subsequently, clinical investigation has pointed up the relation of rheumatic fever to prior infection with the beta-hemolytic streptococcus, and it is thought likely that this organism promotes the development of rheumatic fever through hypersensitivity mechanisms,

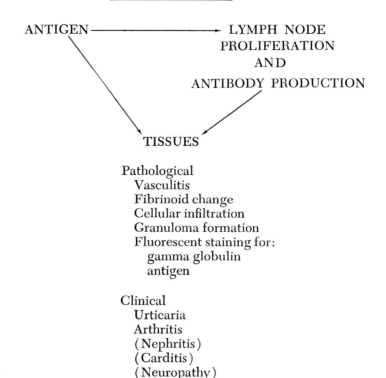

SERUM SICKNESS

ANTIGEN ⟶ LYMPH NODE
PROLIFERATION
AND
ANTIBODY PRODUCTION

TISSUES

Pathological
 Vasculitis
 Fibrinoid change
 Cellular infiltration
 Granuloma formation
 Fluorescent staining for:
  gamma globulin
  antigen

Clinical
 Urticaria
 Arthritis
 (Nephritis)
 (Carditis)
 (Neuropathy)

Fig. 1.

although other possible mechanisms have not been excluded. In rheumatoid arthritis, however, no such defined, exogenous agent as the beta hemolytic streptococcus has been noted (Fig. 2). The basis for thinking of rheumatoid arthritis as a hypersensitivity disease rests upon recognition that many of the other characteristic features of hypersensitivity are present, including the hyperactivity of the lymphoid tissues, the specific serological phenomena of the disease, the presence of gamma globulin in the tissue lesions and the similarities of the histological picture, which Klinge emphasized. The purpose of this paper is to examine the reliability of putting the picture together this way (Fig. 2).

The starting point in the chain of events depicted in the figure is at the level of the lymphoid tissue itself. This brings up the first question to be asked: What is the certainty that lymph tissue hyperactivity actually occurs as a constant feature of the disease? Short[6] has given the incidence of clinically evident lymph node enlargement as 1 out of 3. Recently Dr. William Mayer and I examined postmortem samples of lymph tissue in ten cases. Only six of them could be said to have microscopic evidence of lymph tissue hyperactivity. There was, however, a poor correlation between plasmacytosis and gross lymph node enlargement, and further review made it clear that some of these cases were "burned out" at the time of death. The question of the consistency with which lymphoid hyperactivity occurs is one that

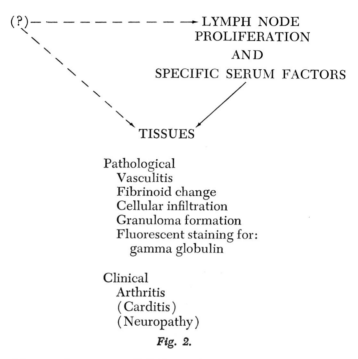

RHEUMATOID ARTHRITIS

(?) — — — — — — — — → LYMPH NODE
                                    PROLIFERATION
                                    AND
                    SPECIFIC SERUM FACTORS

TISSUES

Pathological
    Vasculitis
    Fibrinoid change
    Cellular infiltration
    Granuloma formation
    Fluorescent staining for:
        gamma globulin

Clinical
    Arthritis
    (Carditis)
    (Neuropathy)

Fig. 2.

cannot at this time be answered definitively; it gets us into enormous problems of judgment as to the reliability or sensitivity of the method used to detect the particular feature and the stage of development of the disease at which the assessment is made. For the hypothesis of hypersensitivity one must merely assume that this is indeed an integral and real part of the disease.

The second point in our chain is the manufacture of immunologically specific gamma globulins by the lymphoid tissue. The rheumatoid factor, which is such a frequent hallmark of the disease, is a 19S gamma globulin capable of reacting specifically with 7S gamma globulin molecules. Evidence exists[3, 5] that the rheumatoid factor is, like antibody, made in lymph tissue. At least the rheumatoid factor can be demonstrated there in the stem cells of the lymph follicles and in plasma cells by immunofluorescence techniques. No one has yet succeeded, however, in inducing rheumatoid lymph node tissue to make the rheumatoid factor *in vitro*.

The next link is at the level of the tissue lesion itself. The lesions in rheumatoid arthritis exhibit gamma globulin staining, as they should if they are hypersensitivity lesions. In a series of observations on rheumatoid and nonrheumatoid synovial tissues, Dr. Melvin Kaplan and I found the patterns indicated in Table 1. Most synovia from nonrheumatoid arthritis conditions

TABLE 1.   *BOUND GAMMA GLOBULIN IN PATHOLOGIC SYNOVIA*

SOURCE OF SYNOVIAL TISSUE		BOUND GAMMA GLOBULIN PRESENT	BOUND 19s GAMMA GLOBULIN PRESENT
Patient	Diagnosis		
Sa	Normal synovium	0	0
Sha	Normal synovium	0	0
De	Normal synovium	0	0
Wa	Traumatic arthritis	Trace	0
Sm	Traumatic arthritis	0	0
Ta	Traumatic arthritis	0	0
Ca	Traumatic arthritis	0	0
Th	Osteoarthritis	+	0
Joh	Monarticular arthritis	Trace	0
Ed	Congenital dysplasia, hip	Trace	0
Ke	Traumatic arthritis	+	+
Co	Reiter's disease	++	+
Di	Tuberculous arthritis	+++	++
Jo	Rheumatoid arthritis	++	0
Me	Rheumatoid arthritis	++	+++
Zu	Rheumatoid arthritis	++	+++
Mi	Rheumatoid arthritis	++	+++
Dr	Early rheumatoid arthritis	++	Trace

exhibited little staining for gamma globulin, but synovia from patients with rheumatoid arthritis exhibited much. This staining could be seen in the cytoplasm of the mononuclear cells infiltrating the area and as diffuse staining along the connective tissue bundles. Both 19S and 7S gamma globulin could be identified. Note should be made, however, that a tuberculous synovium and a synovium from a patient with Reiter's disease also fluoresced brightly for gamma globulin, as one would expect of primarily infectious processes to which an immune reaction had occurred.

These observations were extended to determine whether the rheumatoid factor could be identified as a component of the gamma globulins staining the synovia. If, instead of looking broadly for human gamma globulin in these tissues, one exposes the sections to rabbit gamma globulin, thoroughly washes them, and then stains for the rabbit gamma globulin, one can determine where the rheumatoid factor is. Rabbit gamma globulin will be fixed to the rheumatoid factor in essentially the same reaction as that responsible for agglutination by the rheumatoid factor of sheep cells sensitized with rabbit antibody—the familiar sensitized sheep cell agglutination reaction. By this method, the rheumatoid factor can be identified in the cytoplasm of some of the inflammatory cells infiltrating rheumatoid synovia, but not in as many as in those stained directly for human gamma globulin. There is also considerable staining of the perivascular connective tissues, generally of the same tissue areas as those which exhibit 19S gamma globulin staining.

It is now widely recognized that the rheumatoid factor is not the only autoreactive substance found in rheumatoid arthritis. Dr. Kaplan and I occasionally noted in the rheumatoid tissues we examined nuclear staining for gamma globulin, not due to the rheumatoid factor. Also, some rheumatoid sera had the ability to impart to previously nonstaining nuclear tissues staining for gamma globulin. Bardawil and his co-workers[1] have accumulated impressive evidence for the presence in rheumatoid sera of gamma globulins specifically capable of binding with cell nuclei. Weak positive L.E. cell reactions have been described by other workers with as many as 25 per cent of sera of patients with rheumatoid arthritis.

Rheumatoid arthritis, therefore, is a disease manifested by vasculitis, fibrinoid and granulomas consistent with hypersensitivity. The lymphoid tissue in rheumatoid arthritis is productive of autoreactive substances and these, together with other gamma globulins, appear in the lesions of the disease. In classic hypersensitivity the gamma globulins in tissue lesions can, together with antigen, reasonably be assigned a pathogenic role. What role the tissue-bound gamma globulins have in the production of the lesions of rheumatoid arthritis, however, is another question. It must be emphasized that the all-important antigen has not been defined in the rheumatoid arthritis scheme of Figure 2.

Some thought has been given to the possibility that the autoreactive substances in rheumatoid arthritis may have independent pathogenic capacity. However, it has been recognized that these serological entities are not limited to rheumatoid arthritis (cf. 7). Patients with liver disease are found to exhibit autoreactive gamma globulins with especial frequency. A somewhat increased incidence of "rheumatoid" agglutination has been recognized in the sera of patients with sarcoidosis and of patients with syphilis, and evidence is rapidly accumulating that in several chronic bacterial diseases there also are significantly elevated incidences of positive tests for rheumatoid agglutination.

It is not unlikely that most, if not all, of the autoreactive gamma globulins that have been described in various natural diseases of man and in certain experimental diseases in animals are secondary phenomena, and that they do not constitute primary pathogenic substances. Sera containing large quantities of the rheumatoid factor have been transfused into normal recipients without harm to the recipients. The L.E. factor has been transfused into non-lupus patients without untoward effect and has been observed to pass the placenta into the fetus without harm. In a recent series of observations at the University of Rochester, Johnstone has observed antithyroid antibodies to develop in a dog following irradiation-induced thyroiditis; antithyroid antibodies have also been noted to occur in man after the development of thyroiditis apparently due to mumps virus.[2] These observations seem to provide particularly good evidence that autoreactive gamma globulins may develop secondarily to some other primary tissue injury.

The notion that hypersensitivity plays a role in rheumatoid arthritis is based upon the constellation of features we have discussed. No one of these features is definitive of the state, and the all important antigen is unknown. At least some of the gamma globulin in the lesions must be assigned a secondary rather than a primary role.

It is obvious, therefore, that if the concept of hypersensitivity is to be pursued further, this must be in terms of defining the antigen. It would seem that nonliving antigens are an extremely unlikely cause for this because of the persistent, long-term, self-perpetuating nature of the disease. Tissue antigens with autosensitization continue to be a possibility, although for the reasons discussed this is not a favored idea. A living, exogenous antigen—i.e., infection with some micro-organism of low pathogenicity, perhaps one with which mutually compatible symbiosis is the general rule in the healthy population—would fit the known facts admirably.

REFERENCES

1. Bardawil, W. A., Toy, B. L., Galin, S. N. and Bayles, T. B.: Arth. & Rheum., *1*:268, 1958.
2. Felix-Davies, D.: Lancet, *1*:880, 1958.
3. Kaplan, M. H. and Vaughan, J. H.: Proceedings of the Interim Session of the American Rheumatism Association, Rochester, Minnesota, December, 1958.
4. Klinge, F. and Grzimek, N.: Virchow's Arch. f. path. anat., *284*:646, 1932.
5. Mellors, R. C., Heimer, R., Corcos, J. and Korngold, L.: J. Exper. Med., *110*:875, 1959.
6. Short, C. L., Bauer, W. and Reynolds, W. E.: Rheumatoid Arthritis. Cambridge, Mass., Harvard University Press, 1957.
7. Vaughan, J. H.: In Hollander, J. L. (ed.): Arthritis and Allied Conditions. 6th ed. Philadelphia, Lea & Febiger, 1960, pp. 80-96.

Antinuclear Antibodies in
Systemic Lupus Erythematosus

HALSTED HOLMAN
Stanford University Medical Center

The term "antinuclear antibodies" refers to circulating antibodies which react with various chemical constituents of the cell nucleus. These antibodies were first detected in the serums of patients with systemic lupus erythematosus (SLE), though they have subsequently been found in the serum from patients with other diseases. Different antinuclear antibodies have been identified which react with the intact cell nucleus, with deoxyribonucleohistone (nucleoprotein), with isolated deoxyribonucleic acid and with isolated histone. Another antibody reacts with a nuclear substance, probably a glycoprotein, which is extractable from the nucleus and does not contain nucleic acid. Additional antinuclear antibodies may exist which have not yet been clearly characterized. The antinuclear antibody which reacts with deoxyribonucleohistone is responsible for the formation of the LE cell.

The serum substances which react with nuclear constituents are considered to be antibodies because the reactions into which they enter are immunological reactions—i.e., the fixation of complement, hemagglutination, precipitation or passive cutaneous anaphylaxis. In at least two instances the antibodies have been isolated in purified form and have been shown to possess the physical and immunological properties of typical human antibody gamma globulin.

The antinuclear antibodies are autoantibodies because they are capable of reacting with the cell constituents of the patient from whom they are obtained. Distinct from many other types of antibodies, the antinuclear antibodies do not demonstrate an organ or species specificity; they can react with nuclear constituents from cells of many types of animals and micro-organisms.

Serums which contain antinuclear antibodies usually but not invariably contain substances which react with constituents of cytoplasm. The latter substances have not yet been proved to be antibodies.

Though they are present in greatest abundance in the serum of patients with systemic lupus erythematosus, antinuclear antibodies have been found in serum from patients suffering from other connective tissue diseases, such as rheumatoid arthritis and scleroderma, from certain types of liver disease, and possibly from a variety of allergic reactions. They may also appear in other disease states, though this has not been unequivocally established. As a rule, experimental analogues of the antinuclear antibodies have not been detected in animals immunized with nuclear constituents. However, certain efforts to provoke the formation of such antibodies in animals have met with very modest success.

The pathogenic significance of the antinuclear antibodies is unknown. Though they possess the capacity to react with the nuclei of most cells which have been injured, they apparently are not capable of entering cells which are normally viable. Considerable evidence exists that these circulating antibodies are not primarily responsible for cell damage in the patient, though they may contribute to some of the pathological findings after an initial injury to the cell has occurred. It appears that these antibodies are by-products of an abnormal immune system rather than direct pathogenic agents themselves.

Other evidence supports the view that there is a basic immunologic abnormality present in patients with SLE. Such patients demonstrate a peculiar type of skin reactivity to autologous cell constituents which may be an autoimmune variant of delayed hypersensitivity. Furthermore, members of families of patients with systemic lupus frequently demonstrate extensive immunologic abnormalities, though often these members are asymptomatic. These family findings contribute to the view that an aberration in immune response characterizes SLE and is at least partially determined by genetic constitution. It is possible that this immunologic aberration in some way causes tissue damage, but it appears unlikely that the circulating antinuclear antibodies are the vehicle for this damage.

The antinuclear antibodies themselves may coexist with other types of unusual antibodies, e.g., the rheumatoid serologic factor. However, the antinuclear antibodies are usually the low molecular weight type of gamma globulin, whereas the rheumatoid serologic factors are high molecular weight gamma globulins. The relation between the immunologic abnormalities giving rise to these two types of abnormal antibodies remains unknown, but the family studies again suggest that in some way the abnormalities are related to one another.

At this date, the antinuclear antibodies might best be considered highly interesting but pathogenetically relatively insignificant products of an unusual, poorly understood immunologic disorder characteristically but not exclusively present in SLE.

REFERENCES

1. Holman, H.: Systemic lupus erythematosus: a review of certain recent developments in the study of this disease. J. Pediat., 56:109, 1960.
2. Holman, H.: The LE cell phenomenon. Ann. Rev. Med., 11:231, 1960.

Panel Discussion

AMEDEO BONDI, *Moderator*

DR. BONDI: Dr. Kaplan, would you define "hypersensitivity"?

DR. KAPLAN: I think it is very difficult to define "hypersensitivity" in strict terms with respect to one particular type of response. In general, one can say hypersensitivity represents the state of increased reactivity both physiologically and cellularly, to a specific antigenic material to which the animal or man has been previously exposed. Of course, we have no knowledge of prior exposure to a sensitizing agent except in some instances of connective tissue reactions to certain drugs. An endogenous antigenic substance may be implicated in some diseases, but this has not by any means been definitely established, even in patients with SLE or rheumatoid arthritis, since there may be increased reactivity not only with the patient's tissues but also, and even in higher titer, with somebody else's tissues or even with animal tissues. Therefore, there is increased reactivity to an antigen and we presume that this antigen is endogenous, but it is by no means certain. The essential aspect of hypersensitivity is that it is specific and directed only to the antigenic material to which the man or animal has been previously exposed. I am sure that there are better definitions, but we could at least start with this one.

DR. BONDI: Would some other member of the panel, in a broad way, like to either add to or modify this definition?

DR. VAUGHAN: A simple definition, which in its broadest aspects might be controversial, is that hypersensitivity is a process in which tissue injury occurs as a result of immune mechanisms.

DR. HOLMAN: I think that is very reasonable. My personal opinion with regard to hypersensitivity would be yet a third formulation but it is essentially in agreement with these. When a person or an experimental animal contacts a substance which is not normal to itself or to its environment, it reacts, and it reacts in certain circumstances by producing a protein, such as an antibody, which is complementary to this substance and which can react with the substance, presumably inactivating it. In addition, there also may be other types of complementary substances synthesized which we do not currently recognize. Associated with this process there may be a cellular reaction to these substances which results in cell damage in certain circumstances and possibly results in protection of the host in other circumstances. Hypersensitivity might be the general circumstance in which immunity, when defined as something that makes one immune and is therefore presumably beneficial, would be a subdivision; but this is again a personal prejudice and nothing more than that.

DR. BONDI: Dr. Angevine, would you define "hypersensitivity" from a pathologist's viewpoint?

DR. ANGEVINE: I think that when some people discuss this problem they confuse the terms "immunization" and "immunity." The process of immunization is what we are talking about here; sometimes immunity results and sometimes it does not, immunity of course being relative. The immunological reactions we are talking about today do not denote protection at all and this is of some importance. Hypersensitivity (immunization) may occur without immunity, and I think we should

125

use the terms "hypersensitivity" and "immunity" rather than "immunization" and "immunity," because "immunity," on the basis of proper terminology, should be used in terms of protection.

DR. BONDI: From the point of view of immunology, if you want to come down to very simple terms, the basic difference, in effect, is what is good for the body and what is not good for the body. There are all types of antibodies, and the general tendency is to think of all antibodies in terms of the classic antibodies as we have always thought of them in the past. As we study them more we find that they are very diverse in character.

DR. SEEGAL: It seems to me that the relationship of hypersensitivity to immunity is being made more complicated than necessary. If you use the term "immunity" strictly to mean protection from disease, you have a very limited number of antigens that are important. There is the capsule of the Pneumococcus or the type-specific, M protein of the Streptococcus, and only the antibody to that protein will produce immunity; although other antigens may produce an inflammatory reaction in a hypersensitive person, there is no immunity. It seems to me that immunity is not only a fraction of a hypersensitive reaction, but a very small fraction and strictly dependent on the important virulent factor of the disease agent. Is that too narrow?

DR. BONDI: No, I think that is very good. Dr. Angevine, are there any criteria that you apply before calling a given disease an allergic disease?

DR. ANGEVINE: First, you would have to demonstrate whether or not the patient or experimental animal has hypersensitivity. The classic way is to do a skin test or to apply the material to the mucous membranes. Several years ago I thought these tests might parallel one another but they certainly do not. The pathological changes occurring in positive skin tests can also be examined, but although there is edema and other changes, I do not think the cytologic reaction or the character of the histologic reaction helps me very much in the diagnosis of hypersensitivity, although there is a good deal of literature to contradict what I am saying. In addition, there are also immediate and delayed types of reactions to be considered.

DR. WAGNER: I think one of the problems is that when we examine human disease, we see a whole constellation of effects at one time. With the experimental model, you can dissect out and control to a certain degree some of the variables, but in the individual patient you are dealing with the duration of the disease, the intensity of the disease, the therapy, and the age and sex of the patient. All of these things have been shown at one time or another to be influential in the morphological patterns that one sees in these diseases, so I would agree with Dr. Angevine that it is extremely difficult to look at histological material without having any additional knowledge about the patient and say that the lesion is due to hypersensitivity or that it is an allergic type of reaction. There are certain findings which may make us suspicious, but certainly in the human we need additional information from the clinician in terms of the patient's history, physiologic status and therapy in order to determine the type of reaction.

DR. BONDI: Since we have now defined these reactions in general terms, we should be a little more specific and talk about the role of these antibodies in rheumatic fever and rheumatoid arthritis. Dr. Kaplan, you reported that you can detect bound gamma globulin. Before we go any further, would you define this gamma globulin that is bound? How strongly is it bound and what does this finding mean?

DR. KAPLAN: This is, of course, a definition based upon the technique used, and by "bound gamma globulin" we mean gamma globulin which is present in unfixed frozen sections after washing for 20 minutes in several changes of fluid.

By this method, normal heart or pathologic tissues other than the rheumatic tissues do not show any gamma globulin at all despite the fact that gamma globulin is a normal constituent of the interstitial tissue of the extravascular compartment, as well as in the cell.

DR. BONDI: Do I understand correctly, from what you have outlined, that the finding of this bound gamma globulin in tissue by fluorescent antibody techniques is not sufficient for you to draw the conclusion that this is the prime mechanism involved in pathogenesis of rheumatic fever?

DR. KAPLAN: I do not think we can attach any causality to the presence of gamma globulin except to say that it is present in areas where there is a connective tissue alteration. We know that it is at these sites in some cases—in fact, in most cases—but there are some cases in which it is not associated with the connective tissue alteration. It is impossible to go beyond that. We have examined nonspecific inflammation in rabbits, trying to find out whether other types of reaction show such binding but so far have not succeeded in producing binding with simple inflammatory stimuli, such as, for example, agents which will induce production of C-reactive protein.

DR. BONDI: What progress are you or others making in developing antibodies to heart tissue using adjuvants and homologous heart tissue?

DR. KAPLAN: Because of a general interest in the concept of autoantibodies to the heart, we made some observations on this a few years ago. Immunization of rabbits with heterologous heart—for instance, beef or rat heart—stimulates antibodies reactive with the rabbit's heart, this essentially being a cross reaction in which the homologous system is involved. Of course, pursuing this further, it is quite clear that there is an antigen in the heart which is organ-specific and one can show that the antigen will react with no other organ except the heart. This antigen is related to material which is distributed similarly to one of the patterns I showed today, which is the interfibrillar pattern. However, one can certainly see serologic reactions to heart following immunization with other tissues, such as skeletal muscle. Indeed, striated muscle of the heart and skeletal muscle have related antigens, but the cross reaction here does not involve the organ-specific antigen of the heart. One can induce such an antibody with heart tissue but not with skeletal muscle as antigen. I think the point here is that serologic factors similar to the one seen in rheumatic fever and rheumatic heart disease in the postcommissurotomy state can be produced in rabbits when one uses heterologous tissue. Presumably, the heterologous tissue has a foreign antigen to which the haptinic heart component is conjugated and, therefore, that is why it is antigenic. Under these circumstances one gets such autoantibodies, and in studies at the Boston Children's Medical Center we were able to show that immunization of rabbits with heterologous heart will produce mild fibronecrosis, occasionally myocardial necrosis, and occasionally fibrosis. The distribution of gamma globulin in these rabbit hearts is entirely different from that seen in rheumatic hearts; therefore, we hesitate to say that the mechanism involved in experimental lesions which we have produced has any relation at all to whatever is going on in the auricular appendages from rheumatic fever patients, although we know that there are serum factors present in both situations.

DR. LEE: Dr. Kaplan, would you explain why the distribution of gamma globulin in hearts from patients with rheumatic fever had no relation to the distribution of gamma globulin when these hearts or other heart tissues were incubated with these patients' serum?

DR. KAPLAN: Perhaps I did not make myself clear on this. In 18 of the 100 cases examined, the auricular appendages showed gamma globulin within the myofibers and in scattered foci throughout the section. Sometimes myofibers "en bloc" were involved. In 12 of these 18 cases, there was not only involvement of the myofibers but also of the vessel walls and particularly of the arterioles and venules. In addition, there was involvement of the interstitial connective tissue in all 18, and one could see the bound gamma globulin extending from interstitial connective tissue to the myofiber and indeed into the substance of the sarcoplasm of the myofibers. Now, if one argued that the gamma globulin in these hearts was related to serum factors, one might expect that there ought to be serum factors to myofibers, serum factors to vessel wall and serum factors to interstitial connective tissue, but we have not been able to detect any serum factors that we have been convinced of except for a serum factor to myofibers. If one argues that the gamma globulin in the myofibers is due to serum factors, where does the gamma globulin in the vessel walls and the connective tissue come from? This is the essential dilemma.

DR. LEE: That is what I thought you said. Your demonstration of gamma globulin rests on the use of a fluorescent type antiserum. Have you demonstrated that you are definitely marking only 7-S or 19-S gamma globulin? If so, in your serum have you tried to see whether these are the same or different?

DR. KAPLAN: Antisera that can be prepared are specific for 7-S and 19-S gamma globulin on the one hand and for 19-S on the other. These are the only two sera that are available and, although there are rare sera which are specific for 7-S gamma globulin alone, I am sure they are so weak that they are probably not useful in the fluorescent antibody technique. But using these two reactions to detect the presence of 7-S or 19-S with the one sera and the presence of 19-S with the other, I have never seen a heart which contained bound 19-S gamma globulin; however, all of these hearts show gamma globulin which I presume must be 7-S, since they reacted with the 7-S–19-S antiserum but not with the 19-S specific antiserum.

When the fluorescent antibody technique is used, one can also differentiate between serum factors which are 7-S or 19-S, again using the indirect method; the sarcoplasmic and sarcolemmal reactive serum factors belong mostly to the 7-S class, but also in some cases to the 19-S class. The antibody producing the sarcolemmal pattern that I showed which involves the endomysial connective tissue around the myofibers is most frequently a 19-S antibody. Although this factor is rarely found, it is most likely to be present in those patients who have cyclic or chronic rheumatic activity. The usual rheumatic fever patient who recovers without any chronicity usually does not show this, but I do not know what this really means in terms of pathogenesis. But these are the observations.

DR. BONDI: Dr. Vaughan, I am not going to summarize your paper, but essentially your main point was that the serum factors associated with various connective tissue diseases are not necessarily the primary etiologic factors. Do you agree with that?

DR. VAUGHAN: Yes.

DR. A. BLACK: Dr. Vaughan, in your paper you spoke of the rheumatoid factor in the singular and at another time in the plural. I know of at least two factors that have been described by Dr. Ziff. How many factors do you think there are?

DR. VAUGHAN: If I spoke of the rheumatoid factor in the plural, I did not mean to. In spite of Dr. Ziff's work and observations by several other people that it is possible to break down the rheumatoid factor by various physical-chemical maneuvers into separate fractions, I think it is a single biologic entity and this is the way I like to study it and think of it. Although I may be wrong, it is confusing to me to think of more than one factor. I can get a better understanding of the process when I consider the rheumatoid factor as a biologic rather than a chemical entity.

DR. BONDI: Dr. Holley, what do you think? Are we talking about an antibody or not?

DR. HOLLEY: It certainly has a lot of the characteristics of an antibody, but as to whether it is an antibody or not, I do not know. I personally believe that it probably is.

I would like to ask Dr. Vaughan another question. Is there a prehypersensitivity state, and if so what are the characteristics of it ?

DR. VAUGHAN: I certainly would not know how to define a prehypersensitivity state. Hypersensitivity to me in the broadest sense is merely tissue damage induced by an immunological system. I do not see how one can break it down any more than that.

DR. HOLLEY: To phrase the question in a different way, are some people more prone to develop hypersensitivity states? Is there a genetic factor? What are the limiting factors?

DR. VAUGHAN: Various individuals differ in their ability to make antibodies to a given antigen. In a group of experimental animals or humans, there are good antibody formers and poor antibody formers. It is probably true that there are specific immunological differences in the ability of the lymphoid tissue to produce a specific immunological response, be it in the form of delayed sensitivity or in the form of specific antibody production; it may be that lupus is related in some way to the level of overactivity in this particular biologic function, as Dr. Holman has suggested.

DR. BONDI: Is there any problem in differentiating between lupus or rheumatoid arthritis on the basis of these serum factors?

DR. HOLMAN: Both the high molecular weight gammaglobulin—the so-called rheumatoid factor or factors—and the low molecular weight antitissue antibodies can appear in both clinical types of disease whether the appearance is one of chronic deforming arthritis or of an acute multi-system disease or its variants which do not have deforming arthritis. I do not think there is much usefulness in arguing about the specific limits between the two illnesses. There is an abundance of biologic evidence that the two are related, of which the most recently reported is the high percentage of persons suffering from clinical rheumatoid arthritis in the relatives of patients with unequivocal SLE. There are also numerous other factors that everyone is aware of. These diseases at least are related, but where some of the other connective tissue diseases fit into the spectrum I do not know.

I would also like to add one other thing to the definition of hypersensitivity. When we talk about being exposed to a noxious agent and then developing a peculiar type of reactivity to it which we choose to call hypersensitivity, we are not speaking of direct tissue damage as with a toxin. There are two elements that enter into the definition of hypersensitivity, and I don't know how to put them there precisely. One is the fact that tissue reactions, be they directly tissue- or antibody-mediated, take time to develop. The second element is that on the second, third or fourth exposure to the antigen, the appearance of the lesion is accelerated in comparison to the time necessary for the development of the initial lesion, so that the timing aspects of hypersensitivity somehow or other have to be kept in the definition to permit differentiation of hypersensitivity reactions from those due to simple toxins.

DR. HOLLEY: Should any clinical significance be attached to the presence of the LE cell in certain patients with rheumatoid arthritis, or is this of no importance?

DR. V. E. POLLAK: I have had the opportunity to see some patients with this phenomenon. Some of these patients had only relatively recently developed arthritis and could conceivably develop lupus subsequently. There was a group of patients whom I saw at the Chronic Disease Institute, however, who had been there for periods of 10 to 15 years with chronic severe deforming arthritis with LE cells. They had no history or evidence of any other system involvement whatever and I find it very hard to believe that they had systemic lupus.

DR. A. BLACK: Dr. Pollak is discussing a group of patients that we studied some years ago. The group of rheumatoids who had a positive LE preparation, as a general rule, seemed to be patients with more advanced disease, and they had a greater number of subcutaneous nodules. Otherwise they were in no way different from the ordinary patient with rheumatoid arthritis. Two or three of these patients subsequently died and there was no evidence of SLE at postmortem examination. We are in the process of doing a five-year follow-up on some of the survivors now, and as far as we know there is, perhaps with one exception, no evidence of lupus in these patients.

DR. HOLLEY: Dr. Pollak, did you do kidney biopsies on these patients?

DR. V. E. POLLAK: Yes, we did on some of these patients. All of these biopsies were normal, with no evidence of lupus in any of them.

DR. VAUGHAN: I would like to support the notion expressed by Dr. Black. This has certainly been my impression, and I think it is the impression of many people that the patients with rheumatoid arthritis who get the LE change in the serum are those with more severe disease. We have to remember that rheumatoid arthritis is a systemic disease and that it sometimes expresses itself in systemic ways. This may be one of the places where we are confusing ourselves more than we are clarifying the issue—that is, when we speak of rheumatoid arthritis turning into lupus or vice versa. We have to think in terms of rheumatoid arthritis sometimes expressing itself as a systemic disease, but this does not make it lupus erythematosus.

DR. HOLLEY: Maybe we are trying to split hairs.

DR. VAUGHAN: Well, the problem is more than that. It is not splitting hairs, because in keeping this separation you retain the concept that these are two diseases, due to two different basic etiologic factors, but which may at times involve some common parameters of host response.

DR. LEE: The main problem is defining the total picture of lupus erythematosus. It is not so difficult to define what you mean by rheumatoid arthritis, but I think all of us here would probably have different specific definitions for systemic lupus. In addition, there is a tremendous variation in the incidence of positive LE cell tests in patients with rheumatoid arthritis as reported from various clinics all over the world. It varies from 5 to about 30 per cent. First of all, there are differences in techniques for detecting LE cells which result in a greater or lower incidence of positive preparations. In addition, some investigators, using one set of criteria, have taken out of the series certain patients whom they thought had lupus, whereas other investigators, using a different set of criteria, have not done so. Since the criteria for diagnosis vary, the problem remains: What is lupus?

DR. BONDI: Dr. Holman, are antinuclear antibodies present constantly in patients with lupus, or are they present only during exacerbations and absent during remissions?

DR. HOLMAN: The usual experience is that the titers of antinuclear antibodies either greatly diminish or completely disappear with spontaneous or therapeutic remissions.

DR. HOLLEY: Why is it that Dr. Alexander in Scotland has reported that he finds them in 5 per cent of normal subjects and in 15 per cent of patients with other diseases?

DR. HOLMAN: I do not believe the incidence is that high; the difference is probably due to the methods used for detection of the LE cell.

DR. V. E. POLLAK: We have studied antinuclear factors quantitatively by serial titration in a series of about 75 lupus patients and have found in general that there is a reasonably good correlation between the activity of the disease process as judged by common clinical criteria and the titer of antinuclear factors. With successful treatment which usually requires large doses of steroids, the titer of the antinuclear factors gradually comes down. It seems to take a surprisingly long time, and often it is six months before the titer reaches a baseline level. With the technique we are using, we have very rarely been able to demonstrate subsequent complete disappearance of antinuclear factors. In addition, exacerbations of disease are usually accompanied by significant rises in the titer of antinuclear factors. We do not have enough data yet to know whether the rise precedes the exacerbations of the disease. There were, however, some significant exceptions to the correlation between activity of the disease and the titer of antinuclear factors, and this was one of the reasons which induced us to examine the serum of relatives of patients with SLE for antinuclear factors. To date we have studied about 90 relatives of our patients and the incidence of positive LE tests by our technique has been almost 50 per cent, although the vast majority of these relatives have been asymptomatic. Our controls to date have consisted of about 50 healthy subjects, both males and females, and about 100 patients with various disease states. In the normal subjects we were unable to demonstrate nuclear fluorescence except in a small number, and then only with undiluted serum or with serum diluted 1 to 2, whereas in the vast majority of patients with lupus, titers of 1 to 4 or greater were found. Nevertheless, there are some normal subjects in whom antinuclear factors were demonstrable. In patients with other diseases, but not including lupus, positive tests, although not common, occurred occasionally in those with connective tissue diseases such as rheumatoid arthritis and scleroderma. There were also some positive tests in patients with liver disease when it was associated with hypergammaglobulinemia, but not in those with liver disease without hypergammaglobulinemia. In acute infectious diseases and other diseases which appear to be remote from those we are discussing, we have not found a significant number of positive tests.

DR. VAUGHAN: Dr. Holman, you and others have been interested in family studies on serum factors in lupus and rheumatoid arthritis. Would you make a comment about what you think the real meaning of this finding is? I am specifically wondering whether this situation is somewhat analogous to that which occurred in rheumatic fever at the time when rheumatic fever was recognized in high frequency within families and the disease was thought to be related to a significant genetic factor. This, of course, was shown subsequently simply to be due to the fact that there was a high incidence of streptococcal infections in such families.

DR. HOLMAN: I think it would be wrong to overestimate the significance of the family studies thus far, but it is true that five different groups all utilizing various techniques have found a higher incidence of rheumatoid factors in the relatives of patients with SLE than in other population groups. The incidence is 5 to 6 per cent in the average unselected population and about 12 to 15 per cent in the relatives. This is not as high as that Dr. Pollak just mentioned, but we have been using different techniques and this brings out one important point—that the information we are all commenting on here is contingent upon the usefulness of the techniques employed. The number of positive tests depends on the sensitivity of the method and of course, considerable differences can arise if we use the fluorescent antibody technique as opposed to the complement fixation technique; the former is apparently more sensitive and more likely to give false positives if inadequately used.

In regard to the possible similarity or analogy of this situation to the one in rheumatic fever which you mention, it seems that what we have in this instance is one thing not present in the rheumatic fever study; that is, we have evidence of an immunologic disorder aside from the coincidence of the disease. Since I agree, as do other members of this panel, that the serologic factors are not in themselves the pathogenic agents in rheumatoid arthritis and lupus, I would interpret the data only as evidence that there is a deviation from the norm in certain aspects of the immunologic responsiveness in the relatives of these patients. I would hope, but I am only guessing, that, if we abandon our classic studies and pursue some other types of investigation, we might be able to understand more about the pathogenesis than if we continue to apply solely the current concepts of immediate and delayed hypersensitivity to these diseases. The big advantage of the family study is obvious. We have to treat the patients with systemic lupus and, consequently, when a patient is admitted we have only a short period of time before treatment is started to get sera or tissues that are reactive. In the family studies, the subjects are usually healthy, and prolonged follow-up data can be obtained.

Part IV | ETIOLOGY AND
PATHOGENESIS OF
COLLAGEN DISEASES

The Pathogenesis of Rheumatic Fever

LEON SOKOLOFF

National Institute of Arthritis and Metabolic Diseases

Relatively little progress in our understanding of the pathogenetic mechanisms of rheumatic fever has been made in the past decade, in contrast to that of certain other "collagen diseases." Several important elements have been recognized for many years: the fact that rheumatic fever develops in susceptible persons following superficial pharyngeal infections with Group A beta hemolytic streptococci; that rheumatic fever has highly characteristic histologic lesions in the heart and elsewhere; that conventional methods, including cultures and response to treatment with antibiotic compounds, have, by and large, failed to demonstrate its infectious nature; that certain host factors (genetic, sex and mechanical) influence its development and course.

From such observations, a number of hypotheses have been entertained as to the nature of the rheumatic process. Among these are:

1. Rheumatic fever represents a cryptic infection by streptococci or by a filtrable variant of them.

2. Rheumatic fever is a specific infection, perhaps viral, in some manner triggered by the streptococcal disease.

3. Rheumatic fever is an anaphylactic reaction to the streptococcus or some of its growth products.

4. Rheumatic fever results from delayed hypersensitivity to somatic components of the streptococcus.

5. Rheumatic fever is a direct response to toxic elements of the streptococcus.

6. Rheumatic fever is an autoimmune response to the body's own collagenous or other tissues somehow made antigenic by the streptococcus.

There exists, at the present time, an enormous gap between what we know of the disorder and our ability to evaluate these alternative concepts. The experimental reproduction as well as immunologic and biochemical analysis of the clinical condition is greatly limited by the absence of a definitive test for the diagnosis of rheumatic fever. The single most reliable criterion presently available for knowing that we are dealing with a lesion of rheumatic fever is the Aschoff body. The reproduction of rheumatic fever in experimental animals can be validated only by the satisfactory demonstration of Aschoff bodies in them. Furthermore, the most direct approach to the relationship of the streptococcus to the genesis of rheumatic fever lies in the application of the immunofluorescent techniques for demonstrating antigenic components of this micro-organism in such lesions. For these reasons, and also because of recent developments in our knowledge of the subclinical progression of rheumatic heart disease, the present discussion is confined to a review of some recent pathologic studies of the Aschoff bodies.

The ordinary histologic appearances of the Aschoff body are well known. These lesions are submiliary, paravascular lesions occurring in the myocardium. They have two principal characteristics: (1) large cells having a polymorphous nucleus and basophilic cytoplasm, disposed in somewhat lamellar arrangement along (2) coarse, apparently swollen and fragmented perivascular collagen bundles. Minute deposits of fibrin-like or platelet material are seen in the intima of occasional vessels in the vicinity of these lesions but are infrequent.

SIGNIFICANCE OF THE ASCHOFF BODY IN THE LEFT AURICULAR APPENDAGE

The frequent occurrence of submiliary infiltrates in the endocardium of the left auricular appendage was first recognized when mitral commissurotomy was employed in the treatment of rheumatic heart disease. They have subsequently been found in a large proportion of cases in all laboratories of surgical pathology. The lesions are smaller than those ordinarily seen about myocardial vessels in rheumatic carditis and lack their lamellar arrangement. They have generally been classed as Aschoff bodies because of the similarity of the large cells and the fragmentation of the collagen bundles in them. Whether these aggregates constitute evidence of activity of rheumatic carditis as do myocardial Aschoff bodies has been questioned both on morphologic grounds[10] and also because they occur with high frequency in patients who present no other clinical or laboratory evidence of rheumatic activity.[3]

Necropsy data have a bearing on this problem from two different directions:

1. If the appendage lesions have the same significance as the myocardial ones, one might expect to find myocardial Aschoff bodies elsewhere in hearts with such lesions. This was suggested by the studies of Kuschner and Levieff,[8] who showed that ventricular lesions were in fact present in each of a small number of such cases studied carefully. Decker and co-workers[2] likewise observed ventricular Aschoff bodies in four of five such patients. The frequent association of the two lesions suggests that they have a similar significance.

2. In an attempt to determine whether Aschoff bodies are true evidence of activity of the rheumatic inflammation, Tedeschi and Wagner[11] found distinctive histologic features in a small proportion of cases examined in which definite clinical and laboratory findings of inflammatory reaction were present. In these Aschoff bodies, exudative and fibrinoid changes were more conspicuous. In the majority of cases, however, these florid exudative alterations were not seen; in this latter group activity was not clinically apparent. Nevertheless, the appearance of the Aschoff body varies with its own stage of development, and there are reasons for believing that these structures are in fact evidence of active carditis, even when all acute phase reactions are absent. Outstanding among these is that one commonly observes such Aschoff bodies healing with fibrosis and, at least for this reason, they are inflammatory. Furthermore, it must be realized that clinical recognition of rheumatic activity is often lacking during the progressive development of rheumatic heart disease. Perhaps half or more of patients attending adult rheumatic heart clinics have no acceptable history of rheumatic fever, carditis or chorea. In many others, severe heart disease develops decades after an isolated and apparently benign attack of rheumatic fever. Following subsidence of such an acute episode, the healed valvular deformity is presumably subject to sclerotic exaggeration by mechanical and thrombotic

complications. Making due allowance for such influences, the subclinical progression of the heart disease is entirely consistent with, and probably favors, the view that low grade rheumatic activity does persist in these patients and is not detected by current diagnostic tests.

ORIGIN OF THE ASCHOFF BODIES

The origin of the large cells characteristic of the Aschoff body has been a subject of contention among pathologists for many decades. These are frequently designated as Aschoff cells. For the most part, pathologists regard them as connective tissue cells related to and arising from the Anitschkow or so-called "caterpillar" cells. The latter, too, have at times been called Aschoff cells,[10] and in numerous experimental studies such cells have been interpreted as evidence of rheumatic inflammation. Nevertheless, the Anitschkow cells are seen with some frequency in the hearts of nonrheumatic persons. They also occur in the hearts and extracardiac tissues of species other than man in which there is no reason to think of rheumatic inflammation. The fact that the large cells of the Aschoff body appear to originate in the paravascular collagenous connective tissue and are quite similar to the large, polymorphous and multinucleated cells seen in early subcutaneous and other lesions of rheumatic fever in other tissues is one of the bases of theories that rheumatic fever is a generalized "collagen-vascular" disease.

The theory that Aschoff bodies are of myogenic origin has been revived in recent years by Murphy,[9] who regards the large cells in the ventricular lesions as arising from myocardial fibers. This thesis has not found general acceptance among pathologists for reasons already noted, and also because they all differ in appearance from the multinucleated cells known to arise from this muscle under other circumstances. Cross striations are not seen in transitional forms. Furthermore, the cells apparently evolve into fibroblasts. Tonelli[12] and Murphy[9] have suggested that the large cells in the auricular appendage lesion arise from endocardial smooth muscle. Many pathologists have observed Aschoff bodies in extracardiac locations,[14] and for this reason the myogenic theory would appear untenable. The fact that Aschoff bodies have been classified into numerous morphologic types should not be construed, as in the minds of many pathologists, to mean that they may have different histogeneses but rather that they are in different stages of their life history.

A definitive resolution of this problem would be found in the application to the Aschoff body of immunohistologic techniques employing tagged antisera to muscle proteins, as in the method of Klatzo and co-workers.[7] Studies of this sort are under way but data are not yet forthcoming.

THE NATURE OF "FIBRINOID" IN RHEUMATIC LESIONS

A cardinal feature of the concept of collagen diseases has been that they are characterized histologically by fibrinoid change of the collagen bundles. On the basis of such changes in the myocardial Aschoff body, subcutaneous nodules and blood vessels, rheumatic fever has frequently been classified both as a collagen disease and as a lesion of hypersensitivity. It must be understood that the term "fibrinoid" is a morphologic one. It refers to certain tinctorial properties of tissue elements that make them resemble fibrin in certain respects. Those who are not pathologists frequently do not remember that fibrinoid is not a single substance, or even a specific material in the individual collagen diseases. The fibrinoid appearance of the fragmented collagen bundles in the rheumatic lesion apparently is the result of a complex process comprising a number of exudative and proliferative alterations of varying duration and severity. The tissue is swollen and contains increased quantities of acid mucopolysaccharide that can be digested by testicular hyaluronidase; fragmentation of collagen bundles and unmasking or new formation of argyrophile fibrils occurs; binding of serum proteins, particularly of gamma globulin, has been demonstrated; and fibrin or otherwise altered fibrinogen is present to a varying extent. It is more often seen in the subcutaneous nodule than in the Aschoff body, particularly in the early phases of its development. The recognition of the changing and complex character of the exudate in these lesions is necessary in interpreting differences in the findings of several laboratories about the nature of the material[5, 13, 15] and also in drawing appropriate conclusions about the nature and significance of the material in the rheumatic process. It appears unwarranted to conclude that rheumatic fever and other "collagen diseases" are pathogenetically related simply because all have lesions in which fibrinoid alteration of collagen bundles occurs, or to conclude that all are of allergic origin for the same reason.

ATTEMPTS TO DEMONSTRATE STREPTOCOCCAL ANTIGENS, ANTIBODIES OR GAMMA GLOBULIN

The immunofluorescent technique of Coons has been applied to Aschoff bodies of the left auricular endocardium to see whether streptococcal materials, antibodies to them or gamma globulin presumed to be antibody of some sort is concentrated in them. By this means, it would conceivably be possible to identify the offending streptococcal substance or at least to determine whether hypersensitivity mechanisms were involved and to test the hypothetical alternatives already noted. Studies published thus far have not been successful in demonstrating the presence of Group A streptococcal protein, of antibodies to streptolysin O or of streptococcal sonicates.[15] Gamma globulin has been found in the connective tissue of Aschoff bodies by several investigators.[13, 15]

These findings have suggested that antibody of unknown type may be concentrated in the Aschoff body connective tissue and may play a role in the genesis of the lesion. These studies represent a direct approach to the relationship of the streptococcal infection in the rheumatic state and further studies are awaited with interest. Bound gamma globulin has been found by Kaplan[6] in the myocardium unrelated to the Aschoff bodies in some rheumatic patients.

Finally, it probably is the consensus among conservative pathologists that to date no one has reproduced a valid model of the Aschoff body in experimental animals. Recent reports of considerable interest are those of granulomatous reactions resembling the subcutaneous nodules of rheumatoid arthritis and rheumatic fever following implantation of heterologous fibrin into rabbits[1] and of bovine tendon preserved in bovine serum into dogs.[4] These lesions appear to be foreign body reactions to materials whose antigenicity has altered their resorption by recipient subjects. Subcutaneous nodules have a granulomatous-like appearance that has, at times, itself been interpreted as a foreign body type of reaction to autogenous necrotic collagen. The histologic character of the experimental lesions thus has a certain degree of nonspecificity and further studies will be required to allow proper evaluation of them.

It is apparent from these comments that our present knowledge of the pathologic findings is separated by a wide chasm from our understanding of the pathogenesis of rheumatic fever.

REFERENCES

1. Banerjee, S. K. and Glynn, L. E.: Reactions to homologous and heterologous fibrin implants in experimental animals. Ann. N. Y. Acad. Sc., *86*:1064-1074, 1960.
2. Decker, J. P., Hawn, C. V. Z. and Robbins, S. L.: Rheumatic "activity" as judged by the presence of Aschoff bodies in auricular appendages of patients with mitral stenosis. I. Anatomic aspects. Circulation, *8*:161-169, 1953.
3. Enticknap, J. B.: Biopsy of the left auricle in mitral stenosis. Brit. Heart J., *15*:37-46, 1953.
4. Flynn, J. E., Wilson, J. T., Child, C. G., III and Graham, J. H.: Heterogenous and autogenous-tendon transplants. J. Bone & Jt. Surg., *42A*:91-110, 1960.
5. Gitlin, D., Craig, J. M. and Janeway, C. A.: Studies on the nature of fibrinoid in the collagen diseases. Am. J. Path., *33*:55-78, 1957.
6. Kaplan, M. H.: The concept of autoantibodies in rheumatic fever and in the post-commissurotomy state. Ann. N. Y. Acad. Sc., *86*:974-991, 1960.
7. Klatzo, I, Horvath, B. and Emmart, E. W.: Demonstration of myosin in human striated muscle by fluorescent antibody. Proc. Soc. Exper. Biol. & Med., *97*:135-140, 1958.
8. Kuschner, M. and Levieff, L.: Correlation between active rheumatic lesions in the left auricular appendage and elsewhere in the heart. Am. J. M. Sc., *226*:290-295, 1953.
9. Murphy, G. E.: On muscle cells, Aschoff bodies and cardiac failure in rheumatic heart disease. Bull. N. Y. Acad. Med., *35*:619-645, 1959.
10. Saphir, O.: The Aschoff nodule (editorial). Am. J. Clin. Path., *31*:534-539, 1959.
11. Tedeschi, C. G., Wagner, B. M. and Pani, K. C.: Studies in rheumatic fever. 1. Clinical experience of the Aschoff body based on morphological observations. A.M.A. Arch. Path., *60*:408-422, 1955.
12. Tonelli, L.: I noduli di Aschoff como possibile espressione di fenomeni regressivi del tessuto muscolare liscio. Un'interpretazione desunta dallo studio dell'endocardite reumatica in sede auricolare. Arch de Vecchi., *25*:459-479, 1957.
13. Vazquez, J. J. and Dixon, F. J.: Immunohistochemical analysis of lesions associated with fibrinoid changes. A.M.A. Arch. Path., *66*:504-517, 1958.
14. Von Glahn, W. C.: The pathology of rheumatism. Am. J. Med., *2*:76-85, 1947.
15. Wagner, B. M.: Studies in rheumatic fever. 3. Histochemical reactivity of the Aschoff body. Ann. N. Y. Acad. Sc., *86*:992-1008, 1960.

Relationship of Experimental Myocarditis to Rheumatic Fever: Current Concepts*

BERNARD M. WAGNER

New York Medical College

The pathognomonic tissue change of human rheumatic carditis is the Aschoff body. This structure begins its life cycle as an acute, nonspecific lesion and rapidly progresses to the typical mature Aschoff body. The mature lesion then passes into a "healing" phase of unknown duration, ultimately ending as a dense fibrotic area. Gross and Ehrlich,[2] who studied the evolution of the Aschoff body, defined histological criteria for the identification of the lesion in its various stages. These criteria were based on routine tissue preparations and the subjective evaluation of the microscopic findings. Failure to regard the rheumatic process as a changing, dynamic state has led to the idea that a variety of Aschoff bodies exist. General lack of agreement on the minimal criteria needed for the definition of this lesion indicated that other methods of analysis were necessary.

Mitral valvotomy requires in most cases that the left auricular appendage be biopsied. This *intra vitam* tissue presented to the pathologist a unique opportunity to study the rheumatic process in living tissue. Since 1954 we have studied over 800 biopsies.[6, 12] Approximately 20 to 25 per cent showed the presence of Aschoff bodies in various stages of evolution. There were 16 cases which demonstrated histological alterations characteristic of "acute rheumatic carditis." Almost all of the Aschoff bodies were in the loose subendocardial connective tissue. In this location, the lesion is more elongated and the cells more scattered, but the typical nuclear pattern and cytoplasm serve to identify the cells as of the Aschoff variety. In an attempt to extend the parameters of objective criteria to achieve some degree of uniformity, a detailed histochemical and immunochemical study is in progress.[12] These techniques require fresh tissue and the surgical biopsies allow for the application of these methods, eliminating the question of artifacts such as occur when using postmortem material.

In order for these studies to be valid, one must show that the Aschoff bodies in the subendocardium of left auricular appendages are similar to their counterparts in the ventricular myocardium. This has been accomplished by the majority of workers in this field. However, Saphir[5] continues to reject the appendage lesions on the basis of his morphological criteria. It would seem rather unusual to encounter "different" kinds of Aschoff bodies in various parts of the heart. Accepting the fact that the appendage and ventricular lesions are essentially the same, we must ask whether they carry the same significance. Almost all of the clinical-pathological correlations of rheumatic fever are based on autopsy studies with retrospective analysis. In the 16 cases[4] in which the biopsy tissue demonstrated acute rheumatic

* Supported in part by U. S. Public Health Service Grant H-5822.

carditis, postoperative prognosis was not altered. After five years, eight of these patients are completely well. The remainder are well, but follow-up has been less than three years.

What, then, is the clinical significance of the Aschoff body? Does its presence really indicate "active" disease? These questions are difficult to answer. Previous studies have tried to approach these problems.[7]

In addition to trying to establish objective criteria in identifying the Aschoff body in human tissues, these criteria are of equal importance in evaluating experimental material. Has the Aschoff body been reproduced in an experimental model? This crucial question is extremely controversial. All claims for or against the production of the Aschoff body in animals rests on purely morphological evidence. We have already noted the disagreement on human material studies, so we are not surprised at the experimental difficulties. If we could establish a broader base of recognition of the human process, the criteria used would be applicable to the experimentally induced changes.

Other publications have established new criteria of identification.[8, 10, 12] Briefly stated, the earliest recognizable changes are simultaneous events involving collagen fibers, acid mucopolysaccharides and proteins. These may result in the appearance of "fibrinoid." The focal changes are surrounded by cardiac histiocytes (Anitschkow cells) and Aschoff cells. The highly characteristic intranuclear, bar-shaped, serrated chromatin distinguishes these cells from myofibers and fibroblasts. The cytoplasm of Aschoff cells shows esterase and acid phosphatase activity. Gamma globulin and fibrin were frequently localized in the fibrinoid by the fluorescent antibody technique. The basophilia of the cytoplasm is due to the presence of ribonucleic acid. Purified bacterial hyaluronidase fails to remove the metachromasia of the fibrinoid. However, testicular hyaluronidase, which has chondromucinase and proteolytic activity as well, effectively digests the metachromatic components. This strongly suggests that the metachromasia is due to a mixture of highly acidic mucopolysaccharides. All of these findings best fit the notion that the Aschoff body is a granuloma. This hypothesis postulates that the fibrinoid substances are in an area of fiber degeneration. Cardiac histiocytes are transformed into Aschoff cells by unique and unknown stimuli. A surrounding mantle of chronic inflammatory cells completes the picture for a granuloma.

Accepting this hypothesis, we next ask the nature of this most singular type of granuloma. If it represents a response to an antigen-antibody reaction or some form of hypersensitivity, the lesion is highly unusual by comparison with other tissue reactions to similar processes. If the Aschoff body granuloma represents a reaction to a specific micro-organism or toxic biological agent, direct evidence for either or both possibilities is not available. Attempts to localize certain Group A streptococcal antigens in the Aschoff body have not been successful.[12] It is obvious that considerable work is necessary to further explore these areas. Confirmation and extension of the Aschoff body concept as a granuloma may yield important information regarding pathogenesis.

The experimental production of rheumatic carditis depends exclusively on the willingness of the observer to equate the lesions with the human Aschoff body. Animals such as rabbits, rats, mice, guinea pigs and monkeys have been given horse serum,[11] streptococci dead or alive, parts of streptococci[1] with or without other additives, meningococcal endotoxin,[9] E. coli lipopolysaccharide,[9] synovial fluid and blood products by every conceivable route of administration. Some experiments have been short; others have progressed for many months. Of all the animals mentioned, the rabbit has been utilized most extensively. This animal does not develop fatal endocarditis or myocarditis spontaneously. Nor does the rabbit suffer from arthritis or spontaneous Group A streptococcal infections. It is a vegetarian by choice and presents a broad genetic background. With these facts in mind, one might expect some difficulty in producing human rheumatic fever. However, in the literature one encounters terms such as "Aschoff-like," "rheumatic fever-like," "valvular swelling and fibrinoid of the rheumatic type." Indeed, based on the concept that the Aschoff cell is derived from myofibers, striated and nonstriated, Murphy[3] claims reproduction of the Aschoff body in the rabbit. I have been unable to confirm these observations, and I do not agree with the basic assumption as to the myogenic origin of the Aschoff cell. Evidence in support of these statements has been presented elsewhere.

Acute carditis can be produced in the rabbit with little difficulty. The responses are nonspecific and predictable. The lesions produced compare favorably with nonspecific carditis in man. In more chronic experiments, which may or may not be associated with circulating antibodies, myofiber damage occurs in focal areas. An abortive attempt at regeneration results in multinucleated cells.[8] These cells may resemble certain phases of the Aschoff cell when morphological criteria only are used. By defining the human Aschoff body in morphological, histochemical and immunochemical terms while allowing for the importance of location and particular stage of development, we can exclude these multinucleated masses in the rabbit from consideration as related to the Aschoff body.

In conclusion, it is my opinion that the human Aschoff body can be defined in broader terms. Morphology alone, although a powerful tool, will not suffice. The unique features of rheumatic fever require objective specificities. The application of more dynamic methods to a changing process in man seems to indicate that the Aschoff body is a granuloma. These same methods, when applied to experimental carditis, especially in rabbits, establish that the changes produced bear no relationship to rheumatic fever. It is possible that we are dealing with the wrong animal species or that we need inbred lines. Or perhaps the demands we make for similarity between man and animal are too rigid or incorrect. I should think that the thorough elucidation of the rheumatic process in man by appropriate biological methods is an obvious prerequisite in attempting parallel experimental simulation. If this thesis is correct, the experimental production of rheumatic carditis in laboratory animals has not, as of this writing, been accomplished.

REFERENCES

1. Char, D. F. B. and Wagner, B. M.: The cardiac effects of Group A streptococcal sonicates in rabbits. Ann. N. Y. Acad. Sc., 86:1009, 1960.
2. Gross, L. and Ehrlich, J. C.: Studies on the myocardial Aschoff body. I. Descriptive classification of lesions. Am. J. Path., 10:467, 1943.
3. Murphy, G. E.: On muscle cells, Aschoff bodies and cardiac failure in rheumatic heart disease. Bull. N. Y. Acad. Med., 35:620, 1959.
4. Pani, K. C., Wagner, B. M. and Shapiro, S. H.: Serological, electrophoretic and histological observations in mitral commissurotomy Patients. Am. J. M. Sc., 236: 590, 1958.
5. Saphir, O.: The Aschoff nodule. Am. J. Clin. Path., 31:534, 1959.

6. Tedeschi, C. G., Wagner, B. M. and Pani, K. C.: Studies in rheumatic fever. I. clinical significance of the Aschoff body based on morphological observations. Arch. Path., 20:408, 1955.
7. Tedeschi, C. G. and Wagner, B. M.: The problem of subclinical rheumatic carditis. Am. J. M. Sc., 231:382, 1956.
8. Wagner, B. M. and Tedeschi, C. G.: Studies in rheumatic fever. II. Origin of cardiac giant cells. Arch. Path., 20:423, 1955.
9. Wagner, B. M.: Relationships of the Aschoff body to experimental carditis. Fed. Proc., 16:376, 1957.
10. Wagner, B. M.: Hypersensitivity: Role of the Connective Tissue. In Mellors, R. C. (ed.): Analytical Pathology. New York, McGraw-Hill Book Co., 1957, pp. 429-470.
11. Wagner, B. M., Vanace, P. and McGrath, J.: Hypersensitivity myocarditis in rabbits and swine. Fed. Proc., 17:462, 1958.
12. Wagner, B. M.: Studies in rheumatic fever. III. Histochemical reactivity of the Aschoff body. Ann. N. Y. Acad. Sc., 86:992, 1960.

The Rheumatoid Factor in Rheumatoid Arthritis

JOHN H. VAUGHAN

University of Rochester School of Medicine and Dentistry

The agglutinating activity of the sera of patients with rheumatoid arthritis has been shown to be due to a heavy, 19S gamma globulin molecule which differs from the rest of its 19S family by having specific ability to react with smaller 7S gamma globulin molecules. The rheumatoid factor is present in the sera of most patients with rheumatoid arthritis, but not in all. It is not, therefore, a *sine qua non* of the disease. It does not represent a primary pathogenic factor; it has been recognized in the sera of patients without rheumatoid arthritis. One might be led to ask, therefore, why study it further? Actually, in some ways the finding that the factor is not disease-specific has enhanced its potential interest. It represents part of a biological responsiveness not as yet completely understood. Its presence in other diseases indicates that there is in some way a common bond between rheumatoid arthritis and the other diseases.

What are the questions uppermost in our minds about the rheumatoid factor? First, is it antibody? All that we know of it, so far, is consistent with but not mandatory for this assumption. The rheumatoid factor differs from the rest of the 19S gamma globulin molecules only in its specific reactivity. By all other chemical and immunochemical criteria applied to it by Kunkel, it, like classic antibody, could not be differentiated from the remaining gamma globulins of its class.[3] Gamma globulins of species other than man will cross-react with it in much the same way as antigen from one species will cross-react with classic antibody formed to the analogous antigen in another species. The rheumatoid factor from a given individual exhibits its own peculiar profile of reactivity, i.e., in the extensiveness of its cross-reactivity with gamma globulin from other species and in the extensiveness of its predilection for one or another of the human gamma globulin groups. In this respect it is also similar to classic antibody, which notoriously differs from one individual to another in just this way.[4]

The question of whether or not the rheumatoid factor is antibody cannot, however, be decided without full consideration of what its antigen might be. Three possibilities exist: (1.) The rheumatoid factor could be antibody to some as yet undefined antigen, microbial or otherwise, the reactions with human and all other gamma globulins being cross-reactions. There is no information to support this possibility; it is unlikely and will not be considered further. (2.) The rheumatoid factor could be isoantibody. We now recognize that there are gamma globulin serological groups, much the same as there are red blood cell serological groups. An isoantibody, however, does not react autologously, and we know that the rheumatoid factor circulates in complex with autologous gamma globulin. This makes this second postulate untenable, unless some prior mechanism be postulated for getting into our patient some capacity to form a gamma globulin type not genetically his own. Maternal-fetal transfer is the only mechanism for this that comes readily to mind. (3.) Finally, the rheumatoid factor may be a true autoantibody. This would imply that the primary specificity of the factor is for human gamma globulin, reactivity with all other gamma globulins being in the form of cross-reactions. There is no satisfactory explanation as yet for how or why such autoantibody might be formed in the first place, and, in particular, whether denaturation of the gamma globulin is a prerequisite for this (cf. 4).

If the rheumatoid factor is not an antibody, it might be considered a complement or complement-like substance, because of its ability to react with antibody. The group of proteins composing hemolytic complement are capable, as is the rheumatoid factor, of combining with antigen-antibody aggregates. The rheumatoid factor, however, is not any of the presently known hemolytic complement components, and there is nothing to suggest that the rheumatoid factor is essential to complement action. Conglutinin is a complement-like substance in blood which interacts with antigen-antibody complexes. It is poorly understood, but the meager data available do not favor the hypothesis that the rheumatoid factor is related to it. In assigning the rheumatoid factor to such a complement-like classification, in preference to calling it an antibody, one is really taking the stand that the adaptive biochemical pathways responsible for elaborating antibody gamma globulin, with specificity for one or another foreign antigenic configuration, are not responsible for elaboration of the rheumatoid factor. Actually there is no good evidence for making this decision one way or the other.

Several interesting features of the rheumatoid factor, as it exists in rheumatoid arthritis, are independent of the argument as to whether or not the factor is antibody. More and more investigators are now impressed with the finding that most patients with rheumatoid arthritis already exhibit their positive serological reactions when they are first seen with their disease. Rarely do positive reactions develop during the course of observation in the clinic, and in the few instances in which this does appear to have happened the titers developed have not been very high. One orientation to this might be that rheumatoid arthritis is a disease selectively occurring among people with pre-existing positive reactions—more specifically, that the 3 to 5 per cent of the normal population exhibiting positive rheumatoid agglutinating reactions is an overly susceptible population, one more likely to develop the disease. Long-term follow-up studies on seropositive normal people will be needed to assess this possibility. The currently popular studies on the serum characteristics of the members of families of rheumatoid arthritis patients bear on this subject.

Another way to look at the fact that patients are almost always seropositive when first seen is to assume that the real onset of their disease occurred significantly before they were first seen in the clinic. This could allow for the development of seropositivity after the onset of the disease, but before the onset of sufficient symptoms to bring the patient to the doctor. This possibility does not seem unreasonable, for it is common knowledge that careful histories can often elicit vague aches and pains long before the overt expression of disease in a large number of rheumatoid arthritis patients. The reports of the development of weak positive reactions in a few patients some time after first being seen in the clinic may then be taken as evidence of a late serological conversion in a patient whose innate ability to make this particular serological response is poorly developed. The situation could be likened to that of the individual who has a poor ability to make a given antibody in response to a given antigenic stimulation, and who does it late or in low titer, if at all.

Irrespective of these opposing hypotheses, there are certain clinical correlations between presence and absence of the rheumatoid factor which are worth noting. The factor is found more often in patients with severe disease than in those with mild disease. There are apt to be more atrophy of tissues, more joint destruction and subcutaneous nodules in those whose sera have the factor. It would be a mistake, however, to assign to the rheumatoid factor the causative role for these features. Occasional patients have nodules and negative serum reactions, and Good[2] has demonstrated nodules in agammaglobulinemic children with arthritis. It is probable that seropositivity simply reflects "more disease," as do the subcutaneous nodules, and that this is the only relation between the two. Duthie et al.[1] have conducted a six-year follow-up on patients who were classified as seropositive and seronegative at the time of initial examination. Their study strikingly points out the poorer prognosis in those who were seropositive, a finding consistent with the notion that seropositivity reflects "more disease."

The occasional finding of the rheumatoid factor in significant titer in healthy persons, and even, as Dr. Vincent Butler and I have recently found occasionally, evidence of it in concentrated fractions of sera from normal individuals whose original sera had shown no activity, emphasizes that the factor may be a normal serum constituent. Among pathological sera, it is seen not only in rheumatoid arthritis but also in a high percentage of patients with liver disease. It has been reported to be present in significantly increased incidence in patients with various infections. It may be, therefore, that the rheumatoid factor represents part of a normal reaction pattern of the body to certain types of challenge; often this challenge has been infection.

Our present thinking, therefore, is increasingly oriented around the idea that the appearance of rheumatoid factor activity is simply an expression of a type of host responsiveness, that the rheumatoid factor does not represent a primarily noxious agent, and that it is not the product of a faulty cell metabolism. A delineation of the sorts of challenge that can lead to this type of serological response should be meaningful in our further understanding of the cause of rheumatoid arthritis.

REFERENCES

1. Duthie, J. J. R., Brown, P. E., Knox, J. D. E. and Thompson, M.: Ann. Rheumat. Dis., *16*:411, 1957.
2. Good, R. A.: Conference on Host Response Mechanism on Rheumatoid Arthritis, Atlantic City, May, 1959.
3. Kunkel, H. G., Franklin, E. C. and Muller-Eberhard, H. J.: J. Clin. Invest., *38*:424, 1959.
4. Vaughan, J. H.: Am. J. Med., *26*:596, 1959.

The Pathogenesis
of Rheumatoid Arthritis

LEON SOKOLOFF

National Institute of Arthritis and Metabolic Diseases

The etiology and pathogenesis of rheumatoid arthritis remain obscure. It is a chronic inflammatory disease that has many pathologic and clinical characteristics of an infection, but even the most sensitive microbiologic methods presently available have failed to yield pathogenic agents.[23] Hypersensitivity to a variety of antigenic materials has, therefore, been widely considered as a possible pathogenetic mechanism. This hypothesis has been enjoying greater interest in recent years as a result of the development of serologic tests that depend on the presence of macroglobulins having some characteristics of antibodies, and also because of certain anatomic and clinical associations with conditions in which hypersensitivity mechanisms are believed to play a role. In the present discussion, we shall consider a number of the pathologic findings in rheumatoid arthritis as they may be related to its pathogenesis.

THE HISTOLOGIC RELATIONSHIP BETWEEN THE SUBCUTANEOUS NODULES AND THE SYNOVIAL LESIONS

Typically, the joints in rheumatoid arthritis have a pattern of hypertrophic villous synovitis. The articular soft tissues are thickened and elevated in papillary stalks as a result of proliferation of vascular fibrous tissue and infiltration with chronic inflammatory cells. Most of the latter are plasma cells and lymphocytes, some aggregated into nodular clusters and others disposed more diffusely at the surface. Among the connective tissue cells are perivascular fibroblasts. The synovial lining cells become hyperplastic and arranged in a palisade. The lining cells resemble a mesothelium in sections prepared by conventional histologic methods and have a certain phagocytic capacity.[14] Nevertheless, their histogenesis and regeneration following synovectomy indicate that they are modified fibroblasts rather than mesothelium or reticuloendothelium. Despite certain contradictory findings, recent studies of their fine structure seem to support this view.[15, 16, 17]

The pattern of hypertrophic villous synovitis with pannus formation is typical of rheumatoid arthritis, but not pathognomonic of it. It may be seen in quite unrelated conditions in man[21] and it has been reproduced experimentally by a variety of irritants[11] and infectious agents.[9]

By contrast, the subcutaneous nodules have a considerably greater degree of histologic specificity. It is true that they occur rarely in patients who have never presented other evidence of rheumatoid arthritis. Somewhat similar nodules occur in rheumatic fever, less often in systemic lupus erythematosus and scleroderma.

In the subcutaneous nodules of rheumatoid arthritis, three separate elements can be distinguished: focal areas of necrosis of subcutaneous fibrous and granulation tissue; a palisade of cells, usually elongated and rarely multinucleated, about the necrotic material; and an enveloping granulation tissue in which chronic inflammatory cells, predominantly plasma cells and lymphocytes, are seen about blood vessels.

The necrotic centers to a varying extent have a "fibrinoid" appearance, i.e., they are oxyphilic, somewhat refractive and react as fibrin does rather than as collagen with certain stains, notably Van Gieson, Masson, phosphotungstic acid-hematoxylin and Gram stains. It must be emphasized that the composition of the necrotic material varies as the lesion progresses and regresses. It contains large amounts of collagen, lipids, nucleoproteins, acid mucopolysaccharides, serum proteins and, at certain active stages, material that probably is fibrin.[7]

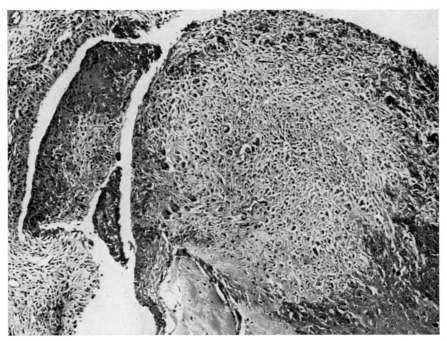

Fig. 1. Granulomatous synovitis in rheumatoid arthritis (interphalangeal joint of finger, S 39057). Focal areas of fibrinoid" necrosis of the superficial portions of the synovial tissue are present. At their base is a palisade of proliferating synovial fibroblasts and multinucleated cells. A portion of the necrotic material has become detached from the lining tissue and lies free in the joint space. (Hematoxylin and eosin, × approximately 50.)

Since the joint lesions are morphologically nonspecific and the extra-articular nodules relatively specific, what is the relationship between the two? If there were no common histologic sequence of events, it would be difficult to conceive that a common pathogenetic factor in rheumatoid disease produced both of these lesions. This question has not often been asked, nor is a completely satisfactory answer forthcoming.

The following hypothesis is offered to account for this: that the type of reaction that is seen in the subcutaneous nodules does actually occur, at least at times, in the joints. In rheumatoid arthritis, focal areas of "fibrinoid" necrosis may be seen in the superficial portions of the synovial tissue. These foci probably contain fibrin, and at their base one observes an ingrowth of fibroblasts and palisades of synovial lining or elongated connective tissue cells quite like those of the subcutaneous nodule (Fig. 1). Their appearance is indistinguishable from that of subcutaneous nodules that have undergone central softening with formation of bursa-like cavities. Collins[4] has referred to the latter as pseudo-synovial spaces.

Thus, the simplest explanation for the differences between such synovial foci and the subcutaneous nodules is that, in the latter, the necrotic material is circumscribed by solid cicatrix, while in the synovial location, the necrotic débris is discharged into the joint space and may appear as a rice body. In the joint, the inflammation thus becomes dissipated in the articular cavity and could give rise to the more diffuse, nonspecific components of the synovitis that also are seen in the granulation tissue about the nodules.

IS THE RHEUMATOID NODULE A GRANULOMA?

Rheumatoid arthritis and rheumatic fever are frequently referred to as granulomatous diseases. The term "granuloma" is interpreted to mean different things by different persons and frequently is believed to imply an inflammatory process in which hypersensitivity is involved. To many, the concept of granulomatous disease is that the basic reactant inflammatory cell is a mononuclear cell (macrophage, histiocyte) or derivative of it. If this is so, it must be demonstrated that the cells forming the palisade in the nodule are of this type. The best cytologic study dealing with this problem is that of McEwen,[18] in which these cells were demonstrated to be unable to phagocytose neutral red as monocytes, macrophages, clasmatocytes and epithelioid cells are characteristically able to do. By this criterion, the rheumatoid nodule is not a granuloma. By the same token, the nodule would not represent a foreign body reaction to autogenous necrotic collagen, as is sometimes suggested. By other criteria, however, the nodule may be called a granuloma—namely, that it is an inflammatory nodule of proliferating connective tissue leading to scar formation. It has, in addition, several architectural features similar to those of other diseases generally accepted as granulomatous: central areas of necrosis bordered by a palisade of elongated cells and, sometimes, by multinucleated cells. Nevertheless, by neither of these criteria can the term "granuloma" suggest that this is a disease of hypersensitivity.

HISTOGENESIS OF THE RHEUMATOID "GRANULOMA"

The appearance of granulation tissue in the developing nodules of rheumatoid arthritis and in the synovial tissue suggests that the cellular palisades represent not so much an epithelioid or histiocytic reaction as an interface between nonspecific, oriented, proliferating granulation tissue (fibroblasts and capillaries) and a fibrin-rich inflammatory exudate. The character of the exudate, including its content of fibrin, necrotic material and compactness, varies with the equilibrium between the necrosis and reparative activity of the granulation tissue. At this interface, aminopeptidase activity can be demonstrated histochemically[8] and there is reason to believe that this protease is a fibrinolysin. The cells originate quite consistently with proliferating capillaries. It is at times hard to tell whether they are in the wall of the latter, outside or different from the cells lining them. They ultimately evolve into fibroblasts.

The perivascular disposition of the chronic inflammatory cells is of the sort designated "perivascular islands" by Gell.[6] Although such lesions appear to be characteristic of tuberculin rather than of other types of hypersensitivity reactions under controlled conditions, they have not been demonstrated to be pathognomonic of tuberculin-type hypersensitivity in other inflammatory reactions.

Several hypotheses have been entertained about the initiation of the vascular and fibroblastic proliferation. According to some, there is an initial necrosis or specific irritation of the subcutaneous or other collagen with secondary vascular changes. Banerjee and Glynn,[1] for example, have noted the similarities of the granulation tissue about implants of heterologous fibrin to that of the rheumatoid nodule.

According to another view, the appearance of the nodules suggests that their development is in some manner mediated by the vascular system.[13, 22] Granulation tissue containing inflammatory leukocytes, lymphocytes and plasma cells has been present in the earliest specimens available for study. It is in such cases that the histologic sequences in the development of the lesion can be studied to best advantage. We have examined 16 subcutaneous nodules early in the course of development, often within two weeks of their clinical detection. In 14 of the 16, conspicuous inflammatory changes were present in the small arteries or about vascular islands of smaller caliber in the granulation tissue. A careful examination of virtually all old standing rheumatoid nodules will demonstrate the presence of healed vascular lesions, but their primary nature cannot be inferred in such instances. In addition, in some old lesions, arteritis may be seen in localized areas of new nodule formation.

Aside from the frequency with which the young subcutaneous nodules are associated with arteritis, there are two principal reasons for believing that the vessels play a role in the genesis of the lesions: (1) There is an intimate morphologic association between the vessels and the necrosis or streaming fibrinoid inflammation of the lesions. The latter changes commonly surround the altered vessels and appear to proceed centrifugally. (2) Furthermore, in such patients, there is a high frequency of arteritis in other tissues. Among 19 patients we have studied who had arteritis in a nodule, nine were subjected to muscle biopsy; five of these nine had arteritis in the gastrocnemius muscle. Such observations suggest that the vascular change in the nodule and in other tissues is an intrinsic rather than a secondary part of rheumatoid arthritis and contributes to the development of the nodule. If the concept proposed above—that the articular changes are inherently those found in the nodule—is correct, the vascular alteration must be an intrinsic part of the development of the joint disease as well.

SIGNIFICANCE OF ARTERITIS IN RHEUMATOID ARTHRITIS

Arteritis was first described as a frequent finding in rheumatoid arthritis in striated muscle and has subsequently been recognized in other organs by many observers. The character of the lesion has varied greatly in different individuals. In some patients it is mild and is recognized only by minute examination of many serial sections of tissue. In a few patients the clinical course is fulminating and the arterial lesions cannot be distinguished from those of polyarteritis nodosa. The observations have raised a number of questions that cannot be answered conclusively at this time. Our views[22] on them may be summarized briefly:

1. The occurrence and severity of the arteritis appear to be increased since the advent of steroid therapy of this disorder. Nevertheless, arteritis has also been seen in patients who have never received such treatment. The steroids are known to aggravate certain other vascular diseases, and may conceivably adversely affect the arteritis that otherwise occurs in patients with rheumatoid arthritis.

2. The arteritis, in the view of some, provides a common anatomic link to other so-called collagen diseases and to polyarteritis nodosa. Furthermore, it has been interpreted as additional evidence that this is a disorder of hypersensitivity. Nevertheless, the changes are morphologically nonspecific and variable in each of these disorders. Comparable changes occur in induced and spontaneous diseases of other species in which a variety of pathogenetic mechanisms are known to occur—anaphylaxis, infection, disturbed electrolyte metabolism and some of unknown etiology.[3, 5, 10, 12, 20] It would appear premature to draw any conclusions about the more ultimate pathogenetic mechanisms involved in the arteritis of rheumatoid arthritis.

The hypothesis that arteritis is an intrinsic part of rheumatoid arthritis and contributes to the development of its other lesions has not won universal acceptance. It has, however, been based on unique material and has the virtue of unifying the various anatomic findings into a single histogenetic account of the disorder.

THE RELATIONSHIP OF THE SERUM "RHEUMATOID FACTOR(S)" TO THE DISEASE

The occurrence of a serum macroglobulin capable of reacting with gamma globulin represents a new and valuable diagnostic tool for rheumatoid arthritis. The thesis that this factor (or factors) represents an antibody or autoantibody and that hypersensitivity mechanisms are involved in the genesis of rheumatoid arthritis has been well reviewed by Vaughan.[24] Mellors and co-workers[19] have presented impressive evidence that this macroglobulin is produced (or concentrated) in plasma cells in the inflammatory lesions of rheumatoid arthritis and to a lesser extent in certain other cells of lymphoid tissue. It was not found in the areas of fibrinoid necrosis. This observation suggests that the rheumatoid factor is not itself a toxic material, although it is conceivable that it is being destroyed in the areas of necrosis. The findings in inflammatory lesions of other etiology in patients with rheumatoid arthritis have not been reported; such studies might clarify whether the development of the rheumatoid macroglobulins in such patients is a generalized metabolic capacity of plasma cells in these individuals or one more intimately related to the rheumatoid disease. The serologic tests, although useful diagnostically and potentially valuable in clarifying the susceptibility of certain persons to develop rheumatoid arthritis, may perhaps have no other significance in the pathogenesis of the disease.

THE OCCURRENCE OF GAMMA GLOBULIN IN THE LESIONS OF RHEUMATOID ARTHRITIS

Gamma globulin has been demonstrated to be concentrated in the areas of necrosis in the subcutaneous nodules. Although localization of gamma globulin occurs in clearly demonstrated antigen-antibody reactions, such as experimental serum sickness, there are a number of tenable theoretical alternatives to the thesis that its occurrence in the nodules is evidence of a hypersensitivity reaction.[25] Apparently gamma globulin has not been demonstrated by comparable methods in the synovial tissue in rheumatoid arthritis. Whether areas of necrosis comparable to those in the nodules were present in the joint tissues studied is not known.

The significance of gamma globulin as evidence of hypersensitivity in rheumatoid arthritis must be examined critically in view of the demonstration of subcutaneous nodules of rheumatoid type in rare patients with arthritis associated with agammaglobulinemia.[2]

From these brief remarks, it is apparent that we have at the moment no real grasp of the pathogenetic mechanisms involved in rheumatoid arthritis. The inconstancy and overlap of the pathologic, serologic and clinical findings in this and the other so-called collagen diseases raise a question as to the definition of rheumatoid arthritis. It may be that this is not a single disorder but a syndrome arising from complex, presently unknown disease processes. Like the proverbial blind men, we comprehend only small portions of the elephant. It may be that when we know more about it, we shall discover that there is no elephant at all.

REFERENCES

1. Banerjee, S. K. and Glynn, L. E.: Reactions to homologous and heterologous fibrin implants in experimental animals. Ann. N. Y. Acad. Sc., 86:1064-1074, 1960.
2. Bridges, R. A. and Good, R. A.: Connective tissue diseases and certain serum protein components in patients with agammaglobulinemia. Ann. N. Y. Acad. Sc., 86:1089-1097, 1960.
3. Campbell, W. G., Jr. and Santos-Buch, C. A.: Widely distributed necrotizing arteritis induced in rabbits by experimental renal alterations. I. Comparison with the vascular lesions induced by injections of foreign serum. Am. J. Path., 35:439-465, 1959.
4. Collins, D. H.: The Pathology of Articular and Spinal Diseases. London, E. Arnold, 1949, p. 195.
5. Deringer, M. K.: Necrotizing arteritis in strain BL/De mice. Lab. Invest., 8:1461-1468, 1959.
6. Gell, P. G. H.: Cytologic events in hypersensitivity reactions. In Lawrence, H. S. (ed.): Cellular and Humoral Aspects of the Hypersensitivity States. New York, Paul B. Hoeber, 1959, pp. 43-66.
7. Gitlin, D., Craig, J. M. and Janeway, C. A.: Studies on the nature of fibrinoid in the collagen diseases. Am. J. Path., 33:55-78, 1957.
8. Glenner, G. G., Burstone, M. S. and Meyer, D. B.: A study of aminopeptidase activity in the stroma of neoplastic tissue with a comparison of histochemical techniques. J. Nat. Cancer Inst., 23:857-872, 1959.
9. Goldie, W. and Collins, D. H.: Erysipelothrix arthritis in rabbits: experimental induction and the response to cortisone. J. Path. Bact., 71:425-439, 1956.
10. Jones, T. C., Doll, E. R. and Bryans, J. T.: The lesions of equine viral arteritis. Cornell Vet., 47:52-68, 1957.
11. Jordan, E. P.: Synovial membrane and fluid in rheumatoid arthritis. Arch. Path., 26:274-288, 1938.

12. Koletsky, S.: Necrotizing vascular disease in the rat. 2. The role of sodium chloride. A.M.A. Arch. Path., 63:405-409, 1957.
13. Kulka, J. P.: The pathogenesis of rheumatoid arthritis. J. Chron. Dis., 10:388-402, 1959.
14. Lang, J.: Vitalfärbung der Gelenkinnenhaut. Zeitschr. f. mikro.-anat. Forsch., 60: 255-259, 1954.
15. Langer, E. and Huth, F.: Untersuchungen über den submikroskopischen Bau der Synovialmembran. Zeitschr. f. Zellforsch., 51:545-559, 1960.
16. Lever, J. D. and Ford, E. H. R.: Histological, histochemical and electronmicroscopic observations on synovial membrane. Anat. Rec., 132:525-533, 1958.
17. Luse, S. A.: A synovial sarcoma studied by electron microscopy. Cancer, 13:312-322, 1960.
18. McEwen, C.: Cytologic studies on rheumatic fever: a comparison of cells of sub-cutaneous nodules from patients with rheumatic fever, rheumatoid arthritis and syphilis. Arch. Path., 25:303-314, 1938.
19. Mellors, R. C., Heimer, R., Corcos, J. and Korngold, L.: Cellular origin of rheumatoid factor. J. Exper. Med., 110:875-886, 1959.
20. Orbison, J. L., Christian, C. L. and Peters, E.: Studies on experimental hypertension and cardiovascular disease. I. A method for the rapid production of malignant hypertension in bilaterally nephrectomized dogs. A.M.A. Arch. Path., 54:185-196, 1952.
21. Sherman, M. S.: Non-specificity of synovial reactions. Bull. Hosp. Joint Dis., 12:110-125, 1951.
22. Sokoloff, L. and Bunim, J. J.: Vascular lesions in rheumatoid arthritis. J. Chron. Dis., 5:668-687, 1957.
23. Utz, J., Phelps, E. T. and Smith, L. G.: Rheumatoid arthritis: viral studies of adult human synovial fluid and tissue using tissue culture techniques. Georgetown Univ. Med. Center Bull., 12:198-200, 1960.
24. Vaughan, J. H.: Serum responses in rheumatoid arthritis. Am. J. Med., 26:596-613, 1959.
25. Vazquez, J. J. and Dixon, F. J.: Immunopathology of hypersensitivity. Ann. N. Y. Acad. Sc., 86:1025-1032, 1960.

The Possible Role of Serotonin in Rheumatoid Arthritis and Other Collagen Diseases

ARTHUR L. SCHERBEL

The Cleveland Clinic Foundation and The Frank E. Bunts Educational Institute

Serotonin, histamine and related amines are widely distributed in the body and are known to produce a number of pharmacologic actions. The primary role of serotonin is unknown but it is believed to have a part in the transmission of nerve impulses.[4] Large amounts of these amines are found in the gastrointestinal tract, lungs and blood platelets.[13] Both serotonin and histamine are believed to have an important function in anaphylactoid and allergic reactions.

Certain specific effects of serotonin and related substances on connective tissue have been described by several investigators. Local injection of serotonin into a rat's paw produces edema similar to that produced by histamine.[5]

Long-term injections of serotonin into the subcutaneous tissue of a rat result in local progressive collagenous and fibrous proliferation within the dermis.[3] Serial injections of histamine subcutaneously or about large joints in guinea pigs result in inflammation and fibrosis of connective tissue.[1]

The present report summarizes briefly our studies on the effects of serotonin, histamine and certain amine inhibitors on connective tissue in experimental animals.[12] It also describes the exaggerated response to these amines when injected intradermally in patients with connective tissue disease, as compared with the reaction in normal control subjects, and the effect of administering an amine inhibitor on the reaction resulting from the injected amine.[10] Finally, it presents the effects of and rationale for administering amine releasers[7, 11] and amine inhibitors[8] to patients with certain connective tissue diseases.

EFFECT OF SEROTONIN AND HISTAMINE ON CONNECTIVE TISSUE IN THE RAT

Our initial experimental studies were designed to determine what effect serotonin and histamine had on connective tissue studied morphologically in rats. Two polyvinyl sponges were implanted subcutaneously in 311 rats. One rat in four served as a control and received injections of physiologic saline solution. Serotonin and histamine were administered subcutaneously adjacent to the sponges in the test animals in doses varying from 10 mg./kg. to 100 mg./kg. for periods of one to 30 days. Treated and control animals were sacrificed in groups at weekly intervals. In the controls, a progressive increase of new connective tissue filled the sponges. The inflammatory reaction, consisting principally of lymphocytes, histiocytes and foreign-body giant cells, was minimal and an occasional heavily granulated mast cell was noted at the periphery. When serotonin was injected, the inflammatory reaction was markedly increased but fibroplasia remained the same as in control animals. When histamine was injected, fibroplasia was significantly increased but the inflammatory reaction was much less than that seen with serotonin. Mast cells were usually degranulated, in contrast to the heavily granulated mast cells in animals that received serotonin.

From these studies it was concluded that serotonin was capable of producing an inflammatory reaction in connective tissue in rats. Short-term studies with the experimental method of implanting polyvinyl sponges subcutaneously suggested that serotonin did not influence fibroplasia. Histamine was also capable of producing an inflammatory reaction in connective tissue but the predominant morphologic change was fibroplasia.

EFFECT OF SEROTONIN ANTAGONISTS ON CONNECTIVE TISSUE IN THE RAT

Two of the most potent serotonin antagonists now available are 1-methyl-D-lysergic acid butanolamide* and cyproheptadine.† Experiments were designed to study the inhibiting action of these compounds on the inflammatory reaction in connective tissue resulting from the administration of serotonin and also to study the effect of these drugs on connective tissue growth in comparison with that of control animals.

* Sandoz Pharmaceuticals.
† Merck Sharp and Dohme Research Laboratories.

Animals receiving both serotonin and one of the serotonin antagonists in an approximate ratio of 10:1 showed greatly diminished inflammatory reactions within the polyvinyl sponges as compared with those animals receiving only serotonin. In addition, connective tissue growth was retarded in comparison with that in the polyvinyl sponges of control animals.

It was concluded from these experiments that the serotonin antagonists (1-methyl-D-lysergic acid butanolamide and cyproheptadine) block the inflammatory reaction resulting from serotonin and that they retard fibroplasia in polyvinyl sponges implanted subcutaneously in rats. These studies, however, did not prove that the observed effects were due to the inhibition of serotonin or related compounds. It is possible that some unknown pharmacologic action was responsible.

SEROTONIN SENSITIVITY IN CONNECTIVE TISSUE DISEASE

Patients with connective tissue diseases respond in an exaggerated fashion to intra-articular, peri-articular or intradermal injections of serotonin and histamine.[10] The reaction to serotonin, as observed in our patients, was characterized by diffuse pain, erythema and swelling over the dorsum of the injected hand; this reaction spread rapidly and occasionally extended proximally into the forearm. Within a few minutes cyanosis occurred in all fingers of this hand and persisted for several hours; the fingers became cold and occasionally were painful. The response to histamine injections was characterized by erythema and swelling of a localized area over the dorsum of the hand. Cyanosis occurred to a lesser degree and lasted for a shorter period than it did with serotonin. Usually normal control subjects responded to injections of serotonin and of histamine with only slight erythema and edema at the site of the injection.

EFFECT OF SEROTONIN ANTAGONISTS ON THE EXAGGERATED SEROTONIN REACTION

The intravenous administration of 2 to 3 mg. of serotonin antagonist (2-brom-D-lysergic acid diethylamide, 1-methyl methergine tartrate) or cyproheptadine during the peak of the serotonin reaction in patients with connective tissue disease rapidly diminished the intensity or reversed it completely within a few minutes. Intradermal injection of 0.2 mg. of a serotonin antagonist also neutralized the serotonin reaction in a localized area a few minutes after its administration. These clinical experiments demonstrated that patients with connective tissue diseases are usually more sensitive to serotonin and related amines than are normal control subjects, and that this exaggerated reaction can be neutralized or diminished *in vivo* by administration of certain serotonin inhibitors.

GENERAL CONSIDERATIONS IN CONNECTIVE TISSUE DISEASE

Much has been written about the inflammatory reaction that occurs in the various connective tissue diseases. It varies in intensity and usually involves mesenchymal tissue in numerous sites of the body. Except for histologic similarities, the lesions are nonspecific and are without pathogenetic basis. In contrast, very little has been written about the nonarticular features of these diseases. Usually these factors are not considered significant in comparison with the musculoskeletal manifestations.

During the past decade we have held the opinion that a biochemical defect suggesting decreased neurohumoral activity within the brain stem is probably present in connective tissue disease. Features relative to the central nervous system include loss of energy, increased emotional instability aggravated by stress reactions, and mental depression. Excessive perspiration involving the palms, face and neck may occur intermittently, as well as bouts of flushing and pallor, intolerance to cold, hyperesthesia, paresthesia and other fluctuating and migratory neuralgic and vasomotor reactions. Muscular atrophy may develop rapidly without apparent disuse of involved muscles, and deep reflexes may become altered; hyper-reflexia occurs early in the disease and hyporeflexia appears later when the disease becomes chronic. These central nervous system features often fluctuate as do the joint manifestations, but not necessarily in a direct relationship to each other. This suggests that neurohumoral abnormalities might also exist in these patients in addition to the numerous other biochemical alterations that are present.

EFFECT OF AMINE OXIDASE INHIBITION IN CONNECTIVE TISSUE DISEASE

In 1952 we discovered that many of the psychic manifestations of rheumatoid arthritis and related diseases could be altered by the administration of small doses of iproniazid, an amine oxidase inhibitor.[6] Initial improvement was usually manifested by elation in mood, increased sense of well-being, strength and emotional stability. In many patients, musculoskeletal pain lessened or disappeared and tolerance to cold increased. Excessive perspiration and vasomotor reactions diminished while muscular strength and deep tendon reflexes increased. When larger doses of iproniazid, sufficient to cause increased stimulation of the central nervous system, were administered, joint swelling and tenderness disappeared but returned when the hyperactivity of the central nervous system subsided.

Following the discovery that administration of iproniazid increased the levels of serotonin and norepinephrine in the brains of laboratory animals,[2] it occurred to us that a similar biochemical mechanism might be responsible for the improvement in manifestations pertaining to the central nervous system in patients with rheumatoid arthritis and related diseases who received iproniazid. It should be emphasized, however, that there is no evidence at present that dysfunction in higher or lower brain centers is related to decreased activity of serotonin or a related substance.

LOCAL EFFECT OF CERTAIN AMINE OXIDASE INHIBITORS ON ISCHEMIC AND INDOLENT ULCERS IN CONNECTIVE TISSUE DISEASE

For certain inflammatory or ulcerating lesions complicating rheumatoid disease, or for ischemic ulcerations complicating Raynaud's phenomenon, application of an ointment (Marsilid 5 per cent or Catron 0.3 per cent in a cream base) is usually effective in stimulating the healing process.[9] The pharmacologic action responsible for stimulation of healing of these lesions is unknown; if amine oxidase inhibition is responsible, perhaps other amines are released which stimulate the healing process. It is also possible that a mechanism of action other than an inhibition of amine oxidase may be responsible, inasmuch as these compounds are capable of altering numerous enzyme systems.

SEROTONIN INHIBITION IN CONNECTIVE TISSUE DISEASES

After observing that serotonin antagonists blocked the inflammatory reaction resulting from serotonin in the connective tissue of experimental animals and that they also blocked the exaggerated serotonin reaction in patients with connective tissue diseases, clinical studies were carried out to determine what effect, if any, these compounds exerted on the various connective tissue diseases.

During the past two years, various serotonin antagonists have been administered intravenously, parenterally and orally to patients of both sexes ranging in age from three to 76 years of age. The connective tissue diseases treated included rheumatoid arthritis, systemic lupus erythematosus, progressive systemic sclerosis, dermatomyositis and hypersensitivity angiitis.

In rheumatoid arthritis, pain in the joints diminished and range of motion increased, with lessening of joint swelling, in many patients. Muscular tightness and spasm decreased and patients usually noted increased muscular coordination. Injection of a serotonin antagonist into inflamed tissue often resulted in almost immediate temporary relief of pain and lessening of joint stiffness. In progressive systemic sclerosis the effect of these compounds appeared to be more significant than in rheumatoid arthritis. Improvement occurred slowly but consistently and was characterized by softening of the skin and loosening of subcutaneous tissue. In patients with subcutaneous calcinosis and draining sinuses, the deposits of calcium became smaller and sinuses healed. When ischemic ulcers of the finger tips were present, they usually healed rapidly.

Other desirable features of treatment with serotonin antagonists included increased appetite, weight gain and an antipyretic action. Undesirable features were increased muscular relaxation, listlessness, an occasional temporary LSD-like reaction (with intravenous administration), and aggravation of a pre-existing depressive reaction. All of these were temporary and rapidly reversible. These effects of the drugs were directly related to dosage, rate and mode of administration.

It was concluded from these clinical studies that serotonin antagonists often produced desirable peripheral effects, characterized by lessening of the mesenchymal inflammatory reaction, pain and muscular spasm, in addition to loosening of the skin and subcutaneous tissue. All manifestations of disease activity returned when medication was discontinued. Undesirable central nervous system manifestations occasionally appeared; these usually were related to relatively large doses of the drug administered intravenously.

DISCUSSION

The experimental and clinical studies briefly summarized here demonstrate a relationship between the nervous and connective tissue systems. It is postulated that certain amines or related substances which are necessary for normal physiologic function in one system of the body may act adversely in another system of the body if the protecting mechanism against this substance or substances becomes inadequate.

Manifestations referable to the central nervous system which are characteristic of these diseases were rapidly alleviated when amine oxidase activity was reduced. This suggested that the enzyme system was present in certain areas of the brain in excess amounts or that the formation of certain inhibiting or regulating substances within the brain was inadequate. If this excess substance is not serotonin or a related substance, it is assumed to be a biochemical abnormality that can be alleviated by decreasing amine activity within the central nervous system.

Theoretically, the peripheral disease manifestations (mesenchymal inflammation and fibroplasia) should increase in severity if the amines are also increased peripherally in mesenchymal tissue. This has not been apparent clinically, although it is safe to state that peripheral disease manifestations do not subside as quickly as do central nervous system manifestations.

Conversely, it is interesting that the serotonin and histamine antagonists which inhibit mesenchymal inflammation are also capable of aggravating existing manifestations of disorder in the central nervous system.

If the known pharmacologic actions of these drugs can be assumed to produce the characteristic clinical response observed in patients with connective tissue diseases, it is apparent that compounds known to release amines have a rapid and desirable effect centrally and an insignificant peripheral effect during the early phase of therapy. It is also apparent that the amine inhibitors which inhibit peripheral disease manifestations, characterized by the inflammation and fibroplasia, do not alleviate the central features of these illnesses and on occasion may aggravate them.

It is not inferred from the evidence presented that connective tissue diseases are due to abnormal neurohumoral dysfunction, but rather it is suggested that a biochemical abnormality of this nature may be one of the many defects which occur in a group of complex diseases.

REFERENCES

1. Bensley, S. H.: Some factors involved in histamine-induced arthritis and rheumatism in animals. In The First Canadian Conference on Research in Rheumatic Diseases, Toronto, Ontario, Canada, March 4, 1955. Toronto, The Canadian Arthritis and Rheumatism Society, 1955, pp. 61-64.
2. Brodie, B. B. and Shore, P. A.: On the role for serotonin and norepinephrine as chemical mediators in central autonomic nervous system. In Hoagland, H. (ed).: Hormones, Brain Function and Behavior. New York, Academic Press, Inc., 1957, p. 161.
3. MacDonald, R. A., Robbins, S. L. and Mallory, G. K.: Dermal fibrosis following subcutaneous injections of serotonin creatinine sulphate (23734). Proc. Soc. Exper. Biol. & Med. 97:334-337, 1958.
4. Page, I. H.: Serotonin (5-hydroxytryptamine); the last four years. Physiol. Rev., 38: 277-335, 1958.
5. Rowley, D. A. and Benditt, E. P.: 5-Hydroxytryptamine and histamine as mediators of the vascular injury produced by agents which damage mast cells in rats. J. Exper. Med. 103:399-412, 1956.
6. Scherbel, A. L.: The effect of isoniazid and of iproniazid in patients with rheumatoid arthritis. Cleveland Clin. Quart., 24:90-97, 1957.
7. Scherbel, A. L.: The effect of Marsilid in patients having rheumatoid arthritis. J. Clin. & Exper. Psychopath., 19 (Suppl.):118-122, 1958.
8. Scherbel, A. L.: Pharmacodynamic effects of UML-491 in animals and man. Cleveland Clin. Quart., January, 1961.
9. Scherbel, A. L., Curtis, G. H. and Harrison, J. W.: Effect of iproniazid ointment on trophic ulcers associated with Raynaud's phenomenon; clinical note. Cleveland Clin. Quart., 25:92-94, 1958.
10. Scherbel, A. L. and Harrison, J. W.: Response to serotonin and its antagonists in patients with rheumatoid arthritis and related diseases. Angiology, 10:29-33, 1959.
11. Scherbel, A. L. and Harrison, J. W.: The effects of iproniazid and other amine oxidase inhibitors in rheumatoid arthritis. Ann. New York Acad. Sc., 80:820-834, 1959.

12. Scherbel, A. L., McKittrick, R. L. and Hawk, W. A.: The influence of serotonin and histamine on the growth of connective tissue in rats. To be published.
13. Udenfriend, S., Weissbach, H. and Bogdanski, D. F.: Biochemical studies on serotonin and their physiological implications. In Hoagland, H. (ed.): Hormones, Brain Function and Behavior: Proceedings of a Conference on Neuroendocrinology Held at Arden House, Harriman, New York, 1956. New York, Academic Press, Inc., 1957, pp. 147-160.

Comparative Histology and Metabolism of Synovial Tissue in Normal and Arthritic Joints[*]

DAVID HAMERMAN, MALLORY STEPHENS and PETER BARLAND

Albert Einstein College of Medicine and the Bronx Municipal Hospital Center

We propose to discuss the results of using cytochemical techniques to localize enzymes in cells of human synovial membrane from normal and arthritic joints. Some of these methods permit visualization of the distribution of enzyme activities in synovial cells while preserving the morphology of the cells and their relation to the joint tissue. Correlation of such cytochemical findings with biochemical studies of tissue slices or homogenates may provide a better understanding of the metabolism of the synovial membrane.[†]

These studies were carried out on synovial membrane from five subjects without arthritis, four subjects with osteoarthritis and five patients with active rheumatoid arthritis.

SELECTION OF CASES

"Normal" (Table 1).   Synovial membrane was obtained from the suprapatellar bursa (with a Polley-Bickel needle[19]) or from an infrapatellar site (at arthrotomy). In one case, specimens from the two sites of the same joint were compared and found to have similar morphological features. In all cases except one (McC.), synovial fluid was obtained for chemical studies. Values in the normal range were found: hyaluronate hexosamine 1.3 mg./Gm.; protein, 25 mg./Gm.; nondialyzable hexose, 0.6 mg./Gm.; and electrophoretic distribution of proteins, albumin 67 per cent, globulins, α-1 6 per cent, α-2 5 per cent, β 8 per cent and γ 14 per cent.[20]

* Supported by a grant from the N. Y. State Chapter, Arthritis and Rheumatism Foundation; by Training Grant 2A-5082, NIAMD (Department of Medicine); and by a grant from The National Foundation (Department of Pathology).

† The terms "synovial tissue" and "synovial membrane" will be considered synonymous for the sake of simplicity. Both designate the specialized connective tissue that forms the inner surface of the fibrous capsule of synovial joints.

TABLE 1. PATIENTS WITH "NORMAL" JOINTS AND OSTEOARTHRITIC
JOINTS SELECTED FOR SYNOVIAL MEMBRANE BIOPSY

	AGE AND SEX	DIAGNOSIS	METHOD TO OBTAIN S.M. AND SITE
Mos.	73M	Normal joint	P.-B., suprapat.
Fel.	52M	Normal joint	P.-B., suprapat.
McG.	39M	Menisceal tear	Arthrot., infrapat.
Bro.	39F	Menisceal degen.	Arthrot., infrapat.
McC.	65M	Knee contractures	Arthrot., infrapat.
Lee	74F	Osteoarthritis	P.-B., suprapat.
DiG.	57F	Osteoarthritis	P.-B., suprapat.
Gom.	61F	Osteoarthritis	Arthrot., infrapat.
Pio.	70M	Osteoarthritis	Arthrot., infrapat.
Kau.	25M	Osteochondritis dissecans	Arthrot., infrapat.

Osteoarthritis. Patients with osteoarthritis (Table 1) (1) complained of knee pain and had evidence of joint deformity; (2) showed x-ray evidence of bony lipping and spur formation of the affected joint; (3) presented no evidence of rheumatoid arthritis or gout. Less than 1 ml. of synovial fluid was obtained from two patients (DiG. and Lee) and these fluids showed normal findings. Two patients (Gom. and Pio.) had large effusions and electrophoresis showed a slightly reduced albumin.

One patient (Kau.) with osteochondritis dissecans of the knee is included in this group.

TABLE 2. PATIENTS WITH RHEUMATOID ARTHRITIS SELECTED
FOR SYNOVIAL MEMBRANE BIOPSY

	AGE AND SEX	DURATION		METHOD TO OBTAIN S.M. AND SITE
		R.A.	KNEE SYMPTOMS	
Fil.	54F	3 days	2 days	P.-B., suprapat.
Nie.	31F	6 yrs.	3 mos.	P.-B., suprapat.
Bau.*	68F	12 yrs.	12 yrs.	Arthrot., suprapat.
Gor.	60F	15 yrs.	10 yrs.	Arthrot., infrapat.
Dio.	40F	3 yrs.	3 mos.†	Arthrot.

* Deceased at time of biopsy.
† Wrist.

Rheumatoid Arthritis (Table 2). Synovial membrane was obtained from involved joints early and late in the course of the disease. In each case the disease was active and four of the patients (Fil., Nie., Bau., Gor.) had subcutaneous nodules, positive latex agglutination tests, and chronic disease of multiple joints. Synovial membrane was obtained from the swollen and painful right wrist of one patient (Dio.) without nodules and with a negative latex test. The left wrist had been inflamed three years before and was now partially ankylosed. Synovial effusions were aspirated in the four classic cases and chemical studies showed abnormal findings: hyaluronate hexosamine, 0.75 mg./Gm.; protein, 59 mg./Gm.; nondialyzable hexose, 1.04 mg./Gm.; and electrophoretic distribution of protein, albumin 37 per cent, globulins α-1 7 per cent, α-2 9 per cent, β 9 per cent and γ 38 per cent.[8, 20]

METHODS

Sections were prepared for cytochemical study without fixation (using either the Bausch and Lomb freezing microtome or a Pearse cryostat,[18] or after overnight fixation in cold formol-calcium.[1] Material was also fixed in formalin for conventional hematoxylin-eosin preparations, and in buffered osmium tetroxide[17] for electron microscopic studies.

With practice, the glistening outer margin of the synovial membrane can be distinguished from the capsular side, even in small samples obtained with the Polley-Bickel needle. Orientation of the specimen for cutting was facilitated when the surgeon "marked" the outer margin of the synovial membrane by placing a small suture needle into the specimen so that the needle entered at the capsule and emerged at the synovial lining.

Frozen sections of formol-calcium fixed tissue were used to demonstrate the activities of LDH,* an enzyme of glycolysis; DPNH-diaphorase, an enzymatic component of the electron transport chain; and acid phosphatase. The methods for LDH and DPNH-diaphorase, employing the tetrazolium salt nitro-BT[12] as an acceptor, have been described elsewhere.[9] The acid phosphatase method was that of Gomori.[7] Sections incubated in media from which substrate was omitted served as controls.

Although formol-calcium fixation preserves the morphological integrity of the tissue, it prevents visualization of the activities of some oxidative enzymes.[13, 14] These may be demonstrated in unfixed tissue. We have made preliminary studies on SDH[9] and IDH, two enzymes of the Krebs tricarboxylic acid cycle; G-6-PDH, an enzyme of the pentose cycle; and TPNH diaphorase, another enzyme of the electron transport chain.

The tetrazolium technique has been reviewed by Novikoff.[14] When a section of synovial membrane is incubated in the appropriate substrate and the tetrazolium salt, nitro-BT, enzymes in the cells oxidize the substrate. Electrons removed from the substrate are transferred, via the electron transport system, to tetrazolium, which becomes reduced and precipitates as dark blue deposits of formazan within the cell.

In the acid phosphatase method,[7, 18] enzymatic hydrolysis of glycerophosphate occurs at pH 5. The liberated phosphate ions are trapped by lead nitrate as lead phosphate. This is converted to black lead sulfide when the section is placed in ammonium sulfide.

RESULTS

Normal Synovial Membrane. Synovial membrane stained with hematoxylin and eosin (Figs. 1, 4) reveals many blood vessels, a number of connective tissue cell types, and, depending in part upon the location in the knee, varying amounts of adipose tissue and collagenous fibers.[4]

Of particular interest is the outer margin of the synovial membrane with its lining cells. The tetrazolium technique not only demonstrates the distribution of oxidative enzymes; it is particularly useful in revealing the morphology of the lining cells. Especially LDH and DPNH-diaphorase activities result in intracellular deposits of formazan that make it possible

---

* Abbreviations used: LDH = lactic dehydrogenase; DPN = diphosphopyridine nucleotide and DPNH its reduced form; TPN = triphosphopyridine nucleotide and TPNH its reduced form; SDH = succinic dehydrogenase; IDH = isocitric dehydrogenase; G-6-PDH = glucose-6-phosphate dehydrogenase; UDP = uridine diphosphate.

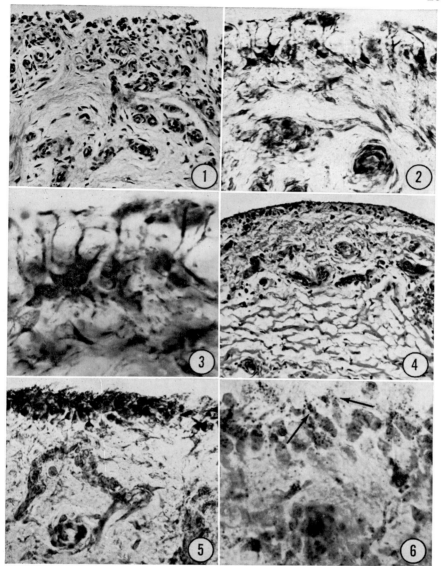

Figs. 1-6. Normal synovial membrane (Figs. 1-3, subject McG.; Figs. 4-6, subject McC.).

Fig. 1. Hematoxylin and eosin (× 140). Areolar synovial membrane with lining cells at upper outer margin.

Fig. 2. DPNH-diaphorase activity (× 230). Note: (1) dark formazan deposits in cell bodies and processes of lining cells; and (2) extensions of processes to the surface.

Fig. 3. Enlargement of lining cells at the left of Fig. 2 (× 480).

Fig. 4. Hematoxylin and eosin (× 140). Somewhat fibrous synovial membrane. Lining cells at outer margin (top).

Fig. 5. DPNH-diaphorase activity (× 230). Note dark formazan deposits in the closely-packed lining cells and in their short processes.

Fig. 6. Acid phosphatase activity (× 480). Note granules (lysosomes) in the lining cells and in their processes (arrows).

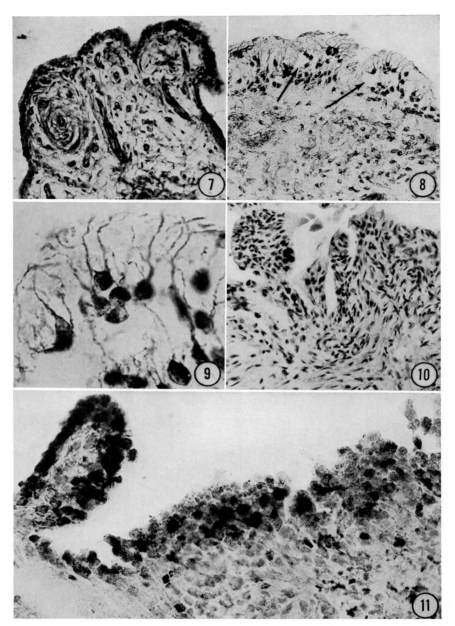

Figs. 7-11. Synovial membrane in osteoarthritis (Figs. 7-9, subject Gom.; Figs. 10-11, subject Pio.)

Fig. 7. Hematoxylin and eosin (× 140). Sparsely cellular synovial membrane with many villi (not shown here) and darkly stained lining.

Fig. 8. DPNH-diaphorase activity (× 115). Note: (1) dark deposits of formazan in lining cells and much lighter staining of other connective tissue cells; (2) orderly arrangement of lining cells and the extension of their fine processes toward the surface; and (3) fusion of the branches of some processes on the surface of the synovial membrane, while other processes enclose apparently clear spaces (arrows).

Fig. 9. Enlargement of lining cells to the right of Fig. 8 (× 480).

Fig. 10. Hematoxylin and eosin (× 140). Fibrotic, hypercellular synovial membrane with multiple villi.

Fig. 11. Acid phosphatase activity (× 230). Note numerous granules (lysosomes) in the lining cells and the variability in their number, size and staining intensity.

162

to trace the delicate processes of the lining cells as they extend toward the joint cavity. From these processes smaller branches arise. At times these branches appear to fuse at the synovial surface to form a limiting outer margin of cell processes (Figs. 2, 3).

The lining cells of normal synovial membrane are also stained by the tetrazolium technique for TPNH-diaphorase. SDH and IDH activities are

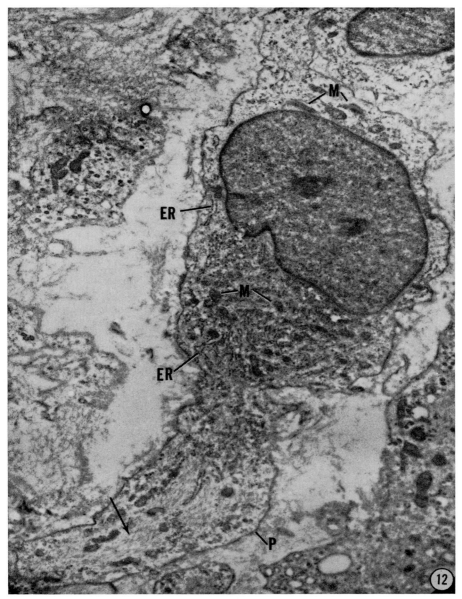

Fig. 12. Electron micrograph of lining cells in the synovial membrane from a patient with osteochondritis dissecans (Kau.) (× 15,000). Note numerous mitochondria (M), abundant ergastoplasm (ER), and part of a cell process (P) with fibrils of unknown nature (arrow).

very faint compared with LDH and DPNH-diaphorase. In preliminary studies G-6-PDH activity is not observed in the lining cells.

Acid phosphatase activity was studied in two cases. It could not be definitely detected in synovial membrane from McG. The membrane from McC. shows moderately strong activity in the lining cells but not elsewhere (Fig. 6). Black granules are seen, often clustered at the end of the lining cells nearest the outer margin.

Synovial Membrane from Osteoarthritic Joints. Sections stained with hematoxylin and eosin usually reveal more collagen than normal and show multiple villi (Figs. 7, 10). Staining for LDH and DPNH-diaphorase activities reveals, as in normal sections, orderly arranged lining cells with delicate processes whose branches appear to fuse at the surface (Figs. 8, 9). The widespread cytoplasmic distribution of DPNH-diaphorase activity and its high level are consistent with the presence of the enzyme in mitochondria and ergastoplasm.[15] Electron microscopy shows the lining cells to possess numerous mitochondria and well-developed ergastoplasm (Fig. 12).

More definitely outlined than in the normal synovial membrane are the apparently clear spaces just beneath the surface enclosed by the processes of the lining cells (Fig. 8). In frozen sections, and also in paraffin embedded sections, these spaces stain metachromatically with toluidine blue. The metachromatic staining is abolished when paraffin sections are incubated in streptococcal hyaluronidase.[10] This suggests that these spaces contain hyaluronate.

TPNH-diaphorase is present in one synovial membrane studied (Pio.). Considerable acid phosphatase activity is observed in the lining cells of two cases studied (Pio., Fig. 11, and Kau., Fig. 12).

Rheumatoid Arthritis. In all five cases, the histology of the synovial membrane stained with hematoxylin and eosin (Figs. 13, 16) is compatible with rheumatoid arthritis:[5] (1) formation of multiple villi; (2) apparent proliferation of lining cells; (3) marked, diffuse infiltration of mononuclear cells, predominantly lymphocytes, but at times chiefly plasma cells, occasionally arranged in "nodes"; (4) dense fibrous tissue coexisting with active synovitis; (5) loss of synovial structure below the lining with replacement by fibrous tissue or round cells.

After five minutes' incubation of synovial membrane from classic cases, intense formazan deposits from LDH and DPNH-diaphorase activities are observed that equal those from normal tissue after 20 to 30 minutes. The lining cells stain much more intensely than the rest of the synovial membrane (Fig. 14). The proliferation of lining cells is evidenced by the great width of the lining cell layer (Figs. 14, 17), by the many lining cells that pack the villi (Fig. 14) and, at times, by the multiple knob-like protrusions of lining cells from the surface of the villi. The increased intensity of staining may be correlated with an increased synthetic activity of the ergastoplasm. Such activity is suggested by our electron microscopic observations. The ergastoplasm appears enlarged into numerous vesicles containing a material of moderate electron opacity.

In all cases the lining cells appear unlike those of the normal or osteoarthritic membranes. Many lining cells are in disordered arrangement and show no orientation toward the surface. Their processes do not intertwine in an orderly fashion to enclose spaces; instead, they criss-cross, and the thick, elongated, densely stained processes give the appearance of a massive

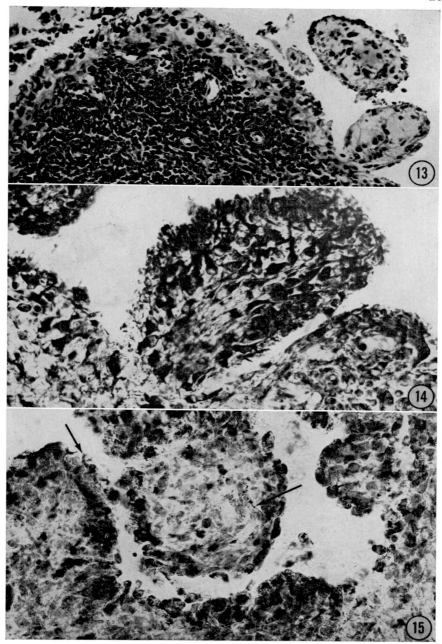

Figs. 13-15. Synovial membrane from a patient (Gor.) with rheumatoid arthritis.
Fig. 13. Hematoxylin and eosin (× 140). Note marked infiltration by inflammatory cells (plasma cells and lymphocytes) beneath the lining. Parts of two villi are seen at the right.
Fig. 14. DPNH-diaphorase activity (× 230). Dark formazan deposits fill the cytoplasm of the lining cells in the villus. Round cells show less activity (lower right).
Fig. 15. Acid phosphatase activity (× 230). Note: (1) small granules (lysosomes) in the cell processes (arrows), and (2) dense accumulations in the outer lining cells.

"log-jam" at the outer edge of the synovial membrane (Fig. 17). Interspersed among the lining cells are lymphocytes and plasma cells.

In two cases studied (Gor., Dio.) TPNH-diaphorase activity is visualized in lining cells. In preliminary studies, IDH does not visualize in one case studied (Dio.); G-6-PDH activity is observed in one case studied (Gor.).

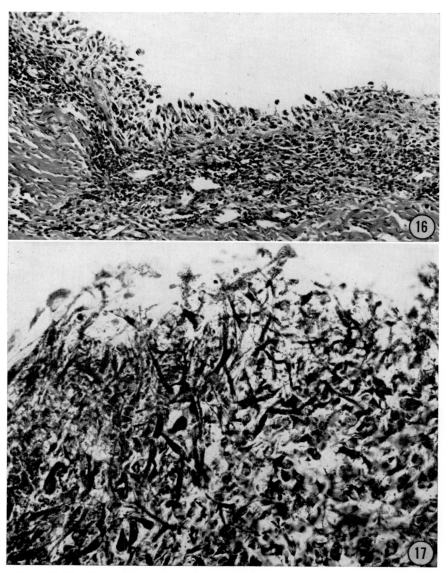

Figs. 16-17.   Synovial membrane from a patient (Bau.) with rheumatoid arthritis.
Fig. 16.   Hematoxylin and eosin (× 140). Multi-layered lining cells along outer margin and marked infiltration of fibrotic synovial membrane by inflammatory cells.
Fig. 17.   DPNH-diaphorase activity (× 230). Note: (1) dark formazan deposits in lining cells; (2) the increased width of the lining cell layer; (3) the disordered arrangement of the lining cells, whose thick, long processes show no evident orientation toward the surface (cf. Figs. 2, 3 and 9); and (4) lightly-stained inflammatory cells interspersed among the lining cells.

Marked acid phosphatase activity is observed in lining cells in two cases studied (Dio., Gor.). Numerous granules of varying size are found in the cytoplasm (Fig. 15).

DISCUSSION

It is known that the synovial membrane synthesizes hyaluronate.[23] Several observations are consistent with the suggestion[9] that the lining cells constitute the major site of synthesis of the hyaluronate of synovial fluid: (1) the location of the lining cells on the outermost part of the synovial membrane; (2) a higher level of oxidative enzymes in the lining cells than in the other connective tissue cells of the synovial membrane; (3) the remarkable enzyme-containing protoplasmic processes of the lining cells, and (4) the presence in some synovial membranes of a hylauronidase-susceptible, metachromatically staining substance in apparently clear spaces enclosed by lining cell processes. Yielding, Tomkins and Bunim[23] showed that synovial membrane slices incubated in glucose C^{14} synthesized radioactive hyaluronate. Biochemical studies also indicate that N-acetyl glucosamine and glucuronate, the repeating dimer of hyaluronate, are formed from glucose with the participation of uridine nucleotides (for reviews, see references 11 and 22). Some enzymes that participate in the synthesis of UDP glucuronate and glucose, and in the formation of glucosamine-6-phosphate from glucose-6-phosphate or fructose-6-phosphate, have been demonstrated in human synovial membrane.[2, 3]

The metabolic activity, as measured by glycolytic rate and oxygen uptake, is very low in normal human synovial membrane and increases markedly in synovial membrane from rheumatoid joints. The highest metabolic activities are found in the hyperplastic villi.[21] The increased rate of LDH and DPNH-diaphorase activities in such villi, suggested by our tetrazolium studies, is consistent with their high metabolic rate. These studies indicate that it is the lining cells that possess the high enzymatic activity.

The observation of G-6-PDH activity in lining cells of one rheumatoid synovial membrane and its absence in a normal case is worth further study. A finding of differences in enzymes of the pentose cycle between rheumatoid arthritis and normal synovial membrane would be of considerable interest. In this connection, caution should be exercised in using staining intensity as a measure of enzyme activity in the cell. Enzyme activity of normal and pathological membranes may be lost at different rates in the fixative, and factors other than enzyme concentration may affect the rate of formazan production.

Acid phosphatase activity in granular form was observed in one of two normal membranes studied, in one case of osteoarthritis, and was most noticeable in two cases of villous rheumatoid synovitis. Studies by Novikoff[15, 16] indicate that the Gomori method for acid phosphatase activity applied to frozen sections of formol-calcium fixed tissues is a reliable means for revealing the cytoplasmic particles called lysosomes. These studies[15, 16] give support to the suggestion of deDuve[6] that lysosomes are related to the uptake and intracellular digestion of proteins, carbohydrates and other materials. The finding reported here of abundant lysosomes in the synovial membrane lining cells, especially in rheumatoid arthritis, may mean that these cells absorb and hydrolyze material in synovial fluid.

ACKNOWLEDGMENTS

The authors are grateful to Dr. A. B. Novikoff of the Department of Pathology for his aid and advice, and to the Department of Orthopedic Surgery, whose members provided synovial membrane at arthrotomy. The photomicrographs were taken by Mr. M. Kurtz.

REFERENCES

1. Baker, J. R.: The structure and chemical composition of the Golgi element. Quart. J. Micr. Sc., 85:1, 1944.
2. Bollet, A. J., Goodwin, J. F. and Brown, A. K.: Metabolism of mucopolysaccharides in connective tissue. 1. Studies of enzymes involved in glucuronide metabolism. J. Clin. Invest., 38:451, 1959.
3. Bollet, A. J. and Shuster, A.: Metabolism of mucopolysaccharides in connective tissue. II. Synthesis of glucosamine-6-phosphate. J. Clin. Invest., 39:1114, 1960.
4. Castor, C. W.: The microscopic structure of normal human synovial tissue. Arth. & Rheum., 3:10, 1960.
5. Collins, D. H.: Is there a pathological definition of rheumatoid arthritis? Acta med. scandinav. Suppl. 341, 5, 1958.
6. deDuve, C.: Lysosomes, a new group of cytoplasmic particles. In Hayashi, T. (ed.): Subcellular Particles. New York, Ronald Press, 1959.
7. Gomori, G.: Microscopic Histochemistry; Principles and Practice. Chicago, University of Chicago Press, 1952.
8. Hamerman, D. and Schuster, H.: Synovial fluid hyaluronate in rheumatoid arthritis. Arth. and Rheum., 1:523, 1958.
9. Hamerman, D. and Blum, M.: Histologic studies on human synovial membrane. 2. Localization of some oxidative enzymes in synovial membrane cells. Arth. & Rheum., 2:553, 1959.
10. Hamerman, D. and Ruskin, J.: Histologic studies on human synovial membrane. 1. Metachromatic staining and the effects of streptococcal hyaluronidase. Arth. & Rheum., 2:546, 1959.
11. Leloir, L. F., Cardini, C. E. and Cabib, E.: Utilization of Free Energy for the biosynthesis of saccharides. In Florkin, M. and Mason, H. S. (eds.): Comparative Biochemistry. New York Academic Press, 1960, vol. 2.
12. Nachlas, M. M., Tsou, K. C., DeSouza, E., Cheng, C. S. and Seligman, A. M.: Cytochemical demonstration of succinic dehydrogenase by the use of new p-nitrophenyl substituted ditetrazole. J. Histochem. & Cytochem., 5:420, 1957.
13. Novikoff, A. B., Shin, W. Y. and Drucker, J.: Cold acetone fixation for enzyme localization in frozen sections. J. Histochem. Cytochem., 8:37, 1960.
14. Novikoff, A. B.: Histochemical and cytochemical staining methods. In Mellors, R. C. (ed.): Analytical Cytology. 2nd ed. New York, McGraw-Hill Book Co., 1959.
15. Novikoff, A. B.: Biochemical and staining reactions of cytoplasmic constituents. In Rudnick, D. (ed.): Developing Cell Systems And Their Control. New York, Ronald Press, 1960.
16. Novikoff, A. B.: Lysosomes and the physiology and pathology of cells. Biol. Bull. 117: 385, 1959.
17. Palade, G. E.: The fine structure of the mitochondria. Anat. Rec., 114:427, 1952.
18. Pearse, A. G. E.: Histochemistry, Theoretical and Applied. 2nd ed. Boston, Little, Brown and Co., 1960.
19. Polley, H. F. and Bickel, W. H.: Experiences with an instrument for punch biopsy of synovial membrane. Proc. Staff Meet., Mayo Clin., 26:273, 1951.
20. Sandson, J. and Hamerman, D.: Non-dialyzable hexose of human synovial fluid. J. Clin. Invest., 39:782, 1960.
21. Thomas, D. P. P. and Dingle, J. T.: Studies on human synovial membrane in vitro. The metabolism of normal and rheumatoid synovia and the effect of hydrocortisone. Biochem. J. 68:231, 1958.
22. Whistler, R. L. and Olson, E. J.: The biosynthesis of hyaluronic acid. Adv. Carbohydrate Chem., 12:299, 1957.
23. Yielding, K. L., Tomkins, G. M. and Bunim, J. J.: Synthesis of hyaluronic acid by human synovial slices. Science, 125:1300, 1957.

Panel Discussion

JOHN H. TALBOTT, *Moderator*

DR. TALBOTT: Dr. Angevine, would you contrast the cardiac alterations in rheumatic fever and rheumatoid arthritis?

DR. ANGEVINE: In the first place, for many years we did not recognize changes in the heart in rheumatoid arthritis, but now there does not seem to be any question that there are very definite lesions. The aortic valve may be involved in rheumatoid arthritis and presents a somewhat different picture grossly and microscopically from that of rheumatic fever. Yesterday, I showed a slide of a lesion in the myocardium undoubtedly associated with rheumatoid arthritis. It simulates the Aschoff body but has much more giant cell reaction than one usually sees. However, I think that when one finds this type of lesion in a particular heart, it has to be interpreted in relation to the patient's disease rather than by putting too much emphasis on the specific morphology.

DR. PEARSON: Dr. Angevine, have you seen features of rheumatoid arthritis either in the heart or elsewhere, plus those of rheumatic fever in the same patient?

DR. ANGEVINE: I think there may be occasional instances, but I do not remember a specific case.

DR. HOLLEY: Dr. Angevine, in the patients with cardiac lesions are you referring to those with both rheumatoid arthritis and ankylosing spondylitis?

DR. ANGEVINE: No, I am not—just those patients with classic rheumatoid arthritis.

DR. TALBOTT: Dr. Holley, since you brought spondylitis into the discussion, and since this had not been mentioned previously, would you comment on the sex chromatin patterns in the female patient with ankylosing spondylitis?

DR. HOLLEY: We have seen only one patient, and the sex chromatin pattern was male.

DR. TALBOTT: Dr. Scherbel, have any studies of the degradation products of serotonin been done in your group of patients with rheumatoid arthritis?

DR. SCHERBEL: Yes, and we have found no significant changes either in the urine or in the tissues. If there is an abnormality in serotonin metabolism or a tissue mediator abnormality, where is this change taking place? First, it is entirely possible that there is an intracellular abnormality in the mechanism involving transfer of the mediator just from one cell to another, and the abnormal products may not saturate the tissue, thus making detection difficult. A second possibility is that the reaction may be a complicated one possibly involving steroids in which slight changes may modify the direction of a given process in the manner Dr. Thornburg so aptly commented on yesterday. The hormone may act on the cell membrane or on the transport system and the particulate matter either within or without the cell. A very active drug may be used, but if tissue binding occurs, the drug may not be able to act on the tissue mediator until it is released. The drug may then become very active and this may explain many of the irregular responses that we observe.

169

DR. COMENS: Dr. Scherbel, it has been shown recently that injection of reserpine or a related compound into animals or into people leads to depletion of serotonin from the brain; along with this there is also depletion of catechol amines from the cardiovascular system. In the patients you treated, I wonder if some of the results are due to release of catechol amines, with subsequent dilation of blood vessels and increase in blood flow, rather than to an antagonistic effect on serotonin itself? Or, if it is a serotonin antagonist, at what level does it block serotonin action?

DR. SCHERBEL: The answers to both of these questions are unknown. When we receive a new drug, we are told by the pharmacologists that it is a potent serotonin antagonist and that it has no effect on histamine, and we must assume that this is correct. The problem may be even more complicated because it is possible that the ratio of these tissue mediators to one another is more important than changes in one mediator alone. For example, when serotonin and histamine are mixed together and injected, a very fulminating reaction occurs in the connective tissue; many amines *may* be involved and it becomes very complicated to decide which one *is* implicated. We thought serotonin might be involved and initiated our studies on this compound. The therapeutic agents being investigated do influence various biological amines, and we do obtain some clinical response with this therapy; although the basis for the results obtained is still tenuous, it has proved to be an interesting mechanism to study.

DR. TALBOTT: Dr. Murphy's concept of the Aschoff body was critically reviewed by both Dr. Sokoloff and Dr. Wagner this morning. Dr. Angevine, would you comment on Dr. Murphy's hypothesis?

DR. ANGEVINE: I have always thought there was something to Dr. Murphy's thesis from a morphological standpoint, and I am fully aware of the disagreement about his findings. There is a recent article from Japan stating that the cells in the Aschoff body are related both to muscle and other mesenchymal cells. I think that this problem will have to be solved by immunological methods. I have looked for cross striations as an indication of the presence of myogenic cells for years, but I have not been able to prove that they are present in the lesion.

DR. TALBOTT: Although Dr. Murphy is not here, a discussion of his work is presented in the September 1960 issue of *Medicine* which sums up his data to the present time.

DR. WAGNER: Much of the problem related to the nature of the Aschoff body and the Aschoff cells is due to the fact that our information is based primarily on morphological evidence, and this has obvious limitations. During the last five years we have studied the Aschoff body by biochemical methods and by the application of fluorescent antibody techniques. To date, we have been unable to demonstrate myosin in the Aschoff cells obtained from auricular appendages, and although we need to study more specimens, the data suggest that the Aschoff cells probably do not come from myofibers. However, I wish to emphasize that multinucleated giant cells may be seen in many nonrheumatic diseases in which cardiac myofiber necrosis occurs. This type of cell has been referred to as a myogenic giant cell, and perhaps it represents an abortive attempt of the body to regenerate muscle.

DR. HAMERMAN: I would like to ask Dr. Wagner and Dr. Sokoloff a general question about the Aschoff body. Is it true that the Aschoff nodule disappears when rheumatic carditis becomes inactive? If it does not disappear with subsidence of clinical activity, are you surprised that there were so few Aschoff nodules in your large series of biopsies of the auricular appendages?

DR. SOKOLOFF: I can not answer that question. It is impossible to determine how long an Aschoff body persists. We know that it can be present or that it can completely heal and leave a scar, but we can not tell how long it has been there. There are no techniques for measuring this.

DR. HAMERMAN: Do you know why so few Aschoff nodules are found, and are they pathognomonic of rheumatic carditis? The relation of Aschoff bodies to rheumatic carditis seems similar to that of defining rheumatoid arthritis in the synovia by the synovial histology. As you pointed out for rheumatic carditis, the synovial lesions are not always typical of rheumatoid arthritis.

DR. SOKOLOFF: I think the Aschoff body is pathognomonic of rheumatic carditis and the lesions are present in 25 to 40 per cent of auricular appendages of patients who have biopsies at the time of surgery. In addition, in postmortem specimens the lesion can be found in other areas of the heart as well as the usual sites of predilection. Quite commonly in an auricular appendage about the size of the tip of the finger, a single section will disclose half a dozen or more Aschoff bodies. They are not rare lesions in these patients.

DR. WAGNER: I think the question Dr. Hamerman asked is a very good one, although it is a vexing one. The question really has two parts: What is the relationship between histologic evidence of activity and clinical evidence of activity? Second, if there is no relationship, what is the significance of the Aschoff body in rheumatic fever? It is only because we are now able to obtain cardiac tissue from living human beings that this problem has come up and forced us to examine these concepts in a very critical way. We decided to follow a group of patients who had active Aschoff lesions diagnosed by the same criteria used for the identification of acute rheumatic carditis—that is, a lesion with the full mantle of inflammatory cells, fibrinoid, and so forth. To our surprise, not very much has happened to these patients. In fact, most of them had an uneventful postoperative course and went home, and this raised many doubts in our minds about the so-called postcommissurotomy syndrome in relation to rheumatic fever. Therefore, I can not draw any conclusions about the significance of these lesions. This will have to be explored further. As Dr. Sokoloff pointed out, there is no way to determine how long the Aschoff body persists, and in this regard I think there is an analogy to tuberculosis. At autopsy, we often find a small calcified anthrocotic node at the hilum of the lung. On section there may be some calcification and perhaps even some caseation. Is this tuberculosis? The patient certainly did not have the clinical disease. This is an incidental finding at autopsy; the patient had tuberculous involvement of the node at one time, but the process is now either healed or healing. I think the same analogy holds true with the Aschoff body; the patient has had rheumatic carditis but the process is now inactive and the lesion is in its evolutionary pattern on the way to oblivion by scar.

DR. ANGEVINE: Several years ago I had an opportunity to study Dr. Wilson's cases in New York. At that time, we were interested in correlating the history of joint pain with the presence of the active Aschoff body. We very seldom found an active Aschoff body unless there had been a relatively recent episode of joint pain. These results were never published. The conclusions were based on the study of many cases and suggest that the presence of active Aschoff bodies is related to active systemic disease.

DR. SOKOLOFF: In regard to the significance of the Aschoff body in the disease process, I want to re-emphasize that rheumatic heart disease, in at least half of the cases, has developed in people who have never had any evidence of rheumatic fever clinically. On the other hand, a person may have an attack of rheumatic carditis at the age of 8, recover in six weeks and die 30 years later of rheumatic heart disease and mitral stenosis; although he has been observed very carefully for recurrent rheumatic fever, there has been no clinical evidence of rheumatic activity, but something has been happening during that time. The only clue that we have as to what is going on is that Aschoff bodies are present in the auricular appendages of such patients. I think this is reasonable presumptive evidence that the rheumatic process has been active during that period.

DR. HOLLEY: Dr. Sokoloff, do you still use the original criteria of Dr. Aschoff to diagnose these lesions or have other criteria been added?

DR. SOKOLOFF: I mentioned the problem of whether there is morphological identity of lesions in the left auricular appendage with those in the myocardium. There may be certain disparities, but the two substantial characteristics that are present in the myocardial lesions are also present in the lesions in the left auricular appendages. I think the cells are morphologically indistinguishable and fragmentation of collagen is also present. Dr. Aschoff did not describe the latter because he did not look at the auricular appendage; no one did until the surgical pathologist began to examine it 10 years ago.

DR. WAGNER: Gross and Ehrlich from the Mount Sinai Hospital in New York reported the histological findings in tissue from the left atrium and left auricular appendage in patients with rheumatic carditis; however, these were fatal cases and this was autopsy material. It is difficult to reconstruct the sequence of events on the basis of the findings in fatal cases.

I would also like to point out that the lesions in the auricular appendage are called Aschoff bodies by the original students of Dr. Aschoff, and I think this is sufficient proof that they are the same as the lesions in the myocardium.

DR. TALBOTT: Dr. Larson, would you discuss the possible role of soluble antigen-antibody complexes in the development of the lesions in acute rheumatic fever?

DR. LARSON: Dr. Seymour Halbert of our institution has given me permission to mention some of the work he has been doing on the cardiac effects following intravenous injection of soluble antigen-antibody complexes into rabbits. When certain complexes are used, electrocardiograms show very bizarre abnormalities, which occur almost immediately after the injection. If appropriate doses are used, ventricular fibrillation ensues and the animals die in about five minutes. This suggests some interesting possibilities with respect to chronic rheumatic activity, in which you can not detect a circulating substance, since it is quite well known that you can not usually measure antigens or antibodies when they are circulating in combination. The suggestion has been made that a circulating soluble antigen-antibody complex may be present in patients with chronic rheumatic activity.

Pathogenesis of Systemic Lupus Erythematosus*

STANLEY L. LEE and SALVADOR B. ZINGALE

State University of New York Downstate Medical Center

A discussion of the pathogenesis of a disease should begin with a description of the etiologic agent or specific metabolic defect, and should explain how the fundamental lesion acts to produce the pathologic physiology and anatomy characteristic of the disease. None of this is possible in the case of systemic lupus erythematosus (SLE). The fundamental lesion is unknown. Any attempt to reconstruct it by analysis from the available clinical and experimental data would be premature. But it may be possible, by such analysis, to choose lines of further investigation which offer some hope for profit.

Extensive studies in the past few years have established a unifying "motif" underlying what seemed previously to be inexplicably varied clinical manifestations. This "motif"—auto-immunity—is not by any means unique for SLE. But its manifestations in SLE are unique, and they provide the largest body of evidence bearing on the origin of this malady.

Attempts have been made recently by two eminent workers[6, 11] to construct pathogenetic bases for SLE from these data. These hypotheses cannot be refuted; however, we do not feel justified in speculating as freely as have these writers. On the other hand, evidence of a nonimmunologic nature seems important enough that any hypothesis must also include it. This evidence, derived from epidemiologic studies and clinical experience with certain drugs, will be reviewed, together with the pertinent immunologic data.

AUTO-IMMUNITY IN SLE

The major studies linking SLE to auto-immune phenomena have been those which have sought to elucidate the LE cell phenomenon.[3, 8, 13, 18, 19, 23, 25, 40, 49, 51] These studies, discussed elsewhere in this volume, have demonstrated a family of antinuclear antibodies in sera from patients with SLE. One or more of these seem to be present in every serum demonstrating the LE cell phenomenon, but the exact correlation between any specific one of these and the ability of a serum to induce the LE cell phenomenon is not yet clear.

The LE cell phenomenon has been the most carefully studied of the auto-immune manifestations of SLE because of its almost ubiquitous occurrence in the disease, but it is not by any means the only such manifestation. The first demonstration of abnormal immune bodies in this disease antedated the discovery of the LE cell by several years.[9] Although the factor responsible for the biologic false positive serologic tests for syphilis found in SLE

* Aided by grants from the National Institute of Arthritis and Metabolic Disease, N. I. H., U. S. P. H. S. (A-3857) and from the Altrua League.

is not truly an auto-antibody, it is clearly a related phenomenon. Antibodies active against red blood cells,[15, 38] leukocytes,[7, 50, 55] platelets,[49] renal glomerular basement membrane,[36, 56] blood coagulation factors[10, 17, 29, 45, 48] and cytoplasmic constituents[2, 12, 20, 32] have all been demonstrated with considerable frequency in sera from patients with SLE.

No one of these abnormal immune bodies, with the possible exception of the anti-deoxyribose-nucleic-acid, is specific for SLE (Table 1). Anti-

TABLE 1.

"ANTIGEN"	SYMPTOMS POSSIBLY CAUSED	OTHER DISEASES
Cell nuclei	none (?)	
DNA-protein	"	Rheumatoid arthritis
DNA	"	Scleroderma
Histone	"	Sjögren's syndrome
		Liver disease
STS antigen	"	Acute infections
Red blood cells	Acquired hemolytic anemia	Lymphomas
		Chronic lymphatic leukemia
		Ulcerative colitis
		Cancer
		"Idiopathic"
Leukocytes	Leukopenia	
Platelets	Thrombocytopenia Purpura	"Idiopathic," after acute infections
Kidney basement membrane	Nephropathy	Glomerular nephritis
		Amyloid disease
		Intercapillary glomerular sclerosis
Blood coagulation factors	Hemorrhagic diathesis	Hemophilia
		Postpartum state
		"Idiopathic"
Cytoplasmic elements	?	Biliary cirrhosis
		Sjögren's syndrome

nuclear antibodies have been demonstrated in rheumatoid arthritis,[2] scleroderma,[3] Sjögren's syndrome[5] and chronic liver disease.[20, 32] Biologic false positive serologic tests for syphilis occur in a wide variety of conditions, as do anti-red-cell, antileukocyte and antiplatelet antibodies. The studies which demonstrated antiglomerular activity in SLE have yielded similar findings in glomerular nephritis, amyloid disease and intercapillary glomerulosclerosis.[35, 36, 57] Circulating anticoagulants are found in patients with hemophilia, in the postpartum state and occasionally without apparent primary disease[4]—although in most cases of SLE with circulating anticoagulant the site of action of the antibody is different from those found in other conditions.[29] Anticytoplasmic activities have been demonstrated in biliary cirrhosis and Sjögren's syndrome.[2, 5, 12]

There are now several diseases in which auto-immune mechanisms can be discerned.[14, 54] In some of these, the relation between cause and effect seems reasonably clear. Thus, in acute thyroiditis, it is assumed that thyroid cellular substance is liberated into the bloodstream by trauma, that this substance is not normally found outside the thyroid gland, that it stimulates the formation of specific antibodies which, transported by the blood, react with remaining portions of the gland and set up a destructive inflammatory reaction.[14, 47] On the other hand, antithyroid antibodies also occur with some frequency in thyroid cancer.[47] There, several possible assumptions can be made to account for the development of the antibodies, but it is impossible to assign them any important role in the pathogenesis of the disease. They are, obviously, by-products.

In acute thyroiditis, then, antithyroid antibodies may well be the direct *cause* of the major manifestations of the disease; in thyroid carcinoma they probably are not important pathogenetically. In both situations, however, the production of antithyroid antibodies is easy to understand; it demands no assumption of abnormality on the part of the antibody-producing mechanism.

The situation in SLE fits neither of the examples just cited, with regard either to the pathogenetic importance of the antibodies or to the mode of their production.

Certain of the antibodies of SLE seem to have pathogenetic significance. Those directed against the formed elements of the blood,[15, 28, 42] against clotting factors[10, 29, 48] and against basement membrane[36, 37] fit into this group. These serologic activities occur all with approximately the same frequency (20 to 30 per cent), although syndromes referable to them have considerably lower frequency.[28] Although any of the syndromes associated with these antibodies may be extremely prominent in individual patients, many patients with SLE go through the entire disease without manifesting any one of them. Further, these syndromes, or similar activities, occur with considerable frequency in conditions not diagnosable as SLE. These antibodies, then, although themselves possibly of importance in producing symptoms, probably do not help to define the underlying disorder responsible for SLE.

The group of antinuclear antibodies found in SLE occupies quite a different position. One or more of them occur with such universality in the disease, and so very infrequently in other conditions, as to suggest strongly that they are somehow related to the fundamental catastrophe which is the basis of SLE. However, all efforts to implicate them in the causation of any of the specific events of the disease have failed.[22, 25, 28] There is good evidence that passive transfer of these antibodies across the placenta is without pathologic significance to the fetus.[22, 42] Experimental evidence indicates that these antinuclear antibodies do not injure intact cells.[23, 27, 41]

Two other peculiarities of the antinuclear antibodies must be mentioned. First, they show an apparent complete lack of species specificity. The anti-DNA of SLE is equally active, for example, against the DNA of human, animal or viral cells.[13, 23, 49] Second, DNA is an extremely poor antigen; it has, so far, been impossible to produce antibodies in an experimental animal using the pure substance as an antigen. DNA-protein or whole nuclei have been used successfully as antigens in the experimental animal, and antibodies reacting with DNA have been obtained, but the antibodies produced have never completely duplicated those found spontaneously in SLE, nor have these animals manifested any indication of systemic disease.[39]

On the basis of these findings, it seems possible to arrive at some working hypotheses concerning the origins and significance of the abnormal antibodies of SLE. These hypotheses are as follows:

1. The antinuclear antibodies of SLE are not specific responses to the antigens DNA, nucleoprotein and histone. Their apparent specificity for DNA and DNA-protein results either from a fortuitous similarity

between the actual antigen and these molecules or from distortions of antibody response to the unknown antigen on the part of the patient. An analogy could be drawn here between antinuclear antibodies in SLE and the heterophil antibody found in infectious mononucleosis or the antibody active against the Wassermann antigen in syphilis.

2. There is a fundamental disturbance of antibody synthesis in SLE which leads to the production of multiple antibodies against normal body constituents. This multiplicity of auto-antibodies in turn leads to multiple system involvement and the typical clinical manifestations of SLE.

Some confirmation for the second of these hypotheses may be adduced from studies conducted in our clinic.[34] This work has demonstrated that patients with SLE respond to the antigens of Brucella much more vigorously than do hospital control patients. This hyper-reactivity was also shown by patients with other rheumatic diseases. Further, in 5 of 11 patients with SLE, antibodies directed against the patient's own red blood cells appeared transiently at the height of response to Brucella vaccination. In no case was there a significant rise in titer of antinuclear antibodies. Thus these patients showed increased responsiveness to the antigen used, and also a certain distortion of the antibody response.

CLINICAL AND EPIDEMIOLOGIC EVIDENCE

Any discussion of the pathogenesis of SLE must take account of the development of SLE-like syndromes, apparently identical with the spontaneous disease, following administration of certain drugs. These were first described following the use of hydralazine in treatment of hypertension.[16, 43] *Hydralazine* lupus is now well authenticated. Recently, identical syndromes following treatment with *trimethadione* in patients with convulsive disorders have been described.[52] We have now under observation a patient in whom an SLE-like syndrome has developed after treatment with *isoniazid* and *para-aminosalicylic acid* for tuberculosis.

In all of these examples, it must be emphasized that the syndromes are indistinguishable from those of "spontaneous" lupus, including the serologic and anatomic manifestations. In most, but not all, clinical evidence of disease disappears quickly once the offending drug is withdrawn. In our experience and in that of others,[52] however, serologic abnormalities often persist for years.

Examination of the structural formulae of the implicated drugs reveals no apparent common denominator. The underlying diseases in the affected patients are likewise diverse. The one aspect common to all drug-induced SLE syndromes is the dose-time factor. In all cases of hydralazine lupus, the drug was administered continuously for a minimum of six to nine months at high dosage. The same pattern obtains for cases due to other drugs. Thus, in the case of drug-induced lupus, the exact nature of the stimulus does not seem too important, but it must be administered at high dosage, continuously and over a considerable period of time.

In a few cases of drug-induced SLE, there has been evidence of hyperglobulinemia predating administration of the offending drug.[52] This may support the thesis of an underlying abnormality of antibody synthesis which can be triggered into the development of SLE by an appropriate stimulus.

Epidemiologic Studies. From the beginning of knowledge about SLE, its preference for the female has been recognized. Reports of SLE occurring in siblings, or in mother and daughter, have appeared from time to time.[1, 21, 26, 30, 31, 33, 44] Recently, in several centers, clinical and serologic studies of relatives of patients with SLE have been begun.[24, 46, 53] None of these studies have so far yielded definitive results; however, preliminary findings all point to a definite increase in incidence of "rheumatic disease" and of serologic abnormalities characteristic of SLE and related conditions. Very incomplete results of one such study[53] are shown in Table 2.

TABLE 2. SLE FAMILY STUDIES

TEST	SLE FAMILY MEMBERS* (143)		CONTROLS** (128)	
	NO. POS.	%	NO. POS.	%
Antinuclear antibodies	7	4.9	1	0.8
LE cells	2	1.4	0	0
VDRL	5	3.5	0	0
Direct anti-globulin (Coombs)	7	4.9	2	1.6
Rheumatoid factor (LPF $\geq 1/160$)	19	13.3	9	7.0
Hyperglammaglobulinemia ($\geq 22\%$ of Tot. Prot.)	19	13.3	18	14.1
Zinc turbidity over 10 Units	39	27.3	24	18.8
History of allergy	29	20.3	30	23.4

* Parents, siblings and children of patients.
** Relatives of patients with nonrheumatic disease chosen for similarity in age, sex, economic and ethnic background.

There seems little doubt that close relatives of patients with SLE share with them certain abnormal antibodies. Whether they also share with the patients the capacity to over-react and to react abnormally to antigenic stimulation is a subject which is now being studied.

Even on the basis of the sketchy data now available, it is clear that there is a familial—probably inherited—abnormality in SLE. Such a familial abnormality has already been demonstrated in rheumatoid arthritis;[58] whether this is the same or merely an analogous defect remains to be shown. From the point of view of pathogenesis, these studies lead to the probable conclusion that SLE occurs in people who have a familial defect of the antibody-forming tissues, and that something about females predisposes them to the disease.

SUMMARY AND CONCLUSIONS

At the beginning of this essay, it was stated that the pathogenesis of SLE is unknown. An attempt to catalogue and correlate what is known, on the basis of the laboratory, clinical and epidemiologic evidence, may make it possible to define the unknown area somewhat. The disease is intimately associated with the production of abnormal antibodies. These antibodies, directed characteristically against many different body constituents, may be the immediate precursors of the multisystem clinical manifestations. SLE differs from other "auto-immune" diseases in the multiplicity of the abnormal antibodies and in the universality of a single group of them—the antinuclear antibodies. These antinuclear antibodies do not seem to be important in the production of symptoms, but may rather refer back to a more fundamental lesion.

There is some evidence that people with SLE react in peculiar ways to certain heterologous antigens. Their relatives seem to have an unusual incidence of immunologic abnormalities related to those found in the disease, and the disease itself occurs not infrequently more than once in a family.

Finally, certain drugs, administered over a long period of time and in high dosage, can give rise to syndromes indistinguishable from spontaneous SLE; there is some suggestion that the same (or a similar) underlying immunologic abnormality exists in people who develop these syndromes.

From these data it seems likely that SLE is a syndrome which depends on at least two fundamental lesions: an inborn disorder of antibody-forming tissues, and the impact of any of several external stimuli. Definite knowledge as to the presence of the intrinsic lesion should be forthcoming soon; its nature remains to be investigated. The extrinsic stimulus may, apparently, be a drug; what it is in spontaneous SLE is still completely unknown.

REFERENCES

1. Agranat, A. L., Bersohn, I. and Lewis, S. M.: Familial disseminated lupus erythematosus. South African M. J., *31*:258, 1957.
2. Asherson, G. L.: Antibodies against nuclear and cytoplasmic cell constituents in systemic lupus erythematosus and other diseases. Brit. J. Exper. Path., *40*:209, 1959.
3. Bardawil W. A., Toy, B. L., Galins, N. and Bayles, T. B.: Disseminated lupus erythematosus, scleroderma, and dermatomyositis as manifestations of sensitization to to DNA-protein. Am. J. Pathol., *34*:607, 1958.
4. Biggs, R. and MacFarlane, R. G.: Human blood coagulation and its disorders. Oxford, Blackwell Scientific Publications, 1957, p. 300 ff.
5. Bloch, K. J., Wohl, M. J., Ship, I. I., Oglesby, R. B. and Bunim, J. J.: Sjögren's syndrome with and without rheumatoid arthritis. Arth. & Rheum., *3*:287, 1960.
6. Burnet, M.: Auto-immune disease. II. Pathology of the immune response. Brit. M. J., *2*:720, 1959.
7. Calabresi, P., Edwards, E. A. and Schilling, R. F.: Fluorescent antiglobulin studies in leukopenic and related disorders. J. Clin. Invest., *38*:2091, 1959.
8. Ceppellini, R., Polli, E. and Celada, F.: A DNA-reacting factor in serum of a patient with lupus erythematosus diffusus. Proc. Soc. Exper. Biol. (N. Y.), *96*:572, 1957.
9. Coburn, A. F. and Moore, D. H.: The plasma proteins in disseminated lupus erythematosus. Bull. Johns Hopkins Hosp., *73*:196, 1943.
10. Conley, C. L. and Hartmann, R. C.: A hemorrhagic disorder caused by circulating anticoagulant in patients with disseminated lupus erythematosus. (Abstr.) J. Clin. Invest., *31*:621, 1952.
11. Dameshek, W.: What is systemic lupus? A.M.A. Arch. Int. Med., *106*:162, 1960.
12. Deicher, H. R. G., Holman, H. R. and Kunkel, G.: Anti-cytoplasmic factors in the sera of patients with systemic lupus erythematosus and certain other diseases. Arth. & Rheum., *3*:1, 1960.
13. Deicher, H. R. G., Holman, H. R. and Kunkel, H. G.: The precipitin reaction between DNA and a serum factor in systemic lupus erythematosus. J. Exper. Med., *109*:97, 1959.
14. Doniach, D. and Roitt, I. M.: Auto-immunity in Hashimoto's disease and its implications. J. Clin. Endocrinol., *17*:1293, 1957.
15. Dubois, E. L.: Acquired hemolytic anemia as the presenting syndrome of lupus erythematosus disseminatus. Am. J. Med., *12*:197, 1952.
16. Dustan, H. P., Tayler, R. D., Corcoran, A. C. and Page, I. H.: Rheumatic and febrile syndrome during prolonged hydralazine treatment. J.A.M.A., *154*:23, 1954.
17. Frick, P. G.: Acquired circulating anticoagulants in systemic "collagen disease." Blood, *10*:691, 1955.
18. Friou, G. J.: The significance of the lupus globulin-nucleoprotein reaction. Ann. Int. Med., *49*:866, 1958.
19. Friou, G. J.: Clinical application of a test for lupus globulin-nucleohistone interaction using fluorescent antibody. Yale J. Biol. & Med., *31*:40, 1958.

20. Gajdusek, D. C.: An "autoimmune" reaction against human tissue antigens in certain acute and chronic diseases. I. Serological investigations. A.M.A. Arch. Int. Med., 101:9, 1958.

21. Glagov, S. and Gechman, E.: Familial occurrence of disseminated lupus erythematosus. New Engl. J. Med., 255:936, 1956.

22. Godman, G. C.: The nature and pathogenetic significance of the L. E. cell phenomenon of systemic lupus erythematosus. In Baehr, F. and Klemperer, P. (eds.): Systemic Lupus Erythematosus. New York, Grune and Stratton, 1959, p. 17.

23. Holman, H. and Deicher, H. R.: The reaction of the lupus erythematosus (L. E.) cell factor with deoxyribonucleoprotein of the cell nucleus. J. Clin. Invest., 38:2059, 1959.

24. Holman, H. and Deicher, H. R.: The appearance of hypergammaglobulinemia, positive serological reactions for rheumatoid arthritis and complement fixation reactions with tissue constituents in the sera of relatives of patients with systemic lupus erythematosus. (Abstr. and discussion.) Arth. & Rheum., 3:244, 1960.

25. Holman, H. R., Deicher, H. R. G. and Kunkel, H. G.: The L. E. cell and L. E. serum factors. Bull. N. Y. Acad. Med., 35:409, 1959.

26. Larsson, O. and Leonhardt, T.: Hereditary hypergammaglobulinemia and systemic lupus erythematosus. I. Clinical and electrophoresis studies. Acta med. scandinav., 165:371, 1959.

27. Lee, S. L.: Unpublished data.

28. Lee, S. L. and Davis, B. J.: The blood in systemic lupus erythematosus. In Baehr, G. and Klemperer, P. (eds.): Systemic Lupus Erythematosus. New York, Grune and Stratton, 1959, p. 37.

29. Lee, S. L. and Sanders, M.: A disorder of blood coagulation in systemic lupus erythematosus. J. Clin. Invest., 34:1814, 1955.

30. Leonhardt, T.: Familial hypergammaglobulinemia and systemic lupus erythematosus. Lancet, 2:1200, 1957.

31. Leonhardt, T.: Hereditary hypergammaglobulinemia and systemic lupus erythematosus. II. Serological studies. Acta med. scandinav., 165:395, 1959.

32. MacKay, I. R. and Gajdusek, D. C.: An "autoimmune" reaction against human tissue antigens in certain acute and chronic diseases. II. Clinical correlations. A.M.A. Arch. Int. Med., 101:30, 1958.

33. Marlow, A. A., Peabody, H. D. and Nickel, W. R.: Familial occurrence of systemic lupus erythematosus. J.A.M.A., 173:1641, 1960.

34. Meiselas, L. E., Lee, S. L., Richman, S. and Zingale, S. B.: The pattern of antibody response in rheumatic diseases. (Abstr.) Arth. & Rheum., 3:455, 1960.

35. Mellors, R. C. and Ortega, L. G.: Analytical pathology. III. New observations on pathogenesis of glomerulonephritis, lipid nephrosis, periarteritis nodosa and secondary amyloidosis in men. Am. J. Path., 32·455, 1956.

36. Mellors, R. C., Ortega, L. G. and Holman, H. R.: Role of gamma globulins in pathogenesis of renal lesions in systemic lupus erythematosus and chronic membranous glomerulonephritis, with an observation on the lupus erythematosus cell reaction. J. Exper. Med., 106:191, 1957.

37. Merrill, J. P., quoted by Peters, J. H. and Freedman, P.: Immunologic aspects of renal disease. New Engl. J. Med., 261:1166, 1959.

38. Michael, S. R., Vural, I. L., Bassen, F. A. and Schaefer, L.: The hematologic aspects of disseminated (systemic) lupus erythematosus. Blood, 6:1059, 1951.

39. Miescher, P., Cooper, N. S. and Benacerraf, B.: Experimental production of antinuclear antibodies. J. Immunol., 85:27, 1960.

40. Miescher, P. and Strassle, R.: New serological methods for the detection of the L. E. factor. Vox Sang., 109:97, 1957.

41. Nathan, D. J. and Snapper, I.: On the interaction of dead leukocytic nuclei, L. E. factor and living leukocytes in the L. E. cell phenomenon. Blood, 13:883, 1958.

42. Nathan, D. J. and Snapper, I.: Simultaneous placental transfer of factors responsible for L. E. cell formation and thrombocytopenia. Am. J. Med., 25:647, 1958.

43. Perry, M. H. and Schroeder, H. A.: Syndrome simulating collagen disease caused by hydralazine (Apresoline) therapy. J.A.M.A., 157:895, 1955.

44. Pirofsky, B. and Shearn, M. A.: Familial occurrence of disseminated lupus erythematosus. New York J. Med., 53:3022, 1953.

45. Ramot, B. and Singer, K.: An unusual circulating anticoagulant in systemic lupus erythematosus. Acta Haemat., 16:158, 1956.

46. Rodnan, G. P., Maclaghlan, M. J. and Creighton, A. S.: Study of serum proteins and

serologic reactions in the families of patients with systemic lupus erythematosus. Annual Meeting American Rheumatism Association, June 1960, Hollywood-by-the-Sea, Florida.

47. Roitt, I. M. and Doniach, D.: Autoimmunization in thyroid diseases. Proc. Roy. Soc. Med., 50:958, 1957.

48. Medal, L. S. and Lisker, R.: Circulating anticoagulants in disseminated lupus erythematosus. Brit. J. Haemat., 5:284, 1959.

49. Seligmann, M.: Études immunologiques sur le lupus érythémateux disséminé. Rev. Franç. d'etu. Clin. et Biol., 3:558, 1958.

50. Seligmann, M.: Leuco-precipitines. II. Mise en evidence d'une réaction de precipitation entre des extraits leucocytaires et le serum de malades atteints de lupus erythemateux disséminé. Vox Sang., 2:270, 1957.

51. Seligmann, M.: Mise en évidence dans le sérum de malades attents de lupus érythémateux disséminé d'une réaction de précipitation avec l'acid désoxyribonucléique. Contes Rendus Acad. Sci. (Paris), 245:243, 1957.

52. Shulman, L. E. and Harvey, A. M.: The nature of drug-induced systemic lupus erythematosus. Annual Meeting, American Rheumatism Association, June 1960, Hollywood-by-the-Sea, Florida.

53. Siegel, M., Widelock, D., Wise, G., Zingale, S. B. and Lee, S. L.: Work in progress.

54. Smart, G. A., Bywaters, E. G. L. and Dacie, J. V.: Discussion on the importance of auto-antibody disease in clinical medicine. Proc. Roy. Soc. Med., Section of Medicine, 52:437, 1959.

55. VanLoghem, J. J., Van Der Hart, M., Hijmans, W. and Schuit, H. R. E.: The incidence and significance of complete and incomplete white cell antibodies with special reference to the use of the Coombs consumption test. Vox Sang., 3:203, 1958.

56. Vazquez, J. J. and Dixon, E. J.: Immunohistochemical study of lesions in rheumatic fever, systemic lupus erythematosus, and rheumatoid arthritis. Lab. Invest., 6:205, 1957.

57. Vazquez, J. J. and Dixon, F. J.: Immunohistochemical analysis of amyloid by the fluorescence technique. J. Exper. Med., 104:727, 1956.

58. Ziff, M., Schmid, F. R., Lewis, A. J. and Tanner, M.: Familial occurrence of the rheumatoid factor. Arth. & Rheum., 1:392, 1958.

The Natural History of
Systemic Lupus Erythematosus

DANIEL L. LARSON

Columbia University College of Physicians and Surgeons

Over the past 20 years, some 500 patients at the Columbia-Presbyterian Medical Center have been suspected of having systemic lupus erythematosus (SLE). The large majority of these patients have been seen in the last 10 years, since confirmatory serologic tests for the presence of "lupus factor" have been available. Of the group of 500 patients, 200 have had a multiple system disease which resembled SLE on clinical grounds; they have shown the characteristic abnormal circulating proteins, and 52 cases showed the pathologic changes of SLE at autopsy examination. The following observations are based on an analysis of the manifestations seen in the 200 patients thought to have definite SLE. The actual incidence of SLE in the general population is thought by many observers to be increasing. Review of the discharge diagnoses given patients from the medical service of the Presbyterian

Hospital during a recent five-month period would seem to bear this out. Of a total of 317 female admissions, 19 (6 per cent) had the clinical diagnosis of SLE. The actual percentage of bed occupancy, however, should be revised upward since some of these patients had more than one admission, and most of them were hospitalized for relatively long periods of time. As might be expected, there were only 4 of 319 male admissions (1 per cent) with a diagnosis of SLE, and in at least one of these the diagnosis is open to considerable doubt.

Early reports on the natural history of SLE would lead one to believe that SLE is an acute fulminating disease with a rapidly fatal termination. Examination of the clinical records at the Presbyterian Hospital, however, would suggest that SLE is a disease of relatively long duration which shares many of the properties of other chronic disorders. If one examines the total duration of some sign, symptom or laboratory finding which could be reasonably attributed to SLE in patients who subsequently develop the full disease pattern, approximately one-third of the patients have their disease ranging from 7 to more than 20 years. Some of these patients may have had only a "biologic false positive" test for syphilis, a convulsive disorder or what was thought to be rheumatoid arthritis before the other features of the disease made their appearance. It is of considerable interest that nine of our patients have been followed for more than 20 years with what is now classic SLE on clinical and laboratory grounds.

The bewildering variety of presenting manifestations of SLE are well known, and the correct diagnosis may be delayed for an inordinately long time. Examination of the length of time after the onset of signs or symptoms of SLE before the correct diagnosis was made in the Presbyterian Hospital series shows that approximately 40 per cent of the patients had their disease for seven years or longer before the diagnosis was established. By far the largest single group of patients had their disease for from one to three years before the correct diagnosis was made, in spite of the increased awareness of the disease and the availability of serologic tests.

There has been considerable interest in the relation of rheumatoid arthritis to SLE, and in the Presbyterian Hospital series, 20 per cent of the patients with SLE also met the criteria of the American Rheumatism Association for the diagnosis of definite rheumatoid arthritis. Ten of these have been examined at autopsy and showed the characteristic findings of both diseases. The clinical course of the patients with both diagnoses tends to be somewhat longer and less stormy than that of the group as a whole, and these patients are in the older age groups. Other than the clinical appearance of rheumatoid arthritis, the most common abnormal physical findings was a systolic heart murmur. This finding usually occurred in association with moderate to severe anemia, and its significance is uncertain. Enlargement of the liver or spleen was not common. Two-thirds of the patients had one or more positive tests for circulating rheumatoid "factor," but the titer usually was in low dilution. The low incidence of renal insufficiency in patients with both diagnoses, as compared with the group as a whole, is reflected in the relatively long clinical course of the patients. The relation between rheumatoid arthritis and SLE remains obscure, but there is some reason to believe they may share some pathogenetic features.

Several authors have drawn attention to the occurrence of thrombocytopenia in the natural history of SLE, and it is quite clear that this complication may antedate other features of the disease by several to many years.

In the Presbyterian Hospital series, the administration of adrenal cortical steroids or corticotropin has often proved to be ineffective or the dosage required to maintain a normal platelet level was prohibitive. For that reason, splenectomy was carried out in seven patients, and another patient was awaiting splenectomy when she died of a subarachnoid hemorrhage. At operation, the spleen was usually of normal size and weight, but in each instance several accessory spleens were identified and removed. Only three of the operative specimens showed periarteriolar fibrosis thought to be compatible with SLE, and there was no correlation between the pathologic findings and the outcome. Only three of the seven patients had a sustained remission in the thrombocytopenia, even though they may have had a temporary rise in platelet levels following operation. Among those who have failed to improve and have been examined post mortem, no remaining accessory spleens have been identified.

There seems to be little doubt that the most important single lesion of SLE as far as survival of the patient is concerned is the renal disease. In the Presbyterian Hospital series, the most common evidence of kidney involvement was persistent proteinuria in the absence of fever or infection. Unfortunately the data on percutaneous renal biopsies are inadequate to correlate with other findings and with the effects of treatment. Approximately one-quarter of the patients became uremic, and this was a major cause of death in the series. A recent survey of the last 48 adult women at the Presbyterian Hospital who had the nephrotic syndrome revealed that 17, or more than one-third, had SLE as the underlying disease process. This clearly establishes SLE as a major cause of the nephrotic syndrome in this age and sex. Among the total of 20 patients with this syndrome, the majority exhibited hypercholesterolemia, half had uremia, and a smaller proportion were also hypertensive. A small group of patients with kidney disease who have developed significant renal insufficiency have been placed on prolonged high dosages of adrenal steroid without noticeable favorable effect on the course of their disease. Undesirable side effects of therapy in this group have been fluid retention, congestive heart failure and serious psychotic breaks.

There is increased recognition of the central nervous system manifestations of SLE, which may take the form of psychotic breaks, convulsions, a combination of both, or a variety of other syndromes. Some of these phenomena take place in patients who are in uremia, or who are on large dosages of corticotropin or adrenal steroids, and as a terminal event. In the Presbyterian Hospital series, there were 50 patients who showed one or more major disorders of the central nervous system. Although psychotic behavior was the most common abnormality, it was often difficult to identify those patients who were showing signs of toxicity to the agents used in treatment as opposed to those who were undergoing reactions to the underlying disease process itself. Of particular importance is the fact that at least two of the patients with alterations in their state of consciousness were thought to be having an exacerbation of their SLE and the dosage of steroids was accordingly increased. Both patients died and were shown to have an unsuspected overwhelming infection of the central nervous system.

In an attempt to explain the central nervous system abnormalities in SLE, it would be tempting to correlate them with lesions seen on histologic examination of the brain and cord. In the Presbyterian Hospital series, the central nervous system was examined histologically in 41 cases. Twenty-two of the patients had shown no clinical evidence of neurologic or psychiatric disease and 19 had shown one or more abnormalities. Among those without clinical disease of the central nervous system, approximately half had major pathologic lesions, focal areas of encephalomalacia being the most common abnormality. On the other hand, in the group of 19 with central nervous system manifestations, nine had no evidence of histologic lesions which could explain the clinical picture. In addition, examination of the cerebrospinal fluid was normal in each case in the absence of evidence of infection or hemorrhage. There was no correlation between the electroencephalogram and the clinical or pathologic picture.

Because of the sex and age incidence of SLE, there is a lively interest in the effects of SLE on pregnancy and the effects of pregnancy on the course of SLE. In the Presbyterian Hospital series, 54 patients with SLE had a total of 117 pregnancies. Of this group of 54 patients, seven were postmenopausal at the time of the onset of their illness and pregnancies in the remote past were not thought to have any bearing on the course of their disease. Twenty-seven of the 54 patients had no new pregnancy after the diagnosis of the disease; some of these were adolescents or unmarried women. Twenty-six of the 54 patients had a total of 36 pregnancies after the diagnosis of SLE had been made. Nineteen of these pregnancies resulted in normal full-term spontaneous deliveries with only minimal evidence of adverse effect on either mother or infant. Several of the infants born of these full-term pregnancies died of unrelated causes, and autopsy examination revealed no evidence that exposure to mothers with high titers of circulating abnormal proteins during the pregnancy resulted in lesions resembling that of SLE. This may be interpreted to suggest that the "antibodies" against nuclear products may well have nothing to do with the pathogenesis of the disease. Ten pregnancies terminated in spontaneous abortions and there were six stillbirths.

In consideration of the advisability of advising termination of pregnancy in a patient with SLE, it becomes apparent that the clinical course of any given pregnant patient is quite impossible to predict. In the Presbyterian Hospital series, three patients were made definitely worse during pregnancy and two had the acute onset of their disease during the course of pregnancy. Of some interest is the fact that three patients were without unusual complaints during pregnancy but had severe flare-ups of their disease in the immediate postpartum period. Six of the patients had more than one pregnancy after the diagnosis of SLE had been established. One patient had five pregnancies after the onset of her disease; she had reactions ranging from complete remissions to severe recurrences of her complaints during the course of the pregnancies. It should be noted that one patient went through an entirely normal pregnancy well after the onset of the nephrotic syndrome due to SLE.

In an examination of the causes of death of patients with SLE, it becomes apparent that it is frequently impossible to assign a single cause. Although patients may have involvement of several organ systems, no one area seems to be seriously enough involved to be responsible for death. More than one-quarter of the patients died of undetermined causes from a clinical point of view, and approximately 10 per cent died of causes which could not be established at autopsy examination. However, the importance of the renal lesions in the course of SLE was emphasized by the fact that more than 20 per cent of the patients died as a result of kidney damage in spite of the use of high dosages of steroids in many instances. The presence of congestive heart failure would appear to be of equal importance as a cause of death.

When it appears, it is usually relatively refractive to the usual measures directed against it. The role of high dosage of steroids in these instances is uncertain. Perhaps of greatest practical importance was the appearance of infections as a major cause of death among patients with SLE. Almost all of these patients were on high dosage of steroids, and in some instances the presence of an infection was not suspected clinically. This emphasizes the importance of reserving steroid therapy for life-threatening situations and the withholding of such therapy in the treatment of minor complaints.

SUMMARY

In summary, it would seem that the incidence of SLE is increasing both relatively and absolutely. The natural history of the disease is such that it frequently exceeds 20 years, and the correct diagnosis is often delayed for a discouragingly long time. The relation between rheumatoid arthritis and SLE has not been clarified, but there seem to be clinical and serologic features which suggest that they may have pathogenetic features in common. Splenectomy does not appear to be particularly effective in treating the thrombocytopenia of SLE, and there is little correlation between the histologic appearance of the spleen and the clinical result of the procedure. Among adult women, SLE has been shown to be a major cause of the nephrotic syndrome. Although neuropsychiatric manifestations are common in SLE, there is poor correlation between these symptoms and pathologic abnormalities in the central nervous system. The fertility of patients with SLE appears to be unimpaired and there is a greater than 50 per cent chance of any one given pregnancy coming to term; however, the clinical course in a given case is impossible to predict. Renal disease and the appearance of congestive heart failure appear to be among the most common causes of death among those patients with SLE in whom a cause of death can be ascribed. Of equal importance is the fact that many patients die of infections; these are usually associated with adrenal steroid therapy and in some instances have gone unrecognized clinically.

Immunological Manifestations
in a Group of Patients
with Discoid Lupus Erythematosus*

J. CLAUDE BENNETT, LAMAR S. OSMENT and
HOWARD L. HOLLEY

Medical College of Alabama

Opinions about discoid lupus erythematous have changed considerably since the original description in 1827. Scott and Rees feel that discoid lupus is entirely mucocutaneous,[19] as does Baehr.[2] Others have felt that the systemic form represents a more advanced pathologic process or that the skin manifestations of discoid lupus represent only one phase of an underlying generalized process.[5, 12] Certainly, patients with discoid lupus often have vague systemic symptoms or signs such as unexplained fever, arthralgia and easy fatigability. Five per cent of patients ultimately having systemic lupus erythematosus (SLE) show only cutaneous lesions for long periods of time. On the other hand, many patients note disappearance of discoid skin lesions and never show any clinical or pathological evidence of lupus after many years.

Positive serological tests for syphilis in both discoid lupus and systemic lupus have been reported.[17] In addition, the Coombs test is frequently positive. However, the percentage of serological abnormalities is higher in the clinically systemic disease than in the localized variety. The term subacute disseminated lupus has been suggested for discoid lupus exhibiting only minor systemic manifestations.

It is entirely possible that the previously used indicators (STS and Coombs test) were not sufficiently sensitive to consistently detect the subtle changes that may have been present. Many new serological methods are now being used to detect the abnormalities associated with not only systemic lupus but also rheumatic fever, scleroderma and other "collagen diseases." These tests are usually in no way specific for any one entity. When they are performed as a battery on patients with various types of "collagen diseases," overlapping of positive results can often be noted. However, each specific condition occupies a rather constant band of the spectrum of laboratory tests. It is entirely possible that all of these tests indicate autoimmune reactions to cellular material, both nucleus and cytoplasm. Evidently, reactive globulins to many cellular constituents may be formed.

The purpose of this paper is to correlate the clinical and laboratory manifestations in a group of patients with discoid lupus with the various newer immunological parameters used to study systemic lupus.[1, 13]

SELECTION OF PATIENTS

Seventeen patients were chosen at random for study. They had had

* This work has been supported by a grant from the National Institutes of Health, (USPH A-3555) and the John R. Irby Fund for the Study of Arthritis.
A portion of this work has been submitted for publication elsewhere.

clinical and histological lesions consistent with discoid lupus for a period of two or more years.

METHODS

Each patient underwent re-evaluation by means of a complete history and physical examination. As laboratory indicators of general health the following studies were routinely done: hematocrit, white blood cell count, indirect platelet count, prothrombin time, whole blood clotting time, blood urea nitrogen, and serum albumin and globulin.

As special indicators of "collagen disease," the following tests were routinely performed: L.E. cell preparations,[14] latex fixation reactions,[20] aggregated gamma globulin precipitations,[8,9] deoxyribonucleic acid (DNA) precipitations,[6] DNA complement fixations,[16,18] the Wassermann test and the Coombs test. Intradermal tests for hypersensitivity were done on each patient with saline-washed homologous leukocytes.[4]

Latex Fixation Reaction.   The latex fixation reaction was performed according to the method of Singer and Plotz, using pooled fraction II human globulin.[14]

Aggregated Gamma Globulin Precipitation Reaction.   Another reaction with a diagnostic relationship to rheumatoid arthritis, but positive in other "collagen diseases," is also apparently dependent on the presence of the "rheumatoid factor."[8,9] Direct precipitation of rheumatoid factor with gamma globulin occurs if the latter has been aggregated by heating at 63° C. for ten minutes or until the solution turns milky white. In our laboratory capillary tubes were prepared with equal parts of the test serum and aggregated gamma globulin. They were observed for particulate matter after standing at room temperature for 30 minutes and overnight.

DNA Precipitation Reaction.   Deicher and his associates have described a precipitive reaction between DNA (deoxyribonucleic acid) and a serum factor in systemic lupus.[6] In our laboratory this procedure was modified for use in capillary tubes. Salmon sperm DNA* was dissolved to 0.5 mg./ml. in 0.15 M sodium chloride. To each serum, in a capillary tube, after inactivation at 56° C. for 30 minutes, an equal volume of the DNA solution was added. Every serum specimen was also reacted with DNA plus deoxyribonuclease (DNase) and DNase activated, using the method of Feinstein by adding magnesium and calcium ions.[10] The final concentration of DNA was the same in each reaction. After all solutions were adjusted to pH 7.6, by buffer, the reactions containing enzyme were allowed to proceed for 15 minutes at 25° C., at which time the test serum was added. The reactions were continued at 25° C. and were read at 30 minutes and 16 hours. Flocculant precipitates appeared in positive DNA reactions. Several normal, rheumatoid and systemic L.E. sera were simultaneously run as controls.

Complement Fixation Reaction.   Complement fixation tests using DNA at a concentration of 0.5 mg./ml. as the antigen were performed according to current methods.[16,18] Five known positive SLE sera were tested simultaneously as a control for accuracy of technique.

Leukocyte Skin Test.   Skin tests, employing the intradermal injection of homologous leukocytes as previously reported from this laboratory,[4] were done on each patient. They were read at 24 hours post injection and were considered positive if at least 5 mm. of induration could be detected. Erythema alone was not considered to constitute a positive reaction.

---

* Obtained from Mann Research Laboratories, Inc., New York, N. Y.

TABLE 1. *IMMUNOLOGICAL REACTIONS AMONG 17 PATIENTS WITH DISCOID L.E.*

PATIENTS	SERUM GLOBULIN	WASSERMANN (STS)	COOMBS TEST	LE PREP	SLE SKIN TEST	LATEX FIXATION	AGGREGATED GLOBULIN ½ hr.	AGGREGATED PPTN. 16 hr.	DNA COMPLEMENT FIXATION	DNA PPTN.	DNA + DNAse PPTN.
I. (N. A.)	3.0 Gm%	0	0	++	0	0	0	+	0	+	0
II. (R. B.)	3.5	0	0	0	0	0	0	+	0	0	0
III. (M. C.)	4.7	0	+	0	0	1:10,240	0	0	0	+	0
IV. (F. D.)	7.4	0	0	0	0	0	+	+++	0	+	0
V. (M. H.)	4.0	0	0	0	0	0	+	++	0	weak +	0
VI. (J. H.)	2.5	0	0	0	+	0	+	++	0	0	0
VII. (E. J.)	3.7	0	0	0	0	0	0	0	0	0	0
VIII. (F. K.)	3.6	0	0	0	0	0	0	0	0	+	0
IX. (B. J. L.)	3.9	0	0	0	0	0	0	0	0	+	0
X. (E. L.)	·	0	0	0	0	0	0	0	0	0	0
XI. (J. Mc.)	4.6	0	0	0	0	1:640	0	0	0	0	0
XII. (W. C. M.)	3.3	0	0	0	0	1:2560	0	0	0	0	0
XIII. (M. P.)	4.0	0	0	0	0	0	+	++	0	+	0
XIV. (A. R.)	4.0	0	0	0	0	0	0	+	0	+	0
XV. (A. L. T.)	3.5	0	0	0	0	0	+	+	0	+	0
XVI. (A. T.)	5.1	+	+	+	+	0	+	+	0	+	0
XVII. (W. C. W.)	2.1	0	0	0	+	1:10,240	0	+	0	weak +	0

RESULTS

Detailed questioning of the 17 patients with discoid lupus revealed the following symptoms: Two patients (IV and XVI) reported significant fever as part of the illness. Three patients (III, IV and XI) had noted weight loss following anorexia. Two patients (XV and XVII) had pain and limitation of joint mobility. Two (IX and XVII) had noted drug reactions to penicillin and one (XVI) to a sulfonamide. Patient No. II gave a history of rheumatic fever as a child.

Abnormal physical findings were few. One patient (IV) had active synovitis of the proximal interphalangeal joints and a second (XVII) had chronic deforming rheumatoid arthritis. Two (V and XI) had hypertensive cardiovascular disease with Grade II eyeground changes. In one (XV) the skin lesions of discoid lupus were generalized. No patient was found to have enlargement of lymphoid tissues, neurological abnormalities or pulmonary involvement.

All of the patients had skin biopsies which were compatible with discoid lupus. Keratin plugs were noted in follicles. A perivascular infiltrate of round cells was noted in the corium underlying areas of liquefactive basal cell layer degeneration.

The abnormal laboratory findings are detailed in Table 1. The sedimentation rates were elevated in 13 instances. This seems without special significance, since this test is almost always elevated in a variety of dermatoses seen in this clinic.[15] Leukocyte counts above 10,000 were noted in three patients (I, IV and XIV) and below 5000 in five (Nos. V, VI, XI, XIII and XV). Four patients were slightly anemic as measured by the packed cell volume determination (III, IV, XV and XVI). Four with platelet counts below 200,000 were found (III, XII, XIV and XVI). Three patients had blood urea nitrogen values above 20, but none were above 24 (III, XVI and XVII). No patient had a clotting time above ten minutes. Two had prothrombin activity of 60 per cent (IV and XV).

Serum globulin levels of greater than 3.5 gm. per cent were present in ten patients and two of these were above 5.0 gm. per cent (IV and XVI). Only one (XVI) had a positive Wassermann reaction and two (III and XVI) had positive Coombs tests. Of two patients with positive L.E. cell preparations (I and XVI) one had noted a paucity of symptoms (I). Three had delayed positive intradermal skin tests to homologous leukocytes (VI, XVI and XVII). The latex fixation test was reactive in four patients (III, XI, XII and XVII). Aggregated gamma globulin was precipitated after reacting overnight with the sera of nine discoid lupus patients. None of the sera fixed complement with DNA. Ten of the sera developed a precipitin with DNA. This was inhibited by prior treatment of DNA with DNase.

DISCUSSION

Du Bois and Martel,[7] in a series of 41 discoid lupus patients, found that 96 per cent had clinical and laboratory findings associated with systemic lupus.

Three of the patients in our series (III, IV, and XVI) had symptoms and physical findings which would suggest a diagnosis of systemic lupus, but only one of these (XVI) had a positive L.E. cell preparation. None of the other 14 patients warranted a diagnosis of systemic lupus at the time of this study. However, only three patients had completely negative serological responses, which is a considerably higher percentage than would be found in a comparable normal group.

In this study, the precipitation of sera with DNA was found to occur with greatest frequency, while no complement fixation using DNA as the antigen was observed. This discrepancy remains to be explained, since it is not noted in systemic lupus.

Several of our patients had sera which reacted with gamma globulin (aggregated gamma globulin precipitation and latex fixation). This has also been found in systemic lupus.[3, 21] Such phenomena may be the result of qualitative or quantitative protein abnormalities.[11]

All except two of the patients having positive DNA precipitation tests had other abnormal serologic reactions as well. This suggests that the DNA precipitation test offers a means of estimating the extent of the systemic pathologic process in patients with lupus erythematosus.

These data have not yet revealed any serologic pattern which would be indicative of impending onset of systemic involvement in discoid lupus. However, the data do indicate that a significant number of discoid lupus patients have serological manifestations characteristic of systemic lupus.

SUMMARY

Seventeen patients with discoid lupus were subjected to intensive study, including several serological tests currently used to detect systemic lupus. After evaluation of symptoms, physical findings and routine and special laboratory results, three patients were considered to have systemic lupus. Eleven of the remaining 14 demonstrated one or more abnormal serological tests. The data seem to indicate that patients formerly considered to have only discoid lupus may actually have subtle immunological manifestations of systemic lupus.

ACKNOWLEDGMENT

The authors wish to thank Mrs. Merry Lynne Johnston and Mrs. Mary Alexander for their valuable technical assistance.

REFERENCES

1. Asherson, G. L.: Antibodies against nuclear and cytoplasmic cell constituents in systemic lupus erythematosus and other diseases. Brit. J. Exper. Path., *40*:209, 1959.
2. Baehr, G.: Diseases of collagen. In Cecil, R. L. and Loeb, R. F. (eds.): A Textbook of Medicine. Philadelphia, W. B. Saunders Company, 1951, p. 483.
3. Bartfeld, H.: Incidence and significance of seropositive tests for rheumatoid factor in non-rheumatoid diseases. Ann. Int. Med., *52*:1059, 1960.
4. Bennett, J. C. and Holley, H. L.: Intradermal hypersensitivity in systemic lupus erythematosus. Arth. & Rheum., *4*:64, 1961. Presented in part at the 1960 meeting, Amer. Rheum. Assoc., Miami.
5. Csermely, E.: Gior. Ital. Dermat., *99*:513-561, 1958. Abstracted in Year Book of Dermatology, 1959-1960. Chicago, The Year Book Publishers, Inc., 1960 p. 228.
6. Deicher, H. R. G., Holman, H. R. and Kunkel, H. G.: The precipitin reaction between DNA and a serum factor in systemic lupus erythematosus. J. Exper. Med., *109*:97, 1959.
7. Dubois, E. L. and Martel, S.: Discoid lupus erythematosus: an analysis of its systemic manifestations. Ann. Int. Med., *44*:482, 1956.
8. Edelman, G. M., Kunkel, H. G. and Franklin, E. C.: Interaction of the rheumatoid factor with antigen-antibody complexes and aggregated gamma globulin. J. Exper. Med., *108*:105, 1958.

9. Epstein, W., Johnson, A. and Ragan, C.: Observations on a precipitin reaction between serum of patients with rheumatoid arthritis and a preparation (Cohn fraction 11) of human gamma globulin. Proc. Soc. Exper. Biol. & Med., 91:235, 1956.
10. Feinstein, R. N.: Activation of the neutral deoxyribonuclease. J. Biol. Chem., 235: 733, 1960.
11. Kunkel, H. G.: Immunologic aspects of rheumatoid arthritis. J. Chron. Dis., 10:418, 1959.
12. Kushniruk, W.: Systemic involvement in chronic lupus erythematosus. Canad. M. A. J., 76:184-193, 1957.
13. Miescher, P.: The antigenic constituents of the neutrophilic leukocyte with special reference to the L. E. phenomenon. Vox Sang., 2:145, 1957.
14. Miescher, P. and Strassle, R.: New serological methods for the detection of the L. E. factor. Vox Sang., 2:283, 1957.
15. Osment, L. S.: The C-reactive protein test in dermatology. South. M. J., 51:746, 1958.
16. Pearson, C. M., Craddock, C. G. and Simmons, N. S.: Complement fixation reactions with DNA and leukocyte material in systemic lupus erythematosus. J. Lab. & Clin. Med., 52:580, 1958.
17. Rein, C. R. and Kostant, G. H.: Lupus erythematosus: serologic and chemical aspects. Arch. Dermat. & Syph., 61:898, 1950.
18. Robbins, W. C., Holman, H. R., Deicher, H. and Kunkel, H. G.: Complement fixation with cell nuclei and DNA in lupus erythematosus. Proc. Soc. Exper. Biol. & Med., 96:575, 1957.
19. Scott, A. and Rees, E. G.: The relationship of systemic lupus erythematosus and discoid lupus erythematosus. A.M.A. Arch. Dermat., 79:422, 1959.
20. Singer, J. M. and Plotz, G. M.: The latex fixation test. I. Application to the serologic diagnosis of rheumatoid arthritis. Am. J. Med., 21:888, 1956.
21. Vaughan, J. H.: Serum responses in rheumatoid arthritis. Am. J. Med., 26:596, 1959.

Hydralazine Lupus Syndrome

PHILLIP COMENS

Washington University School of Medicine

Hydralazine hydrochloride (1-hydrazinophthalazine, Apresoline), an antihypertensive agent, has been used widely since 1951, either alone or in combination with other drugs, for the treatment of essential hypertension.[24, 30] Reports indicate that 10 to 12 per cent of patients being treated with this unique and reactive drug develop a collagen-like syndrome, clinically and pathologically indistinguishable from disseminated lupus erythematosus.[14, 26, 28, 29] The syndrome has been variously called the lupoid syndrome, hydralazine lupus syndrome and hydralazine poisoning, intoxication or toxicity, as well as by many other terms.

Little is known concerning the metabolism of hydralazine or its exact mechanism of action. The known chemical and pharmacological actions, as well as the side effects, are summarized in Table 1, part A. Among the more interesting actions of hydralazine, as a chemical, is its ability to form a stable chelate with certain trace minerals and to act as an anti-enzyme for several biological systems.[31] Pharmacologically, it increases renal blood flow, lowers blood pressure, depresses constricted vascular smooth muscle and abolishes the pressor response to norepinephrine. The more common side

TABLE 1.

A. ACTIONS OF HYDRALAZINE (APRESOLINE)

CHEMICAL ACTIONS	PHARMACOLOGICAL ACTIONS	SIDE EFFECTS
Binds transition metals	Depresses constricted vascular smooth muscle	Palpitation and tachycardia
Inhibits biological acetylation of hexosamines.	Lowers blood pressure	Nasal congestion
Anti-enzyme for histaminase	Abolishes pressor response to norepinephrine	Flu-like symptoms
Reacts with sulfhydryl compounds	Acts like an antihistaminase	Hypertensive headaches
Reagent for carbonyl groups	Increases cardiac output	Tingling and numbness
Neutralizes pherentasin	Increases renal blood flow	Lassitude and weakness
Reacts with glucose and ninhydrin	Glomerular filtration fraction decreased	Generalized edema
	Splanchnic vascular resistance decreased	Diencephalic flush
	Lowers blood cholesterol	Angina pectoris
		Skin eruption

B. VARIOUS FINDINGS IN THE HYDRALAZINE-LUPUS SYNDROME

SIGNS AND SYMPTOMS	LABORATORY TESTS	PATHOLOGY
Normal blood pressure	Positive cephalin-cholesterol flocculation	"Wire-loop" lesions of kidneys
Arthritis	Positive L. E. preparations	Interstitial polymyositis
Fever	Anemia	Muscle lymphorrhagia
Hepatosplenomegaly	Leukopenia	Acute collagenous necrosis of skin; subcutaneous nodules
Skin rash and purpura	Thrombocytopenia	"Onion-peel" lesions of spleen
Weight loss	Elevated sedimentation rate	
Myalgia and polyneuritis	Albuminuria	
Chest and abdominal pain	Hematuria	
Glossodynia	Increased serum globulin level	
Gastrointestinal bleeding	Low serum albumin level	
Depression and psychosis	Positive serologic test for syphilis	
Lymphadenopathy	Abnormal urinary sediment	
Subcutaneous nodules	Altered electrophoretic pattern	

effects of the drug noted on initial administration are tachycardia, headache and anxiety. These are attributed to the effect on the cardiovascular system by histamine-like substances[20] probably due to the antihistaminase action of hydralazine. Many of these symptoms can be controlled by administration of barbiturates or antihistamines; more commonly, by withdrawal of the drug and reinstitution at lower dosage, effects such as these are frequently by-passed. There is no evidence to date to suggest that those who experience these initial side effects are any more prone to develop the hydralazine-lupus syndrome than others receiving the drug.

Originally, only a small percentage of the orally administered dose could be recovered in the urine, partially bound to sulfhydryl radicals.[25] In a recent study[5] the author used single subcutaneous injections of hydralazine tagged in the one position with C^{14} to explore the fate of the compound in normal mice as well as in a few mice chronically receiving hydralazine or manganese. The kidneys were demonstrated to be the probable and primary pathway of excretion.

Because of the striking similarity of this iatrogenically produced disease to disseminated lupus in man, attempts are being made to determine the

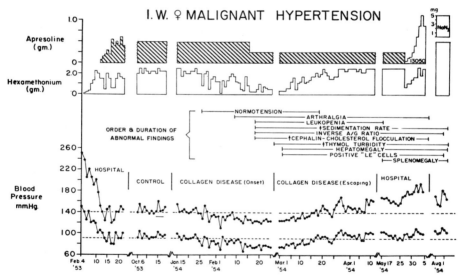

Fig. 1.   Temporal relations of blood pressure, treatment, physical and laboratory findings in a typical case of hydralazine disease. 13050 and NaN3 are experimental antihypertensive drugs unrelated to hydralazine.

etiological factors in an effort to understand the naturally occurring disease. Answers to several questions become of paramount interest: (1) Is this syndrome the same as naturally occurring lupus? (2) What type of reaction is hydralazine disease? (3) What are the long-term effects of hydralazine administration?

Clinical and laboratory findings in hydralazine disease are similar to those of disseminated lupus in their frequency of occurrence.[6] Figure 1 illustrates a typical case of the hydralazine-lupus syndrome in a patient with malignant hypertension who received the drug as antihypertensive therapy over an 18-month period. Only the more common findings are presented, since the clinical picture and the pathological involvement may be as variable as in true disseminated lupus (Table 1, part *B*). The syndrome appears to develop most commonly as the diastolic pressure falls, usually after approximately 16 months of hydralazine treatment and usually in those patients receiving 500 mg. per day or more. However, the syndrome has occurred as early as three weeks after starting therapy and with a dose of only 100 mg. per day of hydralazine;[26] conversely, it has occurred as late as 6½ years after the start of continuous hydralazine therapy. Early, the syndrome may resemble rheumatoid arthritis, but if hydralazine is continued, the lupus syndrome supervenes. When the syndrome is "full-blown," the patient may present any or all of the findings listed in Table 1, part *B*. Pathological studies reveal the same fibrinoid degenerative changes in the skin and typical "wire-loop" lesions of the glomeruli.[1] Patients with hydralazine disease may also manifest a false biologically positive test for syphilis.

Although all patients appear to have complete remissions clinically upon cessation or reduction of hydralazine therapy, L.E. smears may remain positive for as long as one year following discontinuation of the drug, and the syndrome has been reported to persist as long as three to seven years after discontinuation of the drug.[19] Reinstitution of therapy with as little as 150 mg. has been noted to cause a recrudescence of the disease within 24 hours in a small percentage of patients.[34] One wonders whether this represents a recurrence of the reaction or whether in such patients the reaction smolders in a subclinical state. Previous work by the author and others has shown that some 10 per cent of all patients receiving hydralazine, even though they are asymptomatic, may exhibit suspicious L.E. smears.[8] Many patients with abnormal laboratory findings do not develop the syndrome clinically because the dosage of hydralazine is reduced as soon as abnormal tests are noted. Bendersky[1] reported a case in which the patient had a massive intestinal hemorrhage while on hydralazine therapy and yet developed no fever, arthralgia or other evidence of hydralazine intoxication. Postmortem findings revealed "wire-loop" changes in the kidneys and vascular fibrinoid changes in the intestinal wall. There was no evidence to indicate that the patient had malignant hypertension. Others have also reported intestinal bleeding as a result of hydralazine administration.[11] The development of such a syndrome as a complication of hydralazine therapy has aroused considerable interest as a possible means of shedding light upon the pathogenesis of disseminated lupus.

The author has produced the counterpart of this syndrome in dogs by oral administration of hydralazine approaching the maximum human therapeutic dose. These animals showed clinical, laboratory and pathological findings resembling those of systemic lupus.[4] The work has been confirmed by other investigators.[16] Attempts were made by Siguier et al. of Paris to reproduce the syndrome by administering hydralazine to guinea pigs.[33] In 10 of the animals, L.E. cells appeared in the blood, and the accompanying disease proved fatal in two to four months.

Some important differences between hydralazine disease and disseminated lupus as pointed out by other authors[21] are the reversibility or apparent reversibility of the hydralazine syndrome, lack of preponderance in females and the paucity of urinary findings such as hematuria, cylinduria and proteinuria. However, investigational studies presented here suggest that the syndrome is not reversible but merely quiescent. Two other points suggesting a closer association of hydralazine disease and lupus are: (1) The serum of patients with hydralazine disease, as well as sera of hydralazine-fed dogs, reacts in a manner similar to that of lupus patients by the fluorescent tagging antibody technique of Friou.[15] (2) Although it is not specific for lupus, results of the Jones-Thompson test upon the sera of patients receiving hydralazine are similar to those on sera of patients with a known collagen disease.[7]

Is the syndrome one of hypersensitivity, depletion, or dietary inadequacy? The disease is most commonly thought to be due to hypersensitivity or allergic reactions of various types. It has also been called a toxic reaction.

To distinguish allergic from nonallergic drug reactions, the manifestations of the reaction must be different from the pharmacodynamic effects of the drug, withdrawal of the drug must produce remission of the manifestations, and minute amounts of the drug should cause a prompt exacerbation of the symptoms of hypersensitivity.[25] In hydralazine disease the syndrome occurs in patients not receiving a sensitizing dose, and in other instances, patients may be able to resume the drug at lowered dosages without production of symptoms. Usually patients with the history of drug sensitivity present a history of other allergic diseases or manifestations. If hydralazine disease is a drug sensitivity reaction, certainly those patients manifesting the hydralazine syndrome rarely exhibit any other history of allergy or hypersensitivity.

The question of toxicity in contrast to hypersensitivity has been raised. A toxic reaction is rarely manifest after the drug is stopped and rarely immediately when the drug is restarted;[35] in true allergy, occurrence of the reaction is late or onset may follow immediately with institution of the second course. In toxicity there is repetition of the reaction on re-exposure to the drug, but with greater than therapeutic dosages. Case reports indicate that the hydralazine syndrome may have its onset after the drug is discontinued,[32] and a recrudescence may occur within 24 hours with as little as a 150 mg.

Dubois et al. have suggested that the arthralgia and other early symptoms of the syndrome may be a serum sickness type of reaction and that possibly those patients with the hydralazine-lupus syndrome are patients with latent lupus and a superimposed serum sickness reaction.[13] It would be strange indeed if 10 per cent of all hypertensive patients on hydralazine had latent lupus erythematosus. Many, like ourselves, have done pretreatment laboratory studies without finding significant abnormalities. Dustan et al.[14] reported transient pulmonary consolidations in two patients similar to those found in animals killed by experimental serum sickness[15] and similar to those found in association with bronchial asthma, angioneurotic edema and periarteritis nodosa.[18] With the exception of the long incubation period associated with hydralazine disease and the frequent failure to induce a marked exacerbation of symptoms with the second course of therapy, a serum sickness type of reaction remains a possibility.

Some think disseminated lupus may be an expression of an altered state of protein sensitivity or an auto-immune reaction.[10] This concept is supported by the fact that the various diagnostic serological tests used for lupus erythematosus have also given positive results in patients with hypersensitivity and serum sickness reactions. They believe that hydralazine combines with proteins, producing an antigenic complex which in turn results in the formation of specific antibodies. The resulting antigen-antibody conflict would explain the rapid clinical relapses that often take place when the administration of the drug is resumed in patients sensitized by previous treatment. The excellent response of patients with lupus to therapy with corticosteroids is regarded as further support of the hypersensitivity concept.

The dietary theory suggesting deficient intake or disturbed metabolism of some vitamin or mineral seems a likely possibility. We have seen a patient with the syndrome, despite continued hydralazine therapy in the hospital, obtain marked relief with disappearance of the signs and symptoms. Upon returning home, he would again manifest the "full blown syndrome." This is compatible with a dietary change or a deficiency state.

Pyridoxine deficiency in hydralazine disease has been investigated by several workers.[2, 20, 23] Mellinkoff et al. injected rats with 40 mg. of hydralazine per kilogram, which proved a fatal convulsive dose.[22] Pyridoxine had no apparent effect in inhibiting the convulsions; however, a high carbohydrate diet lowered and a high fat diet raised the resistance of white rats to such acute hydralazine intoxication. It is well known that vitamin B_6 is necessary for the intracerebral transamination that produces γ-aminobutyric acid.[2] Even though a definite excess of vitamin B_6 was given, these mice showed no changes in γ-aminobutyric acid levels. Kirkendall and Page[20] suggest that the peripheral neuritis in hydralazine disease is caused possibly by interference with pyridoxine metabolism. They observed favorable results with the administration of intramuscular pyridoxine. However, the hydralazine was discontinued long before improvement was noted. Since the patient actually had been off hydralazine for a period of 14 days, improvement would be expected with or without the pyridoxine. We have given large doses of vitamin B_6 to two patients with the hydralazine syndrome without discontinuation of the hydralazine and noted, not improvement, but a questionable increase in symptoms. The patients also do not manifest the usual findings seen in experimentally induced pyridoxine deficiency. These results, while not conclusive, certainly fail to add strength to the theory that pyridoxine deficiency is an etiological agent of hydralazine disease.

The possibility of depletion of some substance is an interesting area for speculation in regard to the etiology of hydralazine disease, whether this be an absolute depletion of some substance such as a trace mineral or a relative depletion produced by blocking the action of an effective material or the enzyme system involved. Because hydralazine is a potentially good chelating agent, studies of its possible relationship to trace metals were undertaken by the author. Of several metals investigated, manganese was the most interesting, since it appeared to protect rats from single lethal doses of parenteral hydralazine and chicks from joint abnormalities (perosis) which usually occur after 6 weeks of hydralazine feeding.[5] In addition, some of the changes which occurred in dogs fed hydralazine for six months were reversed, at least partially, by subsequent manganese administration. In animals receiving hydralazine for 18 months without manganese supplements the renal lesions were similar to but no more advanced than those found in dogs after nine months of hydralazine feeding, showing apparently that once a certain stage of destruction and change occurred, a static state existed with no further progression of the lesion. On the other hand, dogs in which hydralazine feeding was discontinued after nine months and nothing was given for the next nine months or in which hydralazine was discontinued after nine months and manganese was given for the ensuing nine months showed considerable improvement in the renal lesions at the 18-month biopsy period. (Results of a similar study on dogs undergoing three-month periods of treatment are

TABLE 2. INFLUENCE OF THE MANGANOUS ION ON THE COURSE OF HYDRALAZINE DISEASE IN THE DOG

DOG NO.	MEDICATION	WT.	WBC	Hb	CHOL	ALK. PH.	*L.E.	ALB.	GLOB.	Mn/Na	**GLOM.	TUBULES
1	Control	31	10	16.8	68	.62	—	51.9	48.1	.16	N	N
	Hydral. – 3.5	33	5.8	16.6	49	.38	S	62.5	37.5	.26	1+	N
	Hydr. + Mn. 60 mg.	28	7.8	14.7	65	.13	—	52.1	47.9	.15	1+	N
2	Control	31	11.7	15	68	.82	—	51.6	48.4	.19	N	N
	Hydral. – 7 mg.	24	10.1	10.1	51	.33	+	64.7	35.3	.19	2+	1+
	Hydr. + Mn. 120	26	10.4	14	60	.30	S	44.7	55.3	.12	1+	1+
3	Control	29	13	14	86	.76	—	41.7	58.3	.15	N	N
	Hydr. – 3.5 mg.	37	11	14	68	.30	S	55.9	44.1	.30	3+	1+
	Mn. – 60 mg.	37	11	13	87	.39	—	51.8	48.2	.70	N	+
4	Control	52	8.8	17	75	.40	—	40.9	59.1	.15	N	N
	Hydro. – 7 mg.	48	4.8	10	71	.19	+	51.8	48.2	.15	2+	1+
	Mn. – 120 mg.	38	6.6	15	63	.28	—	48.9	51.1	.5	1+	0
5	Control	29	13	15	89	.5	—	47.8	52.2	.19	N	N
	Hydr. – 3.5 mg.	25	20	11	101	.22	S	45.9	54.1	.28	2+	1+
	Hydr. – 3.5 mg.	23	12	10	49	.33	S	22.4	77.6	.24	2+	1+
6	Control	32	11	14	64	.54	—	44.6	55.4	.16	N	N
	Hydr. – 7 mg.	30	6.8	11	67	.26	+	41.5	58.5	.31	1+	N
	Hydr. – 7 mg.	29	6.4	9	50	.17	+	28.9	71.1	.24	2+	1+
7, 9	Control	28	10	15	82	.63	—	45.5	54.5	.15	N	N
	Control	29	9.6	15	77	.60	—	46.7	53.3	.17	N	N
8, 10	Control	29	9.6	14	75	.65	—	48.0	52.0	.15	N	N
	Control	32	8.3	15	68	.62	—	50.2	49.8	.19	N	N
	Control	34	9.6	15	78	.62	—	51.6	48.4	.20	N	N
	Mn. – 60 & 120	36	10	15	111	.49	—	53.3	46.7	.50	N	N

* S = suspicious (less than 3 typical cells per smear)
** Abnormal renal pathology; on basis of severity 0—4+
N.B. The duration of each period of treatment with the medication indicated was 3 months.

shown in Table 2.) The studies on chicks as well as those on rats demonstrating the inhibition of hydralazine-induced convulsions by manganese tend to suggest that the manganese may be chelating the hydralazine, thereby decreasing the effective amount available to produce convulsions or perosis; but the subsequent dog studies, as well as the isotope studies, suggest the manganese ion to be more deeply involved.

Preliminary studies using isotopically labeled hydralazine in animals were recently presented by the author.[5] Several tissue concentration curves are

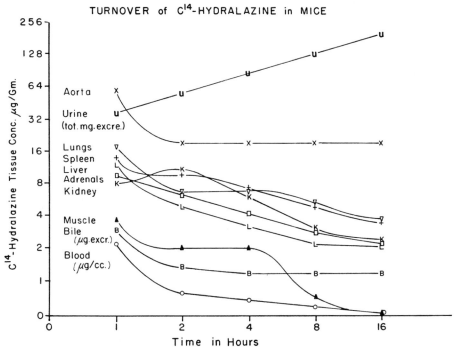

Fig. 2.   The mean concentrations of C[14]-hydralazine in the tissues of 5 pairs of mice at successively doubled intervals after subcutaneous injection. The total amounts present in the urine and bile also are indicated. Blood and brain curves were nearly identical.

shown in Figure 2. Why the aorta retains so much more labeled hydralazine than the other tissues is difficult to understand; the aorta retains approximately three times as much hydralazine 16 hours after injection when the animals are pre-fed with manganese, but pre-feeding with carrier hydralazine seems to have little or no effect. This certainly suggests something more than a casual relationship between manganese and hydralazine. If this is true, it should also be noted that other investigators have shown that manganese is lost from the body of the rodent at 13 to 16 hours after administration and that recent isotope studies by the author reveal a precipitous drop in hydralazine retention by the aorta after the 16-hour period. Recent studies by Cotzias have shown that the manganese pathway in the human is altered by the administration of hydralazine.[9] The presumed enzyme-blocking action of gold in patients with rheumatoid arthritis may be somewhat parallel to giving manganese with possible reversal of the hydralazine syndrome. Because of these findings, the effect of orally administered manganese to patients with lupus erythematosus and hydralazine disease was studied. Figure 3 illustrates results in one patient with the hydralazine-lupus syndrome so treated.

Another theory suggests that the hydralazine syndrome may be due to altered midbrain function, primarily because both the emotional control of hypertensive patients as well as the hypotensive action of hydralazine may be mediated via the midbrain. The actions of hydralazine have been closely compared to those of reserpine on the midbrain. It is also postulated that the lowering of the diastolic pressure indicates that hydralazine has blocked

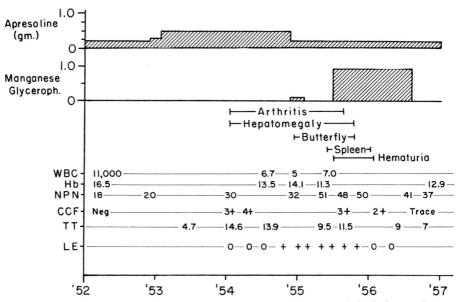

Fig. 3. The clinical and hematological picture in one patient with hydralazine disease before and after the administration of oral doses of manganese glycerophosphate.

the abnormal efferent neural discharges to the brain which cause hypertension.[21] It has been shown that after reaching the blood stream, manganese has a predilection for certain nerve cells at the base of the brain. It has been established as well that reserpine affects the excretion of norepinephrine and epinephrine from the walls of the vascular tissue or in some way blocks the activity of these catechol amines. Hydralazine may work in the same manner. When hydralazine is injected intravenously or intra-arterially, a two-phase drop in the blood pressure is noted. One phase may be the central action on the midbrain, and the second may be a local action of the hydralazine on the arterial wall itself. This would offer some explanation of the dual action of the drug as well as its known local vasodilator properties. The results when the isotopically labeled drug was used certainly suggest a local action in the vascular walls. Radiographic studies now under way may help clarify the answer.

Hydralazine has been shown to block the acetylation of glucosamine,[12] thereby preventing its utilization. Boas and Soffer,[3] as well as others, reported that the serum content of hexosamine and mucoprotein were frequently increased in lupus. Manganese may be chelating the hydralazine, allowing competitive acetylation to progress, producing a tendency to reverse the syndrome of intoxication. We have seen patients with proved pheochromocytoma who were resistant to Regitine respond very nicely to doses of hydralazine. This would certainly tend to suggest a local vasodilatory property of hydralazine as well as to suggest that the primary site of its action is intra-arterial.

A review of the possible etiological factors involved in the production of the hydralazine-lupus syndrome has done little more than to exemplify the fact that, to date, no satisfactory or conclusive evidence has been found to explain or justify any one etiological factor in the production of this complication of hydralazine therapy.

REFERENCES

1. Bendersky, G. and Ramirez, C.: Hydralazine poisoning. J.A.M.A., *173*:1789, 1960.
2. Biehl, J. P. and Vilter, R. W.: Effect of isoniazid on B₆ metabolism; its possible significance in producing isoniazid neuritis. Soc. Exper. Biol. & Med., *85*:389, 1957.
3. Boas, N. F. and Soffer L. J.: The effect of adrenocorticotropic hormone and cortisone on the serum hexosamine level in acute disseminated lupus erythematosus. J. Clin. Endocrinol., *11*:39, 1951.
4. Comens, P.: Experimental hydralazine disease and its similarity to disseminated lupus erythematosus. J. Lab. & Clin. Med., *47*:444, 1956.
5. Comens, P.: Chronic intoxication from hydralazine resembling disseminated lupus erythematosus and its apparent reversal by manganese. In Seven, M. J. and Johnson, L. A. (eds.): Metal Binding in Medicine. Philadelphia, J. B. Lippincott Co., 1960, p. 312.
6. Comens, P.: Complications of malignant hypertension, Miss. Valley M. J., *81*:4, April, 1956.
7. Comens, P.: Unpublished data.
8. Comens, P. and Schroeder, H. A.: The "L-E" cell as a manifestation of delayed hydralazine intoxication. J.A.M.A., *160*:1134, 1956.
9. Cotzias, G. C.: Personal communication.
10. Dameshek, W.: Systemic lupus erythematosus: a complex auto-immune disorder? Ann. Int. Med., *48*:707, 1958.
11. Dammin, G. J., Nora, J. R. and Reardon, J. F.: Hydralazine reaction: case with L. E. cells antemortem and postmortem and pulmonary, renal, splenic, and muscular lesions of disseminated lupus erythematosus. J. Lab. & Clin. Med., *46*:806, 1955.
12. Douglas, C. D. and Hogan, R.: A metabolite of 1-hydrazinophthalazine (hydralazine). Proc. Soc. Exper. Biol. & Med. (In press.)
13. Dubois, E. L., Katz, Y. J., Freeman, V. and Garbak, F. G.: Chronic toxicity studies of hydralazine (Apresoline) in dogs, with particular reference to the production of the hydralazine syndrome. J. Lab. & Clin. Med., *50*:119, 1957.
14. Dustan, H. P., Taylor, R. D., Corcoran, A. C. and Page, I. H.: Rheumatic and febrile syndrome during prolonged hydralazine treatment. J.A.M.A., *154*:23, 1954.
15. Friou, G. J.: Personal communication.
16. Gardner, D. L.: The response of the dog to oral 1-hydrazinophthalazine (hydralazine). Brit. J. Exper. Path., *38*:227, 1957.
17. Gregory, J. E. and Rich, A. R.: Experimental production of anaphylactic pulmonary lesions with basic characteristics of rheumatic pneumonitis. Bull. Johns Hopkins Hosp., *78*:1 (Jan.), 1946.
18. Harkavy, J.: Vascular allergy: pathogenesis of bronchial asthma with recurrent pulmonary infiltrations and eosinophilic polyserositis. Arch. Int. Med., *67*:709-734, 1941.
19. Hildreth, E. A., Biro, C. E. and McCreary, T. A.: Persistence of the hydralazine syndrome. J.A.M.A., *173*:657, 1960.
20. Kirkendall, W. M. and Page, E. B.: Polyneuritis occurring during hydralazine therapy. J.A.M.A., *167*:427, 1958.
21. Lansbury, J. and Rogers, F.B.: The hydralazine syndrome. Bull. Rheum. Dis., *5*:85, 1955.
22. McIssac, W. M. and Williams, R. T.: Studies in detoxication. 70. Metabolism of

 hydrazides and hydroxamic acids derived from salicylic acid. Biochem. J., *66*:369, 1957.

23. Mellinkoff, S. M., Konigsmark B., Namerow H. and Frankland, M.: The effect of diet upon acute hydralazine toxicity in white rats. J. Lab. & Clin. Med., *51*:867, 1958.

24. Morrow, J. D., Schroeder, H. A. and Perry, H. M., Jr.: Studies on control of hypertension by Hyphex: toxic reactions and side effects. Circulation, 8:829, 1953.

25. Perry, H. M., Jr. and Schroeder, H. A.: Studies on the control of hypertension by Hyphex. III. Pharmacological and chemical observations on 1-hydrazinophthalazine. Am. J. M. Sc., *228*:396, 1954.

26. Perry, H. M., Jr. and Schroeder, H. A.: Snydrome simulating collagen disease caused by hydralazine (Apresoline). J.A.M.A., *154*:670, 1954.

27. Pillsbury, D. M., Shelley, W. B. and Kligman, A. M.: Dermatology. Philadelphia, W. B. Saunders Co., 1956, p. 153.

28. Reinhardt, D. J. and Waldron, J. M.: Lupus erythematosus-like syndrome complicating hydralazine (Apresoline) therapy. J.A.M.A., *155*:1491, 1954.

29. Reynolds, H. and Caldwell, J. R.: Hydralazine syndrome—hypersensitivity or toxicity? J.A.M.A., *165*:1823, 1957.

30. Schroeder, H. A.: The effect of 1-hydrazino-phthalazine in hypertension. Circulation, *5*:28, 1952.

31. Schroeder, H. A.: Mechanisms of Hypertension, with Consideration of Atherosclerosis. Springfield, Ill., Charles C Thomas, 1957.

32. Shackman, N. H., Swiller, A. I. and Morrison, M.: Syndrome simulating acute disseminated lupus erythematosus: appearance after hydralazine therapy. J.A.M.A., *155*:1492, 1954.

33. Siguier, F., Betourme, and Bonnet de la Tour, J.: Hydralazine-induced lupus erythematosus. Semaine Hôp. Paris, *34*:773, 1958.

34. Slonim, N. B.: Arthralgia, headache, prostration and fever during hydralazine therapy. J.A.M.A., *154*:1419, 1954.

35. Wood, W. S. and Lepper, M. H.: Drug Reactions. Disease-a-Month. Chicago, Year Book Publishers.

The L.E. Cell: Significance
and Relation to Collagen Disease

RAYMOND W. MONTO, RAFAEL A. RIZEK, CLARENCE E. RUPE and JOHN W. REBUCK

The Henry Ford Hospital and Clinic, Detroit

The lupus erythematosus (L.E.) cell phenomenon has been available for clinical application for over a decade. It is timely that the usefulness of this unique system be reviewed in a large general hospital. Of considerable practical importance in medicine is the evaluation of the L.E. cell in the light of the natural history of systemic lupus erythematosus (S.L.E.) as well as in the interpretation of the "false negative" and "false positive" reactions.[3, 4]

It was the purpose of the present study to examine the records of all the patients from Henry Ford Hospital who demonstrated the L.E. cell phenomenon during the past ten years. As a counterpart, the records of patients with collagen diseases (S.L.E., polyarteritis nodosa, scleroderma, dermatomyositis, rheumatoid arthritis, rheumatic fever and discoid lupus erythematosus) were reviewed in reference to the occurrence of the L.E. cell phenomenon. These

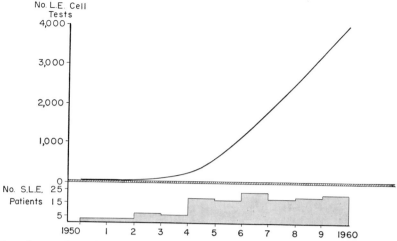

Fig. 1. The number of L.E. cell tests performed in relation to the number of patients diagnosed yearly with S.L.E.

observations have utilized the factor of "time-interval" to clarify the relationship of the L.E. cell to the clinical disorders.

It has been suggested that the finding of one authentic L.E. cell establishes a positive result and a diagnosis of S.L.E. Others have required that five or more L.E. cells in a count of 500 polymorphonuclear leukocytes be present for a positive test.[1] In the patients reported in this review the L.E. cell test was performed on bone marrow specimens until 1955; after this time peripheral blood (two-hour blood clot) preparations were employed.[5]

In 1950 a total of 18 L.E. cell preparations from bone marrows were done at the Henry Ford Hospital; since then, the number of tests has been mounting through the years to approximately 3000 in 1959. This figure will exceed 4000 in 1960 (Fig. 1). Since 1954 the incidence of S.L.E. has averaged 20 to 25 patients a year. This chart must be interpreted in light of our changing concepts of S.L.E., the use of peripheral blood L.E. techniques and a 20 per cent increase in new patient registrations between 1955 and 1960. The performance of the L.E. test in large numbers in diversified diseases other than S.L.E. has afforded an unusual opportunity for the clinical evaluation of this phenomenon.

Table 1 lists the diseases commonly considered to be of connective tissue origin. Two of 51 tested patients with discoid L.E. demonstrated the phenomenon. One of the two subsequently developed S.L.E. and an L.E. cell

TABLE 1. INCIDENCE OF L.E. CELL PHENOMENON IN DISEASES OF CONNECTIVE TISSUE

	TOTAL	TESTED	L.E. PHENOMENON
Discoid lupus erythematosus	102	51	2
Systemic lupus erythematosus	156	156	134
Scleroderma	38	12	3
Dermatomyositis	35	26	3
Polyarteritis	48	39	3
Rheumatic fever	151	28	11
Rheumatoid arthritis	891	455	68

count greater than five. All patients diagnosed as S.L.E. (156) were tested. L.E. cells were not found in 22 cases, a percentage of 14.0. When the patients demonstrating only one to four L.E. cells are included as "negative" the percentage reaches 26.3. Although the L.E. cell phenomenon was noted in scleroderma, dermatomyositis, polyarteritis and rheumatic fever at the frequency seen in Table 1, the number of L.E. cells did not exceed five. In rheumatoid arthritis (R.A.) L.E. cells in varying numbers were found in 68 of 455 patients tested, a percentage of 15.2.

TABLE 2. PATIENTS DEMONSTRATING FIVE OR MORE L.E. CELLS WITH DIAGNOSES OTHER THAN S.L.E.

Rheumatoid arthritis	18	Parkinsonism	1
Pulmonary tuberculosis	1	Aplastic anemia, benign thymoma	1
Chronic dermatitis	1	Chronic hepatitis	1
Chronic lymphocytic leukemia	1	Necrotizing papillitis of the kidney	1
Erythrocytic leukemia	1	Pelvic abscess and pyelonephritis	1
Hodgkin's disease	1	Hydralazine reaction	1

Table 2 lists 29 patients with diseases other than S.L.E. demonstrating five or more L.E. cells. The criteria for rheumatoid arthritis were those of the American Rheumatism Association. It is to be emphasized that we have listed as R.A. those patients presenting a classic clinical picture of R.A. without clinical and laboratory evidence of S.L.E.[2] The largest number (32) of L.E. cells seen in a patient not considered to have S.L.E. occurred in one with R.A.

Diseases other than S.L.E. with incidence of four or less L.E. cells are tabulated in Table 3. There were more than 147 patients in 35 disease categories. R.A. again comprised a major part of this group. The high incidence of connective tissue disorders as well as auto-immune and vascular diseases is noted.

TABLE 3. PATIENTS DEMONSTRATING FOUR OR LESS L.E. CELLS WITH DIAGNOSES OTHER THAN S.L.E.

Connective tissue diseases		Arteriosclerotic heart disease, generalized arteriosclerosis	5
Rheumatoid arthritis	50	Psychoneurosis	3
Rheumatic fever	11	Metabolic diseases (gout, porphyria)	3
Polyarteritis	3	Malignant diseases (leukemia, carci-	
Dermatomyositis	3	noma, sarcoma)	4
Scleroderma	3	Laennec's cirrhosis	2
Undifferentiated collagen diseases	2	Osteoarthritis	2
Discoid L.E.	1	Polyserositis (Armenian disease)	2
Hydralazine reaction	1	Chronic pulmonary fibrosis	1
Idiopathic thrombocytopenic purpura	2	Sarcoidosis	1
Acquired hemolytic anemia	2	Brachial neuritis	1
Pernicious anemia	1	Pancreatitis and duodenitis	1
Infections (septicemia, S.B.E.,		Parkinsonism	1
bronchopneumonia, virus)	11	Menopausal syndrome	1
Miscellaneous skin diseases (erythema		Myeloid metaplasia	1
multiforme, urticaria, chronic		Irritable colon	1
dermatitis, etc.)	7	Endometriosis	1
Miscellaneous kidney diseases (pyelo-		Calcific pericarditis	1
nephritis, chronic glomerulo-		Toxic nodular goiter	1
nephritis, nephrosis)	9	No final diagnosis	6
Miscellaneous vascular disorders			
(Raynaud's, thrombophlebitis)	5		

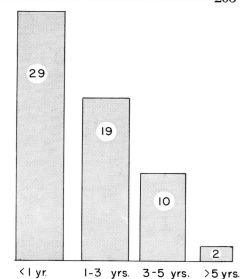

Fig. 2. Patients demonstrating five or more L.E. cells with diagnoses other than S.L.E.—period of observation.

Because of the natural history of S.L.E., it was imperative to obtain observations on the progress of the group of patients not considered to have S.L.E. but demonstrating the L.E. phenomenon. Figure 2 indicates the period of observation on 29 of these patients with five or more L.E. cells, and Figure 3 indicates that on the 147 patients with four or less L.E. cells. During the period of follow-up only one of these patients was considered possibly to have S.L.E. on the basis of necropsy findings. This patient, with generalized Hodgkin's disease, demonstrated "onion-skinning" in the spleen and a plasmacellular interstitial nephritis. In this study, the tissues were not surveyed with antiglobulin fluorescent microscopy. It has been estimated that approximately two-thirds of patients with S.L.E. not under hormonal therapy will demonstrate relapse in a three-year interval. Less than 50 per cent of this group of patients received steroid therapy.

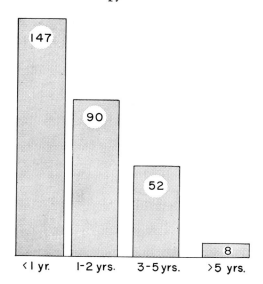

Fig. 3. Patients demonstrating four or less L.E. cells with diagnoses other than S.L.E.—period of observation.

Figure 4 indicates the time interval required for patients with S.L.E. to develop five or more L.E. cells. Of 17 patients with no L.E. cells when the clinical diagnosis of S.L.E. was made, 11 demonstrated five or more cells in six months, two in 9 months, one in 12 months, one in 22 months, and one in 36 months. The time interval required for patients having originally but one to four L.E. cells with the clinical diagnosis of S.L.E.

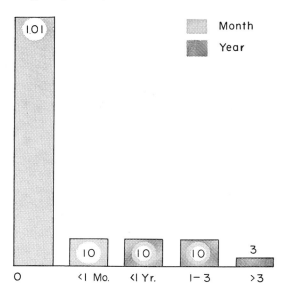

Fig. 4. Time interval required for patients with a diagnosis of S.L.E. to develop five or more L.E. cells.

to develop five or more L.E. cells was as follows: less than one month, three patients; less than one year, three patients; one to three years, six patients; and more than three years, three patients.

SUMMARY AND CONCLUSIONS

The specificity and sensitivity of the L.E. cell phenomenon were evaluated by a large and lengthy retrospective study in a general hospital. The incidence of S.L.E. does not appear to be increasing. The L.E. cell phenomenon was observed in 310 patients; 176 or 57 per cent of these patients were not considered to fulfill the clinical or laboratory criteria of S.L.E. Of this group, 70 patients (40 per cent) were categorized as having a connective tissue disease in which rheumatoid arthritis was dominant. Every patient demonstrating more than 32 L.E. cells was found to have S.L.E. L.E. cells were not found in 22 patients (14 per cent) believed to have S.L.E. Of the patients with five or more L.E. cells, 28 (25.6 per cent) were not believed to have S.L.E. On the basis that five or more cells constitute a "positive" test, in a series of 10,000 preparations less than 0.3 per cent were considered "false positives."

It is concluded that the L.E. cell phenomenon, while a characteristic of S.L.E., lacks both specificity and sensitivity as a diagnostic test. At present, with generally available techniques, the diagnosis of S.L.E. can be made most accurately by considering all factors, both clinical and laboratory, of which the L.E. cell phenomenon is of major importance.

REFERENCES

1. Berman, L., Axelrod, A. R., Goodman, H. L. and McClaughy, R. I.: So-called "lupus erythematosus inclusion phenomenon" of bone marrow and blood. Am. J. Clin. Path., 20:403-417, 1950.
2. Committee of the American Rheumatism Association. Revision of diagnostic criteria for rheumatoid arthritis. Bull. Rheumat. Dis., 9:175-176, 1958.
3. Harvey, A. M., Shulman, L. E., Tumulty, P. A., Conley, C. L. and Schoenrick, E. H.: Systemic lupus erythematosus: review of literature and clinical analysis of 138 cases. Medicine, 33:291-437, 1954.
4. Rupe, C. E. and Nickel, S. N.: New clinical concept of systemic lupus erythematosus. J.A.M.A., 171:1055-1061, 1959.
5. Zimmer, F. E. and Hargraves, M. M.: The effect of blood coagulation on L. E. cell formation. Proc. Staff Meet., Mayo Clin., 27:424-430, 1952.

The Use of Cutaneous Hypersensitivity to Leukocytes in the Diagnosis of Disseminated Lupus Erythematosus[*]

J. CLAUDE BENNETT and HOWARD L. HOLLEY

Medical College of Alabama

In the past four years several factors which produce serological reactions with various nuclear components have been found in patients with systemic lupus erythematosus.[3, 6, 8, 10, 11] Reactions have been described with whole nuclei, nucleoprotein, histone, deoxyribonucleic acid, and more recently, reactions with cytoplasmic components have been studied.[4]

These findings are thought to represent circulating "antibodies" and have provoked much discussion concerning the immunopathology of systemic lupus erythematosus. Although a pathogenic role for these factors cannot be ruled out as yet, it seems more likely that they represent only the effects of some basic defect in those cells responsible for the initiation or control of protein synthesis. It was, therefore, felt that additional information on this disorder might be obtained from a study of intradermal hypersensitivity. Any abnormality in "cellular" reactivity might thereby be detected. Similar studies have been undertaken by investigators at the Rockefeller Institute[9] and by Friedman and co-workers[5] at the Peter Bent Brigham Hospital. Although we are vitally concerned with the physiological meaning of intradermal hypersensitivity in SLE, we shall limit the discussion here to its use as a diagnostic test.

* This work has been supported by a grant from the National Institutes of Health (USPH A-3555) and the John R. Irby Fund for the Study of Arthritis. A portion of this material has been submitted for publication in Arthritis and Rheumatism.

METHODS

In the patients selected for this study the diagnosis of SLE was determined in 17 by the usual clinical criteria and the presence of the LE cell
phenomenon. A positive LE preparation in the absence of clinical criteria
was not accepted as diagnostic. Forty patients with rheumatoid arthritis
were tested in this series. Other patients included eight with related connective tissue disorders, 15 with discoid LE, and 15 with unrelated diseases (Table 1).

Preparation and Administration of Test Substances. Leukocytes were
prepared for administration utilizing a modification of the method of Skoog
and Beck.[12] Approximately 20 ml. of venous blood was drawn from the
forearm of healthy normal donors into syringes, which had first been rinsed
with 10 to 15 mg. of aqueous heparin. A 5 per cent solution of dextran
(molecular weight 150,000 to 200,000) was added, and the suspension was
gently mixed in a sterile 50 cc. glass tube. Upon standing in an ice bath at
4° C. for one hour sedimentation of the red cells became grossly complete.

An erythrocyte fraction was prepared by removal of 0.05 ml. of the
sedimented red blood cells, which was then suspended in 5 ml. of normal
saline. The final erythrocyte concentration was approximately 4×10^6
per 0.1 ml.

The supernatant from the original sedimentation procedure was centrifuged at 2000 R.P.M. for 15 minutes. A leukocyte button (contaminated
with dextran, plasma, platelets and erythrocytes) was thereby obtained.
This was then washed with saline and finally suspended in 1 ml. of normal
saline. White cell counts on this suspension ranged from 5 to 10×10^5 per
0.1 ml., the proportion of contaminating erythrocytes to leukocytes ranging
from 1:1 to 1:10. Less erythrocyte contamination was obtained when
siliconized glassware was used and when the separation was repeated.
Neither separation nor quantitation of platelets was attempted.

The patients in this series were tested with 0.1 ml. intradermal injections of (1) the above described leukocyte preparation, (2) the above
described erythrocyte preparation, and (3) a 0.5 per cent solution of
dextran. These various fractions were prepared under sterile conditions
and were used within 24 hours.

Six patients with SLE were also tested with intradermal injections of
(1) saline suspension of homogenized buffy coat, (2) purified DNA (10,
100, and 500 micrograms per ml.), and (3) nucleoprotein (500 micrograms
per ml.).

RESULTS

Reactions to the leukocytes could be detected as early as 12 to 14 hours
after injection. Early changes consisted of only a small amount of spongy
edema in the immediate area of injection, with erythema extending outward some 10 mm. Definite induration which had a central reddish-purple
coloration was present within 20 to 24 hours. Beyond the induration could
be seen a broad band of erythema and sometimes obvious edema. Within
36 hours the erythema had usually disappeared, but the indurated area was
still prominent. By 72 hours the reaction had disappeared completely.

Induration at the time of maximal reaction covered an area of from 5 to
20 mm. in diameter. The total reaction, including erythema, measured up
to 58.0 mm. Our arbitrary standard for a minimally positive reaction was

selected as 5 mm. of induration. Erythema alone was not considered to constitute a positive reaction.

Skin reactions to the leukocyte injections in normal subjects consisted of only 1 to 2 mm. of edema or up to 5 mm. of erythema. Slight redness or no grossly visible reaction was produced in both the SLE and control patients by either the dextran or erythrocyte injections.

Six patients with SLE were also tested with intradermal injections of nucleoprotein and DNA. No visible reactions were obtained even though these same subjects reacted strongly to the whole homologous leukocytes. These same patients were simultaneously tested with a saline homogenate of buffy coat. This did produce definite induration, but the area of reactivity was only 30 to 50 per cent of that produced by whole leukocytes isolated by the dextran method.

Biopsy specimens obtained at 24 hours post injection have been of some help in interpretation of these cutaneous reactions.[2] Considerable inflammatory exudate was produced in SLE patients by the leukocyte injections and consisted of both mononuclear and polymorphonuclear white cells. These cellular elements seemed to be concentrated around blood vessels and are probably representative of some degree of vasculitis. By the use of Masson's trichrome stain and a phosphotungstic acid-hematoxylin preparation a fibrinoid transudate could be seen around small arteries and arterioles.

Histological study of the injection sites in the control patients failed to reveal any active inflammatory process. Similarly, dextran and erythrocyte injection areas in the patients with SLE showed little or no reaction.

The tabulation of diagnoses in the 95 patients of this clinical series is given in Table 1. In 15 of 17 patients with classic SLE the intradermal test was positive. Only five presumably false positives were obtained from the remainder of the patients. Two of these had long-standing discoid lupus erythematosus with some symptoms suggesting systemic disease. Two had long-standing rheumatoid arthritis and one had rheumatic fever.

TABLE 1. INTRADERMAL SENSITIVITY IN SYSTEMIC
LUPUS ERYTHEMATOSUS

DIAGNOSIS	M	F	LE PREP POS.	SKIN TEST POS.	LATEX POS.	STEROID THERAPY
Systemic lupus erythematosus	1	16	16	15	4	11
Discoid lupus erythematosus	10	5	0	2	0	1
Rheumatoid arthritis	22	18	0	2	30	8
Acute rheumatic fever	2		0	1	0	2
Periarteritis	1		0	0	0	1
Ankylosing spondylitis	2		0	0	0	0
Gout	1		0	0	0	0
Myositis		2	0	0	0	0
Pyelonephritis		1	0	0	0	0
Thyrotoxicosis		1	0	0	0	0
Hypertension		1	0	0	0	0
Leukemia	1		0	0	0	1
Myocardial infarction	2		0	0	0	0
Tertiary syphilis	1		0	0	0	0
Pulmonary fibrosis	1		0	0	0	0
Pneumonia	1		0	0	0	0
Hepatitis	1		0	0	0	0
Sinusitis	1		0	0	0	0
Undiagnosed polysystem disease	4		0	0	2	1

DISCUSSION

The cutaneous reaction which has been demonstrated to occur in patients with SLE when challenged with homologous leukocytes seems to be encountered only infrequently in patients afflicted with other diseases. Only two of the patients who had SLE failed to react to the leukocytes, but both were on large steroid dosages (300 to 500 mg. hydrocortisone per day). Both of the patients with rheumatoid arthritis who had positive reactions to the leukocytes also had latex fixation titers greater than 1:1280. This perhaps is of significance in view of the fact that a considerable proportion of patients with severe rheumatoid arthritis and high agglutination titers often have an abnormal serum globulin which has affinity for nuclear material.[1]

It is not yet clear what type of hypersensitivity reaction has been detected by this test procedure. Biopsy studies of the leukocyte injection site of SLE patients revealed an early polymorphonuclear exudation with a definite vasculitis. This is the sort of histological picture that one would expect to find in the usual Arthus reaction. However, in addition to this process a mononuclear infiltration which tended to localize in "islands" around blood vessels could also be seen. This latter finding, in association with extensive induration, has been observed most commonly in delayed type hypersensitivity.[7] Therefore, the histological characteristics of both the delayed and the Arthus phenomena seem to be present simultaneously. Perhaps this is not too surprising in view of the complexity of the leukocyte as a test antigen.

Six of the SLE patients were also tested with intradermal nucleoprotein and DNA. No reaction was produced by these substances, even though the response to the homologous leukocytes was striking in these same patients. Buffy coat homogenates, to which dextran had not been added, produced a positive but less striking reaction than the whole leukocytes. At the present time we do not know whether the difference is due to some enhancing effect of the dextran or reflects an increased stimulating ability of the whole cell.

Although the intradermal reaction to leukocytes may be of help in the diagnosis of complicated cases of connective tissue disorders, it does have at least one serious drawback; this is that the test as described here is a "one chance affair," in that patients become sensitized to adsorbed dextran. Therefore, interpretation of any future tests would be difficult. It should also be noted that we have observed that normal subjects can be "sensitized" to buffy coat homogenates. This can be seen after the third or fourth weekly intradermal injection of homogenate from the same donor.

The mechanism by which this intradermal hypersensitivity is mediated is as yet unclear. The possibility that it represents an increased rejection of "transplanted" cells has been entertained; but more likely, it is a manifestation of some basic immunopathological defect characteristic of systemic lupus erythematosus.

From the viewpoint of clinical diagnosis the results described above seem to indicate that this intradermal reaction may be of use in the differentiation of disorders included in the connective tissue group.

REFERENCES

1. Bardawil, W. A., Tay, B. Z., Galins, N. and Bayles, T. B.: Disseminated lupus erythematosus, scleroderma, and dermatomyositis as manifestations of sensitization

to DNA-protein. I. Immunohistochemical approach. Am. J. Path., *34*:607, 1958.
2. Bennett, J. C. and Holley, H. L.: Intradermal hypersensitivity in systemic lupus erythematosus. Arth. & Rheum., *4*:64, 1961.
3. Deicher, H. R., Holman, H. R. and Kunkel, H. G.: The precipitin reaction between DNA and a serum factor in systemic lupus erythematosus. J. Exper. Med., *109*:97, 1959.
4. Deicher, H. R. G., Holman, H. R. and Kunkel, H. G.: Anti-cytoplasmic factors in the sera of patients with systemic lupus erythematosus and certain other diseases. Arth. & Rheum., *3*:1, 1960.
5. Friedman, E. A., Bardawil, W. A., Merrill, J. P. and Hanau, C.: "Delayed" cutaneous hypersensitivity to leukocytes in disseminated lupus erythematosus. New Engl. J. Med., *262*:486, 1960.
6. Friou, G. J., Finch, S. C. and Detre, K. D.: Interaction of nuclei and globulin from lupus erythematosus serum demonstrated with fluorescent antibody. J. Immunol., *80*: 324, 1958.
7. Gell, P. G. H.: Cytologic events in hypersensitivity reactions. In Lawrence, H. S. (ed.): Cellular and Humoral Aspects of the Hypersensitive States. New York, Hoeber-Harper, 1959, pp. 43-66.
8. Holman, H. R. and Kunkel, H. G.: Affinity between lupus erythematosus serum factor and cell nuclei and nucleoprotein. Science, *126*:162, 1957.
9. Holman, H. R.: Personal communication.
10. Miescher, P. and Strassle, R.: New serological methods for the detection of the L. E. factor. Vox Sang., *2*:283, 1957.
11. Pearson, C. M., Craddock, C. G. and Simmons, N. S.: Complement fixation reactions with DNA and leukocyte material in systemic lupus erythematosus: correlation with the L. E. cell phenomenon and the clinical status. J. Lab. & Clin. Med., *52*:580, 1958.
12. Skoog, W. A. and Beck, W. S.: Studies on the fibrinogen, dextran and phytohemagglutinin methods of isolating leukocytes. Blood, *11*:436, 1956.

Differentiation of Rheumatoid Arthritis and Lupus Erythematosus by Sheep Cell Agglutination Tests*

ARNOLD BLACK

Chicago Medical School

The differentiation between rheumatoid arthritis (R.A.) and systemic lupus erythematosus (S.L.E.) is not difficult in the majority of cases. However, two situations sometimes arise which create a problem for the discriminating clinician. (1) Many patients with R.A. have L.E. cells in the peripheral blood (3 to 27 per cent).[2] These figures undoubtedly are determined by the sensitivity of the test used and the aggressiveness with which the search is pursued. (2) Many patients with S.L.E. have a significant degree of arthritis (63 per cent)[3] and frequently exhibit a positive test for the rheumatoid factor.[7]

The ultimate designation of these two groups of patients is often dependent on the background of the observer, whether he be hematologist or rheumatologist, and also on his opinion regarding the specificity of the

* Aided by a grant from the Illinois Chapter, Arthritis and Rheumatism Foundation.

L.E. cell phenomenon. One might argue whether a differentiation is very significant in most instances, but it is felt that nosological requirements should be met whenever possible. In addition, the prognostic, therapeutic and genetic aspects of this problem are also pertinent and are discussed elsewhere in this volume.

In 1953 Svartz and Schlossman reported a technique for doing the sheep cell agglutination test for R.A. in which the euglobulin fraction of the serum to be tested was precipitated by the addition of cold distilled water.[4] Subsequently, they evaluated this procedure in patients with S.L.E.[5] Their results indicated that the factor in the S.L.E. serum which agglutinated sensitized sheep cells (in approximately 50 per cent of patients) could be eliminated by preparing the cold precipitable fraction. When the latter material was tested, practically all patients were negative (29 of 30). The authors postulated that the sheep cell hemagglutinating factor of S.L.E. was separated and remained in the supernatant fluid while the rheumatoid factor was in the precipitate.

For the purpose of evaluating a serological differentiation between R.A. and S.L.E., a study was inaugurated using four groups of patients. These were evaluated by sheep cell agglutination tests using two different methods: the cold precipitable fraction as prepared by Svartz and Schlossman[4] and the euglobulin fraction prepared according to the method of Ziff.[6] The following cases were studied: Group I, rheumatoid arthritis, 35 patients; Group II, systemic lupus erythematosus, 28 patients; Group III, rheumatoid arthritis with L.E. cells in the peripheral blood, 17 patients; Group IV, normal controls, 30 patients.

The results are summarized in Table 1 and were reported at an earlier date.[1] In Group I (R.A.), 25 cases (71 per cent) were positive by the euglobulin method. Two of the negative reactors had spondylitis with peripheral joint disease. Eighteen (51 per cent) were positive by the cold precipitation method. All of the latter group were also positive with the euglobulin method, indicating a difference in sensitivity of the two procedures.

In Group II (S.L.E.), the cold precipitation technique was of considerable help. Only four cases (14 per cent) were positive, three such results occurring in the lowest titer (1:16). The other patient was a 35-year-old woman with a two-year history of fever, bilateral pleural effusion, hepatomegaly and rheumatoid involvement of the fingers and wrists with definite x-ray changes. Laboratory results included: positive L.E. phenomenon, total protein of 8.6 gm. with a globulin of 6.1 gm., and a thymol turbidity of 19.8 units. The cold precipitation titer was 1:64 and the euglobulin titer was 1:896.

In this same group, 15 patients (54 per cent) had a positive euglobulin test. Five of these had definite synovitis, although there were five other patients with similar findings who had negative titers.

In Group III (R.A. with L.E. cells), the results were essentially the same as in Group I except that there was a higher incidence of positive results and in higher titers. Most of these patients had severe arthritis of long duration, and nine had subcutaneous nodules. There was never any clinical evidence of S.L.E. in any of these cases.

Both tests were negative in Group IV (normal controls).

We have subsequently evaluated two other patients who have been followed clinically and serologically for some months. One patient, a 45-year-

TABLE 1.*   RESULTS OF SENSITIZED SHEEP CELL AGGLUTINATION TESTS IN FOUR GROUPS OF PATIENTS

CLINICAL GROUP	TOTAL CASES	EUGLOBULIN (ZIFF) METHOD				COLD PRECIPITATION (SVARTZ) METHOD			
		POSITIVE TITERS	TITER LEVELS			POSITIVE TITERS	TITER LEVELS		
			Low 1:28 1:56	Medium 1:112 1:224	High 1:448+		Low 1:16 1:32	Medium 1:64 1:128	High 1:256+
I. Rheumatoid arthritis (R.A.)	35	25 (71%)	6	8	11	18 (51%)	6	6	6
II. Systemic lupus erythematosus (S.L.E.)	28	15 (54%)	10	4	1	4 (14%)	3	1	0
III. Rheumatoid arthritis with positive L. E. preparations	17	16 (94%)	3	5	8	12 (71%)	4	5	3
IV. Normal controls	30	0				0			

* From Black, A., Goldin, M., Poske, R. M. and Malmed, L.: Differentiation between Rheumatoid Arthritis and Systemic Lupus Erythematosus by Sheep Cell Agglutination Tests. Arth. & Rheum., 2:99-103, 1959, by permission.

old woman, has had definite arthritis with synovial proliferation, nodules and radiographic evidence of cystic lesions around the involved joints. She also has had pleurisy, splenomegaly, peripheral neuritis, severe hypochromic anemia, B.F.P. serological test for syphilis, and a large number of L.E. cells in the peripheral blood. Her titers remained high by both methods.

Another patient, a 44-year-old man, presented in February 1960 with a history of definite findings of rheumatoid arthritis of two years' duration, for which he had received only salicylate therapy. One month later he developed purpuric manifestations and was found to have a severe thrombocytopenia. He was placed on steroid therapy on 3/15/60 and this was subsequently increased to a dosage of 60 mg. of prednisone per day before any significant response was noted. At the last observation he was clinically well and his medication was being gradually reduced. A positive L.E. preparation has not been found on repeated examinations. His serological titers are listed:

DATE	STANDARD LATEX TITER	COLD PRECIPITATION TITER
2/20/60	1:128	1:256
4/14/60	1:640	1:64
6/15/60	0	0

These last two cases are presented to demonstrate that there is no clear-cut method which will place a patient in any distinct or specific category of disease all the time. A philosophical approach to the problem must certainly pose the question of whether we are dealing with two distinct disease entities, possibly coexisting in certain situations, or whether this is a spectrum of diseases with one syndrome overlapping the other at various phases. At this time the latter conclusion seems more likely.

From the practical standpoint, certain methodology can be followed. Clinical differentiation between R.A. and S.L.E. is fairly adequate in a considerable number of cases by the accepted methods of history, physical examination and routine laboratory procedures.

The patients who present manifestations of both diseases may fall into any of three categories:

(1) Predominantly S.L.E. with some arthritic manifestations. These will frequently have positive rheumatoid factor titers by the euglobulin or latex test but will practically always be negative with the Svartz technique as demonstrated in the study described above.

(2) Predominantly R.A. with L.E. cells in the peripheral smear. These will most often have a high titer by all tests. However, the clinical picture is one of severe arthritis, most often with the presence of nodules, but not that of a critically ill patient. Steroid therapy is frequently not necessary or, at the most, only in a minimum degree.

(3) Major findings of both diseases with no one specific pattern predominating. These will also have high titers by all serological tests, but the patients are most often quite ill and require therapy with high steroid dosage for some period of their disease. The titers may become negative whenever there is a complete suppression of disease either by therapy or through natural remission. This does not occur in patients described under category 2.

CONCLUSION

An attempt has been presented to assist in the differentiation between R.A. and S.L.E. Although absolute differentiation is not possible in all instances, evaluation of the patient from the standpoint of the clinical as well as the serological pattern will be of significant help in almost every instance.

REFERENCES

1. Black, A., Goldin, M., Poske, R. M. and Malmed, L.: Differentiation between rheumatoid arthritis and systemic lupus erythematosus by sheep cell agglutination tests. Arth. & Rheum., 2:99, 1959.
2. Friedman, I., Sickley, J., Poske, R., Black, A., Bronsky, D., Hartz, W., Feldhake, C., Reeder, P. and Katz, E.: The L.E. phenomenon in rheumatoid arthritis. Ann. Int. Med., 46:1113, 1957.
3. Slocumb, C. H.: Arthralgia and arthritis of lupus erythematosus. Proc. Staff Meet., Mayo Clin., 15:683, 1940.
4. Svartz, N. and Schlossman, K.: Agglutination of sensitized sheep erythrocytes by cold precipitable serum substances in rheumatoid arthritis. Acta med. scandinav., 146:313, 1953.
5. Svartz, N. and Schlossman, K.: Agglutination of sensitized sheep erythrocytes in disseminated lupus erythematosus. Ann. Rheumat. Dis., 16:73, 1957.
6. Ziff, M., Brown, P., Badin, J. and McEwen, C.: A hemagglutination test for rheumatoid arthritis with enhanced sensitivity using the euglobulin fraction. Bull. Rheumat. Dis., 5:75, 1954.
7. Ziff, M.: The agglutination reaction in rheumatoid arthritis. J. Chron. Dis., 5:644, 1957.

Panel Discussion

A. McGehee Harvey, *Moderator*

Dr. Harvey: To initiate the discussion, I would like to make a few comments about the BFP reaction, the biologic false positive test for syphilis. This is a rather unusual phenomenon, and in the past few years, it has been possible to recognize patients with a BFP reaction with ease, because of the development of more specific immunological tests for the presence of syphilis, the Treponema immobilization tests. In addition, because of the mass blood testing that was carried out during World War II and programs that are now carried out in the army, in employment, in pregnancy and in various other situations, there are a large number of people in whom reagin or the BFP reacting material is looked for. Combine this with the fact that certain patients with lupus—about 20 per cent of the patients who later develop the classic syndrome—will have a false biologic test. This gives us an opportunity to try to find out what happens in the development of lupus by being able to pick out these false positive reactors at a time when they are healthy and then to follow their progress over a period of years.

The results of the various studies that have been done in regard to the BFP phenomenon have clearly shown that such subjects can be divided into two different categories, the acute and the chronic BFP reactors. Acute BFP reactions occur primarily in infections—for example, infectious mononucleosis, malaria and atypical pneumonia—but when the disease is over, the reagin disappears from the serum in a matter of weeks or months. There are certain patients left then who have a chronic reaction which persists for many years. The only infection that I am aware of which is associated with a chronic BFP reaction is leprosy.

What is the meaning of the chronic BFP reaction in the other patients? We had the opportunity to follow, for long periods, 184 patients with chronic BFP reactions who were well at the time the reactions were first discovered. These 184 patients have now been followed for an average of eight years, a minimum of four years and a maximum of about 25 years. These patients can be divided into four groups. In the first group there are 52 reactors with no evidence of any related illness and with no other protein abnormalities in the blood. The second group, numbering 81, consists of BFP reactors who have in addition developed some other serum protein abnormality, usually an elevated serum globulin level. Some of these patients also have positive flocculation tests, but they have had no clinical illnesses suggestive of connective tissue diseases. The vast majority of the patients in both of these two groups are still quite healthy. They comprise 82 per cent of the 184 patients. There is a third group of 38 patients who have developed certain clinical features suggestive of a connective tissue disease, and these have been difficult to evaluate. One cannot be certain at this time that the group is homogeneous. In some of them, clinically, lupus seems likely, and they are now being studied intensively for other types of antibodies found in patients with lupus, but a longer period of follow-up will be necessary. Two patients in this group have definitely developed sarcoidosis. In the fourth group there are 12 patients who have very definitely developed systemic lupus and have a positive LE cell test, or in one or two followed to autopsy evidence of lupus was present.

It is interesting to study the sex division of these groups of patients. The chronic BFP phenomenon is predominantly seen in females, 136 of the 184 patients being females; however, in the first group of patients who have not developed symptoms or other protein abnormalities, the sex incidence is about equal. In the second group, who did develop other protein abnormalities, the ratio of females to males is 5 to 1, and in the third group who have some type of clinical illness, the ratio is 6½ to 1. In the fourth group, all are females. Not a single male, in the total group of 184, has developed definite evidence of lupus.

One other point of interest is that one patient who has had the BFP reaction and demonstrable LE cells on repeated examinations is as yet clinically well. In this regard, I would like to ask Dr. Larson to comment on the minimal criteria for the diagnosis of systemic lupus.

DR. LARSON: I am sure that we could discuss the minimal criteria for diagnosis at length and still not come to any serious agreement. It depends on your training, the criteria used for a positive LE cell test and so forth. However, in regard to the so-called false positive LE cell test in patients, the data we have obtained indicate that this is a very long-term disease and that one should not be in a hurry to say that the patient has either lupus or a false positive test. Furthermore, in our experience, a negative LE cell test is of absolutely no clinical significance. This test may be strongly positive at one time and negative at another in patients with lupus in whom on clinical grounds there does not seem to be any question about the diagnosis.

DR. LEE: I think there are several things that are important as criteria for the diagnosis of systemic lupus but I do not think any of them are absolute. One of them is obviously the LE cell phenomenon; another, as was pointed out this morning, is the nephrotic syndrome. The presence of a typical rash of lupus erythematosus would be a third important criterion and a renal or splenic biopsy suggesting or considered typical of the disease would be a fourth important criterion. Those are the major criteria, but there are obviously many, many others.

DR. HAMERMAN: Dr. Lee, would you add thrombocytopenic purpura?

DR. LEE: Not as a major criterion. Thrombocytopenic purpura occurs in a wide variety of diseases, and if you mean idiopathic thrombocytopenic purpura, I do not think that the majority of these patients have lupus.

DR. HARVEY: Dr. Pollak, would you tell us about the usefulness of renal biopsy in the diagnosis?

Dr. Pollak: The renal lesions of this disease are very pleomorphic and many of the lesions which one sees, while consistent with the disease, are not strictly diagnostic. We regard only one particular lesion as being diagnostic; this is the presence of local necrosis with karyorrhexis, fibrinoid and hematoxyphil bodies. Since this lesion does not necessarily appear in all of its features in a large proportion of patients, the renal biopsy may be only suggestive or consistent with the diagnosis of lupus, and it is diagnostic in only a comparatively small proportion of cases.

Dr. Harvey: Are there any further comments on the diagnostic criteria?

Dr. A. Black: I think certain laboratory abnormalities should be listed in the diagnostic criteria for lupus—such things as hyperglobulinemia, perhaps a high thymol turbidity, perhaps urinary abnormalities, certainly the BFP as mentioned by Dr. Harvey, and sometimes it is helpful if leukopenia is present.

Dr. Rose: I think the difficulty in diagnosis of the disease and in selecting the best criteria for diagnosis results from the fact that we do not really have a clear idea of the proper limits of the disease and whether or not it is an entity or only at one end of a continuous spectrum. For example, there is much to suggest that there is a continuous spectrum from discoid lupus at one end to classic systemic lupus at the other, with all grades in between. There is also a continuous spectrum in the general population and the families of lupus patients, from those who have nothing, to those who have serological abnormalities, to those who have the disease. One can also observe a spectrum between rheumatoid arthritis and systemic lupus. Now, if there is continuous variation in the whole range of the spectrum in this way, then diagnostic criteria become in a sense arbitrary, and if arbitrary, then they should be planned according to the purpose that we need the definition for. For each purpose, we need different criteria, and according to our needs we should plan the criteria we adopt in terms of actual measurements of the frequency of the different types of abnormalities in the different classes of patients, rather than in the somewhat haphazard and guesswork fashion that has, on the whole, been the custom so far.

Dr. Harvey: I would agree wholeheartedly. I think this is a very necessary thing to do at the moment, so that when one group report their observations, other people will have some idea of what class of patients they really are talking about. One can then use this data for long-term follow-up and accumulate new information in the proper perspective.

Dr. Black: Dr. Harvey, to what do you attribute the apparent increase in the incidence of lupus?

Dr. Harvey: I do not think that there is any real evidence that it has increased. Do you have such evidence? The concept of what lupus is has expanded, and we are much more alert to the recognition of this wider spectrum of disease. As Dr. Monto pointed out, the number of attempts to find these serologic abnormalities is extremely large and widespread, and I do not think we have a representative population yet from which to determine the incidence of it or any figures from the past to go on.

Dr. Lee: We are presently doing a study to determine what the incidence has been in New York City. This has been a retrospective study from the year 1950 to 1960 in an effort to determine the incidence of systemic lupus within a definite geographic area of known population, and it has been very seriously hampered by the absence of any definite statistical or probability kind of criteria that one can use to make the diagnosis.

Dr. Vaughan: I would like to ask a question about the long course of lupus erythematosus. Many patients with lupus are now recognized to have had connective tissue symptoms for some time in the past, even dating back 20 or 30 or more years, and our inclination is to project that the patients have had the disease this long. Dr. Harvey, have you or others tried to elicit this type of history from a normal population or from a nonlupus population? How reliable is it as an indication of the disease? From the point of view of the serological tests alone it is obvious that many people can have a positive serological test without lupus.

DR. HARVEY: The problem of trying to recreate the clinical pattern of a chronic disease in a retrospective manner obviously has very serious difficulties, and that was the major reason for studying patients with chronic BFP reactions, because in this situation one can start with a healthy subject and get a forward look at the development of the syndrome. It is of interest that, in our series of patients, there are some who had the BFP reaction and episodic illnesses compatible with lupus who did not develop definite serological evidence of it, such as a positive LE test, until some 15 years or more later; so I think there is little doubt that this is a chronic disease.

In regard to the other question, we did such a study in student nurses, who represent a female population, although this group, obviously, is not ideal from the point of view of random selection. We asked them a series of questions about past illnesses and did a battery of tests upon them similar to those that Dr. Holley performed in his patients with discoid lupus. Although none of them had any serologic abnormalities of lupus, there were a number who complained of some pain in the joints, or had this or that clinical phenomenon—not the major manifestations in overt fashion—but things that, if you were looking back in a patient's record retrospectively, I think you would attribute to lupus. Therefore, I think retrospective case analysis is a very difficult way in which to get ideal formation.

DR. LARSON: If I may, Dr. Harvey, corroborate the first comment you just made, we have one patient with a biologic false test for syphilis, who was treated elsewhere for syphilis at the age of eight, at the age of 14 and again at the age of 21; at the age of 29 she was admitted to the hospital with classic lupus, this being 21 years after the onset of the serologic abnormalities.

DR. HOLLEY: I do not think it is commonly realized that lupus may go into remission for many years, and I believe that it is reported that one-third of the patients have such remissions. In our series we now have about 50 patients, and there are three who have been in remission for more than five years without any evidence whatever of the disease. We have been doing multiple serologic tests on the entire group of patients at different periods in their disease, and it is rather interesting to see the changing pattern of the serological phenomena that has taken place during the waning and waxing of the disease.

DR. HARVEY: Are there any further comments on this?

DR. PEARSON: To go to the other end of the spectrum, there have been two or three comments yesterday and today about the possibility of transplacental passage of the LE factor, and some speculation about whether or not it is harmful; apparently the conclusion has been that it does not seem to be harmful. However, we have studied a family in which the mother and two of her children have lupus, and certainly familial lupus is being recognized. The mother had episodes of "nephritis," not recognized as lupus, during each of her pregnancies. The children are adults now, being 16 and 18 years of age. The mother recently died of progressive LE and hypertension with significant renal lesions, and the children developed lupus at the ages of 15 and 17 years. They had minimal symptoms during the interval series of years. Now, is it possible that transplacental passage of some agent took place and that the disease might have lain dormant? Or is this familial lupus not related to transplacental factors?

DR. POLLAK: In regard to what Dr. Pearson just said, I mentioned yesterday that we had studied the relatives of patients with SLE for antinuclear factors, and we have had the opportunity of studying a few newborn infants of these patients. We found the same titer of antinuclear factors in the cord blood as in maternal blood taken at the same time. In only one of these infants have we had the opportunity so far to obtain a follow-up study, and I think the results are of some interest in that after five months, this infant's serum gamma globulin level has fallen to about 40 per cent of the gamma globulin level at birth, which is a perfectly normal phenomenon, yet his titer of antinuclear factors has remained the same throughout this period of time. However, the infant is still well.

The Pathogenesis of Polyarteritis

D. MURRAY ANGEVINE

University of Wisconsin Medical School

It would seem a relatively simple assignment for a pathologist to discuss the pathogenesis of periarteritis nodosa; however, as with most subjects, the deeper one delves the more unanswered questions one finds, and this particular problem as it currently exists is one of rather large proportions. I shall accordingly touch only upon salient features of this condition and emphasize those areas in need of clarification.

This is a disease entity first recognized about 90 years ago in which the medium-sized muscular arteries are involved, with a predisposition for those of the splanchnic area. Few lesions of the terminal arteries or veins are observed and the pulmonary vessels usually escape.

In early reports the nodose or nodular feature of the disease received prominence, but although observed on occasion it certainly is not a conspicuous feature of most cases, perhaps because the disease is being recognized earlier. The irregularly distributed and different-sized infarcts are the significant gross diagnostic sign posts for both the surgeon and the pathologist.

The vessels most frequently involved, in addition to those of the mesenteric area, are those of the kidney and heart. Personally, I have been impressed by the extent and frequency of involvement of the peripancreatic and periadrenal vessels. Vessels in the lung, muscle, brain and skin may also be involved. It is, of course, this "spotty" distribution of vascular involvement that is responsible for the bizarre clinical picture that offers great difficulty in diagnosis.

For a long time most cases were first recognized from the microscopic examination of a surgically removed appendix or kidney or were discovered at the time of necropsy. During the past 15 or more years the clinician has become so aware of the existence of this condition that he frequently suspects it and resorts promptly to biopsy, as evidenced by the relatively low number of positive cases among the large number of muscle biopsies taken from suspected cases. When the tissue is examined by a competent pathologist, the answer should be definitive in the majority of cases.

A word about the biopsy is in order. Because there is always considerable chance of missing an involved artery in the tissue to be examined, it is important that a generous sample be removed and also that the pathologist section the muscle transversely so as to include the maximum number of vessels for examination. Because of the focal nature of this disease it is also advisable that each block of tissue be serially sectioned when the initial sections are negative. Sometimes it is necessary to take more than one piece of tissue for examination.

What is the characteristic microscopic picture by which the diagnosis of the disease is established? Because the condition is progressive, the vascular alterations vary widely between the early stages and the later stages of the disease, so that frequently one sees a variety of histological patterns in the same case.

The initial microscopic alteration indicates an increased permeability of the vessel wall, which suggests that the primary injury involves principally the endothelium and subendothelial space. The earliest observed alteration is edema with escape of fibrinogen into the wall, with the formation of fibrin or material which stains like fibrin. This is followed by fibrinoid necrosis, first of the media and then of the other coats. Fragmentation of the elastica is also a prominent feature which explains the aneurysmal dilatation of some vessels. There is an infiltration of all vessel coats with inflammatory cells, initially neutrophils and frequently eosinophils which later are replaced by those more characteristically present in chronic inflammation.

Since the intima is frequently extensively involved, thrombosis is a common feature. Healing is a conspicuous feature in some cases but unfortunately is accomplished by fibrous occlusion of the arterial lumen and the production of multiple ischemic lesions such as contracted kidneys and myocardial scars that cause extensive renal or cardiac impairment.

It does seem imperative that with the aid of newer techniques an effort must be made to learn more about the precise site or sites of injury. Does it actually occur within the endothelium, or is the target point in the ground substance, the smooth muscle or the collagen fibers?

Let us now examine some of the factors involved in the production of the disease. Since 1925 the concept that the disease is a hypersensitive reaction to some nontoxic agent has increased and is now almost universally accepted; however, the offending antigen frequently remains obscure or cannot be identified. Although I am personally inclined to associate all types of polyarteritis with hypersensitivity, it must be admitted that on the basis of the available evidence such a sweeping assumption may not be entirely justified.

The most significant advance in this direction was that of Rich,[8] who observed polyarteritis in five patients dying of serum sickness. This report stimulated much experimental work, on the basis of which hypersensitivity has been established as the most significant factor in the production of necrotizing arteritis, presumably the result of an antigen-antibody combination at some site probably within the vascular wall. The fact that the disease has resulted from sensitization to such drugs as iodine, Dilantin, penicillin, thiourea and propylthiouracil, as well as the sulfa drugs, also strengthens belief in the role of hypersensitivity. More intensive search for causative agents is indicated in every case.

The case for hypersensitivity as a significant causative factor is strongly supported by the fact that bronchial asthma is frequently complicated by vascular alterations such as occur in polyarteritis.[11] Looking at the problem in reverse, of 300 patients with polyarteritis, 54 (or 18 per cent) had asthma (described as allergic granulomatosis). Wegener's granulomatosis is another condition in which there is a destructive lesion of the respiratory tract, arteritis and nephritis.

The labelling of such entities as granulomatous may be helpful from a clinical standpoint, yet it is difficult to see much advantage from it because the basic pathologic alteration of these two conditions (allergic and Wegener's granulomatosis) is primarily a vascular one. The wide variability of response in different cases would seem to signify quantitative intensities of reaction in certain patients, modified by such factors as duration of illness, nature of antibody response, antigen-antibody ratio and level of sensitization of the host. Many physicians find it advantageous to designate cases associated with allergy as hypersensitivity arteritis or angiitis and to separate them from classic polyarteritis, the principal difference being that in the former (hypersensitivity arteritis) the small vessels—arteries and veins, as well as capillaries—are involved, and the pulmonary vessels are not exempt. Although our cases have never been specifically analyzed on this point, I am reasonably confident that when tissues are extensively examined in all cases, there are frequent exceptions to this pattern.

Because vascular alterations indistinguishable from those of polyarteritis are frequently observed in most connective tissue diseases, some discussion of such alterations is in order.

Friedberg and Gross[3] described four cases of periarteritis nodosa in which there was typical rheumatic carditis as evidenced by Aschoff bodies and considered several other cases of polyarteritis to have an associated rheumatic fever, but these were not included because they did not fulfill rigid criteria for a diagnosis of rheumatic fever. The opinion was also expressed that the association of these two conditions was more frequent than was generally recognized.

Of interest in the light of current therapy are the findings in the vascular system of patients with rheumatoid arthritis, a disease which is not usually associated with hypersensitivity, but for which one might make a strong case. A recent report has attributed three deaths to vascular lesions associated with gangrene of the extremities in patients receiving steroid therapy.[6] The histologic findings presented are indistinguishable from those observed in polyarteritis. For the five-year period 1953 to 1957 inclusive the deaths of 36 patients with rheumatoid arthritis and arteritis attributed to steroid therapy have been reported, and I am aware of several additional cases.

Before incriminating this therapy, the status of the blood vessels prior to the use of steroids must be considered. It is known that a variety of vascular lesions may occur in the synovial membrane, coronary arteries or skeletal muscles of patients with rheumatoid arthritis.

Sokoloff, Wilens and Bunim (1951)[10] described arteritis in the striated muscles of 5 of 57 patients with rheumatoid arthritis who had never received steroids. They pointed out that rheumatoid arteritis is unlike periarteritis in several significant respects. Six years later another report on ten cases noted the increasing frequency of the condition and the possibility that some of the alterations resulted from the deleterious effect of steroid therapy.[9] They emphasized the wide spectrum of lesions and then noted some of their cases to be indistinguishable from periarteritis nodosa.

Bywaters[1] has described peripheral vascular disease in the extremities of seven patients with rheumatoid arthritis who had never received steroids. If steroid therapy does aggravate the vascular lesions (and the evidence suggests that it does), there is need for greater precaution in treatment even though steroids have a known beneficial effect upon polyarteritis.

Although great emphasis has been placed on hypersensitivity in the pathogenesis of arteritis, other significant factors may operate in the various forms of vascular disease under discussion. Such factors as hypertension and the administration of certain steroids or large amounts of sodium might each appropriately be discussed at considerable length.

Knowledge of any disease usually progresses more rapidly when a comparable disease exists in animals or when it can be produced experimentally. The disease occurs naturally in the deer and rat and a necrotizing arteritis has been described in the vessels from various sites in a particular strain (DLB) of inbred mice.[2]

Some observations by Hartmann et al.[4] in our laboratory are of considerable interest in this connection and offer an opportunity for further study. During observations on the carcinogenicity of various fluorinated derivatives of 10-methyl-1,2-benzanthracene (10-Me-BA), all rats injected subcutaneously with the 4'-fluoro derivative died within eight weeks. Conspicuous alterations were observed in the vessels of the lungs and kidneys of these animals.

Such lesions were first observed in the lungs of a rat killed two weeks after injection of 4'-fluoro-10-Me-BA. By the fourth week four of seven animals had advanced lesions of the pulmonary and/or renal vessels, and all but one killed thereafter had similar lesions. The larger branches of the pulmonary and bronchial arteries were involved. The media was edematous and infiltrated with polymorphonuclear leukocytes and fibroblasts. Necrosis usually involved segments of the vessel walls. In the kidneys the conspicuous alteration was hyaline necrosis of the afferent arterioles, occasionally involving a portion of or the entire glomerulus. Such lesions resemble those seen in malignant hypertension.

The renal lesions were most pronounced at four and five weeks, but were absent after seven and eight weeks. This suggests that the lesion is reversible. Hawn and Janeway[5] observed regression of vascular lesions induced in rabbits by the administration of foreign proteins; such regression was correlated with a decreased level of circulating antigen.

The absence of such lesions in rats given the parent hydrocarbon 10-Me-BA or the 3-fluoro derivative would tend to exclude a toxic effect, as would the delay in development of the lesions. Such a delay in development strongly suggests that chemical sensitivity to the 4'-fluoro derivative is the principal etiologic factor. Sensitization to 9,10-dimethyl-1,2-benzanthracene has been reported following topical application in a human volunteer.

Various polycyclic aromatic hydrocarbons have been shown to combine with certain tissue proteins of the mouse in vivo. Should the 4'-fluoro-10-Me-benzanthracene compound likewise combine with one or more proteins in vivo and yield an antigenic foreign protein, auto-immunization would result. I have cited this work at some length for two reasons: (1) Such an experiment may give us another entering wedge with which to explore the pathogenesis of arteritis under controlled experimental conditions. (2) It should also alert us as pathologists to the possibility of an increasing development of arteritis in patients currently receiving a number of chemotherapeutic as well as other chemical agents.

In summary, I hope it is evident that the vascular lesions in a wide variety of conditions result from a reaction of antigen and antibody. Although the basic mechanism may be similar, different degrees of reactivity result in a wide variety of tissue alterations. Some are acute and fulminating, with or without eosinophilia; some have an intense plasma cell reaction indicative of antibody response. Others resemble granulomata with giant cell reaction. Ultimately, as the process subsides, reparative fibrosis predominates.

It seems to me that in our efforts to understand the pathogenesis of this disease we have been focusing too intently upon the morphology of the disease. If forced to place the above conditions into separate categories on the basis of microscopy alone, most of us might fare rather badly. This indicates that there are few, if any, specific anatomic characteristics by which such lesions can be accurately separated. In other words, there are sufficient similarities to suggest that the alterations in each condition, although due to different etiologies, are produced by somewhat similar mechanisms. There is a real need for a new approach to the problem, utilizing some of the modern techniques available.

REFERENCES

1. Bywaters, E. G.: Peripheral vascular obstruction in rheumatoid arthritis and its relationship to other vascular lesions. Ann. Rheum. Dis., *16*:84, 1957.
2. Deringer, Margaret K.: Necrotizing arteritis in strain Bh/De mice. Lab. Invest., *8*:1461, 1959.
3. Friedberg, C. K. and Gross, L.: Periarteritis nodosa (necrotizing arteritis) associated with rheumatic heart disease. Arch. Int. Med., *54*:170, 1934.
4. Hartmann, H. A., Miller, E. C. and Miller, J. A.: Periarteritis in rats given single injection of 4'-fluoro-10-methyl-1,2-benzanthracene. Proc. Soc. Exper. Biol. & Med., *101*:626, 1959.
5. Hawn, C. V. and Janeway, C. A.: Histological and serological sequences in experimental hypersensitivity. J. Exper. Med., *85*:571, 1947.
6. Johnson, R. L. et al.: Steroid therapy and vascular lesions in rheumatoid arthritis. Arth. & Rheum., *2*:224, 1959.
7. Movat, H. Z. and More, R. H.: Nature and origin of fibrinoid. Am. J. Clin. Path., *28*:331, 1957.
8. Rich, A. R.: Role of hypersensitivity in periarteritis nodosa. Bull. Johns Hopkins Hosp., *71*:123, 1942.
9. Sokoloff, L. and Bunim, J. J.: Vascular lesions in rheumatoid arthritis. J. Chron. Dis., *5*:668, 1957.
10. Sokoloff, L., Wilens, S. L. and Bunim, J. J.: Arteritis of striated muscle in rheumatoid arthritis. Am. J. Path., *27*:157, 1951.
11. Wilson, Keith S. and Alexander, Harry L.: The relation of periarteritis nodosa to bronchial asthma and other forms of human hypersensitiveness. J. Lab. & Clin. Med., *30*:195, 1945.

The Natural Course of Polyarteritis Nodosa, with Special Reference to the Respiratory Tract

GEOFFREY A. ROSE

Medical Unit, St. Mary's Hospital, London, England

The introduction of steroid therapy has greatly modified both the clinical course and the pathologist's view of polyarteritis nodosa. As a result, there is little opportunity nowadays to study its natural course and characteristics, except in relation to the fatal cases which escape clinical detection. Obviously these form an atypical sample.

Not long after cortisone was introduced, the Medical Research Council arranged for a retrospective study of all the cases that had been under care at nine British hospital centres during the period 1946 to 1952.[3, 4, 5] In all, 104 histologically proven cases were obtained. The data to be presented here are based mainly on these cases. They probably represent a fairly typical cross-section of polyarteritis nodosa as it was being diagnosed in British hospitals over the period in question.

THE ONSET OF THE DISEASE

The onset of the disease showed an interesting seasonal pattern (Table 1) which very much resembles the familiar seasonal pattern of respiratory infections. It would, however, be a mistake to infer too much from the similarity, for just the same seasonal incidence is shown, for example, by cardiac infarction and by chilblains. It is enough to say that the observation is consistent with the hypothesis that the onset of the disease may be related to preceding respiratory infection.

Around the time when they developed the disease a majority of the patients in the Medical Research Council series had respiratory symptoms of

TABLE 1. THE SEASONAL INCIDENCE OF POLYARTERITIS NODOSA IN 89 PROVEN CASES WITH DATABLE ONSET

MONTH	NO. OF PATIENTS (grouped mean)
January	10
February	10.7
March	12
April	9.3
May	6.7
June	5.7
July	5.7
August	5.7
September	4.3
October	4.7
November	6.7
December	7.7

222

some sort. These could be classified into three groups. First, there were those with chronic respiratory tract infections, amounting to about one-quarter of all patients; clinically and pathologically these appeared simply as straight-forward cases of bronchiectasis, bronchitis or otitis media. Second, there was a group of patients with recent upper respiratory infection, usually occurring about two weeks before the onset of polyarteritis and of streptococcal origin in some, and perhaps in most, instances. Last, in about one-third of all patients the disease itself seemed to start in the respiratory tract—sometimes as an upper respiratory granuloma, but more often in the bronchi or the lung parenchyma.

The patients with specific involvement of the respiratory tract showed a number of interesting features which seemed to mark them off sharply from the remainder. With only one exception, in every patient who at necropsy showed specific respiratory tract lesions there had been clinical evidence that these lesions had been present from the very start of the disease. That is to say, it seems that in polyarteritis nodosa either the lungs are involved at the start or they will not be involved at all. Indeed, the way in which they are spared is sometimes most striking: In a number of cases in which almost every other viscus has been extensively involved, the pulmonary arteries have been quite unaffected. No other organ in the body behaves like this. The skin and joints, for example, are often the first systems to be involved, but it is also common for them to be affected only later in the disease.

EVOLUTION OF THE DISEASE IN CASES WITH LUNG INVOLVEMENT

Cases with specific lung involvement still retain their individuality as the disease evolves. The illness tends to be divided fairly clearly into two phases. In the first the disease is confined to the lungs; in the second it becomes generalised. The interval between the start of the two phases is very variable (Table 2). Sometimes it is many years, especially in patients with

TABLE 2. *INTERVALS BETWEEN ONSET OF RESPIRATORY ILLNESS AND MANIFEST SYSTEMIC POLYARTERITIS IN 30 PATIENTS*

INTERVAL	NO. OF PATIENTS
Under 3 months	11
3 - 5 "	3
6 - 8 "	2
9 - 11 "	2
1 - 2 years	5
3 - 4 "	2
5 - 6 "	3
7 - 8 "	2

asthma; but in about half the cases in this series, it was less than six months. Our present knowledge is practically confined to fatal generalised cases, for only in these is diagnostic proof available as a rule. But it may be that some patients with essentially the same disease never enter a generalised phase. Long-term follow-up studies are badly needed here, particularly, perhaps, in relation to the not uncommon syndrome of asthma with high eosinophilia. (High eosinophilia is very common in polyarteritis nodosa when the lungs are involved, but is never seen when the lungs are spared.[5])

Generalisation of the disease tends to occur when the respiratory illness is most severe. Once this second phase is entered it is uncommon for any sort of remission to occur, and very few patients survive the next six months.

Characteristic granulomatous lesions, often with dense eosinophilic infiltration, have often been described in patients with respiratory tract involvement.[1, 2, 6] Evidence has since been produced[5] that lesions of this sort hardly ever occur apart from lung involvement, and at least a few can be found in nearly all cases with lung involvement. This supports the idea that patients with lung lesions form a special group. If this is so, their characteristic course and pattern of disease demand an explanation.

If polyarteritis nodosa is a hypersensitivity disease, two possibilities arise in relation to this problem. If the antigen is exogenous (bacterial or parasitic infection for example), the portal of entry in these cases seems likely to be the respiratory tract, leading first of all to a purely local reaction. Alternatively, we might be dealing with a state of auto-immunisation to some component of lung tissue. This second hypothesis would leave unexplained the special characteristics of the extrapulmonary lesions in these cases; and it does little to explain the impression of a disease process which is at first held up at some sort of lung barrier but which, having once broken out, spreads widely and unremittingly.

REFERENCES

1. Churg, J. and Strauss, L.: Allergic granulomatosis, allergic angiitis, and periarteritis nodosa. Am. J. Path., 27:277, 1951.
2. Fienberg, R.: Necrotizing granulomatosis and angiitis of the lungs. Am. J. Clin. Path., 23:413, 1953.
3. Rose, G. A.: The natural history of polyarteritis: a report to the Collagen Diseases and Hypersensitivity Panel of the Medical Research Council. 1954. (Unpublished; available from M.R.C.).
4. Rose, G. A.: The natural history of polyarteritis. Brit. M. J., 2:1148, 1957.
5. Rose, G. A. and Spencer, H.: Polyarteritis nodosa. Quart. J. Med. (n.s.), 26:43, 1957.
6. Wegener, F.: Über eine eigenartige chirogene Granulomatose mit besonderer Beteiligung des Arterien-systems und der Nieren. Beitr. 2. path. Anat. u. z. allg. Path., 102:36, 1939.

The Pathogenesis of Progressive Systemic Sclerosis (Diffuse Scleroderma) and Dermatomyositis

A Review of Recent Evidence Indicative of an Immunologic Abnormality in These Disorders*

GERALD P. RODNAN

University of Pittsburgh School of Medicine

PROGRESSIVE SYSTEMIC SCLEROSIS (DIFFUSE SCLERODERMA)

Progressive systemic sclerosis is now recognized to be a systemic disorder of connective tissue with characteristic changes in the skin (scleroderma), synovium and certain internal organs—including the gastrointestinal tract (especially the esophagus), heart, lung and kidney.[6, 34, 62, 72, 77, 82, 84, 97, 98] Although the disease may appear to remain long confined to the integument, in most instances there tends to be steadily, and at times rapidly, progressive involvement of internal organs followed by death from myocardial and/or renal failure. In many cases, however, there are variations in the natural course sufficiently definite to be considered indicative of periods of spontaneous remission and exacerbation in the disease.

Although there is an abundance of theories concerning etiology and pathogenesis, the fundamental nature of progressive systemic sclerosis† remains obscure. We cannot review here the wealth of older and for the most part abandoned concepts;‡ instead, we shall be concerned chiefly with recent studies which suggest the existence of an immunologic basis for this disorder.

Immunologic Abnormalities in P.S.S.

Over the past several years there has accumulated an increasingly convincing body of evidence which tends to support the theory that P.S.S. is related to the major systemic rheumatic diseases and that, in common with such disorders, its etiology and pathogenesis may lie in an abnormal, perhaps basically heritable, immune response.*

* Studies described in this report have been supported by research fellowship HF-5493 and research grant H-2783 of the National Heart Institute, U.S.P.H.S.; Research Grant A-97 of the Health Research and Services Foundation, Pittsburgh; and a research grant from the Western Pennsylvania Chapter, Arthritis and Rheumatism Foundation.

† Hereinafter abbreviated as P.S.S.

‡ The interested reader is referred to extensive earlier reviews by Castle,[13] Boardman,[8] O'Leary and Nomland,[71] and Burch,[11] and the recent summaries of Talbott and Ferrandis[97] and Orabona and Albano.[72]

Familial Nature of P.S.S.   The development of P.S.S. has been observed in sisters[72] and in first cousins,[85] but the occurrence of the disease on a familial basis seems to be rare. Instances have been reported, however, in which a sibling or child of a patient with P.S.S. has developed one or another major rheumatic disease, including rheumatoid arthritis, S.L.E. and dermatomyositis.[42, 61, 85] These observations alone are much too scant to permit any confirmation of a heritable predisposition to the disease.

There are two other observations which would seem to be worthy of additional scrutiny. The first of these is concerned with the familial occurrence of Raynaud's phenomenon,† alone or in association with sclero-

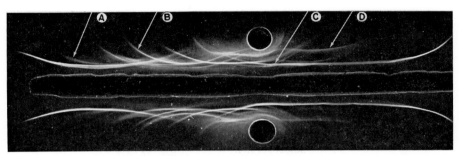

Fig. 1.   Serum immunoelectrophoretic pattern of patient B. Bu.(P.S.S.), illustrating increases in alpha-1 globulin (A), alpha-2 macroglobulin (B), beta-2 macroglobulin (D) and the splitting of gamma globulin (C).

derma.[33, 52, 85] The second is the presence of unexplained hypergammaglobulinemia in a relatively small number of asymptomatic immediate relatives of patients with P.S.S.[85]

Serum Protein Abnormalities.   Hypergammaglobulinemia.   It is not uncommon to find elevations in the concentration of serum globulins in P.S.S. comparable to the values noted in rheumatoid arthritis and systemic lupus erythematosus.[70, 85, 103] Most often and in greatest measure this is due to an increase in gamma globulin; often there is a lesser rise in alpha-2 globulin and the other fractions.

When serum is examined by means of the more sensitive technique of immunoelectrophoresis, one finds a variety of abnormalities, most commonly increases in alpha-1 globulin and alpha-2 macroglobulin, and, in approximately one-half of cases, elevations in beta-2 macroglobulin, and a peculiar increase and splitting in gamma globulin (Fig. 1).[109] These changes are not considered specific for P.S.S., for similar alterations have been noted in other rheumatic and nonrheumatic states.[45]

---

* Early support for the role of immunologic mechanisms (anaphylactic hypersensitivity) as the "common denominator" in the pathogenesis of S.L.E., P.S.S. and other systemic disorders of connective tissue was derived in large measure from certain morphological similarities (including the presence of fibrinoid "degeneration," now believed to be of significantly varying composition[101]) to the lesions of experimental and human serum sickness, polyarteritis and drug hypersensitivity.[80] The prophetic comment of Rich is worthy of note here: "From the standpoint of the entire field of hypersensitivity, there is high promise in an attack on the virtually untouched, fundamental problems relating to the intimate chemical mechanisms through which hypersensitive reactions exert their injurious effects upon the tissues."[80]

† Noted first by Raynaud, himself in 1862.[79]

HEMAGGLUTINATION AND LATEX FIXATION REACTIONS. Kellgren and Ball[56] noted positive sensitized sheep cell agglutination reactions in 16 (41 per cent) of 39 cases of P.S.S. and indicated that high titers "tended to be associated with vascular and articular lesions." Others have reported a similarly high incidence of positive reactions[85, 108] without, however, any close relation to the presence of synovial involvement.[84]

L.E. CELL REACTION. Positive L.E. cell reactions have been found in the course of otherwise typical P.S.S. on a number of occasions,[1, 43, 57, 66, 77, 85, 102] and may well be much more common than presently realized, for the reaction may be inconstant and may require repeated testing.

BIOLOGICAL FALSE POSITIVE SEROLOGICAL TESTS FOR SYPHILIS (BFP REACTIONS). Chronic BFP reactions have been noted only rarely in P.S.S.[77, 81, 85] Here again, however, as in the case of the L.E. cell phenomenon, this reaction may be highly evanescent.

ANTINUCLEAR AND OTHER TISSUE ANTIBODIES. It has now been demonstrated by means of both immunohistochemical and serological techniques that the serum of many patients with S.L.E., P.S.S. and dermatomyositis contains one or more globulins capable of combining with nuclear and cytoplasmic components of autologous, homologous and heterologous tissues, in a manner highly suggestive of an antigen-antibody reaction.[2, 4, 18, 27, 39, 43, 48, 49, 50]

To date, the most elaborate study concerned with P.S.S. and dermatomyositis has been that of Bardawil et al.,[4] who found that nuclear staining by fluorescein isocyanate conjugates of serum globulins from patients with scleroderma and dermatomyositis* was prevented by treatment of tissue sections with deoxyribonuclease, but not with ribonuclease, and concluded that the nuclear material involved in the reaction was deoxyribonucleoprotein. It was observed that nuclear binding with fluorescent conjugate was blocked completely by exposure of the tissue to unconjugated abnormal gamma globulin and that sera of patients with S.L.E. frequently though not invariably demonstrated a capacity for mutual inhibition of the staining reaction. These sera failed, however, to inhibit the binding of gamma globulin from cases of scleroderma. These workers further noted identical nuclear staining by rabbit antihistone antiserum and found these reactions to be inhibited by the serum of some patients, including at least one with scleroderma.[5] Intra-uterine sensitization by fetal or placental tissues and exposure to streptococcal or viral deoxyribonucleoprotein were suggested as possible means for the establishment of these antinuclear antibodies in the patient.

Goodman, Fahey and Malmgren[39] found a positive fluorescein anti-mouse liver nucleus reaction with the serum of two of four patients with scleroderma, and in one a positive antinucleoprotein (calf thymus extract) tanned-cell hemagglutination test. In a report devoted chiefly to observations on S.L.E., Scalettar et al.[89] made incidental note of a patient with scleroderma having positive complement fixation in a serological procedure involving incubation of test serum with crude calf-thymus nucleoprotein. Binding of serum globulin to calf-thymus nucleoprotein in single cases of scleroderma, dermatomyositis and Raynaud's disease has also been observed by Friou.[27]

These serological and immunohistochemical reactions indicative of the presence of antinuclear and anticytoplasmic factors in S.L.E. have not been found to be uniformly positive. (The data in P.S.S. are much too fragmentary

* This group has recently reported the presence of similar antinuclear globulins in approximately one-third of a large number of patients with rheumatoid arthritis.[43]

to comment upon in this regard.) It is possible that at least some of the negative reactions may have been due to difficulties in techniques and/or related to variations in the activity of the disease and the effects of the treatment with adrenal corticosteroids, but the real significance of these antinuclear and anticytoplasmic globulins in the etiology and pathogenesis of the disorders of connective tissue under consideration remains to be determined. The experimental production of cross-reacting antibody-like proteins in rabbits following injection of extracts of foreign nucleoprotein[38] and histone[5] provides evidence for the belief that bacterial and/or viral infection may lead in certain susceptible persons to the production of potentially harmful autoantibodies. A number of workers have pointed out, however, a lack of correlation between positive antinuclear and anticytoplasmic reactions and the symptoms of disease, and they consider this to be evidence militating against direct participation of these factors in the pathogenesis of the disorders in question. The matter is summed up well by Deicher, Holman and Kunkel[18] in the recent statement that "at present, the observed reactions can only be taken to indicate an unusual state of the immune system, the nature of which is still unknown. . . . The significance of these reactions in S.L.E. and other diseases of unknown etiology remains yet to be determined."*

Miscellaneous Serological Findings. Fudenberg[28] described the finding of both warm and cold autoantibodies in an apparently unique example of scleroderma complicated by severe hemolytic anemia. The administration of cortisone was followed by amelioration of the anemia and diminution in the titers of the warm autoagglutinins.

Myerson and Stout[69] observed the presence of marked cryoglobulinemia in a patient with probable P.S.S. and felt that this contributed to the development of cold sensitivity, digital gangrene and retinal artery occlusion in this case.

P.S.S. and Hypogammaglobulinemia. A strikingly high incidence of rheumatic disease has been observed in patients with both the congenital and acquired varieties of hypogammaglobulinemia.[32, 35, 37, 53] In most such instances the syndrome is that of a polyarthritis frequently accompanied by subcutaneous nodules, clinically indistinguishable from rheumatoid arthritis.[32, 35] Less often the rheumatic complaints take the form of systemic lupus erythematosus,[59] scleroderma[9, 100] or dermatomyositis.[32, 44] At first the occurrence of these syndromes in association with marked hypogammaglobulinemia was considered to represent potent evidence against the concept that these disorders were based on a pathologic immunologic response and the presence of abnormal serum gamma globulins.[37] More recent findings have necessitated reversal of this view, for not only is the frequent occurrence of the rheumatic disease in these patients in itself suspicious, but several observers have now reported a high incidence of rheumatoid arthritis, of S.L.E. and of positive serologic tests for rheumatoid factor in the immediate relatives of patients with acquired hypogammaglobulinemia.[29, 37, 59, 85]

---

* The exact means by which immunologic reactions may lead to the lesions of disease are almost completely unknown. Klemperer suggested that "systemic fibrinoid alteration" might be the result of the deposition of abnormal serum proteins (paraproteins) including antibodies.[58] More recently, Dixon and co-workers[20, 21] have directed attention to the importance of circulating antigen-antibody or other globulin-globulin complexes which initiate and are localized in allergic inflammatory arterial and glomerular lesions of experimental serum sickness and glomerulonephritis.

Further, it is now appreciated that while these patients appear unable to form circulating antibody and display a virtual absence of gamma and other antibody globulins in their serum, they retain the ability to develop delayed allergy[36] and possess certain serum beta-2 and gamma globulins which are not demonstrable in normal persons.[10] It would seem reasonable at this time to conclude that hypogammaglobulinemia and the various rheumatic states are indeed inter-related and that both represent manifestations of a more fundamental and profound, probably genetically determined, disorder in globulin synthesis and immunologic responsiveness.

P.S.S. and Sjögren's Syndrome. Sjögren himself made note of the frequent occurrence of polyarthritis in the syndrome* which bears his name.[94] It has now become clear that this disorder may be associated with any one of a number of rheumatic diseases—most commonly rheumatoid arthritis, as well as Felty's syndrome,[19, 41, 96, 99] less often S.L.E.,[30, 46, 67, 68, 78, 96] P.S.S.[7, 14, 30, 42, 47, 63, 73, 76, 78, 86, 87, 93, 95, 96] and polyarteritis.[12, 78]

Of great interest is the recent observation of the concurrence of Sjögren's syndrome and Hashimoto's thyroiditis[46] and of combinations of these with Waldenström's macroglobulinemic purpura,[54, 96] and the demonstration in these conditions of marked hypergammaglobulinemia,[7, 46, 96] antinuclear and anticytoplasmic serum globulins (reacting with salivary, lacrimal, thyroid and other glandular tissues)[7, 23, 54, 55] and a variety of abnormal serological reactions (including positive L.E. cell and sensitized sheep cell agglutination reactions).[7, 46]

Evidence of a familial, perhaps heritable, predisposition to this disturbance is presented in a number of reports of the occurrence of Sjögren's syndrome in two or more members of a kinship.[16, 19, 25, 65]

Experimental Production and Effects of Anticollagen Antibody. Most attempts to induce the formation of antibody to purified collagen have proved unsuccessful, but Rothbard and Watson[88] present evidence for the role of rabbit antirat collagen antibody in the production of renal glomerular lesions in rats prepared by the injection of adjuvant. The histologic changes observed differed from those found following the administration of anti-kidney serum. It was suggested that tissue damage resulted from the interaction of rat antibody with the rabbit antiglobulin bound to its antigen (collagen) in the kidney.

DERMATOMYOSITIS

The clinical and pathologic characteristics of dermatomyositis† are in many cases so closely similar to P.S.S. that a number of competent observers have been led to conclude that the two conditions are expressions of a single disease, affecting the skin and muscle to a different relative degree.[24, 26, 31, 64, 73, 74] Difficulty has also been encountered in the separation of dermatomyositis from S.L.E.[31, 74] Others have considered such resemblance to be superficial and insufficient to prevent clinical differentiation of dermatomyositis.[3, 22]

---

* Salient features of the syndrome include keratoconjunctivitis sicca, xerostomia and enlargement of lacrimal and salivary (parotid) glands; there may also be involvement of tracheobronchial mucosa and vagina, and hyposecretion of the gastric and other exocrine glands.

† Hereinafter abbreviated as D.M.

Theories of Etiology and Pathogenesis*

Heritable Nature of D.M. The occurrence of D.M. has been noted in sisters,[15] in brother and sister,[105] and in "mirror-image twins,"[107] but there is little other information presently available to support the existence of a significant familial or heritable basis for this disorder. Here again, however, as in the case of S.L.E. and P.S.S.,[51, 60, 83, 85] members of the immediate families of patients have been found to have unexplained hypergammaglobulinemia.[85]

Immunologic Abnormality. Hypergammaglobulinemia of moderate degree is a frequent finding in acute dermatomyositis,[70, 75, 85] and positive hemagglutination reactions for rheumatoid factor have been observed on a number of occasions.[56, 75, 108] Christianson observed two patients who developed positive L.E. cell reactions during the course of otherwise "classic" dermatomyositis.[15]

The detection of tissue-binding serum globulins in dermatomyositis by Bardawil et al. is described above.[4] It may be noted that Pagel observed changes similar to human myositis in rabbits given intramuscular injections of muscle antiserum.[74]

Association of Dermatomyositis and Malignant Neoplasms. A number of recent reviews have upheld previous observations of an inordinately high incidence (approximately 15 per cent) of malignant neoplasm in patients with dermatomyositis.[15, 17, 24, 90, 92, 106] The clinical manifestations of these tumors (chiefly carcinomata of widely varying origin) have been found to precede, accompany or, most commonly, follow the development of the D.M., and it has been noted that the latter is characteristically acute in onset and is accompanied by rather florid cutaneous lesions.[106] Further, it has been observed that surgical, radiational or chemical (hormonal) treatment of the neoplasm may be followed by improvement in the dermatomyositis. Explanation of this association is quite unclear. The popular theory that "tumor products" lead to the development of D.M. via an immunologic mechanism receives some support in the report of Grace and Dao,[40] who described a patient with dermatomyositis and carcinoma of the breast in whom there was an immediate skin reaction to tumor extract as well as a positive passive transfer test.

CONCLUSION

Clinical, serological and immunohistochemical studies have provided increasingly convincing evidence of a close relationship between progressive systemic sclerosis, dermatomyositis and other of the systemic inflammatory rheumatic disorders, notably rheumatoid arthritis and systemic lupus erythematosus, although the exact nature of this relationship remains unclear. While the demonstration in many patients of one or more serum gamma globulins possessing properties of antinuclear, anticytoplasmic or antiglobulin antibody has established the existence of an "unusual state of the immune system," the exact role, if any, played by immunologic reactions in the etiology and pathogenesis of these disorders remains to be determined.

REFERENCES

1. Arnold, H. L. and Tilden, I. L.: Fatal scleroderma with L.E. phenomenon. Report of a case. A.M.A. Arch. Dermat., 76:427, 1957.

* For more general reviews the interested reader is referred to Sheard,[91] Talbott and Ferrandis[97] and Walton and Adams.[104]

2. Asherson, G. L.: Antibodies against nuclear and cytoplasmic cell constituents in systemic lupus erythematosus and other diseases. Brit. J. Exper. Path., 40:209, 1959.
3. Banks, B. M.: Is there a common denominator in scleroderma, dermatomyositis, disseminated lupus erythematosus, the Libman-Sachs syndrome, and polyarteritis nodosa? New Engl. J. Med., 225:433, 1941.
4. Bardawil, W. A., Toy, B. L., Galins, N. and Bayles, T. B.: Disseminated lupus erythematosus, scleroderma, and dermatomyositis as manifestations of sensitization to DNA-protein. I. An immunohistochemical approach. Am. J. Path., 34:607, 1958.
5. Bardawil, W. A., Toy, B. L. and Galins, N.: Hypersensitivity to histone induced experimentally in rabbits. Lancet, 1:888, 1958.
6. Beigelman, P. M., Goldner, F. and Bayles, T. B.: Progressive systemic sclerosis (scleroderma). New Engl. J. Med., 249:45, 1953.
7. Bloch, K. J., Wohl, M. J., Ship, I. I., Oglesby, R. B. and Bunim, J. J.: Sjögren's syndrome. I. Serologic reactions in patients with Sjögren's syndrome with and without rheumatoid arthritis. Arth. & Rheum., 3:287, 1960.
8. Boardman, W. P.: Scleroderma, with special reference to its etiology and treatment. Arch. Dermat. & Syph., 19:901, 1929.
9. Bowen, R.: Personal communication quoted in ref. 35.
10. Bridges, R. A. and Good, R. A.: Connective tissue diseases and certain serum protein components in patients with agammaglobulinemia. Ann. N. Y. Acad. Sc., 86:1089, 1960.
11. Burch, G. E.: Etiology and abnormal physiology [of scleroderma]. N. Orleans M. & S. J., 92:12, 1939-40.
12. Cardel, B. S. and Gurling, K. J.: Observations on the pathology of Sjögren's syndrome. J. Path. & Bact., 68:137, 1954.
13. Castle, W. F.: The endocrine causation of scleroderma, including morphea. Brit. J. Dermat., 35:255, 1923.
14. Caughey, J. E. and Richardson, W.: Acrosclerosis, with a report of a case treated with cortisone. New Zealand M. J., 51:227, 1952.
15. Christianson, H. B., Brunsting, L. A. and Perry, H. O.: Dermatomyositis. Unusual features, complications, and treatment. A.M.A. Arch. Dermat., 74:581, 1956.
16. Cloverdale, H.: Some unusual cases of Sjögren's syndrome. Brit. J. Ophth., 32:669, 1948.
17. Curtis, A. C., Blaylock, H. C. and Harrell, E. R.: Malignant lesions associated with dermatomyositis. J.A.M.A., 150:844, 1952.
18. Deicher, H. R. G., Holman, H. R. and Kunkel, H. G.: Anti-cytoplasmic factors in the sera of patients with systemic lupus erythematosus and certain other diseases. Arth. & Rheum., 3:1, 1960.
19. Denko, C. W. and Bergenstal, D. M.: The sicca syndrome (Sjögren's syndrome). A.M.A. Arch. Int. Med., 105:849, 1960.
20. Dixon, F. J., Vazquez, J. J., Weigle, W. O. and Cochrane, C. G.: Pathogenesis of serum sickness. A.M.A. Arch. Path., 65:18, 1958.
21. Dixon, F. J., Weigle, W. O., Vazquez, J. J. and Feldman, J. D.: The immunologic and morphologic consequences of prolonged daily injection of bovine albumin (BSA). Fed. Proc., 19:205, 1960 (Abstract).
22. Domzalski, C. A. and Morgan, V. C.: Dermatomyositis: diagnostic features and therapeutic pitfalls. Am. J. Med., 19:370, 1955.
23. Doniach, D. and Roitt, I. M.: Auto-immunity in Hashimoto's disease and its implications. J. Clin. Endocrinol., 17:1293, 1957.
24. Dowling, G. B.: Scleroderma and dermatomyositis. Brit. J. Dermat., 67:275, 1955.
25. Falls, H. F.: Skeletal system, including joints. In Sorsby, A. (ed.): Clinical Genetics. St. Louis, C. V. Mosby Co., 1953, p. 236.
26. Freudenthal, W.: Generalized scleroderma and dermatomyositis: a histological comparison. Brit. J. Dermat. and Syph., 52:289, 1940.
27. Friou, G. J.: Clinical application of a test for lupus globulin-nucleohistone interaction using fluorescent antibody. Yale J. Biol. & Med., 31:40, 1958.
28. Fudenberg, H.: Scleroderma with symptomatic hemolytic anemia: a case report. Ann. Int. Med., 43:201, 1955.
29. Fudenberg, H., German, J. L., III and Kunkel, H. G.: The occurrence of rheumatoid factor and other gamma globulin abnormalities in the families of patients with agammaglobulinemia. J. Clin. Invest., 39:987, 1960 (Abstract).
30. Futcher, P. H.: Enlargement and round cell infiltration of the salivary glands associated with systemic disease. Bull. Johns Hopkins Hosp., 105:97, 1959.

31. Garcin, R., Lapresle, J., Gruner, J. and Scherrer, J.: Les polymyosites. Rev. Neurol., 92:465, 1955.
32. Gitlin, D., Janeway, C. A., Apt, L. and Craig, J. M.: Agammaglobulinemia. In Lawrence, H. S. (ed.): Cellular and Humoral Aspects of the Hypersensitive States. New York, Hoeber-Harper, 1959.
33. Goetz, R. H.: The pathology of progressive systemic sclerosis (generalized scleroderma). Clin. Proc., 4:337, 1945.
34. Goldgraber, M. B. and Kirsner, J. B.: Scleroderma of the gastrointestinal tract. A review. A.M.A. Arch. Path., 64:255, 1957.
35. Good, R. A., Rotstein, J. and Mazzitello, W. F.: The simultaneous occurrence of rheumatoid arthritis and agammaglobulinemia. J. Lab. & Clin. Med., 49:343, 1957.
36. Good, R. A., Bridges, R. A., Zak, S. J. and Pappenheimer, A. M., Jr.: Delayed hypersensitivity in agamma-globulinemia. In Shaffer, J. M. et al. (eds.): Mechanisms of hypersensitivity. Boston: Little, Brown and Co., 1959.
37. Good, R. A. and Rotstein, J.: Rheumatoid arthritis and agammaglobulinemia. Bull. Rheum. Dis., 10:203, 1960.
38. Goodman, H. C.: Antibodies to nucleoprotein extracts in patients with lupus erythematosus and rabbits immunized with nucleoprotein extracts. Clin. Research, 7:264, 1959 (Abstract).
39. Goodman, H. C., Fahey, J. L. and Malmgren, R. A.: Serum factors in lupus erythematosus and other diseases reacting with cell nuclei and nucleoprotein extracts: electrophoretic, ultracentrifugal and chromatographic studies. J. Clin. Invest., 39:1595, 1960.
40. Grace, J. T., Jr. and Dao, T. L.: Dermatomyositis in cancer. A possible etiological mechanism. Cancer, 12:648, 1959.
41. Gurling, K. J.: Association of Sjögren's and Felty's syndrome. Ann. Rheumat. Dis., 12:212, 1953.
42. Hagberg, B., Leonhardt, T. and Skogh, M.: Familial occurrence of collagen disease. I. Progressive systemic sclerosis and systemic lupus erythematosus. Submitted for publication.
43. Hall, A. P., Bardawil, W. A., Bayles, T. B., Mednis, A. D. and Galins, N.: The relations between the antinuclear, rheumatoid and L.E. cell factors in the systemic rheumatic diseases. New Engl. J. Med., 236:769, 1960.
44. Hansen, A.: Personal communication quoted in ref. 35.
45. Hartman, F.: Études immuno-électrophorétiques des sérums de malades atteints de rhumatisme. In Graber, P. and Burtin, P. (eds.): Analyse Immuno-Électrophorétique. Paris, Masson et Cie, 1960, pp. 191-195.
46. Heaton, J. M.: Sjögren's syndrome and systemic lupus erythematosus. Brit. M. J., 1:466, 1959.
47. Holm, S.: Keratoconjunctivitis sicca and the sicca syndrome. Acta Ophth., 27:Supplementum 33, 1949.
48. Holman, H. and Deicher, H. R.: The reaction of the lupus erythematosus (L.E.) cell factor with deoxyribonucleoprotein of the cell nucleus. J. Clin. Invest., 38:2059, 1959.
49. Holman, H., Deicher, H. R. G. and Kunkel, H. G.: The L.E. cell and the L.E. serum factors. Bull. N. Y. Acad. Med., 35:409, 1959.
50. Holman, H. and Kunkel, H.: Antinuclear antibodies and their detection in systemic lupus erythematosus (SLE). Bull. Rheum. Dis., 10:197, 1959.
51. Holman, H. and Deicher, H. R.: The appearance of hypergammaglobulinemia, positive serologic reactions for rheumatoid arthritis and complement fixation reactions with tissue constituents in the sera of relatives of patients with system lupus erythematosus. Arth. & Rheum., 3:244, 1960 (Abstract).
52. Hutchinson, J.: Congenital defects and inherited proclivities. Arch. Surg., 4:305, 1893.
53. Janeway, C. A., Gitlin, D., Craig, J. M. and Grice, D. S.: "Collagen disease" in patients with congenital agammaglobulinemia. Tr. A. Am. Physicians, 69:93, 1956.
54. Jensen, W. N. and Vazquez, J. J.: The concurrence of Hashimoto's thyroiditis, Sjögren's disease and Waldenström's macroglobulinemia purpura, with observations on autoantibodies in this disease. Tr. A. Am. Physicians, 72:lvi, 1959 (paper read by title).
55. Jones, B. R.: Lacrimal and salivary precipitating antibodies in Sjögren's syndrome. Lancet, 2:773, 1958.

56. Kellgren, J. H. and Ball, J.: Clinical significance of the rheumatoid serum factor. Brit. Med. J., *1*:523, 1959.
57. Kievits, J. H., Goslings, J., Schuit, H. R. E., and Hijmans, W.: Rheumatoid arthritis and the positive L.E.-cell phenomenon. Ann. Rheumat. Dis., *15*:211, 1956.
58. Klemperer, P.: The significance of the intermediate substances of the connective tissue in human disease. Harvey Lect., *49*:100, 1953-54.
59. Kunkel, H. G.: Immunologic aspects of rheumatoid arthritis. J. Chron. Dis., *10*:418, 1959.
60. Larsson, O. and Leonhardt, T.: Hereditary hypergammaglobulinaemia and systemic lupus erythematosus. I. Clinical and electrophoretic studies. Acta Med. Scand., *165*:371, 1959.
61. Leonhardt, T.: Familial occurrence of collagen disease. II. Progressive systemic sclerosis and dermatomyositis. Submitted for publication.
62. Leinwand, I., Duryee, A. W. and Richter, M. N.: Scleroderma. Based on a study of over 150 cases. Ann. Int. Med., *41*:1003, 1954.
63. Leriche, R.: Traitement chirurgical du syndrome de Sjögren (oeil sec et bouche sèche), résultat au bout de vingt-huit mois d'une double section du nerf vertebral; nature de la maladie. Presse méd., *55*:77, 1947.
64. Lewis, T.: Notes on scleroderma (dermatomyositis). Brit. J. Dermat. & Syph., *52*:233, 1940.
65. Lisch, K.: Über Hereditäres vorkommen des mit Keratoconjunctivitis sicca verbundenen Sjögrenschen Symptomenkomplexes. Arch. f. Augenheilkunde, *110*:357, 1937.
66. Longhi, A.: Arch. ital. dermat. sif., *27*:468, 1955 (quoted in ref. 72).
67. McLean, K. and Robinson, H. S.: Sjögren's syndrome. Canad. M.A.J., *71*:597, 1954.
68. Morgan, W. S.: The probable systemic nature of Mikulicz's disease and its relation to Sjögren's syndrome. New Engl. J. Med., *251*:5, 1954.
69. Myerson, R. M. and Stout, R. E.: Cryoglobulinemia associated with gangrene of the digits. Am. J. M. Sc., *230*:499, 1955.
70. Ogryzlo, M. A., Maclachlan, M., Dauphinee, J. A. and Fletcher, A. A.: The serum proteins in health and disease. Am. J. Med., *27*:596, 1959.
71. O'Leary, P. A. and Nomland, R.: A clinical study of one hundred and three cases of scleroderma. Am. J. M. Sc., *180*:95, 1930.
72. Orabona, M. L. and Albano, O.: Systemic progressive sclerosis (or visceral scleroderma). Review of the literature and report of cases. Acta med. scandinav., *160*:suppl. 333, 1957.
73. Ourgaud, A. G.: Syndrome de Sjögren associé à une maladie de Raynaud et à une sclérodermie. Bull. Soc. Ophth. France, No. 9, 816, 1950.
74. Pagel, W. and Treip, C. S.: Viscero-cutaneous collagenosis. A study of the intermediate forms of dermatomyositis, scleroderma, and disseminated lupus erythematosus. J. Clin. Path., *8*:1, 1955.
75. Pearson, C. M.: Rheumatic manifestations of polymyositis and dermatomyositis. Arth. & Rheum., *2*:127, 1959.
76. Piazzesi, W.: Su di un caso di sclerodermia con diplegia faciale e sindrome di Sjögren. Riv. pat. nerv., *77*:584, 1956.
77. Piper, W. N. and Helwig, E. B.: Progressive systemic sclerosis: visceral manifestations in generalized scleroderma. A.M.A. Arch. Dermat. & Syph., *72*:735, 1955.
78. Ramage, J. H. and Kinnear, W. F.: Keratoconjunctivitis and the collagen diseases. Brit. J. Ophth., *40*:416, 1956.
79. Raynaud, M.: On Local Asphyxia and Symmetrical Gangrene of the Extremities. (Translated by T. Barlow.) London, The New Sydenham Society, 1888.
80. Rich, A. R.: Hypersensitivity in disease, with special reference to periarteritis nodosa, rheumatic fever, disseminated lupus erythematosus and rheumatoid arthritis. Harvey Lect., *42*:106, 1946-47.
81. Richter, R. B.: Peripheral neuropathy and connective tissue disease. J. Neuropath. & Exper. Neurol., *13*:168, 1954.
82. Rodnan, G. P., Schreiner, G. E. and Black, R. L.: Renal involvement in progressive systemic sclerosis (generalized scleroderma). Am. J. Med., *23*:445, 1957.
83. Rodnan, G. P., Maclachlan, M. J. and Creighton, A.: Study of serum proteins and serologic reactions in relatives of patients with S.LE. Clin. Res., *8*:197, 1960 (Abstract).
84. Rodnan, G. P., Yunis, E. J. and Totten, R. S.: Experience with punch biopsy of synovium in study of joint disease. Ann. Int. Med., *53*:319, 1960.

85. Rodnan, G. P., Maclachlan, M. J. and Creighton, A.: Unpublished observations.
86. Rodnan, G. P.: Unpublished observations.
87. Rossier, P. H. and Hegglin-Volkmann, M.: Die Sklerodermie als intern-medizinisches Problem. Ein kasuistischer Beitrag. Schweiz. Med. Wschr., 84:1161, 1954.
88. Rothbard, S. and Watson, R. F.: Renal glomerular lesions induced by rabbit anti-rat collagen serum in rats prepared with adjuvant. J. Exper. Med., 109:633, 1959.
89. Scalettar, R., Marcus, D. M., Simonton, L. A. and Muschel, L. H.: The nucleoprotein complement-fixation test in the diagnosis of systemic lupus erythematosus. New Engl. J. Med., 263:226, 1960.
90. Schuermann, H.: Maligne tumoren bei dermatomyositis und progressiver sklerodermie. Arch. f. Dermat. u. Syph., 192:575, 1951.
91. Sheard, C., Jr.: Dermatomyositis. Arch. Int. Med., 88:640, 1951.
92. Sheard, C., Jr. and Knoepfler, P. T.: Dermatomyositis and the incidence of associated malignancy. A.M.A. Arch. Dermat., 75:224, 1957.
93. Shearn, M. A. Sjögren's syndrome in association with scleroderma. Ann. Int. Med., 52:1352, 1960.
94. Sjögren, H.: Zur Kenntnis der Keratoconjunctivitis sicca. Acta Ophth. 11:suppl. 2, 1933. Sjögren. H.: A New Conception of Keratoconjunctivitis Sicca. (Translated by J. B. Hamilton.) Sydney, Australasian Medical Publishing Co., 1943.
95. Šťáva, Z.: Diffuse scleroderma. A clinical study of sixty-five cases. Dermatologica, 117:135, 1958.
96. Stoltze, C. A., Hanlon, D. G., Pease, G. L. and Henderson, J. W.: Keratoconjunctivitis sicca and Sjögren's syndrome. A.M.A. Arch. Int. Med., 106:513, 1960.
97. Talbott, J. H. and Ferrandis, R. M.: Collagen Diseases. New York, Grune & Stratton, 1956.
98. Taubenhaus, M., Eisenstein, B. and Pick, A.: Cardiovascular manifestations of collagen diseases. Circulation, 12:903, 1955.
99. Thompson, M. and Eadie, S.: Kerato-conjunctivitis sicca and rheumatoid arthritis. Ann. Rheumat. Dis., 15:21, 1956.
100. Van Gelder, D. W.: Clinical significance of alterations in gamma globulin levels. South. M. J., 50:43, 1957.
101. Vazquez, J. J. and Dixon, F. J.: Immunohistochemical analysis of lesions associated with "fibrinoid change." A.M.A. Arch. Path., 66:504, 1958.
102. Volpé, R. and Hauch, J. T.: A case of scleroderma with L.E. cells and prolonged remission on cortisone therapy. Canad. M.A.J., 72:597, 1955.
103. Walker, S. A. and Benditt, E. P.: An electrophoretic study of the serum proteins in scleroderma. Proc. Soc. Exper. Biol. & Med., 67:504, 1948.
104. Walton, J. N. and Adams, R. D.: Polymyositis. Edinburgh, E.&S. Livingstone, Ltd., 1958.
105. Wedgwood, R. J. P., Cook, C. D. and Cohen, J.: Dermatomyositis. Report of 26 cases in children, with a discussion of endocrine therapy in 13. Pediatrics, 12:447, 1953.
106. Williams, R. D., Jr.: Dermatomyositis and malignancy: a review of the literature. Ann. Int. Med., 50:1174, 1959.
107. Winckler, K.: Über die Dermatomyositis. Zschr. Haut-Geschlectskrankh., 19:296, 1956.
108. Ziff, M.: The agglutination reaction in rheumatoid arthritis. J. Chron. Dis., 5:644, 1957.
109. Zlotnick, A. and Rodnan, G. P.: Immunoelectrophoresis of serum in progressive systemic sclerosis. Proc. Soc. Exper. Biol. & Med. (In press.)

Rheumatic Features in
Polymyositis and Dermatomyositis*

CARL M. PEARSON

University of California School of Medicine, Los Angeles

Polymyositis and dermatomyositis may be considered to be two clinical variants of a similar pathologic process that have as their primary clinical manifestation muscular weakness, especially of the proximal musculature of the limb girdles and of the neck and pharynx. The basic lesion is a non-suppurative inflammatory or degenerative process which involves the muscle fibers and the adjacent connective tissue stroma. In addition, a variable degree of perivasculitis is often present.

Within recent years it has become more apparent than previously that precise subdivisions of the various connective tissue or collagen diseases into distinct entities is impossible. Rather, in many cases there are gradations and clinical shadings of one disorder into one or more of the others. This is as apparent in myositis as it is in systemic lupus erythematosus (SLE) and somewhat more so than in rheumatoid arthritis and scleroderma. Hence about one-fourth of cases of polymyositis and dermatomyositis will develop dermatologic, gastrointestinal or pulmonary features that are typical for scleroderma (systemic sclerosis), articular signs and symptoms which are usually seen in rheumatoid arthritis, or dermal features similar to those which occur in SLE. Moreover, each of these disorders often shows an abnormal serum protein electrophoretic pattern and the latex fixation test has been positive in two-thirds of our patients in which this test has been done.

The nucleus of this study is a series of 24 patients, diagnosed as having poly- or dermatomyositis, who have been carefully studied and followed during the past four years. Twenty of these were female and four were male. Their ages varied from 2½ to 60 years with an almost equal spread of the majority in the fourth, fifth and sixth decades. When possible, data have also been obtained from two large series in the recent literature by Eaton[5] and by Walton and Adams.[18]

CLINICAL CHARACTERISTICS

The clinical features of myositis are variable, both in their pattern of onset and in their intensity from one case to another, or even at different times in the same patient. If, in addition to the muscular symptoms, the skin is affected with an intense erythema and edema of the face, upper eyelids and upper trunk, the diagnosis can be considered to be dermatomyositis. On the other hand, when dermal signs are absent or atypical in the presence of muscular weakness and biopsy findings of myositis, the condition may be called polymyositis.

The mode of onset of myositis has varied greatly in the present series.

* The author gratefully acknowledges the assistance provided by the Muscular Dystrophy Association of America during the course of these studies.

In general, dermatomyositis has a more acute onset and rapidly progressive course, whereas polymyositis more frequently develops insidiously. There are, however, exceptions in either direction. Although muscular symptoms usually appear early, they are not always the most prominent during the initial stages. This is reflected by the initial diagnoses that have been recorded in 64 cases (Table 1). From this series it can be seen that a rheumatic disorder was seriously considered to be present early in 19 cases and a

TABLE 1. CLINICAL DIAGNOSES RECORDED DURING THE INITIAL COURSE
OF THE ILLNESS IN 64 CASES*

	NO. OF TIMES DIAGNOSED†	
Neuromuscular		
Progressive muscular dystrophy	22	
Polymyositis and dermatomyositis	10	
Myasthenia gravis	8	
Polyneuritis	7	54
Poliomyelitis	2	
Other	5	
Rheumatic		
Rheumatoid arthritis	7	
Systemic lupus erythematosus	7	
"Acute rheumatism"	2	19
"Collagen disease"	2	
Fibrositis	1	
Dermatologic		
Scleroderma	3	
Seborrheic dermatitis	3	10
Exfoliative dermatitis	2	
Other dermatoses	2	
Other conditions		
Streptococcal pharyngitis	2	3
Addison's disease	1	

* From Walton and Adams[18] and present series.
† Multiple diagnoses in some patients.

dermatologic disorder in 10 cases. It should be noted that multiple diagnostic possibilities were considered in some of the cases, and each of these has been listed.

In our own series, 12 of the 24 patients developed rheumatic features. The occurrence of rheumatic manifestations was about equally divided between the 13 cases of polymyositis and the 11 of dermatomyositis. Of the 12 patients with rheumatic features, six had arthritis prior to or at the time of onset of muscular weakness. In two, recurrent articular symptoms quite typical for rheumatoid arthritis antedated weakness by 1½ and 5 years respectively, whereas in the other four an acute or subacute dermatomyositis appeared in conjunction with a polyarthritis. For several days the latter was the foremost feature in three of these cases.

Tabulated in Table 2 is an analysis of the various clinical signs and symptoms that have been observed in 105 cases of myositis. As can be seen, features referable to the musculature are present in *all* cases, variable cutaneous features in about two-thirds, and arthritic or rheumatic manifestations in one-third. In our own series, however, rheumatic signs were present in one-half of the cases studied.

The skin manifestations have been dealt with in detail elsewhere[3, 8, 14] and will not be considered further here.

TABLE 2. ANALYSIS OF CLINICAL SIGNS AND SYMPTOMS IN
105 CASES OF POLY- AND DERMATOMYOSITIS

MANIFESTATIONS	EATON[5] 41 CASES	WALTON AND ADAMS[18] 40 CASES	PRESENT SERIES 24 CASES	TOTAL AFFECTED AMONG 105 CASES
Cutaneous features	22	23	19	64
Raynaud's phenomenon	10	10	3	23
Arthritic or rheumatic features	10	10	12	32
Muscular pain or tenderness	18	16	16	50
Muscular atrophy	19	?	18	37*
Muscular contractures	11	8	16	35
Muscular weakness				
Proximal muscles	38	40	24	102
Distal muscles	24	14	8	46
Neck muscles	14	33	20	67
Dysphagia	22	21	18	61
Facial muscles	5	5	1	11

* From 65 cases. Atrophy was usually slight in degree.

Muscular Symptoms.   The main feature of all the cases was muscular weakness, which eventually overshadowed all other symptoms. It almost invariably affected the proximal musculature of the limbs as well as the pelvic and shoulder girdle muscles. Everyday activities such as rising from a chair, climbing stairs, combing the hair and similar acts became difficult or impossible to perform. Dysphagia was likewise a common feature and was first apparent as an inability to swallow solid food. Later, even sips of water were aspirated. Weakness of the anterior muscles of the neck rendered difficult elevation of the head from the pillow. The distal muscles of the extremities were involved to a lesser degree and in a smaller proportion of cases (Table 2).

Muscular pain and tenderness were mild in all of our cases diagnosed as polymyositis. Several patients with dermatomyositis had tenderness, pain and induration in the muscles. Muscular atrophy, when present, was most readily detected about the shoulder girdle. Contracture was a sign of long-standing or severe involvement of muscles and was due to the presence of shortened fibrous tissue in the muscle. It occurred most commonly in the biceps and wrist flexors.

Rheumatic Symptoms.   Signs and symptoms referable to the joints, bursae and connective tissues were present in 12 of the 24 cases of myositis in the present series (Table 3). This incidence was higher than that noted

TABLE 3. RHEUMATIC FEATURES IN 24 CASES OF MYOSITIS

SYMPTOM OR SIGN	NO. OF CASES AFFECTED
Any rheumatic manifestation	12
Gel phenomenon or clinical "fibrositis"	11
Arthralgias	10
Fluctuating polyarthritis	9
Chronic joint deformity	1
Recurrent bursitis	4
Radiologic features:	
Periarticular radiolucency	3
Joint damage	1

by Eaton[5] and by Walton and Adams,[18] who recorded rheumatic symptoms in about 25 per cent of their patients (Table 2). The difference may in part be explained by the fact that such symptoms were specifically sought for in our series.

In 9 of the 12 patients the rheumatic features were transitory and comprised only a fraction of the total clinical picture. In two of these, however, an acute symmetrical polyarthritis developed in conjunction with muscular weakness and, in each, acute rheumatoid arthritis was diagnosed initially. In the other three cases arthritis was a more prominent feature. The first was a 41-year-old woman who had recurrent polyarthritis for 5½ years before the onset of muscular weakness. Both the small and the large joints were involved without deformity. Progressive muscular weakness eventually led to her death 1½ years later. Corticosteroids were not given in this case.*

In the second patient, a man aged 57 years, a symmetrical polyarthritis was present for five years and involved the knees and the small finger joints. Several subcutaneous nodules were reported to have been present on the extensor surfaces of the forearms early in the clinical disease. A biopsy of one of these in the fourth year of illness was "consistent with a rheumatoid nodule." Eventually flexion deformities developed in the fingers (Fig. 1) and

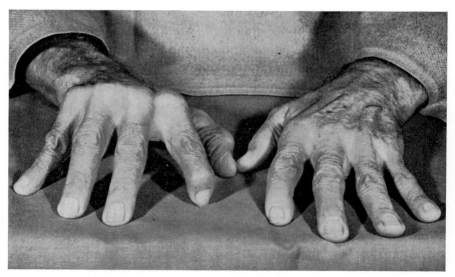

Fig. 1. Deformities in the hand of a 57-year-old man with rheumatoid arthritis for 5 years and clinical myositis for 4 years.

to a lesser degree in the knees and elbows. Radiologic evidence of demineralization, para-articular calcification and some bony destruction was present (Fig. 2). Fluctuating muscular weakness and dysphagia had existed for four years, but these were given little recognition. Muscle biopsy revealed extensive myositis. The weakness was apparently controlled to a certain extent by the corticosteroids which were administered for the arthritis.

The third patient was a 2½-year-old female child who had recurrent knee, wrist and finger joint pain, heat and effusions over a six-month period. An

* For further details see Case I in Reference 11.

episode of muscular weakness of moderate degree occurred during the initial three months and then spontaneously and incompletely subsided. Muscle biopsy at the sixth month showed the residuals of a myositis with minimal continuing activity. Persistent swelling of the joints was present and there was radiologic evidence of demineralization about the clinically involved joints.

In 11 of the 12 cases, the exception being the 2½-year-old child, muscular weakness eventually far overshadowed any rheumatic symptoms. Eleven of

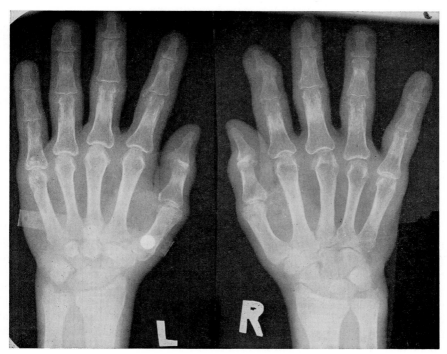

Fig. 2.   Radiographs of the hands seen in Figure 1. There are destructive changes at several proximal interphalangeal joints and soft tissue calcifications, especially in the left index and middle fingers.

the 12 cases (Table 3) showed the morning "gel" phenomenon or clinical features of "fibrositis." Ten patients had arthralgias and nine of these had actual polyarthritis with effusions either at the onset of their disease (seven cases) or later in its course.

The joints were usually affected in a symmetrical fashion with fusiform swellings, redness and heat of the proximal interphalangeal or metacarpal phalangeal joints of both hands, and occasionally effusions in the wrists and knees. In these respects they closely resembled active rheumatoid arthritis. Rheumatoid nodules were present in the subcutaneous tissue in one case, and in another recurrent, red, tender skin lesions appeared in crops on the arms and legs. Biopsy of one of these showed inflammation, edema and fibrinoid necrosis which bore some resemblance to erythema nodosum. Recurrent episodes of bilateral or unilateral subdeltoid bursitis were present in four cases. In one it was the only rheumatic symptom.

PERTINENT LABORATORY RESULTS

Aside from the findings in the muscle biopsy, there are no laboratory results that are specific for myositis. However, several tests are often abnormal and provide valuable assistance in arriving at a diagnosis. The serum levels of several enzymes, which normally are found principally within muscle fibers and other cells, are elevated to a degree which signifies the intensity of muscle necrosis.[4, 10] These enzyme levels return to normal as the myositic process diminishes under the influence of corticosteroid therapy, and they provide a valuable guide for determining the efficacy of the steroid dosage level.

Tests for the rheumatoid factor were positive in six of nine cases with rheumatic manifestations. In six of eight patients the serum protein electrophoretic patterns were abnormal, with a mild reversal of the A/G ratio. Elevated alpha-2- and gamma globulins were the most frequent deviations. These findings have been reported in other series.[2, 6] LE cells were absent in all of ten cases tested. An abnormal electromyogram, with fairly specific features,[7, 9] was present in all of 11 cases studied. Radiologic study of the swallowing mechanism disclosed marked weakness of the pharyngeal musculature with pooling of the barium in the pyriform sinuses and valleculae in those cases that had clinical dysphagia. These functional defects improved significantly on corticosteroid therapy.

HISTOPATHOLOGY OF MUSCLE

Details of the muscle pathology have been outlined in other reports.[1, 12, 18] In summary, the characteristic histologic features of an active myositis are: (1) evidence of isolated or disseminated muscle fiber necrosis of various types; (2) mononuclear or occasionally neutrophilic inflammatory infiltrates, which are usually sparse and focal or paravascular in location but may be more prominent; (3) phagocytosis of necrotic muscle fibers; (4) interstitial edema; (5) basophilia of isolated fibers, usually indicative of attempts at regeneration; (6) considerable variation in the cross-sectional diameter of fibers; and (7) interstitial fibrosis.

These features were present in varying degrees in this series. However, occasionally a careful search was required to find more than one or two of them. In general, inflammation and fiber necrosis were more prominent in the early disease and atrophy and fibrosis in the later, more chronic, stages. No significant differences were noted in the muscle biopsy specimens taken from patients with dermatomyositis as compared with those with polymyositis.

CLINICAL COURSE AND THERAPY

Of the 24 patients in our series five had a visceral malignancy (ovary, breast, lung, esophagus, colon), and two of these had moderate rheumatic features. The increased incidence of malignancy in myositis has been noted repeatedly in the literature[3, 15, 18, 19] and has been seen, as in our series, in cases of both poly- and dermatomyositis. It is somewhat more likely to occur in cases with typical skin lesions.

Therapy with corticosteroids, especially prednisone, has been satisfactory in all of the present series except in those persons with an accompanying malignancy. In all cases there was an initial beneficial clinical response with a decline in serum enzyme levels. However, this response was transitory (several weeks) in the presence of a malignancy. When treatment was begun early in the disease, improvement was prompt and sustained so long as the steroids were continued. Muscular strength gradually returned, pain and dysphagia lessened, and the arthritis or other rheumatic features usually disappeared. In chronic myositis of several years' duration, improvement was less dramatic or complete but was nevertheless definite. In several cases when the corticosteroid dosage was lowered below a "critical" level, which varied from one case to another, or when steroids were discontinued altogether, there was a gradual rise in the serum enzyme levels as well as a slow return of muscular weakness and of arthritic and rheumatic manifestations.

The initial dosage of prednisone averaged 35 mg. daily (range 20 to 70 mg.) and maintenance therapy was necessary in all patients, averaging 15 mg. daily. As mentioned before, patients with an associated malignancy usually become "refractory" to the effect of corticosteroids after a variable period. These persons died from complications of the muscle weakness (aspiration pneumonia, respiratory weakness, etc.) rather than directly from the effects of the tumor. Supportive treatment with salicylates and physical therapy was used when indicated for pain, stiffness and contractures.

DISCUSSION

The occurrence of arthritis of the rheumatoid type, or of other rheumatic manifestations, has been noted more or less incidentally in several reports on myositis. O'Leary and Waisman[8] observed it twice in 40 cases of dermatomyositis, and Sheard[14] found various symptoms in 7 of 25 patients with "actual joint changes in the hand, similar to those of rheumatoid arthritis" in three of them. As recorded in Table 2, Eaton[5] and Walton and Adams[18] saw arthritis or rheumatic symptoms in about 25 per cent of a total of 81 cases. The distribution of the rheumatic features in their cases was similar to that found in the patients in the present series (Table 3).

Talbott et al.[16] have recently described a 52-year-old woman who had the onset of joint symptoms quite suggestive of rheumatoid arthritis 15 years previously. Eight years later muscular weakness and a typical skin rash heralded the appearance of dermatomyositis. Subsequently, while on ACTH or corticosteroids, she showed considerable muscular weakness, contractures and extensive soft tissue calcinosis. Evidence of rheumatoid arthritis was not seen radiologically, but Talbott and Moleres Ferrandis[17] had previously illustrated such a case. Of interest in this respect is one of our patients who had rheumatoid arthritis with subcutaneous nodules for several years, progressive myositis without skin lesions, and radiographic findings of mild rheumatoid arthritis in the hands, plus minimal soft tissue calcification (Fig. 2).

In addition to the rheumatic features of myositis, which most commonly resemble rheumatoid arthritis, a few of our patients have shown mild evidence of scleroderma, both in the skin and in the viscera. Also, the facial rash or the hyperemia surrounding the fingernails resembles that seen in SLE. Reversing the point of focus, one may see localized or even fairly diffuse biopsy evidence of myositis in typical rheumatoid arthritis. The minimal muscular weakness in these cases could readily be explained on the basis of joint inflammation and disuse. We have studied at least five such cases. Likewise, focal myositis and fibrosis are fairly common in typical scleroderma, and a diffuse vacuolar myopathy, with elevation of serum enzymes, was described by us[13] in typical SLE. Four more examples of this syndrome have been seen subsequently.

From an analysis of the present series and of the reported cases it is obvious that both dermatomyositis and polymyositis fit closely into the spectrum of the various connective tissue diseases and often overlap with one or more of them. Rheumatic manifestations are fairly common and principally resemble rheumatoid arthritis. The following subdivisions are offered as natural cleavage groups:

1. Overt myositis with clinical weakness: no features of rheumatic or connective tissue disease ("pure" dermato- or polymyositis; the latter occasionally resembles muscular dystrophy.)
2. Overt myositis: moderate rheumatic, sclerodermatous or lupus features.
3. Overt myositis: overt rheumatoid arthritis.
4. Minimal clinical myositis (biopsy evidence of myositis or vacuolar myopathy only): overt rheumatoid arthritis, scleroderma or SLE.

SUMMARY

Polymyositis and dermatomyositis are clinical variants that have as their most prominent feature weakness which affects the proximal muscles of the limbs, and of the anterior neck and the swallowing mechanism. Among 24 cases analyzed in the present series 12 had various rheumatic manifestations, especially resembling rheumatoid arthritis. In addition, minimal features of scleroderma or lupus were present in an occasional case.

Corticosteroids have been of considerable benefit in the treatment of most cases, except those in which there was an associated visceral malignancy.

The point has been made that myositis fits closely into the spectrum of the various connective tissue diseases. In some cases its clinical features are maximal, whereas in others only biopsy evidence of its presence can be found. A classification has been suggested, based on these findings.

REFERENCES

1. Adams, R. D., Denny-Brown, D. and Pearson, C. M.: Diseases of Muscle; A Study in Pathology. New York, Paul B. Hoeber, 1954.
2. van Bogaert, L., Radermecker, M. A., Löwenthal, A. and Ketelaer, C. J.: Les polymyosites chroniques (essais avec la cortisone). Acta neurol. Belg., 11:869, 1955.
3. Dowling, G. B.: Scleroderma and dermatomyositis. Brit. J. Dermatol., 67:275, 1955.
4. Dreyfus, J. C., Schapira, G. and Schapira, F.: Serum enzymes in the physiopathology of muscle. Ann. N. Y. Acad. Sc., 75:235, 1958.
5. Eaton, L. M.: The perspective of neurology in regard to polymyositis. A Study of 41 Cases. Neurology, 4:245, 1954.
6. Garcin, R.: Considerations générales sur les maladies du collagène. Rev. neurol., 92:419, 1955.
7. O'Leary, P. A., Lambert, E. H. and Sayre, G. P.: Muscle studies in cutaneous disease. J. Invest. Dermat., 24:301, 1955.
8. O'Leary, P. A. and Waisman, M.: Dermatomyositis: study of 40 cases. Arch. Dermat. & Syph., 41:1001, 1940.
9. Nattrass, F. J. et al.: Discussion on the clinical and electromyographic aspects of polymyositis. Proc. Roy. Soc. Med., 49:105, 1956.
10. Pearson, C. M.: Serum enzymes in muscular dystrophy and certain other muscular and neuromuscular diseases. I. Serum glutamic oxalacetic transaminase. New Engl. J. Med., 256:1069, 1957.

11. Pearson, C. M.: Rheumatic manifestations of polymyositis and dermatomyositis. Arth. & Rheumat., 2:127, 1959.
12. Pearson, C. M. and Rose, A. R.: Myositis: the inflammatory disorders of muscle. Proc. A. Res. Nerv. & Ment. Dis., 38:422, 1960.
13. Pearson, C. M. and Yamazaki, J. N.: Vacuolar myopathy in systemic lupus erythematosus. Am. J. Clin. Path., 29:455, 1958.
14. Sheard, C.: Dermatomyositis. Arch. Int. Med., 88:640, 1951.
15. Sheard, C. and Knoepfler, P. T.: Dermatomyositis and the incidence of associated malignancy. Arch. Dermat & Syph., 75:224, 1957.
16. Talbott, J. H., Koepf, G. F., Culver, G. J. and Terplan, K.: Dermatomyositis, disseminated calcinosis and metaplastic ossification. Clinical studies over a period of 7 years in a female with rheumatoid arthritis. Arth. & Rheumat., 2:499, 1959.
17. Talbott, J. H. and Moleres Ferrandis, R.: Collagen Diseases. New York, Grune & Stratton, 1956, p. 232.
18. Walton, J. N. and Adams, R. D.: Polymyositis. Edinburgh, Livingstone, and Baltimore, Williams & Wilkins, 1958.
19. Williams, R. C.: Dermatomyositis and malignancy: a review of the literature. Ann. Int. Med., 50:1174, 1959.

Panel Discussion

Howard L. Holley, *Moderator*

Dr. Holley: I think the enigma presented by these peculiar diseases as to their etiology and ultimate cure has certainly defied all attempts at delineation, to the present. I am not sure that we have even the correct terminology when we call them connective tissue diseases. This panel has to consider the most difficult of all the connective tissue diseases because they have been studied less, probably because of their rarity. Nevertheless they present a problem of increasing concern to the clinician.

Dr. Vaughan, is there any good evidence to support the concept of some workers that dermatomyositis occurring with malignancy is due to autoimmunity set up by the tumor metabolites?

Dr. Vaughan: I think the statistics indicating that a significant number, perhaps 25 per cent, of patients with dermatomyositis have malignancies are probably valid, and one wonders what the relationship between the tumor and the dermatomyositis is. One can create any number of speculative pathogenetic pathways, but there is no way to decide just now what these are. It is "guilt by association" again. This is a disease in which there are a large number of immunological or immune-like phenomena occurring, and therefore it is presumed that the disease is related to the tumor in this fashion.

Dr. Larson: In regard to the last part of your comments, Dr. Vaughan, we have been using the terms "hypersensitivity," "immune reactions," "antigen-antibody" and others yesterday and today and I think it is time to re-examine what we mean by these terms. Immunologically, an immune response is a specific response with a specific antigen and a specific antibody. Nonspecific reactions are also common, such as, for example, the wide variety of polysaccharides that will react with type 14 rabbit antipneumococcus antibody. This is not an immune response, although the term has now become so popular that whenever two large molecules react, the process is called an immunological reaction; this is nonsense.

The second point I wish to make is in regard to the often unwarranted assumption that a pathogenetic mechanism is involved just because these so-called immune responses are present. Using this type of logic, it is quite possible to show that syphilis is due to an alcoholic extract of beef heart. You can see how ridiculous this type of reasoning can become. So when one talks about immune reactions, I think it is very wise to keep the terms definite and to use them in the classic sense.

DR. HOLLEY: I agree with you, Dr. Larson. We have been trying to fit our present knowledge into the category of hypersensitivity and immune reactions, and I am not sure we can do that. Maybe we should be more broadminded.

DR. VAUGHAN: The factors we have been talking about are substances that develop in the sera of individuals with disease. They are gamma globulins. They have the immunologic specific characteristics of antibodies. I do not think it matters too much if one does not dispatch the notion that these are the cause of the disease. To me they are merely an indication that there are immunological phenomena going on, and I do think they are immunological. These particular factors are not the factors responsible for the disease; they only indicate that immunological phenomena are occurring. Their role in the disease is unknown.

DR. HOLLEY: You do not know whether they are the cause of the disease or the result of the disease? Is that what you are saying?

DR. VAUGHAN: The factors that we have been studying certainly are the results of the disease and not the cause of it. What other immunological factors might be present and whatever role they might have in the production of the disease is not clear. In that respect, I would like to ask the other members of the panel to comment about an idea I have heard expressed. That is, that the effectiveness of steroids in dermatomyositis is related to whether or not there is an underlying neoplasm. I have the notion that steroids are not useful in the symptomatic therapy in dermatomyositis unless there is an underlying neoplasm.

DR. PEARSON: I have found just the opposite, Dr. Vaughan. The majority of our patients who have responded have had dermatomyositis or polymyositis not associated with a tumor. In most of these, the disease was of recent onset and often was quite severe. They responded quite well in contrast to the four or five patients who have had a tumor in our series; the latter had a preliminary minimal response and then became worse and died, not of their tumors but of the myositis, despite large quantities of corticosteroids. In addition, two of our patients had either complete resection or total irradiation of the tumor when it was discovered; one of these patients did not have evidence of muscular weakness until six weeks after irradiation was completed and the other one did not respond to the resection of the tumor at all.

DR. SCHERBEL: In regard to neoplasia and dermatomyositis, one of the staff of our clinic has recently reported 40 cases obtained from the literature and from our records during the past 20 years. Dividing these into groups, we found that none of the patients under the age of 40 had a malignancy and that 50 per cent of the patients over 40 had a malignancy; however, the malignancy occurred after the onset of the dermatomyositis in two of the patients—six months after in one, and one year after in the other. One of these had a bronchogenic carcinoma; as soon as the bronchogenic carcinoma was removed, the dermatomyositis went into complete remission. We also had a patient with carcinoma of the prostate who developed dermatomyositis. After the diagnosis was proved by biopsy of the prostate, the patient was treated with intravenous stilphosterol and the dermatomyositis went into complete remission until he eventually had metastases, had a recurrence of the dermatomyositis, and died of the metastases. We have had at least four patients in whom, after removal of the tumor, there was a complete remission of the dermatomyositis, and in two of these a recurrence with the development of metastases. The most common associated tumors we have seen are carcinomas of the lung, breast and prostate.

DR. HOLLEY: The association of dermatomyositis and malignancy also brings up the problem of the possible inter-relationships of connective tissue diseases to each other. For example, does scleroderma sometimes begin as rheumatoid arthritis, or when we see the two in association does it simply represent the simultaneous occurrence of two unrelated disorders? This seems to me to be of some importance since we occasionally see patients who have had rheumatoid arthritis for a number of years before the onset of typical scleroderma.

DR. RODNAN: I am afraid this is an unanswerable question at the present time. It is quite true however, in a considerable number of patients with scleroderma, that rheumatic complaints are the presenting complaints and very often dominate the clinical picture, leading to a diagnosis of rheumatoid arthritis before the advent of the typical cutaneous or visceral changes which allow the proper diagnosis to be made. Biopsy examination of the synovial membrane does not help us in these patients because we find that a great majority of the patients with scleroderma at some time or another will have synovial lesions which resemble those seen in rheumatoid arthritis itself. Furthermore, patients with scleroderma may have some of the serologic abnormalities which are present in rheumatoid arthritis and I think that in the strictest sense we can not tell what the relationship between these two syndromes is. However, there is one lesion of the synovium which is characteristic of scleroderma, namely, a type of collagenous overgrowth which is very similar to that observed in the dermis and certain visceral structures in this disease.

DR. SOKOLOFF: Of some importance is the fact that tenseness, sclerosis and atrophy of the skin, which can be confused with scleroderma, frequently develop in patients with rheumatoid arthritis of the fingers, but probably are part of rheumatoid arthritis. In addition, I have seen patients who had both diseases with unquestionable rheumatoid nodules in addition to the scleroderma.

DR. RODNAN: I think most instances of so-called secondary scleroderma in rheumatoid arthritis are due to confusion between the atrophy of the skin of the digits in rheumatoid arthritis and a true collagenous overgrowth of the dermis.

DR. HOLLEY: Dr. Rodnan, do you really think we make that mistake so often? There is certainly a great deal of difference between atrophy of the skin and the thickening of the skin that is associated with scleroderma.

DR. RODNAN: I agree that it does not happen very often, but I have seen it, and I think this mistake is made occasionally.

DR. WAGNER: There is also a fairly typical lesion of scleroderma in the kidneys of a number of these patients. The blood vessels show a peculiar fibrinoid change in the vessel wall. This has been described in the older literature to be different from the fibrinoid observed in some of the other connective tissue diseases. It appears as a pool or lake of material, and one can observe what appear to be emerging collagen fibers from this amorphous lake of material in serial sections of the vessels. Various people have speculated that perhaps collagen fibers form, *de novo*, directly from this material; this has given rise to the great amount of work that has been done on soluble collagens and to a lot of the information we now have. Is it not possible, then, that scleroderma is primarily a metabolic disease with an overproduction of precursors for collagen production *de novo?*

DR. HOLLEY: Does the use of steroid therapy in systemic sclerosis increase the incidence of this so-called scleroderma kidney lesion?

DR. SOKOLOFF: I do not think anyone can give an answer to that question. We must have an appropriate number of untreated and treated cases to draw a conclusion like that. All of us have seen these lesions. I do not think I have seen a patient with scleroderma who did not have renal lesions to some extent. We have certainly seen very severe lesions in people who have not been treated with steroids, and conversely, we have seen minimal lesions in those who have been treated.

DR. RODNAN: The typical renal lesions were described in the early 1900's, and these patients certainly did not receive steroids. In regard to the fibrinoid lesion in the scleroderma kidney, there are certain staining differences in ordinary histochemical preparations which allow you to suspect the difference between this fibrinoid and that seen in other disorders of connective tissue. Studies at the University of Pittsburgh have shown by immunohistochemical analysis that this is one of the types of fibrinoid that contain an inordinate concentration of fibrinogen rather than gamma globulin. This alone would seem to differentiate it from certain of the other fibrinoid lesions, namely, those observed in the lupus kidney.

DR. SACKNER: Most of the panelists here have discussed the immunologic characteristics of scleroderma. On the other hand, we have attempted to study the pathophysiology of the disturbances of scleroderma, and particularly that of the cardiopulmonary manifestations. We have studied the function of the chest wall, the lungs and the heart by appropriate hemodynamic and pulmonary physiologic testing. With regard to the chest wall, it has long been known that tightening of the skin over the chest may occur in scleroderma patients. If this affected the chest bellows one might expect that these patients would have an alveolar hypoventilation syndrome, but this does not occur. The patients usually have a mild respiratory alkalosis and frequently hyperventilate. In addition, if you record the maximum inspiratory and expiratory pressures at the mouth, the data indicate that the chest bellows is normal.

With regard to the cardiac manifestations and cardiac fibrosis, we have not been able to demonstrate any restriction of diastolic filling such as one might expect if scleroderma produced a syndrome like constrictive pericarditis or like severe interstitial fibrosis secondary to coronary artery disease. On the other hand, in all 12 patients who have been studied, a moderate increase in pulmonary vascular resistance was present, and this was present irrespective of whether the patient had physiologic or roentgenographic signs of pulmonary fibrosis. Some of these patients have been followed and, although most of them have had static pictures, a few have shown pulmonary fibrosis. We wonder if the concept expressed by Dr. Sokoloff in 1956, that Raynaud's phenomenon in the kidney produced the renal changes of scleroderma, might also be the mechanism responsible for the pulmonary changes. Does Raynaud's phenomenon in the lungs explain the increase in pulmonary vascular resistance, and is scleroderma primarily a vascular disease rather than a disturbance of collagenous tissue?

DR. HOLLEY: This is certainly an interesting theory, but I would now like to direct the discussion to some of the other diseases which should be taken up by this panel. Dr. Sokoloff, is the pathological lesion seen in polyarteritis similar to that of delayed hypersensitivity or graft rejection, and if so, how does this relate to the theories of pathogenesis?

DR. SOKOLOFF: The one instance I can think of in which arteritis resembling polyarteritis nodosa has been reported in a condition of delayed hypersensitivity is in tuberculous meningitis. These observations have been made on occasion, and I think most of us have seen it at one time or another, but that is the only circumstance.

DR. ANGEVINE: In regard to the pathogenesis of polyarteritis, I think there are many unrecognized cases, and the conclusions you draw depend to a great extent on your definition of this process. Since Dr. Rose is here and he expressed some skepticism about sensitivity angiitis due to drugs, I would like to hear him express and elaborate his opinion.

DR. ROSE: First of all, Dr. Angevine, do you still adhere to the terminology used in your paper on periarteritis nodosa in a variety of animals, including periarteritis in rats? It seems to me that one must have a very strong case before applying to experimental lesions in animals a term used for a fairly well delineated human disease, and particularly to the arteritis of the rat which is in most cases related to hypertension and is more or less species specific. Other hypertensive animals such as the rabbit and dog do not behave in the same way. In dealing with this situation, it seems to me, one could speak of arteritis or of necrotizing inflammatory arteritis, but there is insufficient evidence to say that we have produced the human disease in animals.

DR. ANGEVINE: I am sure we have not produced the human disease in rats, but in the first experiment we described, the lesion was due to the chemical. This was not the naturally occurring disease in rats; it was one we produced. We also produced the lesions by feeding, but only in the lungs. The rat may be more susceptible; we have not proved that the lesions are due to hypersensitivity, although we are trying to prove that they are. The experiments suggest to me that these lesions are not due to hypersensitivity. Most people seem to feel that the lesions in man are due to hypersensitivity, and I think it is pretty well documented in the literature. So these lesions are ones I am more interested in than the ones in animals.

DR. HOLLEY: How about the lesions produced by hormone administration? Are they similar lesions?

DR. ANGEVINE: This is one of the difficulties, as I tried to point out. There is a basic similarity in all of these lesions. Even in the DLE inbred mice from the N. I. H. the lesions are indistinguishable, as far as I can tell, so we are talking about a vast array of lesions with multiple causes.

DR. WAGNER: In relation to the questions posed, it would be helpful if we had an animal that developed polyarteritis spontaneously—one could study the disease —and I think we have such an animal, an exotic one, the mink. Aleutian mink disease occurs in this country and Australia and costs the mink breeders of the United States about 3 to 5 million dollars a year in loss of stock. It is an interesting disease which usually appears in the fall of the second year of life of the Aleutian or sable or silver mink. It begins with hemorrhagic changes in the gums; then the mink begin to lose weight and their hair falls out. One can produce this disease in the whole flock by immunization, especially if they are immunized with the mink distemper virus vaccine prepared from the tissues of mink who died of distemper. Within an appropriate period of time for antibodies to develop, they begin to have this disease. The genetic history and breeding of these mink are extraordinarily well documented, because the breeder mink are extremely expensive. If you outbreed the mink they lose this tendency to develop periarteritis. I think that this may be an interesting model for further study of the disease since we can genetically control the process and predict its frequency with a reasonable degree of accuracy, and I would suggest that it fairly closely mimics the lesion we call polyarteritis in man.

DR. SOKOLOFF: I want to add one comment about the arteritis of mink. Some years ago it was found that mink were also susceptible to the development of arteritis following the administration of sulfonamides, which had been used in their food as a growth additive.

DR. HOLLEY:　What about polyarteritis in the deer?

DR. PEARSON:　There was an epidemic of polyarteritis in a herd of 900 deer in Germany at the turn of the century, and nearly all of them died of this disease in a period of about four or five years with fairly typical lesions of polyarteritis. Those that survived apparently were resistant for some reason or another, and there has not been a recurrence of the disease subsequently.

DR. HOLLEY:　Is histological examination of tissue of any value in determining the prognosis in polyarteritis nodosa?

DR. WAGNER:　Severe obvious polyarteritis seen in biopsy material, at least to my way of thinking, is always a poor prognostic sign and I think it indicates systemic vascular involvement and important organ involvement. However, it is difficult to give a good answer to that question.

DR. ROSE:　If one looks at the sections from postmortem specimens from a fatal case of polyarteritis nodosa, one sees frequently a very wide range of appearances. Lesions in one place may look fulminating and acute, with necrosis and so on; elsewhere you will see arterioles with just a few lymphocytes around them. I do not see how the clinician, with his very limited access to pathological material during the patient's life, could generalize from the one or two lesions he may see.

DR. SOKOLOFF:　I would agree that the anatomic demonstration of necrotizing arteritis does not necessarily indicate an ominous prognosis. For example, we have seen patients who have had unquestionable necrotizing arteritis and have obtained second biopsies years later. Dr. Klemperer told me of a patient he had with rheumatoid arthritis who had definite polyarteritis nodosa in the pelvic tissues when she had a pelvic operation of some sort; 18 years later arteritis was found in her gallbladder. So we do not necessarily have to prepare the patient for her funeral because we have established the diagnosis of arteritis. I can also show you four or five dozen muscle biopsies which show arteritis from people with rheumatoid arthritis who lived for many years after we made this observation.

　　I want to raise the question, too, of whether one should speak of polyarteritis nodosa in man as a definite disease or whether it is not, in fact, one of a number of diseases—a manifestation of a variety of pathologic processes which can express themselves in necrosis of the artery. We see, for example, people who survive 8 to 18 years in some cases, and others who die in a very few weeks.

DR. BLACK:　Dr. Holley, would you agree that almost all of the diseases we have been discussing in this meeting have overlapping symptoms? We see some patients who have scleroderma and symptoms that overlap into the area of rheumatoid arthritis; we see some that overlap from rheumatoid arthritis into lupus; some from rheumatoid arthritis into rheumatic fever; and there are some forms which are almost impossible to categorize.

DR. HOLLEY:　This is quite true clinically. We often can not differentiate them, and this has been brought up several times in the discussion prior to this panel. Actually they are a group of diseases which may have the same or similar manifestations, but not necessarily the same etiology.

　　Commenting on Dr. Sokoloff's question, I think most of us accept the fact that we are seeing pathological features which merely reflect the limited way that connective tissue can react to adverse stimuli.

Dr. Vaughan: I want to draw a parallel about the whole question of multiple etiological factors in these diseases as opposed to a single etiology with a spectrum of responses. If we had a patient with edema of the ankles, a large liver and ascites, and had only those findings to evaluate the patient, we would be unable to tell whether the findings were due to cirrhosis of the liver, right heart failure, mitral stenosis or any number of other specific and unrelated diseases, and we are certainly dealing with the same sort of thing here.

Dr. Holley: I think we all agree that up to the present time we have studied only the end products of the connective tissue diseases. It would seem timely now to apply our efforts in a different way to the understanding of the basic mechanism of their production. The cause of these diseases and their ultimate cure are not likely to become clear until further research has been carried out regarding the mechanisms of the basic connective tissue alterations. We might ask ourselves whether a better understanding of antibody synthesis by the organism can be delineated and how it has gone askew so that the abnormal sequence of events seen in these diseases takes place. Similarly, one might also want to look at the factors initiating abnormal synthesis of antibodies such as genetic mutation, dysfunction of soluble RNA or the effects of viral infections. We might also ask ourselves whether this involves changes in the integral structure of the antibody itself, the amino acid sequence or the basic structure of the protein. I think it is only through such studies that we will ultimately understand the etiology and pathogenesis of the connective tissue diseases.

Pathogenesis of the
Nephrotic Syndrome

JOSEPH E. IMBRIGLIA

Hahnemann Medical College, Philadelphia

The nephrotic syndrome is a well recognized clinical entity characterized by generalized edema, proteinuria, hypoalbuminemia, hyperlipemia and hypercholesterolemia. This clinical picture may occur as a result of various pathological processes in the kidney,[1, 2, 4, 5, 6] of which the best known are glomerulonephritis, amyloidosis, diabetic glomerulosclerosis, renal vein thrombosis and disseminated lupus erythematosus (Figs. 1-4). It must be remembered that the nephrotic syndrome may arise from many different causes, and in any given case the cause may be difficult to establish; however, prolonged observation and study may make exact diagnosis possible.

Kark et al.[10] have obtained renal biopsies from 98 patients with heavy proteinuria and decreased plasma albumin. Of these, 46 patients were considered to have some form of glomerulonephritis; a further 18 had changes of systemic lupus erythematosus, and 15 had diabetic glomerulosclerosis; lipoid nephrosis was diagnosed in 11, amyloidosis in three and increased renal vein pressure in four, in two of whom the renal veins were thrombosed; nephrosclerosis was found in one case.

Joekes et al.[9] have performed biopsies in 20 adults with the nephrotic

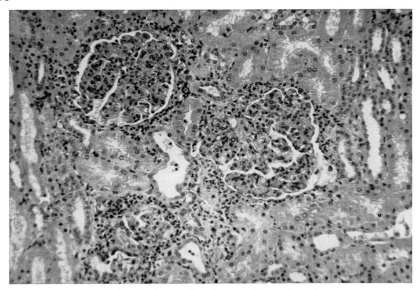

Fig. 1. The glomerulus of acute glomerulonephritis.

syndrome. Of the 20 biopsies, eight were described as glomerulonephritis, three as benign nephrosclerosis, two as renal vein thrombosis, three as focal glomerulonephritis and one as disseminated lupus erythematosus. It is noteworthy that pyelonephritis was not found as a primary cause in either series, although it was noted as a secondary lesion on three occasions by the American workers.

If we combine the data from these two series, it will be noted that the commonest cause of the nephrotic syndrome was intrinsic renal disease, i.e., some form of glomerulonephritis, this accounting for approximately 57 cases

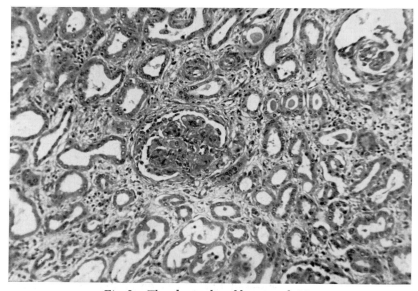

Fig. 2. The glomerulus of lupus nephritis.

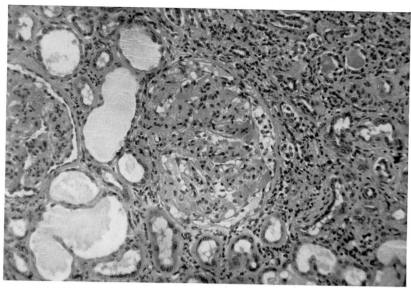

Fig. 3. The glomerulus of Kimmelstiel-Wilson disease.

of the total of 118. Lipoid nephrosis accounted for 14 of the total number of 118 cases. Joekes et al.[9] believe that in three cases which they found no significant changes in the glomeruli, decreased tubular absorption of protein may have been the cause.

An alternative explanation is suggested by the work of Folli et al.,[7] who studied Kark's 11 patients in whom lipoid nephrosis had previously been diagnosed. All of them responded excellently to corticotrophin or adrenal corticosteroid hormones, and all have so far remained well following treatment. In seven of these the glomeruli were studied by electron microscopy

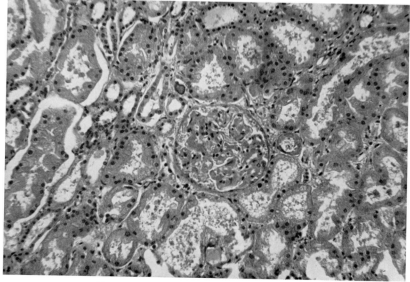

Fig. 4. The glomerulus of amyloid disease.

and in all, striking and consistent abnormalities were found. These changes were limited to the epithelial cells of the glomerular tuft and consisted of replacement of the pedicles (or foot processes) of the epithelial cells by a continuous layer of cytoplasm of irregular thickness. Other but less striking changes were seen in the perinuclear cytoplasm. The changes, which are beautifully illustrated in Folli's paper,[7] are similar to those previously noted in children with nephrosis. This work shows clearly that severe glomerular structural changes can occur which are invisible by conventional techniques but are easily detected by electron microscopy. Possibly the changes in the tubules result from the consequent disturbance of glomerular function.

Folli et al.[7] describe a dramatic instance of this renal disorder; after the nephrotic syndrome had developed in a man of 19 years, renal biopsy revealed the epithelial lesion described above. A second biopsy was made after 31 days of treatment with prednisone, when the patient had lost all his edema. Prednisone was continued, and a third biopsy was taken eight months after the onset of the illness, when he was clinically well. The epithelial cells were almost normal in the second specimen and were completely normal in the third. The authors offer no explanation for these observations.

Spiro,[11] using the electron microscope, has studied renal biopsy specimens of three patients with the nephrotic syndrome (one case of lipoid nephrosis and two cases of amyloidosis); two patients with subacute and chronic glomerulonephritis accompanied by proteinuria were also studied. His observations indicate that the structural common denominator of proteinuria is a defect in the basement membrane of the capillary loops. The defect consists of a loss of continuity of the normally continuous basement membrane of the capillary wall. In the cases studied the basement membrane defect consisted of gaps and pores through which endothelial and epithelial cells were in intimate contact. In amyloid disease the defects were due to replacement of the basement membrane by amyloid substance with a far looser structure. Spiro feels that the defects in the basement membrane may constitute the structural basis of proteinuria; they were of sufficient size to permit relatively free diffusion of protein while excluding cellular elements of the blood. Spiro also observed the transformation of the normal epithelial foot processes, which he feels represents a change that is secondary to the underlying alteration in the basement membrane.

Harkin and Recant[8] have induced the nephrotic syndrome in rats by the administration of an aminonucleoside C-dimethylamino purine, 3-amino-d-ribose. During the early stages of the disorder, no detectable glomerular lesions are noted by light microscopy, although tubular alterations which parallel the progression of proteinuria, hypoalbuminemia, hyperlipermia and edema do occur. The microscopic changes resemble those of pure nephrosis in man. The investigators feel that their experimental observations assume considerable significance in view of the remarkable histologic similarities between aminonucleoside injury in the rat and nephrosis in man.

When kidney sections from aminonucleoside-treated rats were examined by light microscopy, no glomerular lesions were identified in the early and reversible stages of injury. At this stage, swelling of the tubular epithelium and intracellular lipid deposits in the proximal convoluted tubules were seen. These observations were identical to those described in the lipoid nephrosis in children. In the advanced stage, the light microscopic features of the experimental lesions were strikingly similar to those designated as the Ellis type 11 glomerulonephritis.

The electron microscopic studies prior to the advent of proteinuria in the rats, and after 24 hours of treatment with aminonucleoside, revealed enlarged and fused foot processes in great numbers. Four to six such abnormal processes were observed surrounding a capillary in cross section, whereas in the control animal, enlarged processes of this kind were rarely encountered. Thus it seemed that the glomerular alteration was quantitative, in that the number of large processes was increased; it was not qualitative, in that the processes were similar to those seen occasionally in the controls. By the fifth day of aminonucleoside treatment, prior to the development of proteinuria, glomerular lesions were noted in striking contrast to the absence of alterations detectable by conventional microscopy. Progressive merging of fused foot processes into cytoplasmic masses adjacent to the basement membrane constituted the principal change. The investigators state that examination of the sequential changes in experimental nephrosis by electron microscopy indicates that the glomeruli are altered and leak protein, although this is not demonstrable by conventional microscopy.

In the light of present knowledge, the nephrotic syndrome seems best explained as a hyperpermeability of the glomerular capillaries to plasma albumin; according to Allen[3] ". . .'lipoid nephrosis' is in reality a definite variety of subacute or chronic (membranous or lobular) glomerulonephritis with specific histologic alterations of the glomeruli, which are less obvious in children than in adults." Present new methods, therefore, may give us more information about function and structure and about the effects of treatment.

REFERENCES

1. Adams, D. A.: The pathophysiology of the nephrotic syndrome. Arch. Int. Med., *106*:117, 1960.
2. Allen, A.: The Kidney: Medical and Surgical Diseases. London, J. and A. Churchill, 1951.
3. Allen, A. C.: The clinico-pathologic meaning of the nephrotic syndrome. Am. J. Med., *18*:277, 1955.
4. Bell, E. T.: Renal Diseases. Philadelphia, Lea & Febiger, 1950.
5. Derow, H. A.: The nephrotic syndrome. New Engl. J. Med., *258*:77, 124, 1958.
6. Editorial: Lancet, *1*:667, 1959.
7. Folli, G., Pollak, V. E., Reid, R. T. W., Pirani, C. and Kark, R. M.: Electron microscopic studies of reversible glomerular lesions in the adult nephrotic syndrome. Ann. Int. Med., *49*:775, 1958.
8. Harkin, J. C. and Recant, L.: Pathogenesis of experimental nephrosis; electron microscopic observations. Am. J. Path., *36*:303, 1960.
9. Joekes, A. M., Heptinstall, R. H. and Parker, K. A.: The nephrotic syndrome. Quart. J. Med., *27*:495, 1958.
10. Kark, R. M., Pirani, C. L., Pollak, V. E., Muehrcke, R. C. and Blainey, J. D.: The nephrotic syndrome in adults: a common disorder with many causes. Ann. Int. Med., *49*:751, 1958.
11. Spiro, D.: The structural basis of proteinuria in man: electron microscopic studies of renal biopsy from patients with lipid nephrosis, amyloidosis, and subacute and chronic glomerulonephritis. Am. J. Path., *35*:47, 1959.

The Glomerular
Basement Membrane
and the Nephrotic Syndrome

VICTOR E. POLLAK

University of Illinois College of Medicine

Squire, Blainey and Hardwicke have shown that in patients with the nephrotic syndrome the serum albumin concentration is inversely related to the amount of albumin lost in the urine when the urinary albumin loss is expressed in grams per kilogram body weight per day.[25] Albumin loss, however, accounts for only 50 to 80 per cent of the total urinary protein loss, as many other proteins are lost in the urine of patients with the nephrotic syndrome.[14, 24] Despite this, Hardwicke found a good correlation between the serum albumin concentration and the total urinary protein excretion expressed in grams per kilogram of body weight per day.[12] The serum concentrations of cholesterol, phospholipids, triglycerides, fibrinogen, cholinesterase and other substances appear to be inversely related to the serum albumin concentration in nephrotic subjects. In our laboratory 50 grams of salt-poor human serum albumin were infused daily for periods of up to 14 days into nephrotic patients and healthy subjects. The elevated serum concentrations of many proteins and lipids decreased toward or to normal levels in nephrotic patients (Fig. 1) and to below normal levels in healthy subjects, as the serum albumin concentration rose toward normal or above normal limits.[19, 23]

Although proteinuria, hypoalbuminemia and hypercholesterolemia are the well known metabolic hallmarks of the nephrotic syndrome, the many other biochemical aberrations which occur, and their intimate relationship to serum albumin levels and protein loss in the urine, led us to define the nephrotic syndrome as the clinical, metabolic and nutritional consequences of persistent massive proteinuria.[14] In this paper the nephrotic syndrome is considered from the morphological point of view in terms of this basic defect —the massive proteinuria. The evidence that protein is filtered by the glomerulus and reabsorbed by the renal tubules has been reviewed by Rather[22] and Squire,[24] and it seems probable that the basic defect in the nephrotic syndrome is an increase of the normal permeability of the glomerulus to protein. Thus it is pertinent to consider the relationship between the underlying glomerular pathology and massive proteinuria.

The nephrotic syndrome is the metabolic consequence of massive urinary protein loss, which may occur in a wide variety of diseases affecting the glomeruli. The etiology of many of these disorders is still obscure, but the morphological patterns of glomerular pathology have been established by light microscopic study of renal biopsies taken from patients with the nephrotic syndrome at the height of their clinical illness. The histologic diagnoses in the first 98 adult nephrotic patients studied by renal biopsy in our laboratory are listed in Table 1.[14] Other authors have recently reported a

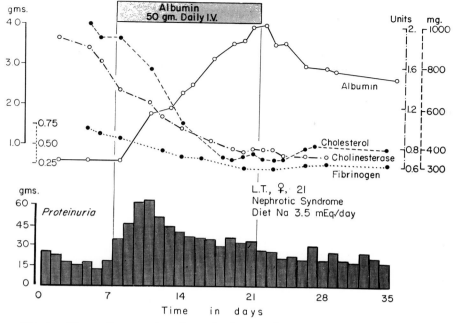

Fig. 1. Observations on the effect of infusing salt-poor human albumin, 50 grams daily, into a patient with the nephrotic syndrome. Note that as the serum albumin level rose to normal the serum concentrations of cholesterol, cholinesterase and fibrinogen fell toward normal or to within normal limits.[19]

total of 83 adult patients with the nephrotic syndrome in whom renal biopsies were done.[2, 3, 13] The incidence of the various underlying morphological abnormalities was similar in our own series and in the series combined from the data of these authors. Glomerulonephritis was the commonest underlying pathologic condition, but "lipoid nephrosis" was observed in 11 of the 98 patients studied in our laboratory. The clinical and light and electron microscopic definitions of "lipoid nephrosis" have been discussed previously.[10] Lupus nephritis, diabetic nephropathy, amyloidosis and increased renal venous pressure were other common underlying pathologic entities.

These findings were all based on light microscopic pathology. In view of

TABLE 1.   HISTOLOGIC DIAGNOSES IN 98 PATIENTS ILL WITH THE NEPHROTIC SYNDROME AND STUDIED BY RENAL BIOPSY

	NO. OF CASES	
I. Glomerulonephritis		46
1. Membranous type	28	
2. Mixed type, membranous and proliferative	12	
3. Proliferative type	6	
II. "Lipoid nephrosis"		11
III. Systemic lupus erythematosus (lupus nephritis)		18
IV. Amyloidosis		3
V. Diabetes mellitus		15
1. Diffuse diabetic glomerulosclerosis	1	
2. Diffuse and nodular diabetic glomerulosclerosis	14	
VI. Severe arterial and arteriolar nephrosclerosis		1
VII. Increased pressure in renal veins		4

the recent application of electron microscopy to the study of glomerular pathology, the relationship of glomerular pathology to massive proteinuria must now be re-evaluated. Using the resolving powers of the electron microscope it is evident that the glomerular capillary wall consists of three layers: a homogeneous basement membrane or lamina densa, about 3000 Å thick in the adult, a thin attenuated layer of endothelial cytoplasm and a complex epithelial cytoplasm with foot processes or pedicles lying in close apposition to the epithelial surface of the lamina densa.[17] These three layers cannot be distinguished by light microscopy, and alterations in any one of the three layers might produce the light microscopic appearance of basement membrane thickening.

Several examples follow which illustrate the relationship between changes in the glomerular capillary wall and massive proteinuria:

Diabetic Nephropathy. In our laboratory two distinct glomerular lesions were separated by light microscopy in renal biopsies: the nodular diabetic glomerulosclerosis of Kimmelstiel and Wilson, and the diffuse diabetic glomerulosclerosis characterized by diffuse thickening of the glomerular basement membrane. A positive relationship was found between the presence and degree of proteinuria and the severity of the diffuse lesion, but there was no correlation with the severity of the nodular lesion.[11] Electron microscopic studies have demonstrated that the earliest and most prominent lesion in diabetic nephropathy was marked diffuse thickening of the basement membrane,[1, 6] thus confirming the relationship between proteinuria and basement membrane thickening.

Lupus Nephritis. The glomerular lesions in lupus nephritis are pleomorphic. Despite this, it was possible to demonstrate a good positive relationship between the degree of basement membrane thickening as judged by light microscopy and the amount of protein excreted in the urine, but there was no correlation between glomerular hypercellularity and proteinuria.[16] When lupus glomerulonephritis was treated successfully with large doses of prednisone, progression of renal histologic damage did not occur, but glomerular basement membrane thickening persisted. Under these circumstances the onset of renal failure was delayed, but the amount of protein excreted in the urine was not changed in many patients.[21] The pathology of lupus nephritis has not yet been defined fully by electron microscopy, but the earliest lesions appear to be patchy thickening of the glomerular basement membrane.[8, 9] Further studies to elucidate the relationship between protein excretion in the urine and the detailed pathology of the glomerulus are needed, but fibrinoid deposits between the endothelial cytoplasm and the basement membrane have been found at an early stage of the disease in some patients.[18] Their effect on glomerular permeability to protein is unknown.

Membranous Glomerulonephritis. In this condition diffuse basement membrane thickening is the characteristic finding by light microscopy. When the lesions of membranous glomerulonephritis were studied by electron microscopy a varied picture was seen. Profound alterations in endothelial cells with an increase of endothelial cell cytoplasm, considerable disorganization of epithelial cells and thickening of the lamina densa have been observed singly or, more frequently, in combination.[9, 18] It remains to be determined whether these varying electron microscopic appearances result from different insults to the kidney or whether they represent different stages of the same disease process. Persistent massive proteinuria is associated with all these lesions. Neither the proteinuria nor the histologic picture—by light and electron microscopy—has been influenced significantly by treatment with cortisone and allied drugs in the majority of cases.[3, 18]

"Lipoid Nephrosis." In "lipoid nephrosis," by contrast, persistent proteinuria is associated with alterations in the epithelial cells. The foot processes are replaced by a continuous layer of epithelial cytoplasm, but the glomerular basement membrane appears normal by both light and electron microscopy. Treatment with cortisone and allied drugs results in a dramatic and predictable decrease in the urine protein loss in almost all patients, and the simultaneous restoration to normal of the foot processes.[10] Observations made in our laboratory on experimental nephrosis of rats produced by a single intravenous injection of the aminonucleoside of puromycin indicate that the earliest pathologic changes are similar to those seen in human "lipoid nephrosis," and that they precede the appearance of protein in the urine.[15] If changes do occur in the basement membrane in "lipoid nephrosis" and the early stages of aminonucleoside nephrosis they must be at a molecular level beyond the resolving powers of the light microscope. In this connection it should be noted that in aminonucleoside nephrosis Farquhar and Palade have demonstrated an increased permeability of the basement membrane to injected ferritin molecules.[7]

Increased Renal Venous Pressure. The nephrotic syndrome may occur as a result of renal vein thrombosis or as a result of other causes of increased renal venous pressure such as congestive cardiac failure and constrictive pericarditis.[4, 5, 20] Definite but mild thickening of the glomerular basement membrane is found by light microscopy in the majority of cases, even within a short period of the onset of increased renal venous pressure.[20] All manifestations of the nephrotic syndrome, including the proteinuria, may disappear entirely if the cause of the increased renal venous pressure can be removed, as has occurred in constrictive pericarditis.[4, 5] Studies have not yet been done by electron microscopy to elucidate the exact nature of the alteration in the glomerular capillary wall, and it is not yet known whether the basement membrane itself is thickened. By analogy with the other conditions discussed, the reversibility of the nephrotic syndrome in these cases suggests that, in at least some instances, true basement membrane changes are not a feature of this disease and that the pathologic changes may be in the epithelial or endothelial cell.

The examples discussed throw some light on the relationship between changes in the glomerular capillary wall and the occurrence of massive proteinuria. Further studies utilizing electron microscopy, immunologic clearance techniques[3] and pathophysiologic experiments are necessary to elucidate this relationship.

REFERENCES

1. Bergstrand, A. and Bucht, H.: The glomerular lesions of diabetes mellitus and their electron-microscope appearances. J. Path. Bact., 77:231, 1959.
2. Berman, L. B. and Schreiner, G. E.: Clinical and histologic spectrum of the nephrotic syndrome. Am. J. Med., 24:249, 1958.
3. Blainey, J. D., Brewer, D. B., Hardwicke, J. and Soothill, J. F.: The nephrotic syndrome. Diagnosis by renal biopsy and biochemical and immunological analyses related to the response to steroid therapy. Quart. J. Med., 29:235, 1960.
4. Blainey, J. D., Hardwicke, J. and Whitfield, A. G. W.: The nephrotic syndrome associated with thrombosis of the renal veins. Lancet, 2:1208, 1954.
5. Burack, W. R., Pryce, J. and Goodwin, J. F.: A reversible nephrotic syndrome associated with congestive heart failure. Circulation, 18:562, 1958.

6. Farquhar, M. G., Hopper, J. and Moon, H. D.: Diabetic glomerulosclerosis: electron and light microscopic studies. Am. J. Path., 35:721, 1959.
7. Farquhar, M. G. and Palade, G. E.: Segregation of ferritin in glomerular protein absorption droplets. J. Biophys. & Biochem. Cytol., 7:297, 1960.
8. Farquhar, M. G., Vernier, R. L. and Good, R. A.: The application of electron microscopy in pathology; study of renal biopsy tissues. Schweiz. med. wchnschr., 87:501, 1957.
9. Farquhar, M. G., Vernier, R. L. and Good, R. A.: An electron microscope study of the glomerulus in nephrosis, glomerulonephritis and lupus erythematosus. J. Exper. Med., 106:649, 1957.
10. Folli, G., Pollak, V. E., Reid, R. T. W., Pirani, C. L. and Kark, R. M.: Electron microscopic studies of reversible glomerular lesions in the adult nephrotic syndrome. Ann. Int. Med., 49:775, 1958.
11. Gellman, D. D., Pirani, C. L., Soothill, J. F., Muehrcke, R. C. and Kark, R. M.: Diabetic nephropathy: a clinical and pathologic study based on renal biopsies. Medicine, 38:321, 1959.
12. Hardwicke, J. R.: Serum and urine protein changes in the nephrotic syndrome. Proc. Roy. Soc. Med., 47:832, 1954.
13. Joekes, A. M., Heptinstall, R. H. and Porter, K. A.: The nephrotic syndrome. A study of renal biopsies in 20 adult patients. Quart. J. Med., 27:495, 1958.
14. Kark, R. M., Pirani, C. L., Pollak, V. E., Muehrcke, R. C. and Blainey, J. D.: The nephrotic syndrome in adults: a common disorder with many causes. Ann. Int. Med., 49:751, 1958.
15. Lannigan, R., Kark, R. M. and Pollak, V. E.: The effect of a single intravenous injection of aminonucleoside of puromycin on the rat kidney. A light and electron microscopic study. J. Path. Bact. (In press.)
16. Muehrcke, R. C., Kark, R. M., Pirani, C. L. and Pollak, V. E.: Lupus nephritis: a clinical and pathologic study based on renal biopsies. Medicine, 36:1, 1957.
17. Mueller, C. B., Mason, A. D. and Stout, D. G.: Anatomy of the glomerulus. Am. J. Med., 18:267, 1955.
18. Pirani, C. L., Folli, G., Pollak, V. E. and Kark, R. M.: Unpublished observations.
19. Pollak, V. E., Kark, R. M. and Dubin, A.: Unpublished observations.
20. Pollak, V. E., Kark, R. M., Pirani, C. L., Shafter, H. A. and Muehrcke, R. C.: Renal vein thrombosis and the nephrotic syndrome. Am. J. Med., 21:496, 1956.
21. Pollak, V. E., Pirani, C. L. and Kark, R. M.: The effect of large doses of prednisone on the renal lesions and life span of patients with lupus glomerulonephritis. J. Lab. & Clin. Med, 57:495-511, 1961.
22. Rather, L. J.: Filtration, resorption, and excretion of protein by the kidney. Medicine, 31:357, 1952.
23. Soothill, J. R. and Kark, R. M.: The effects of infusion of salt-poor human serum albumin on serum cholesterol, cholinesterase and albumin levels in healthy subjects and in patients ill with the nephrotic syndrome. Clin. Res. Proc., 4:140, 1956.
24. Squire, J. R.: The nephrotic syndrome. Adv. Int. Med., 7:201, 1955.
25. Squire, J. R., Blainey, J. D. and Harwicke, J.: The nephrotic syndrome. Brit. M. Bull., 13:43, 1957.

Etiology and Pathogenesis of Glomerulonephritis

WILLARD C. SCHMIDT

Western Reserve University School of Medicine

Glomerulonephritis is a complex of renal diseases in which the damage initiated by various agents is confined primarily to the glomeruli. Clinical and laboratory studies have revealed differences in the symptoms, signs, natural history, and histopathology of varieties of nephritis that have led investigators to distinguish differences in their pathogenesis.[15, 16, 27] These investigations have produced evidence which permits separation of the nephritides into the following entities: acute glomerulonephritis, chronic glomerulonephritis, lupus glomerulonephritis, nephritis associated with anaphylactoid purpura, lipoid nephrosis, focal glomerulonephritis associated with bacteremia, toxemia or metabolic disease, and hereditary chronic nephritis.

This review will be limited to a discussion of one of the more common forms of acute glomerulonephritis, that which follows infection with nephritogenic group A streptococci. It will include a brief description of the natural history and a summary of bacteriological, immunological and pathological studies that support current concepts of the pathogenesis of this disease.

NATURAL HISTORY OF ACUTE GLOMERULONEPHRITIS

The patient with acute glomerulonephritis usually sees a physician because of swelling of his face, hands or feet or because he has passed dark reddish brown or smoky urine. Commonly, these symptoms are preceded by an upper respiratory infection with sore throat. On questioning, the patient often admits to anorexia, and less frequently to nausea, oliguria and vague back or abdominal pain. The blood pressure is often elevated. Examination of freshly voided urine shows proteinuria and increased numbers of erythrocytes, leukocytes, epithelial cells and casts. The intensity of the renal injury in acute glomerulonephritis varies greatly.[7, 24, 30] Some patients experience only moderate malaise, and clinical investigation demonstrates only low grade hematuria, cylindruria and proteinuria. Uncommonly, the initial illness may be severe, with oliguria progressing to anuria, extensive edema, marked hypertension with convulsions, electrolyte disturbances and cardiac failure. However, fewer than 5 per cent of hospitalized patients die in the acute phase.[7] Usually, the disease is not severe and the hypertension and edema subside five to ten days after the appearance of initial signs and symptoms. Proteinuria, hematuria and cylindruria regress more slowly, and traces of albumin and moderate numbers of erythrocytes may be found for weeks or months after the onset of nephritis.

The prognosis in acute glomerulonephritis is good, and although figures vary, it does not seem unreasonable to state that 85 to 95 per cent of patients completely recover.[7, 24, 30] Differences of opinion concerning the likelihood

259

of recovery result from varying conceptions of the pathogenesis of chronic nephritis. Some observers believe that chronic nephritis is a progressive stage of acute nephritis in which the original inflammatory reaction continues, either uniformly or through exacerbations and remissions, eventually to renal failure.[8] Others believe that chronic nephritis rarely occurs as a progressive form of acute glomerulonephritis but is another disease syndrome of unknown, perhaps multiple, etiologies unrelated to group A streptococcal infection.[21, 27]

GROUP A STREPTOCOCCAL INFECTION AND ACUTE GLOMERULONEPHRITIS

Acute glomerulonephritis usually begins one to three weeks after tonsillitis, pharyngitis, sinusitis, cellulitis, pyoderma, or scarlet fever caused by hemolytic or group A streptococci.[17, 21, 30] Sometimes nephritis occurs in epidemics, coincident with large outbreaks of streptococcal infections.[14, 17, 19, 24] Multiple cases of nephritis have also been noted in families in which many members experience monotypic streptococcal infection.[17] Otherwise, sporadic cases of nephritis occur with varying frequency in populations with both high and low streptococcal attack rates. The observation that the attack rate of nephritis is not proportional to the attack rate of streptococcal infections led investigators to the hypothesis that certain strains of group A streptococci are nephritogenic. Rammelkamp[17] and others[26, 29] have summarized and analyzed these epidemiological data and have demonstrated that infection with strains belonging to serotypes 4, 12, 25 and 49 (Red Lake) nearly always occurs before the onset of acute nephritis. Recent bacteriological studies which included streptococcal typing have demonstrated that type 12 streptococcal infection is the most frequent precursor of acute nephritis in the United States, Canada, England and Japan.[21] Type 4 streptococci have been isolated from sporadic cases of nephritis in this country and from patients in nephritis outbreaks in Honolulu and Japan.[21] Type 25 organisms have also been isolated from sporadic cases in this country.[21] Type 49 is known chiefly because of its role in an explosive outbreak of nephritis in a Minnesota Indian reservation,[26] although it has been isolated from a patient with nephritis in Chile.[21]

However, the nephritogenic capacity of strains of group A streptococci is not solely related to type specificity. Many infections caused by types 4, 12, 25 and 49 streptococci do not result in nephritis. The incidence of nephritis following infection with type 12 and type 49 strains described in several reports is summarized in Table 1. The occurrence of nephritis in families infected with nephritogenic streptococci might suggest the participation of a host factor acting in concert with nephritogenic strains. However, the development of nephritis in unrelated persons in the described epidemics would appear to emphasize the role of specific streptococci. Additional evidence of the association of specific types of streptococci with nephritis is the finding of type 12 and type 49 antibodies in the sera of persons who have recovered from acute nephritis. Freedom from recurrences of nephritis is probably due to this type-specific protective antibody or to the statistical improbability of acquiring a second nephritogenic infection from among nearly 50 types of group A streptococci.

In contrast to acute nephritis, the occurrence of antecedent nephritogenic streptococcal infection is often not demonstrable in patients with chronic nephritis. Preliminary studies indicate that sera from these patients do not contain type-specific antibodies to nephritogenic organisms.

TABLE 1. *INCIDENCE OF NEPHRITIS AFTER INFECTION WITH NEPHRITOGENIC TYPES OF STREPTOCOCCI*

LOCATION		YEAR	STREPTO-COCCAL TYPE	ESTIMATED INCIDENCE OF NEPHRITIS (Per cent)
Epidemic Infections				
Bainbridge N. T. S.[24]	USA	1952	12	12*
Pubnico N.S.[19]	Canada	1951-52	12	13†‡
Red Lake Reservation[14]	USA	1953	49	6†
Ft. Warren, Wyo.[17]	USA	1949-52	12	1.6†
New York City[4]	USA	1939-40	12	0†
Sporadic Infections				
Cleveland[17]	USA	1949-51	12	7*
Barkingside, Essex[11]	England	1950-53	12	0†

* Hematuria and clinical nephritis.
† Clinical nephritis.
‡ 33 per cent if calculated on the basis of families infected rather than total population.

Intensive study of strains of streptococci obtained from cases of nephritis has not yet been possible, so that characteristics of the strains that might be responsible for their nephritogenic capacity have not been determined. It has been reported that many strains of type 12 streptococci are capable of unusual variability. Strains producing small white colonies have been described.[18] Typical complete or beta hemolysis on blood agar plates is not characteristic of these strains.[4, 18] They produce narrow hemolytic zones, sometimes with greenish discoloration, and may at times be non-hemolytic. Type 12 strains may grow poorly at 37 degrees and grow well, producing beta hemolysis, at 22 degrees.[4] These atypical growth characteristics may be responsible for the low rates of isolation of streptococci from some groups of patients with nephritis. Most strains of type 12 streptococci produce an enzyme, diphosphopyridine nucleotidase (DPNase),[2] which, because of its ability to destroy DPN, inactivates DPN-dependent enzymes. DPNase activity appears to be responsible for experimental leukotoxic effects of strains of type 12 and other types of group A streptococci, but it is not closely correlated with nephritogenic capacity. Preliminary investigations indicate that types 4 and 12 streptococci, which may be nephritogenic, appear to be more susceptible to infection and lysis by specific bacteriophages than the majority of other streptococcal types.[18] The hypothesis has been suggested that phage infection may convert streptococci to variants of enhanced nephrotoxicity.[18] Also, it is possible that, if phage infection and subsequent streptococcal lysis can occur *in vivo*, abnormal amounts of streptococcal products may be produced that may selectively localize in renal tissue.

PATHOGENESIS OF ACUTE GLOMERULONEPHRITIS

In addition to the epidemiological evidence of the role of nephritogenic group A streptococci in acute nephritis, data pertaining to pathogenesis have been accumulated from pathological studies of nephritic lesions and from investigations with experimental models of nephritis.

Examination of autopsy material has resulted in a composite description of the nephritic lesion. It appears that endothelial proliferation, polymorphonuclear infiltration of the glomerular tuft, escape of erythrocytes and leukocytes into the capsular space and thickening of the basement membrane make up the acute lesion.[21] In chronic nephritis, it is stated that glomerular crescents develop, and obliteration of the capsular space and fibrosis or hyalinization of the glomerulus occur.[21] There are three limitations to autopsy studies: (1) They do not reveal early changes which might, by virtue of indicating the initial lesions, be more helpful in tracing the source of the renal injury. (2) Since investigation of varieties of nephritis has been carried to the point where some of them may be distinguished on clinical or laboratory grounds, it has become apparent that typical pathological lesions are not specific but represent the general response of the glomerulus to multiple injurious stimuli. It is also evident (3) that autopsy studies would seldom include material from cases of streptococcal glomerulonephritis, from which most patients recover completely.

Since the development of the renal biopsy technique, the difficulty of obtaining tissue for study early and at subsequent stages in the course of nephritis has been overcome. Tissues collected during the acute phase of streptococcal nephritis show endothelial swelling and proliferation accompanied by polymorphonuclear infiltration of the glomerulus.[27] Specimens obtained during the first few days of the disease have not yet been described, so that one cannot be certain that the earliest stages of injury have been seen. Renal lesions in biopsies from patients with subacute or chronic nephritis consist of epithelial crescent formation, endothelial proliferation, glomerular fibrosis and hyalinization.[8, 27] Deposition of fibrinoid in glomerular capillaries, foci of interstitial inflammation, as well as some degree of tubular degeneration, dilatation and atrophy have also been infrequently described.[27, 28] In several biopsies, Vernier was able to demonstrate the coexistence of acute and chronic lesions which, when correlated with clinical history, indicate exacerbation of chronic nephritis or the superposition of acute post-streptococcal nephritis upon chronic nephritis.[27] Patients in this category have a much poorer prognosis than those with typical acute glomerulonephritis. The appearance of acute nephritis in patients with previously unrecognized renal disease may be the basis for the belief that in a significant number of patients acute nephritis progresses to the subacute or chronic form.

Studies of biopsy material with the electron microscope indicate that the primary site of renal injury in acute glomerulonephritis is the glomerular endothelium.[27] Proliferation of glomerular endothelial cells and swelling of the cytoplasm of these cells are prominent findings in the acute stage.[27] Accumulation of basement membrane material resulting in thickening of this structure is an additional electron microscopic finding in subacute and chronic nephritis.[27] In contrast, the chief lesion seen with the electron microscope in biopsy material from cases of pure nephrosis is disorganization, smudging or loss of the foot processes of epithelial cells of the glomerulus.[27] An essential step in demonstrating the role of nephritogenic streptococci in the pathogenesis of acute nephritis is the identification of streptococcal products in lesions in renal biopsy material. A recent report,[22] as yet unconfirmed, described the finding, by the use of fluorescent labeled antibody, of streptococcal antigen in a small proportion of biopsy specimens from patients with nephritis.

Because of features of the natural history of glomerulonephritis that resemble known hypersensitivities, immunological reactions of this type produced in animals have been extensively investigated as experimental models of nephritis. Two models have been studied. In one, nephrotoxic nephritis, antibody against components of kidney tissue prepared in a heterologous host or prepared with Freund adjuvant in the homologous host[9] is the reagent used to produce the renal inflammatory reaction. This method is based on the hypothesis that etiological agents in nephritis can produce alterations in renal tissue components that cause them to stimulate the formation of "auto-antibodies" which then react with the tissue components to produce the characteristic nephritic inflammatory reaction. In the second model, foreign protein is injected into animals to stimulate antibody formation; this antibody then reacts with residual antigen, and the reaction products localized in tissue, particularly in renal glomerular cells, produce an inflammatory response. In many features these experimental models resemble nephritis.[21] In particular, recent experiments employing injected foreign antigen-antibody complexes[1] or repeated injection of small doses of antigen over a prolonged period[5] have produced lesions and illnesses remarkably like acute glomerulonephritis. Immunofluorescent methods have demonstrated antigen and gamma globulin which might include specific antibody in these lesions.[6] It is reasonable to hypothesize that streptococcal antigen-antibody systems may operate similarly as nephritis-inducing agents.

However, experiments utilizing streptococci or streptococcal components have met with limited success. Glomerulonephritis in rats following immunization with mixtures of streptococci and homologous kidney homogenates was reported by one investigator,[3] but intensive efforts by others to reproduce these results were unsuccessful.[12] More recently, hypertension, albuminuria and microscopic hematuria were obtained in rabbits injected with living nephritogenic type 12 streptococci or culture filtrates.[18] Histopathologically, however, the lesions resembled those of lower nephron nephrosis rather than glomerulonephritis. Other investigators have obtained renal lesions in mice implanted with intraperitoneal diffusion chambers containing viable streptococci. The membrane walls of these chambers permit diffusion of soluble and perhaps lytic products of streptococcal cells into tissues. Kelly and Winne[13] produced proximal tubular necrosis, thickened basement membrane and glomerular adhesions by implantation of chambers containing nephritogenic streptococci only. Others,[10, 25] using essentially the same technique, found proteinuria, tubular degeneration and casts in mice exposed to diffusates from nephritogenic type 12, and non-nephritogenic type 12 and type 14 streptococci. Glomerular and tubular nephrosis-like lesions with accompanying proteinuria, edema and hypoalbuminemia have also been produced by injecting large doses of viable non-nephritogenic streptococci subcutaneously into rats.[23]

The clinicopathological features of these experimental streptococcal nephropathies are significantly different from those of human post-streptococcal nephritis. At present the experimental renal lesions produced with non-streptococcal antigen-antibody aggregates are closer approximations of the natural disease. It is evident that more must be learned about the characteristics of nephritogenic streptococci and, perhaps, the experimental host in order to reproduce post-streptococcal glomerulonephritis accurately.

REFERENCES

1. Benacerraf, B., Potter, J. L., McCluskey, R. T. and Miller, F.: J. Exper. Med., *111*:195, 1960.
2. Bernheimer, A. W., Lazarides, P. D. and Wilson, A. T.: J. Exper. Med., *106*:27, 1957.
3. Cavelti, P. A. and Cavelti, E. S.: Arch. Path., 39:148, 1945; *40*:158, 163, 1945.

4. Coburn, A. F. and Pauli, R. H.: J. Exper. Med., 73:551, 1941.
5. Dixon, F. J., Weigle, W. O., Vazquez, J. and Feldman, J. D.: Fed. Proc., 19:205, 1960.
6. Dixon, F. J., Vazquez, J., Weigle, W. O. and Cochrane, G. G.: Arch. Path., 65:18, 1958.
7. Earle, D. P.: J. Chron. Dis., 5:3, 1957.
8. Earle, D. P. and Jennings, R. B.: Ann. Int. Med., 51:851, 1959.
9. Heymann, W., Hackel, D. B. and Hunter, J. L. P.: Fed Proc., 19:195, 1960.
10. Hinkle, N. H., Partin, J. and West, C. D.: J. Lab. & Clin. Med., 56:265, 1960.
11. Holmes, M. C. and Williams, R. E. O.: J. Hygiene, 56:43, 1958.
12. Humphrey, J. H.: J. Path. & Bact., 60:211, 1948.
13. Kelly, D. K. and Winne, J. F.: Science, 127:1337, 1958.
14. Kleinman, H.: Minnesota Med., 37:479, 1954.
15. Muehrcke, R. C., Kark, R. M., Pirani, C. L. and Pollak, V. E.: Medicine, 36:1, 1957.
16. Perkoff, G. T., Nugent, C. A., Dolowitz, D. A., Stephens, F. E., Carnes, W. H. and Tyler, F. H.: Arch. Int. Med., 102:733, 1958
17. Rammelkamp, C. H., Jr. and Weaver, R. S.: J. Clin. Invest., 32:345, 1953.
18. Rammelkamp, C. H., Jr.: J. Chron. Dis., 5:28, 1957.
19. Reed, R. W.: Canad. M.A.J., 68:448, 1953.
20. Reed, R. W. and Matheson, B. H.: J. Infect. Dis., 95:191, 202, 1954.
21. Schmidt, W. C. and Rammelkamp, C. H., Jr.: Adv. Int. Med., 9:181, 1958.
22. Seegal, B. C., Hsu, K. C., Fiaschi, E. and Andres, G.: Rass. fisiopat. Clin., 31:1, 1959.
23. Sharp, J. T.: Proc. Soc. Exper. Biol. & Med., 104:428, 1960.
24. Stetson, C. A., Rammelkamp, C. H., Jr., Krause, R. M., Kohen, R. J. and Perry, W. D.: Medicine, 34:431, 1955.
25. Tan, E. M., Hackel, D. B. and Kaplan, M. H.: J. Infect. Dis. (In press.)
26. Updyke, E. L., Moore, M. S. and Conroy, E.: Science, 121:171, 1955.
27. Vernier, R. L., Farquhar, M. G., Brunson, J. G. and Good, R. A.: Am. J. Dis. Child., 96:306, 1958.
28. Watt, M. F., Howe, J. S. and Parrish, A. E.: Arch. Int. Med., 103:690, 1959.
29. Wilmers, M. J., Cunliffe, A. C. and Williams, R. E. O.: Lancet, 2:17, 1954.
30. Winkenwerder, W. L., McLeod, N. and Baker, M.: Arch. Int. Med., 56:297, 1935.

Some Studies in Experimental Glomerulonephritis

BEATRICE CARRIER SEEGAL

College of Physicians and Surgeons, Columbia University

A close counterpart of the acute and chronic glomerulonephritis of man has been reproduced experimentally only by immunologic means. The intravenous injection in the rabbit of large volumes of normal heterologous serum or certain of its fractions causes serum disease characterized in part by glomerular lesions.[5] It has also been demonstrated in the rat that the injection of soluble antigen-antibody complexes results in glomerulitis.[1] In both these instances the renal lesion is relatively mild and healing takes place in a few days. In contrast, the clinical course and histologic picture of acute and chronic glomerulonephritis produced in the rat, rabbit or dog by injection of specific renal antibodies simulates the spectrum of the human disorder in great detail.[15] Whole kidney, glomeruli alone, or even fragments of glomeruli rich in basement membrane have been used to obtain the nephritis-producing or "nephrotoxic" antibodies. Still unexplained is the fact that placenta[17] and lung[6] also evoke the production of a nephrotoxic antibody.

This discussion will be limited to selected studies bearing on the pathogenesis of the disease that results from the injection of specific nephrotoxic sera. The evidence to be presented appears to support the following conclusions: (1) The acute nephritis that immediately follows the injection of nephrotoxic serum is the result of a specific reaction between antigen(s) in the glomerulus and antibodies in the nephrotoxic serum. (2) The severity of the acute nephritis is related to the amount of nephrotoxic antibody globulin which has localized in the glomerulus. (3) The development of chronic nephritis is associated with the continued presence of the injected nephrotoxic globulin in the glomeruli, together with some of the host's own serum globulins. (4) The progression of the chronic nephritis appears to be faster when the initial acute nephritis is more severe. The significance of these conclusions in relation to the mechanism of the experimental disease and some analogies to the human disease will be discussed.

Solomon and his associates[18] first presented evidence that the glomeruli contain the antigen(s) which stimulate the production of nephrotoxic antibody in antirenal serum. They demonstrated that isolated rat glomeruli absorbed the nephrotoxic antibody from rabbit antirat-kidney serum. Pressman[11] used radio-autographs to show that antirat-kidney serum tagged with radioactive sulfur localized in rat glomeruli. Krakower[8] carried the search for the specific antigen further and reported that the glomerular basement membrane of dog kidney was the most effective antigen for producing specific nephrotoxins. Studies by Mellors[10] and by Seegal and her associates,[14] employing fluorescein-tagged antibody, indicated that injected antirat-kidney serum localizes chiefly in glomeruli, notably in glomerular membranes. But, as stated earlier, there is no doubt that the antigen which stimulates the production of nephrotoxic antibody is widely distributed, since both placenta and lung contain it in sufficient amount to produce nephrotoxins. The injection of such specific antilung or antiplacenta serum causes nephritis but no other tissue change. The basis for this phenomenon may be that both these antisera, like the antirenal sera, localize almost exclusively in the glomeruli. This is illustrated, in the case of antiplacenta serum, in Figure 1, which shows a section of kidney from a rat injected one day previously with rabbit antirat-placenta serum. The section has been "stained" with fluorescein-tagged antibody to rabbit globulin prepared in the duck. The bright lines of fluorescence in the glomeruli suggest the localization of the nephrotoxic serum in the basement membranes of these structures. Elsewhere in the body only relatively small amounts of the globulins from the nephrotoxic sera are found in reticuloendothelial cells of certain organs, notably the spleen and adrenal. Control studies with non-nephritogenic antisera have shown either transitory localization of small amounts of the injected globulin in the glomeruli or no demonstrable localization. Further control studies have indicated that the glomerulus does not bind other circulating foreign proteins during the induction of the nephritis. From these reports it may be concluded that nephrotoxic sera localize specifically and chiefly in the glomeruli, because of binding of the nephrotoxic antibody to the antigen in glomeruli.

Two other lines of investigation support the opinion that binding of nephrotoxic serum in the glomeruli is due to a specific antigen-antibody reaction. First, it has been shown[15] that all nephrotoxic sera tested may lose

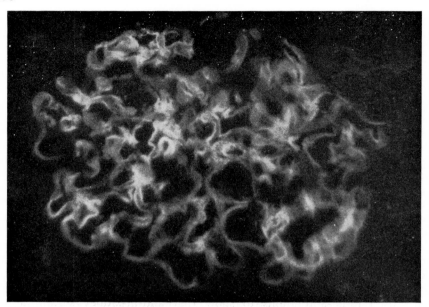

Fig. 1.   Section of kidney of rat injected with rabbit antirat-placenta serum one day previously. Tissue frozen, sectioned in a cryostat and stained with fluorescein-tagged duck antibody to rabbit globulin. The bright lines of fluorescence produced by the bound antibody suggest that the nephrotoxic globulin has localized mainly in the basement membranes of the glomerulus. $\times$ 800.

this property by absorption with either kidney, lung or placenta. Second, Klein and Burkholder[7] have demonstrated, by use of the fluorescent antibody technique, that guinea pig complement is fixed in the glomeruli of nephritic rats. The freshly cut renal tissue from such animals is exposed to guinea pig serum, washed with buffer and then stained with fluorescent antibody to guinea pig complement prepared in the rabbit. Figure 2 illustrates such binding of guinea pig complement in the glomerulus of a nephritic rat.

In order to determine the possible relationship between the amount of nephrotoxic serum bound in the glomerulus and the severity of the ensuing acute nephritis, the relative amount of nephrotoxic globulin found in the glomeruli has been estimated by a technique previously described. This method determines the amount of untagged antibody required to block staining of the glomeruli with fluorescein-tagged antibody to the nephrotoxic globulin.[14] The least amount of untagged antibody required to block staining of the kidney from an animal with severe nephritis is assigned a value of 100, and that required to block the staining of the kidneys from the other nephritic animals is expressed as a percentage of this value. In the experiments reported in Table 1, rats were injected either with decreasing volumes of a single nephrotoxic serum or with different volumes of nephrotoxic sera of varying potency. The animals were killed within two weeks of injection, the relative amounts of nephrotoxic serum in the glomeruli were estimated on fresh frozen tissue, and the severity of the nephritis was evaluated from sections of fixed kidney tissue stained with hematoxylin and eosin and with periodic acid Schiff reagent. It may be seen that 0.5 to 0.7 ml. of antikidney serum 1 produced severe nephritis; this volume was assigned a value of 100

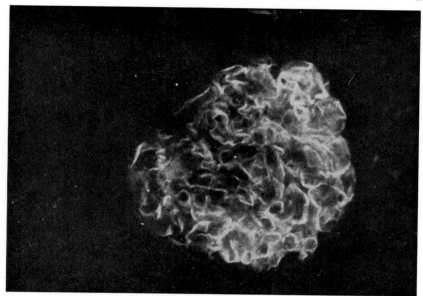

Fig. 2. Guinea pig complement stained in the kidney of a rat injected 2 hours previously with rabbit antirat-kidney serum. After perfusion of the kidney with physiologic saline the tissue was frozen and sectioned and a drop of guinea pig serum, diluted 1:10, added for 30 minutes. After washing, the tissue was stained with fluorescein-tagged rabbit antibody to guinea pig complement. The complement is found in the areas which contained the nephrotoxic serum (see Fig. 1). Courtesy of Dr. Klein and Dr. Burkholder. × 400.

to express the relative amount of the serum globulin demonstrated in the glomeruli. The relative amount of globulin in the glomeruli decreased with diminishing amounts of injected serum and this was associated with a decline in severity of the renal lesions. Nephrotoxic serums 2, 3 and 4 were of different potencies. Whereas 0.4 ml. of serum 2 localized to a value of 100 in the glomeruli of the four rats injected, only about half of this amount of nephrotoxic globulin was demonstrated in the glomeruli of rats receiving the larger volume of serums 3 or 4. Only serum 2 produced severe renal

TABLE 1. CORRELATION BETWEEN SEVERITY OF RENAL LESIONS AND RELATIVE AMOUNT OF NEPHROTOXIC SERUM BOUND IN GLOMERULI (DETERMINED BY PER CENT UNTAGGED ANTIBODY TO NEPHRO-TOXIC GLOBULIN REQUIRED TO BLOCK STAINING WITH TAGGED ANTIBODY)

NEPHRO-TOXIC SERUM INJECTED	AM'T (ml.)	NO. OF RATS	NEPHRITIS PRODUCED; NO. OF RATS			PER CENT UNTAGGED ANTIBODY TO BLOCK
			MILD	MODERATE	SEVERE	
Serum 1	0.5-0.7	5		1	4	100
	0.3-0.4	4		4		50
	0.2	2	2			25
Serum 2	0.4	4			4	100
Serum 3	0.9	4		4		50
Serum 4	1.5	4		4		50

lesions, and moderately severe nephritis followed the injection of serums 3 and 4. From such experiments as these, carried out in rats with many different nephrotoxic serums, it has been concluded that severity of the renal lesion in experimental acute nephrotoxic nephritis is related to the amount of nephrotoxic antibody localized in the glomeruli and is independent of the total volume of whole serum given. Less extensive experiments in rabbits support similar conclusions.

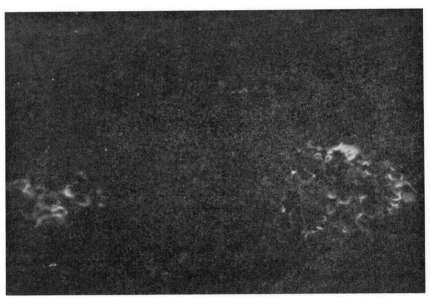

Fig. 3. Section of kidney from a rat injected 21 days previously with rabbit antirat-kidney serum. The kidney was perfused with saline, then frozen, sectioned and stained with fluorescein-tagged duck antibody to rabbit globulin. Localization of the rabbit globulin in the glomeruli is demonstrated. × 400.

Other lines of investigation have been followed in order to obtain evidence concerning the mechanism for the progressive course of the chronic nephritis which follows the acute disease. The continuing inflammatory reaction, in the absence of infection, suggests that experimental chronic nephritis may be maintained by a self-perpetuating antigen-antibody reaction. The persisting nephritis could result from a continuing allergic response to the original antigen-antibody complex or it might arise from a reaction between the injected foreign protein and antibody produced in the host to this protein. Another possibility is that the acute nephritis, under appropriate conditions, induces some change in the renal tissue, which then is able to initiate the development of autoantibodies.

Fluorescent antibody studies have demonstrated that in rats with chronic nephritis, sections of kidney taken ten months following injection of the nephrotoxic globulin still contain some of this substance in the sclerosed glomeruli.[14] Investigation of this problem in rabbits and dogs similarly injected has confirmed the long residence of nephrotoxic serums in the glomeruli of animals with chronic nephritis. It is tempting to speculate that the presence of this latter foreign protein acts as an antigenic stimulus to which the animal responds by production of an antibody which lodges in the glomerulus. Fluorescent antibody studies have shown the presence of native globulin in glomeruli of nephritic animals a few days after injection of the nephrotoxin. This is illustrated in Figures 3 and 4, which are pictures of the kidney of a rat injected with rabbit antirat-kidney serum three weeks previously. The specimen in Figure 3 is stained with fluorescein-tagged duck antibody to rabbit globulin, which indicates the presence of rabbit globulin in the glomeruli; Figure 4 shows that rat globulin also is located there, since this section was stained with fluorescein-tagged rabbit antibody to rat globulin. Examination of renal tissue from other rats in varying stages of chronic nephritis have also shown the existence of rat globulin in the glomeruli. These findings suggest the possibility that an antigen-antibody reaction between the foreign rabbit globulin and the rat antibody to this globulin is present, causing a continuing antigen-antibody reaction which could supply the irritating focus to perpetuate an inflammatory reaction resulting in progressive chronic disease.

Experiments by Sandritter and associates[13] and by Lange[9] in rats have lent support to a theory that autoantibodies cause experimental chronic

Fig. 4. A section of the same kidney seen in Figure 3, stained with fluorescein-tagged rabbit antibody to rat globulin. This globulin is localized in the same general areas which hold the nephrotoxic globulin (Fig. 3). × 400.

nephritis. These investigators joined a nephritic to a normal rat by parabiosis and found that the normal partner developed nephritis. Since fluorescent antibody studies failed to show that the nephrotoxic serum had been transferred from the nephritic kidney to the kidney of the normal parabiotic partner, it was postulated that some other circulating factor in the nephritic rat was responsible for the nephritis occurring in the normal animal. Lange found that rat globulin had localized in the glomeruli of the normal partner and therefore offered the hypothesis that the circulating agent capable of initiating nephritis was presumably autoantibody. Experiments of Rother[12] have failed to demonstrate any capacity of nephritic kidneys from the rabbit to cause autoantibody production in this species. Therefore, no direct evidence has been obtained for the occurrence of autoantibodies to renal tissue during the development of experimental chronic nephritis.

The course of chronic nephritis is greatly accelerated in those animals which show an early, severe, acute nephritis. For example, in series of rats injected with 0.7 ml. of serum 1 or with 0.4 ml. of serum 2 (Table 1), which developed clinically severe acute nephritis, far advanced lesions of chronic nephritis were seen within five months. Rats injected with smaller amounts of serum 1, with 0.9 ml. of serum 3, or with 1.5 ml. of serum 4 required at least eight months to attain the same degree of renal damage. Some nephrotoxic serums cause minimal evidence of early renal lesions, but if animals injected with such antiserums are kept under observation for about 10 months, lesions of mild chronic nephritis will be discovered. The same relationship between the severity of the acute disease and the rate of progression of the chronic nephritis has been observed in dogs. In this species it may take three to four years for the animal to die of renal failure.[15] It is of interest that Earle and Jennings[2] have reported that, in man, the greater the severity of the acute nephritis as determined by renal biopsy data, the greater the likelihood of progression into the chronic nephritic stage.

The facts which seem established by these studies in experimental nephritis are: (1) The glomeruli (glomerular basement membranes?) have a unique capacity to retain heterologous nephrotoxic serum for very long periods of time. (2) The severity of the acute nephritis is greater when more nephrotoxic globulin is bound initially in the glomerulus. (3) A continuing inflammatory response parallels the residence in the basement membranes of the foreign nephrotoxic antibody together with the hosts' own globulins. (4) The rate of progress of the chronic disease is more rapid in the animals which have had severe acute disease. From these findings it appears probable that both acute and chronic experimental glomerulonephritis result from an inflammatory response to the irritating effect of an antigen-antibody reaction. In the early disease it is characteristically due to the reaction between the injected nephrotoxic antibody and some antigen in the glomerulus, and this irritant may persist throughout the course of the disease; however, it also is probable that the foreign protein in the glomerulus which has stimulated antibody production combines with these antibodies to form another antigen-antibody complex capable on its own of causing renal disease. What role, if any, autoantibodies have in this disease is still obscure.

Certain analogies to human nephritis are worthy of comment. In acute nephritis of man serum complement is lowered,[3] suggesting an antigen-antibody reaction. The presence of abnormal amounts of human gamma globulin in the glomeruli has been demonstrated by means of the fluorescent antibody technique in both acute and chronic nephritis in man.[4, 10, 16] This observation suggests that the glomerulus may contain some antigenic substance which is reacting with a circulating antibody. This antigenic substance in the kidney might be altered renal tissue, in which case the hosts' globulins would be of the nature of autoantibodies. On the other hand, the kidney might contain a foreign antigen—for example, some product of the hemolytic streptococcus which had reached the kidney during the streptococcal infection preceding the onset of the nephritis. In this case the antigen should be demonstrable in the glomerulus. We have had the opportunity of examining a few renal biopsies obtained from the clinic of Cassano in Rome during a joint study with Fiaschi and Andres.[16] By means of the fluorescent antibody technique, streptococcal antigen has been found in the glomeruli in three cases of acute or subacute nephritis and in two cases of chronic nephritis during an exacerbation caused by infection with hemolytic streptococcus. Twenty-one other renal biopsies from cases of acute or chronic nephritis failed to show evidence of streptococcal antigen. Whether the streptococcal antigen was present coincidentally or as a factor contributing to the nephritis remains to be determined. However, in conclusion it might be reiterated that there is considerable evidence in experimental nephritis to indicate that a renal lesion similar to that seen in the human disease may result from foreign antigen in the kidney reacting with specific antibody produced by the host, and it seems appropriate to indicate that perhaps here is a disease which is not necessarily the result of damage from autoantibodies.

REFERENCES

1. Benacerraf, B., Potter, S. L., McCluskey, R. T. and Miller, F.: The pathologic effects of intravenously administered soluble antigen-antibody complexes. II. Acute glomerulonephritis in rats. J. Exper. Med., *111*:195, 1960.
2. Earle, D. P. and Jennings, R. B.: Early manifestations of nephritis. M. Clin. North America, *44*:59, 1960.
3. Fischel, E. E. and Gajdusek, D. C.: Serum complement in acute glomerulonephritis and other renal diseases. Am. J. Med., *12*:190, 1952.
4. Freedman, P., Peters, J. H. and Kark, R. M.: Localization of gamma globulin in the diseased kidney. A.M.A. Arch. Int. Med., *105*:524, 1960.
5. Germuth, F. G.: A comparative histologic and immunologic study in rabbits of induced hypersensitivity of the serum sickness type. J. Exper. Med., 97:257, 1953.
6. Goodman, H. C. and Baxter, J. H.: Nephrotoxic serum nephritis in rats. II. Preparation and characterization of a soluble protective factor produced by trypsin digestion of rat tissue homogenates. J. Exper. Med., *104*:487, 1956.
7. Klein, P. and Burkholder, P.: Ein Verfahren zur fluoreszenzoptischen Darstellung der Komplement bindung und seine Anwendung zur histo-immunologischen Untersuchung der experimentellen Nierenanaphylaxie. Deut. med. Wchnschr., *84*:2001, 1959.
8. Krakower, C. A.: Physical and chemical properties of the canine renal glomerulus and its nephrotoxic antigen. Proc. Inst. Med., Chicago, *19*:26, 1952.
9. Lange, K., Wachstein, M. and McPherson, S. E.: Immunologic mechanism for the transfer of experimental glomerulonephritis in parabiotic rats. Proc. Soc. Exper. Biol. & Med., *106*:13, 1961.
10. Mellors, R. C.: Analytical Cytology. New York, McGraw-Hill Book Co., 1959.
11. Pressman, D.: Zone of localization of antitissue antibodies as determined by use of radioactive tracers. J. Allergy, *22*:387, 1951.
12. Rother, K.: Zur Frage der Iso-und Auto-Antigenität kranker Nieren. Zeitschr. f. ges. exp. Med., *127*:611, 1956.
13. Sandritter, W. et al.: Studien zur "Übertragung" der Masginephritis der Ratte. III. Die übertragung der "chronischen" glomerulonephritis durch parabiose genetisch gleichartiger Partner. Zeitschr. f. ges. exp. Med., *132*:453, 1960.
14. Seegal, B. C.: Localization of rabbit and duck antikidney antibodies. Proc. 9th Conf. on Nephritic Syndrome, National Nephrosis Fd., 1958, p. 1.
15. Seegal, B. C. and Bevans, M.: The production of glomerulonephritis by immunologic methods. J. Chron. Dis., *5*:153, 1957.
16. Seegal, B. C., Hsu, K. C., Fiaschi, E. and Andres, G.: La tecnica degli anticorpi fluorescenti applicata allo studio della patogenesi della nefrite umana. Ras. di Fisiopat. Clinica e Terap., *31*:1, 1959.
17. Seegal, B. C. and Loeb, E. N.: Production of chronic glomerulonephritis in rats by injection of rabbit antirat-placenta serum. J. Exper. Med., *84*:211, 1946.
18. Solomon, D. H., Gardella, J. W., Paugh, H., Dethier, F. M. and Ferrebee, J. W.: Nephrotoxic nephritis in rats. J. Exper. Med., *90*:267, 1949.

Preliminary Evidence for the Production of Nephritis in Sheep by an Autoimmune Mechanism*

RAYMOND W. STEBLAY

University of Chicago School of Medicine

Although the pathogenesis of human glomerulonephritis is unknown, certain clinical observations and experimental studies indicate that it may well be an autoimmunologic disorder.

Attempts to relate human nephritis to animal experimental work have chiefly centered around the production of nephritis in certain species by single[4] or repeated[2] intravenous injections of foreign protein, antigen-antibody complexes[3, 7] or antikidney antibodies.[9] The experimental nephritis produced by intravenous injection of hetero-antibody against kidney has been very valuable as an experimental model to study glomerular damage produced by an antibody directed against an antigenic constituent of the glomerulus. Such hetero-nephrotoxic serum nephritis was considered to be highly species specific, but Steblay and Lepper[10] have shown that rabbit antihuman glomerular basement membrane sera will produce nephritis in dogs similar or identical to that induced by rabbit antidog glomerular basement membrane sera. Furthermore, this previously unknown cross reaction permits the use of human tissue antigens in at least one experimental model of nephritis. We are in the process of studying the specificity of human nephrotoxic antigens in various human tissues and species.

While the above experimental models for the production of nephritis have contributed in various ways to our understanding of how antigen-antibody reactions produce glomerular damage, they all fail to provide evidence for the crucial step postulated in the autoimmune theory, namely, the *self*-production of antibodies or antibody-bearing (sensitized) cells or both by the host, specific for an antigen which is a normal constituent of its own glomerular tissue and capable of initiating injury to the antigen-containing tissue.

Many efforts have been made to produce a workable autoimmune model. Diverse autologous, homologous or heterologous kidney preparations with various adjuvants have been injected into several species. In general such efforts have been unrewarding and the few reports of success have not been confirmed. Recently Heymann[5] has reported the production of the nephrotic syndrome in rats by repeated intraperitoneal injection of homologous or autologous rat kidney tissue antigen and Freund's complete adjuvant.

An experimental model which appears to satisfy the above requirements for an autoimmune mechanism is responsible for a growing list of readily reproducible laboratory diseases. These experimental diseases have been produced by injection of certain mammalian tissues incorporated in Freund's

* This investigation was supported (in part) by Grant H-4785 from the United States Public Health Service, by the Chicago Heart Association and by the Schering Corporation.

272

complete adjuvant into certain susceptible species. A list of the tissues used for producing specific organ damage include central and peripheral nervous tissue, uvea, lens, adrenal, testis and thyroid. In some cases (central and peripheral nervous tissue, lens and uvea) heterologous tissue can be used.[12] Regardless of the nature of the antigenic stimulus, whether iso-, homo- or heteroimmunization has been used, the host's own tissue constituents, antigenically related to the injected antigen, serve as the target organ. In the case of successful use of heterologous tissue from several species, it is not yet clear whether the crucial antigens involved are identical although from different species, or closely related—in which case they would constitute true cross-reacting antigens.

In an effort to produce an experimental autoimmune nephritis based on the preceding autoimmune model, glomerular basement membrane (GBM) prepared from kidneys of human and various animal species was incorporated with Freund's adjuvant and injected by various routes into several different species. The purpose of this report is to present evidence for the successful production of glomerulonephritis in sheep by the injection of human, monkey or rat GBM incorporated in Freund's adjuvant.

MATERIALS AND METHODS

Eight young female sheep, ranging in weight from 110 to 140 pounds, were used in the experiment after having been found to be free of disease and to have a normal urine and BUN. Periodic urinalyses and BUN's were determined on the sheep during the course of immunization. At death the BUN was determined, bladder urine was analyzed and the kidneys were examined grossly and microscopically. Kidney and other tissues were fixed in ice-cold 10 per cent formalin and stained with hematoxylin and eosin, periodic acid-Schiff reagent and Masson's trichrome stain.

Human, monkey and rat GBM were prepared by us using a method based on a slight modification of the technique of Krakower and Greenspon.[6] The basement membrane antigen was suspended in saline to desired concentration and used to form a 1:1 water-in-oil emulsion with Freund's adjuvant. The final concentration of GBM ranged from 15 to 25 mg. wet weight per cc. of emulsion. Freund's complete adjuvant consisted of 85 cc. of Bayol F (mineral oil), 15 cc. of Arlacel A (emulsifying agent) and 200 mg. of *Mycobacterium butyricum* (Difco).

Each sheep was injected by a combination of intramuscular, subcutaneous and intradermal routes with 10 to 15 cc. of emulsion every two weeks until death or sacrifice.

RESULTS

The results are summarized in Table 1. Seven sheep received 304 to 1419 mg. of GBM in three to six injections. Each sheep received GBM from a single species. Six sheep died 38 to 90 days after injections began. At time of death all sheep had proteinuria, a greatly elevated BUN and severe chronic glomerulonephritis. Kidney damage was characterized by various stages of glomerular obsolescence. There was marked fibrocellular proliferation of the glomerulus which obliterated Bowman's space and made it difficult to distinguish the various parts of the glomerulus, and the glomerulus from the surrounding interstitial connective tissue. There were

TABLE 1. *CORRELATION OF RENAL HISTOLOGY AND TIME OF DEATH WITH AMOUNT OF ANTIGENS AND NUMBER OF INJECTIONS*

NUMBER OF SHEEP IN GROUP	ANTIGEN*	TOTAL AMOUNT OF ANTIGEN (mg.)	TOTAL NUMBER OF INJECTIONS	TIME OF DEATH IN DAYS AFTER FIRST INJECTION	RENAL HISTOLOGY
1	Human glomerular basement membrane	1171	5	77 (Sacrificed)	Acute glomerulonephritis
4	Human glomerular basement membrane	480-1419	3-6	38-90	Chronic glomerulonephritis
1	Monkey glomerular basement membrane	304	4	67	Chronic glomerulonephritis
1	Rat glomerular basement membrane	794	4	82	Chronic glomerulonephritis
1	Adjuvant only	None	6	100 (Sacrificed)	Normal

* Note: Antigen was suspended in saline to desired concentration and added to Freund's adjuvant to form a 1:1 water-in-oil emulsion.

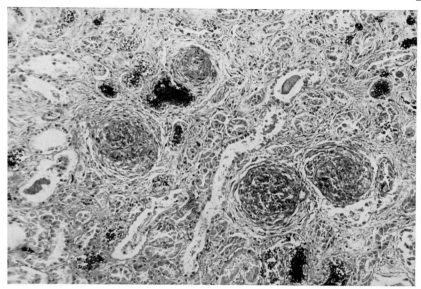

Fig. 1. Kidney of sheep No. 2 which was found dead 42 days after the first of three bi-weekly injections of human glomerular basement membrane and Freund's adjuvant. There is a disruption of the glomerular capillary pattern with fibro-epithelial proliferation completely obliterating Bowman's space and fusing with the conspicuous interstitium, making it difficult to delimit the glomerulus. All stages of tubular retrogressive changes are present, with condensation of the stroma in areas of tubular disappearance. Various types of casts and red cells are prominent in tubules. (Masson's trichrome stain; × 200.)

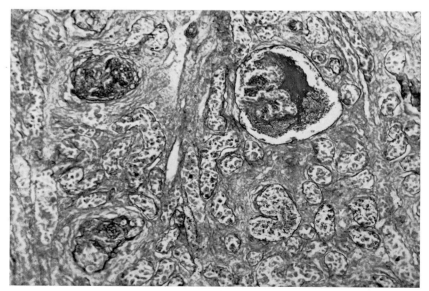

Fig. 2. Kidney from sheep No. 2 above. Interstitial fibrosis is conspicuous and there are various stages of glomerular obsolescence. A recognizable dilated Bowman's space remains in one glomerulus which shows extensive necrosis of the glomerular tuft. (PAS; × 200.)

casts of various types and red blood cells in the tubules. Tubular atrophy and dilatation were present. There was a conspicuous increase of the interstitial connective tissue and some areas of increased interstitial cellular infiltrates (Figs. 1 and 2).

One sheep was sacrificed on the 77th day after receiving 1171 mg. of human GBM in five injections. Examination of bladder urine revealed proteinuria and red and white cells. Grossly, the kidney showed petechiae; microscopically, there were occasional blood cells in the tubules and in Bowman's space, and a mild, diffuse proliferative glomerulitis was present. Because this sheep had been arbitrarily sacrificed early in the course of its disease, only mild early lesions were present.

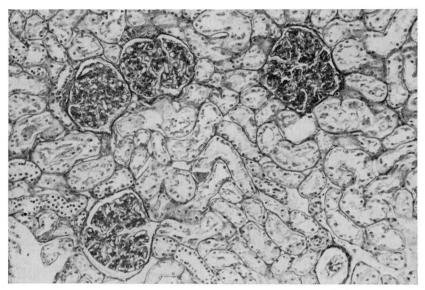

Fig. 3. Kidney of control sheep sacrificed 100 days after the first of six bi-weekly injections of Freund's adjuvant. This demonstrates the normal basis of reference for size and pattern of glomerular and tubular structures. Note the inconspicuous interstitial connective tissue and delicately stained basement membranes of glomeruli and tubules. (PAS; × 200.)

One sheep was given six injections of Freund's adjuvant emulsified with saline as a control. It was sacrificed on the 100th day. No evidence of nephritis was found (Fig. 3). At the time of this writing, three other control sheep have been given a total of seven injections of Freund's adjuvant and are apparently healthy 100 days after injections began. They have no evidence of nephritis and have a normal BUN and urinalysis.

Serum obtained from the sheep given human GBM and sacrificed on the 77th day was fractionated. The gamma globulin was conjugated to fluorescein isothiocyanate and used to stain unfixed sections of human kidney cut 4 microns thick with a cryostat. Proper controls were used as described by Coons.[1] The labelled antisera specifically stained the basement membrane of glomeruli, capsules, tubules, intertubular capillaries and certain extracellular structures in artery walls.[11] It was evident then that circulating antibodies which could localize on human kidney were present

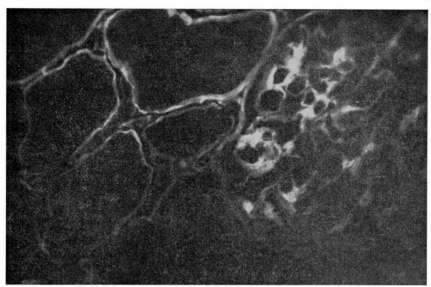

Fig. 4. Human kidney, obtained from a surgical specimen, treated with fluorescein labelled sheep anti-human glomerular basement membrane serum. Basement membranes of capsule, glomerulus, tubules and intertubular capillaries are specifically stained. (× 790.)

in the serum of a sheep with mild kidney damage. Figure 4 shows a section of human kidney tissue specifically stained with fluorescein-labelled sheep antihuman GBM serum. The staining of the glomerular, tubular, capsular and capillary basement membranes may be due to a common antigen in these structures and/or to the presence of small amounts of these structures as contaminants in the GBM preparations.

The serum of the sheep given rat GBM was nephrotoxic for rats. It produced abnormal proteinuria and renal damage within four hours (or earlier) after intravenous injection into the rats.[13] Hence, circulating nephrotoxic antibodies for rats were present in the serum of a sheep immunized with rat GBM. This serum was obtained several weeks prior to death of the sheep from fulminating renal disease.

DISCUSSION

Fatal chronic glomerulonephritis appears to have been produced in sheep by direct injection of heterologous GBM incorporated in Freund's adjuvant. One sheep sacrificed early in the course of its disease showed lesions comparable to acute human glomerulonephritis. The method used to produce this nephritis suggests that it can be classified as an autoimmune disease.

The autoimmune diseases produced in the laboratory may be logically grouped together because of a common technique in producing the diseases. The term "autoimmune," as used in this paper, means that the host's reaction to injected antigen represents an immunologic response directed at a normal constituent of its own tissues. It does not specify or imply whether the response is mediated by sensitized cells and/or antibody. The identification of the responsible vector (or vectors) mediating the autoimmune response remains for experimental demonstration in each appropriate disease. In the case of allergic encephalomyelitis, passive transfer of serum antibodies fails to transmit the disease. Paterson[8] has reported that passive transfer of lymph node cells from sensitized donor rats into recipients which had been made tolerant to the donor cells by neonatal injection would produce encephalomyelitis. It would thus appear that in this particular autoimmune disease the sensitized cell is the vector responsible for mediation of tissue damage.

However, successful transfer of disease by sensitized cells and/or antibodies has not yet been reported in the autoimmune disease (termed "auto-allergic" by Waksman[12]) produced by injection of central and peripheral nervous tissue (except in the case of rat encephalomyelitis discussed above), thyroid, uvea, lens, adrenal or testis.

In the absence of passive transfer of disease by serum antibody and/or sensitized cells, identification of the immunologic basis for the mechanism of the autoimmune diseases rests upon fulfilling other criteria which characterize allergic processes as biologic events according to Waksman,[12] such as the production of lesions by immunizing animals with tissue corresponding to the organs in which lesions later develop, presence of a latent period, specificity of the lesion in that it occurs only in regions where antigen is available in suitable concentrations, histologic appearance of the lesion resembling the tuberculin reaction, diminution of the auto-allergic state with time, anamnestic reaction, and susceptibility of the disease to steroid therapy.

The establishment of an immunologic basis by the above indirect criteria does not specify the relative roles of cells and/or antibodies. However, Waksman has accumulated an intriguing body of observations and arguments to support his contention that the "auto-allergic" diseases probably represent hypersensitivity reactions of the delayed or tuberculin type to tissue antigen.[12]

In our preliminary experiments only heterologous kidney was used as the antigen. Nevertheless, based upon consideration of the kind of criteria used for auto-allergic diseases, the most reasonable explanation for the observed kidney damage is an autoimmune mechanism. Although we wish to classify the "auto-allergic" diseases and the sheep nephritis reported in this paper as having an autoimmune basis, we wish to avoid the implication that the autoimmune mechanism in all these diseases is necessarily mediated by one and the same vector. Only successful passive transfer of these experimental diseases can fully establish their truly allergic nature and simultaneously elucidate the relative roles of antibody or sensitized cells as factors in mediating the disease.

Waksman[12] has pointed out that hetero-antibodies to kidney regularly produce lesions *in vivo*, whereas hetero-antibodies against any of the organs used in experimental auto-allergic diseases consistently fail to do so. He also pointed out that the antigen involved was probably a constituent of the GBM. On the basis of these two observations I would like to point out certain differences between several characteristics of the autoimmune sheep nephritis and their counterparts as described by Waksman[12] in the auto-allergic diseases. (1) The immunizing antigen in autoimmune nephritis was a greatly concentrated preparation of GBM. This is a tissue constituent normally exposed to the blood stream through fenestrations in the glomerular endothelium. The important tissue antigens in the auto-allergic diseases were characterized as being separated from the blood stream by more or less impermeable anatomic barriers. (2) The early lesion in the auto-allergic diseases is described as a perivenous collection of mononuclear cells. By contrast, the early lesion in autoimmune nephritis would seem to arise in the glomerulus. Most likely the origin and appearance of the early lesion are direct consequences of the location and exposure of the antigen to the blood stream in the glomerular capillary wall. (3) In the present experiment, sheep antirat GBM serum produced renal lesions in rats. The renal damage in the rat was presumably due to passive transfer of circulating antibodies present in the serum of the sheep several weeks prior to death of the sheep from chronic glomerulonephritis. It is at present speculative whether the potent nephrotoxic antibodies for the rat played any role in the sheep disease. Heterologous antikidney serum has been known for a long time to be nephrotoxic for the species providing the kidney, but this is the first instance that I am aware of in which the animal which produced the nephrotoxic serum developed nephritis *itself*. In contrast, as Waksman[12] has pointed out, passive transfer of serum from animals with auto-allergic diseases has consistently failed to produce disease in the same or different species.

Whatever the final significance of these preliminary observations may be, it would appear prudent at this time to be cautious before assigning a particular role to sensitized cells and/or antibodies in autoimmune nephritis.

In conclusion, acute and chronic kidney lesions resembling human glomerulonephritis appear to have been induced in sheep by direct injection of human, monkey or rat GBM incorporated in Freund's adjuvant. The serum of one sheep injected with human GBM, which had a mild glomerulitis, contained circulating antibodies which localized on basement membrane structures of human kidney as determined by fluorescent antibody techniques. The serum of another sheep injected with rat GBM was obtained several weeks prior to death of the sheep and contained nephrotoxic antibodies for the rat. It appears that renal damage in the sheep is produced by an autoimmune mechanism. Certain similarities and differences to other experimental autoimmune diseases were noted. Knowledge of the nature of the underlying autoimmune mechanism in this sheep nephritis, whether mediated by circulating autoantibodies and/or sensitized cells, awaits further definitive studies.

ACKNOWLEDGMENTS

I should like to express my gratitude to Dr. Mark H. Lepper, Department of Preventive Medicine, University of Illinois College of Medicine, for helpful suggestions and assistance; to Dr. Ben Spargo, Department of Pathology, University of Chicago, for aid in interpreting the histologic lesions; to Dr. Edward Henderson of the Schering Corporation and to Dr. M. Edward Davis, Department of Obstetrics and Gynecology, University of Chicago, for their interest and support.

REFERENCES

1. Coons, A. H.: Fluorescent antibody methods. General Cytochem. Methods, *1*:399, 1958.
2. Dixon, F. N., Weigle, W. O., Vazquez, J. and Feldman, J.: The immunologic and morphologic consequences of prolonged daily injections of bovine albumin (BSA). Fed. Proc., *19*:205, 1960.
3. Germuth, F. G., Jr., Flanagan, C. and Montenegro, M. R.: The relationships between the chemical nature of the antigen, antigen dosage, rate of antibody synthesis and the

occurrence of arteritis and glomerulonephritis in experimental hypersensitivity. Bull. Johns Hopkins Hosp., 101:149, 1957.

4. Hawn, C. N. and Janeway, C. A.: Histological and serological sequences in experimental hypersensitivity. J. Exper. Med., 85:571, 1947.
5. Heymann, W., Hackel, D. B., Harwood, S., Wilson, S. G. F. and Hunter, J.: Production of nephrotic syndrome in rats by Freund's adjuvant and rat kidney suspension. Proc. Soc. Exper. Biol. & Med., 100:660, 1959.
6. Krakower, C. A. and Greenspon, S. A.: Localization of the nephrotoxic antigens within the isolated renal glomerulus. A.M.A. Arch. Path., 51:629, 1951.
7. Miller, F., Benacerraf, B., McCluskey, R. T. and Potter, J. L.: Production of acute glomerulonephritis in mice with soluble antigen-antibody complexes prepared from homologous antibody. Proc. Soc. Exper. Biol. & Med., 107:706, 1960.
8. Paterson, P.: Transfer of allergic encephalomyelitis in rats by means of lymph node cells. J. Exper. Med., 111:119, 1960.
9. Seegal, B. and Bevans M. The production of glomerulonephritis by immunologic methods. J. Chron. Dis., 5:153, 1957.
10. Steblay, R. W.: In Proceedings of the 10th annual conference on the nephrotic syndrome. New York, National Kidney Disease Foundation, 1959, p. 192.
11. Steblay, R. W.: Similar or identical connective tissue antigens in human placenta and kidney. J. Lab. & Clin. Med. (abstr.), 56:948, 1960.
12. Waksman, B.: Experimental allergic encephalomyelitis and the "auto-allergic" diseases. Internat. Arch. Allergy & Appl. Immunol., Supplement, 14:1, 1959.
13. Winemiller, R., Steblay, R. W. and Spargo, B.: Electron microscopy of acute anti-basement membrane serum nephritis in rats. Fed. Proc., 20:37, 1961.

Interstitial Inflammatory Changes in the Follow-up of Adult Acute Streptococcal Glomerulonephritis by Serial Renal Biopsies*

DANIEL S. KUSHNER, S. HOWARD ARMSTRONG, JR., PAUL B. SZANTO, ALVIN DUBIN and ABRAHAM MARKOWITZ

Hektoen Institute for Medical Research of the Cook County Hospital, Chicago

To the pediatrician, hemorrhagic glomerulonephritis (if the initial acute episode is survived) is a benign self-limited disease. For a quarter century, 90 per cent has remained an accepted estimate of complete healing[7, 10] among children.

No comparable consensus regarding healing exists for the adult. Indeed there are data[17] supporting an inverse relationship between the patient's age at the initial acute episode and incidence of complete clinical recovery.

The purpose of this paper is to summarize those *direct* histological evidences of a continued inflammatory process in a consecutive series of 45

* This work has been made possible by Grants A927 and A1300 from the National Institutes of Health of the United States Public Health Service.

adults who were admitted to the wards of Cook County Hospital with clinical stigmata of acute glomerulonephritis. Serial clinical, biochemical and microbiological studies, supplemented when permitted by serial renal biopsies over follow-up periods ranging from one month to nearly five years, are set forth *in extenso* in another publication.[8]

CLASSIFICATION

As a working schema to facilitate appraisal of the incidence of healing, and with awareness of the arbitrary elements therein, we set up a working classification of these 45 patients as follows:

Class I	10 patients	Clinically acute glomerulonephritis; no evidence of chronicity.
Class II	7 patients	Clinically acute glomerulonephritis with no clinical, but with histopathologic evidence of chronicity.
Class III	4 patients	Clinically acute glomerulonephritis with both clinical and histopathological evidence of chronicity.
Class IV	8 patients	Clinically acute glomerulonephritics for whom there is no histologic data because renal biopsy was declined.
Class V The Melting Pot	16 patients	Suggestive acute glomerulonephritis with serious problems in clinical and/or histological differentiation from hematuric exacerbation of chronic glomerulonephritis.

No significant difference in distribution by age, race or sex was evident between patients in these five classes. This whole series differs from many in having a male-female ratio of 4:3 instead of the usual 2:1.[51] Only eight patients were Caucasian. The resultant 1:4 ratio, taken against our over-all Cook County Hospital ratio of 1:2, is of interest in view of recent information on severity of vascular disease in the Negro.[16]

Clearly, patients in Classes I, II and III present the most valuable information bearing on incidence of chronicity following the adult acute disease. Classes IV and V are necessary methodologic by-products of the study plan.

SOME PROBLEMS OF HISTOLOGIC-CLINICAL CORRELATION

Heirs to traditional histopathologic criteria deriving from over a century of necropsies, today's students of renal biopsies have faced and still face many difficulties in correlation with clinical states of the patients from whom the tissues come.[6] By way of example, epithelial crescents and even glomerular hyalinization (long considered evidences of chronic glomerulonephritis) have recently been demonstrated both in autopsy[6] and biopsy[4] sections from patients with a clinical diagnosis of acute glomerulonephritis.

Important as these findings are, crescents and hyalinization can be considered evidence of inflammation *past*. The chief question is, past by how long: days, weeks, months, years?

We wish to emphasize here evidences of inflammation *present*—evidences which have emerged on sequential biopsies often in the absence of clinical, biochemical, serological or bacteriological correlates.

REPRESENTATIVE RESULTS

A representative sequence is illustrated in Figures 1, 2 and 3. The patient, a white male, was admitted in his seventeenth year with the characteristic

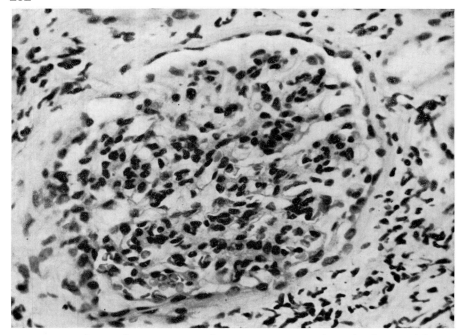

Fig. 1.   Convalescent from acute episode. High power view from the first renal biopsy
(46 days after onset) of the patient described in the text.

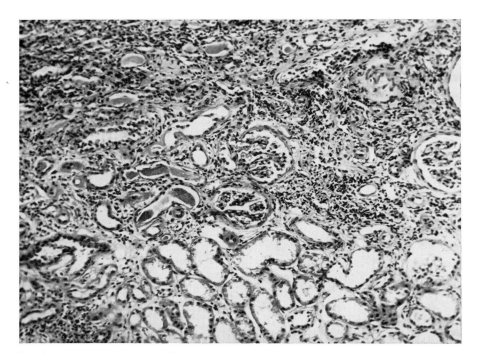

Fig. 2.   Twenty-two months after acute episode. Patient clinically well five months after
streptococcal-related exacerbation. Low power view of fourth biopsy.

findings of acute glomerulonephritis 16 days after an upper respiratory infection. On the basis of five renal biopsies performed in the 43 months between his illness and January 1, 1961, he has been put in Class II (vide supra).

Figure 1 illustrates in high power the typical glomerular hypercellularity in the first of these biopsies, performed 46 days after onset. Microscopic hematuria persisted, and a urinary protein excretion of 550 mg./24 hr. was associated with an alpha$_1$-globulinuria consistent with the proteosuria of Levine and co-workers[9] in acute renal inflammation.

Figure 2 illustrates in low power his fourth biopsy, performed 22 months after onset and 5 months after a serologically demonstrable streptococcal infection associated with transitory proteinuria and proteosuria.

By the time of the fourth biopsy, the urine was once again free of protein, sediment was unremarkable, and endogenous creatinine clearance was 131 ml./min. Notable is the focal interstitial lymphocytic infiltration

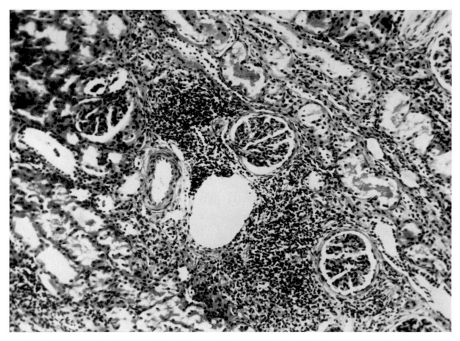

Fig. 3. Twenty-two months after acute episode. Another low power view of fourth biopsy, emphasizing the intensity of the interstitial lymphocyte infiltration coexistent with clinical health.

and fibrosis, together with tubular dilatation and atrophy, in addition to relics of prior glomerular inflammation.

Figure 3 (another low power view of the fourth biopsy) emphasizes the intensity of this focal interstitial lymphocytic infiltration.

For comparison, Figure 4 presents a low power view of a renal biopsy specimen from a patient who has never suffered from clinical evident acute glomerulonephritis and who, following development of the nephrotic syn-

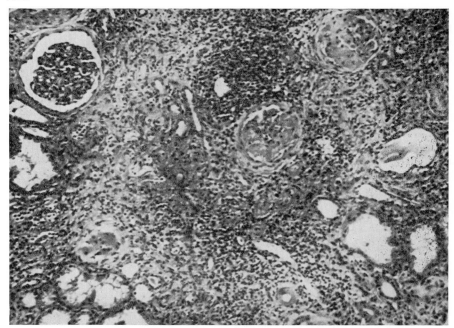

Fig. 4. No acute episode, chronic glomerulonephritis, nephrotic syndrome, impaired renal function. For comparison with the patient of Figs. 1-3.

drome, has been diagnosed as having a typical progressive chronic glomerulonephritis with serious impairment of renal function.

OVER-ALL APPRAISAL OF RESULTS

Identity, qualitative or quantitative, of histologic findings in renal biopsy specimens from all patients in Classes II and III with those in specimens from the patient chosen for illustration (Figs. 1, 2, 3) was neither expected nor found. Nevertheless, on the basis of findings of this sort, in about one-half of the patients in whom by ordinary clinical criteria the disease process was latent or healed, histologic stigmata suggestive of a continued inflammatory process were found. Moreover, asymptomatic pyelonephritis as a possible basis for either interstitial changes or the occasional finding of clumped leukocytes in the sediment was presumed far more frequently than quantitative serial urine culture could confirm.

A 50 per cent incidence of "histological chronicity" raises again a question as old as the first great student of glomerulonephritis. Richard Bright[3] wrote thus concerning the sequelae of hematuric nephritis: "There is great reason to suppose that the seeds of this disease are sown at an early period and that intervals of apparent health produce a false security in the patient, his friends, and in his medical attendants, even when apprehension has been early excited."

Susequent great students have been divided on this question. Volhard[19] and Addis[1] concurred with Bright; Longcope[11] and Ellis[5] have been joined (on the basis of newer developments in the biology of the beta hemolytic streptococcus) by Rammelkamp[18] in believing in an independent pathogenesis of the chronic progressive disease.

In our own work, we have faced but not surmounted the obstacle of sure distinction between an initial acute episode and the hematuric exacerbation of the chronic disease. The magnitude of this problem is illustrated by the proportion of patients reluctantly classified in the "melting pot" (Class V). The hope that clinical uncertainty may be resolved morphologically by use of classic criteria has not been strengthened by serious questions our pathologist collaborator has raised concerning the validity, by classic histologic criteria, of the clinicians' establishment of Class I.

Finally, the data at hand do not as yet indicate a valid choice between two extremes in interpretation of histological abnormalities in those patients who have returned from acute glomerulonephritis to apparent health: (1) merely scars incurred in healing; (2) harbingers of inevitable asymptomatic progression to obvious chronic glomerulonephritis with all its consequences.

Those who tend to a gloomy view may stress the analogy of the interstitial lymphocytic infiltrates with those seen in rejection of renal transplants;[13, 14] those inclined to a cheerful view, with the nonspecific and innocent lymphocytic collections which remain long in areas of old injury to many parts of the body.

Although (for reasons in part published elsewhere[12]) we have used antistreptococcal prophylaxis, our own views have not been gloomy enough to lead us to undertake the steroid regimens described in our subsequent paper in this volume (on patently chronic glomerulonephritis). While steroid therapy is prominent in the regimen used by the Peter Bent Brigham Hospital group for suppression of the rejection phenomenon in homologous renal transplantation, clinical problems encountered with the use of long-term intensive steroid therapy for glomerulonephritis are many, and have been set forth in another publication.[2]

ACKNOWLEDGMENTS

The authors are grateful to Warden Fred A. Hertwig of the Cook County Hospital and to President Daniel Ryan and the Board of Commissioners for provision of basic laboratory facilities.

The authors are grateful to Drs. B. P. Maduros, J. M. Levine, G. L. River, T. N. Gynn, J. P. Pendras, and to A. Poulos, H. A. Dyniewicz, E. Hackett, R. Nelson, A. Costos and J. Cremin for their several contributions to this work.

REFERENCES

1. Addis, T.: Glomerular Nephritis, Diagnosis and Treatment. New York, The Macmillan Company, 1948.
2. Armstrong, S. H., Jr. and Kushner, D. S.: Current status of steroid therapy in chronic adult glomerulonephritis: the unnatural history of Bright's disease. Am. J. Med., 29:377, 1960.
3. Bright, R.: Cases and Observations, Illustrative of Renal Disease Accompanied with the Secretion of Albuminous Urine. Reports of Medical Cases Selected with a View of Illustrating the Symptoms and Cure of Disease by a Reference to Morbid Anatomy. London, Longman, Rees, Orme, Brown and Greene, 1827.
4. Brun, C., Gormsen, H., Hilden, T., Iversen, P. and Raaschou, F.: Kidney biopsy in acute glomerulonephritis. Acta med. scandinav., 161:155, 1958.
5. Ellis, A.: Natural history of Bright's disease; clinical, histologic and experimental observations. Lancet, 1:1, 1942.
6. Grishman, E. and Churg, J.: Acute glomerulonephritis: a histopathologic study by means of thin sections. Am. J. Path., 33:993, 1957.

7. Heymann, W. and Wilson, S. G. F.: Hyperlipemia in early stages of acute glomerular nephritis. J. Clin. Invest., 38:186, 1959.
8. Kushner, D. S. et al. Acute glomerulonephritis in the adult; longitudinal clinical, functional and morphologic studies of rates of healing and progression to chronicity. Medicine. (In press.)
9. Levine, J. M., Dubin, A. and Armstrong, S. H., Jr.: The finding of urinary proteose in certain renal diseases: isolation and identification. J. Lab. & Clin. Med., 53:167, 1959.
10. Loeb, E. N., Lyttle, J. D., Seegal, D. and Jost, E. L.: On the permanence of recovery in acute glomerulonephritis. J. Clin. Invest., 17:623, 1938.
11. Longcope, W. T.: Some observations on the course and outcome of hemorrhagic nephritis. Internat. Clin, 1:1, 1938.
12. Markowitz, A., Armstrong, S. H., Jr. and Kushner, D. S.: Immunologic relationships between the rat glomerulus and nephritogenic streptococci$_a$. Nature, 187:1095, 1960.
13. Merrill, J. P.: Mechanisms of immunity in the rejection of transplanted tissue. Tr. Am. Clin. & Climatol. A., 71:1, 1960.
14. Merrill, J. P., Murray, J. E., Harrison, J. H., Friedman, E. A., Dealey, J. B., Jr. and Dammin, G. J.: Successful homotransplantation of the kidney between non-identical twins. New Engl. J. Med., 262:1251, 1960.
15. Nesson, H. R. and Robbins, S. L.: Glomerulonephritis in older age groups. Arch. Int. Med., 105:23, 1960.
16. Phillips, J. H. and Burch, G. E.: A review of cardiovascular diseases in the white and negro races. Medicine, 39:241, 1960.
17. Ramberg, R.: The prognosis for acute nephritis. Acta med. scandinav., 127:396, 1947.
18. Stetson, C. A., Rammelkamp, C. H., Jr., Krause, R. M., Kohen, R. J. and Perry, W. D.: Epidemic acute nephritis: studies on etiology, natural history and prevention. Medicine, 34:431, 1955.
19. Volhard, F. and Fahr, T.: Die Brightsche Nierenkrankheit. Berlin, Julius Springer, 1914.

Interstitial Changes in Homologous Renal Transplants

JOHN P. MERRILL

Harvard Medical School

The histologic changes which take place following the transplantation of a kidney from one individual to another individual of the same species are best understood in connection with both the gross and functional changes which occur. A kidney transplanted from one dog to another dog has been referred to as a homograft. It is perhaps more properly called an allogenic homograft.[7] The designation "allogenic" stresses the fact that the two individuals, donor and recipient, have different tissue antigens even though belonging to the same species. For this reason the antigens of the donor tissue are capable of causing an immune reaction in the recipient which results in the rejection of the donor tissue. Certain inbred strains of mice and identical human twins exemplify individuals of the same species whose tissue antigens are identical, so that the donor's tissue antigens are not capable of stimulating an immune response in the recipient. Such a transplant is an isogenic homograft.[7] If a kidney is transplanted from one dog to another (allogenic homograft) and the proper arterial and venous anastomoses are successfully effected, a sequence of events occurs which results in the eventual destruction of the grafted organ. The fundamental changes have been well recognized since the early attempts of Alexis Carrel in 1906[4] and C. S. Williamson[18] in the 1920's, when kidney transplantation in dogs became a technically feasible procedure as a result of the development of successful techniques for anastomosing blood vessels. The extensive investigations of Dempster[6] and Simonsen[15] some 30 years later broadened

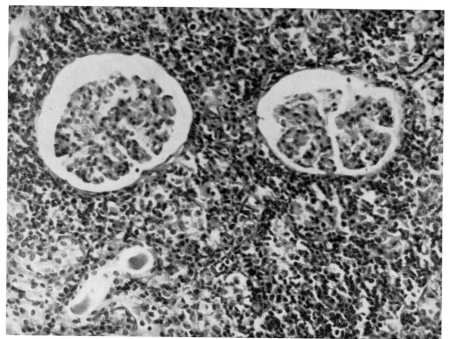

Fig. 1. Histologic changes in renal homograft. See Text. (Dammin, University of Michigan Medical Bulletin, August 1960.)

the scope of knowledge on this subject and also interjected one or two misconceptions which have recently been corrected.

The course of an allogenic renal homograft between two mongrel dogs may be contrasted with what happens when a kidney whose vascular connections have been severed is replaced in the same animal. This latter procedure is an *autograft* and its course is uninfluenced by the immune response. For the first three to four days both the autotransplant and the homograft behave in a similar fashion. When the arterial clamps are released renal blood flow is quickly established and in both instances urine formation begins within minutes to an hour. If the dog is sustained solely by the transplanted kidney the functional events may be more easily followed. Secretion of urine continues in normal quantities for the first few days, the urine containing traces of albumin and occasional casts and red cells. For the first three to four days the course in the dogs with the autografts and homografts is indistinguishable. On the third or fourth day, however, a noticeable difference occurs. The blood urea nitrogen concentration in the dogs with the homografts begins to rise. The urine may contain more albumin, red cells and occasionally red cell casts. The urine volume decreases and the urine becomes isotonic with plasma. The kidney fails to concentrate even with Pitressin stimulation. Finally the secretion of urine ceases completely and the animal dies shortly thereafter of uremia. Serial biopsies of autografted kidneys show few or no changes or, rarely, degenerative tubular lesions secondary to ischemia induced by narrowing of the renal artery.

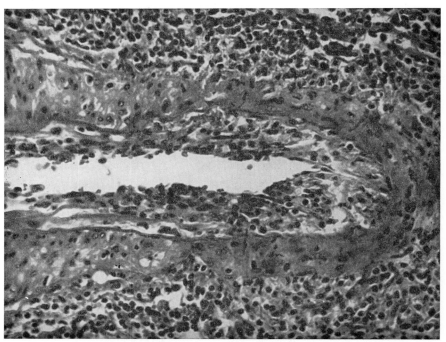

Fig. 2. Vascular lesions in renal homograft. See Text. (Dammin, University of Michigan Medical Bulletin, August 1960.)

The histologic changes in the homograft, however, follow a predictable sequence. Initially these changes are localized largely to the cortex. Classically focal interstitial infiltrations are seen which are localized about the glomeruli and around the small vessels. The small arteries and the thin-walled subcapsular veins are particularly affected. The glomeruli themselves appear normal. Cellular infiltrate consists largely of mononuclear cells of which roughly half are small lymphocytes and the rest larger mononuclear cells of varying forms showing marked pyroninophilia. Clumps of these cells are scattered throughout the interstitium, some having no discernible relation to the glomeruli or blood vessels (Fig. 1). At a later stage one may see proliferation of the endothelium of the smaller arteries sufficient to reduce the size of the lumen. Pyronin-positive cells may also be found lining the lumen of the small vessels. In the larger arteries the lesion resembles polyarteritis nodosum with a focal transmural arteritis (Fig. 2). At this stage the kidney is grossly swollen and has a pale cortex that bulges from the cut surface. From the sixth to the tenth day further changes occur which result in destruction of the tubules. Both hyaline and granular casts are seen in the tubular lumen. The tubules themselves are widely separated by edema, cellular infiltration and occasionally hemorrhage. Some tubules are widely dilated, apparently because of obstructing precipitates. With the advent of further necrosis and interstitial hemorrhage, polymorphonuclear leukocytes makes their appearance. At this time the kidney may develop a fibrous capsule which is densely adherent to the surrounding tissues of the host. Rarely are the larger renal arteries involved except for thromboses subsequent to the surgical intervention. In the small arteries, however, fibrinoid necrosis may involve the whole of the vessel wall and the vascular changes may be similar to those seen in malignant hypertension. These changes are typical of kidneys transplanted in instances in which the transplant represents the first exposure of the recipient animal to the donor's tissue antigens. This is a *primary* or *first-set* homograft.

Medawar, whose fundamental work contributed so much to the knowledge of the immunology of homograft rejection, was the first to point out that when an animal rejected a homograft from another animal he became "immune" or sensitized to the tissue antigens of that animal.[10] As such, the recipient's reaction to a second exposure was an accelerated rejection quite different histologically from that occurring in the first-set graft. The difference in this reaction is well illustrated by the changes that take place when a second kidney from the same donor is transplanted into an animal which has previously rejected a kidney from that donor. After four days the reaction is one of extensive edema and hemorrhage in the interstitial tissue, with a lesser accumulation of pyroninophilic cells. The tubules are more widely separated by edema and have undergone much more severe degenerative changes, including necrosis. Now one finds that the glomeruli themselves are involved, with the tufts showing swelling and increased cellular pyroninophilia and, in some cases, even fibrin thrombi. The function of these kidneys is impaired within the first 24 hours and urine secretion has virtually ceased at the end of the third day. Since the immune rejection response represents sensitization to tissue antigens of the donor as an individual and is not truly organ-specific, a "second-set reaction" to a kidney graft can be obtained if the recipient has been sensitized previously by transplantation of skin from the same donor.[15]

In the human recipient of a kidney transplant the changes are similar but somewhat more variable.[9] In patients in whom no attempt was made to modify the immune response the histologic findings were complicated by infection, which obviously modified the cell type found in the renal interstitium.[9] In the chronically uremic human recipient, homograft rejection does not follow a regular pattern. Although cellular infiltration occurs, prolonged periods of survival of skin and renal homografts have been observed. In the case reported by Michon and Hamburger,[13] in which donor and recipient were closely related (mother to son) and in which the recipient was acutely rather than chronically uremic, the histologic picture more closely resembled that of the experimental animal.

Round-cell infiltration has been the hallmark of homograft rejection in all types of first-set responses studied. Both Simonsen[15] and Dempster,[6] observing the pyronin-positive character of the vascular endothelium, felt that differentiation of vascular endothelial cells of the graft into plasma cells occurred and that these cells represented a reaction on the part of the kidney graft itself against the host. More recent evidence, however, both direct and indirect, suggests that this is not what happens. Thymidine labelling of these plasma cells shows them to be of host origin.[14]

Furthermore, the work of Wheeler, in our group, suggests very strongly that the kidney is not capable of an immune response in itself. Wheeler,[17] transplanting slices of kidney between parent strains and F_1 hybrid mice, found that cellular reaction occurred only when the graft contained antigens against which the host could react and never when the graft was immunologically competent against host antigens. Dempster[6] subjected the donor kidney to small doses of radiation, which should prevent the immune response. This procedure did indeed abolish the infiltration with lymphocytes, although it failed to prevent the rejection of the graft. The recent work of Hume,[8] who irradiated the donor animal with doses of up to 1500 r, indicated that the life of the homograft was not prolonged nor was the histologic picture altered. Since 1500 r of total body radiation given to the host did prolong the life of the homograft, it was felt that the round cell infiltration was entirely a response on the part of the host. It is apparent now that these cells are of host origin and arise in the regional lymph nodes as a result of stimulation by donor antigen. Total body irradiation administered to the host in doses adequate to destroy lymphopoietic tissue markedly prolongs the life of a renal homograft and, in the human, results in absence of the typical histologic picture in the transplanted kidney.[5] This is true also of the administration of radiomimetic agents such as 6-mercaptopurine.[4]

The cellular response of the host is reversible under special circumstances. A kidney transplanted for as long as 72 hours or even eight days in a recipient animal may be retransplanted into the original donor and survive. Surprisingly enough, the cellular reaction becomes more severe during the first week after retransplantation into the donor, probably because of the antigenic stimulation of the homologous cell infiltrate.[2]

The role of the round cell infiltrate in the mechanics of destruction of a homograft is still unclear. Weaver and Algire[16] have shown that it is the presence of the sensitized cell itself which is responsible for the destruction of graft cells. They pointed out that when donor tissue was protected by a millipore chamber impermeable to cells the graft was protected indefinitely. It was destroyed, however, by the introduction into the chamber of sensitized lymphocytes from the recipient animal. We have shown that following the rejection of skin homografts in rabbits both donor and recipient lymphocytes are destroyed when incubated together.[11] Earlier authors have commented on this fact as evident in histologic sections of rejected grafts. The exact mechanism of tissue damage, however, is not clear. The predominance of evidence suggests that contact of donor antigen and sensitized recipient lymphocytes or plasma cells results in destruction of both, and that products of this disintegration may provoke a further immune response and local tissue destruction.[1] It seems reasonable from direct histologic evidence that the vascular endothelium should be primarily involved in this reaction. The other changes may well be secondary to ischemia and thrombosis. Of particular interest in this regard is the fact that while the epithelium of skin grafts seems to be the sensitizing antigen, few cells are found in the epidermis in the accelerated or second-set rejection of skin. In the so-called "white graft," which is the hallmark of the most marked transplantation immunity, the graft is rejected without ever having been vascularized. These results suggest that involvement of the vasculature in the immune state may be so severe as to prevent cells from reaching the site of the presumed antigen.

The rejection of an allogenic homograft is not an "all or none" phenomenon. The antigenic differences between host and recipient, the state of the recipient at the time of grafting, the type of graft and whether or not it is vascularized may all play a role in how rapidly it is rejected. Furthermore, attempts at modifying the immune response by radiomimetic drugs or by x-irradiation may further influence the rate of rejection. A combination of all the factors favorable to the prolongation of a transplanted kidney may result in "partial tolerance" for this kidney even in the human being. We believe that this partial tolerance can be reinforced by subsequent application of x-irradiation and the use of adrenal cortical steroids even when the rejection response has begun. A patient who probably is slowly rejecting his

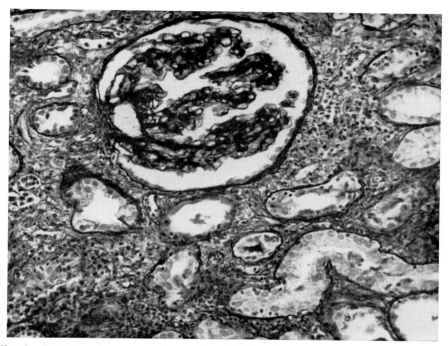

Fig. 3. Rejection phenomenon in transplanted kidney. See Text. (Dammin, University of Michigan Medical Bulletin, August 1960.)

transplanted kidney at the present time is alive and well today two years after a graft.[12] A biopsy of the transplanted kidney shows unequivocal evidence of early rejection (Fig. 3). Subsequent use of whole-body irradiation and adrenal cortical steroids have slowed and modified this rejection so that the renal function is not impaired and the urine contains only small amounts of protein.

This partial tolerance or slow rejection of a kidney whose antigenic structure is similar to but not identical to that of the host in which it resides is strikingly analogous to a number of the so-called "auto-immune" diseases of the kidney, including glomerulonephritis. The fibrinoid necrosis of the small arterioles and the round cell infiltration of the rejected renal homograft are similar to those seen in the human kidney with involvement by lupus erythematosus or polyarteritis nodosum. For the purpose of better understanding both the etiology and the therapy of these diseases in the human, this analogy warrants further careful study.

REFERENCES

1. Amos, D. B.: Ann. N. Y. Acad. Sc., 87:1, 1960.
2. Balankura, O., Goodwin, W. E., Murray, J. E. and Dammin, G. S.: Surg. Forum, 11:24, 1960.
3. Calne, R. Y.: Lancet, 1:417, 1960.
4. Carrel, A. and Guthrie, C. C.: Science, 22:473, 1906.
5. Dealy, J. B., Dammin, G. J., Murray, J. E. and Merrill, J. P.: Ann. N. Y. Acad. Sc., 87:1, 1960.
6. Dempster, W. J.: Brit. J. Surg., 60:163, 1953.
7. Gorer, P. A.: Ann. N. Y. Acad. Sc., 87:1, 1960.
8. Hume, D. M., Jackson, B. T., Zukoski, C., Lee, H. M., Kauffman, H. M. and Egdahl, R. H.: Ann. Surg., 152:3, 1960.
9. Hume, D. M., Merrill, J. P. and Miller, B. F.: J. Clin. Invest., 31:640, 1952.
10. Medawar, P. B.: J. Anat., 79:157, 1945.
11. Merrill, J. P., Hanau, C. and Hawes, M. D.: Ann. N. Y. Acad. Sc., 87:1, 1960.
12. Merrill, J. P., Murray, J. E., Harrison, J. H., Friedman, F. A. and Dammin, G. J.: New Engl. J. Med., 262:1251, 1960.
13. Michon, L., Hamburger, J. and Antoine, B.: Presse méd., 61:1419, 1953.
14. Porter, K. A. and Calne, R. Y.: Transpl. Bull. 26:2, 1960.
15. Simonsen, M., Buemann, J., Gammeltoft, A., Jensen, F. and Jørgensen, K.: Acta path. et microbiol. scandinav., 32:1, 1953.
16. Weaver, J. M., Algire, G. H. and Prehn, R. T.: J. Nat. Cancer Inst., 15:1737, 1955.
17. Wheeler, H. B. and Corson, J. M.: Surg. Forum, 11:472, 1960.
18. Williamson, C. S.: J. Urol., 16:231, 1926.

The Nephropathy of
Systemic Lupus Erythematosus

ABOU D. POLLACK

Baltimore City Hospitals and
School of Medicine, Johns Hopkins University

It has been apparent for some time now that alterations of the kidney are found in almost, but not quite, all patients with systemic lupus erythematosus. The sum total of these changes is so characteristic that there has recently appeared a tendency to encompass them in the term "lupus nephritis." We ought not cavil at this as an expression of convenience. However, it seems incorrect, as some have done recently,[8] to employ "lupus nephritis . . . to focus attention on a specific disease of the kidney . . . the major complication . . . in patients ill with SLE." Although the question of the occurrence of a disease within a disease offers an interesting problem in semantics, I do not myself feel competent to pursue this idea. Almost certainly, all users of the term "lupus nephritis" recognize that the renal changes are variable in configuration and in severity. It has already been stressed that renal or, indeed, other organ changes need not be present, even in overwhelming SLE. No matter how far we may progress in understanding the evolution of the renal changes, the few instances in which lethal SLE fails to present a renal lesion stand as a constant reminder of our ignorance of the pathogenetic principles underlying this disease. If we can clarify the apparent paradox presented by those fatal cases lacking significant morphologic alterations, we will have come a long way toward comprehending systemic lupus erythematosus.

By how much do we understand the morphogenesis of lupus nephropathy? Taken all in all, the constellation of a variety of changes, mainly in the glomeruli, generally permits us to recognize the kidney of lupus. Each change by itself is shared more or less with other nephropathies. This kind of picture-book catalogue, although necessary to diagnosis, provides little insight into the morphogenesis of most of the alterations. It seems fair to say, however, that the glomerular manifestations of the *in vivo* LE reaction are quite specific and now somewhat more comprehensible than the other less characteristic changes.[9]

There is very little that can be added to the descriptions of the several glomerular changes in lupus which are now quite well recognized, and many of these are illustrated in Figure 1. Our ignorance of the genesis of these alterations is indeed frustrating.

Focal necrosis of glomerular loops is of moderate frequency. It is seen generally in the periphery of the glomeruli opposite the vascular stalks. There is a compounding of nuclear and extranuclear débris but infrequent nuclear change of the LE type. The lesion is indistinguishable from that of Loehlein-Baehr in chronic sepsis or from that occasionally seen in periarteritis nodosa. Increased glomerular cellularity, thickening, blunting and fusion of glomerular loops, glomerular adhesions, epithelial and fibrous crescents, hyaline obliteration of glomeruli—these are all found in lupus as they are in glomerulonephritis. Occasionally, in scrutinizing "conventional" glomerulonephritis, one may encounter either one or both of the following distinctive (though not specific) changes which may be considered possible signs of lupus erythematosus: glomeruli with one half showing typical membrane changes,

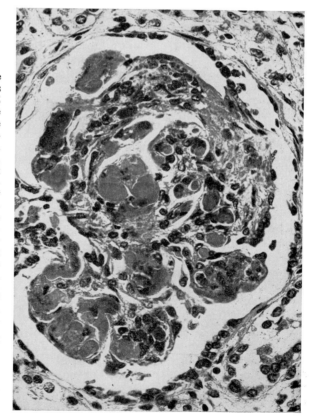

Fig. 1. Many of the renal glomerular alterations which can be found in SLE are exemplified in this single glomerulus. There is extreme disturbance of the architecture. Adhesions are present. Fibrosis is seen at the right. At six and at twelve o'clock there is focal cell proliferation. Many of the capillary loops are occluded by "hyaline thrombi." These are rather homogeneous, eosinophilic plugs occasionally presenting a violaceous cast by virtue of the lysed residue of the LE phenomenon with which they are suffused. LE bodies in various stages of dissolution are seen at twelve o'clock. These in color are purple (hematoxyphil) in contrast to the deep blue of pyknotic nuclei and nuclear débris. Thickening of capillary loops with "fibrinoid" change is seen in the center and at four o'clock.

the other half proliferative and obliterative changes; glomeruli with great focal cellularity, the nuclei sometimes arranged in palisade fashion.

Tubular changes in the kidneys of lupus are not specific. Vascular changes are uncommon. When hypertension supervenes, typical arteriolar sclerosis and necrosis may be present. Rarely, small and medium-sized arteries show necrotizing and inflammatory changes such as one might expect in hypersensitivity. More rarely, these alterations are indistinguishable from those of classic Kussmaul periarteritis nodosa.[1, 7] Very occasional "fibrinoid" globules or clumps may be evident in the walls of small arteries, either as subendothelial "blisters" or as small masses infiltrating the media or adventitia. Small vessels exhibiting necrotic walls marked by whole or disintegrated LE bodies are extremely infrequent. Finally, arteriolar changes of the type found in thrombotic thrombocytopenic purpura have been described.[6]

Hematoxyphil masses in the interstitial tissue are the only specific manifestation of lupus in this renal *terra incognita*. They are found only rarely.

The wire-loop change is inconstant. The greatly thickened, seemingly rigid, glomerular loops owe their bulk not only to thickened basement membranes, but also to acidophilic deposits of so-called fibrinoid substance which is laid down on both sides and within the membranes. This substance is nonhomogeneous and appears to contain, at the least, fibrin,[4] gamma globulin[10] and lipid. The fibrinoid material of lupus glomeruli may be considered a congeries of substances, some formed locally, some diffusing out of the blood, the whole being precipitated mostly beneath the endothelium, less within the basement membranes, and least beneath the epithelium.[2] Occasionally, glomerular capillary loops appear occluded by intensely eosinophilic refractile or sometimes dull-appearing plugs. These have been peculiarly designated "hyaline thrombi." They are never seen except in association with wire-loops with or without added fibrinoid deposit. Plausibly this substance is identical with that laid down in the glomerular loops, but further altered by sequestration and inspissation.

As there are different amyloids, so must there be different "fibrinoids" and different "hyalins." In pursuit of this sense, one might regard the renal glomerular loop manifestations of diabetes mellitus, amyloidosis, subacute membranous glomerulonephritis and lupus erythematosus as expressions of endothelial-basement membrane injury associated with exudation and possibly local elaboration of macromolecular complexes characteristic for each disease. With some of the amyloids, crude tinctorial and histochemical characterization permits relatively specific separation. In lupus erythematosus, on the other hand, an equally dependable stigma is only occasionally present. When the nuclei of damaged cells interact with specific gamma globulin within glomerular loops, LE bodies can be found at these sites. It is also possible that some of these bodies are embolic in origin.[3] When the lumens are occluded by eosinophilic proteinaceous plugs, these, too, may become suffused with the material derived from nuclear protein-gamma globulin interaction. Both moieties of this complex are demonstrable histochemically and immunologically.[5, 10]

CONCLUSION

Multiple renal alterations frequently occur in SLE. Some appear similar to those found in other nephropathies and are therefore nonspecific. Others seem quite characteristic of lupus. When, however, local and systemic conditions are propitious, the LE phenomenon may appear in the kidney, as it can elsewhere. This, the only alteration pathognomonic of SLE, possibly expresses antigen-antibody interaction. However, the spectrum of antibodies which may be present in this disease do not necessarily result from auto-immunization or indeed, from any conventional type of immunization. If, in the course of SLE, whose basic pathogenetic principle still remains hidden, a peculiar perversion of the antibody-producing mechanism occurs, is it not possible that a number of immune bodies may be engendered without provocation by corresponding antigens? It may be profitable to consider once again, in the light of contemporary understanding, the old problem of *dyscrasia.*

REFERENCES

1. Baggenstoss, A. H.: Visceral lesions in disseminated lupus erythematosus. Proc. Staff Meet., Mayo Clin., 27:412, 1952.
2. Farquhar, M. G., Hopper, J. and Moon, H. D.: Diabetic glomerulosclerosis: electron and light microscopic studies. Am. J. Path., 35:721, 1959.
3. German, J. L.: Studies in the pathogenesis of lupus erythematosus. J. Exper. Med., 108:179, 1958.
4. Gitlin, D., Craig, J. M. and Janeway, C. A.: Studies on the nature of fibrinoid in the collagen diseases. Am. J. Path., 33:55, 1957.
5. Godman, G. C.: The Nature and Pathogenetic Significance of the L. E. Cell Phenomenon of Systemic Lupus Erythematosus. In Baehr, G. and Klemperer, P. (eds.): Systemic Lupus Erythematosus. New York, Grune & Stratton, 1959.
6. Laszlo, M. H., Alvarez, A. and Feldman, F.: The association of thrombotic thrombocytopenic purpura and disseminated lupus erythematosus; report of a case. Ann. Int. Med., 42:1308, 1955.
7. Mallory, T. B. and Weiss, S.: Case reports of the Massachusetts General Hospital (Case 24201). New Engl. J. Med., 218:838, 1938.
8. Muehrcke, R. C., Kark, R. M., Pirani, C. L. and Pollak, V. E.: Lupus nephritis: a clinical and pathologic study based on renal biopsies. Medicine, 36:1, 1957.
9. Pollack, A. D.: Some observations on the pathology of systemic lupus erythematosus. In Baehr, G. and Klemperer, P. (eds.): Systemic Lupus Erythematosus. New York, Grune & Stratton, 1959.
10. Vazquez, J. J. and Dixon, F.: Studies on the immunohistochemical composition of inflammatory and degenerative lesions. Am. J. Path., 32:615, 1956.

Panel Discussion

BENJAMIN CASTLEMAN, *Moderator*

DR. CASTLEMAN: In the discussion today of lupus and arteritis, although there was some mention of the overlap between rheumatoid arthritis and the other collagen diseases, no one showed a slide of arteritis associated with lupus. That reminded me of the famous case that was discussed by Dr. Soma Weiss in 1937 at a C. P. C. at the Massachusetts General Hospital. He presented the differential diagnosis of a characteristic case of lupus, but when Dr. Mallory presented the pathological findings, he said the patient had classic arteritis and that there was no evidence of systemic lupus erythematosus. In 1937 we did not know very much about the pathology of lupus, and this patient had very severe arteritis. In the kidney there was very severe necrosis of the vessel walls typical of the findings in polyarteritis nodosa. There were also some of the characteristics we see in lupus, such as "wire looping," which at that time was not recognized. The spleen also showed the characteristic changes around the vessels, but these again were not known to be associated with lupus. We had a similar patient with lupus erythematosus and arteritis two weeks ago and here again in the kidney were the vascular changes that one would assume to be those of an arteritis. There were also some of the healed changes that one sees in an arteritis in a patient who has systemic lupus erythematosus. I thought this should be emphasized since we are beginning to recognize such overlapping in patients with collagen diseases and it is still an area that we do not know very much about. Related to this, what has been the experience of the panel with the use of radiomimetic agents in treatment of polyarteritis and lupus?

Dr. Larson: We have had no experience in our institution.

Dr. Merrill: We have had two patients who have been treated, and Dr. Robert Schwartz of the New England Center Hospital has treated several patients. Of course, the difficulty in evaluating the results has been pointed out, since the clinical syndrome is often unpredictable. However, I can say that I have not recently seen patients with as severe disease as the ones we treated, who have done as well without this type of treatment. I think this is equally true of two patients that Dr. Schwartz treated with 6-mercaptopurine.

In addition, whole body x-irradiation was given to the first identical twin who had a renal transplant in our series, because of severe nephritis with renal failure occurring five years after transplantation. This patient has now lived for a year and a half and is quite well. Again, one cannot be sure in this case what the prognosis would have been without treatment. Our other two patients who developed similar lesions died after three and 12 months. This type of treatment has to be explored. It is heroic treatment, but we can use it if we are careful. However, a large number of patients must be treated and compared with a suitable control group before we can be sure that this type of therapy really influences the course of the disease.

Dr. Lee: I can add one patient to the series. We treated one patient who was quite ill, and although she almost died from the treatment, she subsequently recovered and has done exceptionally well since. However, the possibility that she had a spontaneous remission can not be excluded.

Dr. Castleman: Dr. Merrill, if a kidney is transplanted from one dog to a second dog and interstitial changes characteristic of the rejection reaction appear in the transplanted kidney, are these changes reversible if the kidney is subsequently returned to the donor dog?

Dr. Merrill: Yes. This is the old problem of whether the graft reacts against the host in addition to the host reacting against the transplanted tissue. Some of the original observations in the literature indicated that when the kidney was returned to the host, it subsequently died anyway because the graft host reaction was continuing to go on. However, our group and others have shown that the transplanted kidney may be left in the recipient for as long as eight days and still survive when returned to the original donor, the changes of the homeograft rejection gradually disappearing. However, most of the transplants can be left in the recipient animal only up to 72 hours without having irreversible changes. The interesting thing is that in all series there was a marked increase in the cellular response shortly after the kidney was returned to the donor, but in the kidneys which survived these changes eventually subsided and the cells disappeared.

Dr. Wagner: Dr. Merrill, your slides showed a number of pyroninophillic cells. What are these cells and what do you think the pyronine positivity means?

Dr. Merrill: It is presumed to be related to the synthesis of nuclear protein and possibly antibody. It is difficult to be sure, but from these and other experiments I am convinced that the lymphocytes and plasma cells which appear are probably of host origin and represent antibody-containing cells. The antibody in the graft reaction is in the cell except possibly in the hyperimmune states characterized by the "white graft." I think these cells do contain individual specific antibody, that they appear in these areas in response to the donor antigen, and that they participate in the rejection response in some way .

DR. CASTLEMAN: Dr. Merrill, is there a basis for an analogy between the interstitial inflammatory changes of glomerulonephritis not associated with demonstrable pyelonephritis and the interstitial inflammatory changes in the homologous renal transplants? Is there a common or related immunological basis?

DR. MERRILL: I do not think that all of the cells are necessarily there because they contain antibody, but I do think that the analogy is one that is worth considering, and I do think the histological resemblance is interesting. I have a section of kidney which shows the interstitial lesion of so-called congenital nephritis, and several of our pathologists who are familiar with the changes in the rejected kidney thought this section was from a rejected transplanted kidney. I cannot say that these two pathological processes are identical, but there is enough similarity to indicate that further study and comparison would be worth while.

DR. CASTLEMAN: Dr. Merrill, are the changes in the vessels of the homografts those of an arteritis? Your slides showed an inflammation around the vessels, but has there been actual necrosis with the typical picture of polyarteritis?

DR. MERRILL: There is a lesion which is characterized by fibrinoid necrosis of the vessel wall in the "second set reaction" and we have observed it in animals; however, I did not show this, since for very obvious reasons one does not transplant a second kidney into a human after the first one has been rejected.

DR. CASTLEMAN: Dr. Seegal, in your paper you indicated the possibility that streptococcal antigen reacting with specific circulating antibody might contribute to the pathogenesis of glomerulonephritis. Have you any suggestions as to how the streptococcal antigen would reach the kidney or the basement membrane and remain there?

DR. SEEGAL: The histological findings in sections of the kidney in experimental nephritis can duplicate practically every abnormality seen in the kidney from humans with glomerulonephritis. The antigen-antibody reaction that produces the experimental disease can reproduce the histology and also the clinical picture of acute and chronic nephritis.

Now, if acute nephritis is due to an antigen-antibody reaction, the natural question is: What is the antigen? I think that a product of the streptococcus may lodge in the glomerulus during a preceding streptococcal infection, and in this location serve as the foreign protein to which the body makes antibodies. In support of this theory Dr. David Seegal and I did some experiments many years ago in an attempt to determine why any local area becomes sensitized and why it maintains its sensitivity and reacts over and over again, which is basically the problem in acute nephritis. We found that if we produced a local area of sensitization by injecting antigen into the anterior chamber of the eye, this area, the iris and the surrounding sclera would remain sensitive for years and that a reaction would take place when we gave injections of the specific antigen intravenously at intervals. The next step was to determine why the sensitivity was retained. We found that if you produce any area of inflammation in the eye—as, for example, by simply putting glycerine into the anterior chamber—and then inject the foreign antigen intravenously, you can produce local sensitivity. A reaction in the eye can then be obtained subsequently by parenteral injection of the antigen, although it was never injected into the eye. It is probable that an allergic reaction in itself may bind more antigen at the site of the reaction and hold it there. You then have a situation leading to continued sensitivity. In streptococcal infections there is a tendency to have renal irritation, as evidenced by an increase in the Addis count and some proteinuria irrespective of whether nephritis develops. Toxins of the streptococcus in contact with the kidney probably lead to these abnormalities and in rare instances may be retained by the glomerulus, which certainly binds some materials, including ferritin, in the basement membrane for a period of time. Since we all have a great many antibodies to the streptococcus even normally, the increased amount of streptococcal antigens present during infection perhaps may be held there by the natural antibody that the host makes to them. An antigen-antibody reaction could then cause inflammation early in the course of the disease, resulting in a locus where more streptococcal antigen could be localized, and the result could be a self-perpetuating disease. It is a theory and it can be put to the test by looking for a streptococcal antigen in renal tissue. I have tried to do this myself but very little renal biopsy material has been available to me; however, we have found hemolytic streptococcal antigen in the kidney in a few instances. I hope that those of you with access to renal biopsy specimens will seriously consider the possible fruitfulness of looking for the presence of a streptococcal antigen by the fluorescent antibody technique.

DR. CASTLEMAN: Dr. Schmidt, do you have a comment on that?

DR. SCHMIDT: A number of years ago Dr. Kaplan and I were interested in studying this problem from an experimental standpoint. We isolated streptococcal fractions and injected them into animals. When the group A polysaccharide, which is a small molecule having a molecular weight of about 10,000 or less, was injected in the free form into a mouse and sections of the kidney were examined we found that it went through the tubular cells rapidly and was then excreted.

Dr. Kaplan studied the M protein and found that this substance was taken up by cells in the glomerulus. Subsequently, I studied a nucleoprotein fraction and found that it was also taken up by cells in the glomerulus. However, fairly large amounts of material had to be injected in order to observe this. Therefore, this experimental situation may be entirely different quantitatively from the process that occurs in the natural infection. One of the things we know least about now is what happens to the products of organisms in the host during an infection. How does the host dispose of these and what quantities are present in host tissue? I think the quantities are probably very small and I am constantly looking for new methods that might make it possible to detect these substances more readily. Dr. Seegal's suggestion sounds promising, and I hope other people will send renal biopsy specimens to her so that she can investigate this mechanism further.

DR. WAGNER: It is important that we remember that the renal glomerulus is a filter and that many substances pass through it. Molecules that are small go through faster than those that are big. The latter may be retained for varying lengths of time and may produce damage depending on their inherent biological toxicity or activity. In this regard I would like to ask Dr. Seegal what she thinks about the experiments using soluble antigen-antibody complexes, in which various investigators have claimed that they have produced glomerulonephritis. What do you think the mechanism is?

DR. SEEGAL: Those observations were very encouraging to me because I think that we start with a baseline of antibody to the streptococcus. In a streptococcal infection, the patient probably produces an antigen excess, and there are probably mechanisms available for creating soluble antigen-antibody complexes which results in a situation similar to the experiments.

DR. CASTLEMAN: In this connection, Dr. Steblay has done some interesting experiments in which nephritis was induced in sheep by injection of human glomerular basement membrane and Freund's adjuvant. Dr. Steblay, would you comment on this?

DR. STEBLAY: Although the autoimmune etiology as the cause of nephritis has enjoyed immense popularity, there has been no convincing corresponding laboratory model for this concept. The two chief methods of producing experimental nephritis are, first, to inject antibodies, produced in another species against some part of the kidney, into the original species, and second, to inject antigen-antibody complexes. Neither of these mechanisms satisfies the crucial or necessary step postulated in the autoimmune theory, namely, that the animal must itself make by some immune mechanism antibodies which are specific for and injurious to its own tissue antigens. Therefore, in order to relate the human disease to the experimental model we decided to use human glomerular basement membrane, prepared from isolated human glomeruli, as an antigen. By injecting it in Freund's adjuvant into sheep, we succeeded in producing severe chronic glomerular nephritis which was lethal to the sheep. They died with elevated BUN's and severe renal damage from 40 to 90 days after injection. The sections of these kidneys showed marked fibrocellular proliferation of the glomerulus both inside and outside of Bowman's capsule, and this completely obliterated Bowman's space. There was also some interstitial cell infiltration. I do not want to say that this was caused by a circulating autoantibody or by sensitized cells, but it is caused by an autoimmune mechanism. Sheep serum obtained at the time of death was fractionated and the gamma globulin fraction was conjugated with fluoroescein isothiocyanate, and it was then applied *in vitro* to normal human kidney. This localized in the glomerular basement membrane, the capsular basement membrane and the tubular basement membrane of the human kidney and indicated that the sheep had circulating antibodies which could react with and localize in the glomerular basement membrane. In similar experiments injection of rat glomerular basement membrane into sheep produced the same type of chronic glomerulonephritis. Injection of the serum from these sheep into rats caused nephritis within two hours and the rats died almost immediately.

DR. WAGNER: Did you use Freund's adjuvant alone as a control?

DR. STEBLAY: Yes. No lesions were produced and the sheep remained healthy.

DR. CASTLEMAN: Dr. Seegal, would you comment on this?

DR. SEEGAL: I think these observations are most provocative and very interesting. I have always looked for renal damage in the rabbits in which we injected rat, rabbit or dog kidney to produce antibodies, but I have never seen renal damage in these animals. This reaction may be peculiar to sheep. Do you have any reason to believe that you can produce it in other animals?

DR. STEBLAY: I have never been able to induce it in rabbits, dogs or rats.

DR. SEEGAL: Animal species certainly are different. I have been trying to produce nephritis in guinea pigs for a long time without success. The guinea pig appears to be an animal that does not get nephritis even if you give him antibodies preformed to his own kidney. There is a very great variation in animal species.

DR. WAGNER: Sheep are extremely sensitive to various factors; for example, minerals and trace elements in their diets are very important. In Montana and Washington and other sheep areas there is a disease called "white muscle disease," a peculiar, bilateral, muscular degenerative disease in newborn lambs. It appears to be related to the trace element selenium, and the process can be reversed by proper diet. Sheep ranchers state that the diet must be controlled very carefully, or many diseases occur. Could some similar factor be operating in the sheep which you studied, Dr. Steblay?

DR. STEBLAY: I have repeated this experiment four times, in three different laboratories, with four different sources of sheep and three different types of food, and the results were the same. The kidney sections plus sections of other organs were sent to the Armed Forces Institute of Pathology and the report said the lesion did not resemble any known disease in sheep and that it was a bizzare, severe subacute and chronic glomerulonephritis.

DR. LEE: I do not understand why this is necessarily due to an autoimmune mechanism. It is presumably immune, but you have produced immunity to human kidney or to rat kidney and not to the sheep kidney.

DR. STEBLAY: The essential element in the definition of an autoimmune process is that the animal makes an antibody which is specific for and injurious to some native antigen in its own tissue, regardless of the nature of the antigenic stimulus, be it native or denatured antigen or some antigen foreign to the animal. In other words, the target organ becomes an antigen regardless of the nature of the original antigenic stimulus. Perhaps there is an antigen in the human kidney that is similar to one in the sheep kidney, which may be altered a little in the method of preparation and altered enough so that it is foreign and fools the sheep but not enough so that the antibodies that are formed cannot react with the sheep kidney antigen.

DR. LEE: This is just the point. I do not think that you have demonstrated that the injury in the sheep's glomeruli is due to antibodies to the sheep's glomerulus.

DR. STEBLAY: You may be right. Other experiments such as passive transfer experiments must be done to prove the exact mechanism; however, this may be similar to other autoimmune diseases produced in the laboratory which can not be transferred by serum alone but can be transferred by cells. I can not say definitely whether this type of nephritis in sheep is due to autoantibodies or due to a sensitized cellular mechanism, but it is an immune reaction.

DR. SCHMIDT: Since this is a controversial subject, I would like to point out one more element of controversy. In a recent report, a nephrosis-like syndrome was produced by injection of emulsified homologous rat kidney with adjuvant into rats; however, other people who have tried this have not been successful.

DR. MERRILL: This is a very interesting subject. I heard just yesterday that this same investigator has transferred this by injecting lymphocytes from the original animal into other tolerant rats without nephritis. If this is correct, he has really proved his point.

DR. CASTLEMAN: Do you know, Dr. Kaplan?

DR. KAPLAN: He has been able to transfer this to animals by cross circulation. Also he told me that he has two animals in which he has induced tolerance by transferring white cells from normal rats, and they later developed nephrosis. Dr. Ziff has also produced iso-immune nephrosis by transfer of white cells.

DR. MERRILL: I think it might be of value to clarify the method used in these experiments. My impression is that the disease was induced in animal A by injection of kidney extract. The lymphoid cells containing antibody from animal A were then transferred to animal B, which had been made tolerant to A so that the lymph cells would survive; then animal B developed nephritis. This is certainly a good model if our information is correct.

DR. KUSHNER: I wonder if these types of experimental nephritis are not a somewhat different disease from human glomerulonephritis. I think that the ideal experimental model for acute glomerulonephritis would be one that would start with the type 12 streptococcus. Our group, as well as one other group, has produced a kind of acute glomerulonephritis in rats by suspending virulent type 12 streptococci in porous chambers in the peritoneal cavity or by injection of streptococcal extracts. This is the model that we are all striving to set up; in such a system one could try to demonstrate the exact mechanism. The devastating thing about the McGill group's studies is that their dialysate from nephritogenic streptococci, when applied to a single layer of monkey kidney cells, destroyed the layer of cells in about two hours; this type of nephritis would not appear to depend upon an indirect antigen-antibody reaction but on some direct effect on the cells.

Part V | BIOCHEMISTRY AND
PHARMACOLOGY OF
ANTI-INFLAMMATORY
STEROIDS

Structure-Function Relationships of Anti-Inflammatory Steroids*

GRANT W. LIDDLE and MAURICE FOX

Vanderbilt University School of Medicine

In this paper an attempt is made to summarize knowledge concerning the relationship between chemical structure and biological function of anti-inflammatory steroids. This is done with an admitted anthropocentric bias. The results of steroid assays in experimental animals are frequently in disagreement with those in man. Therefore, even though much excellent assay work has been performed in animals, the emphasis in this paper will be upon human studies. When human data have been unavailable, information obtained from assays in the rat or dog have been included. This discussion will be limited to those biological activities which have been assayed in a reasonably quantitative fashion, i.e., anti-inflammatory, eosinopenic, ACTH-suppressing, hyperglycemic and nitrogen-wasting activities. It has frequently been observed that the effects of corticosteroids on organic metabolism can be dissociated from their effects on inorganic (electrolyte) metabolism. Unless otherwise specified, it will be implied that the anti-inflammatory property of a steroid is closely associated with other organic properties (eosinopenic, ACTH-suppressing, nitrogen-wasting and hyperglycemic activities).

Although cortisone was the first steroid to be shown to have anti-inflammatory activity, it is more convenient from the standpoint of structure-function studies to consider cortisol (hydrocortisone) as the basic anti-inflammatory steroid. Cortisol, rather than cortisone, is the principal hormone of the human adrenal cortex.[38] The anti-inflammatory effect of corticotropin (ACTH) is attributable to the ACTH-induced secretion of cortisol by the adrenal glands. Furthermore, the anti-inflammatory activity of cortisone appears to be contingent upon its transformation by the body to cortisol.[35]

In the normal adult the adrenal glands secrete from 20 to 35 mg. of cortisol per day. Administration of such physiologic quantities of the steroid has little effect other than to suppress the secretion of endogenous corticosteroids. When administered in supraphysiologic doses, however, cortisol also causes eosinopenia, impairment of glucose tolerance, net catabolism of protein, retention of sodium, loss of potassium and suppression of inflammation.

Almost every portion of the cortisol molecule has importance in determining biological activity. One way of illustrating this is to compare the biological activity of cortisol with various naturally occurring analogs, each of which differs structurally in only one respect from cortisol itself.

17-Desoxy-cortisol (corticosterone) has not been shown to have definite anti-inflammatory activity in man.[39] It does, however, possess electrolyte-regulating activity at least equivalent to that of cortisol. It appears that the 17-hydroxyl group selectively enhances the potency of the steroid as a regulator of organic metabolism without enhancing the electrolyte-regulating potency. Corticosterone is the principal steroid secreted by the rat adrenal,

* Supported in part by a grant-in-aid from the U. S. Public Health Service (CY-3107).

and in that species it has approximately one-third the anti-inflammatory potency and one-half the gluconeogenic potency of cortisol.[19]

21-Desoxy-cortisol has very little biologic activity of any sort, indicating that the 21-hydroxyl group is an important determinant of corticosteroid potency.[20, 36]

The crucial importance of the 11β-hydroxyl group is illustrated by comparing cortisol with the following three steroids. 11-Desoxy-cortisol (Reichstein's compound S) is devoid of anti-inflammatory activity in man.[36, 39] In doses up to 400 mg. per day it does not affect nitrogen balance, eosinophil levels or glucose tolerance. It does, however, have some electrolyte-regulating activity.[31] The 11α-hydroxy epimer of cortisol is devoid of biological activity.[33] Cortisone, which differs structurally from cortisol only in that it has an 11-keto rather than an 11β-hydroxyl group, has approximately 70 per cent of the biological potency of cortisol.[26] Normally in the body there is an enzymatically facilitated interconversion between the 11-keto and 11β-hydroxy forms of corticosteroids which results in the net conversion of about 70 per cent of administered cortisone to cortisol.[35] The percentile agreement in these observations supports the concept that the biologic activity of cortisone is contingent upon its conversion to cortisol. Further evidence for this is afforded by the demonstration that when the interconversion of 11-keto and 11β-hydroxyl groups is blocked by the presence of some structure such as a 2α-methyl group, the 11β-hydroxy form of the steroid is fully active while the 11-keto form is biologically inert.[12] When injected intra-articularly, cortisone has been found to be much less effective than cortisol, perhaps because of the inability of the synovium to effect any significant conversion to cortisol.[23, 35]

SYNTHETIC CORTISOL DERIVATIVES

Hundreds of steroids having anti-inflammatory activity have been synthesized during the past seven years. All of them have the basic structure Δ^4-pregnene-11β-ol-3,20-dione (Fig. 1). In addition, each steroid having

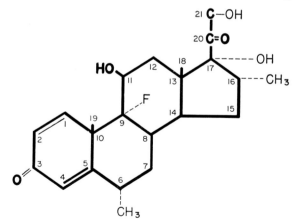

Fig. 1.   The bold lines and letters indicate the structure common to all anti-inflammatory steroids. Substituents which are nonessential but which if present enhance anti-inflammatory potency are represented by light lines and letters.

measurable anti-inflammatory activity in man possesses two or more "potentiating" substituents. In order to illustrate the specific effect of each structural alteration upon biological activity, a series of synthetic steroids each differing from cortisol in only one respect will be considered in the following paragraphs.

Δ^1-Cortisol (1,2-dehydro-cortisol, prednisolone) is approximately four

TABLE 1. EFFECT OF 1,2-DEHYDROGENATION UPON BIOLOGICAL ACTIVITIES OF CORTICOSTEROIDS

| | ORGANIC POTENCY | | ELECTROLYTE-REGULATING POTENCY | |
	1,2-saturated steroid	Δ^1 analog	1,2-saturated steroid	Δ^1 analog
Cortisol	1	4[10]	1	0.8[28]
9α-Fluoro-cortisol	10[9]	20[4]	125[27]	200[29]
16α-Hydroxy-cortisol	< 1[3]	1.5[3]	nil[3]	nil[3]
16α-Methyl-cortisol	2[31]	5[8]	nil[31]	nil[31]
6-Methyl-cortisol	1.3[28]	5[28]	2[28]	0.5[28]

times as potent an anti-inflammatory agent as is cortisol.[10] The electrolyte-regulating activity of cortisol is not enhanced by 1,2-dehydrogenation.[10, 28, 40] This relative freedom from electrolyte effect has been responsible for very wide acceptance of this agent by clinicians. 1,2-Dehydrogenation has been found to enhance the potency of all anti-inflammatory steroids thus far tested. Some of these are listed in Table 1. A partial explanation for the greater potency of Δ^1 steroids is found in the observation that they are metabolized more slowly than their 1,2-saturated analogs. In man the half time of circulating cortisol is about 120 minutes,[34] while that of Δ^1-cortisol is about 200 minutes.[11] This explanation fails to account for the qualitative difference between cortisol and Δ^1-cortisol, that is, the *selective* increase in organic activity without any increase in electrolyte-regulating activity in the case of the Δ^1 derivative.

2α-Methyl cortisol is approximately equal to cortisol in causing eosinopenia, nitrogen-wasting and suppression of ACTH.[27] It is, however, approximately 25 to 50 times as potent as cortisol in promoting sodium retention and potassium excretion.[15, 22, 27] The great potency of this compound as an electrolyte regulator has precluded its use as an anti-inflammatory agent. Introduction of a methyl group in the 2α position has been shown to enhance the electrolyte-regulating potency of a large number of 11β-hydroxycorticosteroids[13, 27] (Table 2). On the other hand, introduction of a methyl group in 2α position has resulted in loss of biological activity of 11-desoxy or 11-keto compounds.[14] For example, 2α-methyl-11-desoxycorticosterone has only 0.08 times the electrolyte-regulating potency of 11-desoxycorticosterone.[27]

Δ^6-*Cortisol* has been shown in man to have ACTH-suppressing, nitrogen-wasting and sodium-retaining potency similar to that of cortisol.[31] Δ^6-Cortisone, however, in doses up to 300 mg. daily,[36] has been reported to have no anti-inflammatory effect in man. In the rat, the Δ^6 modification of cortisone has been shown to result in loss of the lymphopenic and thymolytic effects,[21] while the gluconeogenic effect is reduced by about 50 per cent.[19, 40] The Δ^6

TABLE 2. EFFECT OF 2α-METHYLATION UPON THE BIOLOGICAL ACTIVITIES OF CORTICOSTEROIDS

| | ORGANIC POTENCY | | ELECTROLYTE-REGULATING POTENCY | |
	Nonmethylated steroid	2-methyl analog	Nonmethylated steroid	2-methyl analog
Cortisol	1	0.7[27]	1	25[27]
Δ^1-Cortisol	4[10]	. .	0.8[28]	240[15]
9α-Fluoro-cortisol	10[9]	5[27]	125[27]	250[27]
Cortisone	0.7[35]	0.4[14]	0.7[35]	0.2[27]
11-Desoxycorticosterone	nil[40]	. .	25[27]	1.5[27]

modification has also been found to attenuate to varying degrees the gluconeogenic effects of other corticosteroids while enhancing slightly their sodium retaining activities.[17]

6α-Chloro-cortisol has been studied in rats and has been found to have 5 to 10 times the thymolytic and anti-inflammatory potency of cortisol but to have negligible sodium-retaining effect. Introduction of a chlorine atom in the 6β position, on the other hand, decreases anti-inflammatory activity and enhances sodium retaining potency.[37]

6α-Methyl-cortisol is slightly more effective than cortisol in assays of anti-inflammatory, eosinopenic, nitrogen-wasting and electrolyte-regulating activities in man. In the rat it has been shown to have 2 to 4 times the potency of cortisol as an anti-inflammatory and gluconeogenic agent.[15] It is impossible to generalize concerning the biological consequences of 6α-methylation since of the various compounds modified in this way some show increased and others decreased potency or even dissociation of biological activities when compared with their nonmethylated analogs.[28]

9α-Fluoro-cortisol (fludrocortisone) is more potent than cortisol with respect to all biological activities.[16] Its anti-inflammatory, eosinopenic, ACTH-suppressing, hyperglycemic and nitrogen-wasting activities exceed those of cortisol by an eight- to tenfold factor.[9, 26, 27, 28] In acute assays of electrolyte-regulating activity in both dogs and man, 9α-fluoro-cortisol is about 125 times as potent as cortisol.[27] Under conditions of continued treatment, the effect is even greater. This fact has precluded the therapeutic use of 9α-fluoro-cortisol for any condition other than adrenal insufficiency.[30] In general, it has been found that the introduction of a 9α-halogen substituent increases the biological activity of any corticosteroid.[16, 17, 18] As shown in Table 3, the electrolyte-regulating effect is generally enhanced out of pro-

TABLE 3.   EFFECT OF 9α-FLUORINATION UPON BIOLOGICAL
ACTIVITIES OF CORTICOSTEROIDS

	ORGANIC POTENCY		ELECTROLYTE-REGULATING POTENCY	
	Nonfluorinated steroid	9α-fluoro analog	Nonfluorinated steroid	9α-fluoro analog
Cortisol	1	10[9]	1	125[27]
Δ1-Cortisol	4[10]	20[4]	0.8[28]	200[29]
2-Methyl-cortisol	0.7[27]	5[27]	25[27]	250[27]
Δ1-16α-Hydroxy-cortisol	1.5[3]	5[5]	nil[3]	4*[29]
Δ1-16α-Methyl-cortisol	5[8]	30[8]	nil[8]	@ 12[31]

* Potassium loss only.

portion to the increase in organic effects. Because of this, only those derivatives which have some additional modification that nullifies the electrolyte-regulating effects have been considered suitable for clinical use as anti-inflammatory agents.

14-Hydroxy-cortisol is much less active than cortisol itself in assays of eosinopenic and electrolyte-regulating activity.[31]

16α-Hydroxy-cortisol has about one-half the gluconeogenic potency of cortisol in rats but is entirely free of sodium-retaining activity.[3, 19] A number of other 16α-hydroxycorticoids have been investigated (Table 4), and in every case the substitution of a hydroxyl group in the 16α position has resulted in a slight diminution of organic metabolism-regulating effect and a marked attenuation of electrolyte-regulating activity.

TABLE 4. EFFECTS OF 16α-HYDROXYLATION UPON BIOLOGICAL
ACTIVITIES OF CORTICOSTEROIDS

| | ORGANIC POTENCY | | ELECTROLYTE-REGULATING POTENCY | |
	16-Desoxy steroid	16α-hydroxy analog	16-Desoxy steroid	16α-hydroxy analog
Cortisol	1	0.5[3]	1	nil[3]
Δ[1]-Cortisol	4[3]	1.5[3]	nil[3]	nil[3]
2α-Methyl-9α-fluoro-cortisol	5[27]	2[3]	2500[27]	12[3]
11-Desoxycorticosterone	nil[40]	. .	25[27]	0[2]
Δ[1]-9α-Fluoro-cortisol	20[4]	5[5]	200[29]	4*[29]

* Potassium loss only.

16α-Methyl-cortisol[1] is approximately 2 to 3 times as potent as cortisol in regulation of organic metabolism in man.[8, 31] It is virtually lacking in sodium-retaining activity.[8] The relative anti-inflammatory and electrolyte-regulating potencies of a series of steroids and their 16α-methylated analogs are listed in Table 5. In every case the 16α-methylated derivative is more potent than its nonmethylated analog as an anti-inflammatory agent but much less active as an electrolyte-regulating agent.

TABLE 5. EFFECTS OF 16α-METHYLATION UPON BIOLOGICAL
ACTIVITIES OF CORTICOSTEROIDS

| | ORGANIC POTENCY | | ELECTROLYTE-REGULATING POTENCY | |
	Nonmethylated steroid	16α-methyl analog	Nonmethylated steroid	16α-methyl analog
Cortisol	1	2[31]	1	nil[31]
Δ[1]-Cortisol	4[10]	5[8]	0.8[28]	nil[31]
9α-Fluoro-cortisol	10[9]	12[8]	125[27]	nil[8]
Δ[1]-9α-Fluoro-cortisol	20[4]	30[8]	200[29]	@ 12[29]

TABLE 6. POTENCY FACTORS FOR SUBSTITUENT GROUPS

	ANTI-INFLAMMATORY ACTIVITY	ELECTROLYTE-REGULATING ACTIVITY
Δ[1]	4	0.8
2α-Methyl	0.7	25
9α-Fluoro	10	125
16α-Hydroxyl	0.5	0.005
16α-Methyl	2	< 1
6α-Methyl	1.3 (variable)	2 (variable)

| | ANTI-INFAMMATORY Potency Relative to Cortisol | | ELECTROLYTE-REGULATING Potency Relative to Cortisol | |
	Predicted	Empirical	Predicted	Empirical
Δ[1]-9α-Fluoro-cortisol	40	20	100	200
2α-Methyl-9α-fluoro-cortisol	7	5	3125	2500
Δ[1]-9α-Fluoro-16α-hydroxy-cortisol	20	5	0.5	4*
Δ[1]-9α-Fluoro-16α-methyl-cortisol	80	30	< 100	@ 12
Δ[1]-6α-Methyl-cortisol	5	5	1.6	0.5

* Potassium loss only.

EFFECTS OF MULTIPLE MODIFICATION

The introduction of two or more modifications into the structure of a corticosteroid frequently results in alterations in biological activity which are multiplicative. It is sometimes of interest to attempt to predict the potency of a synthetic steroid by multiplying the effects upon potency observed with individual substituents. In Table 6 the potency factors for individual substituents are listed. In addition, the "predicted" potency and "empirical" potency of some multi-modified cortisol derivatives are presented. Three multi-modified steroids which are in general use as therapeutic agents will be discussed.

Methylprednisolone (Δ^1-6α-methyl-cortisol) is the most widely used of the 6α-methyl corticosteroid derivatives. In man, methylprednisolone is about 5 times as potent as cortisol with respect to anti-inflammatory, ACTH-suppressing, nitrogen-wasting and eosinopenic activities.[7, 28] It has minimal sodium-retaining potency in man[7, 24] and experimental animals.[15, 28] Most of the alteration of biological activity in this cortisol derivative was conferred by the Δ^1 modification. 6α-Methyl-prednisolone is only slightly more effective than Δ^1-cortisol (prednisolone) in regulating organic metabolism and only slightly less effective in regulating electrolyte metabolism.

Triamcinolone (Δ^1-9α-fluoro-16α-hydroxy-cortisol) is about 4 to 5 times as potent as cortisol with respect to anti-inflammatory, ACTH-suppressing, nitrogen-wasting and eosinopenic activities.[5, 31] Triamcinolone is devoid of sodium-retaining activity[3, 5, 29] but does cause some potassium loss.[32] The enhanced organic activity of triamcinolone is due entirely to the Δ^1 and 9α-fluoro modifications. Δ^1-9α-Fluoro-cortisol is 20 times as potent as cortisol itself in regulating organic metabolism whereas triamcinolone is only 4 to 5 times as potent as cortisol. On the other hand, freedom from sodium-retaining activity is due entirely to the 16α-hydroxyl-substituent. Δ^1-9α-Fluoro-cortisol is about 200 times as potent as cortisol itself in promoting sodium retention, whereas triamcinolone has no sodium-retaining activity.

Dexamethasone (Δ^1-9α-fluoro-16α-methyl-cortisol) is about 30 times as potent as cortisol with respect to ACTH-suppressing, eosinopenic, hyperglycemic[6, 41] and anti-inflammatory[8] activities. In dosages of less than 6 mg. per day this steroid causes virtually no sodium retention.[8, 41] With higher dosages, however, significant sodium retention may occur.[31] In contrast to substituents elsewhere in the corticosteroid molecule, the 16-methyl group has the same effect on biological activity regardless of whether it occupies the α or β position.[31]

The very great organic potency of dexamethasone is a function of all three synthetic substituents (Δ^1,9α-fluoro, and 16α-methyl). The relative freedom from electrolyte-regulating activity is attributable to the 16α-methyl group, inasmuch as the nonmethylated analog (Δ^1-9α-fluoro-cortisol) is a very potent sodium-retaining agent.

DISSOCIATION OF GLUCOCORTICOID FUNCTIONS

Up to this point it has been implied that the anti-inflammatory properties of a corticosteroid are inseparable from protein-wasting, hyperglycemic, ACTH-suppressing and eosinopenic activities. Usually a modification of structure which alters one of these biological activities also brings about commensurate alterations with respect to the others. Occasionally partial dissociation of some of these activities has been encountered in animal assays, but usually these observations have not been confirmed when the same steroids were assayed in man.

It has recently been possible, however, to demonstrate clear dissociation of these various properties when certain steroids were administered to human subjects.[25] All of the steroids exhibiting dissociation of various "organic" activities lacked 21-hydroxyl groups. All of them were less potent than their 21-hydroxylated analogs with respect to all biological activities. However, ACTH-suppressing activity was relatively intact, whereas eosinopenic and (with one exception) hyperglycemic activities were greatly attenuated. For example, Δ¹-9α-fluoro-21-*desoxy*-cortisol was approximately 2.0 times as potent as cortisol in assays of ACTH-suppression but only 0.2 and 0.1 times as potent in assay of hyperglycemic and eosinopenic activities, respectively.

Demonstration that various properties of corticosteroids can be separated strengthens the hope that therapeutic agents of increasingly specific action may yet be developed.

REFERENCES

1. Arth, G. E. et al.: 16-Methylated steroids. II. 16α-Methyl analogs of cortisone, a new group of anti-inflammatory steroids. 9α-Halo derivatives. J. Am. Chem. Soc., 80:3161, 1958.

2. Axelrad, J., Cates, J. E., Johnson, B. B. and Luetscher, J. A.: Bioassay of mineralo-corticoids. Relationship of structure to physiologic activity. Endocrinology, 55:568, 1954.

3. Bernstein, S.: The chemistry and biological activities of 16-hydroxylated steroids. Rec. Progr. Hormone Res., 14:1, 1958.

4. Black, R. L., Yielding, K. L., Peterson, R. E., Whedon, G. D. and Bunim, J. J.: Metabolic, hormonal and anti-rheumatic effects of Δ¹-9α-fluoro-hydrocortisone. Ann. Rheum. Dis., 15:76, 1956.

5. Black, R. L., Yielding, K. L. and Bunim, J. J.: Observations on new synthetic anti-rheumatic steroids and critical evaluation of prednisone therapy in rheumatoid arthritis. J. Chron. Dis., 5:751, 1957.

6. Black, R. L., Reefe, W. E., David, J. R., Bloch, K. J., Ehrlich, G. E. and Bunim, J. J.: Dexamethasone: anti-rheumatic properties, hormonal effects and adverse reactions. Arth. & Rheum., 3:112, 1960.

7. Boland, E. W. and Liddle, G. W.: Metabolic and anti-rheumatic activities of 6-methyl prednisolone (Medrol). Ann. Rheum. Dis., 16:297, 1957.

8. Boland, E. W.: 16α-Methyl corticosteroids. A new series of anti-inflammatory compounds; clinical appraisal of their anti-rheumatic properties. Calif. Med., 88:417, 1958.

9. Boland, E. W.: Experiences with 9α-fluoro-hydrocortisone acetate in rheumatoid arthritis. Ann. N. Y. Acad. Sc., 61:591, 1955.

10. Bunim, J. J., Black, R. L., Bollet, A. J. and Pechet, M. M.: Metabolic effects of meta-cortandrolone and metacortandrocin. Ann. N. Y. Acad. Sc., 61:358, 1955.

11. Bunim, J. J., Black, R. L., Lutwack, L., Peterson, R. E. and Whedon, G. D.: Studies on dexamethasone, a new synthetic steroid in rheumatoid arthritis—a preliminary report. Arth. & Rheum., 1:313, 1958.

12. Bush, I. E. and Mahesh, V. B.: Metabolism of 11-oxygenated steroids. 2-Methyl steroids. Biochem. J., 71:718, 1959.

13. Byrnes, W. W., Barnes, L. E., Bowman, B. J., Dulin, W. E., Morley, E. H. and Stafford, R. O.: Adrenal cortical activities of 2-methyl hydrocortisone acetate and 2-methyl-9α-fluoro-hydrocortisone acetate. Proc. Soc. Exper. Biol. & Med., 91:67, 1956.

14. Dulin, W. E., Bowman, B. J. and Stafford, R. O.: Effects of 2-methylation on gluco-corticoid activity of various C-21 steroids. Proc. Soc. Exper. Biol. & Med., 94:303, 1957.

15. Dulin, W. E., Barnes, L. E., Glenn, E. M., Lyster, S. C. and Collins, E. J.: Biological activities of some C-21 steroids and some 6α-methyl C-21 steroids. Metabolism, 7:398, 1958.

16. Fried, J. and Sabo, E. F.: 9α-Fluoro derivatives of cortisone and hydrocortisone. J. Am. Chem. Soc., 76:1455, 1954.

17. Fried, J., Florey, K., Sabo, E. F., Herz, J. E., Restivo, A. R., Borman, A. and Singer, F. M.: Synthesis and biological activity of 1 and 6 dehydro-9α-halo corticoids. J. Am. Chem. Soc., 77:4181, 1955.
18. Fried, J.: Structure-activity relationships in the field of halogenated steroids. Cancer, 10:752, 1957.
19. Fried, J. and Borman, A.: Synthetic derivatives of cortical hormones. Vitamins & Hormones, 16:303, 1958.
20. Goldfien, A., Morse, W. I., Froesch, E. R., Ganong, W. F., Renold, A. E. and Thorn, G. W.: Pharmacological studies in man of 11-, 17- and 21-hydroxyl derivatives of progesterone and their fluorinated analogs. Ann. N. Y. Acad. Sc., 61:433, 1955.
21. Higgins, G. M., Woods, K. A. and Kendall, E. C.: Some observations on the physiologic activity of Δ4, 6-dehydrocortisone (diene). Endocrinology, 48:175, 1951.
22. Hogg, J. A., Lincoln, F. H., Jackson, R. W. and Schneider, W. P.: The adrenal hormones and related compounds. III. Synthesis of 2-alkyl analogs. J. Am. Chem. Soc., 77:6401, 1955.
23. Hollander, J. L., Brown, E. M., Jessar, R. A. and Brown, C. Y.: Hydrocortisone and cortisone injected into arthritic joints. J.A.M.A., 147:1629, 1951.
24. Jenkins, D. and Schemmel, J. E.: Metabolic effects of 6-methyl prednisolone. Metabolism, 7:416, 1958.
25. Kendall, J. and Liddle, G. W.: Dissociation of "glucocorticoid" properties of steroids administered to man resulting from structural alteration at carbon 21. (To be published.)
26. Kupperman, H. S., Blatt, M. H. G., Vessell, M., Gagliani, J., Weisbader, H. and Vosburgh, L.: The comparative effects of metacortandrocin, 9α-fluoro-cortisol and hydrocortisone upon ACTH secretion in man. J. Clin. Endocrinol., 15:911, 1955.
27. Liddle, G. W., Richard, J. E. and Tomkins, G. M.: Studies of structure-function relationships of steroids: the 2-methyl-corticosteroids. Metabolism, 5:384, 1956.
28. Liddle, G. W.: Studies of structure-function relationships of steroids. II. The 6α-methylcorticosteroids. Metabolism, 7:405, 1958.
29. Liddle, G. W.: Effects of anti-inflammatory steroids on electrolyte metabolism. Ann. N. Y. Acad. Sc., 82:854, 1959.
30. Liddle, G. W.: Adrenal insufficiency. In Conn, H. F. (ed.): Current Therapy. Philadelphia, W. B. Saunders Co., 1961, p. 328.
31. Liddle, G. W. and Fox, M.: Unpublished data.
32. Pechet, M. M., Carroll, E. L., Mitchell, M. and Wegner, M. J.: Studies of the activities of steroid hormones on electrolyte balance and the constituents of protoplasm. The effects of 16α-hydroxylation C-21 steroids. J. Clin. Invest., 37:921, 1958.
33. Peterson, D. H. et al.: Microbiological transformation of steroids. IV. The 11 epimer of compound F and other new oxygenated derivatives of Reichstein's compound S. A new route to cortisone. J. Am. Chem. Soc., 75:412, 1953.
34. Peterson, R. E., Wyngaarden, J. B., Guerra, S. L., Brodie, B. B. and Bunim, J. J.: The physiological disposition and metabolic fate of hydrocortisone in man. J. Clin. Invest., 34:1779, 1955.
35. Peterson, R. E., Pierce, C. E., Wyngaarden, J. B., Bunim, J. J. and Brodie, B. B.: The physiologic disposition and metabolic fate of cortisone in man. J. Clin. Invest., 36:1301, 1957.
36. Polley, H. F. and Mason, H. L.: Rheumatoid arthritis—effects of certain steroids other than cortisone and of some adrenal cortex extracts. J.A.M.A., 143:1474, 1950.
37. Ringold, H. J. et al.: A new class of potent cortical hormones, 6α-chlorocorticoids. J. Am. Chem. Soc., 80:6464, 1958.
38. Sweat, M. L.: Adrenocorticosteroids in peripheral and venous blood of man. J. Clin. Endocrinol., 15:1043, 1955.
39. Thorn, G. W. et al.: Pharmacological aspects of adrenocortical steroids and ACTH. in man. New Engl. J. Med., 248:232, 284, 323, 369, 414, 632, 1953.
40. Tolksdorf, S., Batten, M. L., Cassidy, J. W., MacLeod, R. M., Warren, F. H. and Perlman, P. L.: Adrenocortical properties of Δ1, 4-pregnadiene-17α,21-diol-3,11,20-trione (meticorten) and Δ1, 4-pregnadiene-11β,17α,21-triol-3,20-dione (meticortelone). Proc. Soc. Exper. Biol. & Med., 92:207, 1956.
41. West, K., Johnson, P. C., Kyriahopoulos, A. A., Bahr, W. J. and Bloedow, C. E.: The physiologic effects of dexamethasone. Arth. & Rheum., 3:129, 1960.

The Effects of Halogenation on
the Biological Properties of Corticoids

SIBYLLE TOLKSDORF

Biological Research Division, Schering Corporation

The introduction of a chlorine or fluorine atom at carbon 9 of the corticoid nucleus by Fried and Sabo[7] resulted in a striking increase of anti-inflammatory and glucocorticoid activity. It demonstrated for the first time that biological activity of this type can be modified by chemical alteration of the steroid molecule.[6] Subsequent efforts in many laboratories have led to the development of highly potent synthetic steroids for clinical use. Some of these compounds contain a halogen, and all have an oxygen function at carbon 11, which on theoretical grounds[3] has been considered essential for pharmacological action. The $9\alpha,11\beta$-dihalo steroids synthesized by Robinson and co-workers[12, 13] constitute a fundamental departure from this concept because they possess significant anti-inflammatory activity in the absence of an oxygen function at carbon 11. The effect of the replacement of oxygen by halogen on the activity spectrum of these di-halides has been studied and the results are the subject of this report.

MATERIALS AND METHODS

The following steroids have been investigated: (1) a series of $9\alpha,11\beta$-dihalo derivatives of 1-dehydrocortexolone (cortexolone = compound S), specifically dichlorisone, $9\alpha,11\beta$-dichloro-1,4-pregnadiene-17α, 21-diol-3,20-dione (Diloderm, Schering Corporation); (2) 16α- and 16β-methyl dichlorisone; (3) dichlorisone 17, 21-acetonide and its 16α- and 16β-methyl derivatives.

Anti-inflammatory activity was determined in intact female rats by the croton oil granuloma pouch technique.[11, 18] The steroid was deposited locally by a single subcutaneous injection into the dorsal skin lining the pneumoderma. Eosinopenic activity was assayed in adrenalectomized, male C_{57} brown mice.[15, 21] A statistical analysis of these two assay methods has been presented recently.[22] Electrolyte excretion was estimated in adrenalectomized rats,[4] using a flame photometer for the sodium and potassium determinations. Metabolic effects were studied (1) in adrenalectomized rats treated daily subcutaneously for four days and autopsied on the fifth day after a 24-hour fast; (2) in intact rats treated daily subcutaneously for 14 days. The latter procedure also served to assess hormonal effects on body and organ weights and on the blood elements.*

Analytical methods used in the metabolic work included nitrogen determinations by a micro-Kjeldahl procedure, free and total cholesterol,[16] phospholipid,[23] total hepatic lipid by a modified gravimetric method, fasting blood sugar[9, 20] and liver glycogen.[17]

* The rats were the CD strain from Charles River Breeding Labs.

310

RESULTS

All dihalides of 1-dehydrocortexolone showed low eosinopenic activity. The anti-inflammatory activity, on the other hand, was significant and varied in magnitude with the nature of the halogen (Table 1), with the substitution at carbon 16, and with the nature of the side chain (Table 2). The mineralocorticoid activity of the dihalides was insignificant but changed to a diuretic pattern in response to carbon 16 substitution.

TABLE 1.   BIOLOGICAL ACTIVITY OF 9α,11β-DIHALO DERIVATIVES
OF 1-DEHYDROCORTEXOLONE

CONFIGURATION			PREDNISOLONE ACETATE = 1		
9α	11β	21	Eosinopenic Activity		Anti-Inflammatory Activity
Cl	Cl	ol	0.09	(0.03-0.24)*	8.5 (7.8 -9.3)
Cl	Cl	acetate	0.07	(0.03-0.14)	4.0 (3.3 -4.7)
Cl	F	acetate	0.56	(0.16-1.20)	0.83 (0.68-0.98)
Br	Cl	ol	0.01		1.89 (1.20-3.64)
Br	Cl	acetate	0.1		1.2 (0.84-1.79)
Br	Br	acetate	0.12	(0.04-0.31)	0.47 (0.39-0.57)
Br	F	ol	inactive		0.77 (0.45-2.29)
Br	F	acetate	0.015	(0.0003-0.943)	0.28 (0.12-0.42)

* Figures in parentheses are 95% fiducial limits.

Dichlorisone was by far the most active anti-inflammatory steroid in the unsubstituted series (Table 1). Interestingly, this steroid possessed neither the diuretic property of prednisolone nor the extreme salt-retaining property of 9α-chloroprednisolone.

Methylation at carbon 16 exerted unexpected effects on the anti-inflammatory activity of dichlorisone (Table 2). The 16α-methyl group depressed the anti-inflammatory activity of both the 21-alcohol and the 21-acetate by one half. The 16β-methyl group greatly increased the anti-inflammatory activity of dichlorisone alcohol but decreased that of dichlorisone acetate. The 17,21-acetonide system apparently exerted a stabilizing effect on the side chain. Considerable enhancement of activity was observed with the acetonide of dichlorisone and further slight increases were seen in the 16α-methyl and the 16β-methyl derivatives, which were 14 times as active

TABLE 2.   BIOLOGICAL ACTIVITY OF DICHLORISONE DERIVATIVES*

SUBSTITUTION	ANTI-INFLAMMATORY ACTIVITY (PREDNISOLONE ACETATE = 1)		MINERALOCORTICOID ACTIVITY
Dichlorisone, 21-ol	8.5	(7.8-9.3)**	slight Na retention
Dichlorisone, 21-acetate	4.0	(3.3-4.7)	slight Na retention
16α-methyl, 21-ol	5.0	(0.36-8.0)	diuresis of water, K
16α-methyl, 21-acetate	2.1	(0.96-3.0)	diuresis of water, K
16β-methyl, 21-ol	13.0	(8.22-20.57)	
16β-methyl, 21 acetate	0.14	(0-0.28)	
17,21-acetonide	11.1	(10.2-12.1)	no effect
16α-methyl, 17,21-acetonide	13.85	(11.12-17.35)	diuresis of water, Na, K
16β-methyl, 17,21-acetonide	14.04	(11.35-17.08)	slight diuresis of Na

* Eosinopenic activity of all steroids was less than 0.1 × prednisolone acetate.
** Figures in parentheses are the 95% fiducial limits.

TABLE 3.   METABOLIC EFFECTS: ADX* RATS

| | | LIVER | | BLOOD |
| | DAILY | | | |
TREATMENT	DOSE (mg.)	GLYCOGEN (%)	TOTAL LIPID (%)	SUGAR (mg.%)
Prednisolone acetate	0.6	1.27	8.58	108.0
	0.2	0.47	6.45	85.5
Dichlorisone acetate	6.0	0.81	11.35	98.5
	2.0	0.89	10.32	99.2
Controls	. .	0.08	5.96	60.3

5 rats per group.
* Adrenalectomized rats.

as prednisolone acetate. All 16-methylated steroids tested were diuretic in the acute test in adrenalectomized rats.

The low eosinopenic activity characteristic of 9,11-dihalogenated steroids suggested that the known metabolic effects of glucocorticoids might also be suppressed. Dichlorisone acetate was therefore compared with prednisolone acetate in regard to its action on carbohydrate, lipid and protein metabolism.

The data in Tables 3 and 4 show that dichlorisone acetate, at a daily dose of 6 mg., increased liver glycogen concentration tenfold in adrenalectomized and threefold in intact rats, compared with the respective controls. Prednisolone acetate at one-tenth this dose per day produced sixteenfold and sixfold increases in liver glycogen in the two test animals respectively. On the other hand, 6 mg. of dichlorisone acetate raised the fasting blood sugar in both types of rats by 63 per cent over the control values, whereas 0.6 mg. of prednisolone acetate caused a 79 per cent increase in adrenalectomized rats and a 40 per cent increase in intact rats. The conclusion appears justified that the glucocorticoid effects of dichlorisone acetate are less than one-tenth that of prednisolone acetate.

Total hepatic lipids were elevated by both steroids in adrenalectomized (Table 3) and intact rats (Table 5). Analysis of the livers from normal rats

TABLE 4.   METABOLIC EFFECTS: INTACT RATS

| | | | SERUM ANALYSIS (mg.%) | | |
| | DAILY | LIVER | | | |
TREATMENT	DOSE (mg.)	GLYCOGEN (%)	BLOOD SUGAR	CHOLES- TEROL	PHOSPHO- LIPID
Prednisolone acetate	1.8	6.73	144.0	123.9	201.8
	0.6	1.84	120.9	87.9	179.0
Dichlorisone acetate	6.0	0.85	140.8	92.0	156.0
	2.0	0.66	124.9	85.3	146.3
Controls	. .	0.29	86.5	79.9	137.0

Pooled data from 3 experiments. Total of 11 rats per group.

TABLE 5.   METABOLIC EFFECTS: LIVER LIPIDS (%), INTACT RATS

| | DAILY | | | CHOLESTEROL | | | |
TREATMENT	DOSE (mg.)	TOTAL LIPID	PHOSPHO- LIPID	Total	Free	Ester	NEUTRAL FAT
Prednisolone acetate	0.6	9.32	2.95	.351	.196	.156	7.10
Dichlorisone acetate	6.0	9.51	3.42	.427	.195	.232	6.37
Controls	. .	5.83	3.62	.293	.256	.040	2.41

Pooled data from 3 experiments. Total of 11 rats per group.

indicated that this rise was due entirely to the neutral fat fraction (this was estimated by substracting total cholesterol and phospholipid from total lipid). Only minor increases in total serum cholesterol were noted. Prednisolone acetate seemed to increase serum phospholipid levels more than dichlorisone acetate. In general, 6 mg. of dichlorisone acetate produced lipid shifts similar to those produced by prednisolone acetate at one-tenth the dose.

The protein-catabolic effect of adrenocortical steroids is reflected in the body weight changes and increased urinary nitrogen excretion of steroid-treated rats fed ad libitum. Groups of five or six intact male rats (initial body weights 210 grams) were injected for 14 days with dichlorisone acetate (2 mg. and 1 mg. per day respectively) and prednisolone acetate (1 mg. per day) and were autopsied 24 hours after the last injection. Table 6 records

TABLE 6. BODY WEIGHTS, REPRESENTATIVE ORGAN WEIGHTS, AND
HEMATOLOGY OF INTACT, MALE RATS AFTER DAILY
Sc. TREATMENT FOR 14 DAYS

TREATMENT	BODY WT. (gm.)	SPLEEN (mg./100 gm.)	ADRENALS (mg./100 gm.)	LIVER (mg./100 gm.)	THYMUS (mg./100 gm.)	LYMPHS (%)	POLYS (%)
Dichlorisone acetate 2 mg./day	238	245	11.00*	5.89*	69.3*	64.5	28
Dichlorisone acetate 1 mg./day	247	194	10.57*	5.45*	87.9*	66.6	28.6
Prednisolone acetate 1 mg./day	172	126*	11.2*	6.22*	58.9*	26.5*	68*
Controls	293	234	16.5	4.41	210.0	86.5	11.3

* Significant change P = 0.05.

the final body weights, as well as those organ weights which showed significant deviation from the controls. As expected, the prednisolone acetate treated animals lost 37 grams or 2.6 grams per day. In contrast, the dichlorisone acetate treated rats gained 2.0 and 2.6 grams per day respectively and the controls gained 6 grams per day. The relative lack of catabolic as well as of mineralocorticoid properties of dichlorisone acetate was confirmed by analysis of urine from these rats. On the eleventh day of the experiment and without a previous fast, the rats were primed with 5 ml. of 0.2 per cent sodium chloride solution, given intraperitoneally, and placed in individual metabolism cages for six hours (Table 7). During this period, all groups excreted the fluid load; the prednisolone acetate group showed a marked enhancement of sodium, potassium and nitrogen excretion, but the dichlorisone acetate groups did not differ significantly from the controls.

The experiment shows that dichlorisone acetate, at twice the dose of prednisolone acetate, possessed only minor protein-catabolic properties. Unfortunately, anticipated absorption difficulties made it inadvisable to administer dichlorisone acetate at the 10 to 1 dose ratio employed in the previous studies.

TABLE 7. SIX HOUR ELECTROLYTE AND NITROGEN EXCRETION OF
NORMAL FED MALE RATS ON DAY 11 OF SEMICHRONIC EXPERIMENT

TREATMENT	DAILY DOSE (mg.)	NO. OF RATS	BODY WT. (gm.)	URINE VOL. (ml.)	NA (mg./100 gm.)	K (mg./100 gm.)	N (mg./100 gm.)
Dichlorisone acetate	2	6	238 ± 17.5	5.8 ± 1.26	1.80 ± 0.23	5.84 ± 1.49	27.2 ± 5.13
Dichlorisone acetate	1	5	247 ± 11.3	6.7 ± 2.68	2.40 ± 0.25	5.12 ± 0.52	22.4 ± 3.14
Prednisolone acetate	1	6	181 ± 14	5.8 ± 1.47	6.56 ± 3.69	12.48 ± 4.98	47.5 ± 15.12
Controls	.	6	278 ± 10.7	4.9 ± 2.25	1.93 ± 0.69	5.30 ± 1.12	23.8 ± 5.39

Table 6 shows that thymolytic activity and adrenal involution (ACTH suppression) induced by two weeks' treatment with dichlorisone acetate was equal to that produced by prednisolone acetate. Suppression of spleen weight and increase in liver weight by the dichlorosteroid were less pronounced. Changes in formed blood elements were seen only in the prednisolone acetate group; a reversal in the ratio of lymphocytes to polymorphonuclear leukocytes was not induced by dichlorisone acetate.

DISCUSSION

The unique biological profile of the 9,11-dihalo steroids has interesting implications. The substantial topical anti-inflammatory activity of the dihalides calls for a re-evaluation of the importance of the 11-oxygen function. Indeed, Glenn and co-workers[8] have shown that steroids devoid of functional groups at both carbons 11 and 21 possess anti-inflammatory activity in the granuloma pouch. In addition, the fact that dichlorisone acetate has low glucocorticoid activity yet appears to be as potent as prednisolone acetate in regard to ACTH inhibition and thymolytic action emphasizes the complexity of the pharmacology of cortical steroids.

The results obtained in the dichlorisone study also confirm our previous observation[22] of the excellent correlation between eosinopenic and glucocorticoid activity of adrenocorticoids.

Our values for the anti-inflammatory activity of dichlorisone, first mentioned by Robinson et al.,[12] have been challenged by Bowers[1, 2] and by Figdor.[5] These investigators report an activity half that of cortisol for dichlorisone and 1,2-dihydrodichlorisone by the cotton pellet implant method. We have obtained the following data for the latter steroid: eosinopenic activity, less than 0.1; anti-inflammatory activity, 0.93 (0.74 to 1.18); prednisolone acetate = 1; mineralocorticoid activity, sodium retention similar to cortexone acetate (desoxycorticosterone). The discrepancy is based on the two methods of estimating anti-inflammatory activity. The cotton pellet granuloma technique has been notorious for its erratic results, in our own hands (unpublished) as well as in the literature, although it usually gives too high rather than too low potency ratios. An example is the potency of dexamethasone, which has been reported to be 50 times that of prednisolone by the cotton pellet method[19] and 5 times that of prednisolone by the pouch technique,[22] while the clinical efficacy is 5 to 10 times that of prednisolone. In spite of the good predictive value of the pouch method seen so far, it may be suggested that the granuloma pouch response correlates with systemic clinical activity for steroids possessing high glucocorticoid potency, and with topical activity for steroids with low glucocorticoid potency. Thus, dichlorisone (Diloderm) is a potent topical anti-inflammatory agent in man,[10, 14] a fact which would not have been predicted from the cotton pellet results. Another example of this type of correlation is fluorometholone (6α-methyl-9α-fluoro-21-desoxyprednisolone) which assayed in our laboratory as follows: anti-inflammatory activity = 7; eosinopenic activity = 1; prednisolone acetate = 1. It is a moot question whether this distinction is fortuitous, whether it is due to species differences between rodents and man, or whether there are intrinsic differences between the requirements for systemic and those for topical anti-inflammatory action.

SUMMARY

1. A series of 9α,11β-dihalo derivatives of 1-dehydrocortexolone was assayed for anti-inflammatory activity. The most potent steroid was the di-chloro compound, dichlorisone. The effect of 16α and 16β-methylation on the anti-inflammatory activity of dichlorisone was investigated. Introduction of a 17,21-acetonide group increased the anti-inflammatory activity of dichlorisone. 16α and 16β-methylation further increased the anti-inflammatory activity of the dichlorisone acetonide to 14 times that of prednisolone acetate.

2. The eosinopenic activity of substituted and unsubstituted dihalides was in the order of one-tenth that of prednisolone acetate.

3. Dichlorisone caused slight sodium retention in the acute test for electrolyte excretion. C-16 methylation conferred diuretic properties on the dichlorisone derivative.

4. Investigation of the activity spectrum of dichlorisone gave the following profile: anti-inflammatory activity four to eight times that of prednisolone acetate; eosinopenic, glucocorticoid and lipid-metabolic effects one-tenth standard or less; protein catabolic activity less than standard; adrenal involution (ACTH suppression) and thymolytic activity approximately equal to standard.

ACKNOWLEDGMENT

The invaluable assistance of Warren L. Miller, Merl Steinberg, Alexandra D. Stephenson and Felix H. Warren is gratefully acknowledged. For the statistical analysis, I am indebted to Gordon B. Thomas.

REFERENCES

1. Bowers, A.: J. Am. Chem. Soc., *81*:4107, 1959.
2. Bowers, A., Ibañez, L. C., Denot, E. and Becerra, R.: J. Am. Chem. Soc., *82*:4001, 1960.
3. Bush, I. E.: Experientia, *12*:325, 1956.
4. Cook, M. R., Jr. and Elmadjian, F.: J. Am. Pharmacol. A., Sci. Ed., *42*:329, 1953.
5. Figdor, S. K.: Abstracts, p. 66-P, Am. Chem. Soc. Meeting, Chicago, Ill., Sept., 1958.
6. Fried, J. and Borman, A.: Vitamins and Hormones, *16*:304, 1958.
7. Fried, J. and Sabo, E. F.: J. Am. Chem. Soc., *75*:2273, 1953.
8. Glenn, E. M., Richardson, S. L. and Bowman, B. J.: Metabolism, 8:265, 1959.
9. Nelson, N.: J. Biol. Chem., *153*:375, 1944.
10. Nierman, M. M.: Clinical Medicine. (In press.)
11. Robert, A. and Nezamis, J. E.: Acta endocrinol., *25*:105, 1957.
12. Robinson, C. H., Finckenor, L., Oliveto, E. P. and Gould, D.: J. Am. Chem. Soc., *81*:2191, 1959.
13. Robinson, C. H., Finckenor, L. E., Tiberi, R. and Oliveto, E. P. (In press.)
14. Robinson, H. M.: Southern Medicine. (In press.)
15. Rosemberg, E., Cornfeld, J., Bates, R. W. and Anderson, E.: Endocrinology, *54*:363, 1954.
16. Schoenheimer, R. and Sperry, W. M.: J. Biol. Chem., *106*:745, 1934.
17. Seifter, S., Dayton, S., Novic, B. and Muntwyler, E.: Arch. Biochem., *25*:191, 1950.
18. Selye, H.: J.A.M.A., *152*:1207, 1953.
19. Silber, R. H.: Ann. New York Acad. Sc., *82*:821, 1959.
20. Somogyi, M.: J. Biol. Chem., *160*:62, 1945.
21. Speirs, R. S. and Meyer, R. K.: Endocrinology, *48*:316, 1951.
22. Tolksdorf, S.: Ann. New York Acad. Sc., *82*:829, 1959.
23. Zilversmit, D. B. and Davis, A. K.: J. Lab. & Clin. Med., *35*:155, 1950.

Metabolic Effects of Hydrocortisone

E. MYLES GLENN, BARBARA J. BOWMAN and RAYMOND B. BAYER

Department of Endocrinology, The Upjohn Company

Secretions of the adrenal cortex increase the severity of pancreatic diabetes and injection of adrenocortical steroids influences the metabolism of carbohydrates.[5, 13, 17, 18, 19, 25, 26] Earlier investigations attributed these effects to increased production of carbohydrates from noncarbohydrate sources.[26] Later experiments demonstrated that this concept did not adequately explain the influence of adrenal steroids on metabolic processes and suggested that these hormones may have a direct action on carbohydrate metabolism.[14] Although secretions of the adrenal cortex also influence the metabolism of fats and amino acids,[1, 3, 4, 8, 15] it is not precisely known whether these effects are primary or secondary consequences of steroid action. Attempts have been made to define the role of adrenal steroids in metabolism of carbohydrates,[7, 9, 12, 24, 27, 28] but the exact site where they produce their effects is unknown. Several attractive hypotheses have been advanced to explain the alterations of glucose metabolism by steroids; none of them is supported by *direct, definitive* and *specific* experimental proof.[2, 6, 16, 20, 21, 29]

Our approach to the problem of primary metabolic effects of hydrocortisone has been to study the consequences of the administration of the hormone to adrenalectomized fasted rats for the purpose of determining:

1. What are the *first* measurable metabolic changes which occur after injection of hydrocortisone?

2. Which substrates, when injected into experimental animals, markedly alter or *increase* the primary metabolic responses to hydrocortisone?

3. Where does hydrocortisone produce its major effects in animals, in hepatic or extrahepatic tissues?

4. Are results obtained in answer to question 3 a reflection of steroid action at the capillary wall, in the extracellular space, in the cell membrane or at some point within the cell?

We have taken this approach because it is our contention that *in vitro* effects of adrenocortical steroids can neither be interpreted nor understood until more information is available regarding the sequence of events occurring *in vivo* following their injection. These results are in the process of being published in greater detail elsewhere.[11]

GLYCOGENIC EFFECTS OF HYDROCORTISONE

Following subcutaneous or intravenous injection of hydrocortisone (2 mg.) to fasted adrenalectomized rats, liver glycogen does not begin to increase for at least 2 to 4 hours; maximum levels are attained in 8 to 12 hours, decreasing to control values within 24 to 32 hours. Plasma glucose levels increase significantly within 30 to 60 minutes, continue to increase and reach maximum levels in 4 hours (Fig. 1). Significant changes in amino acid or protein blood levels are not apparent during the same time intervals. When varying amounts of hydrocortisone (0.1 to 4.0 mg.) are injected

316

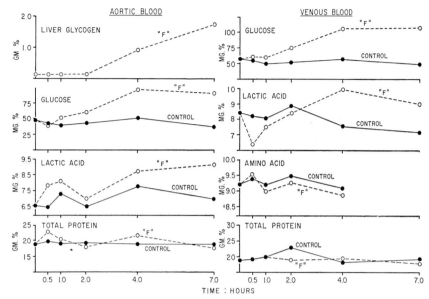

Fig. 1. Time response: effect of hydrocortisone on various blood constituents and liver glycogen. Conditions: 2.0 mg. hydrocortisone, sc. 5 rats/point.

intravenously, a typical S-shaped dose-response relationship is obtained (Fig. 2). Of injected amino acids, fats, tricarboxylic acid cycle intermediates, lactate and glucose, only the latter two substrates straighten out the typical S-shaped response curve and produce a more *immediate* glycogenic response (Figs. 2 and 3). These data strongly suggest that it is either glucose or one of its intermediates upon which hydrocortisone acts to produce glycogenic effects.

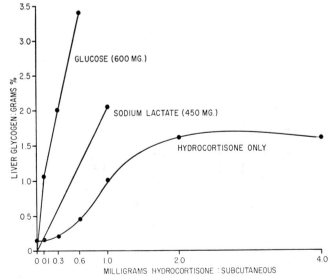

Fig. 2. Dose response liver glycogen deposition following intraperitoneal administration of glucose or sodium lactate. Conditions: 5 rats/point. Glucose and lactate curves represent treated minus control groups.

EACH POINT IS THE MEAN OF FIVE RATS

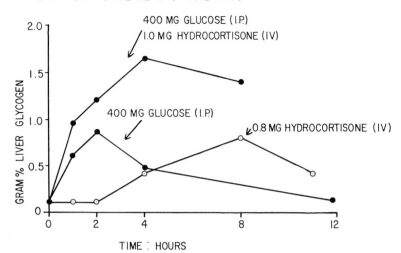

Fig. 3.   Liver glycogen time-response curve following the intraperitoneal administration
of glucose.

If hydrocortisone were primarily involved with increasing the availability
of proteins, amino acids or fats from peripheral tissues to liver, and if these
primary effects were related to the series of events seen after steroid injection, increased glycogenic effects should be observed after injection of
increasing amounts of these substrates. When injected alone in increasing
amounts, amino acids or fat lead neither to accumulation of glycogen in the
liver nor to incorporation of radioactivity from labeled substrates. Intravenous infusion of whole blood (1 to 10 ml.) from fasted adrenalectomized
rats, with or without hydrocortisone, also fails to produce glycogenic effects.
In the presence of hydrocortisone, a wide variety of *labeled* substrates

TABLE 1.   EFFECT OF HYDROCORTISONE ON INCORPORATION OF C^{14}
FROM VARIOUS SUBSTRATES INTO LIVER GLYCOGEN

| | AMOUNT INJECTED | | MG. GLYCOGEN/ LIVER IN TREATED ANIMALS | SPECIFIC ACTIVITY DPM/MG. GLYCOGEN | |
COMPOUND	Labeled	Unlabeled Mgs.		Controls	Hydro- cortisone Treated
Glucose-1-C^{14}	299,440 DPM	20	50.6	0	262
Acetate-2-C^{14}	312,300 DPM	60	50.4	0	72
Pyruvate-1-C^{14}	274,160 DPM	40	60.2	0	241
Acetate-1-C^{14}	789,600 DPM	20	43.6	0	43
Glucose-6-C^{14}	544,000 DPM	20	71.6	0	657
Pyruvate-2-C^{14}	544,000 DPM	20	70.7	0	758
DL-Alanine-2-C^{14}	544,000 DPM	20	93.5	0	644
Succinate-2-C^{14}	1 μc	20	54.7	0	1475
Citrate-1,5-C^{14}	1 μc	20	51.4	0	99
Glycine-2-C^{14}	1 μc	20	59.9	0	773
Formate-C^{14}	2 μc	40	27.0	0	520
Bicarbonate-C^{14}	2 μc	40	29.2	0	150
Palmitate-1-C^{14}	1,986,400 DPM*	..	36.2	0	80
Butyrate-1-C^{14}	2,255,750 DPM	20	65.3	0	298

5 rats per point. All substrates injected IP (palmitate injected I.V.), 2 hours after subcutaneous injection of hydrocortisone and livers removed 5 hours after injection of each
substrate.

* Palmitate-1-C^{14} contained in 5.0 ml. of an intravenous fat preparation (Lipomul).

(including amino acids and fats), are incorporated into liver glycogen because of nonspecific exchange (Table 1). However, only the injection of large amounts of glucose and lactate results in *increased* net synthesis of liver glycogen in the presence or absence of hydrocortisone.

When labeled (4-C¹⁴) or unlabeled hydrocortisone is injected intravenously into fasted adrenalectomized rats, it disappears from the blood within 1.5 to 2.0 hours (Fig. 4). Injection of glucose 3 *hours* after steroid injection leads to increased glycogenic activity (Fig. 5). Steroid blood levels

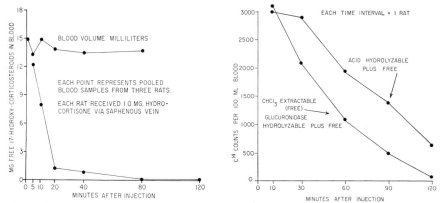

Fig. 4. Disappearance rate of hydrocortisone from blood of adrenalectomized rats. Conditions: For C¹⁴ studies, blood was removed from dorsal aorta, divided into 2 equal parts. One part was extracted with chloroform, then the aqueous residue boiled with 15% hydrochloric acid for 30 min. and re-extracted with chloroform. The other portion of blood was incubated overnight at pH 4.8 with 25,000 units B-glucuronidase (Ketodase). 1.0 mg. hydrocortisone plus 0.4 µc. 4-C¹⁴ per rat via the saphenous vein.

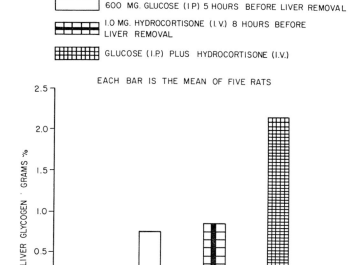

Fig. 5. Influence of intraperitoneal glucose on liver glycogen deposition.

per se, therefore, do not accurately reflect the series of physiological events occurring in the intact animal. After complete disappearance from blood, hydrocortisone *continues* to influence the metabolism of glucose.

HEPATIC AND EXTRAHEPATIC EFFECTS OF HYDROCORTISONE ON GLUCOSE METABOLISM

Injection of hydrocortisone (1 mg.) subcutaneously or via the saphenous or portal veins produces glycogenic effects at a decreasing degree of effectiveness (Fig. 6). It appears that extrahepatic steroid levels may control the degree of glycogenic response to hydrocortisone. Glycogenic effects can be

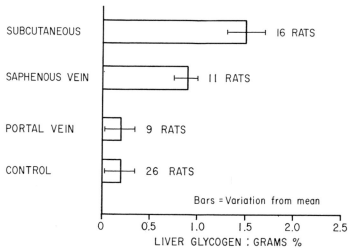

Fig. 6. Liver glycogen: response to 1.0 mg. hydrocortisone by various routes of administration.

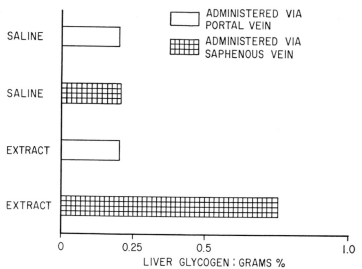

Fig. 7. Glycogenic activity of steroid extracts from the hepatic vein following portal-venous administration of 16 mg. hydrocortisone hemisuccinate. Conditions: 1.0 ml. of ethyl acetate-chloroform extract equivalent to one rat. All rats laparotomized. 5 rats/point.

produced by portal-venous injection of large amounts (10 to 20 mg.) of water-soluble hydrocortisone hemisuccinate. Injection of similar amounts of steroid followed by collection, extraction and chromatography of *hepatic-venous* blood leads to the recovery of measurable amounts of the free alcohol of hydrocortisone. When 16 mg. of hydrocortisone hemisuccinate is injected via the portal vein and hepatic-venous *extracts* are re-injected via the saphenous and portal veins, only via the former route are glycogenic effects produced (Fig. 7). It appears that the amount of steroid *escaping* from liver, *not* the amount *entering* it, determines the effects of hydrocortisone on carbohydrate metabolism. This suggests that hydrocortisone exerts its effects primarily on tissues other than the liver.

HYDROCORTISONE EFFECTS ON GLUCOSE OXIDATION AND MUSCLE GLYCOGEN SYNTHESIS

When large amounts of glucose-1-C^{14} and glycerol-1,3-C^{14} are injected intraperitoneally with carrier, the rate of their conversion to $C^{14}O_2$ is

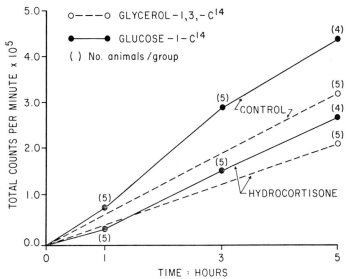

Fig. 8. Effect of hydrocortisone on rate of glucose and glycerol oxidation in fasted adrenalectomized rats. Conditions: Each rat received 500 mg. glucose + 2.0 μc. glucose-1-C^{14} and 300 mg. glycerol + 2.0 μc. glycerol-1,3-C^{14}, I.P. Each point is the mean of duplicate determinations on ( ) rats per point. Total barium carbonate at 5 hrs.:

	GLUCOSE	GLYCEROL
Hydrocortisone	12.875 gm.	9.710 gm.
Controls	12.175 gm.	9.600 gm.

markedly decreased by hydrocortisone (Fig. 8). Hydrocortisone does not inhibit the rate of conversion of labeled amino acids,* fats,† acetate or pyruvate (Fig. 9) to $C^{14}O_2$.

Hydrocortisone does not produce increased glycogen synthesis in gastrocnemius muscle unless large amounts of glucose are also injected (Fig. 10). The time course of both liver and muscle glycogen synthesis is the same after injection of hydrocortisone and glucose (Fig. 11).

* IV. amino acid preparation, The Interchemical Company.
† I.V. fat (Lipomul), The Upjohn Company.

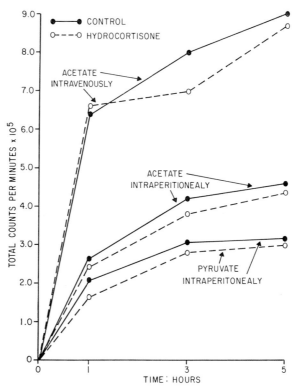

Fig. 9. Effect of hydrocortisone on rate of oxidation of acetate and pyruvate. Conditions: 5 adrenalectomized rats/point. 2.0 mg. hydrocortisone sc. at 8 A.M., 200 mg. glucose I.P. at 10 A.M. 40.0 mg. sodium acetate + 1.0 μc. acetate-1-C^{14} + 1.0 μc. acetate-2-C^{14} or 40.0 mg. sodium pyruvate + 1.0 μc. pyruvate-2-C^{14} and 1.0 μc. pyruvate-1-C^{14}. Collections started at 10 A.M.

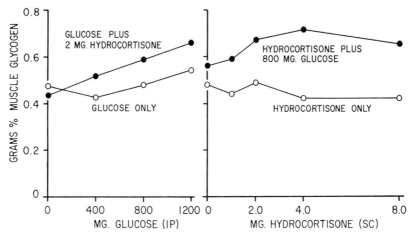

Fig. 10. Dose response of muscle glycogen to glucose and hydrocortisone. Conditions: 5 rats/point.

Injection of hydrocortisone and insulin and oral administration of sucrose to totally depancreatized-adrenalectomized, fasted rats result in greater effects on muscle glycogen deposition than injection of the two hormones alone (Fig. 12).

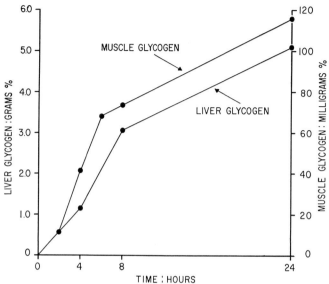

Fig. 11. Time response of rat muscle and liver glycogen. Conditions: Each rat received 4.0 mg. hydrocortisone sc. + 800 mg. glucose I.P. Values obtained by subtracting glucose control group from hydrocortisone + glucose group. 5 rats/point.

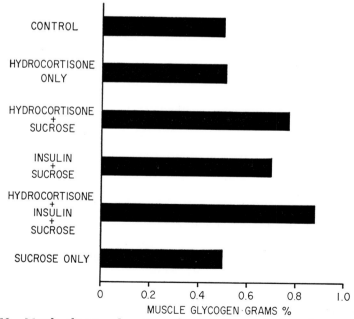

Fig. 12. Muscle glycogen deposition after injection of hydrocortisone and insulin. Conditions: 5 rats/point. Insulin, 0.75 units/rat (sc.); sucrose, 2.0 gm./rat (oral); hydrocortisone, 4.0 mg./rat (sc.).

Hydrocortisone inhibits and insulin increases the rate of oxidation of glucose. If hydrocortisone's effect were opposite to that of insulin on the rate of entry of glucose into the cell, additive effects of insulin and hydrocortisone on muscle glycogen synthesis would not be expected. It is therefore concluded that hydrocortisone inhibits metabolism of glucose *below* its point of entry into the muscle cell.

EFFECT OF HYDROCORTISONE ON DISTRIBUTION OF METABOLIZABLE AND NONMETABOLIZABLE AMINO ACIDS AND CARBOHYDRATES

These experiments were performed on adrenalectomized fasted rats, nephrectomized at least 30 minutes before initiation of experimental procedures. Carbohydrates were injected intravenously or intraperitoneally as 10 per cent solutions, amino acids as 5 per cent solutions. Unless otherwise stated, sugars were given at 100 mg. per 100 grams of body weight, amino acids at 50 mg. per 100 grams of body weight. Two to 4 microcuries of labeled compound were injected with carrier substrate.

Tissues (blood, brain and muscle) were extracted with 5 per cent trichloroacetic acid. Following high speed centrifugation, aliquots of extract were counted in a Packard liquid scintillation spectrometer. The extraction procedure resulted in complete recovery of radioactivity.

Analysis of water content was made on whole blood, gastrocnemius and brain at the same time intervals employed for the investigation of substrates, using wet and dry weight differences. In these studies animals were injected with the same amounts of water or sucrose as animals receiving various other substrates.

Calculations employ the sucrose space (sucrose-UL-C^{14}) as a measure of extracellular volume.

L-Arabinose and D-xylose were measured by chemical[23] and isotope methods of analysis. In both cases, distribution of radioactivity was higher than chemical analysis of distribution. Since the chemical methods measure only specific parts of the molecule and the C^{14} analyses measure both altered and unaltered substrate, we believe that distribution studies with radioisotopes are more accurate.

The concentration of sugar or other substrates in DPM/ml. of blood water (DPM_b), per ml. of muscle water (DPM_m), and per ml. of brain water (DPM_{br}) was calculated from actual water content of tissues. The concentration of substrate per ml. of intracellular water (C_i) was calculated as follows:

$$\text{Muscle: } C_i = \frac{DPM_m - (DPM_b \times E)}{(1.0 - E)} \quad \text{Brain: } C_i = \frac{DPM_{br} - (DPM_b \times E)}{(1.0 - E)}$$

E is the ratio of distribution of injected sucrose (DPM/ml. muscle water: DPM/ml. blood water) as a measure of the extracellular space.

Hydrocortisone does not significantly change the distribution of DL-alanine, D-xylose, L-arabinose and α-amino-iso-butyric acid in muscle or brain; it decreases the distribution ratio of glucose-2-C^{14} in both muscle and brain and decreases the distribution of galactose-1-C^{14} in brain (Table 2). Effects of hydrocortisone on *intracellular* accumulation of glucose-2-C^{14} are shown in Fig. 13. With the possible exception of sucrose space in muscle during the first 4 hours after injection, hydrocortisone did not

TABLE 2. PER CENT DISTRIBUTION OF VARIOUS SUBSTRATES AT
DIFFERENT TIMES AFTER INJECTION: EFFECT OF HYDROCORTISONE

	PER CENT DISTRIBUTION: * Muscle			HOURS AFTER INJECTION Brain		
SUBSTRATE	2	4	6	2	4	6
α-Amino-iso-butyric-1-C14	36.2	49.1	53.4	10.5	17.2	20.4
+ Hydrocortisone (4 mg.)	37.1	50.2	57.1	10.5	17.1	20.0
D-Xylose-1-C14	34.4	42.6	56.9	79.6	77.8	84.2
+ Hydrocortisone (4 mg.)	35.2	43.0	60.0	79.0	78.1	83.4
L-Arabinose-1-C	32.0	34.4	40.4	74.0	84.7	96.7
+ Hydrocortisone (4 mg.)	32.0	34.4	42.0	72.4	83.0	96.0
Glucose-2-C14	53.4	92.0	149.0	177.4	254.5	284.8
+ Hydrocortisone (4 mg.)	40.0	75.1	130.0	160.0	220.0	255.0
Galactose-1-C14	28.0	31.0	36.0	116.1	164.5	204.6
+ Hydrocortisone (4 mg.)	27.8	31.0	38.2	105.0	140.0	170.0
DL-Alanine-2-C14	48.8	60.2	74.4	101.6	105.0	72.0
+ Hydrocortisone (4 mg.)	48.6	59.5	74.4	105.2	97.5	86.0
Sucrose-UL-C14	28.2	28.7	25.0	8.4	9.0	8.4
+ Hydrocortisone (4 mg.)	25.5	24.0	27.5	8.5	8.5	7.0

$$* \frac{\text{DPM/ml. Tissue water}}{\text{DPM/ml. Blood water}} \times 100 = \text{Per Cent Distribution}$$

Total blood water = 81.8%
Total brain water = 80.0%
Total muscle water = 77.5%

significantly alter water content or sucrose space (Fig. 14). When plasma rather than whole blood was analyzed, the distribution ratio of sucrose in muscle and brain was 18 per cent and 6 per cent respectively—values which are considerably lower than those shown when whole blood was analyzed. However, a decrease of 1 per cent for sucrose space in muscle was also obtained after hydrocortisone injection when plasma concentrations were used as a point of reference.

These experiments demonstrate that hydrocortisone, contrary to expec-

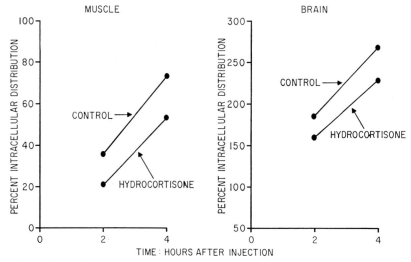

Fig. 13.   Effect of hydrocortisone on intracellular accumulation of glucose-2-C14.
Conditions: 5 rats/point.

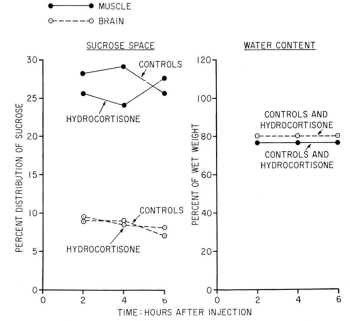

Fig. 14. Summary of effects of hydrocortisone on sucrose space and water content of
adrenalectomized-nephrectomized rats.

tation, does indeed reduce the rate of entry of certain sugars into muscle
and brain cells. This observation can be reconciled with the fact that
hydrocortisone inhibits oxidation of glucose, increases muscle glycogen
synthesis from administered glucose and produces an additive effect on
muscle glycogen synthesis when injected together with insulin, only if it
is supposed that hydrocortisone inhibits the metabolism of glucose below
the cell surface and that the rate of entry of glucose into the cell is blocked
by the intracellular accumulation of unmetabolized intermediates.

SUMMARY AND CONCLUSIONS

1. Of administered amino acids, fat, lactate and glucose, only the latter
two substrates markedly alter the glycogenic response to hydrocortisone.
Changes in blood glucose and lactate levels precede changes in liver glycogen after the administration of hydrocortisone.

2. After complete disappearance from the blood of fasted adrenalectomized rats, hydrocortisone still produces appreciable effects on glucose
conversion to glycogen.

3. Results of administration by different routes suggest that peripheral,
not hepatic, steroid levels control response to steroid and that the major
primary effect of hydrocortisone is on peripheral tissues.

4. Hydrocortisone inhibits the oxidation of glucose and produces increased muscle and liver glycogen synthesis. When administered to totally
depancreatized-adrenalectomized rats, hydrocortisone does not antagonize
the muscle glycogen accumulation caused by insulin.

5. Hydrocortisone decreases the ratio of distribution of glucose-2-C^{14} in
brain and muscle and decreases the ratio of distribution of galactose-1-C^{14}

in brain but does not significantly influence the ratio of distribution of the relatively nonmetabolizable substrates D-xylose, L-arabinose and α-amino-iso-butyric acid, and metabolizable DL-alanine.

6. It is concluded that the primary effect of hydrocortisone is one of inhibiting the oxidation of glucose by the inhibition of some enzymatic process within the cell. It is suggested that the accumulation of carbohydrate metabolites within the cell is responsible for the rate-decreasing effect of hydrocortisone on the entry of glucose into the cell.

REFERENCES

1. Balmain, J. H., Folley, S. J., Glascock, R. F. and McNaught, M. C.: Biochem. J., 56:VI, 1954.
2. Blecher, M. and White, A.: J. Biol. Chem., 235:282, 1960.
3. Bondy, P. K., Ingle, D. J. and Meekes, R. C.: Endocrinology, 45:605, 1949.
4. Brady, R. O., Lukens, F. D. W. and Gurin, S. J.: J. Biol. Chem., 193:459, 1951.
5. Britton, S. W., Silvette, H. and Kline, R.: Am. J. Physiol., 122:446, 1938.
6. Cahill, G., Ashmore, J., Renold, A. E. and Hastings, A. B.: Am. J. Med., 26:264, 1959.
7. Chernick, S. S. and Chaikoff, I. L.: J. Biol Chem., 186:535, 1950.
8. Evans, G. T.: Am. J. Physiol., 114:297, 1936.
9. Freedland, R. A. and Harper, A. E.: J. Biol. Chem., 228:743, 1957.
10. Freeland, R. A. and Harper, A. E.: J. Biol. Chem., 230:833, 1958.
11. Glenn, E. M., Bowman, B. J., Bayer, R. B. and Meyer, C. E.: Endocrinology. (In Press.)
12. Gomori, G. J.: Biol. Chem., 148:139, 1943.
13. Hartman, F. A. and Brownell, K. A.: Proc. Soc. Exper. Med., 32:743, 1934.
14. Ingle, D. J. and Thorn, G. W.: Am. J. Physiol., 132:670, 1941.
15. Ingle, D. J., Prestrud, M. C. and Nezamis, J. E.: Proc. Soc. Exper. Biol. & Med., 67:321, 1948.
16. Kipnis, D.: Ann. N. Y. Acad. Sc., 82:354, 1959.
17. Long, C. N. H. and Lukens, F. D. W.: Proc. Soc. Exper. Biol., 32:743, 1934.
18. Long, C. N. H. and Lukens, F. D. W: J. Exper. Med., 63:465, 1936.
19. Long, C. N. H., Katzin, B. and Fry, E. G.: Endocrinology, 27:971, 1940.
20. Morgan, H. Y., Henderson, M. J., Regen, D. M. and Park, C. R.: Ann. N. Y. Acad. Sc., 82:387, 1959.
21. Park, C. R. and Morgan, H. E.: Diabetes, 9:250, 1960.
22. Robert, A. and Nezamis, J. E.: Acta Endocrinol., 25:105, 1957.
23. Roe, J. H. and Rice, E. W.: J. Biol. Chem., 173:507, 1948.
24. Rosen, F., Roberts, W. R., Budnick, L. E. and Nichel, C. A.: Endocrinology, 65:256, 1959.
25. Russell, J. A.: Am. J. Physiol., 140:98, 1943.
26. Thorn, G. W., Koepf, G. F., Lewis, R. A. and Olsen, E. F.: J. Clin Invest., 19:813, 1940.
27. Weber, G and Cantero, A.: Endocrinology, 61:701, 1957.
28. Weber, G., Allard, C., deLamirande, G. and Cantero, A.: Endocrinology, 58:40, 1956.
29. Winternitz, W. W., Dintzis, R. and Long, C. N. H.: Endocrinolgy, 61:724, 1957.

Pharmacology of Prednisone, Prednisolone, 6-Methylprednisolone and Triamcinolone

DALTON JENKINS

University of Colorado School of Medicine

The therapeutic usefulness of cortisone and cortisol as anti-inflammatory agents is seriously limited by the frequency with which undersirable side effects are encountered. Therefore, it was inevitable that the relationships between the chemical structure and the metabolic and antiphlogistic actions of these hormones be subjected to intensive study aimed at preserving therapeutic activity and eliminating or materially reducing their undersirable effects. Unfortunately, these side effects are primarily overdosage phenomena —exaggerated manifestations of the physiologic actions of corticosteroids. This makes the problem quite complex, for it means that an ideal corticosteroid agent must maintain anti-inflammatory activity while the normal steroid actions on inorganic and organic metabolism are annulled or at least significantly reduced. Whether this dissociation of steroid effects can be achieved remains to be found.

Numerous modifications of the cortisol molecule have been accomplished. The first synthetic compounds to prove useful as anti-inflammatory agents were prednisone and prednisolone. Subsequently, 6-methylprednisolone and triamcinolone were made available for general use. Some aspects of the pharmacology of these four agents are considered here.

MODIFICATIONS OF STRUCTURE AND FUNCTION

Prednisone and prednisolone are the 1,2 dehydrogenated analogs of cortisone and cortisol, respectively.[9] Their synthesis has been accomplished by a number of methods, both microbiological and chemical.[7] The Δ^1 modification produced an increase in glucocorticoid activity without an accompanying increase in mineralocorticoid effects.

A series of methylated derivatives of cortisol has been prepared. The first of these involved the introduction of a 2α-methyl group. This modification produced enhancement of electrolyte regulating effects. However, shifting the methyl group to the C-6 position greatly reduced sodium-retaining activity. Combining the 6α-methylation and 1,2 dehydrogenation to produce 6α-methylprednisolone provided a steroid with somewhat greater glucocorticoid activity and somewhat less mineralocorticoid activity than the parent compound, prednisolone.[22]

It is remarkable that when multiple alterations in the cortisol molecule are combined, each modification exerts its own characteristic effect on biologic activity, largely independent of the other groups. This is well illustrated in the structure of triamcinolone. Fried et al.[7] had previously found that the addition of a fluorine atom at the C-9 position of cortisol increased both glucocorticoid and mineralocorticoid activity, especially the latter. Combining 9α-fluorination with 1,2 dehydrogenation produced a compound (9α-fluoroprednisolone) with great glucocorticoid, anti-inflammatory and salt-retaining activity. The latter property precluded the use of the steroid clinically. However, Bernstein et al.[1] found that C-16 hydroxylation essentially abolished the mineralocorticoid effects of the compound but only partially reduced glucocorticoid potency. The resulting compound, 9α-fluoro-16α-hydroxyprednisolone (triamcinolone) provided anti-inflammatory effects somewhat greater than those of prednisolone without inducing sodium retention.

BIOLOGIC EVALUATION

In order that synthetic steroids can be logically selected for clinical trial, careful evaluation must be carried out in the experimental laboratory. Such studies serve to establish the type of physiologic activity exerted (mineralocorticoid, antiphlogistic, etc.), as well as relative potency. Table 1 compares the activities of prednisolone, 6-methylprednisolone and triamcinolone in the most frequently employed bioassay procedures.

TABLE 1. EVALUATION OF CORTISOL AND SYNTHETIC ANALOGS BY BIOASSAY IN THE RAT

	LIVER GLYCOGEN DEPOSITION (Cortisone = 1)	EOSINOPENIA (Cortisone = 1)	THYMUS INVOLUTION (Cortisone = 1)	GRANULOMA INHIBITION (Cortisol = 1)	SODIUM RETENTION (D C A = 1)
Cortisol	1.6	1.0	2.0	1.0	0c
Prednisolone	4.0	3.3	3.2	3.1b	0c
6-Methylprednisolone	10.00	1.7	. .	6.2b	Excretionc
Triamcinolone	13.0a	3.2	7.0	4.0	Excretionc

a. Bernstein et al.[1] *b.* Dulin et al.[5] *c.* Fried and Borman.[7] All other values from Tolksdorf.[24]

With three different indices of glucocorticoid activity, prednisolone was found to possess three to four times the potency of cortisone and cortisol. Anti-inflammatory effects were similarly enhanced. Prednisolone produced no change in the excretion of sodium in adrenalectomized rats. However, Swingle et al.[23] found that the administration of prednisolone to adrenalectomized dogs in adrenal crisis restored the animals to health and corrected their hypotension, hyponatremia, hyperkalemia, azotemia and hemodilution.

The 6α-methyl group increased the anti-inflammatory effectiveness of prednisolone by a factor of approximately two and glycogenic potency to a somewhat greater degree. Similarly, triamcinolone exhibited a slightly greater granuloma-inhibiting effect than prednisolone, with a more impressive increase in glucocorticoid activity. Both 6-methylprednisolone and triamcinolone promoted the excretion of sodium and water in adrenalectomized (salt- and water-loaded) animals.

These results accurately predicted the increased therapeutic, anti-inflammatory potency of these synthetic corticosteroids as well as their loss of sodium-retaining activity. However, the potency ratios are quite variable for the different indices of glucocorticoid and antiphlogistic activity. And experience has repeatedly shown that the results of corticosteroid bioassays in animals, especially those obtained with synthetic steroid analogs, are not quantitatively applicable to man. Further evaluation in human subjects is always required.

EVALUATION IN MAN

The results of some comparative studies on the metabolic activities of prednisolone, 6-methylprednisolone and triamcinolone in man are shown in Table 2. The potency ratios recorded show a remarkable agreement in view of the variety of procedures used and the number of investigators involved.

TABLE 2.   EVALUATION OF CORTISOL AND SYNTHETIC CORTICOSTEROIDS IN MAN

	HYPER-GLYCEMIA	EOSINO-PENIA	NITROGEN LOSS	PITUITARY ADRENAL INHIBITION	ANTI-RHEUMATIC	SODIUM RETENTION
Cortisol	1	1	1	1	1	1
Prednisolone	4[a]	4[a]-6[b]	7-8[b]	3-4[d]	3-5[f]	±[b]
6-Methylpred-nisolone	5[a]	5[a]	7-9[c]	4-5[e]	4-6[g]	0 or —[c]
Triamcinolone	5[a]	5[a]	7-9[c]	3-5[e]	4-6[h]	0 or —[c]

a. West.[26] b. Pechet et al.[18] c. Jenkins.[11] d. Kupperman et al.[13] e. Kupperman et al.[14] f. Bunim et al.[3] g. Boland.[2] h. Freyberg et al.[6]

These studies demonstrate that mineralocorticoid activity is relatively low in prednisolone and minimal in 6-methylprednisolone and triamcinolone. In large doses (greater than 40 mg. per day), prednisolone often produces definite, although usually transient, sodium retention. In fact, when *equal* doses of prednisolone and cortisol are given to normal subjects, the degree of sodium retention induced by the two agents is approximately equivalent. That sodium retention is not commonly a problem in prednisolone therapy is the result of its increased anti-inflammatory potency, permitting the use of relatively small dosages. When small doses are employed there is usually little or no change in sodium excretion; frequently, a modest, transient sodium diuresis ensues. Sodium retention rarely occurs with 6-methylprednisolone or triamcinolone, even with large doses; usually an increase in sodium excretion is produced. There is good evidence that the increased urinary excretion of sodium commonly elicited by synthetic corticosteroids is not due to an inhibition of aldosterone secretion or to any interference with the renal actions of aldosterone. Liddle et al.[15] have attributed the sodium loss to an elevation of glomerular filtration rate (with an increase in the tubular load of sodium) in the absence of potent effects on renal tubular sodium reabsorption. The net result, in effect, is a dissociation of sodium-retaining activity from glucocorticoid and anti-inflammatory activity.

Cortisol, prednisolone and 6-methylprednisolone produce a characteristic change in urinary potassium excretion. Regularly, potassium loss occurs on the first day of steroid administration; potassium retention, for one or two days, follows the cessation of steroid treatment. In all probability, this immediate but brief increase in potassium output is the result of cellular potassium release (possibly independent of protein breakdown) rather than a primary renal tubular effect, since it accompanies a transient elevation in serum potassium levels, occurs in the absence of sodium retention or, in some instances, in association with an increased urinary sodium output, and precedes nitrogen loss. During maintenance administration of the steroids, there is little effect on potassium excretion unless large doses are given. In the latter case, a secondary increase in potassium output may occur, usually in conjunction with a progressive rise in urinary nitrogen excretion. In small doses (less than 16 mg. per day), triamcinolone usually produces transient changes in potassium output similar to those seen with the other compounds. But with larger doses, triamcinolone usually produces a persistent loss of potassium. In such cases, according to Pechet,[17] potassium loss is greater than that accounted for by a negative nitrogen balance. This implies that the characteristic effect of corticosteroids on the renal handling of potassium persists in triamcinolone even though the capacity to increase the renal retention of sodium has been almost completely eliminated; alternatively, particularly in view of the potent effects of this compound on muscle mass (see Side Effects), it could well reflect a greater effect of triamcinolone on cellular electrolyte metabolism than on protein metabolism.

Eosinopenia, hyperglycemia, nitrogen loss and pituitary-adrenal cortical suppression are included among the so-called glucocorticoid effects of corticosteroids and usually show some degree of correlation with anti-inflammatory potency. Table 2 demonstrates these correlations. It is of interest that the synthetic compounds, when compared with cortisol, appear to exert a somewhat more intense effect on nitrogen balance than on the other indices. This finding alone would serve to predict that some of the undesirable overdosage effects of these analogs would be of equal or even greater intensity than those induced by cortisol. This has been borne out.

Although prednisolone, 6-methylprednisolone and triamcinolone do possess greater potency than cortisol as anti-inflammatory agents, this fact alone is of little importance. The preparation of superior corticosteroids for use in nonspecific therapy requires that the therapeutic ratio be significantly improved and this, in turn, necessitates the dissociation of anti-inflammatory activity and the glucocorticoid effects of these steroids.

CORTICOSTEROID METABOLISM

The cellular mechanisms whereby corticosteroids exert their numerous effects are not known. Therefore, the manner in which alterations of steroid structure increase or lessen steroid activities remains unexplained. Theoretically, a change in potency may result from changes in intrinsic activity of the steroid or from alterations in metabolism of the steroid. Comparison of the approximate glucocorticoid potencies of several steroids with their plasma half-times (Table 3) makes it clear that there is little correlation

TABLE 3. PLASMA HALF-TIMES vs. ANTI-INFLAMMATORY
ACTIVITY OF STEROIDS

	PLASMA HALF-TIMES (mins.)	GLUCOCORTICOID ACTIVITY
Cortisone	30	0.8
Cortisol	110	1
Prednisone	60	4
Prednisolone	200	4
6-Methylprednisolone	190*	5
Triamcinolone	..	5
Dexamethasone	200	25

* Data of Jenkins and Schemmel;[12] other half-times from Peterson.[20]

between biologic activity and the rate at which a given steroid is removed from the plasma. However, the considerable differences in disappearance rates do indicate that modifications of steroid structure must cause significant changes in steroid metabolism. A few such changes have been identified.

Following administration of prednisolone, about 10 per cent of its total urinary excretory product is free, unconjugated prednisolone. This is about five times as great as the amount of free steroid found after the administration of cortisol.[21] In addition, the reduced 20-alcohol derivatives of prednisone and prednisolone are found in urine after the administration of these steroids[8] but tetrahydro- derivatives have not been found. Reduction of the Δ^4-3-ketone group of prednisolone by rat liver homogenates occurs only at a very slow rate.[25] Finally, Nugent et al.[16] have concluded, from studies in normal subjects and in patients with hepatic or renal disease, that the metabolism of prednisolone is largely the result of degradation in organs other than the liver or kidney. This is in direct contrast to the normal mechanisms for the disposal of cortisol. Apparently, 1,2 dehydrogenation stabilizes the A ring of prednisolone. Other facets of the metabolism of the synthetic corticosteroids remain to be explored.

That the metabolism of the analogs of cortisol differs from that of cortisol itself is not surprising. It is possible that these differences serve to stabilize or protect active functional groups essential for anti-inflammatory activity (e.g.: C-3 = O, C-11 = OH, and C-17 = COCH$_2$OH). It is perhaps more likely that the intrinsic capacity of the modified steroids to influence metabolic processes, presumably at an enzymatic level, is augmented. At any rate, the factors responsible for the qualitative and quantitative differences in activity of the various steroids are not yet known.

SIDE EFFECTS

The continuing search for new steroid agents has been stimulated largely by the relatively high incidence of undesirable overdosage effects produced by the natural steroids, cortisone and cortisol. Consequently, the relative incidence of side effects encountered with the synthetic analogs is a factor of some importance in evaluating their usefulness. Table 4 summarizes the

TABLE 4. *RELATIVE INCIDENCE OF CORTICOSTEROID SIDE EFFECTS*

	CORTISONE	CORTISOL	PREDNISONE PREDNISOLONE	6-METHYL- PREDNISOLONE	TRIAMCINOLONE
Equivalent anti-inflammatory dose (mg.)	25	20	5	4	4
Edema	+ + +	+ + +	+	±	0
Moon face	+ +	+ +	+ +	+ +	+ +
Hirsutism	+ +	+ +	+ +	+ +	+ + +
Hyperphagia and weight gain	+ +	+ +	+ +	+	0 or −
Purpura, ecchymoses	+	+	+ +	+ +	+ + +
Striae, flushing	+	+	+	+	+ + +
Muscle weakness	+ +	+ +	+	+	+ + +
Osteoporosis	+ + +	+ + +	+ + +	+ + +	+ + +
Peptic ulcer	+ +	+ +	+ + to + + +	+ + to + + +	+ + to + + +
Diabetes	+ +	+ +	+ +	+ +	+ +
Mental stimulation	+ +	+	+ +	+	0 or −

comparative therapeutic doses and common side effects of cortisone, cortisol, prednisone and prednisolone, 6-methylprednisolone and triamcinolone.*
It is evident that all of the agents produce, in some degree, most of the untoward effects listed. However, it is also apparent that some differences do exist, and it is these differences which now largely control the selection of steroids for clinical use. The major advantage possessed by the synthetic analogs is a significant reduction in edema formation. Unfortunately, they show no decrease in the capacity to induce osteoporosis, to precipitate diabetes mellitus and to aggravate peptic ulcers.

Prednisone and prednisolone have been widely employed and, in many clinics, are still the most frequently used corticosteroids. Prednisone and prednisolone are essentially equal in potency and side effects and are interchangeable. There is general agreement that these agents cause a higher incidence of cutaneous ecchymoses and vasomotor symptoms than either cortisone or cortisol. Whether they are also more prone to produce or aggravate peptic ulcers is subject to some debate.

Side effects due to 6-methylprednisolone appear to be essentially similar in kind and degree to those induced by prednisolone.

The undesirable reactions occurring during triamcinolone administration are of particular interest because this agent has produced some reactions not ordinarily encountered with other steroids. Bright erythema and flushing of the face, neck, forearms and hands occasionally occur. Nausea, bloating, abdominal cramps and pain sometimes appear, without peptic ulcer formation, in the very first days of treatment. Severe headaches, often accompanied by dizziness, lethargy, easy fatigability and somnolence, may occur. When these difficulties are prominent, anorexia and weight loss sometimes supervene. The anorexia may be rather severe. Mild weight loss at the start of treatment, probably due to sodium and water diuresis, occurs frequently. In some patients weight loss is progressive and severe. The factors involved appear to include anorexia, chronic dehydration and the catabolic loss of tissue.[6] Evidence for the latter is seen in the severe muscle wasting which sometimes occurs, accompanied by advanced muscle weakness. The myopathy due to corticosteroids involves mainly the muscles of the thighs, pelvis and low back. Similar degrees of myopathy have been encountered with other steroids,[19] But the incidence is apparently higher with high-dosage triamcinolone treatment. Furthermore, replacement of triamcinolone with other steroids has resulted in gradual recovery. In almost all reported cases of myopathy due to triamcinolone, serum potassium levels have been normal, although Dameshek and Rubio[4] encountered hypokalemia in one patient with severe involvement. Since persistent urinary potassium loss does occur in some subjects during the administration of large doses of triamcinolone,[17] supplemental potassium should be used when this type of therapy is employed. In all likelihood, potassium should be given when high dosages of any active corticosteroid are employed in long-term treatment. On the other hand, potassium administration has usually failed to prevent steroid myopa-

---

* A more precise comparison, giving the statistical incidence of side effects, is difficult because of wide variations in dosage, duration of therapy and the types of patients recorded in clinical reports. In addition, many of the reports concerning the newer agents are based on short-term use. An accurate assessment of steroid toxicity requires time, measured in years.

The scheme employed in Table 4 is modified from Hollander[10] and is largely based on the effects of these agents in patients with rheumatoid arthritis.

thy and, in such cases, the pathogenesis is not known. A direct effect on mechanisms involved in the synthesis or breakdown of muscle proteins may well be involved.

SUMMARY

The production of synthetic cortisol analogs has proved useful, and the chemists responsible for the synthesis of these and related steroids deserve high commendation for their skill and resourcefulness. Much has been learned concerning structure-function relationships of corticosteroids.

An increase in therapeutic potency offers no advantages unless the therapeutic ratio of the steroid is improved. Reduction of mineralocorticoid activity has improved the ratio, but the side effects which reflect glucocorticoid activity and offer the greatest threat to the patient's safety have not been materially altered.

The availability of several synthetic analogs is helpful in some degree since the differences in side effects exerted by these agents have become a major factor in the selection of steroids for use in specific patients or clinical situations.

As yet, an ideal corticosteroid for therapeutic use in inflammatory disorders has not been found.

REFERENCES

1. Bernstein, S. et al.: 16-Hydroxylated steroids. IV. The synthesis of 16α-hydroxy derivatives of 9α-halo steroids. J. Am. Chem. Soc., 78:5693, 1956.
2. Boland, E. W.: The treatment of rheumatoid arthritis with adrenocorticosteroids and their synthetic analogs; an appraisal of certain developments of the past decade. Ann. N. Y. Acad. Sc., 82:887, 1959.
3. Bunim, J. J., Pechet, M. M. and Bollet, A. J.: Studies on metacortandralone and metacortandracin in rheumatoid arthritis; antirheumatic potency, metabolic effects and hormonal properties. J.A.M.A., 157:311, 1955.
4. Dameshek, W. and Rubio, F., Jr.: Drug reactions. (Letter.) J.A.M.A., 167:2117, 1958.
5. Dulin, W. E., Barnes, L. E., Glenn, E. M., Lyster, S. C and Collins, E. J.: Biologic activities of some C-21 steroids and some 6-methyl-C-21 steroids. Metabolism, 7:398, 1958.
6. Freyberg, R. H., Bernstein, C. A., Jr. and Hellman, L.: Further experiences with Δ¹,9α-fluoro-16α-hydroxyhydrocortisone (triamcinolone) in treatment of patients with rheumatoid arthritis. Arth. & Rheum., 1:215, 1958.
7 Fried, J. and Borman, A.: Synthetic derivatives of cortical hormones. Vitamins and Hormones, 16:304, 1958.
8. Gray, C. H., Green, M. A. S., Holness, N. J. and Lunnon, J. R.: Urinary metabolic products of prednisone and prednisolone. J. Endocrinol., 14:146, 1956.
9. Herzog, H. L. et al.: New anti-arthritic steroids. Science, 121:176, 1955.
10. Hollander, J. L.: Clinical use of dexamethazone. J.A.M.A., 172:306, 1960.
11. Jenkins, D.: Comparative metabolic effects of synthetic corticosteroids. In Mills, L. C. and Moyer, J. H. (eds.): Inflammation and Diseases of Connective Tissues. Philadelphia, W. B. Saunders Co., 1961, p. 424.
12. Jenkins, D. and Schemmel, J. E.: Metabolic effects of 6-methylprednisolone. Metabolism, 7:416, 1958.
13. Kupperman, H. S., Blatt, M. H. G., Vessell, M., Gagliani, J., Weisbader, H. and Vosburg, L.: Comparative effects of metacortandracin, 9α-fluorohydrocortisone and hydrocortisone upon ACTH secretion in man. J. Clin. Endocrinol., 15:911, 1955.
14. Kupperman, H. S., Peh-Ping Ho and Epstein, J. A.: Comparative pharmacologic studies on prednisone, 6-methylprednisolone and triamcinolone. Metabolism, 7:463, 1958.
15. Liddle, G. W.: Effects of anti-inflammatory steroids on electrolyte metabolism. Ann. N. Y. Acad. Sc., 82:854, 1959.

16. Nugent, C. A., Eik-Nes, K. and Tyler, F. H.: A comparative study of the metabolism of hydrocortisone and prednisolone. J. Clin. Endocrinol., 19:526, 1959.
17. Pechet, M. M.: The metabolic effects of steroid hormones: effects on renal excretion of sodium and potassium. (Abstr.) Acta Endocrinol. (Suppl), 51:811, 1960.
18. Pechet, M. M., Bowers, B. and Bartter, F. C.: Metabolic studies with a new series of 1,4-diene steroids. II. Effects in normal subjects of prednisone, prednisolone and 9α-fluoroprednisolone. J. Clin. Invest., 38:691, 1959.
19. Perkoff, G. T, Silber, R., Tyler, F. H., Cartwright, G. E. and Wintrobe, M. M.: Studies in disorders of muscle. XII. Myopathy due to the administration of therapeutic amounts of 17-hydroxycorticosteroids. Am. J. Med., 26:891, 1959.
20. Peterson, R. E.: Metabolism of adrenocorticosteroids in man. Ann. N. Y. Acad. Sc., 82:846, 1959.
21. Sandberg, A. A. and Slaunwhite, W. R., Jr., Differences in metabolism of prednisolone-C14 and cortisol-C14. J. Clin. Endocrinol., 9:1040, 1957.
22. Spero, G. B. et al.: Adrenal hormones and related compounds. IV. 6-Methyl steroids. J. Am. Chem. Soc.,78:6213, 1956.
23. Swingle, W. W., Brannick, L. J., Osborn, O. and Glenister, D.: Effect of gluco- and mineralocorticoid adrenal steroids on fluid and electrolytes of fasted adrenalectomized dogs. Proc. Soc. Exper. Biol & Med., 96:446, 1957.
24. Tolksdorf, S.: Laboratory evaluation of anti-inflammatory steroids. Ann. N. Y. Acad. Sc., 82:829, 1959.
25. Tomkins, G. and Isselbacher, K. J.: Enzymatic reduction of cortisone. J. Am. Chem. Soc., 76:3100, 1954.
26. West, K. M.: Relative eosinopenic and hyperglycemic potencies of glucocorticoids in man. Metabolism, 7:441, 1958.

Metabolic and Hormonal Effects of Dexamethasone

JOSEPH J. BUNIM

National Institute of Arthritis and Metabolic Diseases

Dexamethasone is an analog of prednisolone to which have been added a fluorine atom at carbon 9 and a methyl radical at carbon 16, both substituents being in the alpha position. This compound was synthesized independently by two groups of workers in 1958, Arth and his associates[1] and Oliveto and his collaborators.[9] Both teams employed the same raw materials, desoxycholic acid, and the same synthetic process.

In the rat, Arth and co-workers[1] found that the glucocorticoid, mineralocorticoid and anti-inflammatory potencies of dexamethasone were many times greater than those of hydrocortisone as measured by the following parameters: adrenal atrophy, 700 times hydrocortisone; involution of thymus, 400 times hydrocortisone; granuloma inhibition, 190 times hydrocortisone; body weight depression, 100 times hydrocortisone; and glycogen deposition, 17 times hydrocortisone.

In adrenalectomized rats, dexamethasone produced neither sodium retention nor potassium loss.

At the National Institute of Arthritis and Metabolic Diseases, we have studied the metabolic and hormonal effects of dexamethasone on patients with rheumatoid arthritis and on normal subjects.[3, 4] In normal subjects, one mg. of dexamethasone given orally at midnight was sufficient to reduce the plasma level of hydrocortisone to zero by 8 A.M. In the same subjects, 2.0 mg. of Δ^1, 9α-fluorohydrocortisone and 5.0 mg. of 9α-fluorohydrocortisone were required to produce the same results. In 27 patients with rheumatoid arthritis, the dexamethasone/prednisone ratio of antirheumatic potency ranged from 10 to 2.5 and averaged 6.0.

Despite the striking suppression of hydrocortisone production by small doses of dexamethasone, aldosterone production and responsiveness to sodium loss or deprivation remained unimpaired even when 6.0 mg. of this synthetic corticosteroid were given daily. (Table 1).

TABLE 1. *CHANGES IN URINARY ALDOSTERONE EXCRETION RELATED TO SODIUM INTAKE, SODIUM EXCRETION AND DEXAMETHASONE ADMINISTRATION (6 mg. daily) IN A NORMAL SUBJECT**

DATE	SODIUM INTAKE AMOUNT (mEq./day)	NO. DAYS	URINARY SODIUM EXCRETION (mEq./day)	URINARY POTASSIUM EXCRETION (mEq./day)	NO. OF DAYS DEXAMETHA- SONE ADMIN- ISTERED (6 mg./day)	URINARY ALDO- STERONE EXCRETION (μg./day)
4/14-15	87.0	6	75.5	132.6	0	12
4/20-21	8.7	6†	6.1	122.2	0	32
4/21-22	8.7	7	6.9	158.3	1	36
4/24-25	8.7	10	12.5	110.9	4	32
4/28-29	8.7	14	19.3	122.7	8	38
5/2-3	8.7	18	9.2	126.8	12	58
5/7-8	8.7	23	1.4	124.8	5 days after stopping dexamethasone	70

* Potassium intake remained constant at 6.0 Gm. daily.
† Low sodium diet was started on April 15.

Results of metabolic balance studies on a 28-year-old woman with rheumatoid arthritis who was ambulatory are graphically summarized in Figure 1.* As indicated in the chart, three dosage schedules of dexamethasone (MK 125) were followed: 2, 6 and 10 mg. daily. A slight diuresis of sodium occurred at 6 and 10 mg. dosage and significant retention of sodium upon withdrawal. Dexamethasone produced no change in potassium balance at any dosage level. A definite increase in nitrogen excretion is noted as the dose of the steroid is increased. At 10 mg. daily, with an intake of 11.5 grams of nitrogen daily a slightly negative nitrogen balance developed.

The most notable effect of dexamethasone relates to calcium and phosphorus balances. A marked increase in calcium excretion and a negative balance occurred when 6 mg. dosage was reached. At this level, 1.05 grams of calcium was excreted daily. Negative calcium balance persisted for six days after the drug was discontinued. Increased losses of calcium were accounted for almost entirely by increased fecal excretion and were apparent only to a slight extent in urinary excretion. Both urinary and fecal phosphorus excretion increased as the dosage of dexamethasone was increased and a negative phosphorus balance resulted.

* These studies were done by G. Donald Whedon and Leo Lutwak of the National Institute of Arthritis and Metabolic Diseases.

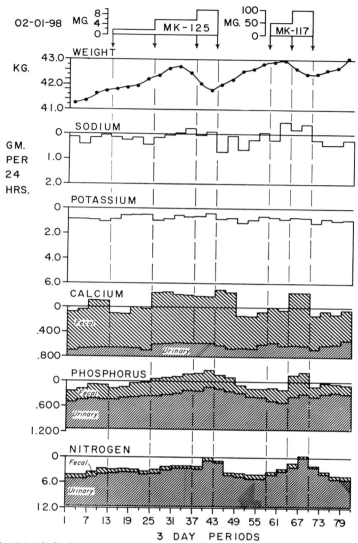

Fig. 1. Metabolic balance studies in a 28-year-old female patient (ambulatory) with rheumatoid arthritis before, during and after administration of dexamethasone (MK-125) and 16α-methyl hydrocortisone (MK-117) in varying dosages. (Bunim: Arth. & Rheum., 1:113, 1958.)

CARBOHYDRATE METABOLISM

The initial impression obtained from bio-assay studies on glycogen deposition in rat liver that dexamethasone might have a significantly lower diabetogenic effect than the other anti-inflammatory synthetic steroids was not borne out in man when dexamethasone was administered for many months. In Table 2 are listed five patients taken from a group of 27 with rheumatoid arthritis treated with prolonged dexamethasone therapy. These five patients showed progressive impairment of glucose utilization during the administration of dexamethasone in doses of 0.5 to 4.0 mg. daily. One of these patients had normal, and another only moderately impaired, function while receiving a related steroid, 16α-methyl prednisone. One had had borderline function while taking triamcinolone. The other two had been receiving aspirin only, prior to dexamethasone, and both had normal function when first studied. Six other patients, not included in Table 2, had diabetic or borderline glucose utilization rates throughout the period of the study. Another group of six continued to have normal rates.

Bastenie and coworkers[2] have demonstrated that although impairment of carbohydrate metabolism occurs almost universally early in the course of corticosteroid administration, in most cases function returns to normal

TABLE 2. PATIENTS SHOWING INCREASING IMPAIRMENT OF THE GLUCOSE UTILIZATION RATE DURING DEXAMETHASONE ADMINISTRATION

CASE	PREVIOUS THERAPY, DAILY DOSE	DEXAMETHASONE, DAILY MAINTENANCE DOSE (mg.)	PRIOR TO DEXAMETHASONE	GLUCOSE UTILIZATION RATE*			
				DURING DEXAMETHASONE ADMINISTRATION			
				1-3 MOS.	4-6 MOS.	7-9 MOS.	10-12 MOS.
J.R.	16-Methyl prednisone 8 mgms.	0.5	Normal (OGTT)†		Borderline (2.7)		
I.M.	16-Methyl prednisone 8 mgms.	3.0-1.0	Borderline (2.6)	Diabetic (2.4)		Diabetic (1.7)	
M.Bl.	Aspirin 3.6 gms.	4.0-3.5	..‡	Normal (3.0)	Normal (2.9)	Diabetic (1.9)	
N.A.	Triamcinolone 8 mgms.	3.5	Borderline (2.6)	Diabetic (1.9)			
C.D.	Aspirin 3.6 gms.	1.0-0.5	..‡	Normal (3.4)	Diabetic (2.3)		Diabetic (2.2)

* Glucose utilization rates were determined by the method of Amatuzio et al. (J. Clin. Invest., 32: 428, 1953). The K values in parentheses represent the rate of disappearance of administered glucose (excess above fasting level) in per cent disappearing per minute.
Normal   2.97 to 4.85
Borderline 2.46 to 2.97
Diabetic   less than 2.46
† OGTT = Oral Glucose Tolerance Test.
‡ Dashes indicate procedure not performed.

in the face of continued corticosteroid therapy. It has been suggested by Fajans and Conn[5] that the islets of Langerhans may respond with increased function to the hyperglycemic effect of the adrenal corticosteroids. Hyperplasia and hypertrophy of the islet cells have been observed by Houssay[7] in animals experiencing corticosteroid suppression of carbohydrate metabolism. Hence, the development of a diabetic state secondary to glucocorticoid excess is probably related directly to the individual's capacity to increase insulin production.[6]

Dexamethasone has been compared to triamcinolone and to hydrocortisone in terms of anti-insulin effect in a diabetic patient.[8] Dexamethasone, 3 mg. daily, produced a greater increase in insulin requirement (40 to 180 U.) than either prednisone, 30 mg. daily (40 to 100 U.), or triamcinolone, 20 mg. daily (40 to 120 U.).

The glucosuric effect of dexamethasone has also been compared to that of other corticosteroids. Frawley[6] found dexamethasone in dosage of 3 mg. daily equivalent to cortisone 100 mg. daily and hydrocortisone 80 mg. daily in the production of glucosuria in a diabetic patient. Slater et al.,[10] also studying a diabetic patient, found a similar ratio in that dexamethasone, 2.4 mg. daily, produced glucosuria comparable to that produced by cortisone, 90 mg. daily.

Since neither fasting hyperglycemia nor glucosuria was demonstrated in our group of 27 patients, it appears that none suffered exhaustion of the "insulin-producing reserve" even after receiving therapeutic doses of dexamethasone for eight to ten months. The variability in extent of the "reserve" in different patients and at different times in the same patient was reflected by different degrees of impairment of the glucose utilization rate.

REFERENCES

1. Arth, G. E., Johnston, D. B. R., Fried, J., Spooncer, W. W., Hoff, D. R. and Sarett, L. H.: 16-Methylated Steroids. 1. 16α-Methylated analogs of cortisone, a new group of anti-inflammatory steroids. J. Am. Chem. Soc., 80:3160, 1958.
2. Bastenie, P. A., Conard, V. C. and Franckson, J. R. M.: Effect of cortisone on carbohydrate metabolism measured by the "glucose assimilation coefficient." Diabetes, 3: 205, 1954.
3. Black, R. L., Reefe, W. E., David, J. R., Bloch, K. J., Ehrlich, G. E. and Bunim, J. J.: Dexamethasone: Antirheumatic properties, hormonal effects and adverse reactions (a 16-month study) Arth. & Rheum., 3:112, 1960.
4. Bunim, J. J., Black, R. L., Lutwak, L., Peterson, R. E. and Whedon, G. D.: Studies on dexamethasone, a new synthetic steroid, in rheumatoid arthritis. A preliminary report. Adrenal cortical, metabolic and early clinical effects. Arth. & Rheum., 1:313, 1958.
5. Fajans, S. S. and Conn, J W.: An approach to the prediction of diabetes mellitus by modification of the glucose tolerance test with cortisone. Diabetes, 3:246, 1954.
6. Frawley, T. F., Shelley, T. and Kistler, H.: Effects of anti-inflammatory steroids on carbohydrate metabolism, with emphasis on hypoglycemia and diabetic states. Ann. New York Acad. Sc., 82:868, 1959.
7. Houssay, B. A., Rodriguez, R. R. and Cardeza, A. F.: Prevention of experimental diabetes with adrenal steroids. Endocrinology, 54:550, 1954.
8. Lichtwitz, A., Hioco, D. and Greale, C.: Intolerances, incidents et accidents provoqués par la dexamethasone (16 MFP). Semaine des Hopitaux, 35:12, 1959.
9. Oliveto, E. P. et al.: 16-Alkylated corticoids. I. 16α-Methylprednisone and 16β-methylprednisone. J. Am. Chem. Soc., 80:4428, 1958.
10. Slater, J. D. H., Heffron, P. F., Vernet, A. and Nabarro, J. D. N.: Clinical and metabolic effects of dexamethasone. Lancet, 1:173, 1959.

Metabolic Effects of the Natural Steroids and the 1,4-Diene Steroids

MAURICE M. PECHET

Massachusetts General Hospital, Boston

Following the demonstration of the therapeutic efficacy of prednisone and prednisolone,[7, 10] the first synthetically prepared steroids possessing enhanced anti-inflammatory activities without a concomitant increase in tubular reabsorption of sodium,[13] a number of analogues of these two steroids were synthesized and tested for anti-inflammatory activity. The analogues which have been subjected to the most extensive clinical trial all contain the chemical structural modification characteristic of prednisone and prednisolone, namely, an extra double bond between carbon atoms 1 and 2 of the steroid nucleus, as illustrated in Figure 1. Since these steroids contain two double bonds, one between carbon atoms 1 and 2 and the other between carbon atoms 4 and 5, they may be referred to collectively as the 1,4-diene steroids.

In this presentation we shall compare the metabolic effects of some of the 1,4-diene steroids with those of the naturally occurring steroids, cortisone and cortisol, in an attempt to correlate physiologic activities with

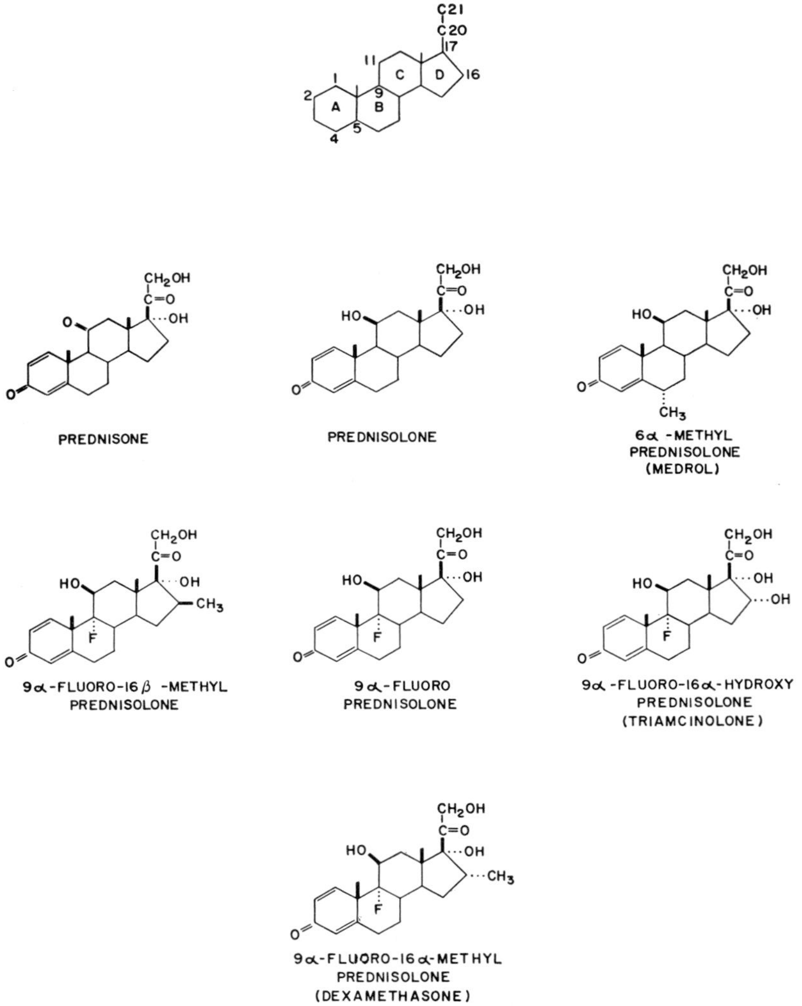

Fig. 1.   Structural formulae of some 1,4-diene steroids.

chemical structure and to inquire into the mechanism involved in the decrease in sodium retention resulting from the introduction of the extra double bond (1,2-dehydrogenation). The presentation will emphasize the metabolic effects of prednisone and prednisolone, since they are the parent members of the 1,4-diene steroid series and consequently have been investigated more extensively; in addition, the metabolic effects of the other members of the 1,4-diene steroid series are, for the most part, similar to those of prednisone and prednisolone, although there are differences of a quantitative nature.

THE EOSINOPENIC EFFECT

In man, prednisone and prednisolone are four to six times as active as the parent compounds, cortisone and cortisol, in causing a reduction in the number of circulating eosinophiles[15] (see, for example, Figure 2). 9α-Fluoro-

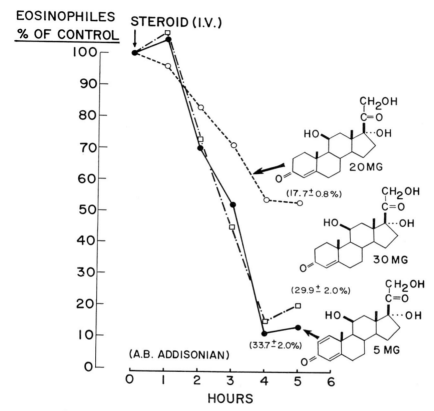

Fig. 2.   The effect of cortisol and prednisolone on circulating eosinophiles four hours after injection. Steroids were given intravenously over 10-minute periods. The average rate of depletion per hour has been determined from the slope of the linear regression and is indicated within parentheses. (Adapted, by permission, from Pechet et al.[15])

cortisol is about two and one-half times as active as cortisol, and 9α-fluoroprednisolone is about sixteen to twenty times as active as cortisol.[24] The effects of 1,2-dehydrogenation and of 9α-fluorination appear to be additive. Replacement of the 6α-hydrogen of prednisolone by a methyl group does not alter the activity of the parent steroid, prednisolone. Replacement of the 16α-hydrogen of 9α-fluoroprednisolone by a hydroxyl group (triamcinolone) decreases (by a factor of four) the activity on circulating eosinophiles of the parent steroid, 9α-fluoroprednisolone. Substitution of a methyl group (dexamethasone) for the 16α-hydrogen of 9α-fluoroprednisolone increases (by a factor of about two) the activity of the parent steroid.

The introduction of a double bond at position 1-2 increases the eosinopenic activity of steroids originally possessing this property, and in one instance this property was conferred by 1,2-dehydrogenation on an eosinopenic-inactive steroid, corticosterone.[15]

NITROGEN METABOLISM

Nitrogen loss, which has been ascribed to anti-anabolism of protoplasm,[1] is characteristically associated with those steroids which exhibit anti-inflammatory activity. The chemical structural requirements for anti-anabolism or catabolism are represented in cortisone and cortisol. An oxygen atom at carbon 11 is essential; in the absence of it, anti-anabolic activity is lacking. Cortisol, which has an oxygen atom at carbon 11, produces nitrogen loss upon administration in appropriate doses, whereas 17α-hydroxydesoxycorticosterone, which lacks the 11-oxygen atom, does not (see, for example, Figure 3).

CUMULATIVE N EXCRETION

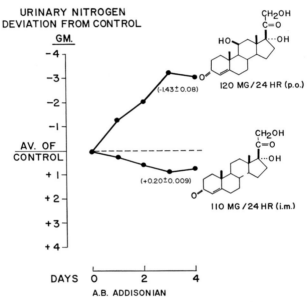

Fig. 3. The effect of cortisol and 17α-hydroxydesoxycorticosterone on nitrogen excretion expressed as the mean daily difference between treatment and control periods. The daily deviation from control is plotted cumulatively. The daily average rate of nitrogen excretion has been determined from the slope of the linear regression and is indicated within parentheses.

1,2-Dehydrogenation of cortisone and cortisol induces a marked enhancement of anti-anabolic activity. As illustrated in Figure 4, the 1,4-diene steroids, prednisone and prednisolone, appear to be seven to eight times as active as the parent steroids in normal subjects.[16] The effects on nitrogen metabolism are more pronounced in addisonian subjects.[15] The effects of prednisone and prednisolone on nitrogen metabolism are not altered by 6α-methylation; Medrol is quantitatively similar to prednisolone. However, the effects of prednisone and prednisolone on nitrogen metabolism are reduced by 16α-hydroxylation; 16α-hydroxycortisol is one-third to one-quarter as active as is the parent, cortisol,[14] and 16α-hydroxy-9α-fluoroprednisolone (triamcinolone) is much less active than its parent, 9α-fluoroprednisolone, and is equal to prednisolone. Conversely, the effects on nitrogen metabolism

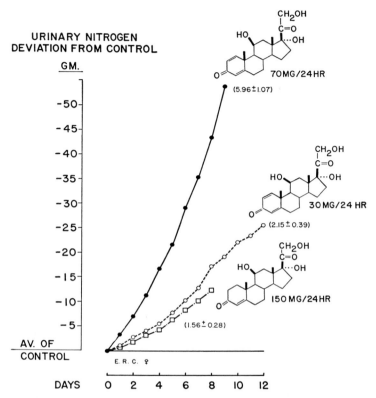

CUMULATIVE N EXCRETION

Fig. 4. The effect of cortisol and prednisolone on nitrogen excretion expressed as the mean daily difference between treatment and control periods. (Adapted, by permission, from Pechet et al.[16])

are enhanced by 16-methylation; 16α-methylprednisolone induces a slightly larger nitrogen loss than does the parent, prednisolone. Substitution of a methyl group at carbon 16 in the β conformation has a similar effect.[12]

CALCIUM METABOLISM

The effects of the 1,4-diene steroids on calcium metabolism vary with the dose and the duration of administration of the steroid. When prednisone and prednisolone are administered in doses of 30 mg. and less, hypercalciuria does not usually result. Cortisone and cortisol in doses four to five times as large may cause a decrease in urinary calcium, and when this occurs, it is generally accompanied by sodium retention and weight gain. When "escape" from sodium retention occurs, "escape" from calcium retention follows. The administration of large doses of 1,4-diene steroids and of the natural steroids, cortisone and cortisol, results in hypercalciuria of a magnitude representing loss of bone tissue. Qualitatively, the effects on calcium metabolism of the various 1,4-diene steroids are similar; quantitatively, some differences are apparent. Initial studies indicate that 9α-fluoro-16α-hydroxyprednisolone (triamcinolone) and 9α-fluoro-16α-methylprednisolone (dexamethasone) exert a more pronounced effect leading to a larger excretion of urinary calcium and especially of fecal calcium.

PHOSPHORUS METABOLISM

The changes in phosphorus metabolism vary with the dose and duration of administration of the steroids. When phosphorus loss does occur during the administration of cortisone, cortisol, prednisone or prednisolone, the loss

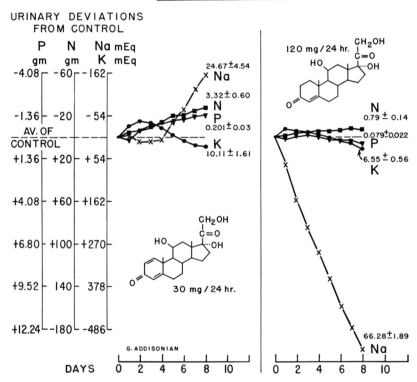

Fig. 5. The effect of cortisol and prednisolone on phosphorus, nitrogen, sodium and potassium excretions expressed as the mean daily difference between treatment and control periods. The daily deviation from control is plotted cumulatively. The daily average rate of phosphorus, nitrogen, sodium and potassium excretion has been determined from the slope of the linear regression and is indicated for each element.

is always *less* than that anticipated from the concomitant loss of nitrogen (see, for example, Figure 5). A retention of phosphorus during steroid-induced nitrogen loss has been attributed to concomitant glycogen formation.[19] To date, triamcinolone (9α-fluoro-16α-hydroxyprednisolone) is the only 1,4-diene steroid which induces a *larger* loss of phosphorus than of nitrogen. Since triamcinolone is one of the most potent steroids in inducing glycogen deposition in animal assays[5, 20, 22] (ten to forty times cortisol), the phosphorus loss induced by triamcinolone should be less than that induced by cortisol or prednisolone rather than more, and should be less than the concomitant loss of nitrogen rather than more. It appears that for triamcinolone the discrepancy in the loss of phosphorus cannot be attributed to concomitant glycogen formation (*vide infra*).

SODIUM METABOLISM

Cortisone and cortisol in large doses generally induce sodium retention, whereas sodium *loss* generally occurs with the administration of prednisone and prednisolone at corresponding therapeutic dose levels. As illustrated in Figure 5, cortisol produced sodium retention of 66.28 ± 1.89 mEq./24 hrs., whereas prednisolone at an equivalent therapeutic dose caused sodium loss of 24.67 ± 4.54 mEq./24 hrs.

Prednisone and prednisolone are four to five times more effective than are cortisone or cortisol in causing an increase in glomerular filtration rate.[15] This enhancement parallels the enhancement of anti-anabolic activity and occurs without apparent change in tubular sodium transport. The sodium loss induced by prednisone and prednisolone is probably the result of the increase in glomerular filtration rate.

The effects of cortisol and prednisolone on sodium metabolism are markedly altered by substitution of a fluorine atom for the 9α-hydrogen atom. As seen in Figure 6, 9α-fluoroprednisolone and 9α-fluorocortisol caused marked sodium retention which is accompanied by potassium loss and hypokalemia. Further chemical alterations of the fluorinated steroids involving hydrogen replacement at carbon 16 by a 16α-hydroxyl group or a 16-methyl group result in nullification of the sodium-retaining properties conferred upon these steroids by 9α-fluorination and may result in promoting sodium loss. Whereas 16α-hydroxylation brings about a reduction in the anti-anabolic activity, 16-methylation gives rise to an enhancement of anti-anabolic activity (*vide supra*). Therefore, 9α-fluoro-16α-hydroxyprednisolone (triamcinolone), although devoid of salt-retaining properties, is a less active anti-anabolic and anti-inflammatory steroid than is the parent, 9α-fluoroprednisolone. The beneficial effects on sodium metabolism result only from the correct conformational chemical alteration of 9α-fluoroprednisolone; the 16α-hydroxy isomer is active, whereas the 16β isomer is inactive.[6] However, both the 16α- and the 16β-methyl isomers of 9α-fluoroprednisolone are active. Heretofore, anti-anabolic activity has been associated with only one of a pair of steroid epimers.

POTASSIUM METABOLISM

The effects of cortisone, cortisol, prednisone and prednisolone on potassium metabolism represent the summation of at least four independent phenomena: (1) the immediate, transient loss of potassium during the first 24 hours of steroid administration and the corresponding transient retention of potassium on withdrawal of the steroid. These changes precede changes in nitrogen and sodium metabolism (see, for example, Figure 6). This potassium "on and off" phenomenon has been attributed to the anti-inflammatory action of steroids.[3] (2) Some loss of potassium occurs when large losses of nitrogen are induced with large doses of steroids. However, the potassium loss is always less than the nitrogen loss (see, for example, Figure 5) except during the administration of triamcinolone, in which case the potassium loss is greater than the nitrogen loss.[18] (3) Potassium loss occurs when sodium is retained, and potassium retention occurs when sodium is lost, independent of changes in nitrogen metabolism (see, for example, Figure 6). This phenomenon probably represents the result of the potentiation by the steroid of the sodium-potassium exchange process at the renal tubular level.[2, 4, 11] (4) During the administration of cortisone, cortisol, prednisone and prednisolone, potassium loss is always less than nitrogen loss (*vide supra*). This has been attributed to a concomitant deposition of glycogen.[19] As noted above, a similar discrepancy in phosphorus metabolism has been attributed to glycogen formation. To date, triamcinolone is the only 1,4-diene steroid which induces a loss of potassium and of phosphorus which

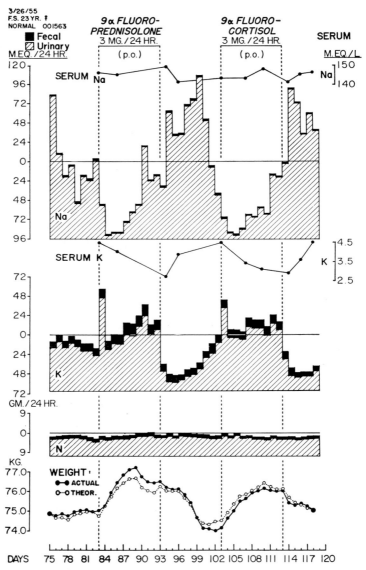

Fig. 6. The effect of 9α-fluoroprednisolone and 9α-fluorocortisol on sodium, potassium and nitrogen balances, serum sodium, potassium, and actual and "theoretical" body weight. (Reported, by permission, from Pechet et al.[16])

is greater than the loss of nitrogen. The magnitude of glycogen formation induced by triamcinolone in animal assays is greater than that induced by other 1,4-diene steroids. Therefore, the loss of potassium and of phosphorus should be less rather than more. The large losses of potassium and of phosphorus associated with triamcinolone administration probably represent the result of the enhanced effect of triamcinolone on intracellular fluid changes.

IN VIVO METABOLISM OF ADMINISTERED STEROIDS

Following the administration of prednisolone to an addisonian subject, six urinary metabolites were isolated and characterized.[8] These and other

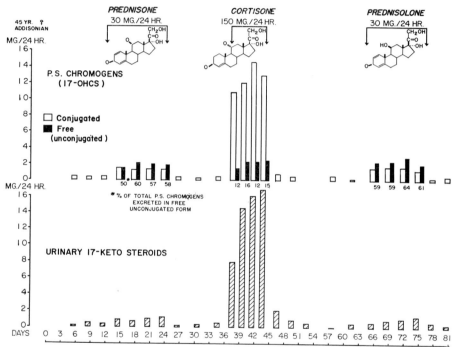

Fig. 7.   The effect of prednisone, cortisone and prednisolone on urinary free and conjugated phenylhydrazine-sulfuric acid chromogens and on urinary 17-ketosteroids in a patient with Addison's disease. (Reported, by permission, from Pechet et al.[16])

studies[9, 21, 23] indicate that the in vivo metabolism of prednisolone is similar to that of cortisol. However, there are differences, albeit of a quantitative nature, in the metabolism of cortisol and prednisolone. As illustrated in Figure 7, during the administration of prednisolone, 17-ketosteroids were excreted at much lower levels than during the administration of cortisol. This is a result of the limited conversion of 1,4-diene steroids to 17-keto-steroids.[17] As illustrated in the same figure, a larger portion (50 to 64 per cent) of the metabolites of prednisone and prednisolone than of the parent steroid, cortisone (12 to 16 per cent), is excreted in the free, unconjugated state. This difference could result from a slower rate of reduction of the two double bonds in the 1,4-diene steroids. These two differences in the metabolism of the 1,4-diene steroids may result in prolonged duration of action of the 1,4-diene steroids and may thereby be related to the enhanced anti-anabolic and anti-inflammatory activities.

SUMMARY

The anti-anabolic and anti-inflammatory properties of steroids are enhanced by 1, 2-dehydrogenation. 6α-Methylation has very little effect on these properties. 9α-Fluorination confers on these steroids strong salt-retaining properties which can be nullified by 16α-hydroxylation and by 16α- or 16β-methylation.

Triamcinolone differs from the other 1,4-diene steroids in that it causes a loss of potassium and of phosphorus greater than the loss of nitrogen. With the administration of cortisone, cortisol, prednisone or prednisolone, changes in potassium and phosphorus metabolism are less than changes in nitrogen metabolism.

Cortisone and cortisol in large doses generally cause sodium retention, whereas prednisone and prednisolone generally cause sodium loss when administered in equivalent therapeutic doses. This loss of sodium-retaining properties by 1,2-dehydrogenation is attributed to the "glomerulotubular" imbalance resulting from the administration of prednisone and prednisolone.

The *in vivo* metabolism of the 1,4-diene steroid prednisolone differs from that of cortisol in the limited conversion of the 1,4-diene steroid to 17-keto-steroids and in the excretion of a much larger portion of the administered 1,4-diene steroid in the free, unconjugated state. These differences may be related to prolonged duration of action and therefore to enhanced anti-anabolic and anti-inflammatory activities.

REFERENCES

1. Albright, F.: Cushing's syndrome. Harvey Lectures, *38*:123, 1942-43.
2. Bartter, F. C.: The role of aldosterone in normal homeostasis and in certain disease states. Metabolism, 5:369, 1956.
3. Bartter, F. C., and Fourman, P.: A non-renal effect of adrenal cortical steroids upon potassium metabolism. J. Clin. Invest., *36*:872, 1957.
4. Berliner, R. W.: Renal excretion of potassium and hydrogen ions. Fed. Proc., *11*:695, 1952.
5. Bernstein, S.: The chemistry and biological activities of 16-hydroxylated steroids. Recent Progress in Hormone Research, *14*:1, 1958.
6. Bernstein, S., Heller, M. and Stolar, S. M.: 16-Hydroxylated steroids. XI. The preparation and epimerization of 16β-acetoxy-17α-hydroxy corticoids. J. Am. Chem. Soc., *81*:1256, 1959.
7. Bunim, J. J., Pechet, M. M. and Bollet, A. J.: Studies on Metacortandralone and Metacortandracin in rheumatoid arthritis. J.A.M.A., *157*:311, 1955.
8. Caspi, E. and Pechet, M. M.: Metabolism of 1-dehydrosteroids in man. I. Isolation of six urinary products after the administration of prednisolone. J. Biol. Chem., *230*: 843, 1958.
9. Gray, C. H., Green, M. A. S., Holness, N. J. and Lunnon, J. B.: Urinary metabolic products of prednisone and prednisolone. J. Endocrinol., *14*:146, 1956.
10. Herzog, H. L. et al.: New anti-arthritic steroids. Science, *121*:176, 1955.
11. Liddle, G. W.: Effect of anti-inflammatory steroids on electrolyte metabolism. Ann. N. Y. Acad. Sc., 82:854, 1959.
12. Oliveto, E. P. et al.: 16-Alkylated corticoids. I. 16α-Methylprednisone and 16β-methylprednisone J. Am. Chem. Soc., 80:4428, 1958.
13. Pechet, M. M.: The metabolic effects of Metacortandracin and Metacortandralone in man: a new series of $\Delta^{1, 4}$ diene steroids. J. Clin. Invest., *34*:913, 1955.
14. Pechet, M. M.: The metabolic effects of steroid hormones: effects on renal excretion of sodium and potassium. Acta Endocrinol. (Suppl.) *51*:811, 1960.

15. Pechet, M. M., Bowers, B. and Bartter, F. C.: Metabolic studies with a new series of 1,4-diene steroids. I. Effects in addisonian subjects of prednisone, prednisolone, and the 1,2-dehydro analogues of corticosterone, desoxycorticosterone, 17-hydroxy-11-desoxycorticosterone, and 9α-fluorocortisol. J. Clin. Invest., 38:681, 1959.
16. Pechet, M. M., Bowers, B. and Bartter, F. C.: Metabolic studies with a new series of 1,4-diene steroids. II. Effects in normal subjects of prednisone, prednisolone, and 9α-fluoroprednisolone. J. Clin. Invest., 38:691, 1959.
17. Pechet, M. M. and Claffey, J.: The metabolic conversion in man of 21-carbon and 19-carbon-1,4-diene steroids to 17-ketosteroids. Clin. Res. Proc., 5:191, 1957.
18. Pechet, M. M., Carroll, E. L., Mitchell, M. and Wegner, M. J.: Studies of the activities of steroid hormones on electrolyte balance and the constituents of protoplasm: the effects of 16α-hydroxylation of 21-carbon steroids J. Clin. Invest., 37:921, 1958.
19. Reifenstein, E. C., Jr., Albright, F. and Wells, S. L.: The accumulation, interpretation and presentation of data pertaining to metabolic balances, notably those of calcium, phosphorus and nitrogen. J. Clin. Endocrinol., 5:367, 1945.
20. Silber, R. H.: The biology of anti-inflammatory steroids. Ann. N. Y. Acad. Sc., 82:821, 1959.
21. Slaunwhite, W. B. and Sandberg, A. A.: The metabolism of 1-dehydro-17-hydroxycorticosteroids in human subjects. J. Clin. Endocrinol., 17:395, 1957.
22. Tolksdorf, S.: Laboratory evaluation of anti-inflammatory steroids. Ann. N. Y. Acad. Sc., 82:829, 1959.
23. Vermeulen, A.: Isolation of Δ1, 4 pregnadiene-3,20-dione-11,17,21-triol from the urine of a patient treated with Metacortandracin. J. Clin. Endocrinol., 16:163, 1956.
24. West, K. M.: Relative eosinopenic and hyperglycemic potencies of glucocorticoids in man. Metabolism, 7:441, 1958.

Biological Evaluation of Some Newer Anti-Inflammatory Steroids

SANFORD L. STEELMAN and EVAN R. MORGAN

Merck Institute for Therapeutic Research

More than a decade has passed since cortisone was found to have anti-inflammatory activity in man. During this period there has been a continuous stream of derivatives with enhanced potency. The assessment of structural requirements for anti-inflammatory activity has also undergone changes. Some of the adverse effects of cortisone and hydrocortisone—in particular, retention of sodium—have been at least partially reduced or eliminated. As with most new classes of therapeutically useful drugs, the research objective continues to be the preparation of compounds with optimal activity and minimal side effects. It is, of course, difficult to experimentally quantify side effects and correlate animal with human data; however, this must be the unending task of the experimental biologist. Toward this goal our emphasis will be on a comparison of the biological properties of the clinically useful as well as some newer steroids.

METHODS

Assessment of anti-inflammatory activity can be accomplished by a variety of methods. The two most common are the cotton granuloma pellet[5, 8] and the granuloma pouch.[6] It has been our experience that both are useful, and the specific activities observed by means of these two methods are generally of the same order of magnitude. The method chosen for our studies was a modification of that described by Silber.[8] The compound was fed in the diet for seven days to male rats whose weight was approximately 125 grams. It is desirable that oral administration be used because this largely eliminates the difficulties encountered in parenteral administration of compounds of limited solubility, such as the esters. By using intact animals one can easily obtain four indices of corticoid activity in a single animal—body weight depression, thymic involution, adrenal weight decrease and granuloma inhibition. Since the primary objective is to find a compound with only anti-inflammatory activity, this method affords a means of quantitatively assessing relative potencies for possible separation of activities.

Two other methods have been used to assess corticoid activity—liver glycogen deposition and ulcerogenesis. The former method was that of Silber.[8] The latter was a modification of the procedure of Robert and Nezamis.[7] Female rats were starved for four days, during which time they were given daily subcutaneous injections of the cortical steroid. The method of evaluation or scoring was based on the estimation in mm. of the length and width of each gastric lesion. Only those which were clearly visible to the naked eye were measured. A statistical analysis of this method revealed that the average total lesion area (length $\times$ width) per animal was the most significant index of activity, although the total number of lesions per animal also correlated quite well. It was observed that there was a linear relationship when the logarithm of the dose of the cortical steroid was plotted against the average lesion area per animal. The utilizable dose response range was 4 to 16 mg./day of hydrocortisone, and the mean index of precision ($\lambda = \frac{s}{b}$) with 6 to 8 animals per dosage level was 0.25 to 0.30.

TABLE 1.   *METHODS FOR BIOLOGICAL EVALUATION*
OF CORTICAL HORMONES

INDEX	ANIMAL	ROUTE OF ADMINISTRATION	PRECISION (λ)*
Granuloma inhibition	Rat	Oral	0.2-0.25
Body weight depression	Rat	Oral	0.1-0.12
Thymic involution	Rat	Oral	0.1-0.15
Adrenal inhibition	Rat	Oral	0.25
Liver glycogen deposition	Mouse	Oral	0.25-0.3
Ulcerogenesis	Rat	S.C.	0.25-0.3

* $\lambda = \frac{s}{b}$

A summary of the methods utilized in our evaluations is found in Table 1. The first four were run simultaneously and represent data on the same animals. This gives them additional validity for comparative purposes. All compounds were also tested in adrenalectomized rats for salt retention activity; those found to retain more sodium than hydrocortisone were eliminated from consideration.

RESULTS

In addition to cortisone and hydrocortisone, there are four principal cortical steroids now being employed clinically—prednisolone (and predni-

TABLE 2. BIOLOGICAL ACTIVITIES OF ADRENAL CORTICAL HORMONES*

COMPOUND	GRANULOMA INHIBITION	BODY WEIGHT	THYMUS	ADRENAL	ULCERO-GENIC	GLYCO-GENIC
Hydrocortisone	1.0	1.0	1.0	1.0	1.0	1
Prednisolone	3.7	3.9	3.3	3.2	2.5	4
6α-Methylprednisolone	5.4	6.4	5.2	4.4	8.0	2
Triamcinolone	3.2	3.6	2.7	3.5	3.0	8
Dexamethasone	154	144	113	121	87	22
Δ⁶-Dexamethasone	150	142	121	125	40	7

* All relative potencies expressed in terms of hydrocortisone.

sone), 6α-methyl prednisolone, 16α-hydroxy-9α-fluoro prednisolone (triamcinolone) and 16α-methyl-9α-fluoro prednisolone (dexamethasone). Table 2 summarizes the various biological activities of these compounds. It can be readily seen that two indices, ulcerogenesis and glycogenic activity, do not parallel granuloma activity. In the case of liver glycogen potencies it should be pointed out that this is an oral assay in the mouse. Although the specific activities of the steroids were less than those reported for the rat, the results of this assay give the general order of magnitude. In the case of one new derivative of dexamethasone, Δ⁶-dexamethasone, the liver glycogen potency was one-third that of dexamethasone, although its anti-inflammatory potency was the same. On the basis of this and other data, it would appear that both the 6α-methyl and the Δ⁶ functions decrease liver glycogen activity in the mouse.

With ulcerogenesis the picture is somewhat different. 6α-Methyl prednisolone has the most unfavorable ulcerogenic to anti-inflammatory ratio, dexamethasone and Δ⁶-dexamethasone having the most favorable ratio. It has been our experience that introduction of a double bond at position 6 does not increase ulcerogenesis but in most instances causes a decrease.

Since the introduction of dexamethasone some two years ago, many derivatives of it have been prepared. A partial list is found in Table 3. None, with the possible exception of 6α-fluoro dexamethasone, was more active. Only Δ⁶-dexamethasone had a significantly better ulcerogenic to granuloma inhibition ratio (U/G). It is perhaps of interest to note that 21-desoxy

TABLE 3. ANTI-INFLAMMATORY AND ULCEROGENIC POTENCIES
OF DEXAMETHASONE DERIVATIVES

COMPOUND	ANTI-INFLAMMATORY* POTENCY	U/G RATIO**
Dexamethasone	1.0	0.6
16β-Methyl-9α-fluoro prednisolone	0.33	0.7
11-Dehydro dexamethasone	0.7	0.8
9α-Chloro-16α-methyl prednisolone	0.3	0.7
6α-Chloro dexamethasone	0.25	. .
6α-Fluoro dexamethasone	1-2.5 (1)	. .
6α-Methyl dexamethasone	1.0	
Δ⁶-Dexamethasone	1.0	0.27
21-Desoxy dexamethasone	0.12	1.4
Dexamethasone 21-phosphate	1.0***	. .
Dexamethasone 21-tertiary butyl acetate	1.0***	. .

* Assuming dexamethasone to be 1.0.
** Ulcerogenic activity divided by anti-inflammatory activity, using hydrocortisone as 1.0. See Table 2.
*** Calculated on a molar basis.

dexamethasone had the highest U/G ratio. This is in agreement with the data of Stafford et al.[9] on fluorometholone, a 21-desoxy compound which is one of the most potent ulcerogenic steroids yet reported. It would therefore seem that in the rat, at least there is a possibility of a partial separation of ulcerogenesis and some of the other activities of corticoids.

Recently Ercoli and Gardi[2] have reported that the 3-enol ethers of cortical, progestational and androgenic steroids have enhanced oral activities. Although specific compounds may show this property, it is apparently not a general phenomenon. Our own experiences with the cortical steroids have been rather disappointing. Only with cortisone and cortisone acetate has there been a significant increase in oral activity. A partial list of compounds tested is given in Table 4. With those compounds evaluated there was no

TABLE 4.   ANTI-INFLAMMATORY ACTIVITIES OF 3-ENOL
ETHERS OF CORTICAL STEROIDS

COMPOUND	ANTI-INFLAMMATORY POTENCY ($\times$ parent compound)
Ethyl ether of cortisone	1.5
Ethyl ether of cortisone 21-acetate	2
n-Propyl ether of cortisone 21-acetate	2-3
Ethyl ether of hydrocortisone	1.0-1.25
Ethyl ether of 16α-methyl hydrocortisone	0.5-1.0
Ethyl ether of 9α-fluoro-16α-methyl hydrocortisone 21-acetate	0.5-1.0
Ethyl ether of 9α-fluoro-16α-methyl cortisone 21-acetate	1.0-1.5
Ethyl ether of dexamethasone 21-acetate	0.5-0.7

change in the ratios of body weight decrease to granuloma, thymus to granuloma, or adrenal inhibition to granuloma. This would suggest that the enol ethers which are rather labile chemically are split to their parent compounds. Parenteral administration usually results in less activity than is observed with the parent compound.

The Δ^6 derivatives of the cortical steroids are illustrative of the difficulties encountered when the chemist and the biologist try to predict the relative potencies of steroids. It has been reported that the introduction of a double bond at position 6 leads to a decrease in activity.[3, 4] Both Δ^6 hydrocortisone and Δ^6-prednisolone are less active than their parent compounds with respect to anti-inflammatory and glycogenic activities. However, a double bond at position 6 in 16α-methyl hydrocortisone increases granuloma activity. Although Δ^6-16α-methyl hydrocortisone has three times the anti-inflammatory activity of 16α-methyl hydrocortisone, its liver glycogen activity is slightly less. The ability to deposit liver glycogen is similarly impaired by the introduction of a double bond at position 6 in a variety of other corticoids. In contrast, Dulin et al.[1] have reported that glycogen deposition activity in the rat is enhanced by the 6α-fluoro group.

On the basis of available information it would also appear that the Δ^6 function decreases ulcerogenic activity. This is true for Δ^6-dexamethasone, but the data on the other compounds is not extensive enough to make it unequivocal.

In summary, it seems reasonable to assume that some additional side effects of cortical steroids can be reduced without sacrifice of anti-inflammatory activity. The evaluation in man is certainly more difficult but not impossible. Only by unrelenting research can we achieve our goal of a truly superior anti-inflammatory steroid.

ACKNOWLEDGMENTS

The authors are indebted to Robert Busch, Edward Chapin, Raymond Oslapas, Maryann Petraitis, Raymond Primka, Mary E. Regn and Walter Worosila for technical assistance.

The compounds used were generously made available to us by members of the Synthetic Organic and Process Research Departments of the Merck Sharp and Dohme Research Laboratories, Rahway, New Jersey. Details of preparative methods will be published in the near future.

Dr. H. C. Stoerk of the Merck Institute for Therapeutic Research kindly conducted the sodium retention assays in adrenalectomized rats.

REFERENCES

1. Dulin, W. E., Schmidt, F. L. and Lyster, S. C.: Proc. Soc. Exper. Biol. & Med., *104*: 345, 1960.
2. Ercoli, A. and Gardi, R.: J. Am. Chem. Soc., *82*:746, 1960.
3. Gould, D. et al.: J. Am. Chem. Soc., *79*:502, 1957.
4. Mattox, V. R., Woroch, E. L., Fleisher, G. A. and Kendall, E. C.: J. Biol. Chem., *197*: 261, 1952.
5. Meier, R., Schuler, W. and Desaulles, P.: Experientia, *6*:469, 1950.
6. Robert, A. and Nezamis, J. E.: Acta Endocrinol., *25*:105, 1957.
7. Robert, A. and Nezamis, J. E.: Proc. Soc. Exper. Biol. & Med., *99*:443, 1958.
8. Silber, R. H.: Am. N. Y. Acad. Sc, *82*:821, 1959.
9. Stafford, R. O., Robert, A., Lyster, S. C., Schmidt, F. L. and Dulin, W. E.: Proc. Soc. Exper. Biol. & Med., *101*:653, 1959.

A Rational Approach to the Synthesis of Some New Anti-Inflammatory Steroids

JOSEF FRIED

The Squibb Institute for Medical Research

In this communication, I wish to describe an intriguing example of the rational use of available structure-activity relationships for converting some compounds of marginal activity into highly potent glucocorticoids.

The point of departure for this work was the finding that 9α- and 12α-halogen substitution had equal effects, both qualitatively and quantitatively, on the corticoid activity of certain 11β-hydroxy steroids. Thus, the 9α-halo-11β-hydroxyprogesterones and the 9α-halocorticosterones had been found to exhibit activities equal for all practical purposes to those of the corresponding 12α-halo derivatives.[4, 5] This prompted the synthesis of the more complex 12α-chlorocortisone,[3] which on the basis of the above considerations was predicted to possess about four times the activity of cortisol. Contrary to expectations, the compound showed no appreciable activity. More recently, Dr. Diassi of our laboratories has been able to synthesize 12α-fluorocortisol, and has found it to be of equally low glucocorticoid activity as 12α-chlorocortisone. The structures and activities in the liver glycogen assay for this group of 9- and 12-fluorinated derivatives are shown in Chart I. The

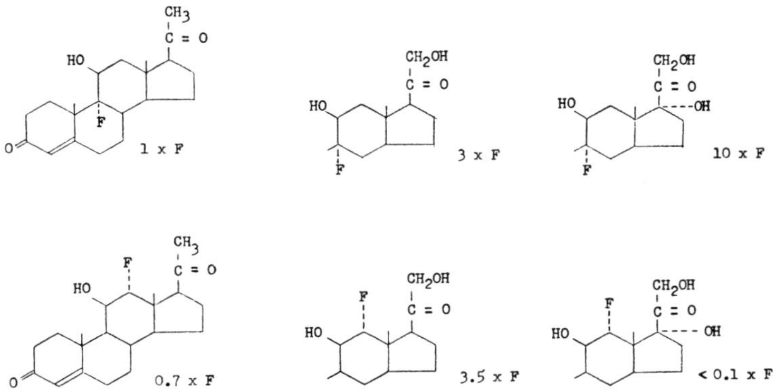

Chart I. Glucocorticoid activity of 9α- and 12α-fluorocorticoids.

discrepancy between the predicted and observed potencies was rationalized by us[1] by assuming that hydrogen bonding between the axial 12α-halogen atom and the pseudo-axial 17α-hydroxyl group was instrumental in suppressing the activity-enhancing effect of the halogen atom. This is illustrated in Chart II. It was also suggested at the time that the correctness of this

Hydrogen Bonding   No Hydrogen Bonding

Chart II. Hydrogen bonding of 12-fluoro-17-hydroxycorticoids.

assumption was amenable to experimental verification, if it were possible to abolish hydrogen bonding by appropriate substitution of the 17α-hydroxyl group. Simple acylation of the 17-hydroxyl group cannot serve for this purpose since such derivatization leads to far-reaching inactivation of 17α-hydroxycorticoids. It has, however, been possible to achieve the desired goal by covering the 17α-hydroxyl group by the introduction of the isopropylidenedioxy group, a chemical feature shown by us[2] to be capable not only of preserving but also of enhancing by a factor of 10 the glucocorticoid activity of the parent compound. For the purpose in mind we prepared both the 9α- and 12α-fluoro derivatives of 16α,17α-dihydroxyprogesterone following the sequence of steps outlined in Chart III for the 12-substituted steroid. The 9α-substituted compound (I, Chart IV) had activity equal to that of cortisol in the liver glycogen assay, while the 12α-fluoro compound (III) had no appreciable activity, as predicted on the basis of the hydrogen bonding hypothesis. Both compounds were then converted into their isopropylidenedioxy derivatives (II and IV) with the result that now both the 9- and 12-substituted derivatives showed activity of equal magnitude, namely

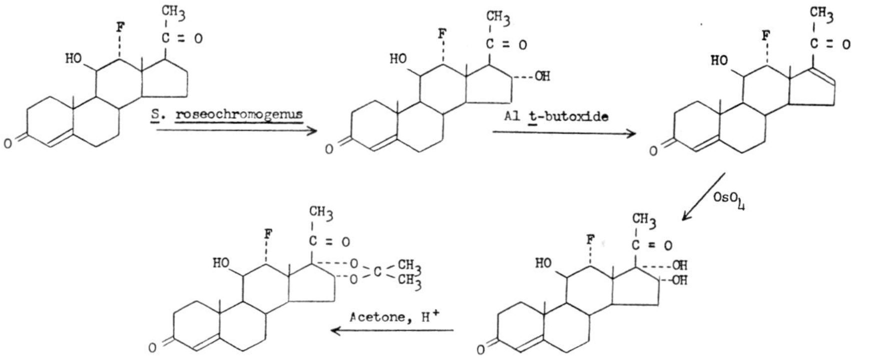

Chart III. Synthesis of 12α-fluoro-Δ⁴-pregnene-11β, 16α, 17α-triol-3,20-dione and acetonide.

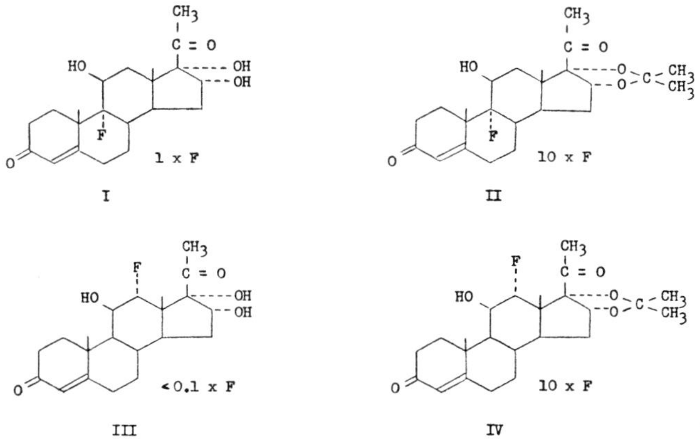

Chart IV. Effect of hydrogen bonding on glucocorticoid activity of 12α-fluorosteroids.

10 times that of cortisol. Thus, by abolishing the hydrogen bond between the 12α-halogen atom and the 17α-hydroxyl group, activity has been restored to the predicted level. Whether the above rationalization represents the "true" state of affairs is not as important as the fact that it suggested the experiment of transforming a compound of marginal activity into a potent corticoid.

REFERENCES

1. Fried, J. and Borman, A.: Vitamins and Hormones, 16:343, 1958.
2. Fried, J., Borman, A., Kessler, W. B., Grabowich, P. and Sabo, E. F.: J. Am. Chem. Soc., 80:2338, 1958.
3. Fried, J., Herz, J. E., Sabo, E. F. and Morrisson, M. H.: Chem. & Ind. (London), 1232, 1956.
4. Herz, J. E., Fried, J. and Sabo, E. F.: J. Am. Chem. Soc., 78:2017, 1956.
5. Taub, D., Hoffsommer, R. D. and Wendler, N. L.: J. Am. Chem. Soc., 79:542, 1957.

Panel Discussion

GLEN E. ARTH, *Moderator*

DR. ARTH: I think that the papers this morning have brought out at least one very important point, and that is that by animal indices various activities of steroids can be separated. One statement made by Dr. Liddle attracted my attention. I think it is the most important thing we could discuss here today and I would like to summarize it. Up to the present time, it has been implied that the anti-inflammatory properties of corticosteroids are inseparable from their protein-wasting, hyperglycemic, ACTH-depressing and eosinopenic activities. Usually a modification of the structure which alters one of these biological activities also brings about a commensurate alteration with respect to the others. Occasionally, partial dissociation of some of these activities has been shown in animal assays, but usually these observations can not be confirmed when the same steroids are assayed in man. It has recently been possible, however, to demonstrate clear dissociation of these various properties when certain steroids were administered to human subjects. All of the steroids exhibiting dissociation of various organic activities lacked the 21-hydroxyl group. All of them were less potent than their 21-hydroxylated analogues with respect to all of their biological activities. In reference to this information presented by Dr. Liddle, it has been possible to dissociate various organic activities in one series of compounds; I would like to ask Dr. Liddle what specific compounds he was referring to.

DR. LIDDLE: We have had the chance to study four compounds in sufficient detail to be sure on statistical grounds that the dissociation of these various activities was significant. One of these is $\Delta 1$-9α-fluoro-21-desoxy-cortisol which I mentioned. Though not showing all of the striking differences that I described, 21-desoxy dexamethasone does show a significant difference between eosinopenic and ACTH-suppressing activity. Another compound which was described by Dr. Fried a number of years ago is 9α-21-difluoro-21-desoxycortisol, and the fourth compound is $\Delta 1$-6α-methyl-9α-fluoro-cortisol-21-mesylate.

DR. ARTH: Has there been definite separation of activities with all these compounds?

DR. LIDDLE: Yes. The most striking dissociation was with the $\Delta 1$-9α-fluoro-21-desoxy-cortisol.

DR. ARTH: Has anybody else had similar or further experiences with these same compounds?

DR. FRAWLEY: We had experience using two of the 21-desoxy-cortisol derivatives, that is, the 6α-methyl, $\Delta 1$, and the 6α-methyl-9α-fluoro, $\Delta 1$ compounds and would agree entirely with what Dr. Liddle has said regarding this dissociation of effects, at least in man.

DR. PECHET: I would like to raise a word of caution about using the term "dissociation." Does one refer to a quantitative difference or a qualitative difference? Using a particular dose we have seen effects which initially would appear to be due to a qualitative difference in certain activities, but on increasing the dose it became obvious that this merely represented a quantitative difference. For example, corticosterone has practically no eosinopenic effect in a dose of about 40 or 50 milli-

356

grams in 24 hours. The Δ1-corticosterone has a very marked eosinopenic effect at this dose. However, if you increase the dose of corticosterone itself up to 80 and 160 milligrams you now begin to see some eosinopenic effect. I would suggest that we be very careful when we use the term "dissociation." Is it qualitative or quantitative?

Dr. LIDDLE: I would like to think we have been very careful and would prefer not to draw the distinction between qualitative and quantitative dissociation, but rather between absolute dissociation and relative dissociation. We have not thought that there was absolute dissociation of these effects, but slight attenuation of one activity and great attenuation of another activity; this may make a great difference as far as the therapeutic index of steroids is concerned. As a matter of fact, the larger the dose of these particular compounds, the greater the dissociation apparently was.

Dr. ARTH: Have these results been obtained using dosages which might be physiologically effective dosages? That is, did the dissociation of effects occur with a dose of these compounds which would give the same anti-inflammatory effect as a given dose of prednisolone?

Dr. LIDDLE: Yes. Insofar as the compound is active it has been tested in doses which are fully active in human subjects, and multiples of the maximally active dose have been used as well.

Dr. ARTH: Are there any other comments on this?

Dr. DI RAIMONDO: We have compared 21-desoxydexamethasone with dexamethasone in terms of pituitary suppression of ACTH in relation to nitrogen-losing effects. At one dose range, when the steroid was given as a single dose we found that the 21-desoxy compound produced less nitrogen loss than dexamethasone in comparable doses with reference to ACTH suppression. However, I am not completely convinced that we have a dissociation of the quantitative and qualitative aspects. I would agree with Dr. Pechet, and I do not think enough attention has been placed on the maximum effects of a drug, particularly when you are dealing with drugs of various potencies, and particularly with reference to nitrogen retention. For example, when one gives the equivalent of 250 mg. of hydrocortisone per day in normal subjects there is a sort of plateau in the nitrogen-losing effects, and unless these factors are taken into consideration one can get unreliable results.

Dr. LIDDLE: I suppose we will just have to publish our data so that everyone can look at it and then invite others to use the same compounds. With the 21-desoxy compound and with the difluoro compound, it has not been possible even to reach maximal effects as far as the eosinopenia is concerned, let alone plateau at maximal effectiveness.

Dr. STEELMAN: Dr. Liddle, what you are basically saying now is that if you increase the dose you get a greater discrepancy between the anti-inflammatory and the other effects. In other words, your dose responses curves are not parallel?

Dr. LIDDLE: That is correct. The parallelism is not good because when we assay the eosinopenic activity of these dissociated compounds there is such poor eosinopenic activity at any dose level that we really do not get a good fall. The same is true of hyperglycemic activity. However, we do not have quantitative data on the anti-inflammatory or nitrogen-wasting effects so that the practical importance of this is obscure.

Dr. PECHET: I believe Dr. Liddle's work is very accurate, but I would like to emphasize this point again, and it is well demonstrated by the initial reports on dexamethasone. When dexamethasone was first studied, a report was made that it had no hyperglycemic effect and that it was devoid of a gluconeogenic effect. We found that it had a very definite effect. Now the difference was, not that the two laboratories were incompetent in doing their investigations, but in the dosages used. We raised the dose up to 15 and 25 mg. for eight days and demonstrated a very definite gluconeogenic effect and a very definite elevation of fasting blood sugar. Subsequently it has been shown that the same effect may occur with smaller doses given over a longer period of time.

Dr. GLENN: In experiments on animals, at least, we have found that the reference to so-called glycogenic activity and anti-inflammatory activity of steroids may be somewhat misleading because the time scale for the assay of these two activities is entirely different. For example, it is possible to show that a given steroid has a certain amount of granuloma pouch inhibiting activity and that it has no glycogenic activity when the glycogenic activity is determined, as it usually is, after administration of the steroid for seven hours and the granuloma pouch after four days of therapy; however, the glycogenic activity may be the same as the granuloma pouch inhibiting activity when the assay is carried out over the same period of time as the granuloma pouch assay. So I think we should be extremely cautious in making statements regarding relative potencies when different time intervals are employed to measure these parameters.

Dr. ARTH: Dr. Tolksdorf, do you have any comments on this?

Dr. TOLKSDORF: I fully agree that it is very treacherous to compare different parameters under different experimental conditions. I would also like to bring up the question of species specificities, which can be extremely misleading. In our study of the dihalo-corticoids, specifically dichlorisone, we found that the assay in the mouse, the monkey and the cow agreed with the human data in respect to the eosinophil and blood sugar responses, but in the dog there was a considerable eosinophil response when the drug was given by intravenous and subcutaneous administration. Even catabolic effects in terms of extreme nitrogen loss occur in the dog.

Dr. ARTH: Dr. Liddle, one of your slides showed that dexamethasone was about 12 times more potent than hydrocortisone in electrolyte-regulating activity. Was this determined in man or dog?

Dr. LIDDLE: Dexamethasone has very little activity in either species, and it is difficult to determine an accurate potency figure. Dexamethasone does have some sodium-retaining activity in doses above 6 mg. per day; however, this is a dose rarely needed in clinical medicine, so for practical purposes it does not have much sodium-retaining activity. In dogs, it does not cause very definite sodium retention, but it does cause some potassium loss in acute assays.

Dr. ARTH: Since dexamethasone is said not to cause sodium retention, what is the mechanism of the edema associated with prolonged administration of this compound in some patients?

Dr. DINGMAN: I shall discuss some of these aspects further when I talk about the effects of the steroids on water metabolism this afternoon. However, edema can be induced by the effects of steroids on water metabolism as well as by their effects on sodium metabolism. For instance, our experiments have shown that most of the glucocorticoids seem to have a fairly reproducible initial effect in suppressing neurohypophysial release of vasopressin. There is an initial water diuresis with administration of most glucocorticoids, but following this the body adjusts quite quickly and there is a phase of water retention. Our data indicate that regulation of the neurohypophysis has been disturbed at this point so that the release of vasopressin is more subject to changes of osmotic pressure and changes in extracellular fluid volume. Edema can also occur without any change in body water by simply a shift of water, and probably sodium also, from the intracellular stores into the extracellular space, and in a patient with poor circulation or a diseased heart this may result in the accumulation of interstitial fluid, which we call edema.

DR. JENKINS: The question about edema and dexamethasone really emphasizes an important point in relation to the discussion we have heard this morning. What has been said, in effect, is that when patients, not normal subjects, take steroids for long periods of time, the effects seen are sometimes a bit different from what might well be predicted from a six- to ten-day acute metabolic study in a normal person. This brings up a very embarrassing situation because this difference makes it very difficult to evaluate steroids in terms of their clinical usefulness. Evaluation of steroids in terms of side effects requires one essential element; that element is time, and that time is measured in years. The effects of steroids, when given to sick people for long periods of time, in varying doses, in varied disease states, and in various environments that the patient is in, are totally and vastly different from those produced by giving the same steroid for a period of seven days to a person whose dietary intake is fixed and whose activity is fixed; it is, therefore, little wonder that sometimes the predictability of our acute studies is not very great. In effect, I think the general experience has been that edema occurs in a smaller number of patients when dexamethasone is used therapeutically than when prednisolone is used therapeutically; however, the incidence is certainly higher than with triamcinolone and probably higher than with 6-methyl prednisolone. This is quite evident, irrespective of what the five-day metabolic studies have shown.

DR. LIDDLE: I think there is one other cause of edema in sick patients, and that is circulatory disease which may be overlooked. Let me illustrate with a case. We recently saw a patient with periarteritis nodosa who was very sick, not eating and had marked hypoalbuminemia but no edema. The question was why he did not have edema with a serum albumin of about 1 gram per cent. When this patient was given dexamethasone he started to eat and then developed edema. This was interpreted to mean that dexamethasone was causing edema in this patient. Actually, this patient had a disease which would have led to edema regardless of his dexamethasone medication.

Effects of Anti-Inflammatory Steroids on Carbohydrate Metabolism*

THOMAS F. FRAWLEY and THOMAS F. SHELLEY

Albany Medical College of Union University

In 1932 Britton and Silvette emphasized the importance of the adrenal cortex in carbohydrate metabolism and demonstrated that this activity could be differentiated from its electrolyte-controlling activity.[3] In 1940 Long showed that the adrenal cortical steroids increased the liver glycogen and glycosuria of partially pancreatectomized animals.[23] During this period Thorn demonstrated the complete relief of hypoglycemia in Addison's disease by the administration of adrenal cortical extracts.[31] The ensuing work of many investigators culminated in a concept of adrenal steroid function related to steroid structure. The naturally occurring C^{21}-adrenal steroids possessing an oxygen atom in the 11 position had carbohydrate activities which were enhanced if a similar accompanying substitution was present in the 17 position. On this basis the carbohydrate activity of known and unknown steroids could be predicted to a certain degree.

However, the many recent modifications of the steroid molecule require some revision of our concepts of the relationship of predictable biological activity to steroid structure. These modified steroids exhibit differences in carbohydrate, pituitary corticotropin suppressive, eosinopenic and anti-inflammatory actions, depending upon the dosage and type of steroid. In the past, knowledge regarding these actions of a given steroid has been derived primarily from studies performed in animals. However, the magnitude of some, but not all, of these actions may be quite different in man than in animals. This is particularly true in the evaluation of the carbohydrate activity of a new steroid. It has, therefore, become increasingly important to assess the activity of various modifications of anti-inflammatory steroids in man as well as animals to determine the extent of their various biological activities.

CARBOHYDRATE-REGULATING ACTIVITY OF ANTI-INFLAMMATORY STEROIDS

This section consists of a summary of the relationship of steroid structure to carbohydrate activity and its determination in animals and man. The standardization of this activity is usually expressed in terms of hydrocortisone activity.

Steroid Structure and Carbohydrate Activity. The major chemical modifications of hydrocortisone are dehydrogenation, halogenation, methylation, hydroxylation and desoxygenation in single or multiple combinations in the same steroid. The modifications increase the carbohydrate activity of steroids in varying degrees. Dehydrogenation of hydrocortisone in the 1-2 position (prednisolone) increases animal and human carbohydrate potency by three

* These studies were carried out with the generous support of the John A. Hartford Foundation, New York, and The Upjohn Company, Kalamazoo, Michigan.

to five times. The fluorination of hydrocortisone in the 9-alpha position increases its activity 12 times. The possession of both modifications as in delta-1, 9-alpha fluorohydrocortisone results in a synergistic effect on carbohydrate activity of about 42 times hydrocortisone in animals and 25 times hydrocortisone in man. This spectacular potentiation of glucocorticoid activity by small structural changes cannot be entirely explained on the basis of delayed rate of conjugation, degradation or inactivation. The reader will find a more complete discussion of this matter elsewhere.[8, 9]

Animal Assay of Anti-inflammatory Steroids for Carbohydrate Activity. A number of effects such as gluconeogenesis, muscle-work performance, resistance to stress and hyperglycemic activity have been used in assaying carbohydrate activity, but the assay of liver glycogen following steroid administration to the adrenalectomized rat or mouse remains as the most universally employed standard for comparison.[8] Other assays of steroid action, such as the involuting effect on the thymus gland and lymph nodes or the effect on the animal's ability to excrete a water load, appear to bear some relationship to, but do not appear to be dependent upon, the carbohydrate activity of the steroid.

Human Assay of Anti-inflammatory Steroids for Carbohydrate Activity. The ideal assay procedure in man has not yet been achieved. Persons having a complete loss of adrenal function are not plentiful enough to serve as assay subjects, and liver glycogen assays in man are impractical. Therefore, other parameters have been measured in normal, diabetic or adrenal-insufficient subjects. For example, the administration of a glucocorticoid to a diabetic subject changes urinary glucose output and/or insulin requirement, and these changes provide an index of the steroid's activity. The glucocorticoids also exhibit anti-insulin effects in adrenal-insufficient and normal subjects. In an attempt to improve upon existing assay methods in man, we are now using a new technique. The steroid in question is given to a normal subject either orally or intravenously prior to an infusion of insulin (0.75 U/kg./hr.). The carbohydrate activity of the unknown steroid is determined by comparing the degree of inhibition of insulin hypoglycemia with that of a standard dose of hydrocortisone. We have also employed the counterpart of this type of assay, viz., the anti-insulin potencies of steroids in organic hyperinsulinism. The carbohydrate activity is related to the degree by which each steroid is able to prevent fasting hypoglycemia.[8]

West has obtained reproducible assays by measuring the blood sugar response following steroid administration and a glucose load to normal subjects.[34] His results agree closely with those of others using different techniques. For example, in our laboratory, using the anti-insulin effect in normal subjects, the glycosuric effect in diabetics and the prevention of fasting hypoglycemia in organic hyperinsulinism, we obtained a carbohydrate potency for dexamethasone of 30 to 35 times that of hydrocortisone. A similar figure was also obtained by West.[35] However, certain objections can be raised to using any oral assay method. There are, for instance, the problems of gastrointestinal absorption of the steroid or the glucose and the inactivation of the steroid as it traverses the liver during its transit from the portal to the systemic circulation.

In conclusion, there is a need for assay methods that will provide a closer correlation between the predictable and the actual carbohydrate effects of steroids in man. This need is particularly urgent because of the increasing number of complex steroids being made available.

Biochemical Effects of Anti-inflammatory Steroids on Carbohydrate Metabolism. Glucocorticoids are capable of producing glycosuria, elevation of blood sugar and reduced glucose tolerance. The glycosuria has been shown to be related to the glomerular filtration of an increased glucose load and only partly, if at all, to steroid suppression of renal tubular glucose reabsorption.[10] Hyperglycemia and the abnormal glucose tolerance appears to be a combination of an increased production and decreased removal of glucose.[1, 2, 33] Research into the cause of the decreased glucose removal has revealed that the steroids decrease the binding of insulin to cells.[29] This could reduce glucose penetration, as there is presumptive evidence from other studies that insulin must be bound before it can exert its effect.[14] Another proposed cause of decreased glucose removal has been the demonstration of decreased glucose phosphorylation in the cell, thus limiting the rate of glucose entry.[22] Biochemical and enzymatic studies with the steroids have revealed both stimulatory and suppressive effects on enzymes participating in carbohydrate metabolism. From recent studies it would appear that certain enzymes necessary for aerobic glycolysis are inhibited,[4, 13] while those involved in the pentose shunt,[17] gluconeogenesis and glycogenesis,[11, 27] are stimulated. These alterations in enzymatic activities may have resulted from effects on the basic electron transport and energy release mechanisms. Recent studies show that certain steroids depress ATP formation,[20] inhibit cytochrome oxidase,[21] may effect TPNH-DPN transhydrogenations[30] and inhibit the oxidation of DPNH to DPN.[39] Effects of this nature might well explain the complex and numerous metabolic actions of the adrenal steroids. ACTH itself has been shown to have glycogenolytic activity in the adrenal cortex and may, in fact, increase steroidogenesis by increasing the availability of TPNH for steroid synthesis.[15] An insulin-like action of ACTH upon the entrance of sugar into adrenal cortical cells has been recently demonstrated.[5]

GLUCOCORTICOIDS AND ALTERED STATES OF CARBOHYDRATE METABOLISM

Excessive glucocorticoid production, which characterizes Cushing's syndrome, produces a diabetic state manifested by hyperglycemia, glycosuria and reduced glucose tolerance. On the other hand, normal glucocorticoid production may be responsible in part for maintaining a diabetic state. This is evidenced by the amelioration in the diabetes of subjects who have undergone hypophysectomy[24] or adrenalectomy,[38] or who have developed spontaneous anterior pituitary insufficiency.[25] The development of diabetes in subjects receiving glucocorticoids is definitely and directly related to the individual's inability to increase insulin production. The large functional reserve of the islet tissue in the majority of patients receiving ACTH or steroids protects them from the development of a significantly impaired carbohydrate tolerance.[37]

Steroid-Glucose Tolerance Tests and Prediabetes. Although, as has been noted above, cortisone and cortisone-like steroids may produce glycosuria and impair glucose tolerance, there are at present no means of predicting their development in a given subject. The induction of a diabetes-like state by such steroids has been the subject of much study, particularly by Fajans and Conn,[6] who developed a cortisone-modified glucose tolerance test as a means of detecting the prediabetic, viz., the person who has a normal glucose tolerance test and an abnormal cortisone-glucose tolerance test. A follow-up of 30 of their test subjects for periods of one to four years revealed that diabetes had developed in 13 per cent of those who had previously exhibited normal glucose tolerance tests but abnormal cortisone-glucose tolerance tests. An additional 10 per cent had developed "probable diabetes." The usefulness of this test procedure in detecting prediabetics has been recently challenged by other workers. Jackson[19] has been impressed with the frequency of "negative" cortisone-glucose tolerance tests in certain persons suspected of having a diabetic tendency. German[12] failed to find any evi-

EFFECT OF CORTISONE ON PYRUVATE DISAPPEARANCE

E.B. 45 M

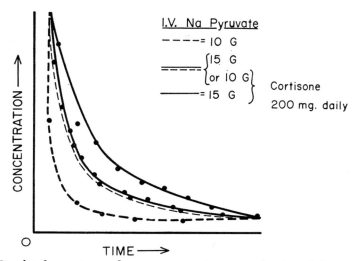

Fig. 1. Translated superimposed curves comparing removal rates of intravenous pyruvate in man. A 10 gram dose of pyruvate disappeared in a cortisone-prepared subject the same as a 15 gram dose in an unprepared subject.

dence that the hyperglycemic responses to cortisone in obese subjects were greater than usual, even though obese subjects are more likely to develop diabetes. Furthermore, the results of West's studies[36] are in complete conflict with those of Fajans and Conn.[6] West examined the hyperglycemic response to cortisone of 26 nondiabetics whose parents were both diabetic. Their responses to cortisone were not significantly different from those of a control group with normal glucose tolerance tests and no family history of diabetes. West concludes: "These findings suggest that individuals with prediabetes are not unusually responsive to the hyperglycemic effects of cortisone when it is administered by the technic of Fajans and Conn."

Steroid Diabetes. The term "steroid diabetes," employed initially by Ingle,[18] described a type of diabetes which developed in rats given corticotropin, corticosterone, cortisone or cortisol. Not all animal species, however, showed equal susceptibilities to these compounds. Steroid diabetes has also been described in man and can be differentiated from diabetes mellitus by differences in both the clinical and biochemical manifestations. These differences have been presented in detail in a previous publication.[8]

One biochemical alteration observed with glucosteroids has been the development of elevated blood levels of pyruvic acid.[7] This has been observed in both short-term and prolonged therapy with glucosteroids. The precise mechanism is unknown, although some recent studies have shed some light on possible mechanisms.[40] Our own studies have consistently led us to believe that the hyperpyruvicemia is due to both a decreased removal and an overproduction of pyruvic acid. Studies have revealed that the disappearance rates of infused sodium pyruvate during hydrocortisone therapy are reduced (Fig. 1). More recent studies performed in our laboratory indicate that hydrocortisone inhibits acetylation of sulfanilamide by the perfused rat liver[41] (Table 1). This is consistent with the extremely important observa-

TABLE 1. EFFECT OF CORTISOL ON PER CENT ACETYLATION OF SULFANILAMIDE IN THE CYCLICALLY PERFUSED RAT LIVER

	% ACETYLATION	
Perfusion time	1 hr.	2 hr.
Control rats	58	82
	68	88
	59	70
Cortisol injected rats	28	40
	17	25

tions of Tomkins and co-workers who found that steroids inhibit the oxidation of DPNH to DPN.[39] DPN is essential for the oxidation of pyruvic acid to acetyl-coenzyme A and CO_2, and any decrease in DPN formation may result in hyperpyruvicemia by decreasing pyruvic acid removal.

The Glucocorticoids and Hypoglycemia. In a previous article we paid considerable attention to this particular aspect of steroid action.[8] Mention was made of the beneficial effects of steroids administered during insulin hypoglycemia. These effects were seen prior to any increase in blood glucose concentration, and a theoretical consideration was given as to the possible beneficial effect of steroids on cerebral metabolism during hypoglycemia. The protective influence of the glucocorticoids against hypoglycemia is well known in such conditions as acute adrenal insufficiency, Addison's disease, hypopituitarism and organic hyperinsulinism.[8]

ESTROGEN-INDUCED ELEVATIONS OF PLASMA CORTISOL

It has been repeatedly observed that the free plasma 17,21-dihydroxy-steroids are elevated during pregnancy or estrogen administration.[16, 28, 32] The elevated steroid levels are mostly due to an increase in the fraction bound to protein considered to be biologically inactive, as neither eosinopenia-inducing activity nor anti-inflammatory activity has been demonstrable.[26] However, as the elevated steroid level may possibly explain the occurrence of a diabetic state in pregnancy, our interest was directed toward detecting an increased biological action on carbohydrate metabolism.

Insulin responsiveness and glycosuria were determined before and after the induction of elevated plasma 17-hydroxycorticoid levels by estrogen administration. In Figure 2, although the plasma level of 17-hydroxycorticoids rose three- to fourfold, there was no change in the fasting blood sugar, and the urinary glucose output may have slightly increased. However, when insulin sensitivity was determined (Fig. 3), a definite reduction in insulin sensitivity had occurred. A similar degree of insulin resistance was induced in this patient when hydrocortisone was administered in a dosage sufficient to raise the plasma 17-hydroxysteroids to 24 mcg. per cent, a level commensurate with that obtained on the thirteenth day of estrogen administra-

ESTROGEN EFFECT ON PLASMA "F", URINE AND BLOOD GLUCOSE

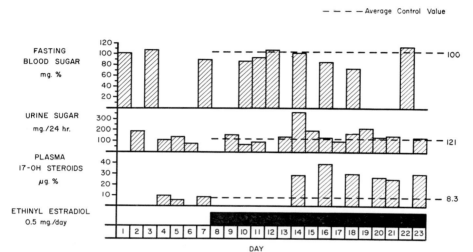

Fig. 2. Estrogen administration to a mild diabetic subject markedly increased plasma 17-hydroxycorticoid levels without altering fasting blood sugar. Urine glucose output showed a questionable increase.

ESTROGEN EFFECT ON HYDROCORTISONE AND INSULIN SENSITIVITY

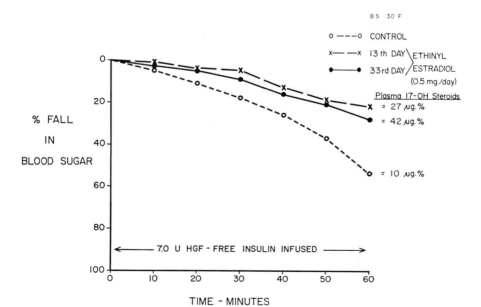

Fig. 3. Estrogen-induced elevation of plasma 17-hydroxycorticoids decreased responsiveness to intravenous insulin.

tion. This study indicates that the elevated plasma steroid level induced by estrogen may have biologic activity.

REFERENCES

1. Ashmore, J., Hastings, A. B., Nesbett, F. B. and Renold, A. E.: Studies on carbohydrate metabolism in rat liver slices J. Biol. Chem., *218*:77, 1956.
2. Bastenie, P. A., Conard, V. and Franckson, J. R. M.: Effect of cortisone on carbohydrate metabolism measured by the "glucose assimilation coefficient." Diabetes, *204*: 205, 1954.
3. Britton, S. W. and Silvette, H.: Effects of corticoadrenal extract on carbohydrate metabolism in normal animals. The apparent prepotent function of the adrenal glands. Am. J. Physiol., *100*:693, 1932.
4. Cori, C. F.: Enzymatic reactions in carbohydrate metabolism. Harvey Lect., *41*:253, 1945-46.
5. Eichhorn, J., Halkerston, I. D. K., Feinstein, M. and Heckter, O.: Effect of ACTH on permeability of adrenal cells to sugar. Proc. Soc. Exper. Biol. & Med., *103*:515, 1960.
6. Fajans, S. S. and Conn, J. W.: An approach to the prediction of diabetes mellitus by modification of the glucose tolerance test with cortisone. Diabetes, *3*:296, 1954.
7. Frawley, T. F.: The role of the adrenal cortex in glucose and pyruvic acid metabolism in man including the use of intravenous hydrocortisone in acute hypoglycemia. Ann. N. Y. Acad. Sc., *61*:464, 1955.
8. Frawley, T. F., Kistler, H. and Shelley, T.: Effects of anti-inflammatory steroids on carbohydrate metabolism with emphasis on hypoglycemic and diabetic states. Ann. N. Y. Acad. Sc., *82*:868, 1959.
9. Fried, J. and Borman, A.: Synthetic derivatives of cortical hormones. Vitamins and Hormones, *16*:303, 1958.
10. Froesch, E. R., Winegrad, A. I., Renold, A. E. and Thorn, G. W.: Mechanism of the glucosuria produced by the administration of steroids with glucocorticoid activity. J. Clin. Invest., *37*:524, 1958.
11. Gay, A., Peris, G. C. and Querido, C.: Influence of hormones on muscle glycogen, II. Maragliano Pat. Clin., *15*:281, 1959.
12. German, J. L.: The glucose tolerance test after cortisone administration in obese and non-obese men. Diabetes, *7*:261, 1958.
13. Golorin, B. P. and Sitinskaya, O. N.: The effects of steroid hormones on renal hexokinase. Vop. Med. Khim., *5*:348, 1959.
14. Haugaard, N., Vaughan, M., Haugaard, E. S. and Stadie, W. C.: Studies of radioactive injected labelled insulin. J. Biol. Chem., *208*:549, 1954.
15. Haynes, R. C., Jr., Koritz, S. B. and Peron, F. G.: Influence of adenosine 3', 5'-monophosphate on corticoid production by rat adrenal glands. J. Biol. Chem., *234*: 1421, 1959.
16. Herrmann, W. L., Schindl, I. K. and Bondy, P. K.: Effect of estrogen on steroid levels in plasma and urine. Proc. Soc. Exper. Biol. & Med., *103*:103, 1960.
17. Huggins, C. and Yoco, F. O.: Influence of hormones on liver. I. Effects of steroids and thyroxine on pyridine nucleotide-linked dehydrogenases. J. Exper. Med., *110*: 899, 1959.
18. Ingle, D. J., Sheppard, J., Evans, J. S. and Kuizenga, M. H.: A comparison of adrenal steroid diabetes and pancreatic diabetes in the rat. Endocrinology, *37*:341, 1945.
19. Jackson, W. P. U.: Prediabetes, a synthesis. Post-Grad. M. J., *35*:287, 1959.
20. Kerppola, W.: Uncoupling of the oxidative phosphorylation with cortisone in liver mitochondria. Endocrinology, *67*:252, 1960.
21. Kerppola, W. and Pitkänen, E.: The action of cortisone on oxidative and glycolytic liver enzyme activities in rats of different age and sex. Endocrinology, *67*:162, 1960.
22. Kipnis, D. M. and Cori, C. F.: Studies of tissue permeability. J. Biol. Chem., *235*:3070, 1960.
23. Long, C. N. H., Katzin, B. and Fry, E. G.: The adrenal cortex and carbohydrate metabolism. Endocrinology, *26*:309, 1940.
24. Luft, R., Olivecrona, H., Ikkos, D., Cornerup, I. and Ljungren, H.: Hypophysectomy in man. Brit. M. J., *2*:752, 1955.
25. Marzullo, E. R. and Handelsman, M. B.: Pituitary necrosis and diabetes mellitus. J. Clin. Endocrinol., *11*:537, 1951.

26. Peterson, R. E., Nokes, G., Chen, P. S., Jr. and Black, R. L.: Estrogens and adreno-cortical function in man. J. Clin. Endocrinol., 20:495, 1960.
27. Rosen, F., Roberts, N. R., Budnick, L. E. and Nichol, C. A.: Corticosteroids and transaminase activity. The specificity of the glutamic-pyruvic transaminase response. Endocrinology, 65:256, 1959.
28. Sandberg, A. A. and Slaunwhite, W. R., Jr.: Transcortin: a corticosteroid-binding protein of plasma. II. Levels in various conditions and the effects of estrogens. J. Clin. Invest., 38:1290, 1959.
29. Skinner, W. and Madison, L.: The permissive role of cortisone in the inhibition of hepatic insulin binding during operative stress. Clin. Res., 7:145, 1959.
30. Talalay, P. and Williams-Ashman, H. G.: Participation of steroid hormones in the enzymatic transfer of hydrogen. Recent Progr. Hormone, Res., 16:1, 1960.
31. Thorn, G W., Koepf, G. F., Lewis, R. A. and Olsen, E. F.: Carbohydrate metabolism in Addison's disease. J. Clin. Invest., 19:813, 1940.
32. Wallace, E. Z. and Carter, A. C.: Studies on the mechanism of the plasma 17-hydroxycorticosteroid elevation induced in man by estrogens. J. Clin. Invest., 39:601, 1960.
33. Welt, I. D., Stetten, D., Jr., Ingle, D. J. and Morley, E. H.: Effect of cortisone upon rates of glucose production and oxidation in the rat. J. Biol. Chem., 197:57, 1952.
34. West, K. M.: Relative eosinopenic and hyperglycemic potencies of glucocorticoids in man. Metabolism, 7:441, 1958.
35. West, K. M.: Personal communication, 1959.
36. West, K. M.: Response to cortisone in prediabetes. Diabetes, 9:379, 1960.
37. Wilson, D. L., Frawley, T. F., Forsham, P. H. and Thorn, G. W.: The functional relationship between the pancreatic islets and the adrenal cortex in man. Proc. Am. Diabet. A., 10:25, 1950.
38. Wortham, J. T. and Headstream, J. W.: Adrenalectomy in human diabetics. Diabetes, 3:367, 1954.
39. Yielding, K. L. and Tomkins, G. M.: Inhibition of the enzymatic oxidation of DPNH by steroid hormones. Proc. Nat. Acad. Sc., 45:1730, 1959.
40. Yielding, K. L., Tomkins, G. M. and Munday, J. S.: The mechanism of the steroid inhibition of pyruvate oxidation. J. Clin. Invest., 39:1041, 1960.
41. Zacharewicz, F. A.: Unpublished observations.

General Effects of Steroids on Protein Metabolism*

JAMES H. LEATHEM

Bureau of Biological Research, Rutgers University

The protein constitution of the body is in a constant state of change, with tissue proteins continuously being broken down and resynthesized. This dynamic state of the body proteins suggests that nitrogen metabolism can be influenced by many factors, including hormones. To evaluate the effect of altered hormonal balances, the same measures which serve in the examination of protein efficiency of foods can be used, i.e., nitrogen balance, plasma proteins, organ protein and the repletion of protein-depleted adults. Nevertheless, evaluation of effects must be made with caution, for the state of the body protein stores and the tissue requirements at the time of hormone administration can influence the results.[5]

* Studies leading to unpublished data presented here were supported by research grant A 462 from the National Institutes of Health, United States Public Health Service.

GONADAL STEROIDS

Estrogens. Estrogens stimulate growth of the uterus, fallopian tubes, vagina and breasts. Uterine growth is accompanied by an increase in nitrogen and nucleic acids. However, estrogens are only mildly anabolic in a broad sense. Nitrogen retention has been observed in patients treated with estrogen, but negative results have also been recorded. In the rat, stilbestrol induces a body weight loss and a negative nitrogen balance due largely, but not entirely, to a reduction in food intake. Plasma albumin levels increase and liver protein is maintained. Withdrawal of stilbestrol is followed by an above-normal nitrogen retention.[3]

Progesterone. Administration of progesterone to men and women appears to favor protein catabolism, although in older subjects a moderate anabolism may be induced. In contrast, progesterone is mildly anabolic in mice, and no answer is immediately available to explain the species differences.[5]

Androgens. It has been evident for a long time that androgens will stimulate growth and protein metabolism in the prostate and seminal vesicle. Furthermore, androgens have a far more general effect on the body proteins than do estrogens as these steroids will cause nitrogen retention and body weight gain, the latter to some extent due to the concomitant salt and water retention.[4] Androgen administration causes an increase in muscle mass. This myotrophic action is best measured on the temporalis muscle of the guinea pig or levator ani of the rat.

The protein anabolic action of testosterone can be observed following castration, adrenalectomy and hypophysectomy, and in diabetes. Reduction in nitrogen and creatine excretion can be obtained with androgen in castrated humans of both sexes, human eunuchoids, postmenopausal women and prepuberal children. Testosterone-induced nitrogen retention is of value in panhypopituitarism, in breast cancer and in the recovery from debilitating disease. However, the androgenic effect is an undesirable "side effect," especially in females, thus prompting a search for "nonandrogenic" androgens. Many compounds have been studied but most have been found wanting. Nevertheless, a powerful anabolic agent with minimal androgenicity which is effective in both laboratory animals and man has recently been reported.[2] This compound is $17(2\text{-methyl-}17\beta\text{-hydroxy-androstra-1,4-diene-3-one})$ (Dianabol, Ciba). This steroid is also anabolic in 2- to 2½-year-old rats provided that nitrogen balance of the test rats was voluntarily at equilibrium prior to treatment.

The modifying influence of protein nutrition on the anabolic action of steroids has had little consideration. In recent studies it was of interest to note the nitrogen-retaining effects of testosterone propionate in rats fed 18 per cent casein, wheat gluten, lactalbumin and gelatin in 100 calorie/kg. amounts. The androgen (0.5 mg. daily) improved nitrogen balance in rats fed lactalbumin and wheat gluten only. Protein concentrations of the heart and muscle were significantly less in hormone-treated rats fed lactalbumin than in hormone-treated rats fed the other proteins.[1]

Anabolic agents gain usefulness when they can be shown to aid adequate nutrition in the recovery from a protein-depleted state. Starvation decreases protein stores, and if the rats are castrated prior to repletion, recovery is aided by testosterone propionate. However, androgen administration to normal rats recovering from chronic starvation did not enhance body weight gain, but a slight improvement of nitrogen balance was obtained with androgens during protein refeeding following a 30-day protein depletion period. Body weight gain was not effected. Borderline enhancement of liver and kidney protein reconstitution by androgen administration was also noted.

ADRENAL STEROIDS

A relationship between adrenal steroids and protein metabolism is well known. Adrenalectomy reduces appetite and body weight gain is prevented. Gluconeogenesis is subnormal in adrenalectomized animals and stress-induced protein catabolism is less than normal. However, body weight gain may be restored to normal by providing saline to adrenalectomized animals. The fed adrenalectomized rat in electrolyte balance excretes a normal amount of urea, indicating that the liver can effect and regulate deaminization without adrenal steroids. Adrenalectomized rats given desoxycorticosterone and fed an adequate diet will gain weight and exhibit a normal liver and kidney protein concentration. However, administration of cortisone acetate in dosages which permit 100 per cent survival is associated with a subnormal 13-gram gain in body weight while pair-fed normal control rats gain 50 grams. Protein efficiency is subnormal—an effect of the hormone noted in normal rats. It is well known that cortisone promotes gluconeogenesis, but failure to obtain a normal body weight gain in adrenalectomized rats is seemingly not due to excessive gluconeogenesis, unless metabolic pathways are altered, as liver glycogen is less in the operated rat than in the pair-fed control. However, protein is apparently diverted to the liver, as the concentration of nitrogen is greater in cortisone-treated animals. Cortisol provided results similar to those obtained with cortisone, but halogenated cortisol returned body weight gain to normal. Subcutaneous and oral routes of administration provided similar results.

When adrenal glands are intact, 200 mg. of cortisone acetate can induce a loss of nitrogen in man. As in Cushing's syndrome, excess C-11 oxygenated adrenal steroids increase nitrogen loss. The skeletal muscle loses nitrogen and water, the skin becomes thin, and the bone matrix is reduced (osteoporosis). Some counteraction of the induced protein catabolism occurs as food intake improves. Further analyses reveal that the increased nitrogen loss is associated with an increased urinary creatine, uric acid and free amino acids. Not only is protein synthesis depressed by corticoids but one also finds evidence of an increased use of protein for gluconeogenesis. Cortisol promotes the concentration of C^{14}-labeled alpha aminoisobutyric acid by the liver, decreases blood proline levels without altering excretion and enhances liver arginase.[6] Each study favors the concept that corticoids promote protein utilization. A site of action in the corticoid influence on gluconeogenesis may be the glutamic-pyruvate transaminase.

In pregnant rabbits resorption and stunting of fetuses occurred during treatment with large doses of cortisone. Similar effects were noted in mice. Suppression of chick embryo growth due to subnormal protein accumulation will follow a single injection of adrenal steroids.

The immature mouse is more sensitive to steroid toxicity during the first ten days after birth than later in life. With ten-day-old mice, 3.2 mg. of cortisone acetate in a single injection permitted 71 per cent to survive, but the same total dosage given in two injections on days 10 and 11 reduced survival to 48 per cent. Death always occurred within 10 days.

The influence of adrenal hormones on protein metabolism has received considerable attention, but relatively little attention has been devoted to the possibility that dietary protein can modify adrenal steroid action. Deletion of dietary protein reduces the effect of NaCl and corticoids in extending the life span of adrenalectomized rats.[5] Proteins also vary in quality, and estimations of the biological value in normal animals and man have been reported. However, the biological values for the various proteins are not invariably maintained when the test animal is adrenalectomized and receiving cortisone acetate. Thus, when one replaces dietary casein with gelatin and survival is reduced in adrenalectomized rats despite corticoid supplementation, these data are anticipated; but when lactalbumin, a protein superior in biological value to casein, also acts as does gelatin, these data are not anticipated. Obviously, dietary protein evaluations are influenced by varied physiological states. Since cortisone is known to enhance the excretion of various amino acids, the dietary protein offered may actually provide an inadequate amino acid pattern for synthesis of tissue proteins. Not only is the diet which is fed during the experimental period of importance but also the diet fed prior to study. Thus, if the body is protein-depleted initially, tissue anabolic potential is changed and the need for corticoids during protein refeeding may differ from normal nutritional states. Using adult male rats, a protein-free diet was fed for 30 days to deplete protein reserves. Then an 18 per cent casein diet was fed ad libitum for 20 days, during which time 1.0 mg. of cortisone acetate was injected. Compared with pair-fed controls, body weight gain was not altered by cortisone acetate and the hormone improved slightly the nitrogen balance. Liver and kidney weights and protein concentrations were, if anything, favorably influenced by cortisone acetate (Table 1). A similar experimental design was used to test

TABLE 1. INFLUENCE OF CORTISONE ACETATE ON PROTEIN REPLETION OF PREVIOUSLY PROTEIN-DEPLETED RATS

	CORTISONE ACETATE (1.0 mg.)	CONTROL (pair-fed)
Body wt. gain (gm.)	113.0	112.0
Nitrogen balance mg/kg (20 days)	11140.0	8760.0
Liver wt. (gm.)	14.6	12.6
Liver water (%)	70.1	67.3
Liver protein (%)	56.2	54.0
Liver total protein (gm.)	2.4	2.2
Kidney wt. (gm.)	2.8	2.5
Kidney water (%)	74.4	74.3
Kidney protein (%)	62.6	58.9
Kidney total protein (gm.)	0.45	0.38

0.1 mg. chlorocortisol and 0.05 mg. triamcinolone acetonide. Rats with and without Cl-F during protein repletion exhibited comparable levels of nitrogen retention; triamcinolone slowed the rate of nitrogen retention.

Adult male rats hypophysectomized after one month of protein-free feeding, then fed a diet containing 18 per cent casein for 20 days, will exhibit a positive nitrogen balance and a body weight gain. Retention of nitrogen and gain in weight are, however, subnormal and replacement therapy is required. Cortisone acetate (1.0 mg.) administration to hypophysectomized rats during the protein repletion period has been tested for possible beneficial effect. Protein efficiency was reduced by cortisone administration, body weight gain was not improved, and nitrogen balance was less positive than in non-treated hypophysectomized rats. The low protein and high lipid composition of the protein-depleted rat liver was reversed by refeeding protein and was not prevented by hypophysectomy in the presence or absence of cortisone. Liver weight increased when cortisone was administered; and, although not great, a significant gain in total liver protein was obtained. On the other hand, cortisone did not modify the decrease in kidney weight and total protein associated with hypophysectomy, thus providing further evidence of metabolic shifts in body nitrogen.

SUMMARY

Steroids are clearly involved in the control of protein metabolism as measured not only by specific tissue responses but also by nitrogen balance. In man, estrogens and androgens are anabolic, whereas progesterone is catabolic. However, the influence of estrogen and progesterone on nitrogen balance in laboratory rodents appears to be the opposite of that seen in man. The precise manner in which these steroids exert their physiological effects remains to be elucidated.

Adrenal corticoids exert an effect on gluconeogenesis, and therefore in adrenal insufficiency protein is not available to replenish carbohydrate stores. In adrenal cortical excess, body proteins are mobilized for gluconeogenesis and a loss in body nitrogen can occur.

Although the endocrine system is involved in protein metabolism, the state of the body protein reserves at the time of hormone administration may determine whether an anabolic or catabolic response is obtained.

REFERENCES

1. Brande, P. F. and Leathem, J. H.: Fed. Proc., 19:168, 1960.
2. Desaulles, P. A., Kraekenbuhl, C., Schuler, W. and Bein, H. J.: Schweiz. Med. Wschr., 89:1313, 1959.
3. Glasser, S. R.: Am. J. Physiol., 179:421, 1954.
4. Leathem, J. H.: In Engle, E. T. and Pincus, G. (eds.): Hormones and the Aging Process. New York, Academic Press, 1956.
5. Leathem, J. H.: Rec. Progr. Hormone Res., 14:141, 1958.
6. Saffran, M. and Saffran, J.: Am. Rev. Physiol., 21:403, 1959.

Enzymatic Basis for the
Gluconeogenic Effect of Cortisol

CHARLES A. NICHOL

Roswell Park Memorial Institute, Buffalo, New York

Discussion of the mode of action of a drug should deal both with the attachment of the drug to a specific enzyme or cellular receptor and with the effects on metabolism and function resultant from such combination. Concerning the corticosteroids, there is little that can be said with regard to the first aspect and much with regard to the second.

The specific locus of attachment of the steroid in target tissues remains a mystery. There is no evidence at present indicating a direct interaction between corticosteroids and any of the several enzymes which are altered in the tissues of animals treated with hormones of this class. Two other possible sites of drug-binding can be considered. The attachment of cortisol to various cellular membranes may occur in a manner that can alter the distribution of metabolites and influence the functional capacity of the specialized cellular compartments. Also, the attachment of cortisol to ribonucleic acids in target tissues could impair protein synthesis and increase the concentration of amino acids, which could then be diverted to pathways of carbohydrate and energy metabolism. Hormones do not endow cells with new enzymes but exert their effects, like other drugs, by altering existing functions. Regardless of the exact locus of cortisol in target cells, the important gluconeogenic effects of the drug must be mediated by changes in the metabolic machinery of hepatic cells. Indeed, without changes in enzymatic activity *in vivo* due to increased availability of substrates or to increased amounts of particular enzymes, the remarkable metabolic effects of corticosteroids would not occur.

The complex changes in carbohydrate and protein metabolism which increase the capacity of an individual to respond to stress are oriented toward the provision of metabolic fuels and the maintenance of homeostasis.[19, 29] Several well defined metabolic pathways mediate both the sequential alteration of substrates supplying the energy-producing tricarboxylic acid cycle and the conversion of noncarbohydrate precursors into glucose and glycogen.[2, 20, 25] It is improbable that individual changes in the activity of each enzyme in a multi-step pathway would be necessary to alter the over-all flow of substrates. Instead, it is logical that effective control of metabolism must involve relatively few rate-limiting reactions. Better understanding of the enzymatic basis for the gluconeogenic effect of the corticosteroids requires the identification of those enzymes which regulate or limit key reactions. Which cortisol-responsive enzymes function as valves in controlling the flow of metabolic fuels?

ALTERED ENZYMATIC ACTIVITY ASSOCIATED WITH
ADRENALECTOMY OR CORTICOSTEROID TREATMENT

A relationship between normal function of the adrenal glands and the level of enzymatic activity in different tissues is inferred when the activity of an enzyme is lowered following adrenalectomy or is increased following treatment with cortisol. The interpretation of the significance of such a relationship, however, is complicated. That this is not a nonspecific effect is indicated by the altered activity of only certain enzymes following adrenalectomy or corticosteroid treatment; other enzymes in the same tissues are not affected.[17, 27, 31] A partial list of enzymes which are lowered in activity following adrenalectomy includes arginase,[7] d-amino acid oxidase,[30] proline oxidase,[31] tryptophan pyrrolase[12, 13] and catalase,[1] as well as glucose-6-phosphatase,[35] phosphoglucomutase,[37] phosphorylase,[37] phosphohexose isomerase[37] and alanine-α-ketoglutarate transaminase.[9] Peculiarities in the responsiveness of enzymes in certain tissues remain puzzling. For example, adrenalectomy lowers the activity of proline oxidase in rat kidney but not in liver,[31] whereas d-amino acid oxidase activity is decreased in liver but not in kidney.[30] A number of the enzymes which are lowered in activity following adrenalectomy, or which are increased in activity following corticosteroid treatment, such as tryptophan pyrrolase[12] and picolinic decarboxylase,[21] are unrelated to pathways of gluconeogenesis. If we consider those enzymes concerned with the availability of glucose which are increased in the liver following treatment with cortisol, then we must direct our attention primarily to a transaminase[28] which mediates conversion of alanine to pyruvic acid and to glucose-6-phosphatase,[3, 33] which controls the release of glucose from the liver.

The number of enzymes altered in activity by adrenalectomy or corticosteroid treatment reflect extensive changes in metabolism. In none of these instances, is there evidence that the activity of the enzyme is altered by direct combination with the corticosteroid. In adrenalectomized rats, the activity of tryptophan pyrrolase can be increased by the injection of tryptophan[12] and the activity of hepatic alanine transaminase can be increased by high levels of dietary protein.[28] Such evidence indicates that the level of enzymatic activity may be related, in certain cases, to the level of substrates available in vivo. Thus, the changes in the activity of many, if not all, of these enzymes may be an indirect effect of the steroid resulting from changes in the availability of substrates which could cause enzyme induction of feedback control of enzyme activity. Such circumstances, however, would not exclude the likelihood that important modification of enzymatic activity would also result from the combination of the steroid with individual enzymes or cofactors.[6]

Certain limitations should be kept in mind when attempting to interpret the altered activity of enzymes in homogenates or particulate fractions prepared from tissues of animals treated with corticosteroids. The enzymatic assays, done under conditions of optimal substrate and cofactor concentrations, reflect a certain enzymatic capacity and give no information concerning the fraction of that capacity that is actually utilized in vivo. Since the actual turnover of a substrate in vivo is a small fraction of the enzymatic capacity measured in vitro, major changes in the rate of metabolism of a compound in vivo could result from increased availability of substrate without involving changes in the actual amount of the enzyme. Thus, it is noteworthy that the activity of only certain enzymes is altered in specific tissues following treatment with cortisol.

The preparation of tissue homogenates or particulate fractions is equivalent to taking apart the cellular machinery to study a single function. Examining a small cogwheel from a watch will not reveal whether the watch was running fast or slow. Dissection of a car's carburetor will indicate neither the potential rate of acceleration nor the potential speed of the vehicle. Similarly, there are limitations in interpreting the significance of changes in the activity of individual enzymes with reference to the functional capacity of cells or organs. The important hormonal control of the rate of metabolism may be apparent only when the integrated cellular machinery is moving. More important than the measure of enzymatic activity *in vitro* is knowledge of the rate of flow of metabolic fuels *in vivo*.

ALTERED ENZYMATIC ACTIVITY IN THE PRESENCE OF CORTICOSTEROIDS IN VITRO

The remarkable increases in enzymatic activity that occur in the liver of a cortisol-treated rat have not been duplicated by incubating corticosteroids with hepatic homogenates or tissue slices. The cortisol-induced increase in the hepatic activity of glucose-6-phosphatase or tryptophan pyrrolase *in vivo* can be impaired by the administration of ethionine or 8-azaguanine.[8, 14, 16] Such observations have been interpreted as indicating that the increase in enzymatic activity is associated with the synthesis of the enzyme protein. The period required for the maximal response of individual enzymes in tissues of cortisol-treated animals varies from several hours, in the case of tyrosine transaminase,[18] to several days in the case of alanine transaminase.[27] It is likely that duplication of such responses in systems *in vitro* will require retention of the capability to synthesize new enzyme protein.

Many confusing observations on the effects of corticosteroids on enzymes or metabolic systems *in vitro* have involved the use of amounts of the steroids so large that there is likely to be little relationship to the effects of physiological or pharmacological concentrations *in vivo*. When cell suspensions or cell cultures respond similarly to cortisol and to other unrelated steroids, this circumstance should be disturbing. Prompt attempts to correlate findings from studies *in vitro* with observations indicating whether similar effects can occur *in vivo* would be helpful.

ALTERED ENZYMATIC ACTIVITY DURING GLUCONEOGENESIS

Glycogenesis may involve only the conversion of available carbohydrate to hepatic glycogen. Gluconeogenesis describes the process of the formation of glucose from noncarbohydrate precursors. The response to severe or prolonged stress mediated by the adrenals involves the formation of glucose by both glycogenolysis and gluconeogenesis. When a similar shift in metabolism is induced by the injection of corticosteroids, glucose formed by reversal of the glycolytic process will be conserved as glycogen in the absence of a high requirement for energy.

Only certain substrates along pathways of gluconeogenesis occupy pivotal positions from which several alternate routes of metabolism are available. Both alanine transaminase and glucose-6-phosphatase mediate the formation and disposition of such pivotal compounds. Each of these enzymes is increased by any of the conditions or treatments that induce gluconeogenesis. Thus, increased activity, similar to that induced by treatment with cortisol, occurs in the livers of rats which are starved or made diabetic by the injection of alloxan.[3, 28] It is apparent that cortisol treatment tends to alter the pattern of hepatic metabolism in the same manner as other conditions or treatments that induce gluconeogenesis. The manner in which cortisol can influence metabolic pathways concerned with the formation of glucose in the liver is beginning to be understood with reference to two cortisol-responsive enzymes.

GLUCOSE-6-PHOSPHATASE

The enzymes acting on glucose-6-phosphate can direct the catabolism of this compound along the glycolytic pathway or the pentose phosphate pathway (Fig. 1). On the other hand, the energy of this intermediate may be conserved by its conversion to glycogen or distributed via the bloodstream as glucose following hydrolysis of the phosphate ester. The shifting balance

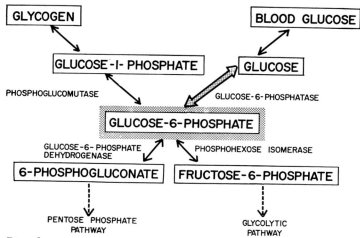

Fig. 1. Pivotal position of glucose-6-phosphate in relation to alternate routes of metabolism.

between the reactions that determine the fate of glucose-6-phosphate in the liver contribute to the regulation of glucose metabolism.[2, 3, 20, 25] The equilibrium of both phosphoglucomutase and phosphohexose isomerase favors glucose-6-phosphate formation, whereas the equilibrium of glucose-6-phosphate dehydrogenase and glucose-6-phosphatase favor removal of glucose-6-phosphate. When measured in the same preparations of rat liver under optimal conditions, the phosphatase is many times more active than the dehydrogenase. The relative rates of these four enzymes under conditions of maximal activity are: phosphohexose isomerase > phosphoglucomutase > glucose-6-phosphatase > glucose-6-phosphate dehydrogenase in both rat liver and human liver.[34] The activity of glucose-6-phosphatase is altered under various conditions in a manner that indicates the likelihood that it has a regulatory function.[3] Adrenalectomy decreases the hepatic activity of this enzyme in fasted rats, whereas injection of corticosteroids increases its activity in normal or adrenalectomized animals. Also, the level of its activity is elevated in fasted, diabetic or thyrotoxic rats.

Glucose-6-phosphate can be formed in various tissues by the action of hexokinase. The occurrence of glucose-6-phosphatase, however, appears to be restricted to the liver and the kidney. Thus, it is unlikely that glucose-6-phosphatase has any role in the responsiveness of lymphoid or connective tissues which are targets of corticosteroid action. The cumulative evidence does indicate that the increased activity of glucose-6-phosphatase is related to the increased capacity of the liver for glucose production.

ALANINE-α-KETOGLUTARATE TRANSAMINASE

Two characteristics of this enzyme prompted investigation in our laboratory of its relationship to gluconeogenesis. First, the activity of this transaminase was found to be increased at least fivefold in the livers of rats injected with cortisol (1 to 5 mg. daily, for four to seven days), whereas the activity in the same tissue of the closely-related aspartate-α-ketoglutarate

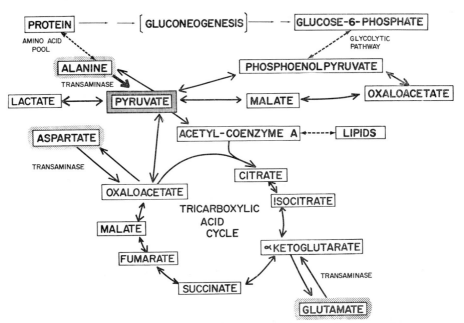

Fig. 2.   Pivotal position of pyruvate in relation to metabolic pathways involving energy production and gluconeogenesis.

transaminase, which mediates a similar transfer of amino nitrogen to the same acceptor compound, was unchanged or was increased very slightly. Second, the keto acid formed from alanine by transamination is pyruvic acid, another pivotal compound for which several alternate routes of metabolism are available (Fig. 2).

The pyruvate formed by glycolysis in the normal catabolism of glucose may be converted to alanine or may enter the tricarboxylic acid cycle following conversion to acetyl-coenzyme A, oxaloacetate or malate. Pyruvate may also be converted directly to lactate or to a lipid via the formation of acetyl-coenzyme A. In the absence of an adequate supply of glucose, as in starvation or replacement of dietary carbohydrate by protein, the intermediates of the tricarboxylic acid cycle, as well as glucose and glycogen, are formed primarily from the gluconeogenic amino acids. Oxaloacetate derived from aspartate or glutamate can be converted to phosphoenolpyruvate and thence to fructose-diphosphate by reversal of the glycolytic process. The step from fructose-1,6-diphosphate to fructose phosphate is carried out by fructose diphosphatase rather than by reversal of the phosphofructokinase reaction. The activity of fructose diphosphatase was reported to be increased in the liver of rabbits which were treated with cortisone.[22] Because of the unfavorable equilibrium for the direct conversion of pyruvate to phosphoenolpyruvate, this reaction is circumvented by the sequential formation of malate, oxaloacetate and phosphoenolpyruvate.[24, 32]

Treatment of rats with cortisol can increase plasma levels of amino acids[4] and stimulate accumulation of amino acids in the liver.[23] Alanine transaminase is increased in target tissues, such as the thymus gland and cortisol-sensitive neoplasms, to a greater extent than in liver.[9, 26] It is apparent that increasing hepatic alanine transaminase will be equivalent to opening a valve allowing the flow of increased amounts of pyruvate needed to maintain energy production via the tricarboxylic acid cycle, as well as glucose production, since neither aspartate nor glutamate can give rise to the acetate unit which combines with oxaloacetate to form citrate. The increased alanine transaminase activity in other tissues which lack the metabolic machinery that mediates gluconeogenesis may well lead to elevated levels of pyruvate and lactate in serum and to impairment of the synthesis of certain proteins through creation of an imbalance in the requisite complement of amino acids.[15] However, the relatively slow cortisol response of hepatic alanine transaminase activity and the lack of any evidence indicating a direct enzyme-steroid interaction would caution, at this time, against any assignment to this enzyme of a causative role in gluconeogenesis.

Observations from our laboratory concerning different treatments which increase, decrease or do not affect the activity of alanine transaminase are listed in Table 1. Comparable increases in hepatic activity occur in each

TABLE 1. EFFECT OF DIFFERENT TREATMENTS ON THE ACTIVITY OF
ALANINE-α-KETOGLUTARATE TRANSAMINASE IN RAT LIVER
AND CORTISOL-RESPONSIVE TISSUES*

TREATMENT	DOSE (mg./day × 7)	HEPATIC ALANINE TRANSAMINASE ACTIVITY
Cortisol	1.0	Increased 5-fold
Fasted 3 days	none	" 4-fold
Alloxan-diabetic	"	" 5-fold
High dietary protein	"	" 4-fold
ACTH	(20 units)	Increased 3-fold
Medrol, prednisolone	0.5	Increased in each case
11-Epicortisol	2.0	Unchanged
9-α-Methoxycortisol	1.0	"
Testosterone	2.0	Unchanged
Growth hormone	2.0	"
Insulin	(2.0 units)	"
Thyroxine	1.0	Increased slightly
Estradiol	0.025	" "
Cortisol	5.0	(Increased 16-fold in thymus gland)
"	2.5	(Increased 14-fold in Walker tumor)
Adrenalectomy of immature rats	none	Unchanged
" " mature "	"	Decreased by 50%
Deoxycorticosterone acetate	3.0	Decreased by 50%

* Experimental details are presented in references 9, 10, 26, 27, and 28.

of the conditions associated with gluconeogenesis. Without exception, all of the potent synthetic glucocorticosteroids which we have tested caused an increase in the activity of this transaminase, whereas analogues of cortisol which are devoid of glycogenic activity had no such effect. This transaminase response to cortisol can also be induced by administration of the adrenocorticotrophic hormone. Adrenalectomy of mature rats decreased the activity of the enzyme by half, whereas no effect was observed following adrenalectomy of young, rapidly growing animals.[9, 10] The remarkable increase in the activity of alanine transaminase in the thymus gland or cortisol-sensitive tumors during administration of glucocorticosteroids or ACTH was accompanied by striking inhibition of growth or even by dissolution of tissue. Such inhibition did not occur with similar treatment of animals bearing cortisone-refractory tumors, and no change in transaminase activity was observed in the tumors.[26] Deoxycorticosterone acetate consistently lowered the activity of this enzyme and caused a slight increase in the rate of growth of the Walker 256 tumor in the treated rats.[26] The relationship between the activity of this enzyme and the growth capacity of cortisol-sensitive tumors is under study.

IN VIVO STUDIES OF ALTERED CAPACITY FOR GLUCONEOGENESIS

The increase in rate of gluconeogenesis in rats which had been treated twice daily for one week with 5 mg. doses of cortisone was calculated by Welt and co-workers[36] from an experiment involving infusion of C^{14}-glucose for several hours. They concluded that such treatment with cortisone resulted in a sevenfold increase over the normal rate of gluconeogenesis. We hope that a similar experimental approach may indicate whether changes in the capacity for gluconeogenesis concern the rate of conversion of alanine to pyruvate *in vivo*. Eisenstein[5] reported that vitamin B_6 deficiency impaired the gluconeogenic response to cortisol as indicated by hepatic glycogen formation; the alanine transaminase response to cortisol was reduced concomitantly in the same tissue. This observation is consistent with the possibility that limitation in the availability of pyridoxal phosphate required for transamination reactions could reduce the rate of gluconeogenesis. Ingle[11] noted that urinary nonprotein nitrogen of corticosteroid-treated animals receiving a high carbohydrate diet was insufficient to account for the extra carbohydrate lost in the urine. The increase in urinary glucose and nonprotein nitrogen that followed injection of corticosteroids, however, continued over a period of several days following initiation of treatment. The rate of increase of hepatic alanine transaminase in response to cortisol follows a similar pattern.

The activity of the aspartate transaminase is approximately 10 to 20 times greater than that of the alanine transaminase per unit weight of liver. Since the alanine transaminase, but not the aspartic acid transaminase, is greatly increased in the liver of cortisol-treated rats, the hypothesis was proposed that the activity of this transaminase may be rate-limiting in gluconeogenesis.[27, 28] Such a hypothesis is useful for the purpose of designing meaningful experiments. Much remains to be done, however, to bridge the gap between measurement of activity *in vitro* and determination of gluconeogenic capacity *in vivo*.

SUMMARY

The elucidation of the enzymatic basis for the gluconeogenic effect of corticosteroids is an intriguing objective toward which an approach has been begun by the study of hepatic enzymes which are altered by corticosteroid treatment or by adrenalectomy. At present, there is no evidence for any combination of cortisol with such enzymes, and the site of steroid binding in target tissues is unknown. The increased activity of glucose-6-phosphatase and alanine-α-ketoglutarate transaminase in liver concomitant with enhanced rate of gluconeogenesis suggests that such enzymatic changes condition the capacity of the liver to produce glucose.

REFERENCES

1. Adams, D. H.: Hormonal factors influencing liver catalase activity in mice. Testicular and adrenal factors. Biochem. J., 50:486, 1952.
2. Ashmore, J., Cahill, G. F., Jr. and Hastings, A. B.: Effect of hormones on alternate pathways of glucose utilization in isolated tissues. Rec. Progr. Hormone Res., 16:547, 1960.
3. Ashmore, J. and Weber, G.: The role of hepatic glucose-6-phosphatase in the regulation of carbohydrate metabolism. Vitamins and Hormones, 17:91, 1959.
4. Bondy, P. K., Ingle, D. J. and Meeks, R. C.: Influence of adrenal cortical hormones upon the level of plasma amino acids. Endocrinology, 55:354, 1954.
5. Eisenstein, A. B.: Relationship of vitamin B6 to gluconeogenic action of cortisol. Endocrinology, 67:97, 1960.
6. Engel, L. L. and Scott, J. F.: Effect of steroid hormones upon diphosphopyridine nucleotide-mediated enzymatic reactions. Rec. Adv. Hormone Res., 16:79, 1960.
7. Frankel-Conrat, H., Simpson, M. E. and Evans, H. M.: Influence of adrenalectomy and of adrenal cortical steroids on liver arginase. J. Biol. Chem., 147:99, 1943.
8. Freedland, R. A. and Harper, A. E.: Metabolic adaptations in higher animals. IV. Effect of ethionine: methionine ratio of the diet on glucose-6-phosphatase adaptation. J. Biol. Chem., 233:1041, 1958.
9. Harding, H., Rosen, F. and Nichol, C. A.: Relationships between corticosteroids and transaminase enzymes. Abstracts, First International Congress of Endocrinology, Copenhagen, 1960, p. 817.
10. Harding, H. R., Rosen, F. and Nichol, C. A.: Corticosteroids and transaminase activity. IV. Influence of age and adrenalectomy on hepatic transaminase activity. (Submitted for publication.)
11. Ingle, D. J.: The production of experimental glycosuria in the rat. Rec. Progr. Hormone Res., 2:229, 1948.
12. Knox, W. E.: Two mechanisms which increase *in vivo* the liver tryptophan peroxidase activity: specific enzyme adaptation and stimulation of the pituitary-adrenal system. Brit. J. Exper. Pathol., 32:462, 1951.
13. Knox, W. E. and Auerbach, V. H.: The hormonal control of tryptophan peroxidase in the rat. J. Biol. Chem., 214:307, 1954.
14. Kvam, D. C. and Parks, R. E., Jr.: Inhibition of hepatic-induced enzyme formation by 8-azaguanine. J. Biol. Chem., 235:2893, 1960.
15. Lardy, H. A.: Hormonal regulation of enzymatic activity. In Kinsell, L. W. (ed.): Hormonal Regulation of Energy Metabolism. Springfield, Ill., Charles C Thomas, 1957, p. 45.
16. Lee, N. D. and Williams, R. H.: Inhibition of the adaptive formation of tryptophan peroxidase in rats by ethionine. Biochim. et biophys. acta, 9:698, 1952.
17. Lin, E. C. C., Civen, M. and Knox, W. E.: Effect of vitamin B6 deficiency on the basal and adapted levels of rat liver tryosine and tryptophan transaminases. J. Biol. Chem., 233:1183, 1958.
18. Lin, E. C. C. and Knox, W. E.: Specificity of the adaptive response of tyrosine-α-ketoglutarate transaminase in the rat. J. Biol. Chem., 233:1186, 1958.
19. Long, C. N. H., Katzin, B. and Fry, E. G.: The ardenal cortex and carbohydrate metabolism. Endocrinology, 26:309, 1940.
20. Marks, P. A. and Freedman, A. D.: Carbohydrate metabolism: metabolic interrelations and control. New York J. Med., 60:3105, 1960.

21. Mehler, A. H., McDaniel, E. G. and Hundley, J. M.: Changes in the enzymic composition of liver. II. Influence of hormones on picolinic carboxylase and tryptophan peroxidase. J. Biol. Chem., *232*:331, 1958.
22. Mokrasch, L. C., Davidson, W. D. and McGilvery, R. W.: The response to glucogenic stress of fructose-1,6-diphosphatase in rabbit liver. J. Biol. Chem., *222*:179, 1956.
23. Noall, M. W., Riggs, R. R., Walker, L. M. and Christensen, H. N.: Endocrine control of amino acid transfer. Science, *126*:1002, 1957.
24. Ochoa, S., Mehler, A. H. and Kornberg, A.: Biosynthesis of dicarboxylic acids by carbon dioxide fixation. I. Isolation and properties of an enzyme from pigeon liver catalyzing the reversible oxidative decarboxylation of 1-malic acid. J. Biol. Chem., *174*:979, 1948.
25. Renold, A. E., Ashmore, J. and Hastings, A. B.: Regulation of carbohydrate metabolism in isolated tissues. Vitamins and Hormones, *14*:139, 1956.
26. Rosen, F., Budnick, L. E., Solomon, D. K. and Nichol, C. A.: Corticosteroids and transaminase activity. III. A relationship between changes in alanine transaminase activity and the growth of Walker carcinosarcoma 256. Cancer Research. (In press.)
27. Rosen, F., Roberts, N. R., Budnick, L. E. and Nichol, C. A.: An enzymatic basis for gluconeogenic action of hydrocortisone. Science, *127*:287, 1955.
28. Rosen, F., Roberts, N. R. and Nichol, C. A.: Glucocorticosteroids and transaminase activity. I. Increased activity of glutamic-pyruvic transaminase in four conditions associated with gluconeogenesis. J. Biol. Chem., *234*:476, 1959.
29. Sayers, G.: Adrenal cortex and homeostasis. Physiol. Rev., *30*:241, 1950.
30. Umbreit, W. W. and Tonhazy, N. E.: Metabolic action of cortisone: d-amino acid oxidase and apparent creatinine formation. Arch. Biochem. & Biophys., *32*:96, 1951.
31. Umbreit, W. W. and Tonhazy, N. E.: The metabolic effects of cortisone. I. The oxidation of proline. J. Biol. Chem., *191*:249, 1951.
32. Utter, M. F. and Kurashashi, K.: Mechanism of action of oxalacetic carboxylase. J. Biol. Chem., *207*:821, 1954.
33. Weber, G., Allard, C., deLamirande, G. and Cantero, A.: Liver glucose-6-phosphatase activity and intracellular distribution after cortisone administration. Endocrinology, *58*:40, 1956.
34. Weber, G. and Cantero, A.: Human liver enzymes of glucose-6-phosphate utilization. Science, *126*:977, 1957.
35. Weber, G. and Cantero, A.: Studies on hormonal factors influencing hepatic glucose-6-phosphatase. Endocrinology, *61*:701, 1957.
36. Welt, I. D., Stetten, D., Ingle, D. J. and Morley, E. H.: Effect of cortisone upon rates of glucose production and oxidation in the rat. J. Biol. Chem., *197*:57, 1952.
37. Willmer, J. S.: Changes in hepatic enzyme levels after adrenalectomy. I. Phosphorylase, phosphoglucomutase and phosphoglucoseisomerase. Canad. J. Biochem. & Physiol., *38*:1095, 1960.

Alterations in Fat Metabolism Induced by Steroids*

GEORGE F. CAHILL, JR.

Peter Bent Brigham Hospital, Boston

Examination of the patient with classic adrenal hypercorticism leaves no doubt that glucocorticoids affect fat metabolism. There is an increase in mesenteric, facial and interscapular fat, and in the moderately severe forms there may be wasting of peripheral fat depots which, when superimposed on depletion of muscle tissue, results in the characteristic "spindly" arms and legs. Patients with lesser degrees of hypercorticism may show a more generalized increase in adipose tissue which appears not too dissimilar from simple nutritional (exogenous) obesity.

The past few years have witnessed much progress in the understanding of adipose tissue metabolism. Contrary to previous thoughts, the greatest bulk of fatty acids are probably synthesized *de novo* from glucose in the adipose cell itself[6, 10] and stored as triglyceride, expanding the lipid vacuole which comprises most of the cell's volume. The conversion of glucose to fatty acid is exquisitely sensitive to the concentration of effective insulin;[16, 26] in fact, insulin is probably the signal to the fat cell to extract glucose from the circulating fluid and to convert it into fat. Another process for expansion of the body's store of lipid is the direct incorporation into adipose tissue of chylomicra. This process also appears to be dependent on the presence of insulin in that it is reduced in the fasted animal and returned to normal by carbohydrate feeding.[1]

Depletion of fat stores is mediated (probably solely) by lipolysis of adipose tissue triglyceride into free fatty acids which are released into the circulation and transported complexed with serum albumin.[7] Many factors seem to be implicated in this mobilization of adipose tissue lipid, but to understand these, the intermediary metabolic reactions of this tissue must be described (Fig. 1).

Recent experiments[2, 4, 27] have shown that adipose tissue triglyceride and free fatty acids are in a continuous state of turnover. In the process of lipolysis, free glycerol[12] is produced in addition to free fatty acids, and since adipose tissue is unable to phosphorylate glycerol effectively,[24, 27] it is unavailable for re-esterification and is released into the circulation and metabolized by liver. For the esterification of free fatty acids, glycerol phosphate is required and is derived from the metabolism of glucose.[2] As stated earlier, insulin is necessary for glucose metabolism in adipose tissue, and therefore, it is insulin which indirectly controls the re-esterification process. Lack of insulin results in less glycerol phosphate synthesis and therefore less esterification, so that free fatty acids accumulate inside the cell and are released into the circulation. Thus, insulin is the signal for adipose tissue to expand itself and, conversely, lack of insulin is the signal to mobilize free fatty acids from adipose tissue stores.[27]

* Supported in part by the National Institutes of Health, United States Public Health Service (H-4569).

From this discussion, it is obvious that there are two possible controlling mechanisms involved in adipose tissue storage. One, already discussed, is the esterification process, which depends on insulin and glucose. The other possible controlling mechanism is the lipolytic process itself. In other words, an increase in the rate of triglyceride breakdown to free fatty acids relative to their rate of re-esterification would also result in net release of free fatty acids. Numerous hormones have been shown to accelerate this process, of which the most important, in a physiological sense, are probably epinephrine and norepinephrine.[3, 14] Other preparations, such as adrenocorticotrophic and growth hormones, have also been shown to mobilize fatty acids, and recently these have also been implicated directly in the lipolytic mechanism.[13, 14] In addition, urine from patients on a low carbohydrate diet contains a small peptide[5] which is also active in increasing lipolysis in adipose tissue both *in vivo* and *in vitro*.

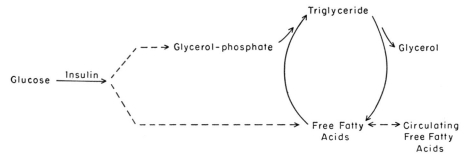

Fig. 1. Simplified scheme of reactions in adipose tissue. Insulin accelerates glucose metabolism, supplying both glycerol-phosphate and newly synthesized fatty acids. These reactions cease in the absence of insulin, and lipolysis of triglyceride to fatty acids then proceeds unopposed by esterification, resulting in a rise in circulating free fatty acids. Lipolytic hormones such as epinephrine accelerate directly the rate of lipolysis of triglyceride to free fatty acids. Recent experiments suggest that steroids may augment fatty acid release by inhibiting glucose metabolism in a manner similar to that associated with low or absent effective insulin.

Animals deprived of pituitary or adrenal hormone[9, 21, 22, 25] fail to demonstrate this increased rate of lipolysis following epinephrine or norepinephrine unless adrenal steroids are previously administered. Likewise, steroid administration to the adrenalectomized animal followed by excision of the adipose tissue and addition of epinephrine to the incubation medium containing the adipose tissue results in a return of the tissue's sensitivity to epinephrine as measured by free fatty acid release.[18] A direct *in vitro* effect of cortisone on the release of free fatty acids has been reported by Jeanrenaud and Renold;[11] however, they were unable to note any alteration in carbohydrate metabolism in the adipose tissue, whether the hormone was administered *in vivo* and the adipose tissue later studied *in vitro* or whether the hormone was added to the flask directly *in vitro*. Their studies, however, showing a direct mobilizing effect of steroids, agree well with the observations of Scow and Chernick[19, 20] in adrenalectomized-pancreatectomized rats and those of Gillman et al.[8] in similarly prepared baboons, where cortisone caused a rapid release of fatty acids from adipose stores followed by development of severe ketosis.

How does cortisone fit into the scheme in Figure 1? Recent experiments by Leboeuf,[13] performed with a smaller and more physiological concentration of glucose in the medium, have shown a definite and significant reduction in glucose metabolism on addition of cortisol to the incubation medium. More important, the increased rate of glucose metabolism, as measured by glucose uptake, oxidation to CO_2, or incorporation into glyceride-glycerol[13, 17] associated with epinephrine stimulation, is markedly depressed by the addition of cortisol. This effect, therefore, results in less re-esterification of the fatty acids mobilized by epinephrine and, hence, a more significant release into the circulation. This inhibition of glucose metabolism by a steroid is a far from novel suggestion; however, direct evidence that such may exist has only recently been shown by Morgan et al.[15] in the isolated perfused rat heart. In this preparation, glucose phosphorylation in the heart excised from the hypophysectomized diabetic animal was returned to the low level of the diabetic by the administration of cortisone.

If the experiments of Leboeuf are physiologically meaningful, the effect of adrenal corticoids is similar to that of decreasing concentrations of effective insulin in limiting production of glycerol phosphate and thereby limiting the re-esterification process. Why then, to return to the patient, the peculiar fat distribution seen in Cushing's disease? One can only speculate, but with some reasonable evidence at hand, that the adipose tissue balance is governed by more than the excessive quantity of glucocorticoids and their fat-mobilizing action. The well known gluconeogenic activity of these steroids results in a constant hepatic infusion of glucose into the blood stream. If the reserve of the beta cells of the islets of Langerhans is adequate, there will be excessive stimulation of insulin release (islet cell hypertrophy has been described in steroid-treated experimental animals[10]) with induction of a persistent "lipogenic" or "fed" state. The fat cell is then caught in the balance of two opposing factors, one favoring lipogenesis and the other favoring fatty acid release. From these facts one can only speculate that the fat cell in one area may be relatively more responsive to the "insulin effect" and in another area to the "cortisone effect." Variations in insulin sensitivity of adipose tissue from area to area have been described;[23, 25] however, no direct studies to date have been proffered which demonstrate anatomical differences in the response to adrenal cortical steroids,* but it is felt that these differences undoubtedly exist, as evidenced by the patient with Cushing's disease.

In this brief discussion on steroids and fat, no mention has been made of the obvious trophic effects of estrogens on mammary and genital fat, or the effects of all the steroids on entities such as circulating lipoproteins, cholesterol, chylomicra, or lipids in other tissues such as liver, heart or vessel wall. These omissions were intentional not only because of space limitations, but more important, because the extensive studies to date have been both qualitative and frequently contradictory.

SUMMARY

Adipose tissue depots reflect a balance between lipogenic factors, namely glucose and insulin, and factors associated with fatty acid mobilization, including epinephrine, norepinephrine, growth hormone and others. Adrenal glucocorticoids appear to be necessary for adequate fatty acid mobilization and their action may possibly be mediated by inhibition of glucose metabolism.

* The typical differences in gynecoid and android fat distributions suggest that adipose tissue is certainly under steroid control, at least in respect to estrogens and androgens.

REFERENCES

1. Bragdon, J. H. and Gordon, R. J., Jr.: Tissue distribution of C^{14} after the intravenous injection of labeled chylomicrons and unesterified fatty acids in the rat. J. Clin. Invest., 37:574, 1958.
2. Cahill, G. F., Jr., Leboeuf, B. and Renold, A. E.: Studies on rat adipose tissue *in vitro*. III. Synthesis of glycogen and glyceride-glycerol. J. Biol. Chem., 234:2540, 1959.
3. Cahill, G. F., Jr., Leboeuf, B. and Flinn, R. B.: Studies on rat adipose tissue. VI. Effect of epinephrine on glucose metabolism. J. Biol. Chem., 235:1246, 1960.
4. Cahill, G. F., Jr., Leboeuf, G and Renold, A. E.: Factors concerned with the regulation of fatty acid metabolism by adipose tissue. Am. J. Clin. Nutrition, 8:733, 1960.
5. Chalmers, T. M., Pawan, G. L. S. and Kekwick, A.: Fat-mobilizing and ketogenic activity of urine extracts: relation to corticotrophin and growth hormone. Lancet, 2:6, 1960.
6. Favarger, P and Gerlach, J.: Recherches sur la synthèse des graisses à partir d'acetate ou de glucose. II. Les rôles respectifs du foie, du tissu adipeux et de certains autres tissus dans la lipogénèse chez la souris. Helvet. physiol. acta, 13:96, 1955.
7. Frederickson, D. S. and Gordon, R. S., Jr.: Transport of fatty acids. Physiol. Rev., 38:585, 1958.
8. Gillman, J., Gilbert, C., Epstein, E. and Allan, J. C.: Endocrine control of blood sugar, lipaemia and ketonaemia in diabetic baboons. Brit. M. J., 2:1260, 1958.
9. Goodman, H. N. and Knobil, E.: Mobilization of fatty acids by epinephrine in normal and hypophysectomized rhesus monkeys. Proc. Soc. Exper. Biol. & Med., 100:195, 1959.
10. Hausberger, F. X.: Action of insulin and cortisone on adipose tissue. Diabetes, 7:211, 1958.
11. Jeanrenaud, J. B. and Renold, A. E.: Studies on rat adipose tissue *in vitro*. VII. Effects of adrenal cortical hormones. J. Biol. Chem., 235:2217, 1960
12. Leboeuf, B., Flinn, R. B. and Cahill, G. F., Jr.: Effect of epinephrine on glucose uptake and glycerol release in adipose tissue *in vitro*. Proc. Soc. Exper. Biol. & Med., 102:527, 1959.
13. Leboeuf, B. and Cahill, G. F., Jr.: In preparation.
14. Lynn, W. S., Jr., MacLeod, R. M. and Brown, R. H.: Effects of epinephrine, insulin and corticotrophin on the metabolism of rat adipose tissue. J. Biol. Chem., 235:1904, 1960.
15. Morgan, H. E., Henderson, M. J., Regen, G. M. and Park, C. R.: Regulation of glucose uptake in heart muscle from normal and alloxan-diabetic rats; the effects of insulin, growth hormone, cortisone and anoxia. Ann. New York Acad. Sc., 82:387, 1959.
16. Renold, A. E., Martin, D. B., Dagenais, Y. M., Steinke, J., Nickerson, R. J. and Sheps, M. C.: Measurement of small quantities of insulin-like activity using rat adipose tissue. I. A proposed procedure. J. Clin. Invest., 39:1487, 1960.
17. Renold, A. E., Cahill, G. F., Jr., Leboeuf, B. and Herrera, M. G.: Effect of adrenal hormones upon adipose tissue. London, Ciba Foundation. (In press.)
18. Reshef, L. and Shapiro, B.: Effect of epinephrine, cortisone and growth hormone on release of unesterified fatty acids by adipose tissue *in vitro*. Metabolism, 9:551, 1960.
19. Scow, R. O., Chernick, S. S. and Guareo, B. A.: Ketogenic action of pituitary and adrenal hormones in pancreatectomized rats. Diabetes, 8:132, 1959.
20. Scow, R. O. and Chernick, S. S.: Hormonal control of protein and fat metabolism in the pancreatectomized rat. Rec. Progr. Hormone Res., 16:447, 1960.
21. Shafrir, E., Sussman, D. E. and Steinberg, D.: The nature of the epinephrine-induced hyperlipidemia in dogs and its modification by glucose. J. Lipid Res., 1:109, 1959.
22. Shafrir, E. and Steinberg, D.: The essential role of the adrenal cortex in the response of plasma free fatty acids, cholesterol and phospholipids to epinephrine injection. J. Clin. Invest., 39:310, 1960.
23. Shapiro, B. and Wertheimer, E.: The metabolic activity of adipose tissue—a review. Metabolism, 5:79, 1956.
24. Shapiro, R., Chowers, I. and Rose, G.: Fatty acid uptake and esterification in adipose tissue. Biochim. et biophys. acta, 23:115, 1957.
25. Wertheimer, E. and Shafrir, E.: Influence of hormones on adipose tissue as a center of fat metabolism. Rec. Progr. Hormone Res., 16:467, 1960.
26. Winegrad, A. I. and Renold, A. E.: Studies on rat adipose tissue *in vitro*. I. Effects of

insulin on the metabolism of glucose, pyruvate and acetate. J. Biol. Chem., 233:267, 1958.

27. Wood, F. C., Jr., Leboeuf, B. and Cahill, G. F., Jr.: Metabolic role of glucose as a source of glyceride-glycerol in controlling the release of fatty acids by adipose tissue. Diabetes, 9:261, 1960.

Panel Discussion

THOMAS F. DOUGHERTY, *Moderator*

DR. DOUGHERTY: Dr. Berliner, do you have any comments on Dr. Frawley's paper?

DR. BERLINER: Yes, there is a comment I would like to make, especially in relation to the binding of cortisol in blood as an effect of estrogens. It has been shown, in an article published in the October 1960 issue of the Journal of Clinical Endocrinology and Metabolism, that tetrahydrocortisone has been found to be free in blood. Estrogen has been shown to have certain effects on the removal of corticosteroids from blood—for instance, inhibition of the conjugation of the corticosteroids, so that increased blood levels of tetrahydrocortisone could occur during estrogen administration. Although tetrahydrocortisone has no biological activity in respect to anti-inflammatory and gluconeogenic activity, it will, however, give a Porter-Silber reaction and make the 17-hydroxycorticosteroid determination in blood high. This is an additional reason why you may have found increased blood 17-hydroxycorticosteroid in the blood without increased biological activity, aside from the binding of cortisol.

DR. FRAWLEY: Yes, I agree that you measure not only bound cortisol but also the metabolites tetrahydro E and tetrahydro F. This would conform to what I said, that the material not only is bound but has very minimal activity.

DR. CLARK: Dr. Frawley, do you think the administration of large amounts of vitamin B_1 would reduce the pyruvate level in your patients?

DR. FRAWLEY: I have not done that, but of course I would think that by adding a decarboxylase enzyme-activating material, one might be able to reduce it. I have not done it and I am not familiar with any animal research in which this has been carried out.

DR. CAHILL: May I ask Dr. Frawley a question? He showed that when hydrocortisone is administered, in addition to 10 grams of sodium pyruvate, the disappearance rate is the same as when 15 grams is given without hydrocortisone, and he interpreted this to indicate that the defect is in decreased pyruvate utilization by the liver in the presence of hydrocortisone. Now, if the hydrocortisone effect were to cause the animal to contribute the equivalent of 5 grams of sodium pyruvate, this would push the curve over to normal. In other words, he could interpret his data completely the other way around—that what the hydrocortisone is doing is to decrease the removal rate, because it causes an increased rate of inflow from the animal itself in addition to the exogenous quantity he is giving.

DR. FRAWLEY: All I can say is that the data do indicate, as you have implied, that the pool of pyruvate is increased but whether the effect is necessarily one of removal or of increased supply is difficult to say; however, I thought it might be due to decreased removal and implied this in some earlier publications without any really good evidence for it. We have, by this pyruvate infusion technique, been attempting to see whether or not the effect was due to decreased removal, but we have not measured the total pyruvic acid pool, which of course would be quite desirable. I thought, in view of Yielding and Tomkins' observations on DPNH and this effect, that it fitted in reasonably well, and this is the reason I concluded it was decreased removal rather than increased supply. However, in support of what you said, we have some data in Addisonian and adrenalectomized patients indicating that cortisol does increase pyruvate, and this indicates that both effects may occur.

Dr. Dougherty: In order to have adequate time to discuss each paper, I now want to direct the discussion to Dr. Leathem's paper. Dr. Nichol, would you start the discussion on this paper?

Dr. Nichol: With regard to the remarkably selective effects of the different classes of steroids which Dr. Leathem discussed, I am wondering whether or not there are techniques or methods indicating the correlation with the localization of the steroids in these tissues?

Dr. Leathem: Is there a particular system about which you want specific information?

Dr. Nichol: I am thinking particularly about the target action of these agents and, since they are rather elusive and in pretty small amounts, it seems to me that we need some methodology in order to study the localization of steroids in target tissues. Would you comment on this in regard to the target tissues you mentioned?

Dr. Leathem: I agree with you entirely. Perhaps I should have concluded my paper by indicating that the lack of better methodology has prevented us from measuring these materials accurately in some instances.

Dr. Stoerk: Dr. Leathem, were the animals that had a striking metabolic response castrated and receiving replacement therapy, or were they normal animals receiving androgens?

Dr. Leathem: The best anabolic action we see with androgens occurs in old animals which are also physiologically old. They eat voluntarily but, in spite of this, only maintain themselves at nitrogen equilibrium rather than in strong positive nitrogen balance. After administration of androgens to these animals, invariably within a period of four days there is an increase in nitrogen retention by about tenfold without a change in food consumption. These were normal but old animals on voluntary food intake. It is usually very difficult to detect an anabolic response with androgens in normal young animals because they are usually in very strong positive nitrogen balance.

Dr. Frawley: Dr. Leathem, do you have any theories as to why changing the type of protein in the diet results in a loss of the anabolic effect of certain agents? I refer specifically to the problem encountered clinically, that certain amino acids produce alterations in carbohydrate metabolism. Possibly, then, denying the animal a source of energy from carbohydrate results in its making it up from protein; therefore, this animal may not be in a position to store protein. What are some of your theories on this?

Dr. Leathem: We have tried to look at the over-all protein picture with the idea of determining how the anabolic agent could be influencing the availability of amino acids internally, but the data may also mean that specific amino acids are more important than others. I can merely cite the effects of gonadectomy, after which, as most of us realize, there is increased nitrogen loss. We can then produce retention of nitrogen by giving testosterone propionate, but we can also produce even greater nitrogen retention by simply adding 1 per cent methionine to the diet of these gonadectomized animals. Now, does this mean that the anabolic agent is operating to retain sulfur amino acids necessary for protein anabolism? The problem, of course is unsolved. We know that the proper complex of amino acids must be available in order for protein synthesis to occur at all, and unless they are present at any one time, the hormone can not have an anabolic effect.

DR. DOUGHERTY: I would like to comment at this point concerning some experiments done at Western Reserve, which demonstrate that in various crops of fibroblasts all grown from single cells—that is, from a clone— there are considerable differences in the amino acid requirements for growth. One of the assumptions we have always made is that certain essential amino acids are necessary for the total body requirements of an animal. However, as far as individual groups of cells are concerned, the amino acid requirements may be considerably different. We have always looked at the sum total, rather than at the individual groups which make up this total amount, and it is possible than an androgen may have one kind of effect on one crop of fibroblasts and not have any effect on another. Then if we study individual cells, the effects on each cell may be quite different, so that possibly in the future this may be the approach we will have to use in the study of hormonal effects, because effects do occur at the cellular level and not at the total animal level.

DR. DI RAIMONDO: There are some clinical corollaries of Dr. Leathem's paper with regard to the protection that high protein diets afford animals that have been placed on large doses of cortisone-like substances. I would like to emphasize that it is very dangerous to put patients who are on large doses of steroids on rigid dietary restrictions. We have had several such patients recently who had severe loss of protein mass and who developed severe weakness in their legs and arms following dietary restrictions. Another point one might consider is that perhaps some of the marked nitrogen-losing effects of triamcinolone are related to the fact that this drug does not stimulate appetite and sometimes even produces anorexia; if these patients are not eating properly there may be exaggerated nitrogen-losing effects.

DR. CLARK: I would like to ask Dr. Leathem whether he has found any differences in the type of protein that is affected by steroids; for example, is collagen primarily affected by the adrenocortical steroids?

DR. LEATHEM: Our basic experimental pattern has been to study total nitrogen balance and to examine five tissues—the heart, kidney, liver, testis and one of the muscles, usually the gastrocnemius. We have not studied the effects on connective tissues *per se*.

DR. CAHILL: May I make one other statement on Dr. Leathem's beautiful work which shows that at times cortisone can be anabolic in nature. In other words, there seems to be a "peck" order in nature as to which way the steroid is going to work. This is reminiscent of the reported experiments with regenerating rat liver, in which cortisone was shown to help the partially resected liver regain its normal weight. This comes up clinically also, in a practical way, because the surgeons always ask us whether high steroid levels will inhibit wound healing in patients with Cushing's syndrome or in those on high dose steroid therapy. These patients often have had massive peripheral mobilization of supportive tissues, and yet, and I am quoting Dr. Thorn, wound healing in these patients is not decreased and, in fact, even may be augmented.

DR. DOUGHERTY: I think this raises a rather important point and that is that the terms "anabolism" and "catabolism" probably should not be used at all, unless they are used with respect to very definite circumstances, or unless you have defined the terms under which you are performing the experiment or describing the clinical situation. For example, we say that thyroxin is a catabolic hormone. Actually, it is, in a sense, catabolic for muscle if you give enough, but if you weigh the thymus you find that there is frequently an increase in the size of this organ. Graves' disease is accompanied by an increase in lymphatic tissue and in these circumstances, thyroxin is not catabolic for lymphatic tissue, but it may be catabolic for another. The big "wastebasket" terms that we have used in the past should be redefined and used only in respect to very specific conditions of experiments or description.

I now want to proceed to the discussion of Dr. Nichol's paper. Dr. Leathem, will you start the discussion?

DR. LEATHEM: Just for my own information, Dr. Nichol, can you clarify the use of the term "alanine transaminase." In the literature there are such terms as SGPT, SGOT, and so forth, and it would be well to define this terminology further.

DR. NICHOL: Thank you for bringing this up, Dr. Leathem. These enzymes are named by the substrates that are involved, and they may be given the name of the substrate on either side of the reaction, such as glutamic pyruvic transaminase or alanine alpha ketoglutarate transaminase. The reason for preferring the name of the amino acid becomes clear when you become involved with some of the other transaminase enzymes, such as tryptophane transaminase and tyrosine transaminase since, to add the names of the alpha keto acids derived from these would make the terminology rather complex.

DR. LEATHEM: I noticed on one of your slides that the animals fed a high protein diet had a fourfold increase in the concentration of alanine transaminase. Do you associate this particular response with an accumulation of glycogen in the liver?

DR. NICHOL: These experiments were done with intact animals fed various high protein diets from the normal level of 18 per cent, going up to 30, 50 and 75 per cent casein in the diet, and there was a corresponding increase in the activity of the alanine transaminase enzyme. This also occurred, but to a lesser extent, in animals that were adrenalectomized. We have not done the correlated glycogen deposition studies in the same animal.

DR. DOUGHERTY: In spite of the fact that Dr. Nichol's paper is primarily on the enzymatic aspects of gluconeogenesis, he made a point that is rather pertinent and important, and that is that one cannot always extrapolate, particularly from the standpoint of rates, from the *in vivo* to the *in vitro* system.

DR. BOLLET: Dr. Cahill, have you had the opportunity to do any *in vitro* studies on fat from different areas in an attempt to find out whether there are differences in responsiveness to steroids?

DR. CAHILL: We have not done these experiments with steroids, but in relation to insulin, the sensitivity of various fat depots throughout the body is markedly different. Reported studies from Jerusalem have shown that intra-articular fat, buccal fat and retro-orbital fat are not insulin-sensitive, and likewise these are the depots that do not increase or hypertrophy during fasting and refeeding. I do not know of any data on the sensitivity of various fat depots to steroids except those data on estrogens; both mammary and vulvar fat are estrogen-sensitive, and this has been shown *in vitro*.

DR. ASBOE-HANSEN: There is a certain redistribution of fat in Cushing's disease, and we also observe hormonally regulated redistribution of fat going on from time to time in other situations. The hormonally regulated interaction between mucin and fat in the connective tissues is something that is involved in this process. In Cushing's disease, for example, I think that there is a generalized trend for mucin to disappear and for fat to proliferate, and exactly the opposite thing occurs in the thyrotropin-stimulated organism. In the myxedematous subject there is accumulation of mucin and reduction in fat, and I think our concepts of this process are far too generalized. There is also the problem that fat disappears from some areas and is deposited in others in patients with Cushing's syndrome. What is the mechanism of this process? I wonder whether Dr. Cahill has any comments on these tissue changes, and especially whether he has any information about mucopolysaccharide metabolism in these diseases? There is an old observation that synovial polysaccharides are polymerized during cortisone treatment *in vivo*, and, on the other hand, that there is a relative cessation of the production of new mucin. What happens in the areas in which fat disappears in patients with Cushing's syndrome?

DR. CAHILL: I have no information on that at all.

DR. DOUGHERTY: About ten years ago we showed in our laboratory, by using an electron microscope, that cortisol enhanced the degree of polymerization of the mucopolysaccharides. Probably the correct term should be "aggregation," not "polymerization," but certainly there was morphological evidence of aggregation of the mucopolysaccharides.

DR. STOERK: Dr. Cahill, one of your slides indicated that cortisone could cause mobilization of fat in diabetic animals, but this is quite in contrast to our studies. We found that administration of cortisone favored deposition of fat in semistarved animals, but that it did not have that effect in the absence of a functioning pancreas; therefore, mobilization and deposition are divergent in that respect, to cortisone.

DR. CAHILL: I agree with that completely. Very simply, we think that cortisone breaks down mainly nitrogenous and probably carbohydrate supporting structures in the periphery; this material goes to liver, the liver makes glucose, and the glucose has to go somewhere; in the presence of an adequate pancreas, the pancreas is stimulated, the glucose is converted into fat and is deposited in adipose tissue. There are any number of factors that can alter this cycle at any point, and once someone introduces fasting plus cortisone, fat is mobilized from the periphery more rapidly than muscles can utilize the fatty acids; if this occurs, then there is fat deposition. If there is not enough cortisone and the animal is fasting and exercising, there will not be fatty acid deposition. In other words, we are measuring the mean effect of about four or five and probably more interacting processes going on at the same time.

DR. FRAWLEY: I want to ask you about your comments this morning regarding the lipolytic activity of epinephrine and norepinephrine. Is it not somewhat surprising to you to find this norepinephrine effect in view of the fact that, generally speaking, it has not shown any metabolic activities other than this? Or perhaps I am wrong and it has shown other activities? It certainly does not stimulate the pituitary; it does not produce hypermetabolism; it does not produce hyperglycemia —all things which epinephrine does. In addition, in one of your publications you make the suggestion that if a patient suspected of having a pheochromocytoma is fat, he probably does not have one. Do you have more than simple speculation to back this up? Some of us have seen fat people with pheochromocytomas depending on whether they have 86 per cent norepinephrine or whether they have 86 per cent epinephrine in their tumor.

DR. CAHILL: I feel very strongly, as far as fatty acid mobilization is concerned, that norepinephrine is probably the most important factor. Sympathetic nerve endings are present in all of the adipose tissue; these release norepinephrine, and I think the continuous turnover of the adipose tissue is a reflection of norepinephrine stimulation causing breakdown of triglycerides and synthesis of more glucose-glycerol phosphate. In other words, the sympathetic nerve endings in the adipose tissue exert a chronic tone for all of us to mobilize fatty acids at all times; it is only because we have normal beta cells which are able to secrete insulin and allow glucose to get in that we do not mobilize fatty acids 24 hours a day but only between meals and at a very slow rate. Therefore, this is perhaps a unique metabolic action of norepinephrine, and as far as fat goes, it is perhaps the most important metabolic role of norepinephrine.

In answer to the other part of your question, we do see fat patients with pheochromocytomas. However, I want to point out one other thing which the surgeons have definitely shown, and that is that when one operates on a patient with a pheochromocytoma and looks around in the abdomen and sees brown, depleted fat, originally called "hibernating fat" by the pathologists, this is a sign of local action of epinephrine or norepinephrine which has diffused out of the tumor into the local adipose tissue, causing local mobilization. On one occasion this finding allowed the surgeon to locate the pheochromocytoma.

Adrenal Steroids
and Water Metabolism*

JOSEPH F. DINGMAN

Tulane University School of Medicine

Physicians in all forms of general and specialty practice utilize many natural and synthetic adrenocortical steroids to produce dramatic and often life-saving clinical effects in a wide variety of disorders including the connective tissue diseases discussed in this volume. Most steroids, unfortunately, produce certain undesirable side-effects which may complicate or thwart continued treatment. A common complication of steroid therapy which results from accentuation of a fundamental physiological action of adrenal steroids on electrolyte and water metabolism is the development of disturbances in fluid balance, edema and even congestive heart failure in susceptible patients. In this discussion, I shall concern myself primarily with the physiological and pharmacological actions of adrenal steroids on the intake, internal distribution and renal excretion of water. The details of their important electrolyte effects and the therapy of fluid retention are discussed elsewhere in this volume.

EFFECT OF ADRENAL STEROIDS ON RENAL EXCRETION OF WATER

The well known diuretic effect of adrenal steroids has been under intensive investigation ever since crude adrenal extracts were first prepared 30

* Supported in part by grants from the United States Public Health Service, the Louisiana Heart Association, The Upjohn Company, Ciba Pharmaceutical Products, and Sandoz Pharmaceutical Co.

years ago. These hormones have been shown to increase the glomerular filtration rate acutely both in adrenal insufficiency and, to a lesser degree, in normal human subjects and animals. The weight of evidence, however, favors the view that the principal effect of adrenal steroids is to decrease the rate of water reabsorption by the renal tubules, particularly in the distal tubular segments where free water is generated; some workers[12, 14] consider this action to be a direct one on the permeability of the tubular cells to water.

Since vasopressin is the most potent humoral substance known to affect distal tubular reabsorption of water, clarification of the action of adrenal steroids on the secretion, metabolism and renal tubular action of vasopressin is required for proper understanding of the hormonal control of water excretion by the kidneys. Although a steroidal antagonism of the action of vasopressin on the renal tubules and delayed metabolism of vasopressin have been demonstrated in animals with adrenal insufficiency,[11] there is good evidence that adrenal steroids do not influence the action of vasopressin on water reabsorption in man and that the metabolism of vasopressin is not abnormal in human adrenocortical insufficiency.

If steroids neither block the renal action of vasopressin nor hasten its metabolic degradation, the only other theoretical site for a steroid-vasopressin antagonism would be at the neurohypophyseal level. We have studied this relationship extensively in recent years,[6, 7, 9] and I might summarize our results as follows:

1. Glucocorticoids such as hydrocortisone, cortisone and prednisone exert a rapid and remarkably reproducible effect in suppressing the action of neural (hypothalamic) stimuli such as intravenous nicotine on vasopressin release from the neurohypophysis (Fig. 1).

2. In normal subjects in a state of constant but submaximal water diuresis this inhibitory effect on neurohypophyseal secretion is frequently accompanied by increased rates of free water excretion and further decreases in urinary osmolality.

3. Patients with primary or secondary adrenocortical insufficiency demonstrate abnormal sensitivity to intravenous nicotine coincident with the typically delayed water diuresis. As in normal subjects, glucocorticoids rapidly suppress the action of nicotine on vasopressin release and simultaneously elevate free water excretion to normal levels in these patients.

4. These effects of glucocorticoids on water diuresis in normal and hypocorticoid subjects are not usually accompanied by significant alterations in the glomerular filtration rate and, although solute diuresis occasionally coincides with the enhanced free water diuresis, we have been able to demonstrate this action of steroids on vasopressin release in subjects retaining sodium maximally in whom the effect of steroids on solute diuresis had been suppressed (Fig. 1).

5. Glucocorticoids appear to suppress selectively the hypothalamic or neural regulation of vasopressin release, since the effect of acute hypertonicity on vasopressin release is not similarly altered (Fig. 1). Also, Kleeman[12] has shown that glucocorticoids apparently do not alter the relatively slight antidiuretic effect of a "volume stimulus" such as venous congestion of the legs, and it is probable that neither osmoregulation nor volume regulation is disturbed by these steroids.

6. In none of our studies in normal subjects and in patients with adrenocortical insufficiency could we demonstrate any abnormality in the action of exogenous vasopressin on the renal tubules.

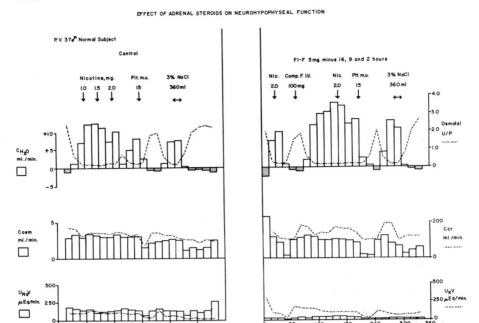

Fig. 1. Sustained oral hydration of 1.3 L. water. Fl-F = fluorohydrocortisone by mouth; Comp. F. = intravenous hydrocortisone; C_{H2O} = free water clearance; Cosm = osmolal clearance; Ccr = creatinine clearance; $U_{Na}V$ and U_KV = sodium and potassium excretion in microequivalents per minute. Nicotine, Pitressin and 3% NaCl administered intravenously. Note the enhanced antidiuretic response to 2.0 mg. nicotine after Fl-F therapy and the suppression of nicotine effect after intravenous administration of hydrocortisone. (Reproduced, by permission, from the Journal of Clinical Investigation.[6])

7. In some instances the sodium-retaining steroid, fluorohydrocortisone, has been shown to sensitize the neurohypophyseal response to nicotine (Fig. 2).

These observations permit certain tentative hypotheses concerning the physiological effects of adrenal steroids in water metabolism and the pathophysiology of edema occurring during steroid therapy. There are sound experimental and theoretical reasons to consider that the central nervous system, particularly the hypothalamus, is dominant in the regulation of neurohypophyseal secretion and that volume regulators and osmoregulators have decreasing priority in that order over this secretion.[3] Glucocorticoids suppress the transmission of neural stimuli to the hypothalamic centers regulating vasopressin secretion but do not alter osmoregulatory or volume-regulatory pathways to the neurohypophysis. A chronic blockade of hypothalamic activity during steroid therapy may render the neurohypophysis completely subject to impulses from the volume regulators and osmoregulators, and vasopressin secretion may then become sustained as long as sodium retention is evident. The fullness of the extracellular fluid compartment will be determined by the relative dominance of these regulators over neurohypophyseal secretion, since sodium retention will activate the osmoregulator initially, and ultimately both regulators will be suppressed when sufficient isosmotic fluid has been retained.

Hydrocortisone and its analogues and even aldosterone produce sodium retention far in excess of fluid retention in normal subjects.[8] The role of potassium in this phenomenon is an important one. The steroid-induced solute retention can be nullified to some degree by an exchange of potassium for sodium in the renal tubule and a shift of sodium into cells to replace the lost potassium; net extracellular retention of solute and the requirement for additional water to preserve extracellular osmotic pressure are decreased thereby. The development of edema with adrenal steroid therapy occurs more readily in chronically ill patients in whom the steroid-induced potassium diuresis is transient and slight and net solute retention therefore more prompt and greater than normal.[4]

Vasopressin is necessary for water retention to accompany the steroid-induced sodium retention. Retention of sodium and solute without water retention has been produced in patients with diabetes insipidus with various

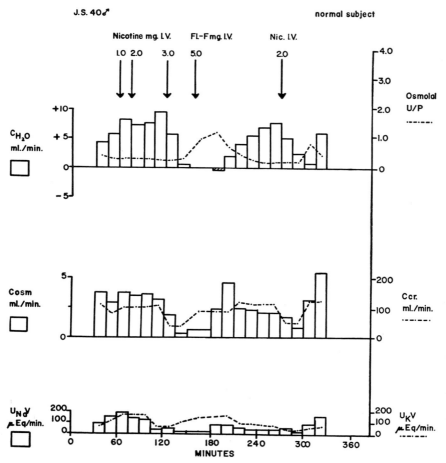

EFFECT OF FLUOROHYDROCORTISONE ON ANTIDIURETIC RESPONSE TO NICOTINE

Fig. 2. Sustained oral hydration of 1.0 L. water. Symbols as in Figure 1. Note lowering of the threshold antidiuretic dose of nicotine after intravenous administration of fluorohydrocortisone. (Reproduced, by permission, from the Journal of Clinical Investigation.[6])

adrenal steroids including aldosterone,[4, 9] water retention nearly proportional osmotically to the degree of solute retention resulting only from combined vasopressin and steroid therapy.

EFFECT OF STEROIDS ON INTERNAL DISTRIBUTION OF WATER

Adrenocortical insufficiency disturbs the intracellular-extracellular fluid balance as well as the distribution of water loads; adrenal steroids correct the abnormal distribution of body water and prevent excessive hydration of cells during water-loading experiments.[10] Glucocorticoids frequently produce a shift of sodium and water from cells to the extracellular fluid in normal subjects;[16] both the sodium and water shifts and the renal retention of sodium and water can predispose to edema formation. Such expansion of the extracellular fluid may represent a physiological checkmate to the renal retention of sodium, since activation of volume regulators may promote sodium and water diuresis despite constant steroid-induced sodium retention.[15]

Recent studies of the action of vasopressin on water transport across biological membranes[13] have shown that transcellular water transfer does not obey simple osmotic laws as we had been taught, but that the cells are relatively impermeable to water in the absence of vasopressin. Vasopressin increases the transfer of water by enhancing the transport of sodium into cells. These findings suggest that vasopressin does, in fact, influence internal sodium balance; but the significance of this action in regard to the renal tubule remains obscure, since many workers have been unable to demonstrate sodium retention with administration of vasopressin to normal subjects. We have obtained data, however, showing an effect of vasopressin in promoting sodium retention along with water retention in patients with diabetes insipidus,[4] an effect which is enhanced by simultaneous administration of aldosterone. These findings warrant further examination of a possible role of vasopressin in renal sodium retention under certain experimental conditions.

Aldosterone also enhances sodium transport into cells,[1] an effect which may be blocked partially by addition of glucocorticoids to the medium.[2] Both vasopressin and aldosterone, therefore, facilitate sodium transport into cells. Vasopressin allows the associated movement of water into the intracellular compartment, and both hormones working together can produce an increase in cellular water and sodium content. Glucocorticoids, within critical concentration ranges, may antagonize the action of aldosterone on sodium transport into cells. This action, in association with an inhibition of vasopressin secretion, may result in an extracellular shift of cellular sodium and water and a salutary diuresis of sodium and water with administration of relatively small doses of glucocorticoids.

ADRENAL STEROIDS AND WATER INTAKE

The total body water content is maintained not only by an action of vasopressin on the kidney to prevent the loss of solute-free water into the urine, but also by a very sensitive intracranial receptor system governing fluid intake located in the hypothalamus in close proximity to the supraoptic nuclei. We have studied several patients with compulsive water drinking in association with hyperadrenocorticism[5] and have demonstrated a derangement in neurohypophyseal response to nicotine in these patients. The ability to concentrate the urine with dehydration and administration of hypertonic saline ruled out diabetes insipidus. Interpretation of these findings in the light of our experiments with steroids and nicotine in normal subjects suggests that the polydipsia may have resulted from a direct effect of steroids on hypothalamic drinking areas or from an indirect effect through alterations in the activity of the supraoptic nuclei.

In general, steroid therapy is associated with increased intake and excretion of water which may continue even in the presence of edema. This phenomenon may be attributed to chronic expansion of the ECF → cellular dehydration → thirst → polydipsia → inhibition of vasopressin secretion through volume and osmo-regulating reflexes → polyuria. Polydipsia may also result from severe potassium depletion during steroid therapy which disturbs the concentrating mechanism of the kidney and leads to near-isosmotic excretion of relatively large volumes of urine.

SUMMARY

Glucocorticoids enhance solute-free water excretion by suppressing the neural control of vasopressin release from the neurohypophysis. Volume regulators and osmoregulators are not similarly affected, however, and the loss of neural regulation may render neurohypophyseal secretion completely subject to the changes in extracellular fluid tonicity and volume occurring during steroid therapy. Mineralocorticoids may enhance the action of neural stimuli on vasopressin release in some instances.

Small doses of glucocorticoids may promote solute diuresis by inhibiting the renal tubular reabsorption of sodium; pharmacological doses may produce sodium retention through an inherent mineralocorticoid action of all adrenal steroids. Vasopressin is necessary for water retention to accompany the steroid-induced sodium retention.

Glucocorticoids produce extracellular fluid expansion by promoting sodium and water shifts as well as by the renal retention of sodium and water. Polydipsia occurring during steroid therapy may be due to alterations in hypothalamic drinking centers, the internal redistribution of body water and the isosthenuria of kaliopenic nephropathy.

REFERENCES

1. Crabbe, J.: Stimulation of active sodium transport across the isolated toad bladder by aldosterone in vitro. Clin. Research, 8:227, 1960.
2. Crabbe, J.: Personal communication.
3. Dingman, J. F.: Hypothalamus and the endocrine control of sodium and water metabolism in man. Am. J. M. Sc., 235:79, 1958.
4. Dingman, J. F.: Role of the neurohypophysis in cardiac edema. In Moyer, J. H. and Fuchs, M. (eds.): Edema, Mechanism and Management. Philadelphia, W. B. Saunders Co., 1960, p. 731.
5. Dingman, J. F., Benirschke, K. and Thorn, G. W.: Studies of neurohypophyseal function in man. Am. J. Med., 23:226, 1957.
6. Dingman, J. F. and Despointes, R.: Adrenal steroid inhibition of vasopressin release from the neurohypophysis of normal subjects and patients with Addison's disease. J. Clin. Invest., 39:1851, 1960.
7. Dingman, J. F. et al.: Studies of neurohypophyseal function in man: Effect of adrenal steroids on polyuria in combined anterior and posterior pituitary insufficiency. J. Lab. & Clin. Med., 51:690, 1958.
8. Dingman, J. F. et al.: Influence of intravenously administered adrenal steroids on sodium and water excretion in normal and addisonian subjects. Metabolism, 7:608, 1958.

9. Dingman, J. F. and Gaitan, E.: Role of the neurohypophysis in retention of water during adrenal steroid administration. Abstract, Proc. Endocrine Society, June 1958.
10. Dingman, J. F., Streeten, D. H. P. and Thorn, G. W.: Effect of cortisone on the abnormal distribution of intravascular water in adrenal cortical insufficiency in man. J. Lab. & Clin. Med., 49:7, 1957.
11. Gaunt, R., Birnie, J. H. and Eversole, W. J.: Adrenal cortex in water metabolism. Physiol. Rev., 29:281, 1949
12. Kleeman, C. R. et al.: Mechanisms of impaired water excretion in adrenal and pituitary insufficiency. II. Interrelationships of adrenal cortical steroids and anti-diuretic hormone in normal subjects and in diabetes insipidus. J. Clin. Invest., 39:1472, 1960.
13. Lamdin, E., Maffly, R. H., Hays, R. M. and Leaf, A.: Some actions of neurohy-pophyseal hormones on a living membrane. J. Clin. Invest., 38:1019, 1959.
14. Raisz, L. G., McNeely, W. F., Saxon, L. and Rosenbaum, J. D.: The effects of cortisone and hydrocortisone on water diuresis and renal function in man. J. Clin. Invest., 36:767, 1957.
15. Strauss, M. B. and Earley, L. E.: An inquiry into the role of "sodium-retaining" steroids in the homeostasis of body sodium in man. Tr. A. Am. Physicians, 72:200, 1959.
16. Ziff, M., Simson, J. and Bunim, J. J.: Effect of ACTH on water distribution in man as measured by antipyrine, T 1824 and bromide. J. Clin. Invest., 31:829, 1952.

Effects of Steroids on

Metabolism of Sodium and Potassium

VINCENT C. DI RAIMONDO

University of California Medical Center, San Francisco

One of the problems in using glucocorticoids as anti-inflammatory agents has been the retention of sodium, chloride and water with concomitant loss of potassium. These changes in electrolyte metabolism are seen most frequently with cortisol, hydrocortisone and ACTH therapy. However, with the advent of the newer synthetic analogues of cortisone and hydrocortisone, e.g., prednisone, prednisolone and more recently 16-hydroxy-9-alpha-fluoro-prednisolone, 6-methyl-prednisolone, and 16-methyl-9-alpha-fluoroprednisol-one, these problems in electrolyte metabolism have practically disappeared. As a matter of fact, the use of large doses of 16-hydroxy 9-alpha-fluoro-prednisolone, 6-methyl-prednisolone, and 16-methyl-9-alpha-fluoroprednisol-one may lead to losses of sodium and water.

PHYSIOLOGY

The adrenocortical steroids that have significant effects on sodium and potassium metabolism include desoxycorticosterone, cortisone, hydrocorti-sone, 9-alpha fluorohydrocortisone, 2-methyl-prednisolone and aldosterone. ACTH increases the secretion of hydrocortisone and, transiently, of aldoster-one. Since the effects of these hormones on sodium and potassium metabolism differ somewhat, let us first consider the effects of aldosterone and desoxy-corticosterone, which, for practical purposes are identical. The changes in sodium and potassium metabolism are mediated primarily by their effects on the kidney, although they do produce changes in intracellular electrolytes and water independent of their effect on the renal tubule. The renal effects in man include sodium, chloride and water retention, and increased excretion of potassium and hydrogen ions. Secondarily, one observes an expansion of plasma and extracellular fluid volume, with or without development of edema and/or increase in blood pressure. In patients with Addison's disease an increase in renal plasma flow and glomerular filtration rate is easily demonstrable. With intense and prolonged therapy, the electrolyte changes reach such magnitude as to result in a hypokalemic alkalosis. If patients are maintained on a low salt diet or have renal disease involving the distal tubules, these changes in electrolyte metabolism do not occur. The loss of potassium is dependent upon the filtered load of sodium which is presented to the distal tubule for exchange with potassium and hydrogen ions. A major effect of the mineralocorticoids is to enhance the exchange of sodium for hydrogen ion and potassium in the distal tubule.[6] If the potassium loss becomes severe, the patients may develop muscle weakness, including the manifestations of periodic paralysis. The renal tubule becomes refractory to Pitressin and the patients may develop a nephrogenic-type diabetes insipidus.[9] Associated with the metabolic alkalosis and hypokalemia the patient may manifest positive Trousseau's and Chvostek signs, the mechanisms for which are not completely understood. With prolonged and excessive treatment with desoxycorticosterone and aldosterone the patient may escape the effects of sodium retention.[7, 8] The exact mechanisms for this escape are not completely understood. However, recent studies done by Biglieri and Forsham[1] on patients with primary aldosteronism suggest that increased glomerular filtration rates with sodium loading may play a role in the escape phenomena. The expansion in extracellular fluid and plasma volume is usually greater than indicated by the increase in weight, suggesting a shift of water from intracellular to extracellular space.[3] A significant increase in intracellular sodium and a decrease in intracellular potassium have been demonstrated during desoxycorticosterone administration. These changes are independent of renal factors.[4]

Although cortisone and hydrocortisone, when given to patients with normal adrenals in doses in excess of 40 mg. per day, produce changes in urinary sodium and potassium similar to those seen with aldosterone, they differ in some aspects.[2] The exact mechanisms for the differences are not known but may be related to the increases in glomerular filtration which these hormones produce. The changes in glomerular filtration occur rapidly and are not necessarily related to an expansion in extracellular fluid. Cortisone and hydrocortisone have little, if any, effect on the exchange of sodium for hydrogen ion in the distal tubules. The urinary potassium excretion is greater than that seen with aldosterone because of the increased tissue breakdown that occurs with release of potassium.

In the doses normally used clinically, prednisone and prednisolone do not produce sodium retention. However, if one uses 30 mg. or more, one can have sodium, chloride and water retention associated with potassium losses. Triamcinolone, 6-methyl-prednisolone and dexamethasone, even when given in large quantities, do not produce sodium retention. They may even produce sodium losses. The exact mechanisms are not understood; however, they may be mediated through increases in glomerular filtration and competitive inhibition of aldosterone at the tubular site.

Since the corticosteroids used clinically as anti-inflammatory agents have metabolic effects, in that they break down proteins, the urinary excretion of potassium is augmented by that released from the destruction of protein. In addition, when huge doses of prednisone or prednisolone are administered to dogs, one can actually produce a diabetes insipidus which is responsive to the administration of exogenous Pitressin.[5]

TREATMENT

Whenever sodium and water retention are particular problems, i.e., in congestive heart failure, etc., one can use the newer synthetic steroids without mineralocorticoid effects. However, even with hydrocortisone, if one restricts sodium the salt-retaining effects can be controlled. Patients will respond to the oral diuretics as well as to mercurials. If the patients develop weakness associated with hypokalemia the treatment includes not only administration of potassium but also restriction of sodium since potassium loss is dependent upon the amount of sodium being delivered to the distal tubule. With restoration of potassium the metabolic alkalosis usually reverses.

REFERENCES

1. Biglieri, E. G. and Forsham, P. H.: Studies on the expanded extracellular fluid and the responses to various stimuli in primary aldosteronism. Am. J. Med. (In press.)
2. Burnett, C. H.: Actions of ACTH and cortisone on renal function in man. In Bradley, S. (ed.): Transactions of the Second Conference on Renal Function, October 19 and 20, 1950. New York, Josiah Macy, Jr. Foundation, 1951, p. 106.
3. Gaudino, M. and Levitt, M. F.: Influence of adrenal cortex on body water distribution and renal function. J. Clin. Invest., 28:1487, 1949.
4. Luft, R. and Sjogren, B.: Metabolic studies with desoxycorticosterone acetate (DCA). Acta endocrinol., 10:49, 1952.
5. Personal communication from Aleksander Ružić, M.D.
6. Pitts, R. F.: Effects of adrenal cortical hormones on renal function. In Adrenal Cortex: Transactions of the Third Conference, November 15 and 16, 1951. New York: Josiah Macy, Jr. Foundation, 1952, p. 11.
7. Ragan, C., Ferrebee, J. W., Atchley, D. W. and Loeb, R. F.: Syndrome of polydipsia and polyuria induced in normal animals by desoxycorticosterone acetate. Am. J. Physiol., 131:73, 1940.
8. Relman, A. S. and Schwartz, W. B.: Effect of DOCA on electrolyte balance in normal man and its relation to sodium chloride intake. Yale J. Biol. & Med., 24:540, 1952.
9. Relman, A. S. and Schwartz, W. B.: The kidney in potassium depletion. Am. J. Med., 24:764, 1958.

Parathyroid Activity
in Hydrocortisone-Injected Rats

H. C. STOERK and R. N. ARISON

Merck Institute for Therapeutic Research

The osteoporosis associated with Cushing's disease or with prolonged steroid therapy is generally thought to be caused by an anti-anabolic action of hydrocortisone upon the collagenous matrix of bone.[1] The increased excretion of Ca and of PO_4 under the influence of excessive amounts of adrenal steroids, according to this idea, is simply a consequence of the aplastic state of the matrix, which—unless newly formed—becomes unavailable for the precipitation of Ca and PO_4 from extracellular fluids. This concept appeared most plausible and has been widely accepted. However, the findings summarized below, at least in part, cast serious doubt on its validity.

We have obtained experimental evidence which indicates that the administration of hydrocortisone or of related steroids is followed by hyperactivity of the parathyroid glands and that this stimulation of the parathyroids is due to a lowering effect on the blood Ca by these steroids. The hypocalcemia caused by hydrocortisone was demonstrated to be the result of a striking inhibition by the steroid of intestinal absorption of Ca. Parathormone (PTH) was found to counteract this steroid action and to enhance the intestinal absorption of Ca.

THE PHOSPHATURIA OF HYDROCORTISONE-INJECTED RATS

The administration of parathyroid extract as well as of hydrocortisone in a variety of species is followed by phosphaturia. In both instances this effect was found to be due to inhibition of tubular reabsorption of PO_4.[4, 9] In view of this similarity of the two hormone actions, the question arose whether they were inter-related. From an extensive study concerning the renal tubular transfer of PO_4, we have previously concluded that the phosphaturia of hydrocortisone-injected rats was mediated by the parathyroids.[2] Experimental data supporting this conclusion are summarized in Figure 1.

Two alternative possibilities were considered to explain this finding. Hydrocortisone may either act to potentiate PTH or may in some way stimulate the parathyroids to secrete more hormone. The first possibility could readily be excluded by the experiments summarized in Table 1. Thus,

TABLE 1.   *FAILURE OF HYDROCORTISONE TO POTENTIATE PARATHYROID EXTRACT (PTE)*

EXPERIMENT	% TRP Ptx.*	% TRP Intact
Controls	97.3	95.2
Compound F, 20 mg./kg.	96.9	91.4
PTE, 200 u./kg.	92.9	93.6
PTE + Compound F	90.2	91.6

* Ptx. = Parathyroidectomized.

the possibility remained that the parathyroids were stimulated by excessive adrenal cortical activity.

Parathyroid activity is known to be devoid of pituitary control[3] but is regulated by the concentrations of Ca in the blood.[10] This regulation is such

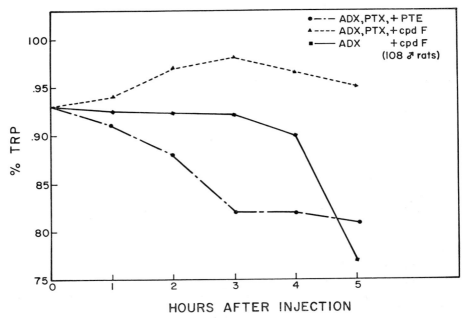

HOURS AFTER INJECTION

Fig. 1. Comparison of tubular reabsorption of PO_4 (% TRP) in groups of (1) adrenalectomized, parathyroidectomized rats injected with PTE, (2) adrenalectomized, parathyroidectomized rats injected with hydrocortisone and (3) adrenalectomized rats with intact parathyroids injected with hydrocortisone. Per cent TRP was calculated by comparing the concentrations of endogenous creatinine and of PO_4 in blood and urine over 5 hours. Striking depression of the % TRP followed the injection of hydrocortisone in non-parathyroidectomized rats (Group 3), while in similarly treated parathyroidectomized rats (Group 2) % TRP remained unchanged. Comparable animals (Group 1) treated with PTE exhibited the usual depression of tubular reabsorption of PO_4.

that a decrease in blood Ca stimulates the parathyroids to secrete more hormone, and a rise in Ca depresses the hormone output.

That hydrocortisone lowers the blood Ca and thereby is capable of stimulating the parathyroids is shown by the following experiments.

THE SERUM Ca-LOWERING EFFECT OF HYDROCORTISONE

Over the past 30 years, a number of reports have pointed to the existence of an action of adrenal cortical activity upon serum Ca antagonistic to that of PTH.[6, 7, 8, 12] It has been known for a long time that parathyroid insufficiency and its attending hypocalcemia are associated with a lowering of the threshold of excitation of motor nerves. A reproducible measurement of its extent was possible by estimating over a range of capacities the number of micro-amperes required to elicit a muscle twitch. Over a wide range of blood Ca concentrations, from very low to normal, an approximate direct proportionality was found between the quantity of current needed for motor

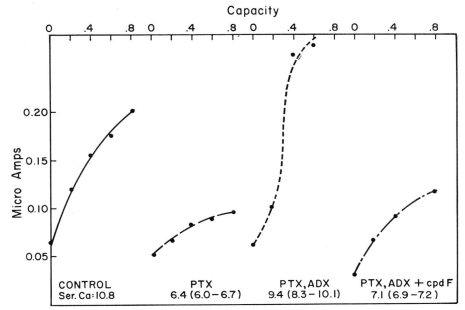

Fig. 2. Increased excitability of motor nerve and hypocalcemia due to adrenal cortical activity. The various experimental groups (6 male rats in each) were subjected to galvanic stimulation. The number of microamps. needed to elicit a muscle twitch is plotted against the capacity. As the latter is increased, more time is required for the current to attain the preset maximum value, and higher currents are required for excitation (accommodation). The degrees of the angles of the various slopes obtained are inversely related to nerve excitability and are approximately proportional to the blood Ca levels.

nerve stimulation and the level of the blood Ca.[11] As illustrated in Figure 2, it was also found that adrenalectomy prevented the hypocalcemia and the increased excitability of motor nerves which invariably follow parathyroidectomy in nonadrenalectomized rats. Conversely, hydrocortisone injected into adrenalectomized, parathyroidectomized rats caused hypocalcemia and its associated hyperexcitability of motor nerves.

It appears, therefore, that hydrocortisone has a serum Ca-lowering effect which can be readily demonstrated after removal of the parathyroid glands (Table 2). It seems not surprising that in the presence of functioning parathyroids, this effect of hydrocortisone can not be measured because of the homeostatic action of increased parathyroid activity. Conversely, the increased quantity of PTH stimulated by the steroid fails to exert its serum Ca-elevating effect since the latter is lowered concomitantly by the action of the steroid. However, the typical effect of increased amounts of PTH

TABLE 2. *SERUM Ca-LOWERING EFFECT OF HYDROCORTISONE*

NO. OF RATS	SERUM Ca (mg.%)		
	Ptx.* Avg. (Range)	Ptx., Adx.**	Ptx., Adx. + Compound F
30	7.5 (6.7- 8.3)	7.0 (6.7- 7.6)	5.7 (5.2- 6.7)
36	8.5 (7.2-10.6)	10.7 (9.0-12.2)	8.7 (6.1-10.3)

* Ptx. = Parathyroidectomized.
** Adx. = Adrenalectomized.

upon the renal tubular transfer of PO_4 can be readily detected and manifests itself in the striking phosphaturia which follows the injection of hydrocortisone or of related steroids.

THE INHIBITION OF INTESTINAL ABSORPTION OF Ca BY HYDROCORTISONE

In an attempt to elucidate the mechanism by which hydrocortisone exerts its lowering effect upon the blood Ca, the intestinal absorption of Ca^{45} was studied.

Groups of intact and parathyroidectomized rats, as well as adrenalectomized rats with and without parathyroids, were divided into subgroups receiving hydrocortisone. The rats were given Ca^{45} HPO_4 by stomach tube, their urethras were ligated and 0.02 ml. of blood was repeatedly taken from the tip of the tail at 5-minute intervals. At the termination of the experiment the rats were killed, their bladders dissected and the specific activity of urine and of blood determined in the scintillation counter. Although the rate of uptake of Ca^{45} into the blood in each individual rat remained surprisingly constant and over 45 minutes approximated a linear relation with time, variations in rates among individual rats of the various groups were too great to encourage a closer comparison of the various experimental groups. However, two experimental groups (Fig. 3) could readily be compared

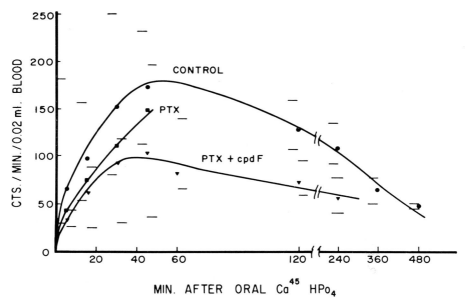

Fig. 3. The three groups of rats summarized above were given equal amounts of $Ca^{45}HPO_4$ by stomach tube. At the time intervals indicated in the abscissa, 0.02 ml. of blood was repeatedly taken from each rat from a cut surface at the tip of the tail. Ca^{45} was determined in the scintillation counter. In 8 intact controls a total of 64 readings was taken at 8 intervals over 480 minutes; in 7 parathyroidectomized rats, 28 over 45 minutes; and in 18 parathyroidectomized rats injected 2 hours before the start of the experiment with 3 mg. of hydrocortisone, 126 samples were counted between 5 and 240 minutes after the introduction of the isotope. The differences in the blood levels of Ca^{45} between parathyroidectomized rats given hydrocortisone and the uninjected, parathyroidectomized controls, at 30 and at 45 minutes, are highly significant (p <0.01).

without necessitating statistical evaluation of large numbers of overlapping values. In parathyroidectomized rats injected with 20 mg./kg. of hydrocortisone, the appearance in blood and urine of orally fed Ca^{45} was strikingly delayed. Parathyroidectomized, steroid-treated rats injected intravenously with $Ca^{45}Cl_2$ exhibited the same rate of disappearance of Ca^{45} from blood as untreated controls.

From these findings it is apparent that hydrocortisone antagonizes a heretofore unknown action of PTH favoring the intestinal (gastric?) absorption of Ca. In the presence of functioning parathyroids this effect is difficult to demonstrate because of the "compensatory hyperactivity" of the parathyroid glands. In parathyroidectomized rats, however, a readily demonstrable, striking inhibition of Ca absorption follows the administration of hydrocortisone. A similar antagonism has most recently been reported to exist between vitamin D and hydrocortisone from *in vitro* experiments dealing with the transfer of Ca^{45} across the intestinal wall.[5]

SUMMARY

Evidence has been presented to suggest that excessive adrenal cortical secretion inhibits the intestinal absorption of Ca. This, in turn, lowers the blood Ca and leads to hyperactivity of the parathyroid glands. Excessive loss of Ca, PO_4 and osteoporosis are at least in part due to this stimulation of the parathyroids by hydrocortisone.

ACKNOWLEDGMENT

We wish to thank Dr. L. B. Achor for advice and instruction with the isotope determinations and Dr. W. H. Ott for statistical evaluation.

REFERENCES

1. Albright, F. and Reifenstein, E. C.: The Parathyroid Glands and Metabolic Bone Disease. Baltimore, Williams & Wilkins Co., 1948.
2. Arison, R. N. and Stoerk, H. C.: Fed. Proc., *14*:159, 1960.
3. Carnes, W. H., Osbold, J. and Stoerk, H. C.: Am. J. Physiol., *139*:188, 1943.
4. Harrison, H. E. and Harrison, H. C.: J. Clin. Invest., *20*:47, 1941.
5. Harrison, H. E. and Harrison, H. C.: Am. J. Physiol., *199*:265, 1960.
6. Leifer, E. and Hollander, W.: J. Clin. Endocrinol., *13*:1264, 1953.
7. Mirvish, L. and Bosman, L. P.: Brit. J. Exper. Biol., *6*:350, 1929.
8. Myers, W. P. L. and Lawrence, W.: Personal communication.
9. Roberts, K. E. and Pitts, R. F.: Endocrinology, *52*:324, 1953.
10. Stoerk, H. C. and Carnes, W. H.: J. Nutrition, *29*:43, 1945.
11. Stoerk, H. C. and Hawkins, J. E.: Unpublished data.
12. Taylor, N. B. and Caven, W. R.: Am. J. Physiol., *81*:511, 1927.

The Effects of Adrenal Cortical Steroids on Bone Calcium and Phosphorus*

IRWIN CLARK and MARILYN L. ROTH

College of Physicians and Surgeons, Columbia University

The effects of the adrenal cortical steroids on the skeletal system vary from species to species. Prolonged administration of these steroids to man often results in osteoporosis,[1] whereas in the rat areas of increased density adjacent to the epiphyses have been observed.[2, 6] Recently it has been reported that the administration of cortisone to rats maintained on a diet low in calcium and phosphorus resulted in progressive rarefaction of bone.[10] Earlier studies with radioactive calcium have demonstrated that the adrenal cortical steroids inhibit the uptake of calcium by bone and increase the urinary excretion of calcium.[3] The following experiments were designed to investigate further the effects of adrenal cortical steroids upon bone phosphorus and calcium metabolism in the rat.

Effects of Adrenal Cortical Steroid Administration on Urinary Radiophosphorus Excretion of Adult Rats 48 Hours after the Administration of P³². It may be seen (Table 1) that subcutaneous administration of the

TABLE 1.   URINARY RADIOACTIVE PHOSPHORUS

HOURS	0-8	9-24	SUM, 0-24
Treatment			
Control*	100	100	100
Hydrocortisone (0.5 mg./100 gm. body weight)	156	72	100
Hydrocortisone (1.0 mg./100 gm. body weight)	196	72	127
Hydrocortisone (4.0 mg./100 gm. body weight)	182	130	148
6-alpha-fluorotriamcinolone (0.1 mg./100 gm. body weight)	213	139	164
6-alpha-fluorotriamcinolone (0.2 mg./100 gm. body weight)	234	190	205

* Control values arbitrarily set at 100 for ease in comparison of data.

steroids increases the urinary P^{32} significantly above the control values at 8 hours. The larger the dose or the more potent the steroid, the greater is the response and the more persistent is its action. Six-alpha-fluorotriamcinolone is about twenty times more active than hydrocortisone as measured by the conventional assays for anti-inflammatory activity. In this experiment the same order of activity seems to be maintained.

The pattern of Ca^{45} excretion observed in rats that had received this isotope 48 hours prior to the administration of adrenal cortical steroids[3, 4]

* Supported by United States Public Health Service Grant No. A-4071.

was similar to that just described for P^{32}. A dose response effect of gluco-corticoid administration on Ca^{45} excretion has been demonstrated.[4] Current investigations are aimed at determining whether P^{32} will behave in a similar fashion.

The Effect of a Single Subcutaneous Injection of Hydrocortisone on Urinary Ca^{40}, Ca^{45}, P^{31} and P^{32} of Intact and Parathyroidectomized Rats Which Had Received the Isotopes 50 Days Before. In an attempt to detect the early changes in calcium and phosphorus excretion, collections of urine were made at 3-hour intervals during the first 9 hours and then from 10 to 24 hours and from 25 to 48 hours. At this time, 50 days after the injection of the isotopes, the soft tissue and serum levels of isotopes are low and the animals excrete a small, consistent fraction of the ingested dose.[9] If there

TABLE 2. URINARY VALUES

HOURS	0-3	4-6	7-9	10-24	25-48	SUM, 0-48
	Intact Rats					
Controls*	100	100	100	100	100	100
Hydrocortisone (3.0 mg./100 gm. body weight)						
Calcium⁴⁵**	285	340	90	106	110	145
Calcium⁴⁰	268	283	102	103	88	105
Phosphorus³²**	145	238	178	208	150	176
Phosphorus³¹	223	316	378	218	181	223
	*Parathyroidectomized Rats****					
Controls*	100	100	100	100	100	100
Hydrocortisone (3.0 mg./100 gm. body weight)						
Calcium⁴⁵**	205	92	22	71	96	96
Calcium⁴⁰	247	128	57	121	136	126
Phosphorus³²**	161	256	463	291	110	173
Phosphorus³¹	235	474	659	275	131	168

* The values for the intact and parathyroidectomized control rats were arbitrarily set at 100 for ease of comparison of data.

** The Ca^{45} and P^{32} were administered 50 days prior to the administration of hydrocortisone.

*** The animals were parathyroidectomized 7 days prior to the administration of hydrocortisone.

is any depression of tubular reabsorption of these ions by the kidneys or any increase in bone turnover, a larger amount of these nuclides will be excreted into the urine. A depression of the reabsorption of either calcium or phosphorus by the tubules of the kidneys will lower the serum levels of these elements, thus necessitating a withdrawal of calcium and phosphorus from the skeleton to restore the serum levels.

It may be seen in Table 2 that the administration of hydrocortisone to the intact animals resulted in a prompt increase in Ca^{45} and Ca^{40} excretion, both of which had returned by 6 hours to the control levels and remained there for the balance of the collection period. The transitory nature of the increased Ca^{45} and Ca^{40} excretion may very likely be the result of the action of the steroid on the kidney tubules.

Hydrocortisone administration also increased the excretion of P^{32} and P^{31} above the control values. In contrast to the calcium excretion data, the phosphorus values remained elevated for the entire 48 hours. It has been reported that cortisone decreases the tubular reabsorption of phosphate in intact or adrenalectomized dogs.[8] Since the renal effect on the calcium excretion had worn off by 6 hours, in all probability the renal effect on phosphorus also had ceased at this time. The elevated P^{31} and P^{32} excretion seen from 7 to 48 hours very likely may be the result of the inhibition of phosphate utilization or re-utilization of normal breakdown products by the skeleton and soft tissues.

The aparathyroid animals (Table 2) that received the steroid also excreted more Ca^{45} and Ca^{40} than their respective controls for the first 3 hours. However, a marked repression of both Ca^{45} and Ca^{40} excretion occurred during the 7 to 9 hour collection period, after which time the excretion of Ca^{45} returned to the control value and the excretion of Ca^{40} increased above the control. The increased excretion of P^{31} and P^{32} again remained elevated throughout the 48 hours as it did with the intact animals. It has been shown[7] that the hyperphosphaturia observed after hydrocortisone treatment is not dependent on the presence of the parathyroid glands.

The relative total excretion values (Table 2—sum, 0-48 hours) indicate that the effects of hydrocortisone are essentially the same on both intact and aparathyroid rats with respect to calcium and phosphorus excretion. Moreover, the similarity between the excretion patterns of calcium and of phosphorus for the first 6 hours would imply a decreased tubular reabsorption of calcium as well as phosphorus. From 7 hours onward the excretion of phosphorus is quite different from that of calcium.

The Effect of Daily Administration (12 Days) of Prednisolone on the Removal of Ca^{45} and P^{32} from Adult Rats Receiving Isotopes 35 Days Before. For 12 days prior to the administration of the steroid and during

TABLE 3. URINARY VALUES

DAYS	1-2	3-4	5-6	7-8	9-10	11-12	SUM, 1-12
Calcium[40] (mg.)							
Control	4.3	4.1	4.4	3.2	2.9	2.6	21.5
Prednisolone	3.8	3.1	4.1	7.9	8.6	5.6	33.1
p-Value	N.S.	N.S.	N.S.	N.S.	< 0.01	< 0.01	N.S.
Calcium[45]* (Counts $\times 10^4$)							
Control	2.4	1.9	1.9	1.9	1.6	1.8	11.5
Prednisolone	1.6	1.8	2.1	2.9	3.4	4.2	16.0
p-Value	< 0.1	N.S.	N.S.	< 0.2	< 0.1	< 0.2	< 0.2
Phosphorus[31] (mg.)							
Control	29.7	34.4	37.4	34.5	32.5	34.0	203
Prednisolone	44.1	42.2	41.9	42.3	48.2	47.7	266
p-Value	< 0.01	< 0.01	N.S.	N.S.	< 0.01	< 0.01	< 0.01
Phosphorus[32]* (Counts $\times 10^4$)							
Control	2.7	2.1	2.1	1.8	1.7	1.8	12.2
Prednisolone	3.9	2.5	3.0	2.4	2.5	2.2	16.4
p-Value	< 0.01	N.S.	< 0.01	< 0.05	< 0.01	N.S.	< 0.01

* The P^{32} and Ca^{45} were injected 35 days before the administration of prednisolone.

the urinary collection period, the rats were maintained on a low calcium, low phosphorus diet in an attempt to minimize the variations in calcium and phosphorus metabolism between individual rats. The animals received 1 mg. of prednisolone per 100 grams of body weight daily for 12 days beginning on the 23rd day. The food intake of the control rats was restricted to approximately that which the treated animals consumed. At the end of the experimental period the steroid-treated rats had lost 57 grams and the control animals had just maintained their weight. Urine was collected from each rat for 48-hour periods during an interval of 12 days.

In Table 3 it may be seen that beginning at about the ninth day there was a significant increase in the excretion of the unlabeled calcium. However, the total excretion values were not significant. Similar results have been reported previously.[3] Again, a repression of urinary radiocalcium was also observed during the first two days.[5] Although there was an increase in urinary Ca^{45} beginning at day 7, it was not highly significant since considerable variation of urinary Ca^{45} existed within the groups. In previous experiments this increase in urinary Ca^{45} had been statistically significant.[3]

The administration of prednisolone resulted in a significant increase in the elimination of both P^{31} and P^{32}. Although most of the isotope is in bone,

TABLE 4. BONE DATA

	CONTROLS (8 Rats)	PREDNISOLONE (8 Rats)	P-VALUES (8 Rats)
Humerus			
Dry and defatted weight (mg.)	354	357	N.S.
Ratio $\dfrac{\text{Ash weight}}{\text{Dry weight}}$	0.64	0.63	N.S.
Ratio $\dfrac{Ca^{40}}{\text{Dry weight}}$	0.39	0.38	N.S.
Ratio $\dfrac{Ca^{45}*}{Ca^{40}}$	1.5×10^4	1.7×10^4	N.S.
Ratio $\dfrac{P^{32}*}{P^{31}}$	2.1×10^3	2.1×10^3	N.S.
Calvaria			
Ratio $\dfrac{\text{Ash weight}}{\text{Dry weight}}$	0.64	0.59	N.S.
Ratio $\dfrac{Ca^{40}}{\text{Ash weight}}$	0.37	0.41	N.S.
Ratio $\dfrac{P^{31}}{\text{Ash weight}}$	0.18	0.19	N.S.
Ratio $\dfrac{Ca^{45}*}{Ca^{40}}$	2.5×10^4	2.5×10^4	N.S.
Ratio $\dfrac{P^{32}*}{P^{31}}$	389	396	N.S.

* The Ca^{45} and P^{32} were administered 47 days before the animals were sacrificed.

the breakdown of soft tissues containing P^{32} cannot be ignored, since these animals lost 57 grams of body weight while their skeletal mass was unchanged as judged by femoral weights (Table 4). The increased elimination of Ca^{45}, however, must come from bone since practically all of the isotope is there.[9]

Analytical data of the humeri and calvaria may be seen in Table 4. No significant changes were found in ash weight or composition of the ash. Furthermore, there were no significant changes in specific activities of the calcium and phosphorus of either the humeri or calvaria. Borle, Nichols and Karnovsky[2] reported an increase in the calcium content of the femur ash. However, in their experiments massive doses of prednisolone (10 mg. per day) were administered for seven days (total 70 mg.), whereas in this experiment the animals received 1 mg. per 100 grams of body weight (total approximately 24 mg. over a 12-day period). In addition, their rats were fed a diet adequate in calcium and phosphorus, whereas in this experiment a diet low in calcium and phosphorus was used. With lower doses such as

2 mg. cortisone per 100 grams of body weight, Follis[6] was unable to find any pathologic changes in the bone in three weeks.

Despite the body weight loss, the humeri of the steroid-treated rats weighed the same as those of the controls. This would imply a lack of any catabolic effect of prednisolone on the rat skeleton and, in fact, would indicate a decrease in osteolytic action as suggested by Follis,[6] since a weight loss of this magnitude does result in a loss of bone weight.

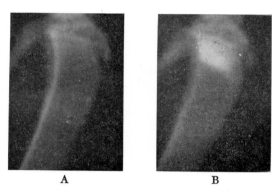

A   B

Fig. 1.   A, Tibia from control rat. B, Tibia from prednisolone-treated rat.

Effect of Prolonged Treatment (60 Days) with Prednisolone on the Mineral Composition of Bone of Growing Rats.   Male Holtzman rats weighing between 125 and 135 grams received 0.5 mg. prednisolone per 100 grams of body weight for 60 days. The histologic changes were similar to those observed by Follis[6] after large doses of cortisone were administered to growing rats. The epiphyses were narrowed and in the metaphyseal area there was a wide zone of densely packed spicules of calcified cartilagenous matrix enclosed by bone. Radiographic examination of the bones revealed areas of increased density in sites where histologic observations indicated an increased number of epiphyseal cartilage fragments in the metaphysis (Fig. 1). However, no changes in the mineral composition of the bone were found (Table 5).

TABLE 5.   BONE DATA

	CONTROLS (12 Rats)	PREDNISOLONE (12 Rats)	P-VALUES
Weight gains (gm.)	192	66	< 0.001
Femur weight (mg.)	515	394	< 0.001
Ratio $\dfrac{Ca^{40}}{Dry\ weight}$	0.24	0.25	N.S.
Ratio $\dfrac{Ca^{40}}{Ash\ weight}$	0.38	0.39	N.S.
Ratio $\dfrac{Ca^{45}*}{Ca^{40}}$	525	385	< 0.1
Ratio $\dfrac{P^{31}}{Dry\ weight}$	0.12	0.11	N.S.
Ratio $\dfrac{P^{31}}{Ash\ weight}$	0.18	0.17	N.S.
Ratio $\dfrac{P^{32}*}{P^{31}}$	10.3	8.5	< 0.1

* Ca^{45} and P^{32} injected 24 hours before the animals were sacrificed.

The calcium and phosphorus specific activities of the femurs of the treated animals, 24 hours after the administration of Ca^{45} and P^{32}, were less than those of the control rats. Again, this indicates a decreased uptake by the bone as has been noted before.[3] The decreased uptake of Ca^{45} and P^{32} by the bones of the steroid-treated rats is compatible with the histologic findings of a marked narrowing of the epiphysis. Since this is the area where the major portion of the isotopes would be deposited initially, obviously any decrease in osteogenic activity will result in a decreased deposition of Ca^{45} or P^{32}.

In summary, the hypercalciuria and hyperphosphaturia observed shortly after a single injection of adrenal cortical steroids to rats is probably the result of a decreased reabsorption of these ions by the kidney tubules.

The persistent hyperphosphaturia observed for 48 hours after a single injection of steroid may be explained by an inhibition of phosphate utilization by soft and hard tissue. The possibility of an increased turnover of phosphorus-containing compounds in soft tissues does exist.

Since the patterns of excretion of both calcium and phosphorus in intact and aparathyroid rats are almost identical, it is apparent that the action of hydrocortisone is not mediated through the parathyroid glands.

The administration of prednisolone for 12 days to adult rats caused no detectable change in the skeletal mass despite a 25 per cent weight loss.

The prolonged administration of prednisolone to growing rats resulted in an inhibition of growth and in a decreased uptake of P^{32} and Ca^{45} by the bones. Moreover, radiographic examination of the bones revealed zones of increased density in support of the histologic findings.

REFERENCES

1. Albright, F.: Harvey Lecture, 38:123, 1942-1943.
2. Borle, A. B., Nichols, G. and Karnovsky, M. J.: Endocrinology, 66:508, 1960.
3. Clark, I., Geoffroy, R. F. and Bowers, W.: Endocrinology, 64:849, 1959.
4. Clark, I.: Fed. Proc., 18:805, 1959.
5. Clark, I. and Geoffroy, R. F.: J. Biol. Chem., 233:203, 1958.
6. Follis, R. H.: Proc. Soc. Exper. Biol. & Med., 76:722, 1951.
7. Laron, Z., Cranford, J. D. and Klein, R.: Proc. Soc. Exper. Biol. & Med., 96:649, 1957.
8. Roberts, K. E. and Pitts, R. F.: Endocrinology, 52:324. 1953.
9. Singer, L. and Armstrong, W. D.: Metabolic Interrelations, New York, Josiah Macy, Jr. Foundation, 1951, p. 259.
10. Storey, E.: Brit. J. Exper. Path., 41:207, 1960.

The Effects of Steroids on Vascular Hemodynamics in Normotensive and Hypotensive States*

MAX H. WEIL

University of Southern California School of Medicine

Biochemical derangements that result from adrenal cortical hyperfunction or from critical reduction of endogenous corticosteroid hormones are sometimes overshadowed by major disturbances in cardiovascular function. Hypertension and congestive heart failure may be predominant clinical features in patients with adrenal cortical hyperfunction, and the appearance of hypotension and shock during an acute illness or following a minor injury may be the presenting signs of previously undiagnosed adrenal cortical insufficiency. When steroid drugs are used as anti-inflammatory agents in patients with diseases of connective tissues, the actions of these hormones on the circulatory system are responsible for several unwelcome side effects, especially with respect to the increased retention of sodium and water. Nevertheless, these drugs are of practical value in the treatment of selected patients with cardiovascular diseases including carditis, congestive heart failure, orthostatic hypotension and bacterial shock. The purpose of this presentation is to summarize current concepts of the cardiovascular actions of corticosteroids. Wherever possible, these are discussed with reference to their clinical use for treatment of patients with cardiovascular disturbances.

CARDIODYNAMIC EFFECTS

Observations on the Normal Myocardium.   Nayler,[44] studying the metabolism of the isolated toad heart, reported that 9-α-fluorohydrocortisone (9-α-FF) has an inotropic action resembling that of digitalis. However, in the isolated perfused guinea pig heart, Nasmyth[43] found that hydrocortisone depressed the amplitude and rate of cardiac contraction. Each of these reports has been cited as evidence for or against the use of steroids in myocardial failure. A third study by Nahas and co-workers,[42] using the isolated perfused heart-lung preparation of the dog does not provide support for either interpretation. Infusion of 10 mg. of cortisol succinate into the cardiopulmonary circuit did not cause any significant alteration in cardiac function as reflected in cardiac output, outflow pressure and electrocardiogram. Present evidence indicates that the acute administration of corticosteroid does not significantly alter myocardial contractility. The protracted use of corticosteroid drugs may alter myocardial function in relationship to alterations in electrolyte and fluid shifts. Loss of intracellular potassium during steroid therapy is especially important in this regard. The reciprocal relationship between potassium concentration and the myocardial action of

* Supported by grants-in-aid from the American Heart Association and the Los Angeles County Heart Association.

410

digitalis glycosides has important and practical clinical implications. In the experimental animal, severe deficiency of potassium has resulted in histologically demonstrable injury to myocardium,[11] and Selye[55] has produced myocardial necrosis in the rat treated with desoxycorticosterone or hydrocortisone. These findings have received considerable attention, but the special conditions of Selye's experiments provide no direct clinical implications for the human patient.

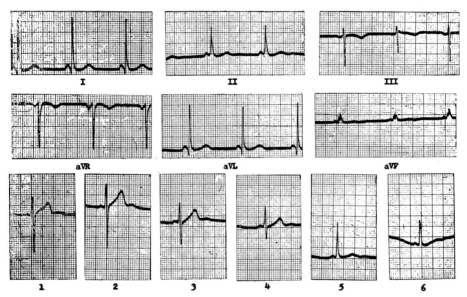

Fig. 1. Electrocardiogram of a 30-year-old Negro woman with Cushing's syndrome, demonstrating shortened P-R interval and early left ventricular hypertrophy. Urinary corticoid excretion was in excess of 20 mg. per 24 hours (Porter-Silber method). The patient also had hypertension (180/120 mm.) and hyperglycemia. She died of embolic complications of pelvic thrombophlebitis. Adrenal hyperplasia and left ventricular hypertrophy were found at autopsy.

Electrocardiographic Effects. Corticosteroids accelerate atrioventricular conduction (Fig. 1). Lown and associates[33] found that the average P-R interval in 34 patients with adrenal cortical hyperfunction was 0.136 seconds, compared with a value which averaged 0.158 seconds in 539 control subjects. The atrioventricular conduction time was inversely related to the concentration of urinary 17-ketosteroids. Corresponding changes were produced by the exogenous administration of glucocorticoid. Conversely, the P-R interval of a group of 50 patients with adrenal cortical insufficiency was significantly prolonged, and ten of these exhibited first degree heart block. Replacement therapy with cortisone decreased the P-R interval but administration of desoxycortisone had no such effect.

The mechanism by which the steroid hormones increase the speed of atrioventricular conduction is not known. Changes in potassium concentration do not explain the effect on the P-R interval. Both Lown[33] and Friedberg[12] and their associates suggest that steroids increase the speed of conduction by increasing the effectiveness of adrenergic stimuli. The possibility of potentiation of sympathetic activity by adrenal steroids will be reviewed in somewhat greater detail in connection with their role in the treatment of shock.

Myocarditis. The benefit derived from corticosteroids during the treatment of inflammatory diseases of the myocardium is associated with anti-inflammatory actions of the hormone. Clinical manifestations of acute rheumatic myocarditis (as well as endocarditis and pericarditis) are dramatically controlled.[66] Although the hormones may be life-saving in cases of pancarditis and myocardial failure, their use in preference to salicylates under less critical circumstances is controversial.[35] Present evidence, which is based entirely on statistical evaluation of clinical observations, favors the viewpoint that the hormones are singularly effective in suppressing the acute inflammatory process that accounts for myocardial failure. However, there is no proof that the natural history of the disease is in any way altered.[26, 36]

Myocardial Infarction. Corticosteroids have been recommended as adjuncts in the treatment of acute myocardial infarction. Reference is made to experiments in which dogs treated with cortisone had (1) decreased mortality, (2) increased vascularity of the myocardium and (3) a smaller area of residual fibrosis in comparison to untreated controls.[14, 25] Detailed studies by three other groups of experienced observers, however, failed to confirm such beneficial effects.[4, 21, 45] Nevertheless, a number of clinical reports have appeared, particularly in the European literature, which favor the use of corticosteroids in the treatment of myocardial infarction with or without shock.[9, 14, 27, 41] These agents reduced fever and leukocytosis and sometimes reversed the conduction defects that were associated with myocardial infarction. It is also reported that in patients with shock, responsiveness to vasopressor agents was improved. The assumption is made that the severe inflammatory response which occasionally accompanies necrosis of cardiac muscle may itself threaten survival. If the systemic response to inflammation is minimized, the metabolic demands on the already injured heart would be correspondingly reduced. In each instance, conclusions were based on analyses of individual cases and no controlled observations were presented. More objective evaluation is needed.

At present, the use of steroids for treatment of myocardial infarction must still be regarded as experimental. Two possible exceptions warrant consideration. Dressler[8] describes a "post-myocardial-infarction syndrome" characterized by protracted or recurrent fever, chest pain of the pleuro-pericardial type and tendency to relapse. A pericardial friction rub is frequently heard and the presence of pleural effusion is roentgenographically demonstrated in many cases. This condition is very similar to the pleuro-pericardial syndrome which follows cardiotomy or traumatic injury of the pericardium. Both bear close resemblance to manifestations of acute connective tissue diseases. If salicylates do not afford relief, steroids usually provide prompt suppression of symptoms. Another possible indication for their use is in the treatment of acute or chronic heart block following myocardial infarction. A reduction in ventricular rate may compromise both coronary and cerebral blood flow, and the potentiality of cardiac arrest, myocardial failure and acute cerebral anoxia (Stokes-Adams syndrome) provide an ominous prognosis. Corticosteroids are reported to be strikingly effective in restoring atrioventricular conduction and abolishing symptoms,[12, 47, 49] but reports of encouraging results are tempered by the limited frequency with which these beneficial responses are actually obtained. In view of the rapidity of response in documented cases, it is more likely that the direct cardiac action of these steroids, discussed in connection with electrocardiographic effects rather than control of inflammation, increases atrioventricular conduction.

Congestive Heart Failure. The mineraloid effect of the adrenal steroid hormone is responsible for renal conservation of sodium and increased elimination of potassium. Reabsorption of sodium leads to a proportionate increase in retention of water. The fluid is retained primarily in the interstitial and intravascular spaces. Overdistention of the interstitial compartment produces edema. The extra fluid in the intravascular space provides an increased distending force which, like overtransfusion, may result in elevation of blood pressure, cardiac enlargement and clinical signs of congestive heart failure.[2, 46, 61] These features are observed in patients with adrenal cortical hyperfunction and can be experimentally demonstrated, especially when a steroid with primary mineralocorticoid action is used.[15, 48, 59] A paradoxical effect has occurred in some patients with congestive heart failure. The administration of glucocorticoid or ACTH resulted in salt and water diuresis, augmented responsiveness to mercurial diuretic and improvement in clinical status.[3, 17, 19, 51, 52]

The mechanism of this paradoxical response in patients with heart failure is not fully understood. Cortisone increases the glomerular filtration rate and sodium loss for a brief period in the dog, but these effects do not usually occur in the human.[6, 13] This form of therapy is most effective in patients with "refractory" heart failure of long duration. In these patients, aldosterone activity is already near maximal. In a final effort to maintain adequate blood flow, there is further increase in vascular volume which results in damaging loss of normal osmolarity of body fluids. It is postulated that diuresis under these circumstances is effected through inhibition of ADH. This is in harmony with the observation that the loss of excess fluid is associated with reversal of the dilutional syndrome.

The vast majority of patients are not in the final stages of cardiac decompensation, and steroids intensify the severity of congestive heart failure.[7, 16] When steroids are used, newer synthetic derivatives such as prednisolone are preferred because of their lesser tendency to cause salt and water retention.[65]

EFFECTS ON HYPOTENSIVE STATES

Postural Hypotension. The autonomic nervous system provides vasomotor reflexes which minimize postural influences on the distribution of blood within the vascular space. Loss of vasoconstrictive reflexes result in postural (orthostatics) hypotension. Hickler and associates[22] were able to control symptoms by the oral administration of 9-α-FF. A reduction in release of norepinephrine by sympathetic nerve endings was demonstrated, but this was unaffected by the steroid therapy. The beneficial effects of fluorohydrocortisone were most likely due to increases in intravascular volume which compensated for excessive loss of blood into dependent vascular beds when the patient assumed the upright posture, but the possibilty that the steroid potentiated the vasomotor activity of sympathetic nerves still capable of function is not excluded.

SHOCK

Role of Adrenal Insufficiency. The property of corticosteroid hormones to reverse shock due to adrenal insufficiency, whether due to previous suppression with steroids or caused by primary adrenal failure during stress, is well documented in patients and confirmed by controlled studies in experimental animals.[10, 18, 23, 24, 34, 53, 60] Following intravenous injection of a soluble preparation of hydrocortisone, dramatic improvement may be confidently expected. These observations in patients with adrenal insufficiency prompted the use of steroids in the treatment of shock due to a diversity of causes. It was assumed that adrenal insufficiency was a major factor in the progression and irreversibility of shock. However, objective studies failed to confirm that adrenal insufficiency was involved in either the causation or the progression of shock in such patients. To the contrary, Melby and Spink[39] found that the plasma cortisol concentration in patients under the stressful conditions of bacteremic shock was markedly elevated. Responsiveness of the adrenal gland to exogenous corticotropin was maintained. Shock was clearly not due to adrenal failure.

Bacterial Shock. Nevertheless, there are now abundant case history data recommending the use of steroids in large doses in the treatment of patients with shock associated with bacteremia.[20, 29, 56, 57, 58] A variety of therapeutic procedures in addition to the administration of corticosteroids are usually involved, so that full agreement as to the ultimate benefit provided by the steroid alone has not been achieved. However, when lethal amounts of endotoxin are injected into mice, rats and dogs to simulate the conditions which are believed responsible for bacteremic shock, recovery from shock is improved by treatment with steroids.[62, 63, 64] Their maximal effectiveness requires early administration of large doses. The quantities required to obtain the maximum number of survivors are many times greater than those needed for optimal replacement of adrenal cortical hormone in the adrenalectomized animal under stress.[28, 63] Since no hormonal deficiency usually exists, the corticosteroids act like drugs. By their physical presence in high concentrations, they appear to protect tissues against the damaging effects of the bacterial toxin.[32, 38] More complete understanding of the mechanism of this protection is presently being sought in our laboratories.

Shock Due to Other Causes. There are conflicting opinions as to effectiveness of steroids in hemorrhagic shock. Knapp and Howard[30] were unable to increase survival of dogs in "irreversible" hemorrhagic shock, but Connolly[5] reported favorable results with the early use of large amounts of cortisol.

In the acute treatment of anaphylactic shock, epinephrine remains the drug of choice. However, the protracted hypotensive state which is associated with severe hypersensitivity reactions is mitigated by the administration of corticosteroids.[67]

Steroids are sometimes used to protect in a "nonspecific" manner against insults that produce hypotension. However, in experiments with mice, corticosteroid increased the acute fatality rate in animals injected with ganglionic blocking drugs. Treatment with the steroid also increased fatalities in mice scalded with hot water.[54, 63] Until additional information becomes available, their use should be limited to shock associated with infection, shock due to hypersensitivity, and possibly hemorrhagic shock unresponsive to transfusion.

Influence on the Effectiveness of Vasopressor Agents. The vasopressor effect of norepinephrine is increased when steroids are administered to an adrenalectomized animal.[50] A lesser degree of potentiation is reported for human subjects with intact adrenal glands.[31, 37] These observations increase understanding of the protracted hypotension of patients with Addison's disease and the dramatic effects of corticosteroid on arterial pressure. In patients with shock unrelated to adrenal insufficiency in whom responsiveness to vasopressor amines is decreased, steroids are sometimes used with the expectation that pressor effect will be potentiated. Spink[58] has reported that in dogs with endotoxin shock large doses of corticosteroid reduced the amounts of metaraminol required to maintain arterial pressure at physiological levels. However, studies on patients in shock after myocardial infarction have not clearly demonstrated that the pressor effect is increased during the hour after large doses of soluble steroids are administered intravenously.[1, 37, 40] Studies in progress at the Los Angeles County Hospital suggest that increased responsiveness to vasopressor agents, especially in patients with bacterial shock, is more closely related to gradual changes in clinical status than to a direct effect of the steroid.

REFERENCES

1. Agress, C. M.: Management of coronary shock. Am. J. Cardiol., *1*:231, 1958.
2. Albert, R. E., Smith, W. W. and Eichner, L. W.: Hemodynamic changes associated with fluid retention induced in noncardiac subjects by corticotropin (ACTH) and cortisone; comparison with the hemodynamic changes of congestive heart failure. Circulation, *12*:1047, 1955.
3. Camara, A. A. and Schemm, F. R.: Corticotropin (ACTH) in heart disease: its paradoxical effect on sodium excretion in resistant congestive failure. Circulation, *11*:702, 1955.
4. Chapman, D. W., Skaggs, R. H., Thomas, J. R. and Greene, J. A.: The effect of cortisone in experimental myocardial infarction. Am. J. M. Sc., *223*:41, 1952.
5. Connolly, J. E.: The use of adrenal cortical compounds in hemorrhagic shock. Journal-Lancet, *79*:460, 1959.
6. Davis, J. O. and Howell, D. S.: Comparative effect of ACTH, cortisone and DCA on renal function, electrolyte excretion and water exchange in normal dogs. Endocrinology, *52*:245, 1953.
7. Dresdale, D. T., Greene, M. A. and Guzman, S. V.: Clinical and hemodynamic effects of cortisone in patients with rheumatic heart disease and congestive heart failure. Am. Heart J., *55*:851, 1958.
8. Dressler, W.: A post-myocardial-infarction syndrome. J.A.M.A., *160*:1379, 1956.
9. Fiegel, G.: Bedeutung der Nebennierenrinden-Steroide in der Hertz Therapie. München. med. Wchnschr., *100*:1769, 1958.
10. Fitz, I. and Levine, R.: Action of adrenal cortical steroids and nor-epinephrine on vascular responses of stress in adrenalectomized rats. Am. J. Physiol., *165*:456, 1951.
11. Follis, R. H., Orent-Keiles, E. O. and McCollum, E. V.: The production of cardiac and renal lesions in rats by diet extremely deficient in potassium. Am. J. Path., *18*:29, 1942.
12. Friedberg, C. K., Kahn, M., Scheuer, J., Bleifer, S. and Dack, S.: Adams-Stokes syndrome associated with chronic heart block: treatment with corticosteroids. J.A.M.A., *172*:1146, 1960.
13. Garrod, O., Davies, S. A. and Cahill, G., Jr.: The action of cortisone and desoxycorticosterone acetate on glomerular filtration rate and sodium and water exchange in the adrenalectomized dog. J. Clin. Invest., *34*:761, 1955.
14. Gerish, R. A. and Compeau, L.: Treatment of acute myocardial infarction in man with cortisone. Am. J. Cardiol., *1*:535, 1958.
15. Gornall, A. G., Grundy, H. M. and Koladich, C. J.: Studies on aldosterone. III. Chronic effect on the blood pressure of rats. Canad. J. Biochem. & Physiol, *38*:43, 1960.
16. Greene, M. A., Gordon, A. and Boltax, J. A.: Clinical and cardiodynamic effects of adrenocortical steroids in congestive heart failure. Circulation, *21*:661, 1960.
17. Gutner, L. B., Moses, J. B., Dann, S. and Kupperman, H. S.: The use of prednisone in congestive heart failure. Am. J. Sc., *234*:281, 1957.
18. Harnagel, E. E. and Kramer, W. G.: Severe adrenocortical insufficiency following joint manipulation: report of patient receiving cortisone orally. J.A.M.A., *158*:1518, 1955.

19. Heidon, G. H. and Schemm, F. R.: The clinical use of corticotropin (ACTH) and adrenal corticosteroids in the therapy of intractable edema. Am. J. M. Sc., 229:621, 1955.

20. Henegar, G. C., Hunnicutt, A. J. and Kinsell, L. W.: Experience with corticotropin and corticosteroids in severe peritonitis. A.M.A. Arch. Surg., 73:2804, 1956.

21. Hepper, N. G., Pruitt, R. D., Donald, D. D. and Edwards, J. E.: The effect of cortisone on experimentally produced myocardial infarcts. Circulation, 11:742, 1955.

22. Hickler, R. B., Thompson, G. R., Fox, L. M. and Hamlin, J. T.: Successful treatment of orthostatic hypotension with 9-alpha-fluorohydrocortisone. New Engl. J. Med., 261:788, 1959.

23. Howland, W. S., Schweizer, O., Boyan, C. P. and Dotto, A.: Treatment of adrenal cortical insufficiency during surgical procedures. J.A.M.A., 160:1271, 1956.

24. Jackson, B. B.: The use of adrenal steroids in the treatment of sudden collapse associated with surgery: a review of five cases. South. M. J., 52:1380, 1959.

25. Johnson, A. S., Scheinberg, S. R., Gerish, R. A. and Saltzstein, H. C.: Effect of cortisone on the size of experimentally produced myocardial infarcts. Circulation, 7:224, 1953.

26. Joint Report by the Rheumatic Fever Working Party of the Medical Research Council of Great Britain and the Subcommittee of Principal Investigators of the American Council on Rheumatic Fever and Congenital Heart Disease, American Heart Association: The evaluation of rheumatic heart disease in children. Five-year report of a cooperative clinical trial of ACTH, cortisone, and aspirin. Circulation, 22:503, 1960.

27. Kaiser, H.: Cortison bei Herz Infarkt. München. med. Wchschr., 102:931, 1960.

28. Kass, E. H. and Finland, M.: Corticosteroids and infections. Adv. Int. Med., 9:45, 1958.

29. Kinsell, L. W.: Nutritional and metabolic aspects of infection. Ann. N. Y. Acad. Sc., 63:204, 1955.

30. Knapp, R. W. and Howard, J. M.: Studies on the effect of hydrocortisone on irreversible hemorrhagic shock in the dog. Surgery, 42:919, 1957.

31. Kurland, G. S. and Freedberg, A. S.: The potentiating effect of ACTH and of cortisone on pressor response to intravenous infusion of l-norepinephrine. Proc. Soc. Exper. Biol. & Med., 78:28, 1951.

32. Levitin, H., Kendrick, M. I. and Kass, E. H.: Effect of route of administration on protective action of corticosterone and cortisol against endotoxin. Proc. Soc. Exper. Biol. & Med., 93:306, 1956.

33. Lown, B., Arons, W. L., Ganong, W. F., Vazifdar, J. P. and Levine, S.: Adrenal steroids and auriculoventricular conduction. Am. Heart J., 50:760, 1955.

34. Marks, L. J., Donovan, M. J., Duncan, F. J. and Karger, R.: Adrenocortical response to surgical operations in patients treated with corticosteroids or corticotropin prior to surgery. J. Clin. Endocrinol., 19:1458, 1959.

35. Massell, B. F.: Diagnosis and treatment of rheumatic fever and rheumatic carditis. Med. Clin. North America, 42:1343, 1958.

36. McEwen, C.: Current status of therapy in rheumatic fever. J.A.M.A., 170:1056, 1959.

37. Mendlowitz, M., Gitlow, S. and Naftchi, N.: Work of digital vasoconstriction produced by infused norepinephrine in Cushing's syndrome. J. Appl. Physiol., 13:252, 1958.

38. Melby, J. C., Bossenmaier, I. C., Egdahl, R. H. and Spink, W. W.: Suppression by cortisol of increased serum transaminase induced by endotoxin. Lancet, 1:441, 1959.

39. Melby, J. C. and Spink, W. W.: Comparative studies on adrenal cortical function and cortisol metabolism in healthy adults and in patients with shock due to infection. J. Clin. Invest., 37:1791, 1958.

40. Miller, A. J. and Moser, E. A.: Arterenol therapy for shock after acute myocardial infarction and pulmonary embolization. J.A.M.A., 169:2000, 1959.

41. Myhrman, G.: The effect of ACTH and cortisone on inflammatory reactions in myocardial infarction. Acta med. Scandinav., 159:239, 1957.

42. Nahas, G. G., Bronson, J. G., King, W. H. and Cavert, H. M.: Functional and morphologic changes in heart-lung preparations following administration of adrenal hormones. Am. J. Path., 34:717, 1958.

43. Nasmyth, P.: The effect of corticosteroids on the isolated mammalian heart and its response to adrenaline. J. Physiol., 139:323, 1957.

44. Nayler, W. G.: Cardiac metabolism: ionic changes; influence of calcium, 9-α-fluorohydrocortisone and cardiac glycosides on the isolated toad heart. Australian J. Exper. Biol. & Med. Sc., 35:241, 1957.

45. Opdyke, D. F., Lambert, A., Stoerk, H. R., Zanetti, M. E. and Kuna, S.: Failure to reduce the size of experimentally produced myocardial infarcts by cortisone treatment. Circulation, 8:544, 1953.
46. Owen, J. A., Engle, F. L. and Webster, T. B.: 9-α-Fluorohydrocortisone-induced hypertension in a male infant with adrenogenitalism, and in six adults with Addison's disease. J. Clin. Endocrinol., 17:272, 1957.
47. Phelps, M. D., Jr. and Lindsay, J. D.: Cortisone in Stokes-Adams disease secondary to myocardial infarction: report of a case. New Engl. J. Med., 256:204, 1957.
48. Plotz, C. M., Knowlton, A. I. and Ragan, C.: The natural history of Cushing's syndrome. Am. J. Med., 13:597, 1952.
49. Prinzmetal, M. and Kennamer, R.: Emergency treatment of cardiac arrhythmias. J.A.M.A., 154:1049, 1954.
50. Ramey, E. R., Goldstein, M. S. and Levine, R.: Action of nor-epinephrine and adrenal cortical steroids on blood pressure and work performance of adrenalectomized dogs. Am. J. Physiol., 165:450, 1951.
51. Riemer, A. D.: The effect of prednisone in the treatment of refractory cardiac edema. Bull. Johns Hopkins Hosp., 98:445, 1956.
52. Riemer, A. D.: Application of the newer corticosteroids to augment diuresis in congestive heart failure. Am. J. Cardiol., 1:488, 1958.
53. Salassa, R. M., Bennett, W. A., Keating, F. R., Jr. and Sprague, R. G.: Postoperative adrenal cortical insufficiency: occurrence in patients previously treated with cortisone. J.A.M.A., 152:1509, 1953.
54. Schottler, W. H. A.: On the therapeutic value of ACTH and cortisone in experimental burns. Endocrinology, 57:445, 1955.
55. Selye, H.: Conditioning by cortisol for the production of acute massive myocardial necroses during neuromuscular exertion. Circulation Res., 6:168, 1958.
56. Spink, W. W.: ACTH and adrenocortical steroids in the management of selected patients with infectious diseases. Tr. Am. Clin. & Climat. A., 71:202, 1959.
57. Spink, W. W.: Adrenocortical steroids in the management of selected patients with infectious diseases. Ann. Int. Med., 53:1, 1960.
58. Spink, W. W.: The pathogenesis and management of shock due to infection. Arch. Int. Med., 106:433, 1960.
59. Swingle, W. W., Baker, C., Eisler, M., LeBrie, S. J. and Brannick, L.: Maintenance of adrenalectomized dogs with 9-alpha-halo adrenal and other steroids. Endocrinology, 57:220, 1955.
60. Swingle, W. W. et al.: Glucocorticoids and maintenance of blood pressure and plasma volume of adrenalectomized dogs subject to stress. Proc. Soc. Exper. Biol. & Med., 100:617, 1959.
61. Walser, M., Seldin, D. W. and Burnett, C. H.: Blood volume and extracellular fluid volume during administration of ACTH and cortisone. Am. J. Med., 18:454, 1955.
62. Weil, M. H.: Experimental studies on the therapy of circulatory failure produced by endotoxin. J. Lab. & Clin. Med. (In press.)
63. Weil, M. H.: Adrenocortical steroid for therapy of acute hypotension with special reference to experiments on shock produced by endotoxin. (Submitted for publication.)
64. Weil, M. H. and Miller, B. S.: Studies on the effects of a vasopressor agent, sympatholytic drugs, and corticosteroid in shock caused by bacterial toxin. Circulation, 22:830, 1960.
65. Weil, M. H. and Shubin, H.: Current concepts on the management of congestive heart failure. Dis. Chest, 38:179, 1960.
66. Wilson, M. G. and Lion, W. N.: Natural course of active rheumatic carditis and evaluation of hormone therapy. J.A.M.A., 160:1457, 1956.
67. Wright, F. W.: Intravenous hydrocortisone in the treatment of a severe urographic reaction. Brit. J. Radiol., 32:343, 1959.

Effects of Steroids
on Specific Enzyme Systems

GEORGE F. CAHILL, JR., and
LEONARD D. GARREN

Peter Bent Brigham Hospital, Boston

In order for hormones to elicit their ubiquitous and prodigious effects on the organism in the small concentrations in which they exist in body fluids, it appears reasonable to suspect that they operate by regulating the catalysts governing the rate of chemical reactions of the cell, namely the enzymes. Despite the massive volume of literature on the effects of hormones, knowledge of the mechanism of their action at an enzymatic level is at best in its infancy. The now classic studies of Sutherland,[24] attributing the hyperglycemic effects of epinephrine and glucagon to an increase in glycogen phosphorylase activity in the liver, and the similar studies of Haynes,[9] demonstrating a rise in adrenal glycogen phosphorylase activity after adrenocorticotrophic hormone administration, have given impetus to this field.

Of the steroid hormones, estrogens have been the subject of the most rewarding investigations. In 1952, Hagerman and Villee[7] reported that minute quantities of estradiol added to slices of human endometrium accelerated oxygen consumption and the incorporation of glucose or pyruvate carbon into CO_2. Later experiments[29, 30] demonstrated an enhanced oxidation of acetate, suggesting activation of the Krebs (tricarboxylic acid) cycle. It was subsequently reported by Talalay and Williams-Ashman[25] and confirmed by Villee and Hagerman[31] that the estrogen-stimulated reaction involved transhydrogenation of reduced triphosphopyridine (TPN) and diphosphopyridine (DPN) nucleotides;

$$H^+ + TPNH + DPN^+ \rightleftharpoons H^+ + TPN^+ + DPNH$$

The mechanism of this reaction is in dispute. Talalay and Williams-Ashman[26] have stated that the transydrogenation is catalyzed by a reversible oxidation and reduction of the estrogen by estradiol dehydrogenase, an enzyme characterized by Langer and Engel.[17] These reactions are illustrated in Figure 1 according to the scheme of Talalay. On the other hand, Villee and his group[8, 31] have accumulated considerable data providing substantial evidence that the enzyme catalyzing pyridine nucleotide transhydrogenation is distinctly separate from the enzyme or enzymes oxidizing or reducing the estrogen.

In either case, the net effect is an increase in available energy to the tissue since the hydrogen from reduced TPN is not available for oxidation and production of high-energy phosphate, whereas that on DPN is available for such to the chain of respiratory enzymes in the mitochondrion. Thus, as illustrated in Figure 2, transfer of hydrogen from TPNH to form DPNH permits at least three principal dehydrogenation reactions to proceed by regeneration of TPN^+ from TPNH. In addition, the hydrogen, now on DPN, is available for energy production. Thus, the anabolic effects of estrogens on tissues such as endometrium, placenta and mammary tissue may be explained.

Studies on the metabolic effects of adrenal steroids on isolated systems

418

Substrate-linked Pyridine nucleotide Transhydrogenase

$$Estrone \; + \; TPNH \; + \; H^+ \longleftarrow Estradiol\text{-}17\beta \; + \; TPN^+$$

$$Estradiol\text{-}17\beta \; + \; DPN^+ \longleftarrow Estrone \; + \; DPNH \; + \; H^+$$

Sum $\qquad TPNH \; + \; DPN^+ \longleftrightarrow TPN^+ \; + \; DPNH$

Fig. 1. Scheme of Talalay and Williams-Ashman whereby reversible oxidation and reduction of the steroid, in this case estradiol, result in oxidizing TPNH and reducing DPN+.

are not as easy to interpret as those on estrogens. Noall, Riggs, Walker and Christiansen[19] have studied the distribution of a non-metabolizable amino acid (alpha-amino isobutyric acid labeled with radioactive carbon) with and without administered glucocorticoid. They found an increased concentration of this amino acid in liver (Fig. 3) and have suggested that increased hepatic trapping of amino acids is the mechanism whereby steroids increase conversion of amino acids to glucose. Their data, however, are not in keeping with the earlier observations of Ingle et al.[12] and Bondy[2] of an increase in plasma amino acids after administration of adrenal hormone, since increased trapping would be expected to be associated with a decrease and not an increase in plasma amino acid concentration.

Recent experiments have suggested that glucocorticoids may augment proteolysis in peripheral tissues, for example, by increasing the activity of leucine amino dipeptidase in muscle.[20] Likewise, there is a diminished incorporation of labeled amino acids into muscle[34] or adipose tissue[10] protein, also possibly explicable by increased proteolysis.

ESTROGEN SENSITIVE DEHYDROGENASES

Endometrium $\Bigg/$ Isocitrate $+ \; TPN^+ \rightarrow \alpha\text{-}ketoglutarate \; + \; CO_2 \; + \; TPNH \; + \; H^+$

Placenta $\Bigg\langle$ Glucose-6-P $+ \;$ " $\; \rightarrow$ 6-P-Gluconate $\qquad + \qquad$ "

Mammary $\Bigg\backslash$ 6-P-gluconate $+$ " $\rightarrow$ Ribulose-5-P $+ CO_2 \; + \qquad$ "

$$Estrone \; + \; TPNH \; + \; H^+ \longleftarrow Estradiol\text{-}17\beta \; + \; TPN^+$$

$$Estradiol\text{-}17\beta \; + \; DPN^+ \longleftarrow Estrone \; + \; DPNH \; + \; H^+$$

$$TPNH \; + \; DPN^+ \longleftrightarrow TPN^+ \; + \; DPNH$$

$$DPNH \; + \; FAD \longrightarrow DPN^+ + \underline{Reduced \quad FAD}$$
$$\searrow \sim P$$

Fig. 2. Three key metabolic reactions in which TPNH is generated and in which regeneration of oxidized TPN+ permits the reaction to proceed in addition to permitting the hydrogen to be transferred to the chain of respiratory enzymes as indicated by FAD (flavin adenine dinucleotide), with the eventual production of high energy phosphate ($\sim$P).

In the liver, there is an increase in the activity of many enzymes or enzyme systems, most of which are intimately involved in gluconeogenesis.[27, 28] These include one or more transaminases, glutamic dehydrogenase, the activity of the "dicarboxylic acid shuttle," fructose-1,6-diphosphatase and glucose-6-phosphatase. The activity of many of these enzymes has been shown to increase by adaptation to increased amounts of substrate, suggesting other than a direct effect of the hormone on the enzyme. Knox and his associates[3, 4, 14, 15] have studied the tryptophan oxidase-peroxidase system and have found the enzyme to be increased by the administration of either

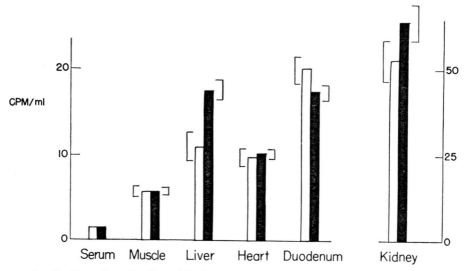

Fig. 3.   Data from Noall et al.[19] demonstrating a significant rise in hepatic trapping of C[14]-α-amino isobutyric acid after administration of cortisone to rats. The open bars represent the counts of C[14] in tissue water in control rats and the darkened bars the counts of C[14] in rats previously treated with cortisone.

tryptophan or glucocorticoid; however, administration of the latter was not accompanied by an increase in intracellular tryptophan, suggesting that steroid induction in this case was *not* due to an increased supply of endogenous tryptophan. However, further experiments from their laboratory have shown induction of activity of this enzyme by other compounds closely related to tryptophan, compounds which need not be substrates for the enzyme itself.[4] These experiments were performed in adrenalectomized animals and therefore in the absence of cortisone or any metabolic equivalent of cortisone.

Kvam and Parks[16] have recently reported that the well known induction of hepatic glucose-6-phosphatase and fructose-1,6-diphosphatase activities by sucrose feeding or hydrocortisone administration does not occur when sucrose is administered to the adrenalectomized animal. In line with this, Weber has reported that the ability of many hepatic enzymes to increase after fasting and refeeding is markedly impaired in the absence of the hypophysis.[32, 33]

Thus, the adrenal corticoids are involved in numerous enzymatic reactions, as summarized in Figure 4. Since the enzymes themselves are proteins, and since maintenance or induction of enzyme activity probably involves either protein synthesis or activation, the latter frequently by a proteolytic mechanism, a fundamental and obviously critical role is fulfilled by these hormones. It has been suggested that adrenal corticoids may exert their metabolic effects, as do estrogens, by transhydrogenation mediated via reversible oxidation and reduction in the 3-position;[11] these suggestions, however, have been severely criticized.[1, 23]

Glutamic transaminase[6, 21] and glutamic dehydrogenase[5, 36] activities have also been shown to be affected by steroids. This is of particular importance since glutamic acid sits at the crossroad of entry of amino acids into the Krebs cycle and therefore occupies a key position in intermediary metabolism. Engel and Scott[5] have recently demonstrated an *in vitro* increase in the activity of crystalline bovine glutamic dehydrogenase in the presence of very small quantities of corticosterone (i.e., 10^{-6} Molar), but they are cautious in extrapolating a physiological interpretation from this observation. This same group has also demonstrated that steroids have an affinity for forming complexes with adenosine,[18, 22] suggesting a physicochemical alteration of the molecular morphology of DPN or TPN in the presence of steroids. On the other hand, Yielding and Tomkins[35] have noted an inhibition of DPNH

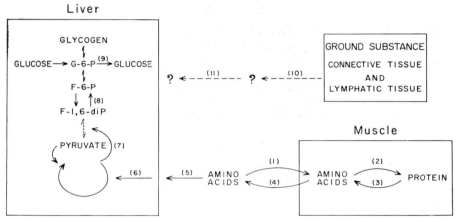

Fig. 4. Scheme from Thorn et al.[28] tabulating the metabolic sites altered or possibly altered after administration of cortisone or its equivalents. These sites are respectively: (1) decreased influx of amino acids into peripheral tissues, (2) decreased peptide bond synthesis, (3) increased splitting of peptide bonds (4) increased efflux of amino acids from peripheral tissues, (5) increased hepatic trapping of amino acids, (6) increased transamination, (7) increased "dicarboxylic acid shuttle," (8) increased fructose-1,6-diphosphatase, (9) increased glucose-6-phosphatase, (10) increased mobilization of other supporting tissues, including mobilization of polysaccharides and (11) possible increased trapping of products mobilized from peripheral tissues other than amino acids.

oxidation in the presence of steroids and have found the site of action to be in the cytochrome system. They also have shown an inhibition of glutamic dehydrogenase activity by estrogens *in vitro*.[36]

One encouraging note in the babel of information on the enzymatic manifestations of the adrenal corticoids is the fact that when these hormones are assayed in a given species, modification of the steroid molecule (for example, introduction of a double bond between carbons 1 and 2) results in a parallel enhancement or inhibition of all the properties attributed to the "glucocorticoids." In other words, the ability to raise the glomerular filtration rate, to decrease circulating eosinophils, to decrease ACTH secretion, to cause osteoporosis, to suppress inflammation, etc., remains proportional for each steroid, particularly when assayed in man, suggesting that the lock into which fits the steroid key is highly specific, and more important, is similar in structure in each of the tissues affected. This inability to segregate the various "glucocorticoid" activities is, of course, in marked contrast to the well established and clear-cut ability to segregate mineralocorticoid from glucocorticoid activities.

Thus, there appears to be a single mechanism, probably enzymatic, which is altered by the glucocorticoids, and in certain reactions this altered process may result in activation of an enzyme; in another reaction it may result in synthesis of an enzyme and in a third, in inhibition or destruction of an enzyme. Precedent for this unitarian theory that an alteration in a single reaction at a cellular level may be amplified into marked alterations in the complete organism is established by any of the hereditary metabolic defects, for example galactosemia, where cirrhosis, cataracts, aminoaciduria and gross physical and mental retardation all result from the lack of a single enzyme, galactose-1-phosphate $\longrightarrow$ uridine diphosphoglucose transferase.[13]

SUMMARY

From this report it is indeed obvious that steroids affect multitudinous enzyme systems. That they exert their known protean physiological actions by a direct effect on all these enzymes and possibly on other unknown enzyme reactions seems rather unlikely. It therefore appears more reasonable to suggest that, despite extensive progress and much important work in this exciting field, the mechanism by which steroids exert their effects on the organism, the cell and the enzymes still remains to be elucidated.

REFERENCES

1. Bloom, B.: An evaluation of hormonal augmented transhydrogenase activity in rat liver cells. J. Biol. Chem., 235:857, 1960.
2. Bondy, P. K., Ingle, D. J. and Meeks, R. C.: Influence of adrenal cortical hormones upon the level of plasma amino acids in eviscerated rats. Endocrinology, 55:354, 1954.
3. Civen, M. and Knox, W. E.: The independence of hydrocortisone and tryptophan induction of tryptophan pyrrolase. J. Biol. Chem., 234:1787, 1959.
4. Civen, M. and Knox, W. E.: The specificity of tryptophan analogues as inducers substrates, inhibitors, and stabilizers of liver tryptophan pyrrolase. J. Biol. Chem., 235:1716, 1960.
5. Engel, L. and Scott, J. F.: Effects of steroid hormones upon diphosphopyridine nucleotide-mediated enzymatic reactions. Rec. Progr. Hormone Research, 16:79-92, 1960.
6. Gavosto, F., Pilesi, A. and Brusca, A.: Increased transaminase activity in the liver after administration of cortisone. Biochim. et biophys. acta, 24:250, 1957.
7. Hagerman, D. D. and Villee, C. A.: Effects of estradiol on the metabolism of human endometrium in vitro. Arch. Biochem. & Biophys., 40:481, 1952.
8. Hagerman, D. D. and Villee, C. A.: Separation of human placental estrogen-sensitive transhydrogenase from estradiol-17 β-dehydrogenase. J. Biol. Chem., 234:2031, 1959.
9. Haynes, R. C.: The activation of adrenal phosphorylase by the adrenocorticotropic hormone. J. Biol. Chem., 233:1220, 1959.
10. Herrera, G. and Renold, A. E.: Personal communication.
11. Hurlock, B. and Talalay, P.: 3α-hydroxysteroids as coenzymes of hydrogen transfer between di- and triphosphopyridine nucleotides. J. Biol. Chem., 233:886, 1958.
12. Ingle, D. J., Prestrud, M. C. and Nezamis, J. E.: Effect of adrenalectomy upon level of blood amino acids in the eviscerated rat. Proc. Soc. Exper. Biol., N.Y., 67:321, 1948.

13. Kalckar, H. M., Anderson E. P. and Isselbacher, K. J.: Galactosemia, a congenital defect in a nucleotide transferase. Biochim. et biophys. acta, *20*:262, 1956.
14. Knox, W. E. and Auerbach, V. H.: The hormonal control of tryptophan peroxidase in the rat. J. Biol. Chem., *214*:307, 1955.
15. Knox, W. E., Auerbach, V. H. and Lin, E. C. C.: Enzymatic and metabolic adaptations in animals. Physiol. Rev., *36*:164, 1956.
16. Kvam, D. C. and Parks, R. E., Jr.: Hydrocortisone-induced changes in hepatic glucose-6-phosphatase and fructose diphosphatase activities. Am. J. Physiol., *198*:21, 1960.
17. Langer, L. J. and Engel, L. L.: Human placental estradiol-17 β-dehydrogenase. J. Biol. Chem., *233*:583, 1958.
18. Munck, A., Scott, J. F. and Engel, L. L.: The interaction of steroid hormones and coenzyme components. Biochim. et biophys. acta, *26*:397, 1957.
19. Noall, M. W., Riggs, T. R., Walker, L. M. and Christensen, H. N.: Endocrine control of amino acid transfer: distribution of an unmetabolizable amino acid. Science, *126*:1002, 1957.
20. Rose, H. G., Robertson, M. C. and Schwartz, T. B.: Hormonal and metabolic influences on intracellular peptidase activity. Am. J. Physiol., *197*:1063, 1959.
21. Rosen, F., Roberts, N. R. and Nichol, C. C.: Glucocorticoids and transaminase activity. I. Increased activity of glutamic-pyruvic transaminase in four conditions associated with gluconeogenesis. J. Biol. Chem., *234*:476, 1959.
22. Scott, J. F. and Engel, L. L.: Molecular interaction between purines and steroids. Biochim. et biophys. acta, *23*:665, 1957.
23. Stein, A. M. and Kaplan, N. O.: Relationship of 3α-hydroxysteroid dehydrogenase to pyridine nucleotide transhydrogenases. Science, *129*:1611, 1959.
24. Sutherland, E. W.: The effect of the hyperglycemia factor and epinephrine on enzyme systems of liver and muscle. Ann. New York Acad. Sci., *54*:693, 1951.
25. Talalay, P. and Williams-Ashman, H. G.: On a coenzymatic function of estradiol-17β. Proc. Nat. Acad. Sci., *44*:862, 1958.
26. Talalay, P. and Williams-Ashman, H. G.: Participation of steroid hormones in the enzymatic transfer of hydrogen. Rec. Progr. Hormone Research, *16*:1-47, 1960.
27. Thorn, G. W., Renold, A. E. and Cahill, Jr., G. F.: The adrenal and diabetes, some interactions and interrelations. Banting Lecture. Diabetes, *8*:337, 1959.
28. Thorn, G. W., Cahill, Jr., G. F. and Renold, A. E.: Some adrenal effects on gluconeogenesis. Bull. de l'Académie Royale de Médecine de Belgique, *25*:74, 1960.
29. Villee, C. A. and Hagerman, D. D.: Effects of estradiol on the metabolism of human placenta *in vitro*. J. Biol. Chem., *205*:873, 1953.
30. Villee, C. A. and Gordon, E. E.: Further studies on the action of estradiol *in vitro*. J. Biol. Chem., *216*:203, 1955.
31. Villee, C. A., Hagerman, D. D. and Joel, P. B.: An enzymatic basis for the physiologic functions of estrogens. Rec. Progr. Hormone Research, *16*:49-69, 1960.
32. Weber, G. and Cantero, A.: Studies on hormonal factors influencing hepatic glucose-6-phosphate. Endocrinology, *61*:701, 1957.
33. Weber, G.: Effect of hypophysectomy on respiration and enzymatic activities of the liver. Abstract 1, International Congress Endocrinology, Copenhagen, 1960, No. 471.
34. Wool, I. G. and Weinschelbaum, E. I.: Incorporation of C^14-amino acids into protein of isolated diaphragms: role of the adrenal steroids. Am. J. Physiol., *197*:1089, 1959.
35. Yielding, K. L., Tomkins, G. M., Munday, J. S. and Curran, J. F.: The effects of steroid hormones on the glutamic dehydrogenase reaction. Biochemical and Biophysical Research Communications, *2*:303, 1960.
36. Yielding, K. L. and Tomkins, G. M.: Inhibition of the enzymatic oxidations of DPNH by steroid hormones. Proc. Nat. Acad. Sci., *45*:1730, 1959.

Comparative Metabolic Effects of Synthetic Anti-Inflammatory Steroids

DALTON JENKINS

University of Colorado School of Medicine

During the past ten years great effort has been expended in a search for effective anti-inflammatory corticosteroids with fewer side effects than the natural steroids, cortisone and cortisol. As a result, an array of synthetic analogs of cortisol has been produced. At least nine structural modifications have been found which enhance anti-inflammatory potency:[12] the 6α-, 9α- and 12α-fluorine atoms; the 9α-chlorine atom; the Δ¹ bond; and the 2α-, 6α-, 16α- and 16β-methyl groups. In addition, five other modifications have resulted in a reduction or virtual elimination of sodium retention: the 16α-hydroxyl, 6α-chloro, and the 6α-, 16α- and 16β-methyl groups. When two or more of these modifications in cortisol structure are variously combined, the potential number of new steroid compounds is obviously great.

Six synthetic corticosteroids have been made available for general use. These are 9α-fluorocortisol, prednisone and prednisolone (the 1,4-diene derivatives of cortisone and cortisol, respectively), 6-methylprednisolone, triamcinolone (9α-fluoro-16α-hydroxyprednisolone) and dexamethasone (9α-fluoro-16α-methylprednisolone). The over-all metabolic effects of these agents appear to be, qualitatively, essentially similar to those of cortisol. The effects on carbohydrate, fat and protein metabolism, on inflammatory processes and on allergic phenomena produced by any one of these steroids are—in terms of net changes, at least—the same effects as those produced by the other synthetic compounds and by cortisol. Quantitatively, the agents differ in relative potency, and the effects of these steroids on electrolyte metabolism (producing sodium retention and potassium loss) show even greater differences. Fluorocortisol is an extremely potent mineralocorticoid; the effects of prednisolone on sodium and potassium metabolism are approximately equal to those of cortisol; 6-methylprednisolone and dexamethasone are less effective than prednisolone; and triamcinolone is practically devoid of sodium-retaining effects while maintaining its capacity to increase potassium excretion. It is, of course, possible that there are fundamental qualitative differences between these compounds in their mineralocorticoid actions. However, at the present, these differences again appear to be mainly quantitative alterations in the well known, typical actions of the natural steroids.

Some of the metabolic effects of the synthetic corticosteroids are compared in this report.

9α-FLUOROCORTISOL

In 1953 Fried and Sabo[5] discovered that the introduction of a chlorine or fluorine atom at the 9α position of cortisol produced a considerable increase in corticosteroid activity, but 9α-fluorocortisol proved to be the most active member of the series. In adrenalectomized dogs the compound is about 20 times more active than cortisol in producing eosinopenia; more striking is the accentuation of mineralocorticoid activity since the compound, in adrenal-ectomized dogs, is approximately five times as active as desoxycorticosterone acetate in producing sodium retention.[8] Similarly, in man the compound has proved to be particularly effective in altering electrolyte metabolism. For example, in normal subjects and in patients with adrenal insufficiency, 9α-fluorocortisol and aldosterone produce approximately equal effects on urinary sodium and potassium excretion.[14] Glucocorticoid effects are also enhanced but the increase is smaller. Boland[3] found that the antirheumatic activity of the compound is about 10 times that of cortisol, and West[16] showed its hyperglycemic potency to be 6 to 12 times that of the parent compound.

Some of the metabolic changes produced by 9α-fluorocortisol in a normal adult male are shown in Figure 1. At a dosage level of 4 mg. per day there was severe urinary sodium retention accompanied by potassium loss. The intensity of sodium retention diminished after four days, despite continued

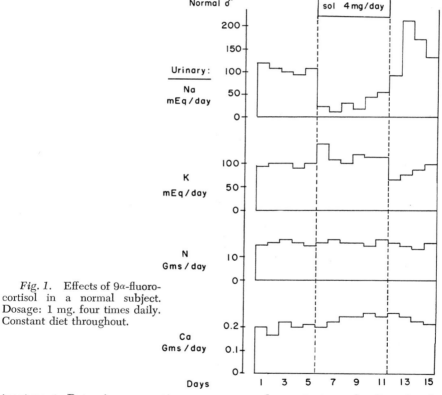

Fig. 1. Effects of 9α-fluoro-cortisol in a normal subject. Dosage: 1 mg. four times daily. Constant diet throughout.

treatment. Potassium excretion was, as usual, greatest on the first day but remained elevated above control levels throughout steroid administration. When the steroid was discontinued, sodium output increased greatly above control levels and, simultaneously, potassium was retained. These effects are consistent with an intense action on renal tubular cation-exchange processes.

Despite the influence on electrolyte metabolism, nitrogen excretion did not materially change during the relatively short course of treatment. This reflects the fact that the 9α-fluoro modification increases the mineralocorticoid activity of steroids to a greater degree than the glucocorticoid effects. Consequently, one might well question whether the prompt but modest rise in urinary calcium output was the result of a significant primary effect on bone. Phosphorous excretion (not shown) did not show any consistent change.

Because of its potent effects on sodium (and water) retention, 9α-fluorocortisol is not employed in the systemic therapy of inflammatory disorders. However, it is most useful in the management of adrenocortical insufficiency as a supplement to maintenance doses of cortisol or cortisone. Although this is only a small area of therapeutic application, the fact that the compound is generally available to these patients is most gratifying.

PREDNISOLONE AND PREDNISONE

The next advance in corticosteroid modification was the introduction of a 1,2-double bond in the steroid nucleus by Herzog et al.[6] The glucocorticoid activity of the Δ^1 derivatives of cortisol and cortisone was found to be three to four times that of the parent compounds as measured by a variety of bioassay techniques. Studies in man showed an anti-inflammatory effectiveness approximately four times that of cortisol. More important, there was no commensurate increase in electrolyte activity. These observations again demonstrated that structural modifications could produce selective changes in steroid functions.

Some effects of prednisolone in a normal adult male are shown in Figure 2. High dosage (80 mg. per day) was deliberately employed in order to magnify the metabolic actions of the compound. The changes shown are representative of the responses exhibited by six normal subjects receiving prednisolone in doses ranging from 20 to 80 mg. daily.

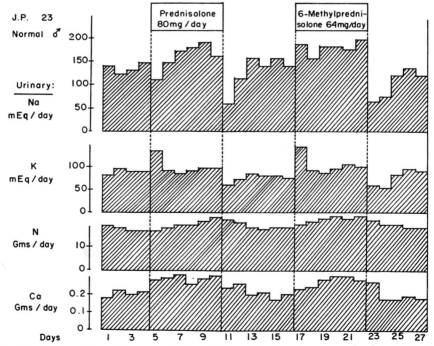

Fig. 2.   Effects of prednisolone and 6α-methylprednisolone in a normal subject. Steroids given orally in four doses daily. Diet constant throughout.

A moderate increase in urinary sodium excretion usually occurs. With large doses there may be an initial period of moderate sodium retention, usually lasting two to five days; this is followed by "escape" to a state of sodium balance or, more often, to a state of modest sodium loss. Urinary potassium output increases sharply on the first day of steroid administration, and then promptly returns toward control levels. This effect occurs regularly. It precedes and is out of proportion to any significant change in nitrogen excretion. Thereafter, with small doses of prednisolone, potassium output remains at control values; with large doses some potassium loss occurs secondarily when nitrogen excretion is definitely increased.

Small doses of prednisolone (15 to 40 mg. daily) produce a small increase in nitrogen excretion. With larger doses nitrogen loss is greater, usually ranging from 2 to 4 grams daily at doses of 40 to 100 mg. However, the effect is not linear. Lipsett et al.[9] found that the nitrogen loss induced by 1000 mg. of prednisone daily was only moderately greater than that induced by 100 mg. daily doses. Pechet et al.[11] pointed out that nitrogen losses produced by prednisolone are greater than those occurring with cortisone or cortisol at comparable therapeutic (anti-inflammatory) doses.

Urinary calcium excretion usually increases moderately. But, as pointed out by Bunim et al.,[4] this effect may be offset in terms of over-all balance by decreasing fecal excretion.

The actions of prednisone and prednisolone are approximately equal and the two agents are interchangeable.

6-METHYLPREDNISOLONE

Corticosteroids methylated in the 6α position were first prepared by Spero et al.[13] in 1956. Lyster[10] showed by bioassay in rats that the effect of the 6α-methyl group is to increase glucocorticoid activity of the parent compound by a factor of approximately three, at the same time causing a reduction of sodium-retaining activity. Studies in man[7] demonstrated that the metabolic effects of prednisolone and its 6α-methyl derivative are quite similar. The latter steroid produced, in normal subjects, somewhat greater increases in urinary nitrogen excretion and sodium output. Similarly, anti-rheumatic potency has been shown to be 15 to 20 per cent greater than that of prednisolone.

In Figure 2 the effects of 6-methylprednisolone are compared with those of prednisolone in the same normal subject, and at comparable anti-inflammatory doses. It is evident that the two agents have very similar effects. Studies of this type have been performed in seven normal adults using doses of methylprednisolone ranging from 30 to 64 mg. daily. The results shown are representative. The steroid is somewhat more potent than prednisolone; qualitatively, the effects of the two agents are very similar.

TRIAMCINOLONE

Bernstein et al.[2] achieved the next step in corticosteroid modification by the introduction of a 16α-hydroxyl group. This alteration virtually eliminated the sodium-retaining activity of the parent compound but, at the same time, reduced anti-inflammatory potency. Thus, 9α-fluoroprednisolone (combining the Δ^1 configuration with the C-9 fluorine atom) was found to have anti-inflammatory activity approximately 15 times as great as that of cortisol and mineralocorticoid effects equal to those of 9α-fluorocortisol. 16α-Hydroxylation (producing triamcinolone) abolished the sodium-retaining activity and reduced antirheumatic potency to a level about five times that of cortisol. Early metabolic studies were reported to show that this steroid produced little or no change in nitrogen or potassium balances and a slight loss of sodium. However, it is unfortunate that very few actual data concerning the metabolic effects of triamcinolone in man have been published.

Figure 3 shows the effects of triamcinolone in high dosage in a normal subject. Sodium excretion is increased throughout the period of steroid

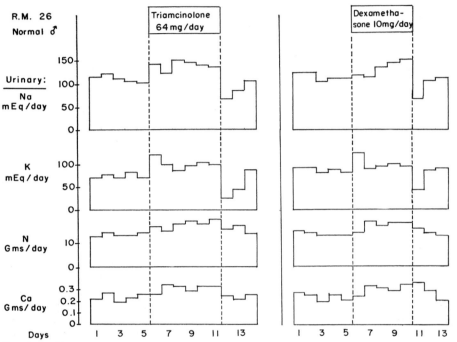

Fig. 3. Effects of triamcinolone and dexamethasone in a normal subject. Steroids given orally in four doses daily. Diet constant throughout.

administration. There is the usual striking loss of potassium on the first day of treatment followed by a persistent, moderate elevation of urinary potassium output. There is a definite increase in urinary nitrogen excretion. Comparable studies have been performed in four normal subjects with doses ranging from 40 to 64 mg. per day with similar results.

Urinary sodium excretion increased in all subjects. Sodium retention was not observed even with the relatively large doses employed; in all probability, triamcinolone has less capacity to induce sodium retention than any of the available synthetic analogs of cortisol. The changes in potassium excretion are of some interest. The initial, relatively large increase in potassium output seen on the first day of treatment is regularly encountered with active corticosteroids. But with trimacinolone, in contrast to prednisolone and 6-methylprednisolone, potassium loss persists. Although with studies limited to changes in urinary excretion, as shown here, precise balance calculations cannot be properly applied, it would appear that the increase in potassium output is in excess of that anticipated on the basis of nitrogen losses. In other words, it would appear that triamcinolone produces either a potent renal tubular excretion of potassium (probably unlikely in view of the apparent absence of tubular sodium exchange) or, more likely, a significant cellular loss of potassium which is out of proportion to cellular losses of nitrogen. In these studies, when 40 mg. or more of triamcinolone was given daily, an increase in urinary nitrogen excretion regularly occurred, comparable to that produced by large doses of prednisolone.

Triamcinolone elicits some side effects with greater frequency than other synthetic corticosteroids. These include muscle atrophy and muscle weakness, often associated with progressive weight loss. Whether these side effects are directly related to potassium depletion during long-term therapy, as the above studies might imply, is not definitely known. However, steroid-induced myopathy is not ordinarily reversed or necessarily prevented by supplemental potassium administration. Furthermore, such changes in muscle mass and function have sometimes occurred with doses considerably smaller than those exhibited in these studies, which are usually not associated with potassium losses of the magnitude shown here. It seems likely that some other alteration in muscle function is the primary event.

DEXAMETHASONE

The most recent addition to the list of corticosteroids available for therapeutic use is dexamethasone. In 1958, Arth et al.[1] described a new series of analogs characterized by a methyl group at the C-16α position. By bioassay, the eosinopenic, glycogenic and anti-inflammatory activities of the steroid proved to be approximately five times that of prednisolone (20 to 25 times that of cortisol).[15] Its antirheumatic activity in man is about six times that of prednisolone or 25 to 30 times that of cortisol.[4]

Bunim et al.[4] carried out interesting metabolic studies with dexamethasone in patients and normal subjects. Sodium diuresis occurred, particularly with larger doses. It is of real interest that, under these circumstances, an increased urinary output of aldosterone was found—as would be expected under conditions of sodium loss provided no inhibition of aldosterone secretion were produced by dexamethasone. Little, if any, change in potassium output occurred. Nitrogen excretion increased. Of considerable interest was the production of negative calcium balance due, primarily, to increased fecal losses. The authors suggested that the effect of dexamethasone on calcium metabolism is greater than that of other corticosteroids. Unfortunately, further studies have not been reported.

Figure 3 shows the effects of dexamethasone, 10 mg. daily, in a normal subject. The results are representative of those obtained in four normal adult males in dosages of 6 to 10 mg. per day. Increased urinary excretion of sodium, potassium, nitrogen and calcium were produced. The effect on potassium was not persistent, in contrast to triamcinolone. Otherwise, the effects of the two agents appeared to be comparable, with the doses used. However, it is to be noted that dexamethasone is six to eight times more potent, in these studies, than triamcinolone, prednisolone and 6-methyl-prednisolone.

SUMMARY

The metabolic effects of the available synthetic corticosteroids are basically similar to those of the parent compound, cortisol. Differences appear to be mainly quantitative rather than qualitative, although, so long as the primary cellular actions of corticosteroids remain unknown, it is difficult to be certain of this in all aspects of steroid actions. 9α-Fluorocortisol is a potent corticosteroid; its predominant actions are on electrolyte metabolism, and the compound is, therefore, primarily useful in substitution therapy of adrenal insufficiency. Prednisolone, 6α-methylprednisolone, triamcinolone and dexamethasone all produce essentially similar effects at comparable anti-inflammatory doses. The usual effects are a mild sodium diuresis, moderate potassium losses (roughly proportionate to nitrogen loss except with triamcinolone, which may induce potassium losses in excess of those accounted for by nitrogen excretion), nitrogen loss and increased calcium excretion. The nitrogen loss induced by the synthetic analogs appears to be greater than that induced by cortisol in comparable anti-inflammatory doses. It is possible that the changes in calcium metabolism induced by dexamethasone are greater than those resulting from the other compounds, but more data are required to substantiate this.

The major changes accomplished so far in the production of synthetic corticosteroids are alterations in mineralocorticoid potency (relative to glucocorticoid actions), and a significant increase in glucocorticoid (including anti-inflammatory) activity. The first has proved useful because the incidence of edema and hypertension during therapeutic use of corticosteroids has been significantly reduced. The second change has contributed important information to better understanding of the relationships between corticosteroid structure and function; it has not materially aided the therapeutic application of these agents since most of the side effects which are undesirable remain intact.

ACKNOWLEDGMENTS

Appreciation is extended to Dr. H. C. Peltier of The Upjohn Co. for prednisone, prednisolone and methylprednisolone; and to Dr. Elmer Alpert of Merck Sharp & Dohme for prednisone, prednisolone, dexamethasone, and 9α-fluorocortisol.

REFERENCES

1. Arth, G. E. et al.: 16-Methylated steroids. II. 16α-Methyl analogs of cortisone, a new group of anti-inflammatory steroids. 9α-halo derivatives. J. Am. Chem. Soc., 80:3161, 1958.
2. Bernstein, S. et al.: 16-Hydroxylated steroids. IV. The synthesis of 16α-hydroxy derivatives of 9α-halo steroids. J. Am. Chem. Soc., 78:5693, 1956.
3. Boland, E. W. and Headley, N. E.: Preliminary clinical trials with 9α-fluorohydrocortisone acetate in rheumatoid arthritis. Ann. Rheumat. Dis., 13:348, 1954.
4. Bunim, J. J., Black, R. L., Lutwak, L., Peterson, R. E. and Whedon, G. D.: Studies on dexamethasone, a new synthetic steroid, in rheumatoid arthritis—a preliminary report. Arth. & Rheum., 1:313, 1958.
5. Fried, J. and Sabo, E. F.: Synthesis of 17-hydroxycorticosterone and its 9α-halo derivatives from 11-epi-17-hydroxycorticosterone. J. Am. Chem. Soc., 75:2273, 1953.
6. Herzog, H. L. et al.: New anti-arthritic steroids. Science, 121:176, 1955.
7. Jenkins, D. and Schemmel, J. E.: Metabolic effects of 6-methylprednisolone. Metabolism, 7:416, 1958.
8. Liddle, G. W., Pechet, M. M. and Bartter, F. C.: Enhancement of biological activities of corticosteroids by substitution of halogen atoms in 9-alpha position. Science, 120:496, 1954.
9. Lipsett, M. D., Greenberg, E. and Pearson, O. H.: Comparison of metabolic effects of high and massive doses of prednisone. J. Lab. & Clin. Med., 56:63, 1960.
10. Lyster, S. C., Barnes, L. E., Lund, G. H., Meinzinger, M. M. and Byrnes, W. S.: Adrenal cortical activities of 6-methyl-1-hydrocortisone. Proc. Soc. Exper. Biol. & Med., 94:159, 1957.

11. Pechet, M. M., Bowers, B. and Bartter, F. C.: Metabolic studies with a new series of 1,4-diene steroids. II. Effects in normal subjects of prednisone, prednisolone and 9α-fluoroprednisolone. J. Clin. Invest., 38:691, 1959.
12. Sarett, L. H.: Some aspects of the evolution of anti-inflammatory steroids. Ann. N. Y. Acad. Sc., 82:802, 1959.
13. Spero, G. G. et al.: The adrenal hormones and related compounds. IV. 6-Methyl-steroids. J. Am. Chem. Soc., 78:6213, 1956.
14. Thorn, G. W., Sheppard, R. H., Morse, W. I., Reddy, W. J., Beigelman, P. M. and Renold, A. E.: Comparative action of aldosterone and 9α-fluorohydrocortisone in man. Ann. N. Y. Acad. Sc., 61:609, 1955.
15. Tolksdorf, S.: Laboratory evaluation of anti-inflammatory steroids. Ann. N. Y. Acad. Sc., 82:829, 1959.
16. West, K. M.: Relative eosinopenic and hyperglycemic potencies of glucocorticoids in man. Metabolism, 7:441, 1958.

Metabolism of Cortisol and Other Steroids by Connective Tissue Cells*

DAVID L. BERLINER

University of Utah College of Medicine

The effects of adrenocortical hormones on the inflammatory reaction have been thoroughly studied and elucidated by Dougherty et al.[10-12] These investigators have shown that corticosteroids act topically in a dose response fashion to inhibit the wave of autocatalytic cell destruction produced in the connective tissue by an inflammatory stimulus[13] and that cortisol is the most potent naturally occurring anti-inflammatory steroid.[14, 15] It has been shown to cause a discernible morphological change in fibroblasts, an alteration associated with a resistance to cellular destruction during inflammation. With these findings as a foundation, it became important to study the interrelationship between fibroblasts and cortisol. A study was carried out to determine the effect of the fibroblast on the cortisol molecule at the time cortisol was acting.

This paper will be concerned with the metabolism of cortisol and related steroids by fibroblasts, a comparison of this metabolism with the over-all fate of the hormone in the organism and the possible biological implications of steroid metabolism.

METABOLISM OF CORTISOL BY FIBROBLASTS

The fibroblasts used in the metabolic experiments were either those of mouse connective tissue (90 per cent of the cells present are fibroblasts)[12] or a pure strain of human fibroblasts grown in tissue culture.[24] Connective tissue cells were able to oxidize the hydroxyl groups at C-11, split off the side chain at C-17 and reduce the double bond at C-4, 5 as well as the ketone at

* This work has been supported by grants from The American Cancer Society (No. 33-0081) and the National Institutes of Health, Cooperative Leukemia Project (No. 34-5917).

TABLE 1.

4-Pregnene-11β, 17α, 20α, 21-tetrol-3-one (20 epi substance "E" of Reichstein)*
4-Pregnene-11β, 17α, 20β, 21-tetrol-3-one (Substance E of Reichstein)**
Pregnane-11β, 17α, 21-triol-3, 20-dione (dihydrocortisol)*
4-Pregnene-17α, 20α, 21-triol-3, 11-dione (20 epi substance "U" of Reichstein)**
4-Pregnene-17α, 21-diol-3, 11, 20-trione (cortisone)*
4-Androstene-11β-ol-3, 17-dione*,**
4-Androstene-3, 11, 17-trione (adrenosterone)*

---

* Loose connective tissue of mice.
** Tissue culture fibroblasts.

These metabolites are compounds isolated and characterized from incubations of 4-C[14] cortisol with tissue culture of fibroblasts of loose connective tissue.

C-20.[1] Chemical conversions of cortisol by tissue culture fibroblasts were of the same type, although there were quantitative differences. Mouse connective tissue cells formed mainly the C-20 alpha isomer, whereas the human fibroblasts produced chiefly the C-20 beta isomer. Table 1 lists the compounds produced by the two types of cell preparations.

Some of the products of cortisol metabolism by fibroblasts were isolated and reincubated with connective tissue preparations. With our methods[2, 3] we were unable to detect oxidation of a C-20 hydroxyl group (on substance E or U of Reichstein) to a ketone. However, these compounds with the glycol side chain could be oxidized or reduced at C-11. Also, cortisone and cortisol were found to be interconvertible. Figure 1 represents the major compounds obtained from the combined *in vitro* studies and illustrates the interconversions found.

Incubations of other steroids with fibroblasts have been performed[4, 5, 23] which indicate that these cells have a general capacity to oxidize and reduce various substituent groups on the steroid nucleus (Table 2).

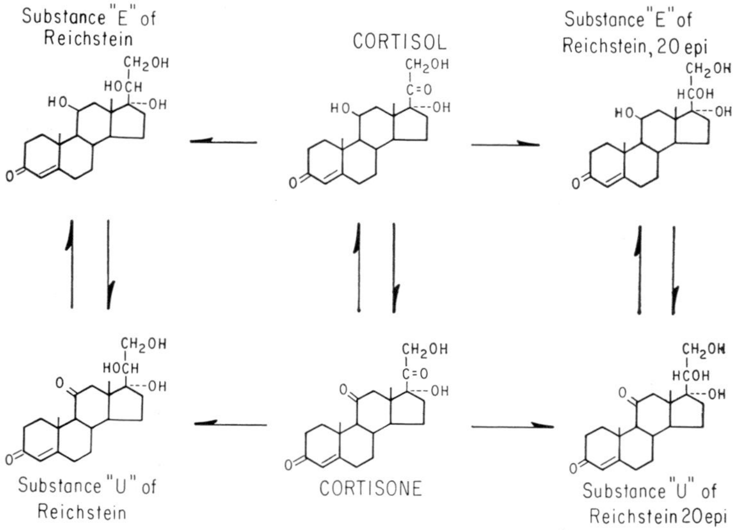

Fig. 1. Cyclic conversions of major cortisol metabolites. Each compound in this scheme was isolated from incubations of cortisol-4C[14] with fibroblasts. The metabolites shown (C[14]-labelled) were then individually re-incubated with fibroblasts of loose connective tissue. Isolation and identification of C[14]-labelled products from the several incubations gave this metabolic scheme. Negligible amounts of C[19] metabolites are not represented here.

TABLE 2.   METABOLISM OF C^{14} STEROIDS BY FIBROBLASTS

STEROID INCUBATED	STEROID ISOLATED
Corticosterone	4-Pregnene-11β, 20β, 21-triol-3-one**
17OH-Progesterone	4-Pregnene-17α, 20-diol-3-one*,***
Progesterone	4-Pregnene-20β-ol-3-one** 4-Pregnene-20α-ol-3-one** Allopregnane-3, 20-dione** Allopregnane-20α-ol-3-one**
4-Pregnene-17α, 21-diol-3, 20-dione (Substane "S" of Reichstein)	4-Pregnene-17α, 20, 21-triol-3, 20-dione*,***

 * Loose connective tissue of mice.
 ** Tissue culture fibroblasts.
 *** Configuration at C-20 not determined at this time.

HEPATIC AND EXTRAHEPATIC METABOLISM OF CORTISOL

Experiments have been carried out in our laboratory to ascertain whether or not the pattern of fibroblastic metabolism of cortisol fits into the general *in vivo* metabolic scheme.

Numerous studies have been reported concerning the metabolism of cortisone and cortisol by the liver.[21] The major metabolic changes appear to be loss of the side chain at C-17, oxidation or reduction at the 3, 11 and 20 positions, reduction of the 4, 5 double bond, and formation of water-soluble conjugates. Kidney slices and homogenates also have demonstrated ability to metabolize corticosteroids,[18] although not to the same extent as the liver. The primary conjugate formed by liver is glucuronide (Fig. 2). The kidneys of mice and dogs have also been shown to conjugate "tetrahydro" steroids with glucuronic acid.[9, 22]

A study on eviscerated rats which were also effectively nephrectomized[6] and on animals which were hepatectomized showed that cortisol can be actively metabolized by extrahepatic and extrarenal cells. The oxidations and reductions observed were similar to those found when fibroblasts were incubated *in vitro* with cortisol. Extrahepatic and extrarenal cells and fibroblasts have a quantitatively lower capacity to reduce ring A of cortisol and other steroids as well (Tables 1 and 2). Furthermore, these cells cannot conjugate steroids to form the water-soluble products.[5, 6]

In Figure 3, we have shown the metabolites which are produced during extrahepatic and extrarenal metabolism and those products of liver and kidney metabolism. Inside the quadrangle are the metabolites produced mainly by extrahepatic tissue; all of these metabolites have been isolated after incubation of cortisol-4-C^{14} with fibroblasts alone (Fig. 3).

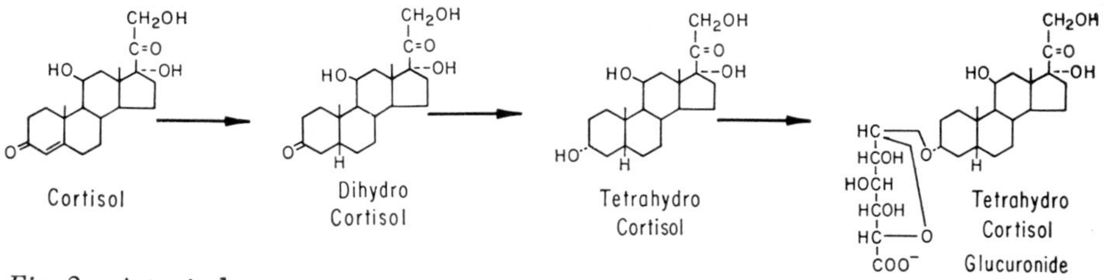

Fig. 2.   A typical reaction sequence representing reduction of ring A and conjugation of a corticosteroid.

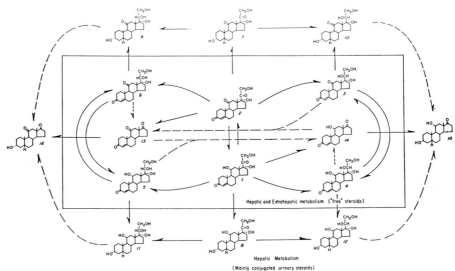

Fig. 3. Hepatic and extrahepatic metabolism of cortisol: (1) 4-pregnene-11β, 17α, 21-triol-3, 20-dione (cortisol); (2) 4-pregnene-17α, 21-diol-3, 11, 20-trione (cortisone); (3) 4-pregnene-17α, 20β, 21-triol-3, 11-dione (substance U of Reichstein); (4) 4-pregnene-11β, 17α, 20β, 21-tetrol,3-one (substance E of Reichstein); (5) 4-pregnene-11β, 17α, 20α, 21-tetrol,3-one (20-epi substance E of Reichstein); (6) 4-pregnene-17α, 20α, 21-triol-3, 11-dione (20 epi substance U of Reichstein); (7) pregnane-3α, 17α, 21-triol-11, 20-dione (tetrahydrocortisone); (8) pregnane-3α, 11β, 17α, 21-tetrol,20-one (tetrahydrocortisol); (9) pregnane-3α, 17α, 20α, 21-tetrol, 11-one (α-cortolone); (10) pregnane-3α, 17α, 20β, 21-tetrol, 11-one (β-cortolone); (11) pregnane-3α, 11β, 17α, 20α, 21,pentol (α-cortol); (12) pregnane-3α, 11β, 17α, 20β, 21-pentol (β-cortol); (13) 4-androstene-3, 11, 17-trione (androsterone); (14) 4-androstene-11β-ol, 3,17-dione (11β-OH-androstenedione); (15) etiocholane-3α, 11β, diol, 17-one (11β-OH-etiocholanolone); and (16) etiocholane-3α, ol, 11, 17-dione (11-keto-etiocholanolone).

All of the compounds listed here are the major ones found; 6β-hydroxylated steroids and others not fully identified are not represented. The configuration 5α or allo is also present in the metabolism of cortisol.[20] The dark lines represent pathways that we and/or other investigators have found to exist. Those indicated by the dotted lines have not been tested as yet in our laboratory.

Recent studies[30] of the metabolism of substance "E" of Reichstein-4C[14] have shown that this compound is metabolized to β-cortol, β-allocortol, β-cortolone, Reichstein's U, and C_{19} steroids.

DISCUSSION

Fibroblasts do not utilize cortisol or its metabolites in the way cells utilize such things as amino acids and carbohydrates to produce structural material, chemical energy, etc. The total effect of fibroblast metabolism on cortisol and its metabolites can be expressed as addition or subtraction of hydrogen (with the exception of side-chain splitting at C-17). The question is: Which chemical events are meaningful to biological activity and which transformations of steroid merely prepare it for excretion? This question leads to the following considerations, which have been experimentally tested.

1. Anti-inflammatory activity of cortisol metabolites. Each of the compounds given in Table 1 and in Figures 1 and 3 was tested for anti-inflammatory activity; none had any significant effect, with the exception of cortisone, which was only 1/77 as effective as cortisol.[13]

2. The action of cortisol may be a product of the oxidation and reduction of key positions in the molecule. Talalay and co-workers have shown that

steroids, as hydrogen donors and acceptors, can participate in the reversible reduction and oxidation of diphospho- and triphosphopyridine nucleotides.[25] However, sufficient proof has not yet been given to make a definite correlation between biological activity of steroids and their ability to stimulate transhydrogenase and dehydrogenase activities.

3. The effect of depressed steroid metabolism on anti-inflammatory activity. *In vivo* studies have shown that 2α-methylcortisol and 2α-methylcortisone are very poorly metabolized[8] and are not nearly as readly interconverted as cortisol and cortisone; i.e., little oxidation and reduction occur at C-11. 2α-Methylcortisol has a higher anti-inflammatory activity than cortisol; 2α-methylcortisone is less active than cortisone.[16] Thus, when oxidation and reduction at C-11 are practically abolished by substitution of a 2α-methyl group the biological activity of the steroid is also altered. The result may indicate that cortisone possesses anti-inflammatory activity only when converted to cortisol.

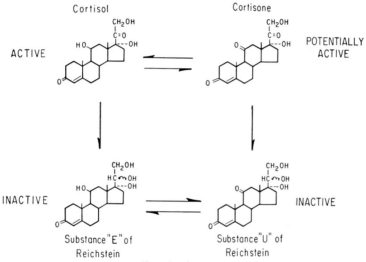

Fig. 4. See text.

It would seem that at least one concept has been established: The metabolism of cortisol abolishes its anti-inflammatory activity when the steroid is converted to any compound other than cortisone, which has a small amount of activity.

The amount of cortisol available to exert an anti-inflammatory activity in the connective tissue can be modified by chemical events in the liver which are influenced by thyroid hormone and ACTH. It has been shown both *in vivo*[19] and *in vitro*[5, 26] that thyroid hormone increases the reduction of ring A of corticosteroids in the liver; cortisol and cortisone, when reduced in ring A, have no anti-inflammatory action.[13] ACTH (given to adrenalectomized mice) causes a reduction in *in vivo* metabolism of cortisol.[7]

The fibroblasts themselves cause structural changes in corticosteroids. The relative rates of conversion locally determine the amount of protection against inflammation available at any one time by controlling the quantities of active and inactive compounds present. Figure 4 represents the biological relationships that exist between the major compounds isolated that are active, potentially active or inactive, measured for anti-inflammatory activity.

REFERENCES

1. Berliner, D. L. and Dougherty, T. F.: Metabolism of cortisol by loose connective tissue "in vitro." Proc. Soc. Exper. Biol. & Med., *98*:3, 1958.
2. Berliner, D. L. and Salhanick, H. A.: Microchemical identification of radioactive and non-radioactive steroids. Anal. Chem., *28*:1608, 1956.
3. Berliner, D. L., Dominguez, O. V. and Westenskow, G.: Determination of C[14] steroids on paper chromatograms. Anal. Chem., *29*:1797, 1957.
4. Berliner, D. L., Swim, H. E. and Dougherty, T. F.: Metabolism of corticosterone 4C[14] by fibroblasts, Strain U12-79. Biochim. et biophys. acta, *38*:184, 1960.
5. Berliner, D. L. and Dougherty, T. F.: Influence of the RES on other cells on the metabolic fate of steroids. In: The Reticuloendothelial System (RES). Ann. N. Y. Acad. Sc., *88*:14, 1960.
6. Berliner, D. L., Grosser, B. I. and Dougherty, T. F.: The metabolism of cortisol in eviscerated rats. Arch. Biochem. & Biophys., *77*:81, 1958.
7. Berliner, D. L., Keller, N. and Dougherty, T. F.: Tissue retention of cortisol and metabolites induced by ACTH, an extra-adrenal effect. Endocrinology (In press).
8. Bush, I. E. and Mahesh, V. B.: Metabolism of 11-oxygenated steroids, 2,2-methyl steroids. Biochem. J., *71*:718, 1959.
9. Cohn, G. L., Hume, M. and Bondy, P. K.: The in vivo conjugation of 17-keto steroids by the dog kidney. Abstract 366, First International Congress of Endocrinology, Copenhagen, 1960.
10. Dougherty, T. F.: The protective role of adrenal cortical secretion in the hypersensitive states. In: Pituitary-Adrenal Function. Washington, D. C., American Association for the Advancement of Science, 1950, p. 79.
11. Dougherty, T. F.: Some observations on mechanism of corticosteroid action on inflammation and immunologic processes. Ann. N. Y. Acad. Sc., *56*:748, 1953.
12. Dougherty, T. F.: Relation of adrenocortical hormones to Hypersensitive State. In: Adrenal Cortex. New York, Josiah Macy, Jr. Foundation, 1950, p. 88.
13. Dougherty, T. F. and Schneebeli, G. L.: The use of steroids as anti-inflammatory agents. Ann. N. Y. Acad. Sc., *61*:328, 1955.
14. Dougherty, T. F.: Studies of the antiphlogistic and antibody suppressing functions of the pituitary-adrenocortical secretions. Recent Progr. Hormone Res., *7*:307, 1952.
15. Dougherty, T. F.: Role of steroids in regulation of inflammation. In Mills, L. C. and Moyer, J. H. (eds.): Inflammation and Diseases of Connective Tissues. Philadelphia, W. B. Saunders Co., 1961, p. 449.
16. Dulin, N. E., Baumann, B. J. and Stafford, R. O.: Effects of 2-methylation on glucocorticoid activity of various C-21 steroids. Proc. Soc. Exper. Biol. & Med., *94*:303, 1957.
17. Fukushima, D. K. and Bradlow, H. L.: Comparative study of the metabolism of Reichstein's substance E and hydrocortisone in man. No. 378. Proceedings, First International Congress on Endocrinology, 1960.
18. Ganis, F. M., Axelrod, L. R. and Miller, L. L.: The metabolism of hydrocortisone by kidney tissue in vitro. J. Biol. Chem., *218*:841, 1956.
19. Peterson, R. E.: The influence of the thyroid on adrenal cortical function. J. Clin. Invest., *37*:736, 1957.
20. Romanoff, L. D., Seelye, J., Rodriguez, R. and Pincus, G.: The regular occurrence of 3α-allotetrahydrocortisol (3α, 11β, 17α, 21-tetrahydroxy, allopregnane-20-one) in human urine. J. Clin. Endocrinol., *17*:434, 1957.
21. Samuels, L. T.: Metabolism of steroids. In Greenberg, D. M. (ed.): Chemical Pathways of Metabolism. New York, Academic Press. (In press.)
22. Stevens, W., Berliner, D. L. and Dougherty, T. F.: Conjugation of steroids by liver, kidney and intestine of mice. Endocrinology. (In press.)
23. Sweat, M. L., Grosser, B. F., Berliner, D. L., Swim, H. E., Nabors, C. J., Jr. and Dougherty, T. F.: Metabolism of cortisol and progesterone by cultured uterine fibroblasts, Strain U12–705. Biochim. et biophys. acta, *28*:591, 1958.
24. Swim, H. E. and Parker, R. F.: Culture characteristics of human fibroblasts propagated serially. Am. J. Hyg., *2*:235, 1957.
25. Talalay, P. and William-Ashman, H. G.: Activation of hydrogen transfer between pyridine nucleotides by steroid hormones. Proc. Nat. Acad. Sc. U.S., *44*:15, 1958.
26. Tomkins, G. M.: Enzymatic metabolism of corticosteroids. Ann. N. Y. Acad. Sc., *82*:836, 1959.

Panel Discussion

WILLIAM A. SODEMAN, *Moderator*

DR. SODEMAN: What evidence is there to indicate that an alteration in the structure of the glucocorticoids, such as reduction of a double bond or of a ketone group, is related to the mechanism of their action on peripheral tissues?

DR. BERLINER: There is no relation. We do not believe that the transformation of one compound to the other has anything to do with the mechanism of action of the steroids, because when we prevent hydrogen transfer, we can either abolish or increase the activity of the steroid, depending on whether we start with cortisone or cortisol. Later on Dr. Dougherty will present some experiments on that, using 2α-methyl cortisol, which cannot be transformed in connective tissues to 2α-methyl cortisone and vice versa; 2α-methyl cortisol is more active than cortisol as an anti-inflammatory steroid, and 2α-methyl cortisone is less active than cortisone.

Also, I would like to comment on something Dr. Cahill mentioned earlier—that estrogens may be involved in transhydrogenase reactions and that this might be their mechanism of action. If this is the mechanism of action of estrogens, why is it that the estrogenic activity of estradiol is not abolished by the introduction of an ethinyl group in the 17 position which blocks hydrogen transfer?

DR. CAHILL: I think that is the major point in the argument against this mechanism. When this fact is mentioned to the people who are endorsing this mechanism, they say oxidation-reduction can occur at some other site, namely, in the phenolic A ring. In other words, this theory appears to be valid for the estrogens, although certainly not conclusive.

DR. BERLINER: The theory you mentioned does not apply only to estrogens, but to testosterone and other steroids. However, it is very fortunate that it can be applied to estrogens, since, if you look at the formula, there is only one place where hydrogenation or transhydrogenation can occur, and that is at the 17 position. Since this can be blocked without decreasing estrogenic activity, I think this makes the transhydrogenation theory unlikely. There is no way in which the phenolic ring A can yield or accept hydrogens. However, all of the other steroids have chemical groups at one or more carbons, such as carbons 3, 4, 11, 17 or 20, which can enter into all kinds of hydrogenation and dehydrogenation reactions, and it would be difficult to disprove this theory using only these compounds.

DR. CAHILL: There is still no evidence to show that the ethinyl side chain is not removed from a few of the steroid molecules, leaving a free unit which can then undergo oxidation-reduction reactions. If you do not believe in this mechanism, how do you think the steroids produce their metabolic effects on peripheral tissues? All the data I showed tended to be negative for every single reaction, and the data you just mentioned are negative for the only good theory we do have, and especially in the case of the estrogens.

DR. BERLINER: Dr. Dougherty will go into detail about this later.

DR. SODEMAN: Dr. Jenkins, do you have any comments about the mechanism of action of steroids?

DR. JENKINS: In his paper, Dr. Cahill made the statement that if all available corticosteroids had essentially similar fundamental actions, dissociation of the various effects would be extremely difficult to achieve, if not unlikely. However, I think that as these steroids become more and more complex with more and more changes in their functional groups, we may very well be moving away from the area where steroid side effects are purely overdosage effects into an area where new molecular configurations are actually producing toxic effects not related to the fundamental action of the steroid molecule itself. It is entirely possible that this is already true when high doses of any of the corticosteroids are given, and also with one or possibly two of the newer steroids now available.

DR. NICHOL: I have two comments concerning Dr. Cahill's paper. I think it was Dr. George Sayers, in a fairly comprehensive review some ten years ago, who expressed the idea that it would be more intellectually satisfying to have one underlying basis for the mode of action of corticosteroids than to try to form an independent hypothesis for each of the different effects observed; and I certainly would be inclined to agree with Dr. Cahill that until we have evidence to the contrary it is much better to consider that a single site of action might be involved. On this basis, the different cells that are affected and the response that they have would depend on the metabolic machinery of those particular cells. I mentioned that there is an increase in the activity of alanine transaminase in the liver when animals are fed a high protein diet. Now, if the steroid acted peripherally and produced changes in amino acid levels, would administration of high protein diets duplicate the effects of steroids on nonperipheral corticosteroid-sensitive tissues? With Dr. Rosen we have done some experiments in our laboratory, in which we have fed high protein diets to rats bearing corticosteroid-sensitive tumors; when we raised the level of protein to 50 per cent, there was marked inhibition of the tumors, in this case Walker 256 tumors, without significant inhibition of body growth. So whatever the cause of this, elevated levels of amino acids can raise the capacity of the liver to produce glucose and also have an effect on a target tissue.

Secondly, I think it would be helpful if we imposed a time scale on these very complex enzymatic responses. Dr. Myles Glenn mentioned this in relation to responses involving carbohydrate metabolism. Only after the time scale was extended did the effects that are concerned with negative nitrogen balance become demonstrable, and in experiments in which animals are injected with corticosteroids and tissues taken for observation of a few hours later, the findings probably have little bearing on the area of metabolism concerned with negative nitrogen balance.

DR. CAHILL: I completely agree that the time sequence is the most important thing, and this tends to localize the effect of corticosteroids in the periphery, because, if I am correct, the earliest action that glucocorticoids have is the restoration of the ability of the vascular bed to respond to epinephrine, and this occurs within minutes.

DR. WEIL: Dr. Cahill, would you elaborate on the fundamental mechanism involved in the relationship of corticosteroids and epinephrine to the vascular system?

DR. CAHILL: Dr. Nichol and I were discussing some of the theories concerning the mechanism of action of corticosteroids. One of the initial effects is increased glucose production by the liver, and it is certainly true that this effect occurs very early and is often demonstrable within an hour and a half after administration of the steroid. I just wanted to point out that there are two effects that occur prior to this—notably, the rise in glomerular filtration rate which occurs within 30 minutes and the effect on peripheral vessels and their response to epinephrine which occurs within one to two minutes. For example, the blood pressure of an Addisonian patient who is not receiving steroids will rise to a maximum of only about 80/60 during administration of norepinephrine or epinephrine, but two or three minutes after administration of intravenous hydrocortisone, while the vasopressor drug is continued at the same rate, the blood pressure will be 120/80 or more. Certainly these effects are not mediated through the liver, and these data suggest that the peripheral action of these compounds is an important one.

DR. SODEMAN: Dr. Weil, does the administration of adrenocortical steroids modify the progression of renal ischemic injury in the shock process?

DR. WEIL: We have some experimental data bearing on this point. If one administers endotoxin derived from a gram-negative bacterium to the dog and produces the characteristic endotoxic type of shock, one of the little-documented features of this circumstance is a reduction of urinary flow; this reduction is disproportionately greater than the reduction in arterial pressure, so that it is not simply a result of reduced perfusion pressure. If one then administers a vasopressor agent to restore the mean arterial pressure to a more physiological level, urinary output may increase slightly; but then, if one adds a corticosteroid such as prednisolone or hydrocortisone, the urinary volume is markedly increased and returns near to the control level. If the steroid is given alone, at least in the series of dogs which I have reference to, this phenomenon is not observed, so the evidence I have bearing on this point indicates that the combined use of a steroid and a vasopressor agent in moderate dosages will maintain urinary flow. This has been seen clinically as well. What the phenomenon is and to what extent it represents protection against renal injury, I do not know.

DR. DINGMAN: Recently, I heard a very interesting report concerning the changes in urinary flow induced by alterations in perfusion pressure to the *in vivo* isolated kidney. By changing the perfusion pressure from a mean value of about 90 mm. up to 150 mm. mean pressure—in other words, within the autoregulating capacity of the kidney—urinary flow could be increased considerably; with a decrease in perfusion pressure, antidiuresis occurred within a few minutes with osmolal UP ratios of about 3. Then, upon raising the pressure acutely, there was a sudden outpouring of hypotonic urine. These workers also showed that renal medullary blood flow could be changed in parallel with the changes in pressure; therefore, the amount of urine flow during hypotensive states seems to depend on the perfusion pressure and changes in renal medullary flow. Possibly the steroids may affect renal circulation, renal vascular resistance and, particularly, renal medullary flow.

DR. WEIL: I do not mean to minimize the importance of adequate perfusion pressure in regard to urine filtration, but on the other hand, I would also say that in experiments in which the isolated kidney is perfused while the pressure and flow are held at control levels, injection of bacterial endotoxin from *E. coli* causes a rapid decrease in the volume of urine that is filtered by the glomerulus.

DR. SODEMAN: In the emergency use of injectable steroids, is the development of either hypertension or congestive heart failure an important risk? Dr. Dingman, do you want to say anything about that?

DR. DINGMAN: I do not think that intravenous administration of steroids *per se* has a special risk over other routes of administration. The development of hypertension and congestive heart failure is related to doses which exceed physiologic amounts and to the duration of therapy. Certainly, we have all treated patients with massive doses of steroids for short periods of time and have observed very little change in blood pressure or in fluid metabolism if the treatment was not continued for too long a period. It takes some time to develop salt and water retention and edema, and many patients tend to escape from this effect even if steroids are continued at high levels. We do not quite understand why certain individuals are susceptible to the development of edema and congestive heart failure and why others are not. I think it may be related to total potassium balance and possibly also to the intracellular protein stores. Some data we have indicate that steroids are more likely to cause salt retention and edema when they are given to sick patients who have lost a lot of weight and who have depletion of total body potassium than when they are given to healthy subjects. The so-called normal control may be given steroids for several days and often does not show any total solid retention or water retention even though there is sodium retention, since if potassium is available, it can be exchanged for sodium in the renal tubule. Even though the retained sodium then may go into the cells, it simply replaces potassium and there is no osmotic effect, and therefore there is no accumulation of fluid.

DR. LEATHEM: I want to comment on the relationship of edema formation by the steroids to the protein levels in the patient. In patients with kwashiorkor, cortisone may have a good diuretic effect and mercurial diuretics may fail completely. Here you have an example of a person in very poor protein balance who has edema because of the low protein level but yet responds magnificently to administration of adrenal corticosteroids.

DR. SODEMAN: Dr. Dingman, how are changes in the water-binding properties of connective tissues brought about by steroids?

DR. DINGMAN: I do not think there is much information available about the effect of steroids on the water content of connective tissue; however, it is possible that the connective tissues serve as some sort of barrier or boundary between the extracellular fluid and the cell medium. We do know from the work of Leaf and his group with the toad bladder, frog skin and frog bladder that vasopressin does affect the water transport of nonrenal cells very considerably. Cells exposed to a fluid medium in the absence of vasopressin do not take up much water, but after addition of vasopressin or even oxytocin the water uptake by these cells can be accelerated; so there is evidence that vasopressin affects other tissues in the body in addition to the renal tubules. At the present time I believe almost everyone is thinking about this generalized effect of vasopressin on cell permeability, which accounts for the fact that water can enter the intracellular compartment more readily. In the absence of vasopressin water is relatively confined to the extracellular space.

DR. SODEMAN: This afternoon we heard about the effects of some of these steroids on calcium metabolism and about the relationship of the parathyroids to this activity. In their papers, both Dr. Clark and Dr. Stoerk discussed some facets of this that are related in some ways, but I gathered that they may differ in their opinions about some of the activities of these agents. I wonder whether they would like to comment about this? Dr. Stoerk, do you have anything to say about Dr. Clark's data?

DR. STOERK: I do not really think that Dr. Clark's data bear on the question we have been dealing with. We have observed in rats a typical parathyroid hormone effect of decreased tubular reabsorption of phosphate, following the injection of any sort of steroid having a hydrocortisone-like action, but only in the presence of the parathyroids and not in parathyroidectomized animals. This, I think, is clear evidence for the mediation of that effect by the parathyroids. Dr. Clark has measured radioactive phosphate excretion in the urine, and unless, as we do, he also measured glomerular filtration rate and allowed for the effects of the greatly increased rate of glomerular filtration following steroid administration to rats, he would not be able to detect this difference. The rest of his observations, interesting as they are, do not bear either on hyperparathyroidism or on osteoporosis, since we have never observed osteoporosis after administration of parathyroid hormone or steroids to rats. Rats are apparently an exception in that regard and develop increased density of bone instead of osteoporosis; osteoporosis associated with ostetis fibrosa occurs only after administration of monstrous doses of the bovine parathyroid extract. Small doses of the hormone produce, if anything, increased density of bone or have no effect whatever.

DR. CLARK: I agree with Dr. Stoerk completely in regard to osteoporosis in rats. We always see increased density after administration of parathyroid hormone.

In regard to the first part of his comments, as he indicated, we did not measure glomerular filtration rate in our rats. However, in the isotope studies we did. The animals were given the isotope 50 days before, and the main source of the radioactivity appearing in the urine could only have been that in bone. Therefore, the only way I can interpret my data is that the parathyroids are not required for this action of steroids. However, we used much larger doses of steroids than Dr. Stoerk did; the doses he used were, I believe, a fraction of the doses that we used.

Part VI | EFFECTS OF
ANTI-INFLAMMATORY
AGENTS ON THE GENERAL
INFLAMMATORY PROCESS

Effects of Anti-Inflammatory Agents on the General Inflammatory Process: General Remarks[*]

PIERRE JEAN

Institut de Médecine et de Chirurgie Expérimentales, Université de Montréal

In recent years, many important new discoveries have been made in the field of inflammation and anti-inflammatory agents. Although we have learned a great many facts about inflammation, it is very difficult to coordinate these into a system of knowledge, because so few of them have been made under strictly comparable conditions. This is one of the greatest handicaps to the acquisition of a more profound understanding of the effects of anti-inflammatory agents on the general inflammatory process.

A large variety of experimental models of inflammation have been used for studying the antiphlogistic activity of salicylates, antihistamines and steroids. Not all the methods devised for measuring inflammation will be reviewed here, but we would like to mention, among others, the granuloma formation around cotton pellets implanted under the skin[4] and the effect of applying chloroform to the skin. Other techniques are based upon the affinity of inflamed tissue for such dyes as trypan blue;[5] here the diffusion of the dye, due to the increase in capillary permeability, is used as an indicator of inflammation. Another method used for measuring inflammation and evaluating the anti-inflammatory action of drugs was suggested by Ungar.[15] It is based on the weight gain of inflamed skin, due to loss of plasma into the tissue after intradermal injection of a phlogogen. Various other techniques are commonly used by different investigators. This diversity gives rise to difficulties in interpreting and correlating the many facts pertinent to the effect of anti-inflammatory agents on the inflammatory process.

It is a well accepted fact that certain steroids, such as hydrocortisone, tend to inhibit inflammation; for this reason, they are called anti-inflammatory or antiphlogistic steroids. They tend to suppress the whole process of inflammation, and therefore the production of everything that is characteristic of it. Inflammation is a complex biologic reaction characterized by an increase in capillary permeability, diapedesis, exudation, antibody formation and granulomatous proliferation. Each investigator sees the site of action of antiphlogistic agents according to his own approach to the general inflammatory process. For instance, Menkin found that cortisone and hydrocortisone suppress the increased capillary permeability induced by an alkaline exudate or its contained leukotaxine.[6] On the other hand, an acid exudate

* The experimental work on which this article is based was supported by grants from the National Science Foundation and the Gustavus and Louise Pfeiffer Research Foundation.

445

(exudin) is inhibited by ACTH, but not by cortisone. In Menkin's experiments, ACTH is reported to have a direct antiphlogistic activity in the focus of inflammation, the mediation of the adrenal cortex not being essential. According to this author, the mechanism of anti-inflammatory corticosteroids and ACTH is to be considered at a cellular level: these substances impair the cellular activity, as shown by a reduction in the incidence of the cell division in the ova of the sea urchin exposed to cortisone, hydrocortisone or ACTH. Thus, the ability of the cell to produce the biochemical factors concerned in inflammation is reduced.[6] Dougherty has expressed the view that anti-inflammatory hormones, when given in large doses, inhibit formation of antibody protein. A rapid synthesis and release of this protein follows the withdrawal of the hormones.[2] Production of parenchymatous cellular degeneration is attributed to the hormonal depression of the inflammatory response.[2] According to Halpern, cortisone should maintain the tonus of the small vessels, which are injured by histamine. It also impedes the reaccumulation of "labile" histamine in the tissues, following depletion by histamine liberators. Cortisone acts by preventing the transformation of "combined" to "labile" histamine.[3] Ungar reported that antiphlogistic hormones accelerate the inactivation of fibrinolysin by its natural inhibitor, antifibrinolysin,[14] resulting in a decrease in the liberation of the phlogogenic mediators. Furthermore, antiphlogistic corticosteroids have been reported to inhibit diapedesis,[1] to diminish fibroblastic activity and to impede mobilization of phagocytic cells.

From this review, it can be seen that anti-inflammatory agents are able to block the inflammatory reaction at various points. In other words, these agents tend to suppress the production of everything that is characteristic of inflammation, just as they tend to suppress the whole process of inflammation.

Let us now consider some of the general conclusions drawn from the experimental work performed in our Institute.

It was observed some years ago that the parenteral injection of egg white into the rat produces a singular, acute inflammatory reaction in certain predisposed "shock organs," such as the snout, the ears, the paws and the genital region. This phenomenon is referred to as an "anaphylactoid" reaction, since it does not depend upon preliminary sensitization with the evocative agent.[7] It is augmented by adrenalectomy and by treatment with desoxycorticosterone (DOC) or somatotrophin (STH), but it is diminished during the alarm reaction of the general adaptation syndrome as well as after treatment with ACTH, cortisone and hydrocortisone. The antiphlogistic action of ACTH is indirect and does not occur in the absence of the adrenals.[7] These investigations led to the concept that two groups of hormones exist, having opposite activities on the inflammatory process: the prophlogistic hormones (STH, DOC) augment the tissue reactivity to injury, while the antiphlogistic hormones (ACTH, cortisone, hydrocortisone) diminish that reactivity.

Later, an experimental arthritis was induced in rats by the topical injection of formalin just beneath the plantar skin of the hind paw. A few minutes after the injection of the irritant, there is intense congestion and diffuse edema of the whole paw, particularly in the metatarsal region. Two days later, the acute reaction tends to localize itself at the joint level. ACTH, cortisone, and the alarm reaction almost completely inhibit this topical-irritation arthritis,[8] and DOC aggravates it. On a purely empirical basis, so-called nonspecific therapeutic procedures (e.g., parenteral injection of foreign proteins, bloodletting) have long been used in the therapy of such inflammatory diseases as rheumatoid arthritis. Probably the most important factor in the therapeutic action of "nonspecific therapy," "fever therapy" and "shock therapy" is the fact that such drastic measures stimulate defense by eliciting a general adaptation syndrome, and more particularly, an increased production of ACTH.

Further information concerning the effects of anti-inflammatory agents on the inflammatory process was obtained by the granuloma-pouch technique. This procedure is described in another paper in this volume. As was to be expected, after using hydrocortisone, either locally or systemically, it was observed that this antiphlogistic corticoid is highly active in preventing the formation of granulomatous tissue. Even more interesting is the fact that the administration of a single threshold dose of hydrocortisone becomes more effective in preventing the development of a large inflammatory focus if given during a certain "critical period,"[9] which is at its maximum on about the third day after the injection of croton oil into the air-space under the skin of the rat. It was observed that, under similar conditions, the inhibitory action of systemic stress upon inflammation also occurs during a sharply delimited "critical period."[11]

The granuloma-pouch technique also helps to dissociate the phlogistic and the necrotizing effects of an irritant. Hydrocortisone inhibits the phlogistic effect of croton oil, but it does not inhibit its necrotizing effect. An inverse proportion exists between the development of an inflammatory barrier around an irritant and the tendency of adjacent tissue to undergo necrosis. The antiphlogistic hormones act, not by erecting a barrier around the cells (and then protecting them against pathogens), but by inhibiting the development of a granulomatous formation in response to an irritant. A mild irritant injected into the pouch induces a great increase in connective tissue due to the granuloma formation. Subsequently, a strong irritant is well tolerated by the skin. If hydrocortisone is given with the mild irritant, it will prevent the transformation of connective tissue into a thick granuloma. Subsequent exposure to a strong irritant results in necrosis of the adjacent skin.[10] The hormone can inhibit one action (inflammation) while aggravating another effect (necrosis) produced by the same agent. Therefore, the granuloma-pouch technique helps to dissociate two closely related phenomena resulting from tissue injury, namely, inflammation and necrosis.

Antiphlogistic agents other than ACTH or corticoids were studied in our Institute. Recently, it was noted that aminoacetonitrile, or "AAN" (NH_2CH_2CN), an osteolathyrogenic compound, tends to inhibit inflammatory reactions.[12] Experiments on adrenalectomized rats maintained on small doses of hydrocortisone and DOC indicate that AAN markedly inhibits the production of inflammatory exudate in the granuloma-pouch. This antiphlogistic effect is an inherent property of the compound, not merely the consequence of an adrenal-mediated stressor action.[13]

In conclusion, it should be pointed out that inflammation is a natural defense mechanism against potentially damaging (necrotizing) agents. Anti-inflammatory agents are useful when we are dealing with pathogens that are not injurious in themselves and whose damaging effect is mainly due to their phlogistic effect.

SUMMARY

Our understanding of the mechanisms of action of the anti-inflammatory agents is hindered by the great variety of experimental models of inflammation and a lack of correlation between the different approaches to the problem.

ACTH, cortisone, hydrocortisone and the alarm reaction have been shown to inhibit the anaphylactoid inflammation, the topical-irritation arthritis and the formation of granulomatous tissue in response to croton oil (granuloma-pouch technique). STH and DOC tend to aggravate these reactions.

It was shown that hydrocortisone and systemic stress act on the inflammatory process at a "critical period."

The antiphlogistic corticoids exert an opposite effect on the inflammatory and necrotizing activities of a single agent.

REFERENCES

1. Delaunay, A., Pages, J. and Martinet, M.: Capsules surrénales et inhibition de la diapédèse. Compt. rend. Acad. sc., 223:218-219, 1946.
2. Dougherty, T. F.: The effect of cessation of treatment with large doses of antiphlogistic adrenocortical hormones on circulating antibody and parenchymatous allergic lesions. In: Jasmin, G. and Robert, A. (eds.): The Mechanism of Inflammation. Montreal, Acta, Inc., 1953, p. 217.
3. Halpern, B. N.: Histamine, antihistaminiques de synthèse et processus inflammatoires. In: Jasmin, G. and Robert, A. (eds.): The Mechanism of Inflammation. Montreal, Acta, Inc., 1953, p. 228.
4. Meier, R., Schuler, W., and Desaulies, R.: Zur Frage des Mechanismus der Hemmung des Bindegewebswachstums durch Cortisone. Experientia, 6:469, 1950.
5. Menkin, V.: Studies on inflammation. I. Fixation of vital dyes in inflamed areas. J. Exper. Med., 50:171-180, 1929.
6. Menkin, V.: Biochemical Mechanisms in Inflammation. Springfield, Illinois, Charles C Thomas, 1956.
7. Selye, H.: Studies on adaptation. Endocrinology, 21:169, 1937.
8. Selye, H.: Further studies concerning the participation of the adrenal cortex in the pathogenesis of arthritis. Brit. M. J., 2:1129, 1949.
9. Selye, H.: The "critical period" in the development of inflammation. Acta physiol. latinoam., 3:188, 1953.
10. Selye, H.: On the mechanism through which hydrocortisone affects the resistance of tissues to injury. (An experimental study with the granuloma-pouch technique.) J.A.M.A., 152:1207, 1953.
11. Selye, H.: The "critical period" for the inhibition of inflammation by a primarily neurogenic stress-situation. Psychosomat. Med., 17:124, 1955.
12. Selye, H.: Lathyrism. Rev. canad. biol., 16:1, 1957.
13. Selye, H.: On the anti-inflammatory action of aminoacetonitrile (AAN). Canad. J. Biochem., 35:1029, 1957.
14. Ungar, G.: The fibrinolytic system and inflammation. In: Jasmin, G. and Robert, A. (eds.): The Mechanism of Inflammation. Montreal, Acta, Inc., 1953, p. 151.
15. Ungar, G., Kobrin, S. and Sezesny, B. R.: Measurement of inflammation and evaluation of anti-inflammatory agents. Arch. internat. pharmacodyn., 123:71, 1959.

Role of Steroids in Regulation of Inflammation*

THOMAS F. DOUGHERTY

University of Utah College of Medicine

The questions which are to be discussed here relative to the metabolism of cortisol are: (1) Is cortisol itself or a metabolic product the active anti-inflammatory agent? (2) Are there qualitative or quantitative differences in distribution of radioactive cortisol in normal and inflamed connective tissue and in blood? (3) Are there differences in metabolic products observed in the tissues of normal and inflamed connective tissue? (4) Are there differences in the amounts of cortisol and its metabolites present in normal and inflamed connective tissue?

It is possible that when answers to these questions are at least partially known we may be able to ascertain the mechanisms involved in the passage of cortisol and its metabolites from blood into tissue and its final metabolism and removal from the organism by hepatic action. It can readily be seen that defects in any one of these metabolic processes could lead to alterations producing exaggerated or diminished inflammatory reactions which could be classified as disease states. In order to obtain information on the grosser aspects of cortisol circulation, metabolism and excretion, labelled cortisol was administered and followed by the application of classic radiobiological methods. Detailed studies concerning the cellular sites of the transformations of cortisol and its analogues included the use of labelled steroids (labelled in the ring, 4C[14]), connective cells and tissue-cultured fibroblasts. These detailed metabolic studies are discussed in the latter sections of this paper.

METABOLISM AND DISTRIBUTION OF CORTISOL 4C[14] IN NORMAL AND INFLAMED CONNECTIVE TISSUE

Radioactive cortisol (4C[14]) was administered intravenously to adrenalectomized mice which were simultaneously given subcutaneous standardized inflaming doses of 1 per cent pyrogen-free gelatin.[13] The gelatin solution was administered to one flank of the adrenalectomized mouse and the other flank was used as a source of noninflamed connective tissue. Samples of inflamed and noninflamed connective tissue of the same animal were taken at the same intervals following induction of inflammation and administration of the 4C[14]-labelled cortisol. The amounts of radioactivity in both control and inflamed connective tissues and the concentration in blood were determined and expressed as CPM/mg. of dry tissue (relative specific activity).

The total radioactivity in the blood diminished rapidly from the time of injection so that by 100 minutes the CPM/mg. of tissue were near background counts. All of the radioactivity in blood was not due to the labelled free cortisol alone but also to metabolites of cortisol.[13]

* This work has been supported by grants from the American Cancer Society (No. 33-0078), the National Institutes of Health (Leukemogenesis, No. 34-5217) and the Department of the Army (No. 35-5201).

When these radioactive molecules were identified by paper chromatography they were separated into three different groups according to their chemical structure. It was observed that free cortisol diminishes rapidly and has a half-life of about 45 minutes. It may be noted that tetrahydrocortisol, which is a metabolite of cortisol produced by the liver prior to conjugation, increased in the blood and remained constant during the whole period of analysis (Fig. 1). This substance is conjugated and excreted. The actual

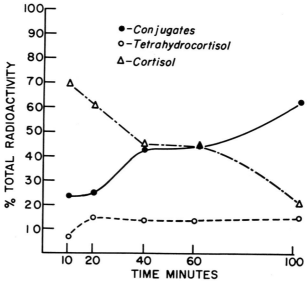

Fig. 1.   Percentage of total radioactivity from different chromatographic peaks. Variations in percentage distribution of cortisol, tetrahydrocortisol and conjugates in blood of mice at various times following intravenous administration of 4C14 cortisol.

amount of cortisol/mg. of tissue was obtained by taking the difference in relative specific activity between the normal and inflamed connective tissue (Fig. 2). The difference in concentration was approximately 0.006 μg./mg. of tissue, which was attained between 40 and 60 minutes after injection. In a sense, then, it can be stated that in order to inhibit an inflammatory response to a mild inflaming stimulus, at least 0.006 μg. of cortisol and its metabolites per mg. of tissue are required. We know, however, that at 45 minutes 50 per cent of the radioactivity measured is in molecules of metabolites which are inactive in antiphlogistic tests. Therefore, only one-half of the total radioactivity represents free active cortisol. It should be emphasized that measurement of radioactivity does not give a true value for the amount of the anti-inflammatory substance since the molecule of cortisol is changed through oxidation and reduction of substituted groups to other non-anti-inflammatory compounds. For this reason it is necessary to identify by chemical means the actual structure of the molecule which is radioactive.

Cortisol is metabolized, in general, in two different ways. The first is that the substituted groups on the gonane nucleus are altered by oxidation and reduction; secondly, metabolites are, in turn, conjugated and excreted.[4] These products of metabolism of cortisol also appear in the blood and in the tissue, so that before the cortisol is conjugated and excreted its metabolic products circulate, pass into the tissues, come back from the tissue into the blood, and, in general, are distributed much as free cortisol itself.[4, 13] In general, it appears that as far as all of these radioactive molecules are concerned, there is no specific mechanism by which the inflamed tissue has a greater capacity to localize the free antiphlogistic hormone.[9, 13] Although, in our study, the radioactivity increased in the inflamed side to an extent much greater than that in the noninflamed tissue, apparently no trapping mechanism for cortisol exists in the inflamed area.

Furthermore, the metabolites of cortisol which were derived from the blood and which went back into the blood again were essentially the same in both inflamed and noninflamed connective tissue.[13] Also, the proportions of free cortisol, tetrahydrocortisol and the conjugates were the same in the tissues at any given time as those found in the blood (Fig. 3). It appears, then, that blood levels of these substances reflect the changes in amounts that occur in the tissues. However, the maximum amount of cortisol in connective tissue is found at a time later than the maximum concentration in blood, and the amount of hormone in the normal connective tissue decreases to a minimum level by the time the half-life of the hormone in blood is reached (Fig. 2).[9, 13]

We have shown that tetrahydrocortisol and its glucuronide do not have anti-inflammatory activity.[8] It is obvious, therefore, that those mechanisms

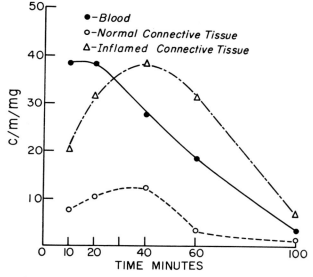

Fig. 2. Distribution of radioactivity in blood and in inflamed and noninflamed connective tissue. Relative specific activity of tissue in each case is plotted against time following simultaneous administration of inflaming substance and 4C[14] cortisol.

by which cortisol exerts its anti-inflammatory effect are influential within the first 40 minutes after the hormone is given. Following this period, blood and tissue levels of both conjugated and nonconjugated cortisol come into equilibrium, and therefore less than half of the total amount of radioactivity measured represents a molecular form which possesses anti-inflammatory action. It is apparent from the evidence which has been presented that free cortisol is not present in an amount adequate to reduce inflammation during the entire period of anti-inflammatory activity, and the actual amount of free cortisol required to inhibit inflammation is present in the connective tissue for a much shorter period of time than the duration of the anti-inflammatory effect.[9] Thus, it appears that free cortisol enters inflamed tissue in a non-specific fashion, brings about inhibition of inflammation, comes into equilibrium with that in the blood, is reduced, conjugated and then excreted. This manner of metabolism suggests that cortisol produces alterations in the connective tissue which persist; in other words, it triggers a mechanism which continues when the hormone as such is no longer present.

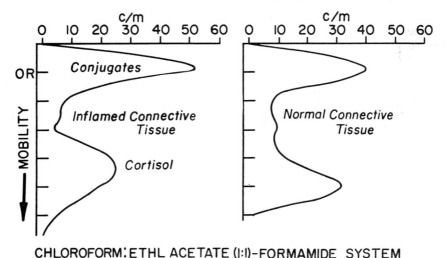

CHLOROFORM: ETHL ACETATE (I:I)–FORMAMIDE SYSTEM

Fig. 3.   Chromatographic distribution of steroids in normal and inflamed connective tissue after injection of cortisol 4C[14] in adrenalectomized mice.

LOCALIZATION OF STEROIDS IN CONNECTIVE TISSUE

The methods for localization of various steroids in connective tissue cells have been described in detail elsewhere.[11] The methods used were applied to air-dried spreads of connective tissue one cell layer thick. Various histochemical and radioautographic methods were used to study such preparations. An important feature of this technique is the fact that the preparations are not treated with any chemical agent, but rather are air-dried, and, therefore, few cellular alterations due to chemical treatment of the tissue are found.

The hydrazide reaction was most prominent in fibroblasts of cortisol-treated animals.[11] Very occasionally histiocytes demonstrated the presence of Seligman-positive granules. Polymorphonuclear leukocytes in the inflamed tissues and lymphocytes in both normal and inflamed tissues were consistently devoid of reactive ketones.[11] The local administration of 4C[14] cortisol resulted in a concentration of radioactivity in fibroblasts and occasional fat cells. Other cells reacted similarly as in the hydrazide reaction and to the neotetrazolium test (NTZ).

It is quite clear that the hydroxy-naphthoic acid hydrazine method for keto steroids may not be completely specific.[11] Either this reagent stains the keto steroids administered, or reactive aldehyde and ketone groupings are formed in the cells. In either case the fibroblast demonstrates a specific uptake of the administered hormone or a metabolic effect of this substance, or both.[11] The cortisol-treated fibroblasts and fat cells show the greatest histochemical effects. As far as the NTZ procedure is concerned, it demonstrates the presence of reducing groups of a wide variety.

In summary, it is probably of some importance to note that, regardless of whether the histochemical methods employed are specific for steroids, they are so for aldehydes and ketones, reactive groups which could be produced within the cell by active steroids. The anti-inflammatory steroids had the greatest effect on fibroblasts from the histochemical point of view and very little on any of the other connective tissue cells. Whether the granules produced indicate the presence of hormone or not, it is evident that the fibroblast is a site of deposition and/or of major action of the anti-inflammatory steroids. Other steroids tested had much less effect, if any, as far as the histochemical tests employed were concerned. Radioautographic evidence indicates that fibroblasts do concentrate $4C^{14}$ cortisol and/or its metabolites.[11] According to this evidence these compounds are not present in lymphocytes, mast cells or histiocytes.[11] A small amount of radioactive deposited material is evident in fat cells.[11] A highly specific change in fibroblasts produced by anti-inflammatory steroids is discussed in the next section.

EFFECT OF CORTISOL ON THE CELLS OF NORMAL AND INFLAMED CONNECTIVE TISSUE

The administration of cortisol produces morphological changes in many of the fibroblasts of loose connective tissue.[9, 11] The alteration is easily recognized and appears to be rather highly specific. It consists of a pulling in of cytoplasmic processes with a rounding up of the fibroblast so that it is an epithelioid cell (Fig. 4). Such changes occur in nests of fibroblasts, so that if one looks over a field of connective tissue fibroblasts, one finds that this morphological alteration produced by cortisol does not involve every single cell but occasional groups of cells. Such rounded up cells are easily recognized since they also have an increase in the amount of basophilia of the cytoplasm, and frequently vacuoles are present in the cell. Such changes in loose connective tissue fibroblasts are observed following either local administration or intravenous administration of the cortisol. These cells are very similar to the rounded up fibroblasts which are found about the edges or on the walls of wounds and which migrate into the inflamed area to repopulate the tissue that was destroyed by the initial stages of inflammation.

The amount of hormone required to produce the epithelioid cells is in the dosage range which produces an inhibition of the inflammatory response.[11] Fibroblasts are among the very first cells showing degeneration in the connective tissue when it becomes inflamed.[7, 15] They are destroyed rapidly, and in preparations in which cytological changes are easily evaluated it is seen that there are many different types of degenerative alterations in these cells in the alterative or initial stage of cell damage—the first stage of inflammation. Rounded up fibroblasts, however, appear to be very resistant to such waves of cellular destruction (Fig. 5), and they may remain intact even though they are surrounded by fibroblasts in various stages of degeneration. Similar epithelioid formations have been observed in tissue-culture fibroblasts treated with cortisol.[18]

Preparations of living loose connective tissue of mice have been made and studied by phase-contrast, time-lapse cinemicrography.[12] Preparations of inflamed connective tissue made at various times following the instigation of inflammation were treated and studied in the same fashion as the noninflamed tissues. Preparations of both types have been treated with cortisol to evaluate the differences among the cells, their movements, phagocytosis, etc., in hormone-treated and non-hormone-treated noninflamed and inflamed connective tissue.

The most striking feature concerns the effects of cortisol on the connective tissue cells. The fibroblasts become epithelioid and cease their motility (Fig. 6). Pinocytosis stops and the constant movement of mitochondria ceases as well. The whole cell becomes very quiescent and may act as though it were frozen in a bizarre shape. Of course, the polymorphonuclear leukocytes and the numerous macrophages characteristically found in inflamed connective tissue are not observed in the preparations in which inflammation is inhibited by administration of cortisol. Polymorphonuclears and macrophages are almost completely absent, although macrophages may

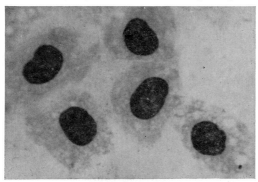

Fig. 4. Eipthelioid fibroblasts 6 hours afte.· local injection of 25μg. cortisol. Air dried. May Gruenwald Giemsa stain. × 1200.

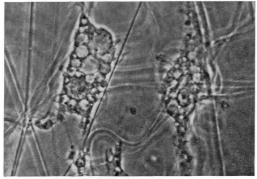

Fig. 5. Epithelioid fibroblasts. Living cells from loose connective tissue of cortisol-treated mouse. Note collagenous and elastic fibers in the field. The five spike-like processes are pulled in and the cell does not exhibit the rapid pinocytosis which characterizes it. Large vacuoles contain reducing substances. Taken from gelatin inflamed cortisol-treated area. Dark field phase contrast microscopy × 1200. (From the film "Inflammation.")

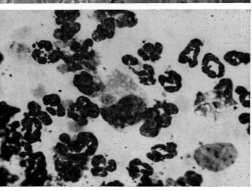

Fig. 6. Epithelioid fibroblast of mouse, surrounded by fibroblasts in various stages of degeneration and polymorphonuclears invading site of histamine induced inflammation. The only intact fibroblasts which persist in the most inflamed areas are the epithelioid cells which are formed following prior cortisol treatment. May Gruenwald Giemsa. × 800.

be found in small numbers here and there. These cells are extremely motile in the nontreated inflamed tissue. Macrophages have been found in other studies to be like lymphocytes, susceptible to the karyorrhectic effects of cortisol.[7] Those few macrophages which survive this effect of the hormone appear to be acted upon in the same way as the fibroblast. They are extremely sluggish in their movement if they are motile at all. Phagocytosis does not seem to occur. On the other hand, eosinophils do not appear to be influenced by cortisol action in this manner. Their motility is as vigorous as that found in non-hormone-treated preparations. Such effects of cortisol last for two to three hours following local administration. After this time the cells begin to move, first of all in a very sluggish fashion and then more rapidly, until they seem to regain their former capacity for active threshing about of their cytoplasms.

These observations of living cells in connective tissue lend support to the idea suggested by Eyring and Dougherty[17] that in inflammation there is an increase in the activation of the cell and that cortisol, by stabilizing the cell membrane, brings about an inactive state. This will be further discussed below, with respect to the mechanisms by which cortisol inhibits the inflammatory response.

METABOLISM OF CORTISOL BY CONNECTIVE TISSUE CELLS

Strips of connective tissue were removed from the mouse and incubated in appropriate buffer (phosphate buffer at pH 7.4) for periods of three hours. Such preparations were shown to produce certain conversions of the cortisol molecule to other steroids.[3] Pure cultures of fibroblasts oxidize the 11 position, reduce the 20 position and remove the hydroxyl group at C-17 with subsequent cleavage of the side chain.[20] The various compounds produced are Reichstein's substance U, Reichstein's substance E, cortisone, and 17-keto steroid compounds.[3, 20] Further details of these transformations are discussed in this volume by Berliner. Fibroblasts do not possess any significant capacity to reduce the A ring of the gonane nucleus.[3] Similar conversions resulted from incubations of normal loose connective tissue strips.[3] Lymphocytes, which also are found in connective tissue in second largest number after fibroblasts, produced cortisone, but the other products of conversion given above were not found in detectable amounts.[10] It appears, then, that fibroblasts are the cells which produce most of the connective tissue conversion products. When connective tissue strips which were inflamed were incubated with cortisol, very few of the conversion products were obtained.[2] This is attributed to the fact that most of the fibroblasts in such inflamed preparations are destroyed by a wave of cellular destruction which accompanies the initial stage of inflammation. The few remaining fibroblasts possibly could bring about conversions; however, the amounts could not be detected by the available methods of study. It should also be emphasized that fibroblasts do not possess the ability to form water-soluble conjugates of cortisol or any of the conversion products of this hormone produced by the hepatic cells.

PARTICIPATION OF RETICULOENDOTHELIAL CELLS IN STEROID AND STEROL METABOLISM

It is worth mentioning that it has been shown in our laboratory and by others that fibroblasts in tissue culture have the capacity to synthesize cholesterol from acetate, and the suggestion is strong that the synthesis of cholesterol by connective tissue is essentially due to the activity of fibroblasts and not of histiocytes.[9]

STRUCTURE-ACTIVITY RELATIONSHIPS OF ANTI-INFLAMMATORY STEROIDS

Although the data to be presented here were published several years ago and have been amply confirmed so far as the structure of the normally produced anti-inflammatory steroids is concerned, there are several features of some importance related to the cytological method used in these studies.[14] Analyses were not made of the antiphlogistic action of various synthetic steroid hormones other than in those instances in which the basic anti-inflammatory structure of the physiologically occurring hormones was studied. Although this method has been used for determination of steroid anti-inflammatory activity, the goal of investigation in our laboratory has been primarily the elucidation of the action of physiologically occurring antiphlogistic hormones and the relation of their metabolism to their anti-inflammatory activity.

The method used in this laboratory has been described in detail in numerous publications (see reference 14). Therefore, only the results will be given here, except in those instances in which certain features of our method of study point up differences among hormones or differences among the cellular features in areas of inflammation. The method of assay allows a quantitative estimation of potency ratios and, thus, structure activity relationships with particular attention to various substituted groups may be deduced. In addition, the method used includes notation of changes in cellular morphology, fluctuations in cell population and alterations in tissue structure which can be evaluated in the sequence in which the phenomena of inflammation occur. This first study on the structure-activity relationships of normally occurring steroid hormones was performed on more than 900 mice of the CBA strain. Standard doses of inflaming substances were first quantified in such a fashion that graded degrees of inflammation were produced; the effects could then be compared with those found in other experimental investigations in which graded doses of anti-inflammatory hormones were administered and could be evaluated in a highly quantitative fashion. Inflaming substances included allergic inflammation in which animals were previously sensitized to horse serum and the inflammation was produced by subsequent injection of the substance.[7] Histamine[7, 14] as well as bacterial[14, 15] and chemical poisons[15] were used, as well as gelatin, which produced a very mild degree of inflammation and could be better evaluated.

The normally occurring hormones studied were cortisol, cortisone, corticosterone, substance S and compound A.[14] Analogs of these substances were used in order to ascertain the relative importance of the various substituted groups on these steroids. The basis for comparison of antiphlogistic potency of the hormones tested was the anti-inflammatory activity of hydrocortisone. The amounts of hormone used were graded from 0.0001 μg. to 10 μg. except in certain cases. For example, for substance S and corticosterone larger doses were administered. The linear regression line for the different doses of hydrocortisone showed that the curve was linear over the dosage range from .001 γ to .01 γ. Previously it had been shown that when doses from .01 γ to approximately 1 γ were given, the antiphlogistic curve did not regress further.[7] Above 10 μg. the inflammatory response may actually return, so that rather than being inhibited at this point the inflammation may actually be increased or may not differ significantly from the control values.[7] These assays were all performed in adrenalectomized animals; therefore, no dilution with endogenously secreted hormone was possible.

According to this method of assay, cortisone is approximately 76 times less potent than hydrocortisone.[14] Several analogs of cortisol in which the A ring was reduced demonstrated no activity. Subsequent investigations by several workers have confirmed this finding.[19] Corticosterone was only slightly antiphlogistic and had a large standard deviation of the slope, indicating that the compound is very variable in its antiphlogistic influence. Linear regression lines for the numbers of cells in inflamed areas could not be obtained for dehydrocorticosterone (compound A); this compound has no anti-inflammatory activity. It is suggested, then, that the absence of a hydroxyl group at the 17 position markedly reduces antiphlogistic effectiveness. On the other hand, the absence of a hydroxyl group or oxygen at 11 did not completely eliminate the anti-inflammatory effect, and the linear regression curve for inflammatory response was parallel for substance S of Reichstein to that for cortisol.

One of the most striking findings in studies using this procedure was that the preservation of fibroblasts is maintained by the anti-inflammatory steroid hormones, among which cortisol provides the greatest degree of protection against fibroblastic destruction.[7] The fibroblastic destruction is so extensive in all other preparations that for those individuals who have had little experience with cytological characteristics, it provides difficulty in the performance of this test as a routine assay procedure.

The importance of the substitutions at 11 and 17 has been emphasized in recent years since it has been suggested that cortisone is not an effective anti-inflammatory hormone but is converted to cortisol,[4] which, in turn, is antiphlogistic. Further evidence on this point has been obtained in our laboratory and supports the suggestion of others that cortisone is not in itself antiphlogistic. For example, 2-methyl cortisol is a potent anti-inflammatory agent,[16] whereas 2-methyl cortisone is not.[16] It has been shown that these two steroids are poorly metabolized in *in vivo* studies.[5] Apparently the methyl group at C-2 inhibits the oxidation and reduction at C-11.[5] Recent studies in this laboratory have shown that connective tissue cannot oxidize or reduce, respectively, 2-methyl cortisol and 2-methyl cortisone at C-11.[2]

DISCUSSION

Inflammation is not a single event but a concatenation of events, each triggered by a previous alteration, which eventually results in the infiltration and final destruction of the integrity of connective tissue. It is probable that various factors may intervene to inhibit this chain reaction, so that the eventual dissolution of connective tissue and, concomitantly, a parenchymal cells, may not occur. In this case any of the steps leading to the complete inflammatory reaction may be emphasized because the progression has been stopped at that point. Thus one may find minor changes in capillary permeability, stickiness of endothelium and edema as the predominant features without marked destruction of cells and fibers or disorganization of ground substance.

Indeed, it is evident that an inflammatory response is confined to variable but limited volumes of tissue. When it is not, other changes—frequently the initial enhanced capillary permeability of the first stage of inflammation—take place over a large part of the body, and the response is frequently called shock.

We have often discussed the fact that cortisol, unlike some other inhibitors of inflammation, can check the phlogistic response at any stage from the swelling and increased permeability of endothelium to final dissolution of connective tissue.[6] The action of this hormone, then, is exerted at a very primitive initiating level among those processes which begin the progress of events leading to typical inflammation.[6] When the action of cortisol is analyzed with respect to anti-inflammatory potential, it becomes clear that cortisol acts in a dose-response fashion,[14] that it acts as such within the area of inflammation[6] and not by a circuitous mechanism, and that it inhibits to various degrees the maximum development of any of the stages of inflammation, depending upon the nature and amount of the phlogogenic stimulus.[7, 14, 15] It should be emphasized that endogenously secreted cortisol is capable of limiting the inflammatory response in the same fashion and that without this supply the inflammatory response is increased.[15]

There are few theories as to the basic mechanisms by which cortisol inhibits inflammation, and there is little to add since the author's first review of the subject in 1954.[6] It appears that an essential action of cortisol is its inhibition of the progressive destruction of fibroblasts in an area of potential inflammation[6] and that the fibroblast is the most common cell in connective tissue which sequesters and metabolizes this steroid.[11]

One of the first events in inflammation is the focal destruction of fibroblasts at a site of injury. This is not generally appreciated except by those who have observed the phenomenon, and it cannot be measured by indirect methods of anti-inflammatory assay.

It has been suggested that the degree of inflammation is enhanced by the autocatalytic destruction of fibroblasts, in which the destruction of one cell adds to the amount of phlogogenic substances (histamine, serotonin, etc.) and leads to the destruction of others.[6, 17] This chain reaction of cell breakage is interrupted by the action of cortisol, which increases resistance of some fibroblasts. The epithelioid fibroblast described previously is a morphological form of the cell that is highly resistant to the wave of cytological destruction. This form of the fibroblast has long been known to surround areas of inflammation and to serve as a source of cells for fibroblastic repopulation.

The fact that the anti-inflammatory effect of cortisol persists when detectable radioactive molecules of this substance are no longer present in connective tissue may be related to the fact that cortisol brings about changes in the fibroblasts which render them more resistant, or that once a threshold has been reached, the amount of hormone required to maintain resistance decreases to undetectable levels.

In any case, it is clear that cortisol is metabolized by fibroblasts. The metabolic transformations are of two general categories when one considers their functional significance. First, it should be understood that the evidence is becoming clear that the active form of the corticosteroid molecule which inhibits inflammation is cortisol. Alterations of this molecule have been shown to yield inactive or poorly active antiphlogistic compounds. Among the fibroblastic metabolites are cortisone and those compounds reduced in position 20 (Reichstein's substances E and U).[3] The transformation of cortisol to cortisone is reversible (see Berliner in this volume),[1] and thus some of the cortisone can be reduced to cortisol with a reversal to an active state. Cortisone is converted from an inactive to an active molecular form and thus possesses antiphlogistic activity. However, the compounds reduced at C-20 cannot revert to cortisol and are thus inactive metabolites since they possess no anti-inflammatory activity of their own. Thus, a cyclic transformation of cortisol is performed by fibroblasts in which one transformation is reversible and others act as a drain away from antiphlogistic action to form nonactive compounds and reach the ultimate irreversibility when oxidation of C-17 takes place. The side chain is then removed and C-19 compounds are formed. The reason that cortisone is less than half as active as cortisol is that cortisone can also be reduced in C-20 and oxidized at C-17. Thus, only a small portion of cortisone molecule can revert to the active cortisol molecule.

Transformations of cortisol by fibroblasts and other cells depend not only on the presence of proper enzyme systems but also on the availability of cofactors (DPN, TPN, DPNH and TPNH). We have emphasized the importance of this point with respect to the maintenance of a particular molecule in an active antiphlogistic form (cortisol).[4] The less the metabolism of cortisol, the greater the anti-inflammatory activity; conversely, the greater the metabolism of cortisol to inactive and irreversible inactive products, the smaller the number of active molecules. The availability of a particular cofactor (oxidized or reduced) will determine the amount of metabolism to active or inactive steroid hormones. Even if a sufficient amount of cortisol is produced by the adrenal cortex in individuals having inflamed tissue, if the hormone is inactivated at the fibroblastic site of action more rapidly than under usual normal conditions, antiphlogistic influence could be insufficient to inhibit the inflammation (peripheral fibroblastic-induced adrenocortical insufficiency). It is evident that inflammatory disease (acute or chronic), once initiated, could be potentiated or ameliorated as a result of (a) deficiency of hormone supply, (b) alterations in fibroblastic metabolism which could arise from enzymatic defects or cofactor imbalances, and (c) a combination of (a) and (b). According to this theory, the peripheral cells may influence the disease process by their own capacities to metabolize cortisol. Thus, the fundamental defects in chronic inflammatory diseases may not be at the hormone supply level, but may be due to altered (either quantitative or qualitative) hormone metabolism at the fibroblastic level.

REFERENCES

1. Berliner, D. L.: Metabolism of cortisol and other steroids by connective tissue cells. In Mills, L. C. and Moyer, J. H. (eds.): Inflammation and Diseases of Connective Tissues. Philadelphia, W. B. Saunders Co., 1961, p. 431.
2. Berliner, D. L. and Dougherty, T. F.: Metabolism of cortisol by mouse connective tissue. Fed. Proc., *17*:189, 1958.
3. Berliner, D. L. and Dougherty, T. F.: Metabolism of cortisol by loose connective tissue, *in vitro*. Proc. Soc. Exper. Biol. & Med., *98*:3, 1958.
4. Berliner, D. L. and Dougherty, T. F.: Influence of the RES and other cells on the metabolic fate of steroids. Ann. N. Y. Acad. Sc., *88*:14, 1960.
5. Bush, I. E. and Mahesh, J. B.: Metabolism of 11-oxygenated steroids to 2-methyl steroids. Biochem. J., *71*:718, 1959.
6. Dougherty, T. F.: The mechanisms of action of adrenocortical hormones in allergy. Progr. Allergy, *4*:219-260, 1954.
7. Dougherty, T. F.: Relation of adrenocortical hormones to the hypersensitive state.

In: Adrenal Cortex. Transactions of the Second Conference. New York, Josiah Macy, Jr., Foundation, 1950, pp. 88-114.

8. Dougherty, T. F.: Unpublished results.
9. Dougherty, T. F. and Berliner, D. L.: Some ways by which ACTH and cortisol influence functions of connective tissue. In Page, I. (ed.): Connective Tissue, Thrombosis and Atherosclerosis. New York, Academic Press, Inc., 1959, p. 143.
10. Dougherty, T. F., Berliner, M. L. and Berliner, D. L.: Hormonal influence on lymphocyte differentiation from RES cells. Ann. N. Y. Acad. Sc., 88:78, 1960.
11. Dougherty, T. F., Bigler, R., Schneebeli, G. L. and Salhanick, H. A.: On the localization of steroid hormones in connective tissue. Ann. N. Y. Acad. Sc., 64:466, 1956.
12. Dougherty, T. F. and Schneebeli, G. L.: Film: Inflammation. Department of Anatomy Laboratory, University of Utah.
13. Dougherty, T. F., Brown, H. E. and Berliner, D. L.: Metabolism of hydrocortisone during inflammation. Endocrinology, 62:455, 1958.
14. Dougherty, T. F. and Schneebeli, G. L.: The use of steroids as anti-inflammatory agents. Ann. N. Y. Acad. Sc., 61:328, 1955.
15. Dougherty, T. F. and Schneebeli, G. L.: Role of cortisone in regulation of inflammation. Proc. Soc. Exper. Biol. & Med., 75:854, 1950.
16. Dulin, N. E., Bauman, B. J. and Stafford, R. O.: Effects of 2-methylation on glucocorticoid activity of various C-21 steroids. Proc. Soc. Exper. Biol. & Med., 94:303, 1957.
17. Eyring, H. and Dougherty, T. F.: Molecular mechanisms in inflammation and stress. J. Am. Scientist, 43:457, 1955.
18. Holden, M. and Adams, L. B.: Inhibitory effects of cortisone acetate and hydrocortisone on growth of fibroblasts. Proc. Soc. Exper. Biol. & Med., 95:365, 1957.
19. Holtkamp, D. E., Bates, D. E., Heming, A. E., Paetsch, C. E., Lawrence, C. J. and Duell, H. E.: Synergy of hydrocortisone and phenylephrine in local antiphlogistic activity. Acta endocrinol., 21:268, 1956.
20. Sweat, M. L., Grosser, B. I., Berliner, D. L., Swim, E. H., Nabors, C. J., Jr. and Dougherty, T. F.: The metabolism of cortisol and progesterone by cultured uterine fibroblasts, strain U12-705. Biochim. et biophys. acta, V. 28, 1958.

Mechanism of Steroid Inhibition of Connective Tissue Growth

G. ASBOE-HANSEN

University of Copenhagen

Connective-tissue growth is characterized initially by edema and subsequently by mucinous and fibrous organization of the water. The regeneration process has been studied in the normal growing organism, in healing wounds and fractures, in acute and chronic edemas of human patients, and in induced edemas in man and experimental animals.

Connective tissue cells produce the overwhelming amount of extracellular substance determining to a large extent the growth process.

MAST CELLS

Mast cells are large mesenchymal cells characterized by globular cytoplasmic granules containing acid mucopolysaccharides that are responsible for their metachromatic stainability. These mucopolysaccharides are partly sulfuric and of the heparin type, partly sulfate-free and of the hyaluronic acid type. The granular material may be liberated to the surrounding connective-tissue ground substance. In addition to mucopolysaccharides, mast cells contain and synthesize histamine. In rats and mice, serotonin (5-hydroxytryptamine) has been demonstrated as a cytoplasmic component.

FIBROBLASTS

Fibroblasts are the origin of collagen. Collagen prestages are manufac‑ tured by these cells and are liberated to the extracellular compartment where the molecules become polymerized and oriented to collagenous fibrils. Some evidence exists that this orientation may take place even in the cytoplasm of the fibroblasts.

GROUND SUBSTANCE

In loose connective tissue the ground substance is a gelatinous material. The connective-tissue ground substance, the synovial fluid, and the fluids of the eye and the inner ear contain, in addition to salts and water, a variety of proteins as well as neutral sugars and acid mucopolysaccharides. Some of these constituents are supplied by the blood. Most substances are on their way from blood to cells or from cells to blood. Mucopolysaccharides are formed by the local connective-tissue cells. Hyaluronic acid is the only muco-polysaccharide present in the synovia, and in the humors of the eye and the labyrinth. Hyaluronic acids lends to the ground substance certain of its im-portant physiochemical properties., e.g., its viscosity, gelatinous character and water-binding capacity. Evidently, the presence of chondroitin sulfate is highly important to any collagen formation. The lack of this mucopolysac-charide in the above-mentioned mesenchymal spaces (joints, eyeballs, canals of the inner ear) may explain the lack of fibrosis in these sites in normal circumstances.

TISSUE RESPONSE

In fresh edemas of the corium, e.g., urticarial wheals, mast cells are degranulated and hardly demonstrable.

In chronic edemas of the legs due to venous stasis, the number of mast cells is significantly increased, and the extracellular ground substance is ample and contains considerable amounts of nonsulfated as well as sulfated mucopolysaccharides.

In myxedema, the mast cells of skin connective tissue are numerous and show various phases of granularity. The ground substance is mucinous and contains ample amounts of hyaluronate as well as chondroitin sulfate.[1]

Within a few minutes after injection of physiologic saline solution or Tyrode's fluid into skin, degranulation of the mast cells takes place.

Cheek pouches of living hamsters have been injected with physiologic saline or Tyrode's solution with the injection needle in the loose connective tissue of the double-membrane. In other experiments the cheek pouches were surgically split, and the fluids dropped on the moist connective-tissue surface. After some minutes the mast cells lost their granules, and a cytoplasmic structure resembling a honeycomb or a sponge became visible in stained cells viewed with an ordinary microscope or without staining with the phase-contrast microscope. Around the cells a zone of unstructured material was demonstrated. This substance, staining metachromatically with toluidine blue, was broken down by testicular or bacterial hyaluronidase. The degranulated cells were able to regranulate.

Water brought about an irreversible disintegration of the cells, probably caused by osmotic forces.

Physical trauma, e.g., rubbing the pouch between two fingers, produced edema and a degranulation or disruption of the mast cells.[26]

Shock, systemically administered histamine, histamine-liberator substances and serotonin (5-hydroxytryptamine) produced edema and mast-cell degranulation.[7, 8]

In other experiments the base of one cheek pouch was ligated by a silk suture, and venous stasis was produced. After 24 hours, the pouch appeared as a grape-like sac filled with a mucinous gelatinous fluid. If it was cut up, the material did not flow out. The gel took a metachromatic stain with toluidine blue, indicating acid mucopolysaccharide. Bacterial or testicular hyaluronidase changed the viscous material into a watery fluid. Twenty-four hours after ligation the edema fluid was demonstrated by paper chromatography to contain considerable amounts of glucosamine, but practically no galactosamine. After 48 hours it contained 80 per cent glucosamine and about 20 per cent galactosamine.

After intraperitoneal injection of S^{35}-labeled sodium sulfate, 4 μC per gram body weight, the content of S^{35} in the tissue and in the edema fluid was determined. Twenty-four hours after the ligation the amount of S^{35} in the tissue was found to be 55 per cent higher than that of blood plasma, whereas the content in the edema fluid was 36 per cent lower than the plasma content. The first day there was an abrupt decrease in the number of mast cells. From the second to the seventh day the number and granularity of the mast cells increased along with an increasing content of sulfomucopolysaccharide measured as S^{35}.[9]

In incised wounds, the primary edema is bound by hyaluronic acid, forming a mucinous gel. After the first few days the sulfomucopolysaccharide content increases, the metachromasia becomes more intense, and along with the increasing content of sulfate there is an increase in collagen and in tensile strength of the wounds.[21] The fibrous organization leads to scar formation.

In rabbit aortae, intravenous injections of epinephrine or norepinephrine bring about lesions of the media and intima. The lesions are characterized by necrotic areas in the media with calcification and an increase in the content of hexosamine and water, in the hexosamine:hydroxyproline ratio (roughly representing the mucopolysaccharide:collagen ratio), in the metachromatic stainability of the ground substance, and in the uptake of S^{35}-labeled sulfate. There is no lipid accumulation unless the lipid level in the blood is raised.[20] The vascular injury is probably provoked by repeated anoxic injuries due to epinephrine-induced constriction of the vasa vasorum. The accumulation of acid mucopolysaccharides demonstrated in these experiments is probably one step of the repair process started by the anoxic edema.

In early fetal life the connective tissues are mucinous and are characterized by an ample content of acid mucopolysaccharides. With aging during pre- and postnatal life collagen deposition becomes more and more predominant. Clausen found that the hexosamine:hydroxyproline ratio steadily decreases from young to old embryos, through infancy, childhood, adult life and old age.[13]

The biological half-life of hyaluronic acid is about two days whereas that of chondroitin sulfuric acid is several times longer.[11, 14]

Mast cells are the only cells in the connective tissues that contain acid mucopolysaccharides, and they are able to release these substances to the ground substance. The concentration of tissue water is a stimulus to mucopolysaccharide release. Mast cells may be able to release histamine independently of simultaneous mucopolysaccharide release. Histamine may induce an increase in capillary permeability and produce edema; the edema provokes release of mucopolysaccharides that bind the water, changing it into a hydrated gel. The presence of acid mucopolysaccharides stimulates the deposition of collagen fibrils and thus connective-tissue growth. It appears that fibroblasts as well as mast cells are actively and indispensably involved in the above-mentioned processes.

Growth, regeneration and repair depend on well regulated processes in connective tissues. Hormones influence and control such processes and the main target seems to be the mucinous system. Collagen, once deposited, is an almost inert substance in certain organs, e.g., the skin and tendons.

EFFECTS OF ADRENAL GLUCOCORTICOID STEROIDS

The above-mentioned processes of regeneration and growth are inhibited by the influence of glucocorticoids, and simultaneously it is possible to demonstrate sufficient morphologic and biochemical changes to explain this effect.

Mast cells diminish, become vacuolated and acquire irregular outlines. The granules, which normally stain metachromatically with, for example, toluidine blue, may now take an orthochromatic stain; they clump together to form major or minor aggregates. Widely different granule sizes are observed. The number of demonstrable mast cells is reduced.[3]

Cortisone has also been found to inhibit mast cell activity in tissue cultures of embryonic skin and spleen.[22]

Normal function of the mast cells is also interfered with. The uptake of S[35]-labeled sulfate by mast cells in living mammals is inhibited by cortisone and cortisol (hydrocortisone). This has been shown by autoradiography and by biochemical methods. In induced precancerous papillomas of mouse skin most mast cells take up large amounts of radioactive sulfate, and the contrast in autoradiographs between the cells and the ground substance is considerable. However, after cortisone treatment of the animals this difference is equalized because of a decreased uptake of S[35] by the mast cells.[4] This phenomenon is associated with an inhibition of the skin carcinogenesis. After local injection of cortisol acetate in the connective tissue below the tumors, similar structural changes were noticed in the mast cells,[5] and simultaneously regression of existing papillomas was observed.

In keloids and other fibroses, similar changes have been induced by local injections of cortisol acetate, and at the same time, regression of the fibrosis and flattening of the keloids were observed.[6]

Morphologic phenomena corresponding to those mentioned above have been observed in mast cells in the cheek pouches of living hamsters.[27]

Cortisone inhibits the accumulation of liberated histamine in the connective tissue.[16] The metachromatic staining of the extracellular substance is reduced.[2] The content of hexosamine has been found to decrease, indicating a lowered content of mucopolysaccharides.[25]

Cortisone inhibits the synthesis of chondroitin sulfuric acid in connective-tissue ground substance, especially in healing wounds and in cartilage slices.[12, 19] Capillary permeability is inhibited. Thus, the amount of extracellular water is influenced and, thereby, regeneration.

Fibroblasts seem to be influenced by cortisone and cortisol, although varying results have been obtained *in vitro* by different research groups. In some experiments adrenal steroids inhibited the growth and migration of fibroblasts in cultures,[10, 18] and collagen formation by the cells was found to be reduced.[15]

In experimental wounds a reduced number of fibroblasts have been found in rabbits treated with cortisone. At the same time, wound healing was delayed. The inhibition affected the development of vessels as well as formation of ground substance and fibrils.[23] The oxygen uptake by wound tissue was reduced,[24] and the tensile strength of experimental, sutured wounds in rats was reduced during administration of cortisone.[17] It is believed that the inhibition is due to direct action upon the cells in the wound tissue and upon the connective-tissue ground substance.

The absorption of blood in bone fractures is retarded in cortisone-treated subjects, and the formation of collagen fibrils is delayed.[23]

The development of peritoneal and pleural adhesions after physical and chemical injury is inhibited by local deposition of cortisol acetate in the serosal cavity.[28]

REFERENCES

1. Asboe-Hansen, G.: Acta dermat.-venereol., *30*:221, 1950.
2. Asboe-Hansen, G.: Scand. J. Clin. & Lab. Invest., *2*:271, 1950.
3. Asboe-Hansen, G.: Proc. Soc. Exper. Biol. & Med., *80*:677, 1952.
4. Asboe-Hansen, G.: Cancer Res., *14*:94, 1954.
5. Asboe-Hansen, G. and Zachariae, L.: Acta path. & microbiol. scand., *37*:145, 1954.
6. Asboe-Hansen, G., Brodthagen, H. and Zachariae, L.: Arch. Dermat. & Syph., *73*:162, 1956.
7. Asboe-Hansen, G. and Wegelius, O.: Acta physiol. scand. *37*:350, 1956.
8. Asboe-Hansen, G. and Wegelius, O.: Nature, *178*:262, 1956.
9. Asboe-Hansen, G., Dyrbye, M. O., Moltke, E. and Wegelius, O.: J. Invest. Dermat., *32*:505, 1959.
10. Barber, M. and Delaunay, A.: Ann. Inst. Pasteur, *81*:193, 1951.
11. Boström, H. and Gardell, S.: Acta chem. scand., *7*:216, 1953.
12. Clark, I. and Umbreit, W. W.: Proc. Soc. Exper. Biol. & Med., *86*:558, 1954.
13. Clausen, B.: To be published.
14. Dorfman, A.: In Asboe-Hansen, G. (ed.): Connective Tissue in Health and Disease, Copenhagen, Munksgaard, 1954.
15. Gerarde, H. W. and Jones, M.: J. Biol. Chem., *201*:553, 1953.
16. Goth, A., Allman, B., Merrit, B. and Holman, J.: Proc. Soc. Exper. Biol. & Med., *78*:848, 1951.
17. Howes, E. L., Plotz, C. M., Blunt, J. W. and Ragan, C.: Surgery, *28*:177, 1950.
18. Kaufman, N., Mason, E. J. and Kinney, T. D.: Am. J. Path., *29*:769, 1953.
19. Layton, L. L.: Arch. Biochem., *32*:224, 1951.
20. Lorenzen, I.: Proc. Soc. Exper. Biol. & Med., *102*:440, 1959.
21. Moltke, E.: Acta endocrinol., *25*:179, 1957.
22. Paff, G. H. and Stewart, R.: Proc. Soc. Exper. Biol. & Med., *83*:591, 1953.
23. Ragan, C., Howes, E. L., Plotz, C. M., Meyer, K., Blunt, J. W. and Lattes, R.: Bull. N. Y. Acad. Med., *26*:251, 1950.
24. Scarpelli, D. G., Knouff, R. A. and Angerer, C. A.: Proc. Soc. Exper. Biol. & Med., *84*:94, 1953.
25. Sobel, H., Zutrauen, H. A. and Marmorston, J.: Arch. Biochem., *46*:221, 1953.
26. Wegelius, O. and Asboe-Hansen, G.: Exper. Cell Res., *11*:437, 1956.
27. Wegelius, O. and Asboe-Hansen, G.: Acta endocrinol., *22*:157, 1956.
28. Zachariae, L.: Local effect of hydrocortisone on connective tissue. (In Danish, with English summary.) Copenhagen, Coster, 1956.

Metabolic Changes During Inflammation and the Effect of Anti-Inflammatory Agents*

ALFRED JAY BOLLET

University of Virginia School of Medicine

Anti-inflammatory drugs are still the foundation of treatment of most of the rheumatic diseases. Although the general pharmacologic effects of these agents have been fairly well delineated, the basic mechanisms underlying such effects remain unknown. Knowledge of these mechanisms would be of considerable aid in the search for new and better therapeutic weapons. In general, pharmacologic agents act by inhibiting one or more metabolic processes; it is a reasonable assumption, therefore, that an inhibitory effect, probably at an enzyme level, underlies the basic action of anti-inflammatory drugs. Analysis of the metabolic effects of anti-inflammatory drugs should help to elucidate their mechanisms of action.

Fundamental to the study of the action of anti-inflammatory compounds is knowledge of the changes in tissue metabolism which bring about the inflammatory process. The object of this paper is to analyze present knowledge of the metabolic alterations which occur during inflammation, with special reference to changes in the connective tissue, the primary site of the inflammatory process. The known mechanisms of action responsible for the therapeutic and toxic effects of anti-inflammatory drugs used in the treatment of rheumatic diseases are also analyzed, in regard to general metabolic effects and effects on connective tissue.

METABOLIC ALTERATIONS DURING INFLAMMATION

In view of the multiplicity of biochemical alterations during inflammation, consideration of the mechanism of drug action requires a preliminary determination of the phenomena basic to the inflammatory process. Exudation, necrosis and proliferative changes all occur in inflammatory states; in addition, there are systemic changes including fever, leukocytosis and alterations of plasma proteins (acute phase phenomena). It seems logical to assume that the local proliferative changes and the acute phase phenomena are secondary to the existence of the inflammatory state. Necrosis produced by toxins, trauma or disease can induce an inflammatory response, but inflammation can occur without necrotizing injury. Substances released by necrotic cells in the inflammatory exudate, extensively studied by Menkin,[23] contribute to the course of events, but they appear after the inflammation is established.

The primary event in an inflammatory process would seem to be the increase in permeability of small vessels, resulting in exudation. Inflammation

* The work described in this paper was primarily supported by a grant from the U. S. Public Health Service (A-3421).

can be considered to begin as a change in the state of the connective tissue components which determine the physiological properties of the small blood vessels. This implies that, whatever the organ affected, it is alteration in the connective tissue of the blood vessels which is fundamental to the development of the inflammation, and that investigations of the alterations which occur during inflammation and of the mechanism of action of anti-inflammatory agents should include studies of connective tissue. Metabolic activity and levels of enzymes vary in different tissues[3, 4, 10] and it cannot be assumed that metabolic changes occurring in connective tissue can be inferred from studies made in other organs.

Increase in vascular permeability could result from alterations in the characteristics of the endothelial cells, in the size or distribution of the pores which apparently exist between these endothelial cells, in the properties of the cement substance between the cells, in the properties of the underlying basement membranes or in the tissues surrounding the basement membrane. Unfortunately, the chemical nature of the cement substance and the basement membrane are not fully delineated. Mucopolysaccharides, which contribute to the fundamental properties of connective tissue, are present in vessel walls and may play a role in the maintenance of normal permeability characteristics; knowledge of the chemistry and metabolism of these compounds is increasing at a rapid pace.[29] An additional possibility which has received very little consideration is that the normal permeability characteristics of vessel walls are determined by an active process requiring energy, in a fashion similar to the permeability characteristics of cell walls. Alterations in the metabolism of the cells comprising the vessel walls would then produce alterations in vascular permeability; drugs which influence the metabolic activities of these cells could thus influence vascular permeability.

Changes in Connective Tissue. Testicular hyaluronidase, which depolymerizes several mucopolysaccharides—namely, hyaluronic acid and chondroitin sulfates A and C—has been administered to animals in attempts to demonstrate that alterations in these compounds can produce exudation. The data in the literature are contradictory. Zweifach and Chambers report a lack of effect of intravenously injected hyaluronidase, although petechial hemorrhages were produced by local injection.[39] Elster, Freeman and Dorfman have reported evidence of a generalized increase in capillary permeability in rats following the intravenous injection of sufficiently large doses of hyaluronidase,[13] confirming earlier studies of the effects of hyaluronidase and spreading factor.[2, 12] As a result of these studies, the breakdown of the mucopolysaccharides of ground substance has been suggested to be a factor in the production of inflammation.[21] However, it has not been conclusively shown that hyaluronidase exists in mammalian tissues other than the testes; indeed, the nature of the enzymatic steps in the breakdown of mucopolysaccharides in connective tissue has not been elucidated. Several studies have revealed increases in the concentration of mucopolysaccharides in serum and increased excretion in the urine in many types of inflammation, suggesting alterations in the metabolism of these compounds.[6, 19]

METABOLIC ACTIONS OF ANTI-INFLAMMATORY AGENTS

The most commonly used antirheumatic, anti-inflammatory agents are the adrenal steroid hormones and related synthetic analogues, salicylates and a variety of chemically and pharmacologically similar compounds, and the phenylbutazone-antipyrine family of compounds. Consideration should also be given to the action of gold salts, which are effective in suppression of the inflammation seen in rheumatoid arthritis.[14, 15] Many analyses of the metabolic effects of salicylates have been done, and there have been a few studies of the basic actions of the steroid hormones; investigation of the mechanisms of action of the other anti-inflammatory agents has been notably lacking.

General Metabolic Effects

Steroid Hormones. The over-all metabolic effects of the steroid hormones are too well known to require review; attention will be given here only to studies of mechanisms of steroid action, including demonstration of inhibition of a respiratory pathway, changes in levels of transaminases, chelating effects and inhibition of mucopolysaccharide synthesis by connective tissue.

The report by Yielding and Tomkins[38] of the inhibition of diphosphopyridine nucleotide (DPNH) oxidation by mitochrondria and microsomes is of considerable interest. This effect was specific for DPNH, not involving oxidation of TPNH. The inhibition occurred between DPNH and cytochrome C, could be reversed by alpha tocopherol, was demonstrable in very low catalytic concentrations of steroid, but was not limited to the anti-inflammatory steroids. Jenson and Newhard[17] demonstrated that cortisol had a similar inhibitory effect on DPNH oxidation by fragmented heart sarcosomes, but 6-methyl prednisolone, which is also an anti-inflammatory compound, did not have this effect. In view of the fact that this inhibitory effect on the respiratory pathway is not specific for the anti-inflammatory steroids, it is unlikely that it is related to this action of these compounds.

Rosen and co-workers[30] have demonstrated that cortisol administration causes an increased activity of the glutamic-oxaloacetic and glutamic-pyruvic transaminases in the liver of rats, and Bollet and Shuster[4] have shown a similar effect on the glutamic-pyruvic transaminase of connective tissue. These changes might explain several of the metabolic effects of steroid administration, including gluconeogenesis, hepatic glycogen deposition, protein breakdown, and negative nitrogen balance. Cortisol does not effect the activity of these enzymes *in vitro,* indicating that these changes are secondary to actions elsewhere. The exact mechanism responsible for this alteration in transaminase activity and its relevance to suppression of inflammation are unknown at present.

Wiesel[37] demonstrated that gluconeogenic steroids can chelate potassium ions and are capable of binding copper; he noted that cortisone causes a redistribution of copper in the body, with an increased renal and urinary concentration and a decreased concentration in other tissues and in serum. In addition, he observed that salicylates are capable of chelation of copper and iron, and that a nonsteroid chelating agent, 8-hydroxyquinolone or oxine, is anti-inflammatory in rats. Wiesel suggested that the anti-inflammatory effect of the steroid compounds occurs because of the chelation of an essential metal activator of an undefined enzyme.[37]

Salicylates. Salicylates affect oxygen consumption, high energy phosphate bond formation, carbohydrate metabolism, protein metabolism, mucopolysaccharide synthesis, pituitary-adrenal functions, antigen-antibody interactions and metal-binding; *in vitro* effects on some enzymes have been demonstrated. The literature on salicylate effects has been summarized recently by Smith[32] and Done.[11]

Greatest attention has been given to the effects of salicylate on cellular respiration. Oxygen consumption increases when salicylate is given; this effect also occurs in tissue slices *in vitro,* indicating a direct peripheral effect on cellular respiration. Salicylates inhibit the synthesis of high-energy phosphate bonds during the oxidation of a variety of substrates. This uncoupling of oxidative phosphorylation is also produced by many other compounds, including dinitrophenol, thyroxin and tetracycline. The uncoupling effects of thyroxin and tetracycline are no longer noted when the membrane of the mitochrondria is removed with digitonin, whereas salicylates and dinitrophenol still uncouple the oxidative phosphorylation which occurs in the remaining mitochrondrial particles.[32] Phenylbutazone also can uncouple oxidative phosphorylation. However, several salicylate derivatives which are not anti-inflammatory have this effect,[1] whereas gentisic acid and resorcylic acid, which are anti-inflammatory, do not uncouple oxidative phosphorylation;[25] this, in addition to the inability to dissociate the mechanism of action of salicylate from that of dinitrophenol, an agent which has no anti-inflammatory effect, militates against an influence on oxidative phosphorylation being fundamental to the anti-inflammatory effect.

The block in oxidative phosphorylation and resulting impaired synthesis of ATP probably explain the increase in oxygen uptake which occurs in isolated tissues, intact animals and patients receiving salicylates. The increased glucose uptake by cells which is produced by salicylates is probably also on the basis of reduced ATP synthesis, since the maintenance of normal impermeability of cell walls is dependent upon an available supply of high-energy phosphate. The decreased blood and urine sugar levels which occur when salicylate is given to diabetic patients[28] and alloxanized, pancreatectomized or cortisone-treated animals[32] are probably the result of this altered membrane permeability. The inhibition of the incorporation of C^{14}-labelled acetate into glycogen and the rapid depletion in total liver glycogen which occur in rabbits, rats and mice given salicylates are presumably also secondary to the decrease in ATP synthesis.[33]

A negative nitrogen balance occurs in rats receiving 75 mg. of salicylate per 100 grams of body weight and is also reported to occur in rheumatic fever patients who have salicylate levels of 20 to 70 mg. per cent. Although an increased protein breakdown may occur in these patients, a decrease in protein synthesis is likely since salicylates *in vitro* cause a decrease in protein synthesis from C^{14}-labelled glycine, glutamate and lysine in rat diaphragm. This effect, too, is probably related to the lack of synthesis of the ATP needed for peptide-bond formation.[32]

Salicylates have been shown to have a stimulatory effect on the adrenal gland. Adrenal medullary output is increased, possibly accounting for some of the effect of salicylates on carbohydrate metabolism.[32] It has been suggested that the anti-inflammatory effect of salicylates is due to the stimulation of adrenal cortical secretion, but this has been contradicted by several studies,[26, 34, 36] including the observation that the anti-inflammatory effect of salicylate is demonstrable in adrenalectomized animals and in humans with greatly suppressed adrenal function.[26]

The metabolic effects which have been mentioned appear to be related to some pharmacologic and toxic effects of salicylates, but it is uncertain what relation they have to anti-inflammatory effects.[9] Much of the toxicity of salicylates is apparently due to uncoupling of oxidative phosphorylation, paralleling the effects of dinitrophenol, including hyperthermia, increased oxygen consumption, decreased respiratory quotient and decreased liver glycogen. Hyperpnea, induced by a central action of salicylates, accounts for the respiratory alkalosis which occurs in salicylate toxicity. Inhibition of fatty acid oxidation, a phenomenon which has been demonstrated *in vitro* and is secondary to the decreased generation of high-energy bond formation, probably explains the late metabolic acidosis which occurs in salicylate intoxication.[9] In view of the lack of correlation of an uncoupling action on oxidative phosphorylation with anti-inflammatory activity, it seems unlikely that this phenomenon is related to the mechanisms of the anti-inflammatory effect, although Smith[32] has suggested that the decreased ATP synthesis might produce an anti-inflammatory effect by altering the normal ATP-dependent impermeability of cell membranes to water and electrolytes.

Trethewie and Rumberg[35] demonstrated that salicylates inhibit the release of histamine from guinea pig lung tissues during anaphylactic shock, and that high salicylate concentrations inhibit antigen-antibody interaction *in vitro*. Salicylates also block the passive cutaneous anaphylaxis reaction *in vivo*.[20] The relationship of these effects on immune phenomena to the anti-inflammatory properties of salicylates remains unclear.

Other Agents. Although phenylbutazone is a widely used antirheumatic agent, studies of its metabolic effects are sparse; report of an uncoupling action on oxidative phosphorylation has been mentioned.[32] The mechanisms of the therapeutic and toxic effects of gold compounds are unknown, although speculation has centered about the likelihood of inhibition of enzymes by inactivation of sulfhydryl groups.

Effects on Connective Tissue Metabolism

Steroids. The adrenal steroid hormones are known to inhibit the proliferation of fibroblasts in tissue culture and in intact animals, as demonstrated by the inhibition of induced granuloma formation and wound healing.[16, 27] At a metabolic level, several investigators have demonstrated an inhibition of the incorporation of radioactive sulfate into the mucopolysaccharides of connective tissue under the influence of cortisone or cortisol *in vitro*[18] and *in vivo* in rats.[7] Shiller and Dorfman[31] demonstrated decreased incorporation of both $S^{35}O_4$ and C^{14}-acetate into the hyaluronate and chondroitin sulfate of the skin of rats given cortisone, indicating impairment of synthesis of the entire polysaccharide rather than simply prevention of incorporation of sulfate into previously synthesized polysaccharide molecules, as had been suggested by Bostrom and Odeblad.[7] Shiller and Dorfman[31] also showed that the rate of decay of radioactivity in the mucopolysaccharides of rat skin was somewhat decreased by the influence of steroids. Inhibition of mucopolysaccharide synthesis by steroids was also demonstrated by McCluskey and Thomas;[22] following depletion of cartilage matrix by papain, they found that restoration of normal rigidity and reaccumulation of the basophilic ground substance was largely prevented by cortisone, cortisol and prednisone. Recovery following the papain effect was prevented locally by intra-articular injection of these compounds without systemic effects, indicating that inhibition of chondroitin sulfate synthesis occurred by direct action on the cartilage. In our own laboratory, we have shown that cortisol does not inhibit the enzyme which synthesizes glucosamine-6-phosphate from fructose-6-phosphate and glutamine *in vitro,* although it does cause a decrease in the activity of this enzyme following intramuscular administration.[4]

Salicylates. A direct effect of salicylate on connective tissue was demonstrated by Bostrom and Manssom,[7] who showed an inhibition of S^{35} incorporation into cartilage slices *in vitro* by salicylate in a concentration of 55 mg. per cent. Aspirin and benzoic acid had very little effect, and a variety of related compounds with no anti-inflammatory properties had no influence. We have shown that salicylate can inhibit *in vitro* the enzyme which synthesizes glucosamine-6-phosphate, an initial step in mucopolysaccharide metabolism.[5] An effect on this enzyme could be the mechanism of the effect observed by Bostrom and Mansson. Aspirin had only a minimal effect on this enzyme, and a compound with no anti-inflammatory properties did not influence it. A lack of *in vitro* effect of aspirin might be related to the rapid deacetylation which is known to occur after absorption.

An influence of salicylate on the anti-hyaluronidase activity of serum has been studied extensively but the physiologic significance of this action is doubtful, particularly in view of the lack of evidence of participation of a hyaluronidase in mammalian mucopolysaccharide metabolism.[24]

Hershberger, Hanson and Ranney[16] demonstrated that phenylbutazone as well as cortisone can depress the incorporation of S^{35} into cotton-pellet granulomas in rats, indicating a similar effect of these two types of anti-inflammatory compounds on connective tissue metabolism. This is one of the few studies concerning the metabolic effects of phenylbutazone. We have found that phenylbutazone and related compounds apparently also inhibit the transamidase which synthesizes glucosamine-6-phosphate; this may account for the block in S^{35} incorporation into the granulomas.

Gold compounds can also inhibit the enzyme which synthesizes glucosamine-6-phosphate *in vitro* in homogenates of connective tissue.[4] Inhibitory concentrations were in the range of those found in the plasma of patients receiving therapeutic doses of gold. These concentrations of gold had no effect on the activity of the same enzyme in liver homogenates. Parenteral administration of gold sodium thiomalate to rats caused a decrease in the level of activity of the glucosamine-6-phosphate synthesizing enzyme in connective tissue but not in the liver.

CONCLUSION

Of the metabolic effects of the anti-inflammatory agents which have been studied, the one which seems to be the most consistent is an inhibition of mucopolysaccharide synthesis by connective tissue. In view of the location of the primary changes in an inflammatory reaction in the connective tissue of the vascular tree, the observed changes in mucopolysaccharide concentrations which occur in serum and urine as a result of inflammation, the key role of mucopolysaccharides in determining the functional properties of connective tissue, and the experimental production of increased vascular permeability by substances with hyaluronidase activity, the observation of an effect of these agents on mucopolysaccharide metabolism may be of physiologic significance.

It seems warranted to state that future work on the primary changes in inflammation should center on the vascular connective tissue, including the mucopolysaccharide components and that further study of the effects of therapeutic agents on the inflammatory process should include analysis of influences on mucopolysaccharide metabolism.

REFERENCES

1. Adams, S. S. and Cobb, R.: A possible basis for the anti-inflammatory activity of salicylates and other non-hormonal anti-rheumatic drugs. Nature, *181*:773, 1958.
2. Aylward, F. X.: Physiological properties of Reynals' testicular diffusion factor. Proc. Soc. Exper. Biol. & Med., *49*:342, 1942.
3. Bollet, A. J., Goodwin, J. and Brown, A. K.: Metabolism of mucopolysaccharides in connective tissue. I. Studies of enzymes involved in glucuronide metabolism. J. Clin. Invest., *38*:451, 1959.
4. Bollet, A. J. and Shuster, A.: Metabolism of mucopolysaccharides in connective tissue. II. Synthesis of glucosamine-6-phosphate. J. Clin. Invest., *39*:1114, 1960.
5. Bollet, A. J.: Effects of anti-rheumatic agents on connective tissue metabolism. Presented at Annual Meeting of the American Rheumatism Association, June 10, 1960.
6. Bollet, A. J.: Unpublished observations.
7. Bostrom, H. and Odeblad, E.: The influence of cortisone upon the sulphate exchange of chondroitin sulphuric acid. Arkiv. f. Kemi, *6*:39, 1953.
8. Bostrom, H. and Mansson, B.: The action of salicylate and related compounds on the sulphate exchange of chondroitin sulphuric acid. J. Pharm. & Pharmacol., *7*:185, 1955.
9. Brody, T. M.: Action of sodium salicylate and related compounds on tissue metabolism *in vitro*. J. Pharm. & Exper. Therap., *117*:39, 1956.
10. Bucher, T., Schmidt, E. and Schmidt, F. W.: Serum patterns of key-pathway enzymes. Ninth Middle East Medical Assembly, May 8-10, 1959.
11. Done, A. K.: The nature of the anti-rheumatic action of salicylates. Clin. Pharm. & Therap., *1*:141, 1960.
12. Duran-Reynals, F.: A general permeability-increasing effect of a factor from mammalian testicle on blood capillaries. Yale J. Biol. & Med., *11*:601, 1939.
13. Elster, S. K., Freeman, M. E. and Dorfman, A.: Hyaluronidase on the passage of fluid and of T-1824 through the capillary wall. Am. J. Physiol., *156*:429, 1949.
14. Empire Rheumatism Council: A multicenter controlled trial of gold salts in rheumatoid arthritis. Presented at Annual Meeting of the American Rheumatism Association, July 11, 1960, by Prof. E. G. L. Bywaters.
15. Freyberg, R. H.: Gold therapy for rheumatoid arthritis. In Hollander et al.: Arthritis. Philadelphia, Lea & Febiger, 1960.
16. Hershberger, L. J., Hansen, L. and Ranney, R. E.: Growth and S[35] uptake of cotton granulomas in rats. Proc. Soc. Exper. Biol. & Med., *101*:328, 1959.
17. Jensen, P. K. and Neuhard, J.: Steroid inhibition of the oxidation of reduced diphosphopyridine nucleotide by fragmented heart sarcosomes. Presented at First International Congress on Endocrinology, Copenhagen, July, 1960.
18. Layton, L. L.: Effect of cortisone upon chondroitin sulfate synthesis by animal tissues. Proc. Soc. Exper. Biol. & Med., *76*:596, 1951.
19. Loewi, G.: Urinary excretion of acid polysaccharide in rheumatoid arthritis and other diseases. Ann. Rheum. Dis., *18*:239, 1959.
20. Mark, V. and Smith, M. J. H.: Anti-inflammatory activity of salicylates. Nature, *187*: 611, 1960.
21. Mayer, R. L.: Hyaluronidase and inflammation of the skin. Ann. N. Y. Acad. Sc., *52*: 1041, 1950.
22. McCluskey, R. T. and Thomas, L.: The removal of cartilage matrix *in vivo* by papain: prevention of recovery with cortisone, hydrocortisone and prednisolone. Am. J. Path., *35*:819, 1959.
23. Menkin, V.: Biology of inflammation. Science, *123*:527, 1956.
24. Meyer, K.: The biological significance of hyaluronic acid and hyaluronidase. Physiol. Rev., *27*:335, 1947.
25. Packer, L., Austen, F. K. and Knoblock, E. C.: Effect of salicylates on respiration and phosphorylation in heart mitochondria. Proc. Soc. Exper. Biol. & Med., *100*: 239, 1959.
26. Peterson, R. E., Black, R. L. and Bunim, J. J.: Salicylates and adrenocortical function in man. Arth. & Rheum., *1*:29, 1958.
27. Ragan, C., Howes, E. L., Plotz, C. M., Meyer, K., Blunt, J. W. and Lettes, R.: Effect of ACTH and cortisone on connective tissue. Bull. N. Y. Acad. Med., *26*:251, 1950.

28. Reid, J. and Lightbody, T. D.: The insulin equivalence of salicylate. Brit. M. J., *1*: 897, 1959.
29. Roseman, S.: Mucopolysaccharide metabolism. Am. J. Med., *26*:749, 1959.
30. Rosen, F., Roberts, N. R. and Nichol, C. A.: Glucocorticosteroids and transaminase activity. I. Increased activity of glutamic-pyruvic transaminase in four conditions associated with gluconeogenesis. J. Biol. Chem., *234*:476, 1959.
31. Schiller, S. and Dorfman, A.: The metabolism of mucopolysaccharides in animals: the effect of cortisone and hydrocortisone on rat skin. Endocrinology, *60*:376, 1957.
32. Smith, M. J. H.: Review article: Salicylates and metabolism. J. Pharm. & Pharmacol., *11*:705, 1959.
33. Smith, M. J. H.: The effects of salicylate on the metabolism of acetate in the rat. J. Biol. Chem., *234*:144, 1959.
34. Thrift, C. and Traut, E. F.: Effect of salicylates on circulating eosinophils and urinary 17-ketosteroids in man. Ann. Rheum. Dis., *17*:108, 1958.
35. Trethewie, E. R. and Rumberg, C.: The effect of salicylate on the *in vitro* antigen-antibody reaction in anaphylaxis. Australian J. Exper. Biol. & M. Sc., *37*:77, 1959.
36. Ulloa, A., Gautney, M. C., Holley, H. L. and Hill, S. R., Jr.: Therapeutic doses of salicylates; effect on adrenal cortical secretory activity in normal subjects. A.M.A. Arch. Int. Med., *105*:914, 1960.
37. Wiesel, L.: Metal chelation in the mechanism of action of glucogenic corticosteroids. Metabolism, *8*:256, 1959.
38. Yielding, K. L. and Tomkins, G. M.: Inhibitors of the enzymic oxidation of DPNH by steroid hormones. Proc. Nat. Acad. Sc., *45*:1730, 1959.
39. Zweifach, B. W. and Chambers, R.: The action of hyaluronidase extracts on the capillary wall. Ann. N. Y. Acad. Sc., *52*:943, 1950.

Inhibition of Antibody Production by Cortisone

EDWARD E. FISCHEL

The Bronx Hospital, New York City

More than a decade has passed since attention was focused on the effects of cortisone on the inflammatory reaction in rheumatic and other diseases by Hench and his colleagues. An anti-inflammatory action of a hormone had not been clearly anticipated in the great bulk of endocrinologic work previously done. Although an extensive literature existed on the relationships of various hormones to antibody production and immunity, considerable perspective has been gained, in part by a consideration of the anti-inflammatory activity of corticosteroids. Several articles have served to review this subject,[4, 6, 13, 20, 25] and the papers in this volume constitute an additional review. I should like to consider some previous studies on antibody production which may contribute to understanding of the probable interrelationships of protein metabolism and the inflammatory process.

It has been well demonstrated that administration of cortisone or adrenocorticotropin during immunization will be followed by a diminished amount of circulating antibody. This effect was shown for the primary antibody response to egg albumen by Germuth.[14, 15] Our own experience in this

* Supported in part by grant H-2144 from the National Heart Institute, by the Helen Hay Whitney Foundation and by the New York State Chapter, Arthritis and Rheumatism Foundation.

TABLE 1.   PER CENT OF CONTROL ANTIBODY PRODUCED IN RABBITS
TREATED WITH ACTH OR CORTISONE DURING THE
PRIMARY RESPONSE

	9TH DAY	14TH DAY	28TH DAY
ACTH 1.5 to 3.0 mg.		52%	43%
Cortisone 2.5 mg.		61%	
Cortisone 10.0 mg.	44%	37%	

100% represents the mean antibody nitrogen of the respective control groups immunized simultaneously with each of the test groups.
(Data from J. Exper. Med., 93:37, 1951.)

regard, with Bjørneboe and Stoerk,[1] was first accomplished with a particulate antigen, multivalent, killed pneumococcal vaccine. In both studies, antibody was measured by the quantitative agglutination method of Heidelberger and Kabat (cf. 18). Table 1 illustrates the mean per cent of inhibition achieved in our work with differing dosages during the course of the primary response. Parenthetically, it should be emphasized that these percentile differences are being used merely for illustrative purposes. The true data, as published, showed a considerable degree of variation within groups and some overlap between groups. Since great variation occurs when antibody protein nitrogen is determined, it is difficult to accept data with still greater variation introduced by geometric dilution methods, or methods employing multiple undefined antigens or pooled sera for antibody titration.

While antibody was significantly diminished in the corticoid treated groups, particularly with the larger dose of cortisone, there were still appreciable amounts of antibody produced in these groups, probably enough antibody to contribute to the development of serious hypersensitivity reactions if cortisone was not biologically effective in other ways.

To determine whether cortisone would have an effect on the amount of circulating antibody after immunization had been well established, rabbits were immunized for two weeks and then divided into comparable groups. Some groups received cortisone; others did not. Immunization with polyvalent pneumococcal vaccine was continued. Table 2 summarizes briefly

TABLE 2.   SUMMARY OF CHANGES IN AMOUNTS OF ANTIBODY PROTEIN
WHEN CORTISONE IS ADMINISTERED AFTER IMMUNIZATION
IS WELL ESTABLISHED

2 WEEKS	SUBSEQUENT TREATMENT	3 WEEKS	4 WEEKS
100%	No cortisone	141%	237%
100%	Cortisone 5 and 2.5 mg. daily	79%	36%

Per cent of mean AbN/ml at 2 weeks in groups of animals bled at the times indicated.

the magnitude of changes in the mean concentration of antibody protein one and two weeks after instituting cortisone therapy.[1] Again the administration of cortisone was accompanied by a marked diminution in the level of circulating antibody.

It could not be determined from these experiments whether cortisone was causing an accelerated catabolism of antibody protein or, on the other hand, an inhibition of its formation. To test the former possibility, passive immunization was employed. Antibody protein was administered intravenously to four rabbits[10] two of which received 10 mg. of cortisone daily

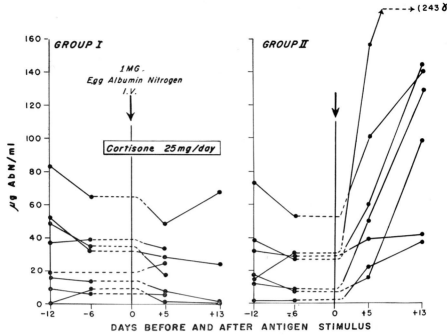

Fig. 1.   The effect of cortisone on antibody levels of rabbits before and after the induction of a secondary response.

beginning three days prior to the intravenous injection. Therefore, there was no mechanism present for anabolism or synthesis of antibody in these rabbits. Antibody protein is unusual in that it carries its own label or marker. The disappearance rate of the protein from the serum could be traced by determining the concentration of specifically reacting protein remaining in the blood stream. The disappearance curves of antipneumococcal antibody in the cortisone-treated animals were similar to the curves of the untreated animals, indicating that no increased catabolism of antibody protein occurred. An independent experiment of a similar nature, employing antibody to egg albumen, was reported by Germuth et al.[15]

Since it did not appear likely that the effect of cortisone during active immunization was related to accelerated catabolism of antibody protein, a system was employed in which the rate of breakdown of antibody was minimal and the rate of synthesis was maximal. This occurs during the elicitation of the secondary response or specific anamnestic reaction. Rabbits were immunized with crystalline egg albumen and, after two months, achieved relatively stable amounts of circulating antibody (Fig. 1). Then, after cortisone therapy was begun in one group, a booster injection of crystalline egg albumen was given to both groups. It is readily evident that the control group responded with the characteristic secondary response, a remarkable increase in specific antibody protein evident on the fifth day and more striking on the thirteenth day. The cortisone-treated animals did not show the same response. The synthesis of antibody protein appeared to be distinctly inhibited.[11]

This sequence of studies was done at a time when work by several investigators with other protein synthesizing systems indicated that cortisone inhibited the incorporation of labelled amino acids into tissue protein.[22] Under most circumstances, it appears that cortisone has a distinct anti-anabolic effect on proteins, generally inhibiting the synthesis of protein. In the case of antibody protein, a specialized instance of protein synthesis, the same effect is suggested by the experiments cited.

It is pertinent, then, to ask whether the action on protein metabolism might be related to the well documented anti-inflammatory activity of cortisone. Inflammation is generally a clinical or morphological term. That which we call inflammation probably results from several biochemical and physiological processes. In a sense, antibody production may be thought of as a chemical result of an inflammatory reaction to a foreign substance. Depending on its primary irritant or toxic qualities, an antigen may give rise to a grossly visible inflammatory reaction. Less visible processes occur during inflammation, as shown by the appearance of acute phase substances in serum. After the injection of a relatively bland foreign protein, crystalline egg albumen, the more classic manifestations of inflammation may be absent, but we have found that one of the acute phase reactants, an elevation of serum complement, may be striking.[7] This suggests that a chemical manifestation of inflammation does occur shortly after antigens are injected.

The more classic manifestations of inflammation resulting in gross cellular proliferation are readily observed during the course of immunization with adjuvants. Certain substances such as alum, killed tubercle bacilli and various vehicles and irritants act as adjuvants to enhance antibody production. This property is related, in large part, to the ability of the adjuvant to elicit a particular cellular reaction of a granulomatous type.[8, 12, 24] In work on acute disseminated encephalomyelitis in monkeys, Kabat, Wolf and Bezer[19] demonstrated that suppression by cortisone of the experimental disease was associated with a suppression of the granulomatous response at the site of antigen-adjuvant emulsion. In order to determine whether this latter effect could be related to the degree of inhibition of antibody, guinea pigs were inoculated with crystalline egg albumen emulsified with Freund's adjuvant and killed tubercle bacilli.[9] Cortisone, in doses of 5 or 25 mg. daily, was given to two groups of animals and a third group served as untreated controls. Figure 2 illustrates the differences found in the three groups. A wide

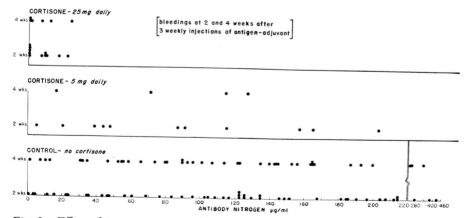

Fig. 2. Effect of cortisone on amount of anti-egg albumen nitrogen in guinea pigs immunized with crystalline egg albumen in Freund adjuvants.

range of antibody concentration occurred in the control group and in the group treated with 5 mg. of cortisone. These groups also had the characteristic granulomatous lesions at the sites of antigen-adjuvant injection and in regional lymph nodes and lungs. The group of guinea pigs treated with 25 mg. of cortisone had a marked suppression of antibody and there was little gross reaction at the site of antigen-adjuvant inoculation. In systemic immunization, the germinal centers of the spleen and lymph nodes are reactive centers which proliferate when exposed to antigen.[17] Corticosteroid inhibits this reaction[1] and causes atrophy of lymphoid tissue.[4] This may also be regarded as a kind of anti-inflammatory action of cortisone which results in inhibition of antibody synthesis.

The relationship of inflammation and antibody production is also seen in Ward and Johnson's work demonstrating the adjuvant action of endotoxin on antibody formation.[29] This action is potent enough under certain circumstances to counteract the inhibitory effect of cortisone administration.[29]

Other effects of cortisone are also of interest in antibody synthesis. There have been several studies indicating that the metabolism of some antigens is interrupted by cortisone,[5, 21] and we have expressed this as a failure of assimilation of antigen into the body economy,[11] recognizing that simple phagocytosis may not be affected appreciably. This block may result from the lack of functioning of the antibody mechanism. In this respect the studies of Dougherty and Hayes (cf. 4), McMaster and Edwards[23] and Ward and Johnson[29] are of interest. These investigators demonstrated that the inhibition to antibody synthesis is readily reversed when cortisone is discontinued, with an apparently augmented response to residual antigen. In some respects this is reminiscent of the rebound of inflammatory activity that occurs in certain chronic diseases when cortisone is discontinued.

There are other avenues of investigation which also suggest interrelationships of protein metabolism and inflammation in the production of antibody. It is striking, for example, that somatotrophic hormone, an anabolic hormone with an action biologically antagonistic to cortisone, appears to augment an inflammatory reaction[26] and probably augments antibody production also, as measured by hemagglutination titers.[16]

Among the agents which appear to have antibody suppressing effects similar to those of cortisone, a pyridoxine analog (resulting in acute pyridoxine deficiency)[27] and x-ray[3, 28] are notable. X-ray shares other actions with cortisone which are worth considering. Both x-ray and cortisone result in a reduction of lymphoid tissue and, curiously and perhaps coincidentally, both may lead to the production of capsular opacities in the lens.[2]

The role of cortisone in antibody production should also be considered at other levels of biologic integration, from cell culture and tissue transplantation studies to studies of human antibody production with their associated difficulties of dosage, timing, type of antibody system employed and method of assessment of effects. These have been considered critically by various authors and in the reviews previously cited.

In summary, it is apparent that the inhibition of antibody production by cortisone may be related on the biochemical level to its anti-anabolic action on protein metabolism and, on the cellular level, to its inhibition of inflammatory response. It is tempting to suggest that these are, indeed, closely related activities, protein synthesis probably being a requisite for the accumulation and multiplication of inflammatory cells, and certain of these cells, in turn, being required for antibody protein synthesis.

REFERENCES

1. Bjørneboe, M., Fischel, E. E. and Stoerk, H. C.: J. Exper. Med., *93*:37, 1951.
2. Black, R. L., Oglesby, R. B., von Sallmann, L. and Bunim, J. J.: Proceedings, Annual Meeting American Rheumatism Association, Hollywood-by-the-Sea, Florida, June, 1960.
3. Dixon, F. J., Roberts, J. C. and Weigle, W. D.: J. Exper. Med., *105*:417, 1957.
4. Dougherty, T. F.: Progr. Allergy, *4*:319, 1954.
5. Fagraeus, A. and Berglund, K.: Acta path. et microbiol. scandinav., Supp. 13, 20, 1952.
6. Fischel, E. E.: In Shwartzman, G. (ed.): The Effect of ACTH and Cortisone on Infection and Resistance. New York, Columbia University Press, 1953.
7. Fischel, E. E.: Unpublished.
8. Fischel, E. E., Kabat, E. A., Stoerk, H. C. and Bezer, A. E.: J. Immunol., *69*:611, 1952.
9. Fischel, E. E., Kabat, E. A., Stoerk, H. C., Skolnick, M. and Bezer, A. E.: J. Allergy, *25*:195, 1954.
10. Fischel, E. E., Stoerk, H. C. and Bjørneboe, M.: Proc. Soc. Exper. Biol. & Med., *77*:111, 1951.
11. Fischel, E. E., Vaughan, J. H. and Photopoulos, C.: Proc. Soc. Exper. Biol. & Med., *81*:344, 1952.
12. Freund, J.: Ann. Rev. Microbiol., *1*:291, 1947.
13. Germuth, F. G., Jr.: Pharmacol. Rev., 8:1, 1956.
14. Germuth, F. G., Jr. and Ottinger, B.: Proc. Soc. Exper. Biol. & Med., *74*:815, 1950.
15. Germuth, F. G., Jr., Oyama, J. and Ottinger, B.: J. Exper. Med., *94*:193, 1951.
16. Hayashida, T. and Li, C. H.: J. Exper. Med., *105*:93, 1957.
17. Hellman, T.: In Moellendorf, W. (ed.): Handbuch der mikrskopischen Anatomie des Menchen. Berlin, Julius Springer, 6:233, 1930.
18. Kabat, E. A.: Kabat and Mayer's Experimental Immunochemistry. 2nd ed. Springfield, Ill., Charles C Thomas, 1961.
19. Kabat, E. A., Wolf, A. and Bezer, A. E.: J. Immunol., *68*:265, 1952.
20. Kass, E. H. and Finland, M.: Ann. Rev. Microbiol., 7:361, 1953.
21. Kass, E. H. and Kendrick, M. I.: Fed. Proc., *11*:472, 1952.
22. Marshall, L. M. and Friedberg, F.: Endocrinol., *48*:113, 1951.
23. McMaster, P. D. and Edwards, J. L.: Proc. Nat. Acad. Sc., *43*:380, 1957.
24. Ramon, G.: Rev. Immunol., *4*:5, 1938.
25. Rose, B.: In Shaffer, J. H., LoGrippo, G. A. and Chase, M. W. (eds.): Mechanisms of Hypersensitivity. Boston, Little, Brown and Co., 1959.
26. Selye, H.: J. Endocrinol., *10*:347, 1954.
27. Stoerk, H. C., Eisen, H. N. and John, H. M.: J. Exper. Med., *85*:365, 1947.
28. Taliaferro, W. H.: Ann. N. Y. Acad. Sc., *69*:745, 1957.
29. Ward, P. A. and Johnson, A. G.: J. Immunol., *82*:428, 1959.

Effect of Adrenocorticosteroids on Various Types of Antigen-Antibody Reactions[*]

EDWARD E. FISCHEL

The Bronx Hospital, New York City

Allergic reactions are complex phenomena made up of a number of pathogenetic mechanisms. It may be anticipated, therefore, that the effect of corticosteroids on allergic reactions will depend on their effect on these mechanisms. The common denominator of allergic reactions is the union of antigen with antibody. In many instances, such as the tuberculin reaction, the evidence for the presence of antibody is only presumptive or indirectly demonstrable as an acquired and uniquely specific reactivity of tissues with the antigen.

Antigen-antibody interaction in the test tube is a precisely definable, specific physicochemical reaction.[21, 24, 29] The effect, or lack of it, of corticosteroids on allergic reactions in tissues appears to be unrelated to an effect of the hormones on the actual combination of antigen with antibody. This was well demonstrated by Malkiel and Hargis,[34] who showed no deviation of quantitative precipitin curves when antibody was derived from animals treated with ACTH or cortisone, despite the diminution of antibody production that occurred with hormone therapy. As discussed previously,[12] the administration of corticosteroids during active immunization diminishes the amount of antibody produced. Since the induction of allergic reactions depends in large part on the amount of antibody present (cf. 24) it might be anticipated that corticosteroids, when administered to actively sensitized animals during immunization, would tend to diminish the severity of most allergic reactions by reducing the amount of antibody available. This would occur particularly if relatively large amounts of antibody are needed for reaction, as in the active Arthus phenomenon. Germuth's studies have amply demonstrated this.[15, 17]

In order to obviate the effect of steroids on antibody production and to study the effect of steroids on allergic reactions per se, it is necessary to study the reactions in animals to which a known quantity of antibody is administered, i.e., passive sensitization. Amounts of antibody are used which give predictable and reproducible reactions in control animals when these are challenged with antigen. Appropriate time intervals and criteria of reactivity have been developed, and biological models of allergic reactions are available for study. Two prototypes of allergic reactions have been standardized in this way—anaphylaxis, both generalized[2, 25] and local,[39] and the Arthus reaction.[3, 13]

In anaphylaxis, the predominant reaction appears to be related to the "fixation" of antibody to strategic tissue.[1] After the injection of specific antigen, there is a release of histamine, a contraction of smooth muscle and

* Supported in part by grant H-2144 from the National Heart Institute, by the Helen Hay Whitney Foundation and by the New York State Chapter, Arthritis and Rheumatism Foundation.

478

increased permeability of the local vascular bed. Corticosteroids appear to have little effect on the release of histamine from sensitized cells,[45] unless it may be to augment its release.[36] Once released, the regeneration of histamine by tissue may be inhibited,[19] but the reactivity of smooth muscle to histamine is not affected. Therefore, the lack of dramatic effect of ACTH or cortisone on systemic anaphylaxis in the guinea pig may be readily comprehended.[7, 18, 20, 30, 33] Our own experience with this system is seen in Table 1.[11] With increased amounts of antibody and varying latent periods

TABLE 1. LACK OF EFFECT OF ADRENAL CORTICAL HORMONES ON ANAPHYLAXIS INDUCED IN GUINEA PIGS BY PASSIVE SENSITIZATION

SENSITIZING DOSE OF ANTIBODY NITROGEN—I.V.	LATENT PERIOD AND SHOCKING DOSE—I.V.	TREATED GROUP		UNTREATED GROUP
		Hormone Given before Shock	*Severity of Shock*	*Severity of Shock*
240 µg.	1 hr. 0.16 mg. Ea N.	2 mg. ACTH 8 hrs. before	+ + + + + + + + + +	+ + + + + + + + + + + + + +
30 µg.	48 hrs. 0.16 mg. Ea N.	2 mg. ACTH q 6 h for 2 days	+ + + + + + + + + + + + + + + + + +	+ + + + + + + + + + +
32 µg.	48 hrs. 0.06 mg. Ea N. (gp. 300–400 Gm.)	cortisone 2.5 mg. I.M. for 3 days	+ + + + + + + + + + + + +	+ + + + + + + + + + +
25 µg.	48 hrs. 0.16 mg. Ea N.	cortisone 25 mg. I.M. for 4 days	+ + + + + + + + + + + + + + + + + + + + + +	+ + + + + + + + + + + + + + + + + +
12.5 µg.	48 hrs. 0.16 mg. Ea N.	cortisone 25 mg. I.M. for 4 days	+ + + + + + + + + + + +	+ + + + + + + + + + + + + + + + + + + + + + +

before shock there is no real difference in the severity of anaphylaxis in guinea pigs treated with ACTH or cortisone and those untreated, except perhaps at the lowest level of antibody used for sensitization. In a comparable study by Humphrey,[23] lesser doses of cortisone (5 mg./kg. contrasted to our level of 25 mg. per 250 gram guinea pig) diminished the severity of shock in six animals who had received about twice the amount of antibody for sensitization (0.16 mg. AbN/kg.). The weights of the guinea pigs are not indicated, although this has a rather important bearing on the response to anaphylactic shock as produced by the method of Kabat and Landow.[25]

Local passive cutaneous anaphylaxis in the guinea pig is not appreciably affected by corticosteroids,[39] and this system appears to depend more on vascular permeability than does systemic anaphylaxis. Passive cutaneous anaphylaxis is an exquisitely sensitive reaction, induced with very small amounts of antibody. While the reaction may be inhibited by antihistaminic agents, it is not appreciably affected by cortisone.

In the mouse, a different result has been observed by several investigators. Anaphylaxis is inhibited by cortisone,[9, 35, 44] although passive sensitization has not been employed and the factor of inhibited antibody synthesis is not entirely excluded.

The inhibition of mouse anaphylaxis by cortisone may be related to the active immunization or to species differences which concern the more complex mechanism of anaphylaxis in the mouse. This phenomenon has been well explored by Dougherty.[9] The reaction is slower and perhaps more dependent on vascular permeability, cellular aggregation and other mechanisms which are known to be modified by corticosteroids in nonallergic inflammatory reactions. It is noteworthy that antihistaminic agents are not as effective in mouse anaphylaxis as in guinea pig anaphylaxis (cf. 44).

Another classic example of tissue damage resulting from the combination of antigen and antibody in tissues is the Arthus reaction. Reduced to its basic components, it appears that the passive Arthus reaction is simply a reaction to the formation of antigen-antibody complexes *in vivo*[8, 16] or even *in vitro*, as the classic studies of Opie[37] demonstrated in 1924. The antigen-antibody complex may act as finely dispersed foreign bodies, but perhaps it also involves complement and the chemical toxicity associated with it as shown for anaphylaxis.[38] Unlike anaphylaxis, the development of the Arthus reaction does not appear to require the fixation of antibody to tissue.[1] The severity of the reaction is directly related to the amount of antibody available for reaction.[13] When amounts of antibody are employed which result in minimal reactions, or more severe ones, the administration of cortisone does not appear to alter the severity of the passive Arthus reaction.[10] Although the edema is inhibited,[23] the late necrotizing effect is unchanged. Witorsch, Kahn and Kibel, recently working in our laboratory, had occasion to repeat this type of study with large doses of hydrocortisone, 25 mg. per day per rabbit, and were unable to note any consistent change in the Arthus reaction. This was so when, after sensitization of the skin with antibody, the challenge injection of antigen was administered either locally into the same site or intravenously (reversed passive Arthus reaction).

In Germuth's study, passively induced Arthus reactions were similarly unaffected.[17] As previously stated, the actively induced Arthus reaction was diminished, and this could be attributed to the diminution of antibody levels in the cortisone-treated animals. Examples and variants of anaphylaxis and Arthus reactions are encountered in various clinical and experimental conditions. It is curious that in hay fever, although the symptomatic response to cortisone may be dramatic, the elicitation of positive skin tests by ragweed antigen is unaltered, even during the period of maximal clinical improvement or if passive transfer is performed.[31, 32, 48] Serum sickness, experimental and clinical, and nephrotoxic nephritis may be viewed as systemic extensions of the Arthus reaction. In the latter instance, in which nephrotoxic nephritis is induced "passively" by the administration of antibody, no change has been noted with cortisone.[27, 42] The effect of corticosteroids on many of the various models of allergic reactions, both active and passive, have been reviewed by Dougherty,[9] Germuth[15] and others.[11, 40]

A third prototype of allergic reactivity can only be mentioned at the present time. The tuberculin reaction is an intriguing kind of allergic reaction which is difficult to study quantitatively. In most instances cortisone appears to inhibit the tuberculin reaction,[6, 14, 20, 46] although it rarely suppresses it entirely. In passive transfer studies of tuberculin sensitivity, Cummings and

Hudgins[5] reported that cortisone had no effect on this type of sensitivity when the donor animals were treated, but appeared to diminish the severity of the reaction when recipient animals were treated. In another study of passively transferred delayed hypersensitivity, using 2,4, dinitrochlorobenzene as the antigenic determinant, Seebohm, Tremaine and Jeter[41] demonstrated no inhibition of sensitivity if either the donor or the recipient guinea pig received ACTH or cortisone.

In carefully controlled cell culture studies, Holden, Seegal and Adams[22] observed that the specific toxic effect of tuberculin on tissues from tuberculin-sensitive animals was not modified by cortisone.

The phenomenon of delayed hypersensitivity or cell-fixed sensitivity is operative in the homotransplant reaction. Cortisone does depress inherited and acquired resistance to tumor grafting[47] and skin homografts.[4, 28] In another type of hypersensitivity reaction that is probably of the tuberculin type, experimental disseminated encephalomyelitis in monkeys, cortisone given prior to the injection of brain-adjuvant emulsions protected monkeys from developing the disease.[26] Cortisone may have been operative by preventing the formation of granuloma at the injection site.[26] As noted previously,[12] cortisone affected the development of circulating antibody in this type of experiment.

In this discussion we have been chiefly concerned with the effect of large amounts of corticosteroids in intact animals. This is somewhat analogous to the use of corticosteroids clinically in various diseases unassociated with true adrenal insufficiency. It has been well demonstrated that the adrenalectomized animal, like the patient with Addison's disease, is highly susceptible to many noxious agents and can be readily thrown into cardiovascular collapse with associated salt and water imbalance. In such instances, relatively small amounts of corticosteroids will restore a great degree of normal physiological reactivity to the organism. Such doses of corticosteroids may be termed "physiological" in contrast to the larger "pharmacological" doses which are of interest clinically for their anti-inflammatory activity.

While corticosteroids in larger or pharmacological doses may affect some allergic reactions in animals as well as in man, it is unfortunate that the corollary has been accepted by some clinicians, namely, that the response of an obscure inflammatory process to corticosteroid administration indicates that it may be of allergic origin. The lack of logic here is readily apparent. Aside from the combination of antigen with antibody, there is no aspect of the allergic reaction that does not occur with other causes of inflammation or tissue damage, whether due to infection, or to chemical or physical trauma. The anti-inflammatory effect of cortisone has been well demonstrated at several levels of integration, and it appears to be superfluous to introduce a specific anti-allergic effect above and beyond the known anti-anabolic, anti-inflammatory effects that have been well presented by others.

REFERENCES

1. Benacerraf, B.: Atti del VI Congresso Int. Microbiol. Roma, 2:85, 1953.
2. Benacerraf, B. and Kabat, E. A.: J. Immunol., 62:517, 1949.
3. Benacerraf, B. and Kabat, E. A.: J. Immunol., 64:1, 1950.
4. Billingham, R. E., Krohn, P. L. and Medawar, P. B.: Brit. M. J., 1:1157, 1163, 1951.
5. Cummings, M. M. and Hudgins, P. C.: J. Immunol., 69:331, 1952.
6. Derbes, V. J., Dent, J. H., Weaver, N. K. and Vaughan, D.D.: Proc. Soc. Exper. Biol. & Med., 75:423, 1950.
7. Dews, P. B. and Code, C. F.: J. Immunol., 70:199, 1953.

8. Dixon, F. J., Vazquez, J. J., Weigle, W. O. and Cochrane, C. G.: Arch. Path., 65:18, 1958.
9. Dougherty, T. F.: Progr. Allergy, 4:319-360, 1954.
10. Fischel, E. E.: Bull. N. Y. Acad. Med., 26:255, 1950.
11. Fischel, E. E.: In Shwartzman, G. (ed.): Symposium: The Effect of ACTH and Cortisone upon Infection and Resistance. New York, Columbia University Press, 1953, ch. 6.
12. Fischel, E. E.: Inhibition of antibody production by cortisone. In Mills, L. C. and Moyer, J. H. (eds.): Inflammation and Diseases of Connective Tissues. Philadelphia, W. B. Saunders Co., 1961, p. 472.
13. Fischel, E. E. and Kabat, E. A.: J. Immunol., 55:337, 1947.
14. Gell, P. G. H. and Hinde, I. I.: Brit. J. Exper. Path., 32:516, 1951.
15. Germuth, F. G., Jr.: Pharmacol. Rev., 8:1, 1956.
16. Germuth, F. G., Jr., Maumenee, A. E., Pratt-Johnson, J. A., Senterfit, L. B., Van Arnam, C. E. and Pollack, A. D.: In Shaffer, J H., et al.: Mechanisms of Hypersensitivity (reference 43).
17. Germuth, F. G., Jr., Oyama, J. and Ottinger, B.: J. Exper. Med., 94:139, 1951.
18. Germuth, F. G., Jr., Ottinger, B. and Oyama, J.: Proc. Soc. Exper. Biol. & Med., 80:188, 1952.
19. Halpern, B. W., Biozzi, G., Briot, M. and Benacerraf, B.: Compt. rend. Soc. de biol., 147:1180, 1953.
20. Harris, S. and Harris, T. N.: Proc. Soc. Exper. Biol. & Med., 74:186, 1950.
21. Heidelberger, M.: Lectures in Immunochemistry. New York, Academic Press, 1956.
22. Holden, M., Seegal, B. C. and Adams, L. B.: J. Exper. Med., 98:551, 1953.
23. Humphrey, J. H., Brit. J. Exper. Path., 32:274, 1951.
24. Kabat, E. A.: Kabat and Mayer's Experimental Immunochemistry. 2nd ed. Springfield, Ill., Charles C Thomas, 1961.
25. Kabat, E. A. and Landow, H.: J. Immunol., 44:69, 1942
26. Kabat, E. A., Wolf, A. and Bezer, A. E.: J. Immunol., 68:265, 1952.
27. Knowlton, A. I., Loeb, E. N., Stoerk, H. C. and Seegal, B. C.: Proc. Soc. Exper. Biol. & Med., 72:722, 1949.
28. Krohn, P. L.: Brit. J. Exper. Path., 35:539, 1954.
29. Landsteiner, K.: The Specificity of Serological Reactions. Cambridge, Mass., Harvard University Press, 1946.
30. Leger, J., Leith, W. and Rose, B.: Proc. Soc. Exper. Biol. & Med., 69:465, 1948.
31. Leith, W., Graham, M. J. and Burrage, W. S.: J. Allergy, 22:99, 1951.
32. Loveless, M. H.: Bull. New York Acad. Med., 27:495, 1951.
33. Malkiel, S.: J. Immunol., 66:379, 1951.
34. Malkiel, S. and Hargis, B. J.: J. Immunol., 69:217, 1952.
35. Nelson, C. T., Fox, C. L., Jr. and Freeman, E. B.: Proc. Soc. Exper. Biol. & Med., 75:181, 1950.
36. Noah, J. W. and Brand, A.: The effect of corticosteroids upon in vitro blood histamine release. In Shaffer, J. H. et al.: Mechanisms of Hypersensitivity (reference 43).
37. Opie, E. L.: J. Immunol., 9:259, 1924.
38. Osler, A. G., Randall, H. G., Hill, B. M. and Ovary, Z.: Some relationships between complement, passive cutaneous anaphylaxis and anaphylatoxin. In Shaffer, et al.: Mechanisms of Hypersensitivity (reference 43).
39. Ovary, Z.: Progr. Allergy, 5:459, 1958.
40. Rose, B.: Hormones and allergic responses. In Shaffer, J. H. et al.: Mechanisms of Hypersensitivity (reference 43).
41. Seebohm, P. M., Tremaine, M. M. and Jeter, W. S.: J. Immunol., 73:44, 1954.
42. Seegal, B. C. and Hasson, M. W.: Fed. Proc., 13:443, 1954.
43. Shaffer, J. H., LoGrippo, G. A. and Chase, M. W.: Mechanisms of Hypersensitivity. Boston, Little, Brown and Co., 1959.
44. Solotorovsky, M. and Winsten, S.: J. Immunol., 72:177, 1954.
45. Spain, W. C., Fontana, V. J. and Strauss, M. B.: J. Allergy, 23:242, 1952.
46. Stoerk, H. C.: Fed. Proc., 10:352, 1951.
47. Stoerk, H. C.: Depression by cortisone of inherited and acquired resistance to infection and to tumor grafting. In Shwartzman, G. (ed.): Symposium: The Effect of ACTH and Cortisone upon Infection and Resistance. New York, Columbia University Press, 1953, pp. 72-83.
48. Stollerman, G. H., Rubin, S. J. and Plotz, C. M.: Proc. Soc. Exper. Biol. & Med., 76:261, 1951.

Panel Discussion

DAVID M. SPAIN, *Moderator*

DR. SPAIN: I want to start the discussion by asking a few questions on some subjects about which the speakers have an apparent difference of opinion. Dr. Dougherty referred to the fibroblast as one of the target points and one of the key factors with respect to the inhibition of the inflammatory response by steroids, and Dr. Asboe-Hansen referred to the mast cell as one of the key factors. I had great difficulty in making up my mind from looking at the slides whether some of the cells were fibroblasts or degranulated mast cells. Dr. Rebuck, would you comment on this first? Then we will hear from the various authors later.

DR. REBUCK: From the material that we saw, I think the cells were tissue mast cells in Dr. Asboe-Hansen's slides and fibroblasts in Dr. Dougherty's slides.

DR. DOUGHERTY: I do not think there is any real difference of opinion as far as site of action of cortisol is concerned; there is no real evidence that cortisol has very much inhibitory effect on mast cells, and there is no reason to assume that mast cells are present in large numbers in all areas in which inflammation occurs; they may or they may not be. However, it is a fact that over 90 per cent of the cells in loose connective tissue, regardless of where it is found in the body, are fibroblasts, as determined by actually counting these cells. This same technique has been used by others, and they have obtained the same figures.

DR. ASBOE-HANSEN: I do not really disagree with that. However, we may be examining this process at different stages from the point of view of cortisone effect. The first thing that happens in inflammation after edema develops is mucinous organization of it; in that stage we find mast cells regularly in certain stages of activity. Of course, after that, collagen formation begins and then fibroblasts take over the activity; this is the longest phase of the inflammatory reaction by far, and therefore the fibroblast is the dominating cell. There is no doubt about that. However, I do not think fibrosis would occur without the initial mucinous phase. In the acute stages of inflammation we do not see mast cells very often because these cells are in an edematous environment and they are degranulated; however, in chronic inflammation these cells are recognizable.

DR. SPAIN: Dr. Dougherty, you stated that there is more cortisol in the inflamed area because of greater transport as a result of the increased vascularity or permeability of that area, and yet everybody invokes decreased capillary permeability as one of the key factors in the inhibition of inflammation by this compound. Are these two points of view necessarily in conflict?

DR. DOUGHERTY: I do not think so at all. If one plots a curve of the rate of increase and decrease of the amount of C^{14} labelled cortisol (and this of course includes its metabolites) in the inflamed tissue, and expresses it in relative specific activity (that is, in microcuries per milligram of dry tissue), one finds that there is more at the inflamed site than at any other. There does not seem to be any specific trapping mechanism for the cortisol because the rate of disappearance is the same although the quantity differs. Therefore, it does not appear that there is something special that happens in inflamed tissue to attract the cortisol; rather, it is a reflection of increased blood flow and increased permeability of the inflamed area, and it does not matter whether the substance involved is trypan blue or

483

cortisol or something else. As Dr. Menkin showed about 1936, essentially the same thing happens if you give trypan blue to an animal and produce inflammation; the dye localizes in the inflamed area, and in his experiments, when crude adrenal cortical extract was given there was a reduction in the rate of uptake of trypan blue. This was the first demonstration of the anti-inflammatory action of the steroids as far as I am concerned, and the next one was our own.

DR. SPAIN: If a decrease in capillary permeability accounts for the decrease in cellular elements, edema and fibrin formation in inflammation, how do you explain the increased influx of cortisol into the area?

DR. DOUGHERTY: It is possible that there is a differential change in permeability.

DR. SPAIN: Would anybody else care to make a comment on this?

DR. MENKIN: Yes. We observed the increased capillary permeability to trypan blue in 1936 and published it in 1940, and I think Dr. Dougherty is essentially right. Initially there is increased permeability at the site of inflammation and there will be a great accumulation of corticoids. We found that by the method that was described. It is only after the cortisol appears at the site of inflammation that its effect on the capillary occurs.

DR. REBUCK: In this connection I want to ask Dr. Dougherty what his latest ideas are about the failure of the lymphocytes to migrate after administration of steroids. What is the mechanism and how does protecting or modifying the fibroblast diminish mononuclear exudation?

DR. DOUGHERTY: Within loose connective tissue, there are certain cells native to that tissue, such as fibroblasts, mast cells and fat cells, a few plasma cells and eosinophiles, and only very few lymphocytes. In the mouse there are 2.4 per cent macrophages per square millimeter of tissue. In the very first stages of inflammation there is migration of non-native cells, the polymorphonuclears and lymphocytes, from the blood to the localized inflamed area. The lymphocytes, as Dr. Rebuck has shown, certainly come later and have a very definite set time of appearance. My explanation for the fact that we do not have mononuclear infiltration and mononuclear cells changing over to macrophages in such areas is that if we inhibit the production of inflammation, we inhibit the migration of non-native cells in the same way that other events of inflammation, such as early transudation and exudation, are inhibited. However, polymorphonuclear infiltration normally occurs early in the process, in contrast to lymphocytic infiltration, and since it takes some time for the steroid effect to occur, migration of lymphocytes is inhibited to a greater degree than polymorphonuclear infiltration.

DR. SPAIN: Dr. Favour, in connection with that, do you believe that steroids reduce the phagocytic activity of the mononuclear cells, and if so, how would that relate that to the quantitative reduction in the number of cells? Are these two separate functions or similar functions?

DR. FAVOUR: There are probably many processes occurring at the same time. Dr. Dougherty has outlined the first line of defense—that is, migration of these cells through the capillary into the inflamed tissue—and in this regard I think it is worthwhile to call your attention to the outstanding experiments of Dr. Ebert, in which small windows were placed in rabbits' ears. Under the window there was a thin layer of connective tissue and capillaries, which could be easily observed. When, for example, tuberculin was injected into a sensitive animal, the white blood cells became "sticky" and would stop at the site of injury; the cells would then pass through the capillary wall into the interstitial tissue. The first cells, as we have talked about, were the polymorphonuclear cells, but sooner or later a very large number of cells accumulated, including lymphocytes and macrophages, and it became very hard to tell what the proportions were. Evidently not only is there a change in the capillary wall which permits this, but something happens to the cells themselves causing them to stop and to migrate through the capillary wall at the site of inflammation, and this process can be inhibited *in vivo* by corticosteroids. If these cells are studied outside the host, the phagocytic and migratory properties of leukocytes can also be inhibited readily by corticosteroids. So I am sure that steroids have a cellular effect as well as an effect on the capillary.

Dr. Spain: Dr. Dougherty, in one of your slides it was very difficult for me to say whether some of the cells were fibroblasts undergoing alterations or whether they were macrophages neglecting to become fibroblasts.

Dr. Dougherty: These were fibroblasts. I studied with a man who knew what fibroblasts were, and I have looked at these cells for many years. I know what a fibroblast is, and I can assure you that these cells were fibroblasts.

Dr. Favour: Is there any way besides just looking at these cells by which you can prove they are fibroblasts, such as by analysis of what they produce or by other methods?

Dr. Dougherty: Are fibroblasts in tissue culture fibroblasts, if you start off with a single fibroblast to begin with?

Dr. Favour: Yes, but these are not single cells you are talking about.

Dr. Dougherty: But we have done this with fibroblasts grown in cell culture from single cells, as I have mentioned.

Dr. Favour: But your descriptions are of inflammation in subcutaneous tissue, and you do not know whether the cells were all fibroblasts or cells which migrated into the area from the outside.

Dr. Dougherty: These cells have the morphological appearance of fibroblasts. Chemically they may be different. We can not ignore the experiments in which cells that are morphologically identical to fibroblasts have entirely different amino acid requirements for growth. Are these cells fibroblasts? This is the situation. All I can say is that if I take cells which have the morphological characteristics of fibroblasts and put cortisol on them, I get such and such a reaction. For convenience we can call these cells fibroblasts. In other words, I could just simply state that if you put cortisol on cells called fibroblasts in tissue culture you will get a certain result, and along with it there is a metabolic alteration in the steroid molecule. Not only that, but we take time-lapse cinemicrographs of these cells; the effects are all on record, and it is very easy for people to see them. The cells pull in their processes, round up and take this shape, and this is as much as I can tell you.

Dr. Spain: Dr. Rebuck, do you have some other comments?

Dr. Rebuck: Yes. I want to ask Dr. Fischel a question about the effects of steroids on antibody formation and antigen-antibody reactions. In any group of animals, say 100 rabbits, there are some that will not form any antibodies to an antigen, there are some that are poor antibody formers, and finally there are the majority who are good antibody formers. Now, do steroids have different effects on these groups?

Dr. Fischel: In the data I showed, from a group of about 70 guinea pigs, there were great differences in antibody production, from practically none to 500 micrograms per ml. I do not know which animals we picked for the cortisone experiment, but certainly after cortisone there was an unusual distribution in the 0 to 20 microgram group. In addition, in other experiments with animals that were immunized, further immunization was done after 14 days at a time when some of them were good antibody producers and some were poor antibody producers, and cortisone did modify the subsequent further response to immunization. The animals responded as you might have expected from the results of the previous immunization —that is, the previously good antibody formers had a greater response than the poor ones.

DR. REBUCK: I was hoping that your data would show that some of the animals would escape this depression and would make more antibodies; this seems to happen clinically once in a while.

DR. FISCHEL: I was never convinced that this effect was well demonstrated clinically. The only clinical studies I know of suggested that cortisone did not have much effect on antibody production except in humans who were producing large amounts of antibody in certain types of leukemia. Generally speaking, when antibody production is determined by mouse protection tests, as with the pneumococcus or with diphtheria toxoid, no great effect has been shown in the human; however, it is possible that this system does not lend itself to good quantitation or that the dose of cortisone used in the studies was not very large.

DR. FAVOUR: The dose you used in the rabbits was quite large, was it not, in comparison to the amounts that are often used clinically in patients?

DR. FISCHEL: I refuse to compare this with patient data, because if you want to do something in an animal—for example, to inhibit wound healing or to inhibit any other biochemical process—you do not give the steroid on a weight basis or even on the basis of surface area. For example, it requires a much greater dose of steroids to get the same biological effect in the guinea pig than in the rabbit.

The Cellular Response to Inflammation and Its Modification by Glucocorticoids[*]

CUTTING B. FAVOUR

Georgetown University School of Medicine

This presentation on inflammatory responses is concerned with the separate functions of four cell types which play a prominent role both in nonspecific as well as in various allergic inflammatory processes. These cells are the phagocytic polymorphonuclear (PMN) and monocytic (MON) cells, which are important in nonspecific inflammation, and the lymphocyte and nonphagocytic plasma cell, which take part in allergic inflammation. The general functions of these cells are listed in Table 1.

Although it is instructive to single out the role played by each of these cells in inflammatory responses and to relate the separate effect of excess glucocorticoids on each to clinical observations, it should be remembered in the presentation which follows that in the intact host these cells do not function independently of each other nor of other body systems. Insofar as

[*] Work done under grants E-3775 and 2E-182 from the U. S. Public Health Service.

TABLE 1.

PMN	MON	LYMPHOCYTE	PLASMA CELL
Primary phagocytosis	Secondary phagocytosis Granuloma formation	Delayed allergy Homograft rejection	Humoral immunity and allergy

these cell types are morphologically and functionally different one from another, however—and they do differ in many ways—this method of analysis gives considerable insight into the cellular basis for inflammatory reactions.

THE POLYMORPHONUCLEAR LEUKOCYTE

Functions of the PMN. Phylogenetically, the polymorphonuclear leukocyte is a primitive mesenchymal cell form. It is found in invertebrates, "down" to the level of the echinoderms of the seashore as well as in the insects which have colonized the land.[34] The neutrophilic series of granulocytes also appears early during intrauterine life. It is first seen in the fourth month of the human fetus[118, 122] and by the time of birth is a fully active cell form.

The mature PMN (Table 2) is a differentiated end-stage cell which

TABLE 2. PROPERTIES OF MATURE NEUTROPHILS

Ameboid motion Chemotaxis Phagocytosis High metabolism Ratio of glycolysis to lactate production, 1:2	Nonreproductive No antibody production No passive transfer of allergy	Contain: Lysozyme Anti-staph factor Proteolytic enzymes Lipolytic enzymes

cannot reproduce. PMN do not make antibodies.[27] Neither are PMN able to passively transfer delayed-type allergy.[68] Furthermore, they can be washed free of serum and when so washed they do not contain plasma protein within their cytoplasm.

The PMN is characterized by marked ameboid activity, responsiveness to chemotaxis,[86] a sticky surface,[115] and the power to phagocytose and usually to digest a wide range of particulate materials. Phagocytosis and digestion are accompanied by an increased O_2 uptake and anaerobic CO_2 production.[83] Any one of a variety of circumstances which interfere with their metabolism will inhibit these various interrelated activities. If the functional deficit is severe, it may be the cause of one of the "low resistance" syndromes.[35] Among these inhibitors are the presence of small amounts of alcohol,[63] a low vitamin C level,[93] the reduction in circulating antibodies, a fall in the serum complement and excessively high glucocorticoid levels. On the other hand, the evolution of the PMN antedated the appearance of the specific immune systems which supply antibodies which are bactericidal in the presence of complement, as well as antibodies which promote phagocytosis. Furthermore, PMN antedated the evolution of the endocrine system of higher animals, which has come to have a powerful though not absolute regulatory control over their function.

Under ordinary circumstances the primordial functions of the PMN, unaided by specific antibodies, are a major factor in the control of tissue invasions by the saprophytic resident microflora of the healthy animal. Even virulent infections may be controlled by this inherent function of PMN. This capacity has been called "surface phagocytosis,"[119] by which is meant the power to corner virulent micro-organisms against other cells and phagocytose them without the help of antibody. Ingested bacteria usually are destroyed whether or not the ingestion process is aided by the opsonizing effect of humoral antibody. This is not always so, for mucins which may accompany bacteria when they are ingested tend to inhibit digestion.[85] Furthermore, some bacteria such as the anthrax organism possess a tissue-damaging factor which inhibits phagocytosis.[22] The polysaccharide of the pneumococcus capsule is thought to have a similar property.[37]

This destructive process within PMN is accomplished by a variety of cellular ferments. Among those which have been found in PMN are lysozyme,[39, 56, 92] an antistaphylococcus factor, and a number of proteolytic enzymes.[108] Inert particles or bacteria which resist digestion eventually outlive the short life span of the individual PMN to be taken up again either by PMN or by some other cell of the reticuloendothelial system.[94] Among bacteria which are readily destroyed after phagocytosis are pneumococci,[119] staphylococci, beta-hemolytic streptococci and coliform bacilli.[47] Among organisms which can survive intracellularly are tubercle bacilli,[12] typhoid bacilli,[48] brucella bacilli, α-hemolytic streptococci and numerous protozoan parasites. Micro-organisms which are not readily destroyed by PMN are handled by other cells of the RES as noted below.

Effect of Glucocorticoids on Function of Neutrophils. One of the important PMN functions to be altered by excess glucocorticoidal levels is suppression of pseudopodial activity (Table 3). The ability of PMN to adhere to

TABLE 3.   EFFECT OF GLUCOCORTICOIDS ON NEUTROPHILS

Depress:	Increase:
Stickiness	PMN in blood
Diapedesis	PMN survival
Ameboid activity	Antipyretic effect
Phagocytosis	
Digestion	
Glycolysis	

capillary walls and to migrate into areas of nonspecific allergy inflammation is suppressed by the systemic use of glucocorticoid.[20, 42, 43, 45, 88] Topical application of cortisone has the same effect.[99] This inhibition of diapedesis has been most beautifully demonstrated with the use of ear-window studies in rabbits. Glucocorticoids are seen to suppress leukocyte diapedesis in local anaphylactic[25] as well as tuberculin reactions.[26] *In vitro* suppression of PMN migration by the presence of excess glucocorticoids has also been demonstrated in capillary tube experiments in which a dose-response curve can be demonstrated.[66] Optimal migration of PMN takes place at 0.4 to 1.0 gamma/ ml. of hydrocortisone. Higher levels of 10 to 100 gamma/ml. cause a proportionally greater inhibition of cell migration. This hormone-induced failure of PMN to leave the circulation at their normal rate has been suggested as the reason for the leukocytosis of excessive glucocorticoid therapy.[25]

Migratory activity of PMN is also closely related to phagocytic activity. Glucocorticoids at very high levels have been shown to inhibit the phagocytic index where bacteria and carbon particles have been used as test agents. This inhibitory effect is seen even in the presence of hyperimmune serum active against the bacterial species under study.[21] It is interesting that the phagocytic index is also reduced as a result of adrenalectomy.[9] This reduction is reversed by adrenal cortical extract.[10] It is not known to what degree the phagocytic index is altered at glucocorticoid levels close to the physiologic range. The few adverse effects on infections of moderate glucocorticoid treatment in a wide variety of clinical problems suggest that it is the higher blood levels which significantly lower resistance in man.

The digestive power of PMN, once they have taken up bacteria or other particulate material, likewise may be altered by high levels of glucocorticoids in the cellular environment. Bacteria which normally would be destroyed may lie dormant, later to disseminate infection throughout the host. Again, the extent of this effect is related to the magnitude and duration of high steroid dosage. Excess steroid levels for long times are the circumstances in which clinical infections have progressed.

These various studies all support the thesis that the reduced metabolism of PMN caused by excess glucocorticoids is causally related to a general reduction in cellular chemotaxis, migration, phagocytosis and digestive power brought about by high levels of these compounds. The inherently high glycolytic activity of PMN tends, further, to accentuate these effects over less obvious changes brought about by the effect of glucocorticoids on cellular function of tissues with different metabolic pathways and rates of metabolism. On the other hand, although the effect of glucocorticoids on PMN is great, it may not be as dramatic as it is on other cellular systems, the lymphocyte in particular, as we shall see later on in this review.

The extrapolation of these laboratory findings to human infections is complicated by genetic differences in the capacity of individuals to develop protective responses, differences which are not under hormonal control. Furthermore, inflammatory changes which are augmented by the delayed-type allergy may be suppressed more vigorously by glucocorticoids than is predictable from direct *in vitro* studies with phagocytes. In this respect it has been relatively easy to design laboratory experiments employing mice,[54] guinea pigs[109] and rabbits[82] which show that cortisone will adversely affect the course of tuberculosis in animals, whereas, in fact, the exacerbation of tuberculosis in humans receiving excess glucocorticoids is rare.[40]

Antipyretic Effect of Glucocorticoids. Support for the cell-injury theory of fever production in which the PMN is thought to be the source of endogenous pyrogen comes from the effect of glucocorticoids on febrile conditions. Glucocorticoids in liberal doses are antipyretic.[59, 100] The mechanism of this action is not clear, however, for both the occurrence of leukopenia and the *in vitro* liberation of endogenous pyrogens which follow exposure to typhoid toxin are not affected by cortisone therapy.[1] On the other hand, tolerance to an exogenous pyrogen which develops upon repeated exposure to this agent is prevented by cortisone administration.[6] It has been suggested that glucocorticoids block the effect of endogenous pyrogen on the thermoregulatory center.[62, 119] The minute amounts of endogenous factors which will initiate a febrile response complicate the study and interpretation of these results. In man, for example, the amount of material liberated by injury to the leukocytes present in 500 ml. of blood is enough to raise the body temperature of a compatible recipient to 105° F. for several hours.[95]

The Antitoxic Effect of Glucocorticoids. Although glucocorticoids do not block the direct effect of a toxin such as diphtheria toxin[2, 33] once it has reached tissue cells, they do have nonspecific antitoxic effects in many inflammatory states which are not fully understood. Decreased capillary permeability,[81, 121] lessened leukocyte chemotaxis[28] and diminished cellular diapedesis[25] into areas of inflammation, as well as the suppression of delayed-type allergic reactions,[26, 95] are mechanisms by which glucocorticoids may bring about these nonspecific antitoxic responses.

THE MONOCYTE

Phagocytic Mononuclear Cell.   We have seen that the major function of the PMN is to promote phagocytosis of bacteria and other small particles which get into the body fluids. Metchnikoff originally called these "microphages" to distinguish them from "macrophages" which ingest larger particles and are slower to reach inflammatory sites.[76] Macrophages have since been given a number of names depending on their location in the body: the monocyte of the blood, the Kupffer cell of the liver, the histiocyte of inflammation and the resting-wandering cell of the tissues. The primary functions of these cells are migration, phagocytosis and granuloma formation (Table 4).

TABLE 4.   PROPERTIES OF MONOCYTES

Ameboid motion	Reproductive	Contain:
Chemotaxis	No antibody production	Proteolytic enzymes
Phagocytosis	No passive transfer of	Lipolytic enzymes
Granuloma formation (sequestration)	allergy	Organic acids

They do not form antibodies[27, 102] and they do not passively transfer delayed-type hypersensitivity.

Infectious agents and particulate materials which are not destroyed by PMN generally undergo secondary phagocytosis by the mononuclear phagocytic system. Like that of the PMN, their considerable digestive capacity appears to depend upon changes in intracellular pH,[105] organic acid production[52] and the possession of a variety of digestive enzymes.[7] Their equally great capacity to protect the tissues and to function as scavengers which remove injured cells has earned them the reputation of being the most powerful phagocytes in the body.[113] Some idea of their effectiveness is gained from studies on the fate of intravenous infusion of viable bacterial suspensions in experimental animals. By means of a catheter placed in the venous outflow tract from various organs in the body,[65, 84] it has been found that the liver (active phagocytosis by Kupffer cells) will remove 85 per cent of a suspension containing 10,000 organisms per ml. in the course of one passage of blood through this organ. Other body structures have substantially less filtering power. Usually virulent organisms are cleared from the blood less readily only to return later to the blood stream, as in clinical sepsis.

Another function of macrophages is their ability to imprison microorganisms and particulate materials which they cannot destroy. This holding action of macrophages led Goodpasture[49] to classify such resistant organisms as "intracellular" infections to differentiate them from "extracellular" infections in which the micro-organism is destroyed at the time of primary phagocytosis. According to this view, the pneumococcus and various avirulent coliform organisms are "extracellular" infections. Examples of "intracellular" infections are typhoid, tuberculosis, brucellosis, malaria, subacute bacterial endocarditis and some beta-hemolytic streptococcus infections. Micro-organisms of this category may lie dormant in macrophages safe from humoral immunity. From these reservoirs chronic or recurrent infections may develop. This principle is well illustrated in clinical typhoid infections in which the organism has been observed to survive mitosis in macrophages, going intact into both daughter cells.[48] One of the clinical consequences of this type of sequestration is the substantial relapse rate in typhoid fever whether or not treated by antibiotics. The principle also applies to tuberculosis, where the power of the mononuclear cell to destroy tubercle bacilli appears to be, in part, under genetic control.[80] Time-lapse movies of embryo tissue cultures, devoid of immunity, have been used to show how invasion of the tissue cells by virulent avian tubercle bacilli is prevented so long as enough macrophages are available to hold bacilli within their cytoplasm. Eventually, the macrophage system in these cultures declines in numbers as the cells die off. Only then are fibroblasts invaded by tubercle bacilli.[36]

Granuloma Formation. Like the PMN, the mononuclear cell also is of primitive origin.[34] It is found in insects and other lower phyla, where its function is similar to that well known in vertebrates. It appears during the fourth lunar month in the human fetus[118] and is fully active at birth. One of its most important functions is its capacity, when in groups, to form granulomata. Again, this is a primitive trait well known in lower animals which are devoid of the specific humoral and hypersensitivity immune systems of man. In the earthworm, for example, granulomata form about noxious agents. When these masses are large, they gravitate to rear segments which eventually are sloughed and replaced by regenerated tissue or by whole anatomical segments.[15] In man something akin to this rejection process is represented by the silicotic granuloma and the encapsulated echinococcosis cyst. Although encapsulation or sloughing off occurs in the skin and in walls of viscera of man, organized regeneration of whole structures in the primitive sense does not occur. Healing by scar tissue formation is the usual mechanism for replacement of lost tissue. In each of these processes the macrophage is an active part of the much more complex host reaction which constitutes granuloma formation in higher animals.

Effect of Glucocorticoids on Monocytes. The effect of excess glucocorticoids on monocytes is much like their effect on PMN. These changes are listed in Table 5. An important result of excess glucocorticoids is a decrease

TABLE 5. EFFECT OF GLUCOCORTICOIDS ON MONOCYTES

Depress:	Increase:
Mitoses	Intracellular parasite survival time
Diapedesis	
Phagocytosis	
Digestive power	
Granuloma formation	

in mitotic activity which has been observed both *in vitro*[41] and *in vivo*.[98] It is of equal interest that a decrease in phagocytic activity by macrophages follows adrenalectomy[50] and that this activity can be restored by the administration of physiologic amounts of adrenocortical extract.[50, 114] Another result of excess glucocorticoids is decreased monocyte phagocytic[23] activity much like that noted in PMN exposed to high glucocorticoid levels. In the intact animal this decreased function is manifest as greater vulnerability of the host to relatively "avirulent" micro-organisms, more so in rabbits and rats than in guinea pigs, monkeys and humans.[8, 77] A similar species difference in the effect of glucocorticoids on monocytes has been observed in tissue culture studies. Guinea pig monocytes are 10 to 100 times as resistant to the suppressive effect of hydrocortisone as are monocytes taken from rats and mice.[41] Other examples of reduced monocyte activity in the host as a result of excess glucocorticoid levels are a diminished monocyte destruction of tubercle bacilli[82] *Treponema pallida*,[116] fungi, viruses and other micro-organisms[71] and a reduced capacity of the pulmonary phagocytes to destroy extravasated erythrocytes in the lungs.[60] Glucocorticoids in excess do not affect all monocytes in a given cell population to the same degree, however. Individual monocytes among a group being suppressed may function normally in the presence of 100 mcg. of cortisol per ml., which is a level above that usually attained in clinical practice.[41]

THE LYMPHOCYTE

Lymphocytes, which like plasma cells are nonphagocytic, seem also to be of more recent origin phylogenetically than are the more primitive phago-cytic cell systems of the reticuloendothelial system. Lymphocytes as we know them in mammals have not been described in the invertebrates which have been studied. On the other hand, they are well known in vertebrate species from fish to man.[34] In the human fetus lymphocytes appear soon after erythropoiesis starts, some time in the fourth month of gestation, which is soon after the first appearance of phagocytes. Lymphocytes seem to be a different cell line than other lymphoid cell systems well before they reach their characteristic appearance as mature cells. When time-lapse movies are taken of immature lymphocytes,[10] they are found to exhibit a characteristic mode of locomotion which is different from that of other RE cells. Other morphological and functional differences between developing lymphocytes and the plasma cell in particular have been reviewed recently.[36] The metabolic activities and function of lymphocytes are given in Table 6.

Function of Lymphocytes. Although antibody formation has long been suggested as a function of lymphocytes,[23, 53, 55] the evidence for this contention is inconclusive. The small mature lymphocytes, over which there is no disagreement regarding morphology and identity, do not make antibodies.[64] Peripheral blood leukocytes which include mature lymphocytes do not make antipneumococcal antibodies[31] nor antibodies to diphtheria toxin.[74] On the other hand, thoracic duct lymphocytes—about the identity of which there is some doubt, since 5 per cent are immature forms of uncertain type—have been found to produce antibodies to *Salmonella typhosa* and to horse serum antigens used to immunize the cell donor.[117] Lymph node cells containing

TABLE 6.   PROPERTIES OF MATURE LYMPHOCYTES

Nonphagocytic	Reproductive
High O_2 consumption	Passive transfer of delayed allergy
Ratio of glycolysis to lactate production, 1:3	

less mature leukocytes of even less certain identity have been shown to yield tissue fragments which will passively transfer antibody-producing capacity to a nonimmunized recipient.[110, 111]

The best substantiated function of the small compact cells of the lymphoid series to which this discussion is limited is their capacity to transfer delayed-type allergy. This function is thought to be mediated by a "transfer factor"[73] which they liberate. Crude Fuelgen staining techniques of cell extracts after treatment with desoxyribonuclease to destroy nucleic acids suggest that "transfer factor" is not a nucleoprotein. By extrapolation from negative transfer studies done with other cell types found in the peripheral blood, it is believed that the lymphocyte is the cell which releases transfer factor.

This general concept that mature lymphocytes mediate delayed-type allergy and do not form antibody of the classic type is supported by correlative information drawn from clinical medicine. Lymphatic leukemia is not ordinarily accompanied by hypergammaglobulinemia. In fact, the reverse may be true.[106] Furthermore, patients with chronic lymphatic leukemia have a poor or absent antibody-forming capacity.[72]

Effect of Glucocorticoids on Lymphocytes. Some of the effects of glucocorticoids on lymphocytes are given in Table 7. Review of these changes

TABLE 7. EFFECT OF GLUCOCORTICOIDS ON LYMPHOCYTES

Depress:	Unchanged:
Number in tissue and blood	Donor cell activity
Glycolysis	Transfer of delayed allergy
Active delayed-allergy	Lactate production
Passive transfer of delayed allergy	

indicates that, in general, the inhibition of cell function parallels the reduction in cell metabolism brought about by these steroids.

Peripheral blood lymphocytes are one source of lymphoid cells which have been obtained in sufficient purity to make direct comparisons between the metabolic activity of lymphocytes, PMN and malignant cells. Aerobic metabolic studies on normal human peripheral blood lymphocytes of the small mature type have shown that they have a rate of glucose utilization and lactate production which is approximately half that of PMN.[99] A similar lower rate of lactate production by lymphoid cells has been observed by others.[5, 58] This relatively low rate of lymphocyte lactate production is accompanied by an O_2 consumption half again as much as that of PMN.[99] On the other hand, lymphocytes incubated at the normal range of glucose concentration, 80 to 120 mg. per cent, produce approximately 3 moles of lactate to 1 mole of glucose utilized. This is a relatively higher ratio of lactate production to glucose utilized than that of PMN studied under comparable conditions. In this type of cell system glucocorticoids have a lesser suppressive effect on glucose utilization by lymphocytes than they do on PMN. In spite of this reduced glycolysis, lymphocytes continue to produce lactate at the usual rate, even though exposed to glucocorticoids.[99] Glucocorticoids also have been shown to inhibit the incorporation of glycine-2-C^{14} into the protein and into the nucleic acids of thymus cells.[4, 11] The small glucocorticoid inhibition of glucose utilization and the greater glucocorticoid inhibition of protein synthesis by intact cells would appear to cause these cells to use other cellular resources (possibly cellular protein) for continued lactate production. According to this concept, the dissolution of the lymphoid cell by glucocorticoids is a phenomenon of rapid energy starvation taking place in a cell during a period when it has an obligatory high metabolic rate.

Although this is an attractive hypothesis with which to explain the mechanism of action of glucocorticoids on lymphoid tissue, this thesis needs further validation. We know, for example, that 17-d-ethyl-10-nortestosterone in the physiologically high concentration of 10^{-5} moles also inhibits glycine-2-C^{14} incorporation into thymus cells. This compound has no glucocorticoid effect, either *in vivo* or *in vitro*.[11]

In view of these metabolic alterations, it is not surprising that large doses of glucocorticoids have the effects they do on rapidly multiplying cell systems such as the lymphocyte series. Under these conditions glucocorticoids are powerful metabolic inhibitors,[3] they reduce mitosis,[23] they decrease the rate of P^{32} incorporation in lymphocytic nucleic acid[17, 57, 70] and they inhibit the synthesis of nucleic acids.[11, 69]

THE PLASMA CELL

Plasma cells, which, like lymphocytes, are nonphagocytic, also seem to have had a more recent origin phylogenetically than have the more primitive phagocytic reticuloendothelial cells (Table 8). In general plasma cells and lymphocytes are found in close association with each other. Both cell types

TABLE 8. *PROPERTIES OF PLASMA CELLS*

Nonphagocytic	Reproductive
	Antibody formation
	Primary
	Secondary

have been described in fish, salamanders and frogs, as well as in mammalian species.[34] The only exception to their presence together is the disorder of hypogammaglobulinemia in man,[14] where the virtual absence of plasma cells is in contrast to the presence of a morphologically and functionally[46] intact lymphocyte system. The fact that this condition often is a sex-linked hereditary disorder in males suggests that it may be a throwback to an earlier stage of evolution during which the lymphocytic system was as far as the RES had gone in development. To date, no animal, other than the few humans with this finding, has been found with a similar deficit.

In the human fetus, plasma cells do not appear until the time of birth and antibody formation and isoagglutinin production do not appear until the first months of life. The later development of the plasma-cell-antibody system than that of the lymphocyte system is due in part to the lack of antigenic exposure during intrauterine life. This discrepancy is also an inherent one, since germ-free animals retain the neonatal pattern of lymph tissue development into adult life.[90]

The aspect of plasma cell activity with which we are concerned in this discussion is the relation between their level of metabolic activity and their capacity to form antibodies. Other aspects of their part in antibody formation are too well known to need elaboration in this discussion.

The morphological sequences in lymphoid tissue undergoing response to an immunizing stimulus are listed in Table 9. In the first phase of lymphoid tissue hypertrophy, there is a rapid building of desoxyribose nucleic acid (DNA) in the cell nucleus and of ribose nucleic acid (RNA) in the cell cytoplasm.[13] Both processes are known to be associated with the synthesis of cellular proteins.[16] This increase in cellular RNA is directly related to protein synthesis by cells.[89, 110, 111] When protein formation proceeds anaerobically, it is dependent on the presence of glucose.[11] As is true for cancer cells and other rapidly multiplying tissues, it is during the early phase of development, some time between 12 and 48 hours, that tissues are most vulnerable to a variety of altered biochemical activities. The involution of lymphoid tissue caused by large amounts of glucocorticoids[3, 91] is one example of such an inhibiting effect. Other agents have similar effects. Among these are nitrogen mustards,[67, 104] large doses of desoxycortisone[18, 51, 107] and exposure to high energy radiation both *in vivo*[24, 75] and *in vitro*.[97]

During the early phase of lymphoid tissue hypertrophy, fluorescent tagging techniques have shown that antigens are localized in the cytoplasm and in the nucleus of lymphoid follicle cells as well as in other RES cells.[19] Thereafter, antigen tends to disappear from tissue sites and seems to be absent when antibody formation is still active.

When follicle cells are removed for *in vitro* study 48 hours after an antigenic stimulus, by which time maximum DNA and RNA activity is present, they do not have the morphological characteristics of plasma cells.[32, 64] These cells are thought by some not to make antibodies *in vitro*,[32, 102] although others disagree.[64] Since it is a technical feat to dissect follicle cells free of surrounding lymphoid tissue for incubation experiments of this type, it is not surprising that divergent results have been reported.

In contrast to the studies of follicle cells, there is wide agreement that some of the perifollicular cells which also multiply rapidly following an antigenic stimulus go through the evolution of pre-plasma cell to plasma cell and are the source of antibody.[32, 64, 102] By various methods of analysis, antibody production is found to increase up to four to six days after an antigenic stimulus. It is at this time that plasma cells are found, by fluorescent tagging methods, to contain abundant antibody, and maximum antibody production is present. When labeled amino acids are fed to an animal during this period of active antibody formation, radioactivity appears within an hour in freshly formed antibody molecules.[112] It is also at this time, after antigenic stimulus, that plasma cell RNA activity is at a peak.[29, 87] The RNA activity of follicle cells reaches a peak earlier. Ordinarily the evolution of follicle cells into the small mature lymphocyte is essentially complete by

TABLE 9.   CELLULAR CHANGES FOLLOWING ANTIGENIC STIMULUS

	LYMPHOCYTES	PLASMA CELL
Maximum DNA	12-48	12-48
Maximum RNA	2-4 days	4-6 days
Maximum mitosis	1-3 days	after 3 days
Maximum vulnerability	12-48 hours	12-48 hours
Maximum antibody		4-6 days
Maturity	1-3 days	after 3 days

four to six days, when they stop undergoing mitoses and reach the peripheral blood stream.

Effect of Glucocorticoids on Plasma Cells. The principle effects of glucocorticoids on plasma cells are listed in Table 10. In general these changes are the result of suppressed cellular metabolism at a stage of rapid cell development and, accordingly, are manifested chiefly as modifications of the rate but not necessarily the amount of antibody produced. Ordinarily, the better established antibody production is in a given host, the less is the effect of high glucocorticoid levels on circulating titers. Sometimes a lesser glucocorticoid dose will also reverse the ill effects of an antibody response. Antibody production can be obliterated, however when gluco-corticoids in very large doses are given simultaneously with antigen[38] (Table 10). When patients with hypersensitivity lesions of the periarteritis type which are presumed to be due to circulating antibody combining with antigen in sufficient quantity to form precipitates in the presence of antigen excess in the tissues are treated early enough with glucocorticoids to

TABLE. 10.   EFFECT OF GLUCOCORTICOIDS ON PLASMA CELLS

With primary antigenic stimulus
  Suppress mitoses
  Suppress antibody formation
With secondary antigenic stimulus
  Few mitoses to suppress
  Less effect on antibody formation

suppress antibody levels below critical levels, the lesions of this disease can be prevented.[44] When glucocorticoids are administered well after antibody formation is under way, there is usually much less effect. Normally, antibody titers in human diseases, when treatment is not started until after the invading agent is established, are little changed when the therapeutically large doses of corticoids are given. This means that prolonged and excessive glucocorticoid therapy may have only a limited effect on ordinary acquired immunity to common infections. This, of course, is a desirable circumstance. On the other hand, such treatment may have an equally limited effect on a pathological process associated with circulating antibodies, as, for example, in thrombocytopenia.

This effect of glucocorticoids on the lymphoid cells which infiltrate allergic reactions early in their course, greater than on the development of pyrinophilic plasma cells which arise in allergic reactions after four to five days, has been well documented in studies on the evolution of Arthus-type reactions in rabbits.[43] In the same way the clinical use of glucocorticoids is much more effective in shrinking lymphoid tissues[23] and in suppressing delayed-type hypersensitivity,[76, 78, 79] as, for example, poison oak dermatitis, than it is in reversing an established antibody response[43, 95] or a disease process due to a circulating antibody.

This correlation between the relatively greater effect of glucocorticoids on lymphoid cells than on other less rapidly maturing reticuloendothelial cells and the relatively greater effect of glucocorticoids on allergic rather than on nonspecific inflammation and established immunity is of general interest to the bedside physician. The clinician, who at times must compro-mise in the treatment of vexing disorders, can be comforted somewhat with the knowledge that the lower doses of glucocorticoids usually will suppress hypersensitivity responses mediated by lymphocytes to a greater degree than they will reduce the normal protective functions of the phagocytic and antibody-producing cells of the reticuloendothelial system.

SUMMARY

Four cell types of the reticuloendothelial system important in inflamma-tory responses are the polymorphonuclear (PMN) and mononuclear (MON) phagocytes, which take part in nonspecific inflammation, and the lymphocyte and plasma cell, which take part in allergic inflammation.

The chemotactic, phagocytic and digestive capacity of the phagocytic cells is associated with a high rate of metabolism which is readily suppressed by a variety of antimetabolic agents, of which important examples are the glucocorticoid hormones.

Direct *in vitro* studies indicate that glucocorticoids reduce the glycolytic activities of neutrophils and of lymphocytes to a degree which is proportional to the concentration of these agents above physiological levels in the body. Under aerobic conditions neutrophils compensate by a proportionate fall in lactate production. Lymphocytes continue to produce lactate despite a reduced glycolytic rate. Exhaustion of energy sources within lymphocytes, which appear to have a fixed high rate of metabolism, may account for their unusual vulnerability to glucocorticoids.

Another function of lymphocytes which conditions the effect of glucocorticoids on them is their somewhat shorter and, consequently, more actively anabolic maturation time than that of plasma cells. This difference is even greater when the comparison is made between rapidly growing lymphocytes and leisurely maturing plasma cells associated with an established immune response. Since mature lymphocytes mediate delayed-type hypersensitivity and since maturing plasma cells (particularly those present after a second antigenic stimulus) mediate antibody production, it is not surprising that the effect of excess glucocorticoids is much greater on inflammation due to delayed-type hypersensitivity than it is on antibody production or even on nonspecific inflammation.

Other than the capacity to suppress general cell function by exploiting differences in metabolism dependent on active glycolysis,[14, 17, 19, 20, 22] glucocorticoids do not have a specific anti-inflammatory capacity.

REFERENCES

1. Atkins, E., Allison, F., Smith, M. R. and Wood, W. B., Jr.: Studies on the anti-pyretic action of cortisone in pyrogen induced fever. J. Exper. Med., *101*:353, 1955.
2. Atlas, L. T., Levine, M. I., Osgood, C. K. and Favour, C. B.: The effect of cortisone on the survival of guinea pigs inoculated with diphtheria toxin. Bacteriol. Proc., 12, 1952.
3. Baker, B. L., Jugle, D. J. and Li, C. H.: Histology of lymphoid organs of rats treated with adrenocorticotropin. Am. J. Anat., 88:313, 1951.
4. Barron, E. S. G. and Kit, S.: Studies on the mechanism of action of adrenal cortical hormones. The inhibition of protein synthesis in lymphatic cells by some corticoid hormones. Tr. A. Am. Physicians, 65:293, 1952.
5. Beck, W. S. and Valentine, W. N.: The carbohydrate metabolism of leukocytes: a review. Cancer Res., *13*:309, 1953.
6. Bennett, I. L., Jr. and Beeson, P. B.: Effect of cortisone upon reactions of rabbits to bacterial endotoxins with particular reference to acquired resistance. Bull. Johns Hopkins Hosp., 93:290, 1953.
7. Bergel, S.: Weiteres zur lipoids fallenden Funktion der Lymphozyten. Beitr. z. Path. u.z. allg. Path., 73:404, 1925.
8. Berlin, B. S., Johnson, C., Hawk, W. D. and Lawrence, A. G.: The occurrence of bacteremia and death in cortisone-treated mice. J. Lab. & Clin. Med., 40:82, 1952.
9. Blanchard, E. W.: An experimental study of the opsonins of the blood; effect of bilateral adrenalectomy. Physiol. Zool., 4:302, 1931.
10. Blanchard, E. W.: An experimental study of the opsonins of the blood; further studies of their relationship to adrenal cortical function. Physiol. Zool., 7:493, 1934.
11. Blecher, M. and White, A.: Effect of various steroids and metabolic inhibitors on the incorporation of glycine-2-C^{14} into total proteins and nucleic acids of normal and malignant lymphocytes *in vitro*. J. Biol. Chem., 233:1161, 1958.
12. Bloch, H.: Studies on the virulence of tubercle bacilli; the relationship of the

physiological state of the organisms to their pathogenicity. J. Exper. Med., 92:507, 1950.

13. Brachet, J.: The nucleic acids. In Chemistry and Biology. New York, Academic Press, 2:475, 1955.
14. Bruton, O. C.: Agammaglobulinemia. Pediatrics, 9:722, 1952.
15. Cameron, G. R.: Inflammation in earthworms. J. Path. & Bact., 35:933, 1932.
16. Caspersson, T.: The relation between nucleic acid and protein synthesis. In Symposium on Nucleic Acid. London, Cambridge University Press, 1947.
17. Clark, I. and Stoorck, H. C.: The uptake of P^{32} by nucleic acids of lymphoid tissue undergoing atrophy. J. Biol. Chem., 222:285, 1946.
18. Congegny, P.: Involution of lymphoid tissue by large doses of desoxycorticosterone. Proc. Soc. Exper. Biol. & Med., 63:248, 1946.
19. Coons, A. H., Sedue, E. H. and Kaplan, M. H.: Localization of antigen in tissue cells; the fate of injected foreign protein in the mouse. J. Exper. Med., 93:173, 1951.
20. Coste, E., Piquet, B., Gomiche, P. and Cayla, J.: Cortisone corticotrophin (ACTH) and infections. Ann. Med., 52:747, 1951.
21. Crepea, S. B., Magnin, G. E. and Seastone, C. V.: Effect of ACTH and cortisone on phagocytosis. Proc. Soc. Exper. Biol. & Med., 77:704, 1951.
22. Cromartie, W. J., Watson, D., Bloom, W. and Heckly, R.: Studies on infection with *Bacillus anthracis;* immunological and tissue damaging properties of extracts prepared from lesions of *B. anthracis* infections. J. Infect. Dis., 46:26, 1947.
23. Dougherty, T. F. and White, A.: Functional alterations in lymphoid tissue induced by adrenal cortical secretion. Am. J. Anat., 77:81, 1945.
24. Dougherty, T. F. and White, A.: Pituitary-adrenal cortical control of lymphocyte structure and function as revealed by experimental X-radiation. Endocrinology, 39:370, 1946.
25. Ebert, R. H. and Wissler, R. W.: *In vivo* observations of the effects of cortisone on the vascular reaction to large doses of horse serum, using the rabbit ear chamber technique. J. Lab. Med., 38:497, 1951.
26. Ebert, R. H.: *In vivo* observations on effect of cortisone on experimental tuberculosis, using the rabbit ear chamber technique. Amer. Rev. Tuberc., 65:64, 1952.
27. Ehrich, W. E., Harris, T. N. and Martens, E.: Absence of antibody in the macrophages during maximal antibody formation. J. Exper. Med., 83:373, 1946.
28. Ehrich, W. E.: Functional significance of the various leukocytes in inflammation. J. Mt. Sinai Hosp., 15:337, 1948-49.
29. Ehrich, W. E., Drabkin, D. L. and Forman, C.: Nucleic acids and production of antibody by plasma cells. J. Exper. Med., 90:157, 1949.
30. Ehrich, W. E.: Adaptation phase in inflammation. In Jasmin, G. and Robert, A. (eds.): Mechanism of Inflammation. Montreal, Acta, Inc., 1953.
31. Erslev, A.: Antibody in lymphocytes from hyperimmunized rabbits. J. Immunol., 67:281, 1951.
32. Fagraeus, A.: Antibody production in relation to the development of plasma cells. Acta med. scandinav. (Suppl.), 264, 1948.
    Fagraeus, A.: Plasma cellular reaction and its relation to the formation of antibodies *in vitro.* J. Immunol., 58:1, 1948.
33. Favour, C. B., Atlas, T. L., Levine, M. I. and Osgood, C. K.: The effect of cortisone on the survival of guinea pigs inoculated with diphtheria toxin. Lab. Invest., 3:1, 1954.
34. Favour, C. B.: Comparative immunology and the phylogeny of homotransplantation. Ann. N. Y. Acad. Sc., 73:590, 1958.
35. Favour, C. B.: Treatment of low-resistance syndromes. J. Am. Geriat. Soc., 7:184, 1959.
36. Fell, H. B. and Brieger, E. M.: Effect of phagocytosis on the growth and survival of avian tubercle bacilli in embryonic chicken tissue cultivated *in vitro.* J. Hyg., 54:359, 1947.
37. Felton, L. D. and Bailey, G. H.: Biological significance of the soluble specific substances of pneumococci. J. Infect. Dis., 38:131, 1926.
38. Fischel, E. E.: Adrenal hormones and the development of antibody and hypersensitivity. In Shwartzman, G. (ed.): The Effect of ACTH and Cortisone upon Infection and Resistance. New York, Columbia University Press, 1953, pp. 56-71.
39. Flemming, A.: On a remarkable bacteriolytic element found in tissues and secretions. Proc. Roy. Soc. (London), 93:306, 1922.
40. Fred, L., Levin, M. H., Rivo, J. B. and Barrett, T. F.: Development of active pul-

monary tuberculosis during ACTH and cortisone therapy. J.A.M.A., *147*:242, 1951.
41. Furness, G.: Effect of cortisone on the macrophages of different species of animal. J. Bacteriol., 77:461, 1959.
42. Gell, P. G. H. and Hinde, I. T.: Observations on histology of Arthus reaction and its relation to other known types of skin hypersensitivity. Internat. Arch. Allergy, 5:23, 1954.
43. Gell, P. G. H.: Histology of allergic lesions in rabbits and the effect of cortisone. Internat. Arch. Allergy, 6:326-336, 1955.
44. Germuth, F. G., Nedzel, G. A., Ohinger, B. and Oyama, J.: Anatomic and histological changes in rabbits with experimental hypersensitivity treated with compound E and ACTH. Proc. Soc. Exper. Biol. & Med., 76:177, 1951.
45. Glaser, R. J., Berry, J. W., Loeb, L. H. and Wood, W. B., Jr.: Effect of cortisone in streptococcal lymphadenitis and pneumonia. J. Lab. & Clin. Med., 38:363, 1951.
46. Good, R. A.: Agammaglobulinemia, a provocative experiment of nature. Bull. Ninn. Hosp., 26:1, 1959.
47. Goodpasture, E. W.: Use of embryo chick in investigation of certain pathogenic problems. South. M. J., *26*:418, 1933.
48. Goodpasture, E. W.: Concerning the pathogenesis of typhoid fever. Am. J. Path., *13*:175, 1937.
49. Goodpasture, E. W.: Cell-parasite relationship in bacterial and virus infection (Alvarenga Prize lecture). Tr. & Stud. Coll. Physicians Philadelphia, 9:11, 1941.
50. Gordon, A. S. and Katsh, G. F.: The relation of the adrenal cortex to the structure and phagocytic activity of the macrophagic system. Ann. N. Y. Acad. Sc., 52:1, 1949.
51. Gregoire, C.: Sur le mécanisme de l'atrophie thymique déclenchée par les hormones sexuelles. Arch. internat. pharmacodyn., 70:45, 1945.
52. Harris, H. and Barclay, W. R.: A method of measuring the respiration of animal cells *in vitro*, with some observations on the macrophages of the rabbit. Brit. J. Exper. Path., 36:592, 1955.
53. Harris, T. N. and Harris, S.: Suppression of transferred lymph node cells in neonatal rabbits by the injection of leukocytes. Ann. N. Y. Acad. Sc., 87:156, 1960.
54. Hart, P. D'A. and Rees, R. J.: Enhancing effect of cortisone on tuberculosis in the mouse. Lancet, 2:391, 1950.
55. Hayes, S. P. and Dougherty T. F.: Studies on local antibody production; demonstration of agglutination by lymphocytes. J. Immunol., *73*:95, 1954.
56. Hiatt, R. B., Flood, C., Karush, A. and Engle, C.: The role of the granulocyte as the source of lysozyme in ulcerative colitis. J. Clin. Invest., *31*:721, 1952.
57. Hull, W. and White, A.: Effect of adrenocorticotrophic hormone on phosphorus metabolism of lymphoid tissue. Endocrinology, 51:210, 1952.
58. Jedeikin, L. A. and White, A.: *In vitro* and *in vivo* effects of steroids on glucose oxidation and respiration by normal and malignant lymphoid tissue. Endocrinology, *63*:226, 1958.
59. Kass, E. H. and Finland, M.: Effect of ACTH on induced fever. New Engl. J. Med., *243*:693, 1950.
60. Kass, E. H. and Finland, M.: The Effect of ACTH and Cortisone upon Infection and Resistance. New York, Columbia University Press, 1953.
61. Kass, E. H. and Finland, M.: Adrenocortical hormones in infection and immunity. Ann. Rev. Microbiol., 7:361, 1953.
62. Kass, G. H.: Hypothermia following cortisone administration. Am. J. Med., *18*:146, 1955.
63. Kelepser, R. G. and Nungester, W. J.: The effect of alcohol upon the chemotactic response of leukocytes. J. Infect. Dis., 65:196, 1939.
64. Keuning, F. J. and van der Slikke, L. B.: Role of immature plasma cells, lymphoblasts, and lymphocytes in the formation of antibodies, as established in tissue culture experiments. J. Lab. & Clin. Med., 36:167, 1950.
65. Kerby, C. P., Holland, H. C. and Martin, S. P.: Quantitative estimation of the removal of bacteria from the blood by the various organs of the immunized animal. J. Immunol., *64*:123, 1950.
66. Ketchel, M. M., Favour, C. B. and Sturgis, S. H.: *In vitro* action of hydrocortisone on leucocyte migration. J. Exper. Med., *107*:211, 1958.
67. Kindred, J. E.: Histologic changes occurring in hemopoietic organs of albino rats after single injections of 2-chloroethyl vesicants; quantitative study. Arch. Path., *43*:253, 1947.

68. Kirchheimer, W. F., Hess, A. R. and Spears, R. G.: Attempts at passive transfer of tuberculin type of sensitivity with living granulocytes. Am. Rev. Tuberc., *64*:516, 1951.
69. Kit, S. and Barron, E. S. G.: Effect of adrenal cortical hormones on incorporation of C^{14} into the protein of lymphatic cells. Endocrinology, *52*:1, 1953.
70. Kit, S., Bacila, M. and Barron, E. S. G.: The incorporation of P^{32} into the nucleic acid in lymphatic cells *in vitro;* effect of adrenal cortical hormones (compound F). Biochim. et biophys. acta, *13*:516, 1954.
71. Kligman, A. M., Baldridge, G. D., Rebell, G. and Pillsbury, D. M.: The effect of cortisone on the pathologic responses of guinea pigs infected cutaneously with fungi, viruses and bacteria. J. Lab. & Clin. Med., *37*:615, 1951.
72. Larson, D. L. and Tomlinson, L. J.: Quantitative antibody studies in man; antibody response in leukemia and other malignant lymphomata. J. Clin. Invest., *32*::317, 1953.
73. Lawrence, H. S.: The delayed type of allergic inflammatory response. Am. J. Med., *20*:428, 1956.
74. Lawrence, H. S. and Pappenheimer, A. M., Jr.: Transfer of delayed hypersensitivity to diphtheria toxin in man. J. Exper. Med., *104*:321, 1956.
75. Leblond, C. P. and Segal, G.: Differentiation between the direct and indirect effects of roentgen rays upon the organs of normal and adrenalectomized rats. Am. J. Roentgenol., *47*:302, 1942.
76. Long, D. A. and Miles, A. A.: Opposite action of thyroid and adrenals in allergic hypersensitivity. Lancet, *1*:492, 1950.
77. Long, D. A.: The influence of corticosteroids on immunological response to bacterial infections. Internat. Arch. Allergy, *10*:5, 1957.
78. Long, J. B. and Favour, C. B.: The ability of ACTH and cortisone to alter delayed type bacterial hypersensitivity. Bull. Johns Hopkins Hosp., *87*:186, 1950.
79. Lurie, M. B., Zappasodi, P., Dannemberg, A. M., Jr. and Swartz, I. B.: Constitutional factors in resistance to infection; the effect of cortisone on the pathogenesis of tuberculosis. Science, *113*:234, 1951.
80. Lurie, M. B., Abramson, S. and Heppleston, A. G.: On the response of genetically resistant and susceptible rabbits to the quantitative inhalation human type tubercle bacilli and the nature of resistance to tuberculosis. J. Exper. Med., *95*:119, 1952.
81. Lurie, M. B., Zappasodi, P., Dannemberg, A. M., Jr. and Cardona-Lynch, E.: The effect of cortisone and ACTH on the pathogenesis of tuberculosis. Ann. N. Y. Acad. Sc., *56*:779, 1953.
82. Lurie, M. B.: On the role of hormones in experimental tuberculosis. Adv. Tuberc. Res., *6*:18, 1955.
83. Marinelarena, R.: The effects of various chemical substances and bacteria on the glycolytic and respiratory activities of leukocytes. Thesis, University of Michigan, 1950.
84. Martin, S. P., Kerby, G. P. and Holland, B. C.: A method for measuring removal of bacteria from the blood by the various organs of the intact animal. Proc. Soc. Exper. Biol. & Med., *72*:63, 1949.
85. McCleod, C.: The mode of action of mucin in experimental meningococcus infection; effect of mucin upon the defense mechanism of the mouse. Am. J. Hyg., *34*:Sc. B. 50, 1941.
86. McCutcheon, M.: Chemotaxis in leucocytes. Physiol. Rev., *26*:319, 1946.
87. McNeil, C.: Cellular changes in rabbits during antibody formation; multiple antigen injection. J. Immunol., *65*:359, 1950.
88. Michael, M., Jr. and Whorton, C. M.: Delay of the early inflammatory response by cortisone. Proc. Soc. Exper. Biol. & Med., *76*:754, 1951.
89. Mirsky, A. E.: Chromosomes and nucleoproteins. Adv. Enzymol., *3*:1, 1943.
90. Miyakawa, M.: The lymphatic system of germ-free guinea pigs, Ann. N. Y. Acad. Sc., *78*:221, 1959.
91. Murphy, J. B. and Strum, E.: The lymphoid tissue and antibody formation. Proc. Soc. Exper. Biol. & Med., *66*:303, 1947.
92. Myrvik, Q. and Weiser, R. S.: Studies on antibacterial factors in mammalian tissues and fluids. J. Immunol., *74*:9, 1955.
93. Nungester, W. J. and Ames, A. M.: The relationship between ascorbic acid and phagocytic activity. J. Infect. Dis., *83*:50, 1948.
94. Nungester, W. J.: Mechanism of man's resistance to infectious diseases. Bact. Rev., *15*:105, 1951.

95. Osgood, C. K. and Favour, C. B.: The effect of adrenocorticotrophic hormone on inflammation due to tuberculin hypersensitivity and turpentine and on circulating antibody levels. J. Exper. Med., 94:415, 1951.
96. Payne, R.: The association of febrile transfusion reactions with leuko-agglutinins. Vox Sanguinis, 2:233, 1957.
97. Puck, T. T., Marcus, P. J. and Cucuira, S. J.: Clonal growth of mammalian cells in vitro. J. Exper. Med., 103:273, 1956.
98. Ragan, C., Howes, E. L., Plotz, C. M., Meyer, C. K. and Blunt, J. W.: Effect of cortisone on production of granulation tissue in the rabbit. Proc. Soc. Exper. Biol. & Med., 72:718, 1949.
99. Rauch, H. C., Loomis, M. E., Johnson, M. E. and Favour, C. B.: In vitro suppression of polymorphonuclear leucocyte and lymphocyte glycolysis by cortisol. Endocrinology. (In press.)
100. Rebuck, J. W. and Mellinger, R. C.: Interruption by topical cortisone of leucocyte cycles in acute inflammation in man. Ann. N. Y. Acad. Sc., 56:715, 1953.
101. Recant, L., Ott, W. H. and Fischel, E. E.: Antipyretic effect of cortisone. Proc. Soc. Exper. Biol. & Med., 75:264, 1950.
102. Reiss, E., Martens, E. and Ehrich, W. E.: Agglutination of bacteria by lymphoid cells in vitro. Proc. Soc. Exper. Biol. & Med., 74:732, 1950.
103. Rich, A. R., Lewis, M. R. and Wintrobe, M. M.: The activity of the lymphocyte in the body's reaction to foreign protein, as established by the identification of the acute splenic tumor cell. Bull. Johns Hopkins Hosp., 65:311, 1939.
104. Robertson, J. S.: An analysis of the effects of $\beta\beta'$-dichloro-diethyl methylamine hydrochloride and of formalin on the weight of the lymphoid organs of intact and adrenalectomized mice. J. Path. & Bact., 61:619, 1949.
105. Rous, P.: The relative reaction within living mammalian tissues. J. Exper. Med., 41:460, 1925.
106. Rundles, R. W., Coonrad, E. V. and Arends, T.: Serum proteins in leukemia. Am. J. Med., 16:842, 1954.
107. Selye, H.: The general adaptation syndrome and the diseases of adaptation. J. Clin. Endocrinol., 6:117, 1946.
108. Sieracki, J. C.: The neutrophilic leukocyte. Ann. N. Y. Acad. Sc., 59:690, 1955.
109. Spain, D. M. and Molomut, N.: Effect of cortisone on the development of tuberculous lesions in guinea pigs and their modification by streptomycin therapy. Am. Rev. Tuberc., 62:337, 1950.
110. Sterzl, J.: The demonstration and biological properties of the tissue precursor of serum antibodies. Folia Biologica (Prague), 1:193, 1955.
111. Sterzl, J. and Hrubesoua, M.: The transfer of antibody formation by means of nucleoprotein fractions to nonimmunized recipients. Folia Biologica (Prague), 2:21, 1956.
112. Taliaferro, W. H.: Functions of the spleen in immunity. Am. J. Trop. Med. & Hyg., 5:391, 1956.
113. Tompkins, E. H.: Reaction of the reticuloendothelial cells to subcutaneous injections of cholesterol; experimetal animals: mice. Arch. Path., 42:299, 1946.
114. Tompkins, E. H.: The response of monocytes to adrenal cortical extract. J. Lab. & Clin. Med., 39:365, 1952.
115. Tullis, J. L.: Blood Cells and Plasma Proteins. New York, Academic Press, 1953, p. 265.
116. Turner, T. B. and Hollander, D. H.: Cortisone in experimental syphilis. Bull. Johns Hopkins Hosp., 87:505, 1950.
117. Wesslen, T.: Studies on the role of lymphocytes in antibody formation. Acta dermat. et venereol., 32:265, 1952.
118. Wintrobe, M. M.: Clinical Hematology. Philadelphia, Lea and Febiger, 1956, pp. 29-78.
119. Wood, W. B., Jr., Smith, M. R., Perry, W. D. and Berry, J. W.: Studies on cellular immunology of acute bacteremia; intravascular leucocytic reaction and surface phagocytosis. J. Exper. Med., 94:521, 1951.
120. Wood, W. B., Jr.: The pathogenesis of fever. Am. J. Med., 18:351, 1955.
121. Wyman, L. C., Fulton, G. P. and Shulman, M.: Direct observations on the circulation in the hamster cheek pouch in adrenal insufficiency and experimental hypercorticalism. Ann. N. Y. Acad. Sc., 56:643, 1953.
122. Zanaty, A. F.: Erythrokonten und Erythropoese bei der biermerschen Anamie und bei den Embryonen. Virchows Arch. f. path. Anat., 293:794, 1934.

Modification of the Leukocyte
Response in Man by ACTH

JOHN W. REBUCK, R. W. SMITH, JR.
and RAYMOND C. MELLINGER

Henry Ford Hospital, Detroit

The leukocyte response in man was studied in a series of *in vivo* samplings of the cellular exudates obtained in adults with skin window preparations.[7] The lesions were prepared by scraping away the epithelium from an area 3 mm. in diameter on the volar surface of the forearm; the trauma of the technique marked the beginning of the inflammatory cycle and served as the inflammatory excitant. In addition, a nonpyogenic antigen (triple typhoid vaccine, diptheria toxoid, old tuberculin or egg white) in 0.05 ml. amounts was applied, and the lesion was covered with a sterile cover slip and surgical tape. Leukocytes of the inflammatory exudate migrated to the under surface of the cover slip within an hour, after which time the cover slip was removed and consecutive new cover slips were placed over the same lesion at timed intervals at approximately 3,5,7,9,12,14,16,21 and 24 hours of inflammation. The cover slips collected from each lesion were air-dried and stained like blood smears or histochemically. The lesions were prepared in duplicate in 12 healthy control volunteers, in 11 patients before and concurrent with the administration of corticotropin in customary clinical dosages,[10] and in 12 human volunteers in whom one of the sister lesions contained topical cortisone[8] (Compound E) 25 mg. per ml. in normal saline or topical hydrocortisone (Compound F).

The 24 lesions in the control volunteers and the majority of the 22 lesions studied in patients before the administration of corticotropin were characterized by an early phase (1 to 8 hours) of increasing neutrophilic leukocytic migrations coupled with mobilization of the few available tissue macrophages in the area. In the middle phase (8 to 14 hours) the neutrophilic leukocytes were joined by increasing numbers of lymphocytes (Fig. 1) which started a gradual hypertrophy of their cell bodies (Fig. 3) while the neutrophils conversely underwent loss of their peripheral cytoplasm and shrinkage of their nuclei. The hypertrophying lymphocytes and tissue macrophages avidly ingested the neutrophilic cytoplasmic fragments. In the third phase (14 to 24 hours) the lymphocytic nuclei enlarged gradually, with breaking down of their coarser chromatin blocks into finer and finer chromatin pieces while their cell bodies continued to increase in size until finally it was difficult to distinguish the macrophages arising from the lymphocytes from those of tissue origin. As macrophages predominated in almost pure culture at 24 hours, the neutrophils completed their process of disintegration.

In the 22 lesions studied concurrent with the administration of corticotropin, in all but two there was a marked depression of lymphocytic participation in the middle phase (8 to 14 hours). Figure 1 depicts the seventh hour of inflammation in the lesion of a patient with periarteritis nodosa prior to therapy with corticotropin. Somewhat precociously, the

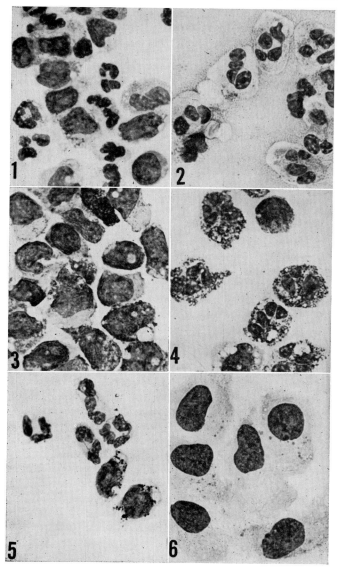

Fig. 1. Pretreatment. Seven hours of inflammation in man. Exudate rich in lymphocytes and neutrophils. May-Grunwald-Giemsa. × 1100.

Fig. 2. Same patient as Figure 1, treated with ACTH. Seven hours of inflammation. Note lack of lymphocyte migration. May-Grunwald-Giesma. × 1100.

Fig. 3. Pretreatment. Ten hours of inflammation in man. Lymphocytes positive for verdoperoxidase. Peroxidase-May-Grunwald-Giemsa. × 1100.

Fig. 4. Same patient as Figure 3, treated with ACTH. Ten hours of inflammation. Depletion of lymphocytes. Peroxidase-May-Grunwald-Giemsa. × 1100.

Fig. 5. Depression of leukocytic phagocytic ability in patient treated with ACTH. Note small number of ingested carbon particles. Twelve hours of inflammation in man. May-Grunwald-Giemsa. × 1100.

Fig. 6. Massed histiocyte response at 5.75 hours of inflammation in a patient with Boeck's sarcoid treated with ACTH. May-Grunwald-Giemsa. × 1100.

lymphocytes have already made their appearance in the lesion; nine lymphocytes are depicted here. In addition, an eosinophil and seven neutrophils can be seen. The neutrophilic leukocytes have lost the cytoplasm outside their nuclear lobes, and their nuclear lobes present some pyknosis. Figure 2 depicts the seventh hour of inflammation in the same patient concurrent with corticotropin therapy. In addition to the lack of lymphocytic migration, a peculiar edematous change has been produced in the responding neutrophilic leukocytes. In another patient studied prior to corticotropin therapy the inflammatory response depicted in Figure 3, the tenth hour of inflammation, was marked by the presence of increasing numbers of lymphocytes with the cell bodies of a few undergoing growth. This preparation has been prepared histochemically for verdoperoxidase and shows the customary positivity of lymphocytes for this reaction which they elaborate after a brief sojourn in the field of inflammation;[9] the dark verdoperoxidase-positive granules are best seen in the lymphocytes in the lower right portion of this illustration. Figure 4, in the same patient at the same tenth hour of inflammation concurrent with corticotropin therapy, depicts the typical lymphocytic depletion of the middle inflammatory phase. One lymphocyte which is peroxidase-positive is found amid the swollen, vacuolated neutrophils, which are also verdoperoxidase-positive. Phagocytic activity of the exudative cell types can be tested for at any stage in the inflammatory cycle by application of a small amount of India ink to the experimental lesion. In the control lesions and in those prior to therapy (not illustrated), the neutrophilic leukocytes, lymphocytes, enlarging lymphocytes, monocytes (if present), and macrophages are all quickly filled with the carbon particles.[9] In still a third patient studied, concurrent with corticotropin therapy (Fig. 5) the twelfth hour of inflammation is marked by a paucity of lymphocytes (although two are shown here) together with a marked suppression of phagocytic ability on the part of those exudative cells which are still capable of responding. The occasional lymphocytes to be found have ingested a few carbon particles, but the neutrophils show greatly depressed phagocytic powers. Not only, then, is there a depression of potential macrophages but the phagocytes that do respond show decreased phagocytic ability. In a small series of lesions studied in patients with Boeck's sarcoid, large masses of macrophages composed most of the exudative cells at 5.75 hours of inflammation, a time of neutrophilic predominance in control lesions. The peculiar massed macrophage response at 5.75 hours of inflammation persisted with corticotropin therapy (Fig. 6).

A similar study was made of the cytology of the sister lesions in the 12 human volunteers treated with topical cortisone or hydrocortisone. The same retardation and incompleteness of the leukocytic sequences were manifest in marked depression of lymphocytic participation at the 8 to 14 hour period of inflammation. Similarly, there was inhibition of phagocytic activity of the neutrophilic leukocytes as well as depression of phagocytic cells or those potentially phagocytic—that is, the lymphocytes, enlarging lymphocytes and resultant macrophages.

Riis,[11] employing the skin window method of study, noted a reduced emigration of macrophages in cases of myeloid leukemia treated with corticotropin or corticosteroid medication, although the hormone therapy did not appear to be the sole cause of macrophage reduction. Similarly, in a patient with prurigo, the lesions after corticotropin showed a lower number of macrophages than those before therapy, although no reduction was noted in a patient with Felty's syndrome similarly followed. Boggs[2] observed that long-term prednisone therapy did not alter the character of the exudate in patients with chronic lymphocytic leukemia, a finding to be expected from the prior observations of Dougherty that cortisol, which is a normal regulatory hormone of lymphatic cell growth and differentiation, is catabolized and converted to ineffective lymphocytolytic products by the lymphocytic leukemic cell.[3] It has been shown definitely that cortisone does kill lymphocytes *in vitro*[12] but in our affected preparations there was no evidence of lymphocytolysis; instead there was failure of lymphocytic migration to the inflammatory site. Eyring and Dougherty[4] and Berliner and Dougherty[1] have suggested that inflammation produces an autocatalytic cell destruction in which the breakdown of one cell leads to the breakdown of another through destructive products liberated by the broken cell. Cortisol can stop the catalytic process of cell destruction by making the fibroblasts resistant to the destructive effect of substances that bring about their swelling and lysis. Our observations after corticotropin therapy (Figs. 2 and 4), and especially in the sister lesions treated with topical hydrocortisone, that the neutrophils were edematous and failed to lose their cytoplasm peripheral to their nuclear lobes may similarly be said to demonstrate production of resistant neutrophilic leukocytes. Priest and his associates[6] reported increased basophilic granulocytic migrations in patients with ulcerative colitis; one of the few exceptions was in such a patient under therapy with corticosteroids. Nicol and Bilbey,[5] in their recent report on the effect of various steroids on the phagocytic activity of the reticuloendothelial system, found that cortisone acetate had a strong depressant effect on the phagocytosis of particulate carbon in mice.

From the foregoing there emerges the view that since lymphocytic dissolution is directly effected by cortisol, although deficiency of cortisol at the inflammatory site may lead to reduction in phagocytic activity conversely, unphysiologic excess at the local inflammatory site in man leads to suppression of lymphocytogenous macrophage participation and over-all depression of leukocytic phagocytic activity. Finally, we have presented a method which will facilitate the extended studies of related hormonal effects on host defense mechanisms in man which are so sorely needed.

REFERENCES

1. Berliner, D. L. and Dougherty, T. F.: Influence of reticuloendothelial and other cells on the metabolic fate of steroids. Ann. N. Y. Acad. Sc., 88:14-29, 1960.
2. Boggs, D. R.: The cellular composition of inflammatory exudates in human leukemias. Blood, 15:466-475, 1960.
3. Dougherty, T. F.: In Rebuck, J. W. (ed.): The Leukemias: Etiology, Pathophysiology and Treatment. New York, Academic Press, 1957, pp. 293-298.
4. Eyring, H. and Dougherty, T. F.: Molecular mechanisms in inflammation and stress. Am. Scientist, 43:457, 1955.
5. Nicol, T. and Bilbey, D. L. J.: The effect of various steroids on the phagocytic activity of the reticuloendothelial system. In Heller, J. H. (ed.): Reticuloendothelial Structure and Function. New York, Ronald Press Co., 1960, pp. 301-320.
6. Priest, R. J., Rebuck, J. W. and Havey, G. T.: A new qualitative defect of leukocyte function in ulcerative colitis. Gastroenterology, 38:715-731, 1960.
7. Rebuck, J. W. and Crowley, J. H.: A method of studying leukocytic functions *in vivo*. Ann. N. Y. Acad. Sc., 59:757-805, 1955.
8. Rebuck, J. W. and Mellinger, R. C.: Interruption by topical cortisone of leukocytic cycles in acute inflammation in man. Ann. N. Y. Acad. Sc., 56:715-732, 1953.
9. Rebuck, J. W., Monto, R. W., Monaghan, E. A. and Riddle, J. M.: Potentialities of

the lymphocyte, with an additional reference to its dysfunction in Hodgkin's disease. Ann. N. Y. Acad. Sc., 73 (3):8, 1958.

10. Rebuck, J. W., Smith, R. W., Jr. and Margulis, R. R.: The modification of leukocytic function in human windows by ACTH. Gastroenterology, 19:644-657, 1951.
11. Riis, P.: The Cytology of Inflammatory Exudate. Copenhagen, Munksgaard, 1959.
12. Trowell, O. A.: The lymphocyte. Internat. Rev. Cytol., 7:235-293, 1958.

The Anti-Inflammatory Problem:
The Effects of Corticoids
and of ACTH (Corticotropin)*

VALY MENKIN

University of Kansas City School of Dentistry, Kansas City, Missouri

In 1940 the writer first published his findings on the suppressive effect of adrenal cortical extract on the increase in capillary permeability induced by an exudate or its contained leukotaxine.[2] In 1942 the same suppression was shown to occur with Compound E, which eventually came to be known as cortisone.[3] These were the first experimental observations on the anti-inflammatory property of cortisone. In 1950, subsequent to the brilliant discovery by Hench and Kendall at the Mayo Clinic of the usefulness of cortisone and ACTH in arthritis,[1] our earlier studies on this problem were resumed. We then found that neither adrenal cortical extract nor cortisone repressed appreciably the increase in capillary permeability induced by an acid exudate (Fig. 1).[4] This, however, was readily suppressed by ACTH (Fig. 2).[5] There are thus at least two factors concerned in the mechanism of increased capillary permeability in inflammation:† (1) leukotaxine, predominantly present in the initial or alkaline stage of development of the inflammatory reaction, and (2) another factor termed exudin, present in the later or acid stage (but independent of the pH). Exudin is found to be readily inhibited by ACTH.[5] Crude exudin located in the pseudoglobulin-albumin fraction of acid exudates is thermolabile, nondiffusible and has a nitrogen content of about 10 per cent. Its liberation by injured cells reasonably explains the continuous seepage of fluid into the extracapillary spaces throughout the duration of an acute inflammation. In contrast to leukotaxine, exudin fails to induce any appreciable migration of leukocytes. Recently, observations have been undertaken in order to obtain further insight into the nature of exudin. Differential centrifugation of acid exudates indicates the presence of exudin in the soluble phase or "S_1" fraction.[14] This component displays the biological properties of exudin. It induces increased capillary

* These studies were aided by grants from the U. S. Public Health Service, Bethesda, Maryland.

† Conceivably there are also other factors involved in the mechanism of increased capillary permeability, such as, for instance, the PF/Dil factor described in serum by Miles and associates,[18, 20] or the globulin recently studied by Spector.[19]

permeability as measured by the local accumulation of trypan blue into treated cutaneous areas in rabbits. The augmented permeability is suppressed by ACTH but not by cortisone.[14]

These studies on the purification of exudin by differential centrifugation have been pursued[16] (see scheme of extraction). In brief, an acid exudate is centrifuged at 2000 r.p.m. The resulting supernatant is centrifuged at 3190 $\times$ g for about 20 minutes. The sediment termed "mitochondrial" fraction is discarded. The second supernatant is centrifuged at 21,600 $\times$ g in an angle centrifuge for about one hour. The final resulting supernatant, termed the "S_2" fraction, contains exudin.[16] It is dialysed through cellophane tubing (size 20/32) against distilled water in a refrigerator at about 9° C. for several days. The indiffusible "S_2" fraction is adjusted to a pH varying from about 3.2 to 4.5 with N acetic acid. A precipitate results, which can be

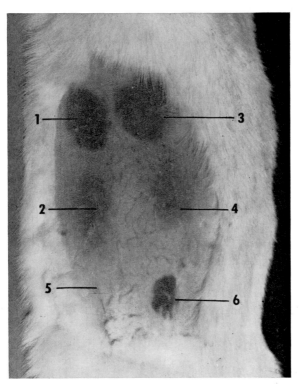

Fig. 1. Rabbit 4-94. Inability of cortisone and adrenal cortical extract to affect acid exudates. The darkly stained areas in the figure represent the accumulation of injected trypan blue from the circulating blood owing to the increased local capillary permeability.

Area 1: 0.4 cc. of a rabbit exudate at pH 6.25 obtained from a 41-hour inflamed peritoneal cavity of Rabbit 4-98 by the intraperitoneal injection of 2 cc. of physiological saline containing 0.5 cc. of glacial acetic acid.

Area 2: 0.5 cc. from mixture of 0.5 cc. of Rabbit 4-98 exudate at pH 6.25 plus 10 mg. cortisone suspended in 0.5 cc. of saline.

Area 3: 0.5 cc. of above rabbit exudate from Rabbit 4-98 at pH 6.25.

Area 4: 0.5 cc. from mixture of 0.5 cc. of above rabbit exudate at pH 6.25 plus 0.5 cc. of Upjohn adrenal cortex extract.

Area 5: 0.5 cc. of 10 mg. of cortisone suspended in 0.5 cc. of saline.

Area 6: 0.5 cc. of Upjohn adrenal cortext extract.

(From Menkin: Am. J. Physiol., *166*:509, 1951.)

dissolved at about pH 7 with dilute NaOH. This fraction displays the biological properties of exudin, as described above. Heating to boiling fails to induce coagulation and leaves the ability to increase capillary permeability essentially unaltered. The ninhydrin reaction is positive, but it may at times be biuret negative. DU spectrophotometric absorption indicates a peak at 260 to 265 mμ that still tends to persist at 278 to 280 mμ.[15, 16] This is consistent with the possibility that this fraction of exudin contains nucleo-

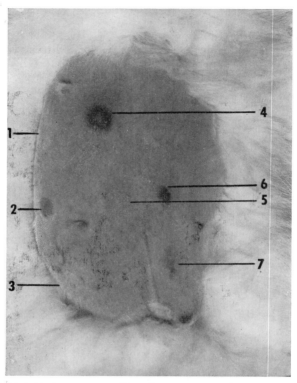

Fig. 2. Rabbit 4-49. Suppressing effect of ACTH on exudin. The darkly stained areas in the figure represent the accumulation of injected trypan blue from the circulating blood owing to the increased local capillary permeability.

Area 1: 1.44 mg. ACTH in 0.4 cc. of physiological saline.

Area 2: 0.2 to 0.3 cc. of canine exudate at about pH 6.5.

Area 3: 0.5 cc. of physiological saline.

Area 4: 0.5 cc. of canine exudate at pH 6.7 to 6.8.

Area 5: 0.5 cc. from mixture of 1.8 mg. of ACTH in 0.5 cc. of physiological saline plus 0.5 cc. of canine exudate at pH 6.7 to 6.8.

Area 6: 0.35 cc. from mixture of 0.5 cc. of canine exudate at pH 6.7 to 6.8 plus 0.5 cc. of Upjohn adrenal cortext extract.

Area 7: 0.5 cc. of Upjohn adrenal cortex extract.

(From Menkin: Am. J. Physiol., *166*:518, 1951.)

tide and peptide linkages. Chromatographic studies also substantiate both the presence of peptides and of nucleotide-like material in the active "S$_2$" fraction. The collected chromatographic data appear in Table 1. Inactivation by aminotripeptidase and also by ribonuclease adds further support to the view that exudin is a *nucleopeptide*.[16]

SCHEME OF EXTRACTION OF EXUDIN BY DIFFERENTIAL CENTRIFUGATION

Exudate (acid pH)
↓
Centrifuge 2000 rev./min. (10 min.)
↓
Supernatant
↓
Centrifuge 3190 g (20 min.)
↓
Supernatant
↓
Centrifuge 21,600 g (1 hr.)
↓
Supernatant ("S₂" fraction)
↓
Dialyse against H₂O in refrigerator (2 days)
↓
Indiffusible "S₂" fraction
↓
Adjust to pH 4 to 4.5 with acetic acid
↓
Centrifuge
↓
Precipitate
↓
Redissolve with dilute NaOH at pH 7.0 (approx.)
↓
Nucleopeptide (*Exudin*)

TABLE 1. CHROMATOGRAPHIC STUDIES OF HYDROLYSED NUCLEOPEPTIDE FROM "S₂" FRACTION

NUMBER OF CHROMATOGRAMS	9	8
	Amino acids identified and frequency of recovery ( )	Purine, pyrimidine and derivatives identified and frequency of recovery ( )
	taurine (5)	guanine (5)
	tyrosine (4)	adenine (5)
	cystine (3)	uridine (5)
	tryptophane (3)	cytidine (4)
	glutamine and glutamic acid (3)	uridylic acid (3)
	a-alanine (3)	cytidylic acid (2)
	threonine (2)	uracil (1)
	serine (2)	adenosine (1)
	valine (2)	guanine deoxyriboside (1)
		5-methyl-cytosine (1)
		thymine (1)

Besides being obtained as a nucleopeptide as stated above,[16] exudin can be obtained also by repeated precipitations with ammonium sulfate at one-third saturation.[4] It can at times be crystallized by the addition of N acetic acid to the pseudoglobulin-albumin fraction of an exudate.[8] The suppressing effect of ACTH on exudin seems to be a direct effect.[12, 13] This does not controvert the classic view that ACTH acts via the adrenal cortex. In inflammation, however, there is such an extensive increase in local capillary permeability that some of the ACTH injected into the blood stream enters the site of an acute inflammation, and once there it can act directly on exudin. Furthermore, the same type of activity is seen in adrenalectomized rats injected with exudin and ACTH.[12, 13] The question of any impurity, such as vasopressin, in the commercial ACTH preparation utilized has recently been eliminated by the use of Li's α-corticotropin.[12] With his presumably pure fraction of ACTH we have obtained essentially the same inhibitory effect as with commercial ACTH.[12, 13]

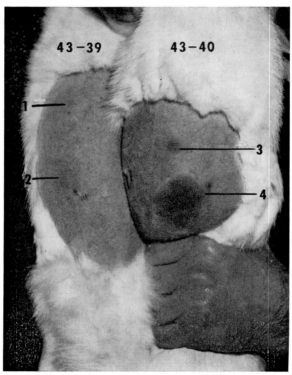

Fig. 3. Rabbits 43-39 and 43-40. The skin of the abdomen of two rabbits. Rabbit 43-39 received 32 mg. of corticotropin (ACTH) in 4 cc. of saline intravenously several minutes prior to the intracutaneous injection in Area 1 of 0.5 cc. of exudate taken from the pleural cavity of another rabbit, which in turn had received four intravenous injections of cortisone (Merck) aggregating to about 115 mg. of the hormone. In Area 2, 0.5 cc. of exudate from the pleural cavity of an untreated control rabbit was injected. Following the intracutaneous injections of exudate 6 cc. of 1 per cent trypan blue in saline was injected intravenously, and the accumulation of dye in the respective area was subsequently studied by the amount of local staining of the treated tissue. In Rabbit 43-40 the same procedure was followed as in Rabbit 43-39 without, however, any preliminary intravenous injection of corticotropin (ACTH), and only 4 cc. of saline was administered in the circulation. It is clear that the cortisone-containing exudate in Area 3 is much less stained than the control Area 4. Evidently the cortisone in the exudate in Area 3 has to a great extent suppressed the increase in capillary permeability, as gauged by the passage of trypan blue in the area when compared to Area 4. The suppressing effect is very pronounced in the ACTH-treated rabbit (Rabbit 43-39) with the additional elimination of any exudin present in the inflammatory exudate by corticotropin (ACTH) in the animal. (From Menkin: Brit. J. Exper. Path., 34:412, 1953.)

Cortisone penetrates from the systemic circulation into the site of an acute inflammation.[6] This can be demonstrated by testing the exudate of a rabbit repeatedly injected intravenously with cortisone, and comparing in another rabbit its reducing effect on the local passage of trypan blue with that of a control exudate (Fig. 3). With the accumulation of the corticoids in an inflamed area there is likewise a suppression of diapedesis.[6] It can also be demonstrated that repeated injections of ACTH into the circulating blood reduce the potency of exudin present at the site of inflammation (Fig. 4).[7]

With the above information at hand, a study was undertaken in an endeavor to determine the anti-inflammatory mechanism. First, it was shown that cortisone tends to suppress cell activity in an invertebrate form.[9] This was done by observing the reduction in the incidence of cell division after

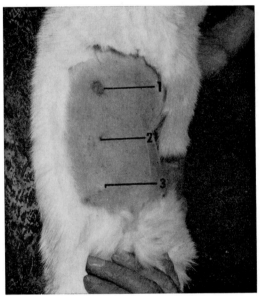

Fig. 4. With the presumable penetration of corticotropin (ACTH) (Armour) into the area of inflammation, the effect of exudin in increasing capillary permeability is suppressed. Rabbit 20-30 was injected intracutaneously in the surface of the abdomen with exudin extracted from the exudate of Dog 1-91 following reinjection of the irritant in its pleural cavity. The exudin was diluted with physiological saline (1:1) and 0.5 cc. of the mixture was injected into the skin of R-20-30 in Area 1. Subsequently, the dog received daily intravascular injections of corticotropin (ACTH) (30 mg. per injection). After three and four such injections of corticotropin (ACTH), the exudate was withdrawn from the pleural cavity and exudin extracted from the respective material obtained in the intervals stated. In Area 2, one sees that after three intravascular injections of ACTH there is hardly any increased capillary permeability induced by the recovered exudin. This suppressing effect is even more pronounced following four intravascular injections of corticotropin (ACTH). The local increase in capillary permeability to trypan blue is wholly inhibited (Area 3). This suppressing effect is not seen in the exudin recovered from the exudate of a dog not injected with corticotropin (ACTH). (From Menkin: Brit. J. Exper. Path., 34:420, 1953, and Internat. Arch. Allergy, 4:131, 1953.)

exposure of sea urchin ova to corticoids prior to their fertilization.[9, 17] The data and interpretation on an invertebrate system, however, cannot be readily transferred to as complicated a process as inflammation in vertebrate animals. Nevertheless, the observation on sea urchins (*Arbacia punctulata*) provided an idea. Is it possible that the anti-inflammatory mechanism is

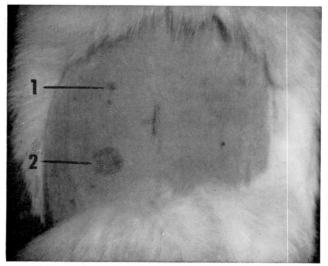

Fig. 5. Rabbit 21-19. Effect of compound F on the increase in capillary permeability caused by leukotaxine. Area 1: Leukotaxine from exudate following two local injections of compound F into the inflamed area. Note the essential suppression of any increased capillary permeability. Area 2: Leukotaxine from the exudate of an untreated inflamed area shows a pronounced increase in capillary permeability. (From Menkin: Science, *120*:1026, 1954, and Internat. Arch. Allergy, *4*:131, 1953.)

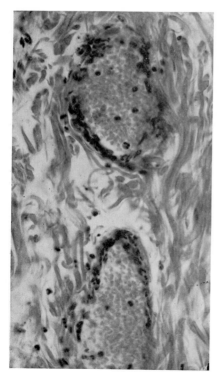

Fig. 6. The effect of leukotaxine in inducing the margination of polymorphonuclear leukocytes about one hour subsequent to the injection of the substance in turn extracted from a sample of canine exudate. The dog had received an injection of turpentine in the right pleural cavity followed by two successive daily injections of saline, each 3 cc. × 400. (From Menkin: Nuevos Conceptos sobre Inflamacion, p. 206. Translation of Newer Concepts of Inflammation, 1st ed., but with an added chapter. Edited and translated by Carlos Tanturi, Buenos Aires, 1955.)

primarily referable to a suppression of cellular activity of injured cells at the site of inflammation, so that now they are incapable of adequately forming the chemical factors that essentially constitute inflammation? Experiments were set up to determine whether detectable or measurable amounts of active leukotaxine or of leukocytosis-promoting factors could be formed by injured cells following repeated injections of hydrocortisone directly into the site of an acute inflammation.[10, 11] Recovered leukotaxine was diminished in its activity (Figs. 5, 6, 7). The leukocytosis-promoting factor was likewise demonstrated to be reduced in its potency.[10, 11] The *in vitro* mixture of hydrocortisone (Compound F) and the LPF fails to reduce the activity of the leukocytosis-promoting factor. This would indicate that the corticoid does not interact with the LPF, but rather that the formation of this factor by the injured cell is actually impaired.

In conclusion, the anti-inflammatory mechanism can be considered at a cellular level. By suppressing the capacity of the injured cell to form the chemical factors involved in inflammation, the inflammatory process is definitely reduced. From the point of view of the writer, it is the factors that are liberated by the injured cells which constitute inflammation. The corticoids appear to suppress the activity of the injured cells in forming these chemical mediators.

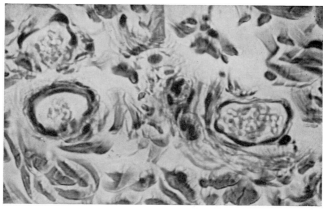

Fig. 7. The effect of two direct injections of compound F into the inflamed area (total amount of injections was 40 mg. of the commercial hydrocortisone into Dog 260T) on the potency of leukotaxine to induce leukocytic migration. Following the two injections of the corticosteroid not only was the increased capillary permeability caused by leukotaxine scarcely to be observed, but there was also no diapedesis of leukocytes (cf. the effect with that in the control, Figure 6). The experimental sample of exudate utilized for leukotaxine extraction was equal in amount to that employed in the control, the effect of which is shown in Figure 6 (× 410). (From Menkin: Science, *120*:1026, 1954.)

REFERENCES

1. Hench, P. S., Kendall, E. C., Slocumb, C. H. and Polley, H. F.: Proc. Staff Meet., Mayo Clin., *24*:181, 1949.
2. Menkin, V.: Am. J. Physiol., *129*:691, 1940.
3. Menkin, V.: Proc. Soc. Exper. Biol. & Med., *51*:39, 1942.
4. Menkin, V.: Am. J. Physiol., *166*:509, 1951.
5. Menkin, V.: Am. J. Physiol., *166*:518, 1951.
6. Menkin, V.: Brit. J. Exper. Path., *34*:412, 1953.
7. Menkin, V.: Brit. J. Exper. Path., *34*:420, 1953.

8. Menkin, V.: Internat. Arch Allergy, *4*:131, 1953.
9. Menkin, V.: Proc. Soc. Exper. Biol. & Med., *82*:189, 1953.
10. Menkin, V.: Science, *120*:1026, 1954.
11. Menkin, V.: Biochemical Mechanisms in Inflammation. Springfield, Ill., Charles C Thomas, 1956.
12. Menkin, V.: Am. J. Physiol., *189*:98, 1957.
13. Menkin, V.: J. Physiol. Path. Gen., *49*:761, 1957.
14. Menkin, V.: Am. J. Path., *34*:921, 1958.
15. Menkin, V.: Fed Proc., *18*:494, 1959.
16. Menkin, V.: Leucotaxine and exudin in relation to inflammation. In Polypeptides Which Affect Smooth Muscles and Blood Vessels. New York, Pergamon Press, Inc., 1960.
17. Menkin, V. and Pepper, M.: Biol. Bull., *107*:316, 1954.
18. Miles, A. A. and Wilhelm, D. L.: Brit J. Exper. Path., *36*:71, 1955.
19. Spector, W. G.: J. Path. & Bact., *72*:367, 1956.
20. Wilhelm, D. L., Mill, P. J. and Miles, A. A.: Brit. J. Exper. Path., *38*:446, 1957.

Steroid Alterations in the Histopathology of Chemically Induced Inflammation

DAVID M. SPAIN

Beth-El Hospital, Brooklyn, New York

Inflammation, as defined by Menkin, is "the complex vascular, lymphatic, and local tissue reaction elicited in higher animals by the presence of micro-organisms or of nonviable irritants." In a broader sense, it is a continuing process and not a single episodic state, so that the histologic appearance at any given time fails to impart a comprehension of the complex dynamics of the continually changing picture. Intimately and, in fact, inseparably related to inflammation is the repair process which has its origins and induction in this inflammatory event.

In the broadest sense, all inflammation is chemically induced. In the narrow sense, it is used in this report to mean that the obvious noxious agent is a nonviable chemical such as oil of turpentine. The use of this type of chemically induced inflammation in studying steroid inhibition has the advantage of not involving antigen-antibody or hypersensitivity mechanisms. Interference with these on the part of the steroids therefore cannot play a significant role in the alterations observed, as would be the case with induced bacterial inflammation. By now the effects of such steroids as cortisone, hydrocortisone, prednisolone and more recently developed compounds on the histopathology of inflammation are well known, having been verified in many different experimental ways and in innumerable human disease entities. Very little can be added to these descriptions. Still requiring considerable clarification are the mechanisms whereby steroids produce these alterations in the histopathology of the inflammation regardless of the method of induction. A fundamental difficulty inherent in this problem is that despite many excellent studies by Menkin as well as by others, a clear understanding of such phenomena occurring in inflammation as the triple reaction alterations in capillary permeability, liquefaction of necrotic tissue and its removal, and the role of such substances as histamine, hyaluronidase, leucotaxine, exudin, necrosin, other polypeptides, globulin factors, nucleosides, nucleotides and 5-hydroxytryptamine still eludes us.

The studies which we originally undertook relative to the influence of cortisone in the inflammatory and repair processes began a decade ago and utilized oil of turpentine to induce inflammation and puncture wounds to study repair.[7]

In the first series of studies, concentrations of turpentine were of such magnitude as to produce an overwhelming inflammatory response which masked any differences that might have been present between the control and cortisone-treated animals. This is mentioned only to emphasize that steroid anti-inflammatory inhibition is only relative to the magnitude and virulence of the noxious agent involved.

In the next series, 0.025 ml. of oil of turpentine was injected subcutaneously over the sternum of mice. Various groups of mice were untreated or pretreated for three days with doses of cortisone ranging from 0.0025 mg. to 1.0 mg. per mouse. Treatment at the various dose levels was continued daily until sacrifice. In these groups and in later studies mice were sacrificed at 2 hours, 6 hours, 24 hours, 48 hours and seven days after induction of inflammation. In later studies mice also received hydrocortisone and prednisolone.

In the wound healing studies similar schedules of cortisone dosage were used. In addition, some animals were not placed on steroids until 48 hours after wounding. Each animal received two standardized circular and symmetrical wounds on its back (technique previously described). Animals were sacrificed daily for seven days.

In other studies estrogens and STH were administered simultaneously to the cortisone-treated animals in both the inflammation and the repair studies. In still others, various materials were applied locally to the wounds in cortisone-treated animals. These materials—a drop of the animal's own blood, hyaluronidase and fibrinogen—were applied as soon as the wounds were induced.

In brief, the following were the histologic findings with the various conditions just mentioned. Beginning with the early phase (two hours) of the inflammation induced by oil of turpentine, a distinct difference was noted between the control and treated animals. In the untreated animals some edema, fibrin, scant numbers of leukocytes and capillary hyperemia with some margination were present at the site of injury. In the treated animals at the same time, only the alterations in the tissue as a result of the injury were noted. These were evidenced by loss of striations and a baked appearance of the striated muscle in this area. Six hours after induction of inflammation there was considerable intensification of the process in the control animals, with a considerable increase in the number of leukocytes. A distinct zone of leukocytes, fibrin and hyperemia was now bordering the injured area. The cortisone-treated animals now exhibited changes similar to those seen in the untreated animals at the two-hour period. As time went on, the treated animals continued to lag in all of the characteristic elements seen histologically in the inflammatory process. This was manifested not only by lesser numbers of granular leukocytes but by diminished numbers of lymphocytes and macrophages as well as considerably less liquefaction necrosis. By the seventh day the injured areas in the control animals were well walled off and sharply delineated from the surrounding uninjured tissue. The wall consisted of an inner dense zone of inflammatory exudate and an outer zone of granulation tissue. In the treated animals the delineation between the original area of injury and surrounding tissue was not nearly so well defined. The leukocytic zone and its granulation tissue layers were sparse and incomplete. Striated muscle peripheral to this revealed areas of coagulation, necrosis and sparse inflammatory cellular infiltrate.[8]

In those animals that received graded doses of cortisone there was no dissociation at the various dose levels between the histologic appearance of the inflammatory process, the extent of wound healing and reduction in splenic size. With the exception of the circulating eosinophil counts, there was in general a relationship between the level of the steroid dose and the degree of inhibition. The method used in these studies and the variations among animals in the same group, however, precluded more precise quantitation.[10]

In the wound healing studies no apparent differences were noted in the degree of fibroblastic proliferation until 48 to 72 hours had elapsed. For this reason, Lattes et al.,[3] after similar studies, concluded that the early phase of the wound healing process was not inhibited by cortisone. However, in the animals in which we delayed giving cortisone until 48 hours after wound induction, there was only slight eventual inhibition of wound healing in contrast to those treated initially. This would indicate that the steroid influence on wound healing affects mechanisms in the earliest phases of the process.

Examination through the seventh day revealed considerable difference in the number of fibroblasts, vascularity and compactness between the treated and untreated animals. The treated animals had altered metachromasia of the ground substance.

No antagonism to the influences of cortisone on inflammation and repair was produced by the simultaneous treatment with either estrogens or STH. Repetition of these studies with hydrocortisone and prednisolone revealed intensified effects.

In addition to reduction in the number of macrophages, further studies in which carbon black particles were injected into the peritoneal cavity revealed a diminution in the phagocytic activity of the macrophages in those animals under the influence of cortisone. In other studies, pledgets of Gelfoam saturated with cholesterol, cholesterol esters and unsaturated fatty acids were placed beneath the skin of mice and rabbits; there was delayed resolution in the cortisone-treated animals, and diminished numbers of macrophages were present at the site of these lesions.

Numerous investigators during the past decade have reported observations based upon different experimental methods that are generally similar to those just described.[1, 2, 5, 6] Considerable clarification, however, is required concerning the precise points at which steroids act to produce these alterations. One of our own studies was of interest relative to this problem. When the animal's own blood was applied as a dressing to the wound immediately upon induction, the rate of wound healing did not appear to be as inhibited by the effects of steroids in comparison with those animals in which this was not done. The application of collodion hyaluronidase or fibrinogen did not affect the rate of wound healing in cortisone-treated animals.[9] It would appear, therefore, that the inhibition of granulation formation is directly related to the suppression of the appearance of cellular or humoral elements at the site of wounding in response to induction of inflammation. It would also indicate that interference with repair begins at the very inception of the process and not several days later, as suggested by others. Further support for this may be inferred from the fact, already mentioned, that delayed cortisone treatment failed to alter significantly the rate of the repair response already established.

SUMMARY

The anti-inflammatory steroids suppress quantitatively all the known elements characteristically seen in the morphology of the acute inflammatory process.

A qualitative alteration is also shown by a depression in phagocytic activity.

There is a direct relationship between the inhibition of the inflammatory and the repair processes. Inhibition appears to be related to the magnitude of the steroid dose administered.

REFERENCES

1. Crepea, S. B., Magnin, G. E. and Seastone, C. V.: Effect of ACTH and cortisone on phagocytosis. Proc. Soc. Exper. Biol. & Med., 77:704, 1951.
2. Dougherty, T. F. and Schneebell, G. L.: Role of cortisone in regulation of inflammation. Proc. Soc. Exper. Biol. & Med., 75:854, 1950.
3. Lattes, R., Blunt, J. W., Jr., Rose, H. M., Jessar, R. A., de Guise, V. and Regan, C.: Lack of cortisone effect in the early stages of inflammation and repair. Am. J. Path., 29:1, 1953.
4. Menkin, V.: The effect of adrenal cortical extract and certain cortical steroids on the inflammatory process. Proc. Soc. Exper. Biol. & Med., 51:39, 1942.
5. Menkin, V.: Further studies on mechanisms of increased capillary permeability in inflammation with the aid of cortisone and ACTH. Proc. Soc. Exper. Biol. & Med., 77:592, 1951.
6. Michael, M. and Whorton, C. M.: Delay of the early inflammatory response by cortisone. Proc. Soc. Exper. Biol. & Med., 76:754, 1951.
7. Spain, D. M., Molomut, N. and Haber, A.: Biological studies on cortisone in mice. Science, 112:335, 1950.
8. Spain, D. M., Molomut, N. and Haber, A.: Studies of the cortisone effects on the inflammatory response. J. Lab. & Clin. Med., 39:383, 1952.
9. Spain, D. M. and Molomut, N.: Studies on the mechanisms of cortisone inhibition of granulation tissue formation. Am. J. Path., 27:755, 1951.
10. Spain, D. M. and Molomut, N.: Effect of cortisone on inflammation in mice. Am. J. Clin. Path., 22:944, 1952.

Panel Discussion

Cutting B. Favour, *Moderator*

Dr. Favour: During the last several days numerous speakers have said that the mechanism of cortisone effect is unknown and then immediately have given an explanation of how cortisone works. The members of this panel are also interested in what cortisone does at the cellular level. I think your orientation so far has been that cortisone affects the influx of cells into various lesions, that it affects these cells individually, and that it affects their function individually. It also controls the liberation of various substances by the cell and controls what these liberated materials may do. Various mechanisms responsible for this process have been postulated, and although they do not explain what goes on at the enzymatic level, they do explain to a degree what goes on at the cellular level. Perhaps we can devote most of our time to these mechanisms.

Dr. Rebuck, why do you think the sarcoid cell does not function properly? What is wrong with this large mononuclear cell that does not allow it to phagocytose certain substances and does not allow it to go through some of the evolutionary phenomena that we see normally in the phagocytic process?

Dr. REBUCK: I think that it does function and I think this is borne out clinically except for the tubercle bacillus, which macrophages have difficulty with at all times. The patient with Boeck's sarcoid has no trouble in defending himself against invasion or infection. I think the defect is that he has an overabundant macrophagic response. As I indicated, there is a hyperactive response to even the smallest lesion, and all these granulomata lead ultimately to scar formation, and eventually there is loss of vital tissue.

Dr. SPAIN: I cannot agree that there is necessarily a hyperactive macrophagic response. If we do not know the nature of the noxious agent or what abnormal substance is present in the body, how can we say there is an over-reaction to it?

Dr. REBUCK: The alveolae are always subject to many intrusions by foreign substances, and I think that in this disease there is a granulomatous response to antigens, which would probably elicit a nongranulomatous response, or at least an insignificant one in normal subjects.

Dr. FAVOUR: Dr. Jean, do you have some comments? What kind of mononuclear cells do you see in the granulomatous walls of the pouches that you create? Do you find the same sequence of cell types that Dr. Rebuck described?

Dr. JEAN: Yes, we see practically the same cell types that Dr. Rebuck showed in his slides.

Dr. FAVOUR: Is this also true of the cells free in the fluid of the pouches?

Dr. JEAN: They are seen primarily in the tissue wall.

Dr. REBUCK: Lest you think that this sequence was first revealed by our studies, I want to point out that the first studies of cellular changes in experimental inflammation were those of Metchnikoff published in Virchow's Archives in 1888. He described the same sequence of events.

Dr. MENKIN: I have been interested for many years in the cellular sequence that Dr. Rebuck showed so well today, and particularly in the mechanism responsible for the acidosis which occurs as the inflammatory reaction progresses. Opie had shown that leukoprotease was a predominant enzyme in the polymorphonuclear leukocytes and that lymphoprotease predominated in the mononuclear phagocytes, and we wondered whether the hydrogen ion concentration was an important conditioning factor for the activity of these cells. Therefore, we studied the pH in relation to the cytological picture. About 1934 we confirmed the fact that polymorphonuclear leukocytes were the predominant cells in the initial stage of inflammation, and found that the pH is alkaline in this phase, being about 7.2 to 7.4. As the reaction progresses the inflammatory exudate becomes acid, and at about pH

7.0 the polymorphonuclear and mononuclear cells are present in approximately equal numbers. As the pH comes down to about 6.8, the polymorphonuclears simply succumb to the effect of the acid pH, and the mononuclear leukocytes, which are much more resistant to an acid pH, predominate. Then, as the pH falls even lower, to about 6.0, all of the leukocytes die and then there is pus; so pus is virtually a function of the hydrogen ion concentration. Now, this is not merely a spurious correlation, because when leukocytes are suspended in buffers of various pH *in vitro* and stained with supravital neutral red stain, the polymorphonuclear leukocytes do not survive when the pH is acid. We have found that this local acidosis is due to glycolysis at the site of inflammation—a true acidosis due to accumulation of lactic acid.

DR. FAVOUR: Dr. Fischel, how do antigen-antibody reactions produce the local lesion of polyarteritis? Can we use presently available information concerning antigen-antibody reactions and postulate whether this lesion is a result of either the immediate or delayed type of reaction as immunologists classify them?

DR. FISCHEL: Clinically periarteritis nodosa certainly looks like an allergic reaction, but if it is, I do not know what the antigen is. I think the experimental disease in animals has been studied by several men on this panel and others who were here in the last few days. If we draw an analogy from various experiments, such as Dixon's recent studies, or even go back to Opie's work in 1924 on the reaction of tissues to antigen-antibody complexes, we find that these complexes act as foreign bodies in a sense and produce an inflammatory reaction. The nature and severity of the process appears to be dependant on the nature of the antigen and its primary toxicity. In addition, I am sure that if this antigen-antibody complex incorporates serum complement into its meshes we have additional tissue destroying factors which may be important, but this is all just a hypothesis and I do not know of any definite, well defined explanation.

DR. FAVOUR: This is Dr. Germuth's general thought, too. In experiments in which he used, in a sense, a sort of gel diffusion technique, allowing antigen and antibodies to diffuse towards each other in the cornea of animals, there was injury to the cellular bundles of the cornea at the site where these met and presumably formed an antigen-antibody complex. This occurred even before leukocytes came into the area, so presumably the complex or resulting reaction was directly toxic. However, we do not know whether this takes place in human disease; we only know that this is true in special experiments in animals.

DR. REBUCK: May I comment on that? I heard Dr. Dixon speak about this point two weeks ago, and his data may help explain the phenomenon of nonspecifically induced polyarteritis nodosa, which we have observed through the skin window. Dixon's concept relates to whether the soluble antigen-antibody complexes which can be formed only in the poor antibody former produce glomerulonephritis only because of their filtration through the glomerulus in large quantities, or whether the presence of a directing antibody directs the complex to the target organ, such as an antileukocytic antibody directing soluble complexes to the leukocyte, or such as an antithyroid antibody directing these complexes to the thyroid, and so on. This theory would also help to explain how the so-called directing antibodies to the thyroid, to leukocytes and other tissues which are now being found in plenitude in so many conditions are themselves fairly permanent. It is only in the presence of the soluble complexes that they become destructive.

DR. FISCHEL: Dr. Rebuck, I think that the localization of an antigen-antibody complex can be determined by local tissue factors, so that the glomerulus is not necessarily the only place that a macromolecular substance can get stuck. If you irritate another area of the body, localization occurs there secondarily and it will set up its own primary site for further localization.

DR. REBUCK: We were surprised to see the lesions of polyarteritis through our skin windows, since they would not be expected in this area; also, as you know, we observed LE formation in the windows in patients suffering from lupus. This mechanism may be the explanation for this phenomenon.

DR. FAVOUR: I would like to call your attention to a report regarding the fate of macrophages. In studies of the pathogenesis of silicosis, it was found that particles of quartz would kill macrophages after phagocytosis had taken place. In silicosis the macrophage apparently comes to the lung, phagocytoses a particle of quartz and is killed; if it contains an antigen which it may have acquired somewhere else in the host at another time, the antigen is released. Groups of plasma cells then appear around the disintegrating macrophage, and this phenomenon presumably accounts for the hypergammaglobulinemia present in these patients and their ability to make antibodies to all sorts of antigens which are not in any way related to the disease. Since this is so, it is apparent that one might be able to use silica as an adjuvant for antibody formation. Stimulation of antibody formation in animals which had received a standard antigen was reported. If Freund's adjuvant is also added, there is still a further adjuvant effect. In other words, the macrophage is prevented from holding the antigen, and perhaps the host is exposed to more antigen than it would otherwise be. The existence of such a mechanism is going to complicate our interpretation of some of the immune responses that occur in a number of these diseases. Maybe we should expect excess antibody formation in a number of diseases in which an inflammatory process is present, the antibodies formed really having nothing to do with the pathogenesis of the lesions; this may account for some of the confusion which has arisen in regard to the antibodies associated with certain of these diseases that do not in any way seem to explain the pathogenesis of the disease. Does anyone on the panel have any other thoughts on the cause of hypergammaglobulinemia which is associated with chronic granulomatous lesions?

DR. SPAIN: I think there are any number of diseases in which there is stimulation of the reticuloendothelial system, and it is frequently associated with hypergammaglobulinemia. I think that silica probably acts by the same mechanism—the more irritation there is, the more the RE system is stimulated, and the more cells will be produced and destroyed. It is purely a nonspecific thing seen in many situations.

DR. FAVOUR: Dr. Dougherty, how do your data on the cellular sequence in inflammation fit in with those of Dr. Rebuck?

DR. DOUGHERTY: We found the same sequence, and there is nothing new about it. However, one of the things which I think is very important, and one which we have to study further to add to the sequence, is something Dr. Rebuck found in relation to ulcerative colitis, and that is that the basophils predominate in this lesion. For instance, I would like to find out what the proportional increase in basophils in blood is at this time.

Another important point related to the appearance of the cells in an inflammatory lesion is that when ACTH is administered to a patient, one of the accompanying features is a lymphopenia. Consequently, there is a mechanical factor involved in the alteration of the cellular sequence after ACTH; if there are fewer circulating lymphocytes there are fewer lymphocytes available to go to the area of inflammation.

I also think the other point he made—the lack of peroxidase staining characteristic of cells from ACTH-treated people—is worth consideration.

Finally, he made the very interesting observation that cortisol tends to reduce the capacity of the macrophages to phagocytize various substances.

I think these are points of some significance. I would like to call your attention to the fact that to get an increased tissue concentration of cortisol, human beings do not require administration of exogenous ACTH. The ordinary stress of inflammation certainly induces and increases the output and retention of endogenous cortisol, so the changes in the lesions that Dr. Rebuck and I have described after cortisol administration are not only related to treatment with these compounds, but also represent what may happen when cortisol is secreted endogenously from the adrenal gland. We must remember that they do the same thing. Therefore, it is an interesting point that cortisol would inhibit phagocytosis at the time that there is an increase in the tissue level. The inhibition appears to be due to an anesthetic effect of cortisol on the macrophage. A little larger dose destroys it, but doses which are within the tolerance of the cells practically inhibit its activity completely.

DR. REBUCK: I am not so pessimistic about our understanding of the mechanisms of the actions of corticosteroids, and I think we can reconstruct part of this process. First, as Dr. Dougherty pointed out, the formation of potential mononuclear cells in the lymphocytopoietic organs is inhibited by these compounds. Second, they are depressed in numbers in the transport system—the blood. Third, as shown by Dr. Menkin's work, margination and diapedesis are inhibited. Fourth, these steroids have a direct effect, as so many of you have shown, on the mononuclear cells already present in the area of inflammation. Fifth, the area of potential damage, the fibroblastic bed, as Dr. Dougherty has shown, is somewhat protected by these compounds, so that the biochemical response to cellular injury, as shown by Dr. Menkin, is depressed, and this in turn would reduce the chemotactic influence of an inflammatory lesion, so that there would be less stimulus for influx of these cells. Consideration of these facts and Dr. Asboe-Hansen's concept of the depression of tissue mast cell degranulation allows one to obtain a reasonable concept of what is happening in the inhibited inflammatory area.

Part VII | THERAPEUTIC USE OF STEROIDS AND OTHER DRUGS IN SPECIFIC INFLAMMATORY STATES

Evaluation of Corticosteroid
Therapy in the Rheumatic Diseases

JOSEPH J. BUNIM

National Institute of Arthritis and Metabolic Diseases

Appraisal of the corticosteroids is difficult even after eleven years of intensive study and extensive experience by numerous observers on a worldwide scale. And it is bound to be controversial. There are several reasons for conflicting opinions.

The philosophy of the physician is an important factor. A clinician whose overriding credo is *"Primum est non nocere"* (above all, do no harm) will be oppressed by the major hazards of prolonged corticosteroid therapy and by the difficulty of withdrawing the hormone. On the other hand, a practitioner who believes that the risks entailed in administering a potent drug should be weighed against the risks taken in withholding it, when confronted with a disabling, crippling or fatal disease for which no cure is available, will be impressed with the many beneficial attributes of the corticosteroids.

The severity of a disease that a given physician treats is another factor that introduces bias in evaluation. In the better known medical centers and research institutions, the severely ill or refractory patients constitute the "average" cases (circumstantial selection). Such patients are usually seen quite late after onset when a substantial component of the disease may have become irreversible or when excessive maintenance dosage may have been established well before admission, or the severity of the illness may be such that high dosage becomes obligatory. In the former instance (late treatment), the results may be compromised, and in the latter (high dosage), the incidence of serious adverse effects and mortality rate may be alarming. Reports issued from such institutions—and these outnumber the rest—will be discouraging. On the other hand, to the private practitioner who institutes treatment relatively early often achieving a gratifying therapeutic response and most of whose cases are of mild or moderate severity and hence require low or moderate dosage, these reports are almost unbelievable; again, controversy ensues.

The values attributed to certain therapeutic results vary with physicians and patients depending on the patient's socio-economic needs and temperament and the doctor's thoroughness and tenacity in following *all* the patients who have been under his care at one time or another so that he can estimate the end results. In the modern economic setting of this country, to enable a skilled worker with rheumatoid arthritis to return to his job as soon as possible so that he may continue to support his family, meet the bills on the many commodities he has bought on credit, pay for his hospital and medical care and purchase the very steroids that make all this possible, may render the risks of bleeding peptic ulcer or fractured vertebrae quite acceptable, whereas in the modern economic setting of a country like Great Britain which contrasts sharply in every regard mentioned above, such a risk might be forbidding. It is not surprising, then, that American and British colleagues often disagree in their evaluations of steroid therapy.

525

It should be added, incidentally, that steroids are currently used very widely in England.

The foregoing to the contrary notwithstanding, there are many principles and conclusions related to evaluation of hormonal therapy on which most of the workers in this field, both here and abroad, do agree.

1. Corticosteroids have an important place in the treatment of almost all cases of acute or subacute dermatomyositis, most cases of severe systemic lupus erythematosus (SLE), carefully selected cases of rheumatoid arthritis and acute rheumatic carditis, some cases of polyarteritis nodosa and few of scleroderma.

2. They are effective anti-inflammatory agents that act promptly and uniformly.

3. They do not substantially alter the natural course of the disease in rheumatoid arthritis, rheumatic fever, polyarteritis nodosa and scleroderma.

4. They do not induce remissions, so that when they are discontinued before the activity of the disease has spontaneously subsided, relapse will occur.

5. Therapeutic gains made early in the course of treatment often diminish as therapy is prolonged, and the risk of adverse effects may no longer be warranted.

6. Inflammatory changes are reversible by corticosteroids, whereas fibrotic and destructive changes are not.

7. Most of the undesirable effects are reversible when the drug is discontinued; some even while the compound is continued, such as peptic ulcers and infections, provided specific treatment is administered concomitantly.

8. In some cases discontinuance of corticosteroid administration is difficult or intolerable. This is often related to duration of therapy and size of dosage.

9. Synthetic corticosteroids are superior to the naturally occurring hormones (cortisone and cortisol) in that their administration is associated (a) with little if any sodium retention or potassium loss when they are given in conventional dosage and (b) with lower incidence of hypertension, congestive heart failure and possibly psychosis.

10. Among the several synthetic preparations in common use (prednisone, prednisolone, methyl prednisolone, triamcinolone and dexamethasone) no one compound has a significant therapeutic advantage when compared to the others, although individual patients may tolerate or respond more satisfactorily to one than to another.

11. None of the corticosteroid preparations thus far produced is free of major adverse effects such as peptic ulcer, gastrointestinal hemorrhage, visceral perforation, activation of infection, necrotizing angiitis or fractures.

12. Potency *per se* offers no real therapeutic advantage.

13. The amount of drug given daily (dosage), more than any other single factor, will determine frequency of adverse effects.

14. Certain undesirable effects are disease-related. Patients with rheumatoid arthritis develop peptic ulcers, fractures or polyarteritis nodosa much more frequently during the course of prolonged steroid therapy than patients with asthma or ulcerative colitis.

USEFULNESS OF CORTICOSTEROIDS IN INDIVIDUAL DISEASES

Elsewhere in this volume, reports appear on the effects of steroids on the separate rheumatic diseases. These reports by competent authorities include data drawn from direct experience to support appraisal of the hormones. In an attempt to avoid duplication, the writer of this section will not encumber the reader with tables of data of results of treatment collected over the past decade and published elsewhere by others or by his group. What follows is the present impression of one observer (subject to many inherent limitations) based both on published reports and his own experience of the usefulness of corticosteroids in the several rheumatic disorders. The diseases will be discussed in the order of diminishing importance of steroids in their treatment.

DERMATOMYOSITIS

There is no uniformly effective measure for this serious disease. Without the benefit of steroids, life expectancy is limited to several years in a high proportion of cases. Corticosteroid therapy may be life-saving. The required dosage in this disease is generally higher than in rheumatoid arthritis. Since the prognosis is usually grave, the increased risk entailed in dosages high enough to control symptoms is warranted. At the beginning of treatment, 40 to 60 mg. of prednisone or its equivalent may be necessary. As activity of the disease is suppressed—and this may require weeks—dosage may be gradually reduced to safer levels such as 15 or 20 mg. daily or less if possible. As is true in other rheumatic diseases, response to corticosteroids is proportional to the extent and activity of the inflammatory process in diseased structures. Thus, in the early and acute cases marked improvement may result as fever and symptoms subside and muscle pain, tenderness and weakness diminish or disappear. The patient may be tided over a critical period of several weeks or months until such time as spontaneous remission may supervene. However, in cases in which extensive necrosis, degeneration and atrophy of muscle have occurred, muscle weakness and wasting will persist and steroids will produce little if any improvement.

SYSTEMIC LUPUS ERYTHEMATOSUS

In the severe, fulminating or critical cases, especially those complicated by intercurrent bacterial infections, corticosteroids are of the greatest value. As in cases of dermatomyositis, initial dosage requirements in lupus may range between 40 and 60 mg. of prednisone or its equivalent daily. Certain manifestations respond uniformly, promptly and often dramatically to hormonal therapy. These include fever, rash, arthritis, pericarditis, pleuritis and peritonitis. Some workers believe that early administration of steroids may prevent development of inflammatory lesions in the cardiac structure. Since the advent of hormonal therapy, it has become possible for women with systemic lupus erythematosus receiving corticosteroids to survive pregnancy and give birth to normal offspring.

The meticulous observations by Pollack, Pirani, Kark and Muehrcke, whose report appears elsewhere in this volume, on the beneficial effect of prolonged (six months or more) corticosteroid administration in high dosage (50 mg. prednisone daily or equivalent) on incipient renal lesions in systemic lupus erythematosus have introduced new hope in the management of lupus nephritis. Until then, it was the consensus of most clinicians that steroid therapy could not retard, let alone arrest, the progression of glomerulonephritis in this disease and that renal disease therefore was the commonest single cause of death in lupus. The clinical experience of the Illinois group and histological evidence they have collected dispel this hopelessness. Further observations and longer follow-up by this and other groups will be of considerable importance and interest.

RHEUMATIC FEVER

From the point of view of the clinician responsible for the care of patients with acute rheumatic carditis, the conflicting opinions of those directly concerned with clinical trials of corticosteroids in this disease need not be disconcerting, for there is more real agreement on important practical therapeutic principles than is apparent. The issue that has not yet been conclusively resolved is whether or not corticosteroids are more effective than aspirin in preventing residual cardiac damage one or two years after steroids had been given in adequate dosage for about 12 weeks soon after onset of the first attack. What seems of greater importance to this writer is the area of agreement: (1) Corticosteroids are not indicated in cases of rheumatic fever that are not complicated by carditis. (2) They cannot reverse well established cardiac lesions and therefore are not used in chronic rheumatic heart disease. (3) In early, acute rheumatic carditis, they are almost uniformly effective in suppressing inflammatory reactions in cardiac structures and elsewhere. (4) In congestive failure due to acute rheumatic carditis, they may be life-saving because the response is prompt, effective and usually dependable. (5) Patients who are severely ill with active carditis and who do not respond to aspirin should be given adequate dosage of corticosteroids without much delay. (6) Major adverse effects of *short-term* (12 weeks) administration of corticosteroids are uncommon. (7) Combined steroid and salicylate therapy is not contraindicated.

RHEUMATOID ARTHRITIS

Controversy as to the usefulness of corticosteroid therapy in rheumatoid arthritis is greater than in the three preceding diseases discussed. This is understandable because rheumatoid arthritis does not threaten or appreciably shorten life, though it often makes it unbearable. There are serious limitations to the usefulness of hormonal therapy in this particular disease. Spontaneous remissions in cases of more than one or two years' duration are infrequent, and steroids do not induce remissions. The major adverse effects, at times fatal, occur more frequently during prolonged corticosteroid administration in rheumatoid arthritis than in other diseases. The destructive joint changes that occur in severe rheumatoid arthritis are not prevented, reduced or suppressed by long-term therapy. Considerable improvement in functional capacity is achieved with steroid treatment but in a high proportion of cases, these benefits diminish as administration is prolonged beyond one year. Yet most experienced clinicians in this field believe that corticosteroids have an important place in the management of selected cases of rheumatoid arthritis, approximately 10 to 20 per cent of cases seen at the average arthritis clinic. Steroids are of value for patients whose arthritis is active and severe, is not controlled by conservative measures and salicylates or by gold compounds, and is controlled by relatively "safe" dosage of corticosteroids.

Steroid Excretion
Patterns in Rheumatoid Arthritis[*]

S. RICHARDSON HILL, JR. and HUGH DEMPSEY

University of Alabama Medical Center

Subtle abnormalities in adrenal cortical secretion of 17-hydroxycorti-costeroids have been demonstrated in patients with connective tissue diseases.[13, 17] Patients with rheumatoid arthritis show diminished urinary 17-hydroxycorticosteroid levels, over a 24-hour period, because of a lower output of these hormones during the early morning hours. That these changes are not unique for rheumatoid disease has been shown by qualitatively similar changes in steroid excretion observed in patients with nonrheumatoid chronic diseases.[14] The cause of these minor, but possibly significant, changes in adrenal cortical secretion would appear to be of considerable importance since the demonstration of the dramatic effect of C^{21}, 11-17 oxygenated corticosteroids and corticotropin in rheumatoid arthritis.[12, 31] This is especially true after consideration of studies in animals which suggest a relationship between an altered hormonal balance and certain connective tissue diseases.[3, 4, 6, 10, 11, 24, 25, 29, 30] Indeed, precise delineation of a relationship between the adrenal gland and inflammatory disorders still remains a major biological problem in our present understanding of diseases of connective tissue.

The following possibilities of abnormal adrenal function, as related to connective tissue disease, would appear worth investigating: (1) central nervous system-pituitary corticotropin release mechanisms; (2) quantitative and qualitative adrenal cortical responsiveness to corticotropin (ACTH), growth hormone or other stimuli; (3) pathways of steroid metabolism; (4) tissue responsiveness to adrenal-elaborated steroids; and (5) adrenal medullary response.

CENTRAL NERVOUS SYSTEM-PITUITARY CORTICOTROPIN RELEASE

This aspect has been investigated previously by comparing the diurnal pattern and 24-hour levels of total urinary 17-hydroxycorticosteroids and 17-ketosteroids of rheumatoid patients with those of control subjects and of subjects with nonrheumatoid chronic disease.[14] These data revealed minor, but suggestive, differences between these groups. More precise studies, to examine the speculation of a disturbed pituitary-adrenal relationship in rheumatoid arthritis, are now being carried out in our laboratory. These have been designed to provide evidence which might distinguish between anterior pituitary and adrenal cortical function as a cause of such subtle changes. Serial plasma 17-hydroxycorticosteroid (17-OHCS) levels have been determined before and after the infusion of SU-4885 (an amphenone

* This study was aided by grants A-1265, A-3555 and CY-5301 from the National Institute of Arthritis and Metabolic Diseases, National Institutes of Health, Bethesda, Maryland.

TABLE 1. PLASMA FREE 17-HYDROXYCORTICOSTEROID INCREASES
FOLLOWING THE ADMINISTRATION OF ACTH, SU-4885 AND PYROGEN
TO NORMAL SUBJECTS, PATIENTS WITH NONRHEUMATOID CHRONIC
DISEASE AND PATIENTS WITH RHEUMATOID ARTHRITIS

GROUP	ACTH RESPONSE*		SU-4885 RESPONSE†		PYROGEN RESPONSE‡	
	No.	Mean 4-hr. increase over control (µg. %)	No.	Mean 6-hr. increase over 2-hr. level (µg. %)	No.	Mean 4-hr. increase over control (µg. %)
Normal subjects	7	32.8	7	7.8	6	16.3
Nonrheumatoid chronic disease	9	25.9	4	4.2	9	22.5
Rheumatoid arthritis	5	24.3	4	3.8	8	13.6

   * Depot ACTH, 80 units, given intramuscularly.
   † SU-4885, 1.0 gram dissolved in 500 cc. 5% normal saline, given over a 2-hour period.
   ‡ Lipopolysaccharide pyrogen, 0.5 µg., given intravenously.

analog which inhibits adrenal cortical 11-beta-hydroxylase activity) in order to measure anterior pituitary corticotropin release as a result of suppression of the negative feedback mechanism[1, 8, 9, 18, 21] in normal subjects and in patients with rheumatoid and nonrheumatoid disease. In the same manner, plasma 17-OHCS levels have been determined in similar groups before and at intervals following the infusion of a purified lipopolysaccharide pyrogen, from *Salmonella abortis equi*, to determine pituitary function by means of a standardized stressful situation.[8, 19, 21] These data have been compared with observations obtained under similar circumstances before and after ACTH administration. The results are shown in Table 1. The measurements from all of the subjects—controls, rheumatoids and those with nonrheumatoid chronic disease—fell well within the normal range, indicating normal pituitary adrenal cortical activity within the range of the methods of the study. Further evidence of normal pituitary-adrenal relationships is provided by the uniform plasma 17-OHCS levels observed during the day, in both normal subjects and patients with rheumatoid arthritis,[32] as shown in Table 2.

ADRENAL CORTICAL RESPONSIVENESS

In order to determine the degree of adrenal responsiveness in rheumatoid disease, the urinary 17-ketosteroid and total 17-hydroxycorticosteroid responses to ACTH, infused on two consecutive days, were measured in

TABLE 2. SERIAL FREE PLASMA CORTICOIDS IN NORMAL SUBJECTS AND
PATIENTS WITH RHEUMATOID ARTHRITIS, BEFORE AND
FOLLOWING ACTH INFUSION

GROUP	NO. STUDIED	MEAN AGE	CONTROL			1ST ACTH*	
			7:00 A.M.	1:00 P.M.	5:00 P.M.	7:00 A.M.	1:00 P.M.
Normal subjects	18	23	13.7† ± 1.13	9.7 ± 1.18	5.3 ± 0.86	14.3 ± 2.04	33.5 ± 1.82
Rheumatoid arthritis	10	51	18.6 ± 3.72	10.9 ± 2.39	9.97 ± 2.18	14.7 ± 2.57	34.2 ± 6.06

   * 25 units of lyophylized ACTH in 1000 ml. 5% dextrose in water given intravenously over 8 hours.
   † Mean values in µg.% ± one standard error of the mean.

TABLE 3. MEAN URINARY 17-KETOSTEROID AND 17-HYDROXYCORTICO-
STEROID LEVELS IN RESPONSE TO INFUSIONS OF ACTH IN
NORMAL SUBJECTS AND PATIENTS WITH RHEUMATOID
AND NONRHEUMATOID CHRONIC DISEASES

| | | | CONTROL | | 1ST ACTH* | | 2ND ACTH* | |
| | | | 17-KS (mg./24-hr.) | 17-OH (mg./24-hr.) | 17-KS (mg./24-hr.) | 17-OH (mg./24-hr.) | 17-KS (mg./24-hr.) | 17-OH (mg./24-hr.) |
GROUP	NO. STUDIED	MEAN AGE						
Normal subjects	10	26	18.4† ±1.59	8.2 ±0.75	23.4 ±2.04	21.1 ±1.96	26.9 ±3.23	32.9 ±3.63
Rheumatoid arthritis	30	49	15.3 ±1.38	6.3 ±0.57	19.2 ±1.72	17.1 ±1.45	21.8 ±1.34	22.5 ±1.91
Ankylosing spondylitis	10	35	14.3 ±1.39	5.7 ±0.55	20.2 ±1.86	17.4 ±2.15	21.9 ±1.37	24.1 ±1.90
Nonrheumatoid chronic disease	11	50	12.3 ±1.20	5.7 ±1.94	17.3 ±2.84	16.3 ±2.48	22.7 ±1.73	25.2 ±2.97

* 25 units lyophylized ACTH dissolved in 1000 ml. 5% dextrose in water given intravenously over an 8-hour period.

† Refers to mean value ± one standard error of the mean.

control subjects and in patients with rheumatoid arthritis, ankylosing spondylitis and nonrheumatoid chronic debilitating diseases.[15] The results of this study are shown in Table 3. The mean urinary 17-hydroxycorticosteroid levels were similar in all groups on the control and on the first day of ACTH administration, although the highest levels were observed in the group of normal subjects. On the second day of ACTH administration, the mean 17-hydroxycorticosteroid levels of rheumatoid and ankylosing spondylitis patients were significantly lower (p less than 0.01 and 0.05, respectively) than those observed in normal subjects and more closely resembled the levels found in the patients with nonrheumatoid chronic diseases. No differences were noted in the mean 17-ketosteroid levels.

Free plasma 17-hydroxycorticosteroid levels estimated in rheumatoid patients not only revealed a diurnal pattern resembling that of normal subjects, as described above, but also demonstrated the same pattern of elevation following the infusion of ACTH[32] (Table 2).

One further aspect of adrenal responsiveness should be considered. It has been shown[27, 30] that the effects of glucocorticoids (mainly 17-hydroxy-

TABLE 4. URINARY 17-HYDROXYCORTICOSTEROID AND ALDOSTERONE
LEVELS IN NORMAL SUBJECTS, PATIENTS WITH RHEUMATOID ARTHRITIS
AND PATIENTS WITH NONRHEUMATOID CHRONIC DISEASE

| | | | CONTROL | | 1ST ACTH* | | 2ND ACTH* | |
| | | | 17-OH (mg./24-hr.) | ALDO-STERONE (μg./24-hr.) | 17-OH (mg./24-hr.) | ALDO-STERONE (μg./24-hr.) | 17-OH (mg./24-hr.) | ALDO-STERONE (μg./24-hr.) |
GROUP	NO. STUDIED	MEAN AGE						
Normal subjects	14	26	6.7† ±0.76	6.5 ±0.86	21.6 ±1.28	6.2 ±1.32	34.9 ±3.32	9.8 ±1.47
Rheumatoid arthritis	13	50	6.0 ±0.57	9.8 ±0.88	15.9 ±2.45	13.5 ±1.60	24.9 ±3.66	10.3 ±1.20
Nonrheumatoid chronic disease	11	48	6.0 ±1.27	9.1 ±1.16	19.3 ±2.44	11.0 ±2.09	28.7 ±3.49	9.7 ±1.64

* 25 units lyophilized ACTH dissolved in 1000 ml. 5% dextrose in water given intravenously over 8 hours.

† Mean value ± one standard error of the mean.

corticosterone) and mineralocorticoids (mainly aldosterone) are mutually antagonistic in their action on inflamed connective tissue. Detailed observations on the effects of these hormones on tissue have led to the designation of glucocorticoids as "antiphlogistic" and of mineralocorticoids as "phlogistic." A relationship between possible abnormal proportions of these two types of adrenal cortical hormones secreted and rheumatoid disease states in man has been implied from such studies. In order to investigate the validity of the postulated changes in the adrenal elaboration of these hormones, urinary 17-hydroxycorticosteroids and aldosterone levels have been determined in control subjects, in rheumatoid patients and in nonrheumatoid chronic disease patients. These substances were measured during basal conditions and during two days of ACTH administration.[15] The mean 24-hour urinary levels from the three groups studied were compared and are shown in Table 4. The mean control urinary 17-hydroxycorticosteroid levels were

MEAN URINARY C19 ANDROGEN PROFILE
NORMAL AND RHEUMATOID MALES

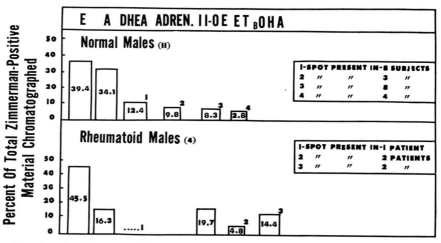

Fig. 1. The following abbreviations have been used: E for 3-alpha-hydroxy-etiocho-lane-17-one (etiocholanolone); A for 3-alpha-hydroxyandrostane-17-one (androsterone); DHEA for 3-beta-hydroxy-delta-5-androstene-17-one (dehydroepiandrosterone); ADREN. for delta-4-androstene-3,11,17-trione (andrenosterone); 11-OE for 3-alpha-hydroxyetio-cholane-11,17-dione (11-ketoetiocholanolone); ET for etiocholane-3,11,17-trione; beta OHA for 3-alpha, 11-beta-dihydroxyandrostane-17-one.

similar in all groups. During ACTH administration, the mean levels of this hormone rose in all groups, although the magnitude of this response was again least in rheumatoid patients. On the second day of ACTH, the rise in this latter group was strikingly less (p less than 0.05) than the rise observed in the normal subjects and resembled the rise observed in the group of non-rheumatoid chronic diseases. The mean aldosterone levels in rheumatoid and nonrheumatoid patients were higher (p less than 0.01 and 0.05 respectively) during basal conditions than those of normal subjects. Patients with rheumatoid arthritis continued to show higher mean aldosterone levels (p less than 0.01) during the first day of ACTH than did the normal controls; these values again more closely resembled those observed in the patients with non-rheumatoid chronic diseases.

Much of the above data, while indicative of minimal although definite changes in adrenal responsiveness, tend to be as characteristic of chronic debilitating nonrheumatoid disease as they are of rheumatoid arthritis.

STEROID METABOLISM

Few detailed quantitative studies of steroid metabolism have been reported; some evidence has been presented to imply an abnormal metabolism of adrenal cortical steroids in connective tissue diseases. These studies have been based either on the determination of half-lives of exogenous steroids,[17] or on the presence of abnormal steroid metabolites in the urine.[2, 5, 16] Other workers, however, have shown a normal turnover of hydrocortisone in

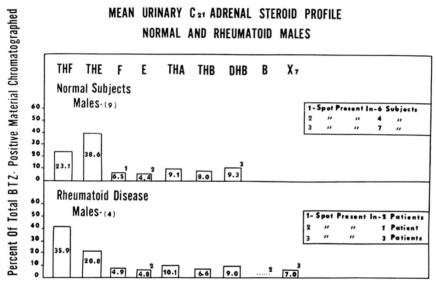

Fig. 2. The following abbreviations have been used: THF for 3-alpha, 11-beta, 17-alpha, 21-tetrahydroxy-pregnane-20-one (tetrahydrocortisol); THE for 3-alpha, 17-alpha, 21-trihydroxy-pregnane-11,20-dione (tetrahydrocortisone); F for 11-beta, 17-alpha, 21-trihydroxy-4-pregnene-3,20-dione (hydrocortisone) E for 17-alpha, 21-dihydroxy-4-pregnene-3,11,20-trione (cortisone); THA for 3-alpha, 21-dihydroxy-pregnane-11,20-dione (11-dehydrotetrahydrocorticosterone); THB for 3-alpha, 11-beta, 21-trihydroxy-pregnane-20-one (tetrahydrocorticosterone); DHB for 11-beta, 21-dihydroxy-pregnane-3,20-dione (dihydrocorticosterone); B for 11-beta, 21-dihydroxy-4-pregnene-3,20-dione (corticosterone); X_7 is as yet unidentified blue-tetrazolium-positive material present on chromatography.

patients with rheumatoid arthritis.[22, 23] Until recently, detailed structural analysis of the urinary excretion of adrenal cortical steroid metabolites was not possible, because of limitations in methodology. Using a chromatographic procedure, part of which is based on the techniques developed by Wilson and her associates,[33] detailed analyses of urinary adrenal cortical C^{19} and C^{21} steroids are now in progress in our laboratory. Although these studies are still in a preliminary stage, the chromatographic patterns of adrenal cortical steroid metabolites present in the urine show characteristic "profiles." The

C^{19} and C^{21} profiles observed in patients with rheumatoid arthritis, compared with profiles from normal subjects, reveal several interesting features. The mean values for the C^{19} androgen profile observed in male rheumatoid arthritics (Fig. 1) reveal slight relative increases in etiocholanolone (E) and in 11-ketoeticholanolone (11-OE), and depression of the proportion of androsterone (A) when compared with those of normal healthy males. Even more striking are the changes in the mean relative proportions of C^{21} adrenal cortical steroids observed in rheumatoid males. On comparison with data obtained in normal males, the C^{21} profile of patients with rheumatoid disease revealed a relative increase in the mean levels of tetrahydrocortisol

URINARY CATECHOL AMINE LEVELS

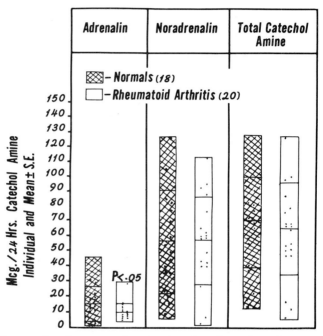

Fig. 3.   Bar graphs of urinary adrenalin, noradrenalin and total catecholamines; the length of the bar represents the range of values; the midline of each bar represents the mean value of the group, and the lines on each side of the mean represent one standard error. Each dot represents one individual's determination.

(THF) and a decrease in the proportion of tetrahydrocortisone (THE) (Fig. 2).

The finding of altered urinary C^{19} and C^{21} adrenal cortical steroid profiles, in the absence of a precise demonstrable disorder in central nervous system-pituitary corticotropin release or in adrenal responsiveness, might suggest a defect in the metabolic pathways of free adrenal steroids in rheumatoid patients. Confirmation of the consistency of such changes in steroid metabolism in a large series of patients would seem to be of considerable biological importance in broadening our understanding of diseases of connective tissue. Delineation of the exact nature of such a metabolic defect, whether in tissue utilization, degradation, conjugation or excretion of adrenal cortical hormones, seems a fruitful and necessary area for future investigation.

TISSUE RESPONSE TO ADRENAL CORTICAL STEROIDS

Almost no information is available concerning this aspect of human connective tissue diseases.

ADRENAL MEDULLARY FUNCTION

Recent studies have demonstrated increased urinary adrenalin and decreased noradrenalin in patients with rheumatoid arthritis.[20] Confirmation of these studies would be of considerable importance in regard to certain metabolic features of rheumatoid disease.[7] Levels of 24-hour urinary excretion of adrenalin, noradrenalin and total catecholamines were measured in patients with rheumatoid disease and compared with those of healthy ambulatory normal subjects of comparable age and sex.[28] The results are shown in Figure 3. The mean adrenalin levels were slightly lower (p less than 0.05) in the rheumatoid disease group, compared with normal controls, whereas the noradrenalin and total catecholamine levels were similar in both groups. These data do not support previous studies of increased urinary excretion of adrenalin and decreased excretion of noradrenalin in rheumatoid arthritis patients.

SUMMARY

It would seem clear, from a consideration of the available data, that the adrenal cortical steroids do not play a major role in the etiology of rheumatoid disease. No consistent, specific evidence of a disturbance in central nervous system-pituitary corticotropin release, or of failure of adrenal cortical responsiveness, can be found in patients with rheumatoid arthritis, using a variety of investigative techniques. Preliminary studies on adrenal cortical steroid metabolism, using urinary C^{19} and C^{21} steroid profile determinations, suggest a rewarding investigative aspect of the problem of connective tissue disease.

ACKNOWLEDGMENTS

The authors wish to express their thanks to Drs. H. Upjohn and H. C. Peltier of The Upjohn Company for supplies of ACTH; to Dr. C. H. Sullivan of Ciba Pharmaceutical Products, Inc., for supplies of SU-4885 ditartrate; and to Dr. F. H. Schultz of the Wander Company for supplies of Salmonella lipopolysaccharide, used in these studies. They are grateful for help in the preparation of these studies to Miss Mary Sheffield and to the many unnamed medical students who served as normal control subjects.

REFERENCES

1. Chart, J. J., Sheppard, H., Allen, M. J., Bencze, W. L. and Gaunt, R.: New amphenone analogues as adrenocortical inhibitors. Experientia, *14*:15, 1958.
2. Devis, R.: Méthods chimiques et applications cliniques du fractionnement chromatographiques des stéroïds urinaries. Ann. Endocrinol., *12*:451, 1951.
3. Desaulles, P.: Comparison of the effects of aldosterone, cortexone and cortisol on

adrenalectomized rats under various salt loads. In Muller, A. F. and O'Connor, C. M. (eds.): International Symposium on Aldosterone. Boston, Little, Brown & Co., 1958.

4. Desaulles, P., Schuler, W. and Meier, R.: Vergleich der Wirkung des Aldosterone auf das Fremdkörpergranulom der Ratte mit derjenigen von Cortexon, Corticosteron, Cortison und Hydrocortison. Experientia, 11:68, 1955.

5. Dorbiner, K.: Adrenal function and steroid excretion in disease. In White, A. (ed.): Symposium on Steroids in Experimental and Clinical Practice. Philadelphia, The Blakiston Co., 1951.

6. Dixon, A. St. J. and Bywaters, E. G. L.: The effect of intra-articular injection of cortisone acetate and hydrocortisone acetate in rheumatoid arthritis. Clin. Sc., 12:15, 1953.

7. Dresner, E.: Some current concepts of the etiology of rheumatoid arthritis. J. Chron. Dis., 5:612, 1957.

8. Farmer, T. A., Jr., Hill, S. R., Jr., Pittman, J. A. and Herod, J. W., Jr.: Studies on the plasma 17-hydroxycorticosteroid response to ACTH, SU-4885 and lipopolysaccharide pyrogen. J. Clin. Endocrinol. (In press.)

9. Farmer, T. A., Jr., Pittman, J. A. and Hill, S. R., Jr.: Studies on adrenocortical and anterior pituitary responsiveness. Clin. Res., 8:82, 1960.

10. Gerarde, H. W. and Jones, M.: The effect of cortisone on collagen synthesis in vitro. J. Biol. Chem., 201:553, 1953.

11. Cross, F. Loustalot, P. and Meier, R.: Production of hypertension by aldosterone. Acta endocrinol., 26:417, 1957.

12. Hench, P. S., Kendall, E. C., Slocumb, C. H. and Polley, H. E.: Effect of hormone of adrenal cortex (17-hydroxy-11-dehydro-corticosterone: compound E) and of pituitary adrenocorticotropic hormone on rheumatoid arthritis. Preliminary Report. Proc. Staff Meet., Mayo Clin., 24:181, 1949.

13. Hill, S. R., Jr. and Holley, H. L.: The role of the endocrine glands in the rheumatic diseases. In Hollander, J. L. (ed.): Arthritis. 6th ed., Philadelphia, Lea & Febiger, 1960.

14. Hill, S. R., Jr., Holley, H. L., Ulloa, A., Starnes, W. R., Hibbitt, L. L. and McNeil, J. H.: Studies on adrenal cortical activity in patients with rheumatoid arthritis: the diurnal pattern of twenty-four hour levels of urinary total 17-hydroxycorticosteroids and 17-ketosteroids. Arth. & Rheum., 2:114, 1959.

15. Hill, S. R., Jr., Ulloa, A., Starnes, W. R. and Holley, H. L.: ACTH stimulation in rheumatoid arthritis: studies on urinary aldosterone and corticosteroid excretion. (To be published.)

16. Kellie, A. E. and Wade, A. P.: Urinary steroid excretion in rheumatoid arthritis: changes in ketonic and non-ketonic fractions during hormone therapy. Brit. M. J., 2:594, 1953.

17. Kelly, V. C. and Fly, R. S.: Production and metabolism of adrenocorticosteroids in connective tissue disease. Ann. N. Y. Acad. Sc., 86:1115, 1960.

18. Meakin, J. W., Tantongco, M. S., Crabbe, J., Bayles, T. B. and Nelson, D. H.: Evaluation of pituitary-adrenocortical function in patients with rheumatoid arthritis following steroid therapy. Ann. N. Y. Acad. Sc., 86:1109, 1960.

19. Melby, J. C.: Assessment of adrenocorticotrophic activity with bacterial pyrogens in hypopituitary states. J. Clin. Invest., 38:1025, 1959.

20. Michotte, L. J.: Reversal of the urinary excretion ratio noradrenaline/adrenaline in rheumatoid arthritis. Acta med. Scandinav. (Suppl.), 341:101, 1958.

21. Morrow, J., Farmer, T. A., Jr., Holley, H. L., Dempsey, H. and Hill, S. R., Jr.: The pituitary-adrenal response to ACTH, SU-4885, and lipopolysaccharide pyrogen. (To be published.)

22. Peterson, R. E., Black, R. L. and Bunim, J. J.: Independence of therapeutic effect of salicylate and adrenocortical activity. Arth. & Rheum. 1:271, 1958.

23. Peterson, R. E., Wyngaarden, J. B., Guerra, S. L., Brodie, B. B. and Bunim, J. J.: The physiological disposition and metabolic fate of hydrocortisone in man. J. Clin Invest., 34:1779, 1955.

24. Pirani, C. L., Stepto, R. C. and Sutherland, K.: Desoxycorticosterone acetate and wound healing. J. Exper. Med., 93:359, 1949.

25. Ragan, C., Howes, E. L., Plotz, C. M., Meyer, K. and Blunt, J. W.: Effect of cortisone on production of granulation tissue in rabbit. Proc. Soc. Exper. Biol. & Med., 72:718, 1949.

26. Selye, H.: The physiology and pathology of exposure to stress. Montreal, Acta, Inc., 1950.

27. Selye, H.: The anticortisol action of aldosterone. Science, *121*:368, 1955.
28. Skelton, B. L., Skinner, A., Holley, H. L., Dempsey, H. and Hill, S. R., Jr.: Urinary total and fractional catecholamine levels in patients with rheumatoid arthritis. (To be published.)
29. Sobel, H., Zutrauen, H. A. and Marmorston, J.: The collagen and hexosamine content of the skin of normal and experimentally treated rats. Arch. Biochem., *46*:221, 1953.
30. Taubenhaus, M., Taylor, B. and Morton, J. V.: Hormonal interaction in the regulation of granulation tissue formation. Endocrinology, *51*:183, 1952.
31. Thorn, G. W. et al.: Studies on the relation of pituitary-adrenal function to rheumatic disease. New Engl. J. Med., *241*:529, 1949.
32. Ulloa, A., Hill, S. R., Jr. and Holley, H. L.: ACTH stimulation in rheumatoid arthritis: studies on urinary and plasma 17-hydroxycorticosteroid and 17-ketosteroid levels. (To be published.)
33. Wilson, H., Borris, J. J. and Garrison, M. M.: Chromatographic procedure for the determination of urinary corticosteroids and C^{19} steroids. J. Clin. Endocrinol., *18*:643, 1958.

The Effects of Steroids in Rheumatoid Arthritis: Acute Results and Management

DAVID H. NEUSTADT

University of Louisville School of Medicine

The purpose of this discussion is to summarize the indications and objectives, the factors requiring consideration in deciding which of the various steroidal agents is best suited for a particular patient, methods of application and management, and the clinical effects of acute administration of corticosteroids in treating rheumatoid arthritis.

The terms "acute" and "short-term" administration are used interchangeably and are arbitrarily limited to represent a total duration of therapy ranging from several days to a maximum of three months.

INDICATIONS AND OBJECTIVES

Certain relevant questions may be raised: Is "short-term" steroid therapy advisable or even "fair" for a patient suffering from a "long-term," painful and potentially disabling disease? Will a brief respite from the torments of the disease only tantalize the patient who is faced with the prospect of a return of the same or possibly worse symptoms following withdrawal of the therapy? Should a short course of steroid therapy be initiated if continuous therapy is not possible either for economic reasons or because the patient may have a definite predisposition to certain serious complications which may develop during prolonged therapy? Will the physician and/or the patient be able to resist the temptation of continuous therapy?

Corticosteroid therapy is, of course, neither necessary nor prudent (for any length of time) for all patients with rheumatoid arthritis. Regardless of one's answers to the above questions, certain selective indications for a short trial of steroid administration seem relatively clear-cut. These include: (1) facilitation of rehabilitative measures, (2) treatment of acute "flares" or episodes of severe inflammatory arthropathy occurring in a chronic but usually "low grade" rheumatoid arthritis, and (3) treatment of severe systemic manifestations such as pericarditis or pleuritis, which may occasionally develop during the course of rheumatoid arthritis.[11, 16]

Other indications, less definite or urgent but nevertheless deserving of consideration, are: (1) reassurance and demonstration to a dejected or discouraged patient that resources are available to control symptoms adequately, and (2) an attempt to restrain the disease and to restore function in a patient who, despite a carefully regulated management program, is developing disturbing disability interfering with gainful employment and other important duties and responsibilities.

Finally, another possible indication for short-term therapy which, in my opinion, is of dubious importance is bridging the difficult gap for a patient in whom it is hoped that a partial or complete remission may eventually result from the administration of gold salts[19] or antimalarial therapy.

None of these indications are absolute; each must be carefully evaluated by the physician and a judgment made after an analysis of the needs and problems of each individual patient.

The most frequently cited indication for a short course of steroid therapy is as an aid to the institution of a planned program of physiotherapeutic and rehabilitative measures. The correction of reversible disabling features, such as an early flexion contracture at a knee, in a patient who has significant pain from an active inflammatory component was an almost insurmountable problem prior to the availability of steroids. Administration of corticosteroids will suppress the symptoms, permitting the application of measures designed to extend and straighten the affected joint. Appropriate splinting or bracing can be subsequently adapted. During teaching of judicious therapeutic exercises to strengthen muscles, to restore function or prevent dysfunction in joints and to increase endurance, the concomitant administration of steroids may be of great value. Although recurrence of inflammatory phenomena may follow steroid withdrawal, the gains derived are frequently worth while and durable.

Another useful application of short-term steroids is for episodic "flare-ups" in patients who have occasional almost violent attacks resembling those occurring in gout. These patients usually have a relatively mild, slowly progressive but chronic course of active rheumatoid arthritis. Intermittent corticosteroid therapy will frequently prevent periods of temporary disability and unemployment. Although the exacerbations may be relatively brief, the agents must be gradually and slowly withdrawn to prevent an abrupt "rebound."

Although clinically significant involvement of pulmonary and cardiac structures is not common in rheumatoid arthritis, the occasional occurrence of such complications as pericarditis and/or pleurisy may be a major threat to the patient and is usually beneficially influenced by corticosteroids.

Some patients struggling with this difficult and unpredictable disease may become disappointed and depressed (along with the physician). To prove to the patient that certain resources are available to control symptoms, a short course of steroids may be given, should it become absolutely necessary.

The commonest indication for the administration of corticosteroids in rheumatoid arthritis is inadequate control of the disease leading to an incapacity for work and increasing disability. Sometimes, even during hospitalization, the disease may continue to progress relentlessly, making steroids almost mandatory for relief of the symptoms. Unfortunately, it is this group of patients from whom the withdrawal of hormonal therapy is the most difficult.

Some physicians are of the opinion that remissions can be induced with certain forms of therapy such as gold salts[19] and antimalarial compounds. The most enthusiastic promoters of these forms of therapy, however, agree that the expected amelioration is not dramatic and that improvement may not result for several months. If such therapy is planned, steroids may be given in a small dosage to partially suppress the bothersome symptoms and to bridge this "waiting period." Unfortunately (although the intent is laudable), this "waiting period" may become infinite.

The objective in using short-term steroids for any of the described indications is to suppress the inflammatory manifestations (at least temporarily), to induce clinical improvement, to prevent dysfunction and restore function, and to keep the patient active and employed without the risk of the potential untoward effects which may occur during protracted administration. Certainly there is no definite evidence that steroid therapy can significantly retard or permanently influence the natural course of the underlying disease process.[4, 7, 12]

CONTRAINDICATIONS AND DISADVANTAGES

As there is no absolute indication for the use of steroids in rheumatoid arthritis, there is, on the other hand, no absolute contraindication. The contraindications for short-term steroid therapy are in no way different from those given consideration when long-term steroid therapy is contemplated. The well known, so-called contraindications are relative, and a decision to administer steroids must be made after taking into consideration many factors and weighing the relative risks against the possible benefits for each particular patient. Of course, some patients in whom prolonged therapy might be considered extremely hazardous would not be barred from short courses or these agents.

The chief potential disadvantages of acute administration of steroids, in my opinion, are the subsequent problem attending withdrawal and the possibility that a short course of therapy may extend into continuous therapy with all its inherent difficulties. Unfortunately, the point at which corticosteroid therapy passes from "short-term" to "long-term" is not measurable.

CRITERIA FOR CHOICE OF VARIOUS STEROID AGENTS

There are, currently, seven adrenal corticosteroid substances commercially available for use in rheumatoid arthritis: cortisone, hydrocortisone, prednisone, prednisolone, 6-methyl prednisolone, triamcinolone and dexamethasone. Many additional compounds have been synthesized,[6] and a number are presently undergoing clinical trials.

The decision as to which one of the steroidal agents should be selected for initiating therapy must be based on such factors as effectiveness, nature and frequency of adverse effects, ease of administration, cost to the patient, and certain characteristics peculiar to each agent which must be considered with regard for any special features presented by the individual patient who is to receive the therapy.

Although cortisone and hydrocortisone have had the most extensive clinical usage and are now the least costly (of the available preparations), these steroids have a strong tendency to provoke sodium and fluid retention and increased potassium excretion when given in therapeutic dosage. Therefore, with the exception of the rare circumstance when it is relatively certain that only a few days of therapy will be necessary, or in treating children, these compounds should be avoided in favor of one of the newer synthetic analogues.

Similar antirheumatic benefit can be obtained by employing any one of the agents in sufficient dosage.[15] Thus the difference in potency of the compounds is of little practical importance. Occasionally one of the corticosteroids may show a superior therapeutic advantage in an individual patient, but this can be demonstrated only on a trial and observation basis.

Due regard for untoward effects, while of the highest importance in selecting a steroid for "indefinite" or relatively prolonged therapy, is of reduced significance when considering short-term therapy. Undesirable side effects are uncommon and usually minor during brief treatment periods.

Certain distinctive features peculiar to the various substances must also be given consideration when attempting to select the most suitable agent for a particular patient. Both prednisone and prednisolone have a somewhat greater tendency than the newer compounds to produce electrolyte disturbances and edema formation.[15] Therefore, in treating any patient with a pre-existing cardiorenal or hepatic disorder, these agents should be avoided. Prednisone and prednisolone also have a more pronounced "stimulating" or euphoria-producing effect; if this effect is desired, prednisteroids may well be the best choice. Triamcinolone has shown the least tendency to cause edema, and in fact, may in some instances exhibit a diuretic effect for the first few days.[8] This property is especially helpful for the edema-prone patient. Triamcinolone is also the most effective of the various compounds for the patient with rheumatoid arthritis associated with psoriasis.[10] Characteristic of this steroid, in a certain percentage of patients, is an appetite depressant effect which may be turned to advantage for the occasional overweight rheumatoid patient; conversely, it should not be chosen for the undernourished and underweight patient. Dexamethasone, the most potent agent on a weight basis, has shown a remarkable propensity to stimulate appetite and cause weight gain in a substantial proportion of patients treated with this agent.[15] This newest steroid is therefore a logical one to administer to the thin patient with a poor appetite. Methylprednisolone has shown no consistent effect on appetite, and for the "in-between" or average patient will serve satisfactorily.[13, 15]

METHOD OF ADMINISTRATION, DOSAGE SCHEDULES AND MANAGEMENT

Optimally, the corticosteroid agent should be administered orally in divided doses, approximately every five to six hours. For practical purposes this schedule is modified to allow the first dose to be taken on arising, the second and third after the noon and night meals, and the final dose before retiring. Two techniques recommended for initiating therapy are noteworthy. The steroid may be given in a large (suppressive) initial dosage, which is then gradually diminished in small decrements until the lowest maintenance dosage is reached; or a small initial dosage may be given which is then increased in accord with the response of the patient until control is obtained. In most instances, however, when rapid defervescence of symptoms is desired, it is best to start with large doses and decrease gradually in a stepwise fashion. This is in contrast to the preferred practice of giving initial small doses when indefinite steroid therapy is planned.

Regardless of the analogue chosen, it is unnecessary to restrict any dietary products or to give supplementary (nutritive) substances when the drug is given in therapeutic dosage unless a concurrent medical illness requires these measures.

The routine use of prophylactic antacids has been recommended,[2] but, in my opinion, it is not usually necessary and may possibly mask early significant gastrointestinal symptoms and lull the physician into a false sense of security.

All corticosteroid compounds require careful regulation of dosage. Dosage must be determined according to the response of the patient. No arbitrary limits can be set as to minimum dosage. Despite the presumed safety factor with short-term therapy, the least dose that will accomplish the ultimate goal is optimal.

Prior to the initiation of steroid treatment a careful and complete medical examination should be made, with special attention to any conditions which might contraindicate steroid treatment or predispose to complications from steroidal treatment. Meticulous supervision, with frequent assessments to evaluate progress, adjust dosage and search for any possible unwanted side side effects, is of extreme importance.

When an exercise and rehabilitative program is given, it is best carried out in a hospital where close observation can minimize the risk of any serious steroid side effects.

THERAPEUTIC RESPONSE

Rapid resolution of inflammatory effects can be obtained with all steroid agents in the majority of patients, and especially in those who receive steroid therapy for the first time. Although some patients derive superior therapeutic advantage from one steroid as compared with another, this is not a consistent occurrence and the differences in benefit are usually minimal.

The antirheumatic potency of the currently available steroids and three new preparations now undergoing clinical trials is shown in Table 1. Clinical anti-inflammatory effect is determined by the average (total daily) maintenance dosage required to sustain satisfactory control of the disease, based on data derived from observations on a large series of patients with rheumatoid arthritis who have been receiving steroid therapy for extended periods.[14] Since the dosage required will vary from time to time, even in the same individual, owing to spontaneous fluctuations in the activity of the disease, the usual range of dosage is also included. The results of granuloma-inhibition tests, indicating anti-inflammatory potency and the liver glycogenic activity of the various compounds, are also shown in Table 1.[6, 17, 20]

Notable differences in anti-inflammatory potency and biological activity of the various steroids resulting from seemingly minor chemical modification of parent compounds have led to intensive attempts to develop new analogues with the expectation of a possible dissociation between enhanced rheumatic

TABLE 1.   ANTI-INFLAMMATORY POTENCY AND BIOLOGICAL ACTIVITIES
OF CORTICOSTEROIDS, INCLUDING SOME 6-FLUORO- AND 16-METHYL
C-21 COMPOUNDS AND A 21-METHYL STEROID

STEROID COMPOUND	AVERAGE DAILY DOSAGE (mg.)	USUAL DOSAGE RANGE (mg.)	LIVER GLYCOGEN X F	GRANULOMA POUCH X F
Hydrocortisone	40	(25-60)	1	1
Prednisolone[6]	11	(6-14)	3-4	3-4
Methylprednisolone[17, 20]	7.5	(4-12)	10	6
Triamcinolone[17, 20]	7	(4-12)	13-36	4
Dexamethasone[6, 17, 20]	1.5	(.75-2.5)	250*(20**)	165-200
6α-Fluoro-dexamethasone[6]	1.25	(.5-1.75)	675*	420
6α-Fluoro-16α-methylpredniso-lone[6]	3.5	(2-6)	150	50
6α,9α-Difluoro-21-methyl-prednisolone[14]	10	(6-14)		60

* In rats. ** In adrenalectomized mice.

benefit and unwanted adverse effects.[1, 6, 9, 18] Observations derived from 19 patients who have received 6-fluoro-dexamethasone for an average treatment period of 50 days suggest that this new compound is even more potent than its antecedent, which had been the most potent steroid yet devised, on a mg. for mg. basis.[14] Experience with this drug is still insufficient for any true appraisal of its efficacy or its potential regarding adverse reactions. It is of interest, however, that the remarkable and frequently troublesome stimulating effect on the appetite and the associated weight gain which occur during dexamethasone therapy seem so far to be lacking. Clinical trials with the other new steroids listed in Table 1 are also too limited to permit any definite conclusions.

SIDE EFFECTS

Although serious undesirable side reactions are seldom encountered during short-term steroid administration, and therefore are of less concern, certain unwanted effects may occur early in therapy. Some of these effects are chiefly limited to the so-called "special purpose" steroids, dexamethasone and triamcinolone. The appetite-stimulating effect of dexamethasone may cause weight gain which can become excessive and burdensome during prolonged therapy; however, for the debilitated and anorexic rheumatoid arthritic, this property may be useful for short periods of time. On the other hand, the not infrequent appetite-depressing effect of triamcinolone may be of value for the occasional patient with exogenous obesity. The unusual effects of triamcinolone, characterized by pronounced weakness and loss of subcutaneous and muscle tissue, do not usually occur during the first few weeks of triamcinolone therapy.[5, 15]

Other side effects which may occur early in administration are of minor consequence regarding morbidity but, although considered as only a nuisance by some, may be of cosmetic significance. These effects include the well-known physical evidence of hypercortisonism with moon facies, supraclavicular and suprasternal fullness from fat pads, hypertrichosis and acne. "Buffalo" hump, an advanced problem of fat redistribution, is rarely encountered during short-term administration. Ecchymotic and purpuric skin lesions may occur but not to the extensive degree noted during protracted treatment. Other minor effects which occur in a small percentage of patients include such nonspecific diverse effects as insomnia in some, drowsiness in others, and erythema of the face and hot flushes (erythema and hot flushes are confined chiefly to triamcinolone). Although digestive disturbances occur frequently, the problem of the incidence and frequency of steroid ulcer or gastrointestinal catastrophes resulting from steroid ingestion has not as yet been resolved.[3] Osteoporosis with compression fracture is rarely a major threat in patients receiving short-term treatment. The possibility of masking manifestations of a serious infection is remote in short-term therapy when the agent is given in therapeutic dosage.

Objectionable withdrawal symptoms following hormonal therapy of less than three months' duration are usually minimal, in my experience, when the preparation has been gradually tapered prior to discontinuance.

ACKNOWLEDGMENTS

Dexamethasone was supplied by Merck Sharp & Dohme, Inc., West Point, Pennsylvania; triamcinolone was supplied through Dr. Christopher H. Demos by Lederle Laboratories Division, American Cyanamid Company, Pearl River, New York; methyl prednisolone and 6α-fluoro-dexamethasone through Dr. Harold Upjohn, by The Upjohn Company, Kalamazoo, Michigan; 6α-fluoro-16α-methylprednisolone through Dr. Glenn Irwin by the Eli Lilly Company, Indianapolis, Indiana; 6α, 9α-difluoro-21-methylprednisolone through Dr. Leonard Brahen by the Charles Pfizer Company, Brooklyn, New York.

REFERENCES

1. Bernstein, S. et al.: J. Am. Chem. Soc., 78:5693, 1956.
2. Boland, E. W.: J.A.M.A., 174:835-841, 1960.
3. Bowen, R., Jr., Mayne, J. G., Cain, J. C. and Bartholomew, L.: Proc. Staff Meet., Mayo Clin., 35:537-544, 1960.
4. Bunim, J. J., Ziff, M. and McEwen, C.: Bull. Rheumat. Dis., 5:73, 1954.
5. Dubois, E. L.: J.A.M.A., 167:1590-1599, 1958.
6. Dulin, W. E., Schmidt, F. L. and Lyster, S. C.: Proc. Soc. Exper. Biol. & Med., 104:345-348, 1960.
7. Empire Rheumatism Council: Ann. Rheumat. Dis., 16:277, 1957.
8. Freyberg, R. H., Berntsen, C. A., Jr. and Hellman, L.: Arth. & Rheumat., 1:215-229, 1958.
9. Fried, J. and Sabo, E. F.: J. Am. Chem. Soc., 76:1455, 1954.
10. Hollander, J. L., Brown, E. M., Jessar, R. A., Udell, L., Copperband, S. and Smukler, N. M.: Arth. & Rheumat., 2:513, 1959
11. McCrae, T.: Arthritis deformans. In Osler, W. and McCrae, T. (eds.): Modern Medicine, Its Theory and Practice. 2nd ed. Philadelphia, Lea & Febiger, 1915, chapter 25.
12. Medical Research Council and Nuffield Foundation: Brit. M. J., 2:695, 1955.
13. Neustadt, D. H.: Metabolism, 8(Part 2):497, 1958.
14. Neustadt, D. H.: Unpublished data.
15. Neustadt, D. H.: J.A.M.A., 170:1253-1260, 1959.
16. Short, C. L., Bauer, W. and Reynolds, W. E.: Rheumatoid Arthritis Cambridge, Mass., Harvard University Press, 1957, p. 78.
17. Silber, R. H.: Ann. N. Y. Acad. Sc., 82:821-828, 1959.
18. Spero, G. B. et al.: J. Am. Chem. Soc., 78:6213, 1956.
19. Thompson, H. E. and Rowe, H. J.: Ann. Int. Med., 36:992, 1952.
20. Tolksdorf, Sibylle: Ann. N. Y. Acad. Sc. 82:829-835, 1959.

Comparative Effects of Certain Synthetic Analogues of Hydrocortisone and Cortisone in Rheumatoid Arthritis*

EDWARD W. BOLAND

University of Southern California School of Medicine

The need for drugs with therapeutic indices higher than those of the natural adrenal cortical hormones became obvious soon after the clinical introduction of cortisone and hydrocortisone as treatment agents for rheumatoid arthritis. Apart from their main deficiency, that of exerting suppressive rather than curative action, the hormones were found to have other serious limitations. [4, 22] These may be listed as follows: (1) the frequent intervention of undesirable physiologic side effects, which often limit effective dosage and interfere with successful management; (2) their tendency to aggravate certain coexisting pathologic conditions, thereby setting up contraindications or hazards for their use; (3) the development of relative refractoriness after prolonged treatment in some patients, with resulting deterioration of improvement; and (4) their frequent failure to halt disease progression even though symptomatic improvement may be maintained during administration. Investigators found that these and other impedient features prevented the long-term maintenance of satisfactory improvement in more than one-half of rheumatoid patients receiving the hormones systemically on an uninterrupted treatment basis. [5, 6]

In 1953, Fried and Sabo[20, 21] discovered that the anti-inflammatory and other physiologic functions of hydrocortisone were altered decidedly when halogen atoms were substituted at the ninth carbon position of the steroid nucleus. This observation dispelled the widely held notion that the natural hormones could not be improved. It brought hope that chemists might modify the molecular structures of hydrocortisone and cortisone so as to eliminate or attenuate certain of their unwanted actions and yet retain their anti-inflammatory properties. It gave promise that steroids might be created synthetically which would be more helpful in controlling rheumatoid arthritis and other conditions responsive to steroids.

During the past seven years the formulae of hydrocortisone and cortisone have been altered in a number of ways, and hundreds of complex synthetic compounds have been produced. Some have displayed variances in anti-inflammatory potency and/or have exhibited quantitative differences in one or several biologic properties. A number of synthetically modified analogues have been introduced commercially for the treatment of rheumatoid arthritis and other amenable conditions. Some have possessed advantages in one respect or another, but none has been divested of the major deterrent features of corticosteroid therapy, and some have produced peculiar objectionable

* This study was supported, in part, by a grant from the Ahmanson Foundation.

reactions of their own. Herein, an attempt will be made to summarize the relative therapeutic merits of seven synthetic analogues—prednisone, prednisolone, methylprednisolone, triamcinolone, dexamethasone, fluprednisolone and paramethasone.

PREDNISONE AND PREDNISOLONE (Δ^1-CORTISONE AND Δ^1-HYDROCORTISONE)

The introduction of a double bond between the first and second carbon positions of cortisone and hydrocortisone enhances anti-inflammatory potency and glycogen deposition activity without increasing electrolyte activity correspondingly.[23] Prednisone and prednisolone are the most widely known preparations containing this modification. Mainly because the incidence of salt and water retention is low with clinically effective dosages, the predni-compounds have been attractive therapeutically.

Several pertinent clinical observations have been made with prednisone and prednisolone as therapeutic agents for rheumatoid arthritis:[7, 8, 15, 16, 18]

1. Their milligram antirheumatic potencies are, on average, approximately four times greater than that of hydrocortisone (range in individual cases: 2.4:1 to 5.3:1); accordingly, the dosages required are smaller. In the author's practice the usual dosage range has been about 10.0 to 15.0 mg. a day for severe cases, 7.5 to 12.5 mg. for moderately severe cases, and 5 to 7.5 mg. for moderate cases. For practical purposes, prednisone and prednisolone are equally potent and effective and may be used interchangeably.

2. When dosages of equivalent antirheumatic potency are given to patients not previously treated with steroids, prednisone and prednisolone promote the same pattern of initial improvement as does hydrocortisone. Statistical results of the improvement status during the first few months of therapy have been similar with the three compounds, but the results of longer term therapy have been significantly better with the predni-steroids.

3. Satisfactory rheumatic control, lost after prolonged hydrocortisone or cortisone therapy, may be regained in an appreciable number of patients by changing medication to prednisone or prednisolone. Among 70 of the author's patients whose conditions deteriorated below adequate levels during hydrocortisone administration, nearly one-half recovered their previous improvement after transfer to the derivatives in dosages slightly larger in terms of antirheumatic strength.[21] With further prolongation of steroid therapy, the improvement again waned in certain patients, but in others successful management was retained for periods longer than three years. In some instances the improved state was attributable to the more effective doses permitted by correction of salt and water retention, but in other instances there was no adequate explanation.

4. When administered in doses of similar antirheumatic strength, the general incidence of adverse reactions from prednisone and prednisolone is about the same as from hydrocortisone. The compounds differ, however, in their tendencies to induce certain side effects. The incidence and degree of salt and water retention and blood pressure elevation are much less with prednisone and prednisolone. Conversely, these analogues are more likely to promote digestive complaints, peptic ulcer, vasomotor symptoms and cutaneous ecchymoses. The occurrence rate for digestive complaints and for roentgenographically demonstrable peptic ulcers may be substantially reduced, probably to a level as low as during hydrocortisone therapy, by

the simultaneous administration of nonabsorbable antacids with each divided dose of the drugs.[13] Other unwanted effects, such as facial "mooning," fat pads, nervous symptoms, hypertrichosis, acne, skin tabs, disturbances of glucose tolerance and, probably, osteoporosis, appear with similar frequency when comparable antirheumatic doses are prescribed.

Most clinical investigators prefer prednisone or prednisolone to hydrocortisone or cortisone for rheumatoid patients who require steroid therapy. This preference is prompted by the analogues' reduced tendency to cause salt and water retention and potassium loss, their ability to restore improvement in a significant percentage of patients in whom control has been lost during hydrocortisone or cortisone therapy, and their better long-term statistical results.

METHYLPREDNISOLONE (6 α-METHYLPREDNISOLONE)

The addition of a methyl group at the C-6 position tends to lower somewhat the electrolyte activity of certain compounds (for example, hydrocortisone and prednisolone).[25, 28] The results of clinical evaluations with 6 alpha-methylprednisolone (methylprednisolone) indicate that 6 alpha-methylation slightly increases anti-inflammatory potency but fails to influence other metabolic activities significantly.[14, 24]

Observations made during the administration of methylprednisolone in patients with rheumatoid arthritis have led to the following deductions:[14, 26]

1. Direct comparisons of methylprednisolone and prednisolone dosages required to maintain similar degrees of clinical improvement indicate that, on average, methylprednisolone is about 15 to 20 per cent more potent per milligram.

2. The character and degree of improvement in rheumatic manifestations resulting from methylprednisolone administration as initial therapy do not differ from those anticipated from prednisolone given in similar or slightly larger milligram doses. Among patients being maintained on either drug, transfer of medication to the other does not interfere significantly with the state of improvement.

3. The type, incidence and degree of adverse reactions noted from methylprednisolone are essentially the same as from prednisolone, although its proclivity for inducing salt retention may be somewhat lower.

From the standpoint of practical therapeutic application, methylprednisolone has proved to be a satisfactory antirheumatic agent, but when compared to prednisolone it has not clearly exhibited either advantages or disadvantages. Since the two steroids promote similar responses in previously untreated patients, maintain clinical improvement equally well on long term administration and provoke adverse effects which, for the most part, are similar in kind, degree and frequency, their therapeutic indices seem to be about equal.

TRIAMCINOLONE (16 α-HYDROXY, 9 α-FLUOROPREDNISOLONE)

The addition of a hydroxyl radical at the sixteenth carbon position has resulted uniformly in lessening glucocorticoid potency and in reducing corticoid activity drastically. This modification was the first to make possible the systemic application of 9 alpha-fluorinated compounds as anti-inflammatory agents because the substituent deprives 9 alpha-fluorohydrocortisone and 9 alpha-fluoroprednisolone of their excessive electrolyte effects while only partially reducing their strong anti-inflammatory properties.[2] Triamcinolone, the most widely known 16-hydroxylated derivative, has proved to be the least likely among commercially available corticosteroid analogues to induce edema.

Clinical experiences with triamcinolone may be summarized as follows:[12, 19]

1. Comparative dosage studies have established that, on a weight for weight basis, the antirheumatic potency of triamcinolone is about 15 to 20 per cent greater than that of prednisolone and approximately equal to that of methylprednisolone.

2. The improvement resulting from the initial administration of triamcinolone is similar to that observed with other steroid compounds that possess powerful antirheumatic activity. In the author's experience, the percentage of patients maintained satisfactorily for long periods has been distinctly smaller than with prednisolone and methylprednisolone. Inferior results have been due principally to the intrusion of undesirable reactions, peculiar to the drug, which have made transfer of medication to another steroid necessary or prudent. Continuance of triamcinolone therapy was considered inadvisable in 20 per cent of patients who received the steroid as initial treatment and in 24 per cent of patients whose medication was transferred from prednisolone.

3. When comparable antirheumatic dosages of prednisolone and triamcinolone are employed, the incidence and degree of certain individual unwanted reactions from the drugs differ considerably. Triamcinolone seldom causes appetite stimulation, and, compared with prednisolone, its tendency to cause weight gain and abnormal fat deposition (mooning of the face, supraclavicular and cervicodorsal fat pads) is less. The two steroids, however, seem to have about the same propensity for inducing such objectionable reactions as hirsutism, acne, striae, vasomotor symptoms, glycosuria and dyspepsia. Although conclusive data are not available, the same is probably true for osteoporosis, peptic ulceration and its complications, phlebitis and nervous reactions. Cutaneous ecchymoses and thinning of the skin occur more commonly and more severely than with prednisolone given in equally effective antirheumatic doses.

Triamcinolone tends to promote unique unwanted effects of its own. Among these may be listed anorexia, weight loss (sometimes with notable wasting of subcutaneous and muscle tissue), muscle weakness, leg cramps, nausea, cutaneous erythema, dryness and burning sensation, generalized fatigue, dizziness and "general toxic feeling." The incidence of some of these reactions has been substantial (anorexia, 10 per cent; muscle weakness, 16 per cent; pronounced weight loss, 18 per cent).

These peculiar side effects have occurred with sufficient frequency and prominence to discourage the routine use of triamcinolone for rheumatoid patients. It would appear that the drug may be employed to best advantage as a "special purpose" steroid, as when salt and water retention (from other steroids, in hypertension, cardiac decompensation, etc.) or excessive appetite and weight gain are problems in management.

DEXAMETHASONE (16 α-METHYL, 9 α-FLUOROPREDNISOLONE)

In animal studies, compounds of both the hydrocortisone and cortisone series have manifested alterations in physiologic properties, including intensification of anti-inflammatory action, when a methyl radical is substituted at the sixteenth carbon position.[1, 27] The increase in antirheumatic potency has varied considerably and has been most pronounced with compounds which also contain a fluorine atom at the ninth alpha carbon position. Methylation at C-16, like 16-hydroxylation, abolishes the severe salt-retaining action of 9 alpha-fluorination and permits compounds containing a 9 fluoro substituent to be administered systemically. Although eleven different 16-methylated steroids have been tested clinically, only one, dexamethasone, has been made available commercially.

Clinical evaluations with dexamethasone may be summarized as follows:[3, 9, 10, 17]

1. Its antirheumatic activity is, on average, approximately seven times greater than that of prednisolone, a finding which establishes it as one of the most powerful antirheumatic steroids yet synthesized. In practical management, 0.75 mg. of dexamethasone promotes a therapeutic response equivalent to about 4 mg. of triamcinolone or methylprednisolone, 5 mg. of prednisolone or 20 mg. of hydrocortisone.

2. Among patients not previously treated with steroids, dexamethasone prescribed in remarkably small initial daily doses (1.0 to 2.5 mg.) promotes an immediate response and subsequent early improvement similar to that induced by other anti-inflammatory steroids administered in much larger milligram doses.

3. The improvement lost during prednisolone therapy may be regained in some patients by transferring medication to dexamethasone. In one group of 55 patients who suffered from severe stubborn disease and were poorly controlled on prednisolone, transfer to dexamethasone resulted in the recovery and maintenance of adequate improvement for two years in approximately one-sixth.

4. The over-all incidence of adverse reactions is not lower with dexamethasone than with prednisolone, either among patients receiving steroid therapy for the first time or among patients transferred from prednisolone to dexamethasone.

5. Compared with prednisolone administered in dosages of corresponding antirheumatic strength, the development of individual unwanted effects was similar in some respects and different in others. From observations made among 92 rheumatoid patients treated with dexamethasone (average daily dose of 1.2 mg., range 0.5 to 2.25 mg.) by the author for one year, the following similarities and differences were evident:

Peripheral edema occurred uncommonly with dexamethasone and, even then, it was mild. The occurrence rate was 7 per cent, an incidence less than that for prednisolone and greater than for triamcinolone. The steroid had little or no tendency to produce or to aggravate hypertension.

Among the more common, and certainly the most objectionable, side effects were excessive appetite (21 per cent), excessive weight gain (26 per cent), abdominal girth (20 per cent) and abdominal bloating and distention (16 per cent). These reactions were sufficiently severe in 21 per cent of the patients to warrant transfer of medication to another steroid.

Ecchymotic skin lesions developed in 59 per cent of patients and thinning of the skin in 28 per cent; often these reactions were severe, and they became more pronounced as treatment was prolonged. In the author's experience, fragility of the capillaries and friability of the skin developed more commonly and more intensely with dexamethasone and triamcinolone than with other steroids.

Digestive symptoms suggestive of peptic ulcer were uncommon with dexamethasone, being noted in only 2 per cent of patients treated with it, but roentgenographically demonstrable ulcers were disclosed on routine roentgen examinations in 9 per cent, an incidence equal to that observed in prednisolone-treated patients who were subjected to routine x-ray studies.

Although dexamethasone has greater biologic potency than prednisolone, it would appear that its therapeutic index is not higher. The over-all results among patients receiving dexamethasone as initial treatment have not been greater, and it has been necessary to transfer one-fifth of patients to another steroid because effects such as appetite stimulation, weight gain, abdominal girth and distention, cutaneous ecchymoses and thinning of the skin became unduly troublesome. In the authors opinion, dexamethasone should not be selected as the steroid of first choice for rheumatoid arthritis but, rather, should be reserved for special circumstances, i.e., when the therapeutic response to other steroids is not satisfactory or when appetite stimulation and weight gain are particularly desired.

FLUPREDNISOLONE AND PARAMETHASONE

During the past year the author has attempted to assess the therapeutic efficiency of two newer analogues of hydrocortisone, each containing a 6 α-fluoro substituent. In general, compounds with a fluorine atom at C-6 have demonstrated in animals an intensification of anti-inflammatory, glycogen deposition and eosinopenic activities, though not to as great a degree as 9 α-fluoro compounds. In contrast to 9 α-fluorination, however, the addition of fluorine at C-6 exerts little or no influence on electrolyte metabolism.

Fluprednisolone (6α-fluoroprednisolone) has been administered to 54 of our rheumatoid patients for continuous periods of one year or longer.[11] Its antirheumatic potency is approximately two and one-half times greater than that of prednisolone. With maintenance dosages ranging from 2 to 7 mg. a day, the steroid has proved to be a satisfactory antirheumatic agent, and its therapeutic index appears to be at least equal to that of prednisolone. Preliminary evaluations indicate that fluprednisolone may be even less likely to cause salt and water retention than prednisolone and may perhaps show less tendency to induce appetite stimulation, weight gain and abnormal deposition of fat.

The second compound, paramethasone (6α-fluoro, 16α-methylprednisolone), differs chemically from fluprednisolone only by the addition of a methyl radical at the 16-alpha carbon position. Dosage comparison studies indicate that the steroid has slightly greater antirheumatic potency than fluprednisolone (average, 2.8 times prednisolone). Observations made among 48 patients with rheumatoid arthritis treated uninterruptedly for longer than nine months suggest that paramethasone differs little from fluprednisolone on the basis of percentage of patients held under adequate control and the incidence of undesirable effects.

SUMMARY

An attempt has been made to evaluate, in general terms, the relative therapeutic efficiencies of seven chemically modified derivatives of hydrocortisone and cortisone. It is obvious that none of them approximate ideal treatment agents for rheumatoid arthritis or other diseases responsive to steroids. It would appear that prednisone, prednisolone and methylprednisolone have similar therapeutic indices and should be preferred for the ordinary rheumatoid patient requiring steroid therapy. Conversely, triamcinolone and dexamethasone, because of unique reactions which they are prone to cause and their greater proclivity for causing certain troublesome "side effects," are less desirable for general use and may be better employed as "special purpose" steroids. Preliminary observations suggest that in therapeutic effectiveness fluprednisolone and paramethasone are at least equal to prednisolone. It may be hoped that with further research and with the accumulation of more precise information as to the influence of structural changes on their physiologic properties, steroids possessing a wide dissociation between wanted and unwanted properties will eventually evolve.

ACKNOWLEDGMENT

Grateful acknowledgment is made to the pharmaceutical companies that generously supplied the steroids used in this study. Prednisone, prednisolone and dexamethasone were supplied by Merck Sharp and Dohme Research Laboratories, Rahway, N. J. Methylprednisolone and fluprednisolone were supplied by The Upjohn Co., Kalamazoo, Mich. Triamcinolone was supplied by the Lederle Laboratories, Pearl River, N. Y. Paramethasone was supplied by the Eli Lilly Co., Indianapolis, Ind.

REFERENCES

1. Arth, G. E., Johnston, D. B. R., Fried, J., Spooncer, W. W., Hoff, D. R. and Sarett, L. H.: 16-Methylated steroids: I. 16α-methyl analogues of cortisone, a new family of anti-inflammatory steroids. J. Am. Chem. Soc., 80:3160, 1958.
2. Bernstein, S. et al.: 16-Hydroxylated steroids. IV. The synthesis of the 16α-hydroxy derivatives of 9α-halo steroids. J. Am. Chem. Soc., 78:5693, 1956.
3. Black, R. L., Reefe, W. E., David, J. R., Bloch, K. J., Ehrlich, G. E. and Bunim, J. J.: Dexamethasone: antirheumatic properties, hormonal effects and adverse reactions. Arth. & Rheumat., 3:112, 1960.
4. Boland, E. W.: Clinical use of cortisone, hydrocortisone and corticotropin. J.A.M.A., 150:1281, 1952.
5. Boland, E. W.: Oral hydrocortisone in the treatment of rheumatoid arthritis. Med. Clin. N. Amer., 38:337, 1954.
6. Boland, E. W.: Present status of hydrocortisone as a therapeutic agent in rheumatoid arthritis. Ann. New York Acad. Sc., 61:349, 1955.
7. Boland, E. W.: Prednisone and prednisolone therapy in rheumatoid arthritis. J.A.M.A., 160:613, 1956.
8. Boland, E. W.: Prednisone and prednisolone in rheumatoid arthritis: an evaluation of their therapeutic efficiency. Med. Clin. N. Amer., 41:553, 1957.
9. Boland, E. W.: 16α-Methyl corticosteroids: A new series of anti-inflammatory compounds: clinical appraisal of their antirheumatic potencies. Calif. Med., 88:417, 1958.
10. Boland, E. W.: The treatment of rheumatoid arthritis with adrenocorticosteroids and their synthetic analogs: An appraisal of certain developments of the past decade. Ann. N. Y. Acad. Med., 82:887, 1959.
11. Boland, E. W.: Chemically modified adrenocortical steroids: An appraisal of their relative therapeutic efficiencies in rheumatoid arthritis. J.A.M.A., 174:835, 1960.
12. Boland, E. W.: Unpublished data.
13. Boland, E. W. and Headley, N. E.: Effectiveness of antacids in reducing digestive disturbances in patients treated with prednisone and prednisolone. Calif. Med., 89:262, 1958.

14. Boland, E. W. and Liddle, G. W.: Metabolic and antirheumatic activities of 6-methylprednisolone (Medrol). Ann. Rheumat. Dis., *16*:279, 1957.
15. Bollet, A. J., Black, R. L. and Bunim, J. J.: Major undesirable side effects resulting from prednisolone and prednisone, J.A.M.A., *158*:459, 1955.
16. Bunim, J. J., Black, R. L., Bollet, A. J. and Pechet, M. M.: Metabolic effects of metacortandralone and metacortandracin. Ann. N. Y. Acad. Sc., *61*:358, 1955.
17. Bunim, J. J., Black, R. L., Lutwak, L., Peterson, R. E. and Whedon, G. D.: Studies on dexamethasone, a new synthetic steroid in rheumatoid arthritis—a preliminary report: adrenal cortical, metabolic and early clinical effects, Arth. & Rheumat., *1*:313, 1958.
18. Bunim, J. J., Pechet, M. M. and Bollet, A. J.: Studies on metacortandrolone and metacortandracin in rheumatoid arthritis: antirheumatic potency, metabolic effects and hormonal properties. J.A.M.A., *157*:311, 1955.
19. Freyberg, R. H., Berntsen, C. A., Jr. and Hellman, L.: Further experiences with delta-1, 9-alpha-fluoro-16-alpha-hydroxy-hydrocortisone in treatment of patients with rheumatoid arthritis. Arth. and Rheumat., *1*:215, 1958.
20. Fried, J. and Sabo, E. F.: Synthesis of 17α-hydroxycorticosterone and its 9α-halo derivatives from 11-epi-17α-hydroxycorticosterone. J. Am. Chem. Soc., *75*:2273, 1953.
21. Fried, J. and Sabo, E. F.: 9α-fluoro derivatives of cortisone and hydrocortisone. J. Am. Chem. Soc., *76*:1455, 1954.
22. Hench, P. S. and Ward, L. E.: Rheumatoid arthritis and other rheumatic or articular diseases. In Lukens, F. D. W. (ed.): Medical Uses of Cortisone. New York, The Blakiston Co., Inc., 1954, p. 177.
23. Herzog, H. L. et al.: New antiarthritic steroids. Science, *121*:175, 1955.
24. Liddle, G. W.: Studies of structure-function relationships of steroids. 2. The 6α-methyl-corticosteroids. Metabolism, 7:405, 1958.
25. Lyster, S. C., Barnes, L. E., Lund, G. H., Mainzinger, M. M., and Byrnes, W. W.: Adrenal corticoid activities of 6-methyl-Δ1-hydrocortisone. Proc. Soc. Exper. Biol. & Med., *94*:159, 1957.
26. Neustadt, D. H.: Effects of methylprednisolone (Medrol) in rheumatoid arthritis: a preliminary study. Metabolism, 7:497, 1958.
27. Silber, R. H.: The biology of anti-inflammatory steroids. Ann. N. Y. Acad. Sc., 82:821, 1959.
28. Spero, G. B. et al.: Adrenal hormones and related compounds. IV. 6-Methyl steroids. J. Am. Chem. Soc., 78:6213, 1956.

Gold Salt Therapy in the Treatment of Rheumatoid Arthritis

L. MAXWELL LOCKIE

University of Buffalo School of Medicine

During the past twenty-five years the management of the rheumatoid arthritis patient has improved greatly. The introduction of cortisone and its derivatives by Hench et al. has given a tremendous impetus to research and interest in this field. In addition, the greatly increased use of gold salts as an important therapeutic measure in the program of treatment has given the patient a 20 per cent better chance of improvement than heretofore.

A study to determine the exact effectiveness of gold salt therapy was undertaken with a group of 3120 private patients who had rheumatoid arthritis. The first patients were treated in 1933, and at the beginning gold was given only to those whose response to other treatment was poor. Since 1940 all patients with reversible rheumatoid arthritis not suffering from contraindicating conditions were given gold salt therapy as part of the broad program of management. The total individual dose has ranged from 10 mg. to 12,000 mg. administered intramuscularly. Of those who followed the program faithfully only 7 per cent failed to respond, and 57 per cent experienced either complete remission or major improvement.

It is important that the physician elicit and record a detailed history from the patient who presents symptoms of arthritis, make a complete physical examination, perform relevant basic laboratory procedures and obtain joint x-rays if indicated. As a result of this study, he should be able to determine the type of joint involvement and then outline a plan of management appropriate to the type of arthritis and for the individual patient. It is to be remembered that laboratory studies provide data of the patient's physical condition but are not specifically diagnostic. Roentgenograms are often necessary in the differential diagnosis. The program of management should be outlined in detail, both to the patient and to a responsible member of the family, in order that all concerned may obtain a clear understanding of the essential procedures involved. Often it is best to furnish a written outline since many details must be covered, freely discussed and thoroughly understood.

In our experience, an initial period of complete bed rest in the hospital has afforded the best opportunity to start this program. It permits close contact so that the physician is able to instruct the patient in many details which must be carried out properly if maximal improvement is to be expected. The patient is confined to bed, except to go to the physical therapy department in a wheel chair. A bed board of ¾-inch plywood is placed under a rubber or inner spring mattress. Pillows are not permitted under the knees, but one is put into the bed at the foot so that the bed clothes rest on the pillow, thus avoiding pressure on the toes and preventing deformities of the feet. The patient is encouraged to relax in a recumbent position much of the day, allowing one pillow only for the head. For six periods of 30 minutes each the patient is allowed to sit up straight in bed, such as at meal times. No bathroom privileges are permitted, nor is the patient allowed up in a bedside chair if maximal improvement is to be gained. These seemingly trivial instructions are extremely important. Shorter hospitalization than three weeks does not produce the best result. Following hospital discharge, the patient gradually resumes previous duties as tolerance permits.

The patient is instructed in minute detail regarding physical therapy and the very important non-weight-bearing exercises. These are simple in design so that the program can be continued at home at the convenience of the patient, and so that he can avoid going outside to an office or hospital for this treatment in extremes of weather. The salicylates usually control symptoms satisfactorily and can be taken safely over a long period. The adrenocorticosteroids are used orally, or intra-articularly, in selected patients.

The author is impressed at this time that the most effective treatment for reversible rheumatoid arthritis is to use gold salts injected intramuscularly as part of an over-all program of management. It was in 1913 that Feldt described the bacteriocidal properties of gold containing the sulfhydryl group. In 1927 Lande and Pick independently used gold salt therapy in patients with rheumatoid arthritis, and in the following year Forestier began to use it intensively. His report in 1929 provided great interest and soon gold salt therapy was used generally. The patient who receives weekly intra-muscular injections will have 0.4 to 0.8 mg. per cent in the blood plasma. Usually 7 to 10 mg. per week is excreted in the urine. Gold can be detected up to 36 months in the plasma and urine following the last injection.

The antiarthritic action of gold salts is not yet understood. Objective evidence of improvement develops slowly, usually requiring a minimum of six to eight weeks. First there is a gradual abatement of the inflammatory phase of the arthritis, accompanied by a fall in the erythrocyte sedimentation rate. This is followed by lessening of pain and stiffness in the joints, and in a few weeks by improvement in general health. The drug is of greatest benefit in treating patients who have an active arthritic process during the early or moderate stage of rheumatoid arthritis. Gold therapy should not be reserved as a last resort, for by then the period of its greatest usefulness is likely to be past. In recent years rheumatologists have come to prescribe gold as early as possible in the course of rheumatoid arthritis. It is especially beneficial in preventing further joint damage, as is noted in the study of our patients, only 7 per cent of whom failed to show measurable improvement.

In the presence of certain coexisting conditions, e.g., acute disseminated lupus erythematosus, severe kidney or liver impairment or pregnancy, gold is not to be prescribed. It can, however, be administered safely in the presence of peptic ulcer, mental disturbances, hypertension or diabetes. Age alone is not a contraindication, for children can be given gold in suitably reduced dosage over periods of years; the same applies to elderly patients, even those over the age of 80. In both of these widely separated age groups it has proved effective.

Usually Myochrysine (gold sodium thiomalate) is used, for it is water soluble, easy to handle and available in 10 cc. rubber-stoppered multiple-dose vials containing 50 mg. per ml. It is injected deeply into the deltoid muscle through a 24-gauge ¾-inch needle. That area is preferred to the gluteal region for it is more convenient and it assures definite intramuscular deposition. Occasionally, Solganal (aurothioglucose) is used in similar manner, but it is an oil suspension, the needle must be much larger; the results appear to be comparable although the number treated in this group with Solganal is much smaller than that treated with Myochrysine. The gold is given intramuscularly at seven-day intervals, the initial dose consisting of 10 mg., the second dose of 20 mg., and thereafter a dose of 40 mg. each week. If no signs of sensitivity appear, treatment is continued until 500 mg. has been administered. At this juncture the future weekly dosage of gold is determined on the basis of the patient's clinical status. Patients with moderate or severe arthritis usually require further weekly injections of 40 mg. until a dosage of 800 mg. has been administered. The treatment is then carried on with 20 mg. per week for a variable period, depending on clinical improvement, before cutting down to 10 mg. weekly. Thereafter, doses of 10 mg. are given at varying intervals, determined by the patient's condition, until a final schedule of 10 mg. once every four weeks, for an indefinite period, is achieved. One patient received 12,010 mg. of gold salts from 1942 to 1958 without reaction.

At each visit, prior to injection, the patient is questioned concerning such early signs of sensitivity as glossitis, stomatitis or dermatitis. The blood studies and urinalyses are carried out at monthly intervals. Gold sensitivity may appear at any time during the course of therapy. Many patients will have a mild glossitis, stomatitis or dermatitis, but with a decrease in the amount of gold given at weekly intervals, these symptoms usually disappear. In this group, especially, the effectiveness of therapy is amazing. While these reactions are mild and do not require that gold be discontinued, they do warn the physician that the patient must be watched carefully in order that the symptoms do not worsen. If deemed advisable, the gold may be omitted temporarily for a few weeks and then resumed with a smaller dosage. Occasional patients may develop severe reactions, but the number of such individuals is small when compared with the large group whose rheumatoid arthritis can be treated uneventfully with intramuscular injections of gold. When the toxic manifestations are not easily controlled, the use of BAL (British anti-lewisite) will prevent further involvement. Fifty per cent of those patients who have experienced mild reactions can subsequently receive gold therapy without the appearance of further toxic manifestations, provided that the dosage is suitably reduced and that it is given under careful supervision.

A very interesting series of observations is apparent following the tabulation of the results of the study of these patients. It was decided to analyze those who had received a minimum of 300 mg. of gold salts intramuscularly as a part of this broad program of management and who were seen at weekly intervals for a minimum of three months. There were 369 patients in this group, compared with 566 controls, i.e., those who were following the same program except that they received weekly subcutaneous injections of a vaccine consisting of 4 million organisms of hemolytic streptococci, in place of gold salts.

GROUP COMPARISON

RESPONSE TO TREATMENT	GOLD-TREATED, MINIMUM OF 300 MG. GOLD SALTS	CONTROLS
Major	213 (57%)	219 (38%)
Minor	130 (35%)	270 (48%)
None	26 (7%)	77 (13.5%)
	369 patients	566 patients

The figure for the gold-treated group of 57 per cent who received complete remission or showed major improvement was startling to us. This compared with 38 per cent in the control group. The 19 per cent difference is approximately the same as reported recently by the British Empire Council in the 24-clinic 18-month double-blind study in Great Britain, in which gold-treated patients were compared with a control group. Only 7 per cent of our gold-treated group failed to show improvement, but there were 13.5 per cent among the controls.

The above data confirm the clinical impression that intramuscular injection of gold salts, as one vital component of a rounded, conscientiously followed program for the treatment of rheumatoid arthritis, affords cooperative patients a 20 per cent advantage in terms of complete recovery or of major improvement. Modern gold salt therapy, wisely administered, may be continued safely over a period of many years.

Long-Term Maintenance Therapy with 4-Aminoquinoline Compounds in Rheumatoid Arthritis

ARTHUR L. SCHERBEL

The Cleveland Clinic Foundation

Since the time of Hippocrates, volumes have been written regarding the treatment of rheumatoid arthritis, but as yet no ideal therapeutic agent has been discovered. As a rule, most drugs are only temporarily effective or else they produce toxic manifestations when administered for long periods. Nevertheless, during the past decade, an increasing number of reports have appeared in the medical literature emphasizing the effectiveness of antimalarial compounds in the treatment of certain patients with rheumatoid arthritis.[1, 5, 13] As the duration of treatment and the number of patients increase, evidence is accumulating that long-term medical treatment for some patients with rheumatoid arthritis is now possible.

The first antimalarial compound used in the treatment of rheumatoid arthritis was quinacrine hydrochloride, but this often produced toxic reactions that were serious or even fatal.[10] Primaquine diphosphate, an 8-amino-quinoline compound, was also found to be effective in rheumatoid arthritis, but serious side effects again limited its widespread use.[16] More recently, three 4-aminoquinoline compounds—chloroquine phosphate, hydroxychloroquine sulfate and amodiaquin—have been investigated, and all have some effect on rheumatoid arthritis. Some authors, however, have warned against the use of amodiaquin because it apparently has caused hepatic damage and leukopenia in some patients.[3, 9] Chloroquine phosphate and hydroxychloroquine sulfate are currently the most widely used antimalarial compounds in the treatment of rheumatoid arthritis and related disorders. Chloroquine phosphate is 7-chlor-4 (4-diethlamino-1-methylbutylamino) quinoline diphosphate (Fig. 1, A). Hydroxychloroquine sulfate is 7-chloro-4-(4-(N-ethyl-N-beta-hydroxyethylamino)-1-methylbutylamino) quinoline sulfate (Fig. 1, B).

DOSAGES OF DRUGS

Chloroquine phosphate is available in scored tablets of 125 mg. and 250 mg. The usual dose for adults is 250 mg., administered orally after a meal each day. It is recommended that the dose of 250 mg. should not be exceeded, to avoid or lessen side effects and possible toxic reactions. The usual dose for children has varied between 62 mg. and 125 mg. daily; in most instances, children weighing less than 40 pounds have received 62 mg.

Hydroxychloroquine sulfate is available in scored tablets of 200 mg. In equal doses, hydroxychloroquine sulfate appears to be approximately one-half to one-third as effective as chloroquine phosphate (600 mg. of hydroxychloroquine sulfate results in approximately the same effect as 250 mg. of chloroquine phosphate), and the incidence of drug reactions is approximately one-half that of chloroquine sulfate. Previously we observed that larger doses did not hasten initial improvement but often increased the incidence of side effects.[12] Although drug reactions are fewer with hydroxychloroquine sulfate than with chloroquine phosphate, they are similar and may be just as severe.

RESPONSE TO THERAPY

The initial response to chloroquine compounds is delayed and usually unimpressive as compared with the usual rapid response to corticosteroid or phenylbutazone therapy. In many instances, medication has been stopped

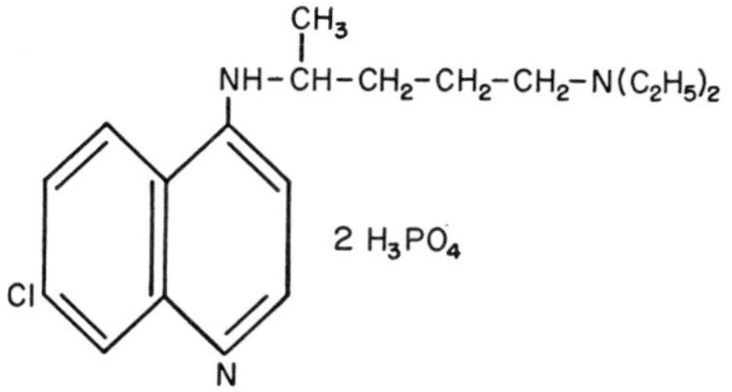

A   Chloroquine phosphate

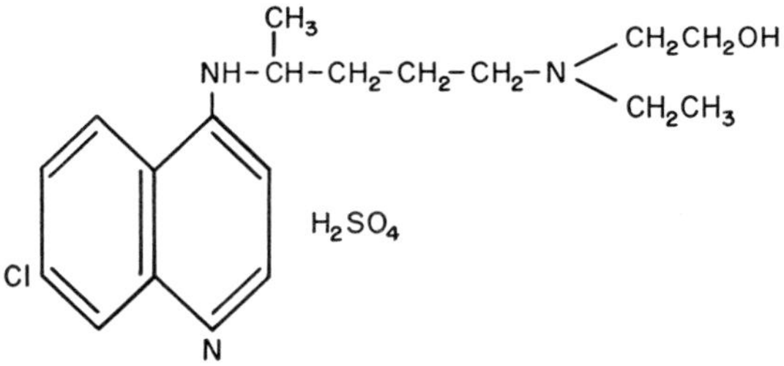

B   Hydroxychloroquine sulfate

Fig. 1.

prematurely when the expected improvement was not readily apparent. In those patients (approximately 65 to 75 per cent) who showed initial improvement, recovery appeared irregularly and required periods ranging from a few weeks to more than a year, during which time the disease fluctuations slowly decreased or disappeared. In those patients who eventually attained major improvement, exacerbations became less severe and of shorter duration, and remissions lasted for longer periods. Eventually periods of exacerbation became modified and appeared as transient weakness, exhaustion or depression, which usually persisted for a few days and subsided spontaneously. In the approximately 35 per cent of patients who responded unsatisfactorily to treatment, two-thirds failed to improve initially and one-third relapsed after attaining satisfactory improvement. More than half of the patients who showed unsatisfactory initial response had been receiving large doses of corticosteroids prior to the institution of antimalarial therapy.

The response to treatment was usually gratifying in patients with juvenile rheumatoid arthritis. Among 73 patients treated during the past five years, moderate to great improvement occurred in 61. Furthermore, only 10 per cent of the patients in this group relapsed after major improvement had occurred, as contrasted with 20 per cent of adults who received these compounds.

DURATION OF TREATMENT

It has become increasingly apparent that the majority of patients who respond to antimalarial therapy will probably require maintenance therapy indefinitely to prevent relapse. Of 78 patients who became asymptomatic while receiving a chloroquine compound in 1955, recurrence of musculo-skeletal symptoms occurred in 44 three months to two years after treatment was discontinued. The duration of the initial treatment had ranged from 18 months to 26 months. Major improvement again occurred in 40 of these patients the second time a chloroquine compound was administered.

Among 563 patients with major improvement who began antimalarial treatment three years ago or longer, 356 (approximately 65 per cent) are continuing treatment at present because of minor joint manifestations and persistence of increased serum glycoproteins above 160 mg. per 100 ml. of blood.[15] Inasmuch as the incidence of remissions in this group of patients is no greater than that expected from the natural course of the disease,[11] it is assumed that antimalarial therapy may alleviate certain disease manifestations, but that it does not induce or hasten a complete and permanent remission.

DRUG REACTIONS

The 4-aminoquinoline compounds alter numerous enzyme systems, and it is likely that the pharmacologic actions responsible for producing side effects or certain toxic reactions are also responsible for the effects of these drugs in suppressing certain disease manifestations of rheumatoid arthritis. Some type of drug reaction occurred in approximately one-half of the patients treated with an antimalarial compound, but in almost 70 per cent the reactions were transient and disappeared spontaneously after a few weeks of therapy. In another 25 per cent of the patients, the reactions subsided when medication was stopped temporarily or the dose was reduced or one antimalarial compound was substituted for another. In the remaining 5 per cent, medication was discontinued completely because of the severity of the reaction. Nevertheless, in our series of more than 1500 patients who have received an antimalarial compound for periods varying from a few months to five years, there have been no deaths attributable to the drugs, and all drug reactions have been completely reversible following discontinuation of medication.

Neurovascular reactions occurred frequently and were usually self-limiting despite continuation of medication. In 440 consecutive reactions, approximately 50 per cent involved the nervous or vascular systems; two-thirds of these disappeared spontaneously during the first month of treatment.

The most frequent reactions included vascular headaches simulating migraine, difficulty in visual accommodation, vestibular dysfunction, tinnitus, nervousness, insomnia and mental confusion. More than one-third of the patients with neurovascular reactions had throbbing unilateral headaches with or without visual auras. In most instances, these subsided spontaneously within a few weeks after therapy was started.[11] Patients susceptible to migraine usually had more frequent and severe headaches during the first few months of treatment.

Difficulty in visual accommodation occurred commonly and disappeared after a few weeks. Haloes around lights or persistent blurring of vision did not occur in any patients at the beginning of therapy. In five of 1500 patients, visual disturbances appeared six months or longer after treatment was started. Four of these were receiving chloroquine phosphate, 250 mg. daily, and one had received hydroxychloroquine sulfate, 600 mg. daily. In each of these five cases, corneal deposits appeared which were detected only by means of a corneal microscope. In every instance the corneal lesions disappeared completely within three to six weeks after medication was discontinued.

Zeller and Deering[17] and Calkins[4] have reported that corneal changes resulting from chloroquine therapy appear to be reversible on cessation of drug therapy. Hobbs and his co-workers[7, 8] described corneal and also retinal lesions which they believe resulted from the administration of chloroquine compounds. These investigators did not advocate that antimalarial agents should not be used but emphasized that these ocular lesions may occur without relationship to dosage, and hence they recommend periodic biomicroscopic examinations and discontinuation of therapy if such lesions appear.

Vestibular dysfunction, characterized by a sensation of imbalance, appeared intermittently and was usually noted when the head was turned quickly. This symptom was usually transient, but in rare instances the patient felt sufficiently uncomfortable to justify discontinuation of medication. Tinnitus of temporary duration also occurred occasionally. In a few patients, extrapyramidal tremors appeared but subsided when treatment was stopped.

Gastrointestinal reactions appeared in approximately 15 per cent of all patients and included anorexia, nausea, abdominal distension, heartburn, vomiting, abdominal cramps and diarrhea. In about 50 per cent of these patients, gastrointestinal symptoms subsided spontaneously after two to three weeks without discontinuation of medication. In 35 per cent of this group, symptoms subsided when the dosage of the compound was reduced or hydroxychloroquine sulfate was substituted for chloroquine phosphate. In the other 15 per cent, who had persistent anorexia resulting in weight loss, vomiting or diarrhea, medication was usually discontinued. Gastrointestinal symptoms occurred approximately 50 per cent less often with hydroxychloroquine sulfate than with chloroquine phosphate. Among 106 patients who were studied extensively while receiving an antimalarial compound as the sole therapeutic agent, only one was found to have a duodenal ulcer.

Drug reactions involving the skin or hair occurred in less than 1 per cent of patients who received a chloroquine compound. The reactions varied greatly in duration and severity. Dryness, the most common skin reaction, was more noticeable in winter. Other manifestations included itching, urticarial reactions, morbilliform and maculopapular eruptions, desquamating and exfoliating lesions, increased pigmentation, alopecia and graying of hair. Increased pigmentation and graying of the hair appeared more frequently in patients who were exposed to sunshine.

In the simple maculopapular or morbilliform eruptions, generalized desquamation usually began over the face and shoulders and extended down over the trunk and extremities during a period of one or two weeks. In patients who exhibited skin reactions, joint symptoms usually improved noticeably prior to the onset of the skin lesions. Chloroquine therapy should be discontinued immediately if itching or skin lesions appear.

Bleaching or graying of the hair may occur following the administration of either chloroquine compound. We observed three patients with extensive bleaching of the hair who were receiving excessive doses of chloroquine phosphate varying between 750 mg. and 2.0 grams per day for three months or longer. Two other patients receiving hydroxychloroquine sulfate, 600 mg. daily, noted patchy alopecia and graying of the hair six months after beginning treatment. Bleaching of the hair may be followed by return to the normal color despite continuance of the drug.[6] The same phenomenon has been observed in patients with alopecia, which may subside spontaneously while medication is continued.

Excessive pigmentation of the exposed areas of the skin occurred routinely in most patients during the summer with the use of either drug. In some patients it did not disappear completely during the winter.

Psoriasis may improve or become worse when chloroquine compounds are administered. Of 41 patients with this disease, eight improved and ten became worse. In four of the ten who became worse, severe exfoliative dermatitis occurred and persisted for two or three months.

DISCUSSION

It is well known that rheumatoid arthritis is a complicated, progressive, fluctuating disease or group of diseases of unknown etiology involving multiple systems of the body. No single therapeutic agent is available which can effectively control all the disease manifestations without the possibility of producing serious toxicity reactions, especially when long-term administration is necessary. The chloroquine compounds are only mildly to moderately effective therapeutic agents in rheumatoid arthritis, but they produce surprisingly few serious toxic reactions, all of which have been completely reversible when they were recognized and the medication was stopped.

This fact alone convinced us as early as 1957 that the chloroquine compounds were the therapeutic agents of choice in most patients with peripheral rheumatoid arthritis. Furthermore, these drugs can be administered with other therapeutic agents when necessary; this presents another advantage. Bagnall[2] recently stated that the chloroquines appear to have replaced the use of gold in long-term management of classic rheumatoid arthritis of peripheral joints. At present, we have observed no evidence of liver, renal or bone-marrow toxicity in any of the patients treated with a chloroquine compound.

There are, of course, several undesirable features which are characteristic of these drugs; usually there is a delay in onset of clinical improvement which ranges from weeks to a number of months; often maximal improvement is delayed as long as twelve months. Approximately one-third of patients respond unsatisfactorily either initially or by relapse following satisfactory improvement for a variable period. In addition, mental depression, which we believe to be a characteristic feature of rheumatoid arthritis, is not readily nor effectively alleviated by the chloroquine compounds.

To utilize the chloroquines effectively in rheumatoid disease, it is important to become familiar with the characteristic drug response and to realize at the beginning of treatment that the primary purpose is long-term control of the disease, similar to the effect of a uricosuric agent in chronic progressive gouty arthritis. This means that some other antirheumatic agent may be necessary to alter disease manifestations at the start of therapy. In highly active disease, a chloroquine compound is more effective if it is administered initially with a small dose of intravenous ACTH, with nitrogen mustard or with phenylbutazone.[14] In these cases the chloroquine compounds appear to be more effective if the disease is suppressed initially by a more rapidly acting antirheumatic agent or agents administered simultaneously with the antimalarial drug of slower action. As improvement continues, the compounds with more rapid effect are withdrawn in orderly fashion. When a depressive reaction is severe, an antidepressant drug is temporarily administered along with the other therapeutic agents. This usually hastens improvement and appears to potentiate the desirable effect of the chloroquine compounds in rheumatoid arthritis.[16]

By these means the limitations of the chloroquine compounds can be circumvented without danger of increasing toxicity reactions, and in most instances all therapeutic agents other than the chloroquine compound can be eventually withdrawn. In some cases, the chloroquine compound can be withdrawn after 18 to 24 months, but in certain patients the antimalarial agent may need to be continued indefinitely. Despite the low incidence of chronic toxicity, the patients receiving these drugs should be re-evaluated every two or three months and the eyes should be examined with a corneal microscope for evidence of corneal edema or deposits. It has been our policy to re-evaluate patients at intervals of four to six weeks until the disease manifestations have become stabilized; afterwards they are seen at intervals of three months.

With such a regimen, it is now possible to continue long-term therapy in certain patients with persistently active or progressive disease without danger of serious toxicity. In those patients who respond relatively rapidly and completely to treatment, only a chloroquine compound need be administered; in those patients with highly active and deep-seated disease, a combination of drugs can be utilized, followed by orderly withdrawal of all other drugs when the antimalarial compound is exerting its maximal therapeutic effect.

REFERENCES

1. Bagnall, A. W.: Value of chloroquine in rheumatoid arthritis; four-year study of continuous therapy. Canad. M. A. J., 77:182-194, 1957.
2. Bagnall, A. W.: Antimalarial compounds in rheumatoid disease. Canad. M. A. J., 82:1167-1169, 1960.
3. Bepler, C. R., Baier, H. N., McCracken, S., Rentschler, C. L., Rogers, F. B. and Lansbury, J.: A 15-month controlled study of the effects of amodiaquin (Camoquin) in rheumatoid arthritis. Arth. & Rheum., 2:403-413, 1959.
4. Calkins, L. L.: Corneal epithelial changes occurring during chloroquine (Aralen) therapy. A. M. A. Arch. Ophth., 60:981-988, 1958.
5. Freedman, A.: Chloroquine and rheumatoid arthritis; short-term controlled trial. Ann. Rheumat. Dis., 15:251-257, 1956.
6. Goldman L. and Preston, R. H.: Reactions to chloroquine observed during treatment of various dermatologic disorders. Am. J. Trop. Med., 6:654-657, 1957.
7. Hobbs, H. E. and Calnan, C. D.: The ocular complications of chloroquine therapy. Lancet, 1:1207-1209, 1958.
8. Hobbs, H. E., Sorsby, A. and Freedman, A.: Retinopathy following chloroquine therapy. Lancet, 2:478-480, 1959.
9. Pomeroy, H., Warren, C., Mills, D. and Clark, G. M.: The effect of amodiaquin

(Camoquin) on the course of rheumatoid arthritis. Arth. & Rheum., 2:396-402, 1959.

10. Prokoptchouk, A. J.: Traitement du lop erythemateux par l'acriquine. Vestnik. venerol i dermat. 2/3:23-26, 1940; abst. Zentralbl. Haut. u. Geschlectskr. 66:112, 1940-1941. (As reported in Sulzberger, M. B. and Baer, R. L. (eds.): Year Book of Dermatology and Syphilology. Chicago, The Year Book Publishers, Inc., 1952, p. 92.)

11. Ragan, C.: Rheumatoid arthritis: the natural history of the disease and its management. In Ashford, M. (ed.): The Musculoskeletal System. New York, The Macmillan Company, 1952, chapter 9, pp. 206-219.

12. Scherbel, A. L., Harrison, J. W. and Atdjian, M.: Further observations on the use of 4-aminoquinoline compounds in patients with rheumatoid arthritis or related diseases. Cleveland Clin. Quart., 25:95-111, 1958.

13. Scherbel, A. L., Schuchter, S. L. and Harrison, J. W.: A rational approach to the treatment of rheumatoid arthritis: IV. Comparison of effects of two antimalarial agents, hydroxychloroquine sulfate and chloroquine phosphate, in patients with rheumatoid arthritis. Cleveland Clin. Quart., 24:98-104, 1957.

14. Scherbel, A. L., Schuchter, S. L. and Harrison, J. W.: A rational approach to the treatment of rheumatoid arthritis: V. Chemotherapy in rheumatoid arthritis; a concept. Cleveland Clin. Quart., 24:105-115, 1957.

15. Shetlar, M. R., Foster, J. V. and Everett, M. R.: Determination of serum polysaccharides by tryptophane reaction. Proc. Soc. Exper. Biol. & Med., 67:125-130, 1948.

16. Steck, I. E., Zivin, S., Joseph, N. and Montgomery, M. M.: Influence of primaquine on clinical findings and joint potentials in rheumatoid arthritis. American Rheumatism Assoc., Proceedings of Annual Meeting, 1952, Ann. Rheumat. Dis., 11:310-313, 1952.

17. Zeller, R. W. and Deering, D.: Corneal complication of chloroquine (Aralen) phosphate therapy. J.A.M.A., 168:2263-2264, 1958.

Absorption of Various Steroids from Joints

ROGER L. BLACK

National Institute of Arthritis and Metabolic Diseases

Early in the corticosteroid era, the efficacy of intra-articular instillation of hydrocortisone acetate in the treatment of rheumatic disease was explored and reported (1951) by Hollander and his group.[4] Since then, the advantages of this therapeutic approach have been amply confirmed by numerous other workers.[1, 2, 5, 7, 17] The earlier compounds studied included cortisone, hydrocortisone and their acetates. More recently the acetates of prednisone, prednisolone, 6-methyl prednisolone, triamcinolone and dexamethasone have been evaluated.[6] The tertiary butyl acetates of hydrocortisone, prednisolone and dexamethasone as well as triamcinolone acetonide[6] and prednisolone trimethylacetate[11] have also been tried as intra-articular agents.

In contrast to the other corticosteroid compounds mentioned, cortisone acetate and its analogue prednisone acetate have been found to be ineffective when employed intra-articularly. It was apparent that local factors were responsible for the relative impotency of these steroids, which are effective when employed systemically, and the study of the intra-articular disposition and fate of injected corticosteroids became of practical importance.

A considerable variation exists among the available corticosteroids with respect to the rate of disappearance from the synovial fluid after injection. Gallagher and his co-workers[3] found that radioactive labelled cortisone cleared from the synovial cavity at the same rate as sodium. Wilson and her collaborators[12] showed that the injected acetates of cortisone and hydrocortisone disappeared from the synovial fluid at the rate of 86 per cent in the first hour. Peterson, Black and Bunim[9] demonstrated that the free alcohol forms of these compounds were cleared from the synovial fluid at a similar rate (½ time = 1 to 2 hours). On the other hand, less soluble salts clear more slowly. Will and Murdoch[11] were able to recover prednisolone from aspirated synovial fluid as long as 14 days after intra-articular injection of prednisolone trimethylacetate.

The possible routes by which injected corticosteroids may leave the synovial space are limited. The compound may be: (1) absorbed directly into the circulation, (2) stored in the synovial tissue or (3) metabolized by the synovial tissue.

Evidence for systemic absorption of intra-articularly administered hydrocortisone was reported in 1954 by Young, Ward and Henderson.[15] This group found clinical improvement in involved but uninjected joints in 31 (21 per cent) of 148 rheumatoid arthritis patients who had received injections of hydrocortisone in the joints. The systemic improvement occurred from 2 to 20 hours after the injection and lasted for a one- to two-day period. Most of the patients (90 per cent) enjoying such relief, however, were among the group receiving the higher (50 mg. or more) steroid doses. The obvious conclusion from these observations was that part of the steroid reached the general circulation promptly after injection. Wilson and her collaborators[13, 14] ascertained by chromatography the presence of hydrocortisone in a non-injected knee 30 minutes after the administration of hydrocortisone into the contralateral knee. Oka[8] studied the problem even more directly. In his experiment, delta-1,9α-fluorohydrocortisone was administered orally (2 mg. per 24 hours) to six patients with rheumatoid arthritis or osteoarthritis, thereby suppressing the endogenous production of adrenocortical hormone. Plasma hydrocortisone levels were measured at or near zero micrograms per 100 ml. prior to the intra-articular injection of 25 to 100 mg. of hydrocortisone acetate but rose promptly after injection, being maximum at three hours and returning to the near-zero levels in 24 hours. That such direct absorption of the soluble compounds occurs is hardly surprising, however, in view of the well known permeability of the synovial membrane. Indeed, Rodnan and MacLachlan[10] have recently demonstrated the prompt absorption of such large molecules as albumin and globulin after intrasynovial injection.

The therapeutic effect of intra-articular corticosteroids has been prolonged by the use of less soluble esters. Hollander et al.[6] have reported the average duration of relief as six to eight days following injection of the various acetates (hydrocortisone, prednisolone, 6-methyl prednisolone, triamcinolone and dexamethasone). Relief persisted for an average of 12 to 15 days following the administration of the tertiary butyl acetate esters of hydrocortisone, prednisolone and dexamethasone. Triamcinolone acetonide also produced relief for a two-week period.

As mentioned previously, Will and Murdoch[11] measured residual steroid concentration in joint fluid aspirated at varying intervals following the intra-articular administration of prednisolone trimethylacetate. Whereas predniso-lone acetate could not be identified in aspirated specimens 24 hours after its injection, the trimethylacetate compound was identified in synovial fluid obtained as long as 14 days after administration. This 14-day specimen also contained free prednisolone, suggesting slow release of the alcohol form of the steroid. Thus, solubility of the injected steroid is clearly an important factor in the rate of clearing from the synovial fluid.

A second route of escape from the synovial fluid is into storage in the synovial tissue. Zacco et al.[16] have presented evidence that the acetates of hydrocortisone and cortisone, following injection into the joint, may be stored for several hours in the cells present in synovial fluid. In their study, spec-imens of synovial fluid were collected at varying intervals following the local injection of hydrocortisone or the acetate of cortisone or hydrocortisone. The samples were centrifuged, and both the supernatant fluid and the solids were assayed for 17-hydroxysteroids. The acetate esters tended to be concentrated in the cells, the free steroid in the fluid. This same group studied synovial lining obtained during surgery at various intervals following intra-articular injection. These lining cells were found to store hydrocortisone acetate for longer periods (several days) than cortisone acetate.

Finally, injected corticosteroids may leave the joint cavity by undergoing metabolic change, with subsequent absorption of the newly formed meta-bolic products. This has been explored by Wilson and her co-workers,[13, 14] after injection of cortisone or hydrocortisone into the inflamed knees of patients with rheumatoid arthritis. Postinjection synovial fluid was subjected to chromatography. The pattern following cortisone injection indicated the presence of hydrocortisone as well as several other unidentified steroids in the joint fluid from one patient. Hydrocortisone yielded three other corti-costeroids. The conversion of cortisone to hydrocortisone was of special interest, since not all subjects studied by the Wilson group possessed this ability. Peterson, Black and Bunim[9] explored this problem further, utilizing isotopic techniques. In one subject cortisone-4-C^{14} placed in the knee failed to result in the presence of labelled hydrocortisone in the synovial fluid withdrawn at intervals up to four hours subsequently. Later hydrocortisone-4-C^{14}, with 1 mg. of hydrocortisone and 5 mg. of cortisone, was injected into the knees of two rheumatoid arthritis patients. Serial specimens of synovial fluid over a four-hour period showed a steady rate of disappearance of both hydrocortisone and cortisone. There was no "dilution" effect in the specific activity (counts per minute per microgram) of the recovered hydrocortisone which would have been observed had conversion of cortisone to hydrocorti-sone taken place.

It has been suggested that cortisone *per se* is inactive as an anti-inflammatory agent. Its ready conversion to hydrocortisone in the liver and kidneys may account for the therapeutic effects following the systemic administration of cortisone. On the other hand, the relative incapacity of the synovium to effect the conversion may account for the lack of anti-inflammatory activity of intrasynovially administered cortisone.

REFERENCES

1. Austen, F. K. and Calkins, E.: Serial studies of synovial fluid in evaluating intra-articular agents. Ann. Rheum. Dis., *14*:283, 1955.

2. Chandler, G. N., Wright, V. and Hartfall, S. J.: Intra-articular therapy in rheumatoid arthritis: comparison of hydrocortisone tertiary butyl acetate and hydrocortisone acetate. Lancet, 2:659, 1958.
3. Gallagher, T. F., Nellman, L., Bradlow, H. L., Zuckner, J. and Freyberg, R.: Dynamics of radioactive cortisone distribution in rheumatoid arthritis. Ann. Rheum. Dis., 12:347, 1953.
4. Hollander, J. L., Brown, E. M., Jr., Jessar, R. A. and Brown, C. Y.: Hydrocortisone and cortisone injected into arthritic joints: comparative effects of and use of hydrocortisone as a local anti-arthritic agent. J.A.M.A., 147:1629, 1951.
5. Hollander, J. L., Brown, E. M., Jr., Jessar, R. A., Udell, L., Smukler, N. and Bowie, M. A.: Local anti-rheumatic effectiveness of higher esters and analogues of hydrocortisone. Ann. Rheum. Dis., 13:297, 1954.
6. Hollander, J. L. et al.: Nine years of experience with intrasynovial steroid therapy. Arch. Inter-American Rheumatol., 3:171, 1960.
7. Kehr, M. J.: Comparison of intra-articular cortisone analogues in osteo-arthritis of the knee. Ann. Rheum. Dis., 18:325, 1959.
8. Oka, M.: Absorption of hydrocortisone from the joint cavity into the circulation. Ann. Rheum. Dis., 15:327, 1956.
9. Peterson, R. E., Black, R. L. and Bunim, J. J.: Disposition of intra-articularly injected cortisone and hydrocortisone. Arth. Rheum., 2:433, 1959.
10. Rodnan, G. P. and MacLachlan, M. J.: The absorption of serum albumin and gamma globulin from the knee joint of man and rabbit. Arth. & Rheum., 3:152, 1960.
11. Will, G. and Murdoch, W. R.: Persistence of intra-articular steroid: experience with prednisolone trimethylacetate. Brit. M. J., 1:94, 1960.
12. Wilson, H., Glyn, J., Scull, E., McEwen, C. and Ziff, M.: Rate of disappearance and metabolism of hydrocortisone and cortisone in the synovial cavity in rheumatoid arthritis. Proc. Soc. Exper. Biol. & Med., 83:648, 1953.
13. Wilson, H., Fairbanks, R., McEwen, C. and Ziff, M.: Studies on the metabolism of adrenal cortical steroids in the synovial cavity in rheumatoid arthritis. Ann. N. Y. Acad. Sc., 61:502, 1955.
14. Wilson, H., Fairbanks, R., Scialabba, D., McEwen, C. and Ziff, M.: Metabolites of hydrocortisone and cortisone in synovial fluid in rheumatoid arthritis. J. Clin. Endocrinol., 16:86, 1956.
15. Young, H. H., Ward, L. E. and Henderson, E. D.: The use of hydrocortisone acetate (compound F acetate) in the treatment of some common orthopaedic conditions. J. Bone & Jt. Surg., 36A:602, 1954.
16. Zacco, M., Richardson, E. M., Crittenden, J. O., Hollander, J. L. and Dohan, F. C.: Disposition of intra-articularly injected hydrocortisone acetate, hydrocortisone and cortisone acetate in arthritis. I. Concentrations in synovial fluid and cells. J. Clin. Endocrinol., 14:711, 1954.
17. Zuckner, J., Machek, O., Caciolo, C., Ahern, A. M. and Ramsey, R.: Intra-articular injections of hydrocortisone, prednisolone, and their tertiary-butylacetate derivatives in patients with rheumatoid arthritis and osteoarthritis. J. Chron. Dis., 8:637, 1958.

Intra-Articular Corticosteroid Therapy: a Nine-Year Follow-up

DANIEL J. McCARTY, JR. and
JOSEPH L. HOLLANDER

University of Pennsylvania School of Medicine

Hydrocortisone acetate was first injected intra-articularly into rheumatoid joints in our clinics more than nine years ago.[3] Since that time published reports of more than one hundred investigators throughout the world[4, 12, 13, 15] have supported our findings.[1, 7, 8, 9, 10] It would appear justified at this time to consider this mode of symptomatic therapy as a standard adjunct in the treatment of arthritis, to be integrated with the over-all plan of therapy.

Our experience now comprises more than 100,000 injections made into the joints of nearly 4000 patients. Although follow-up study at this writing is not complete, certain trends are worthy of comment. The indications and contraindications for intrasynovial steroid therapy have been published previously and have not changed in our longer experience.

Techniques for joint injection have also been described extensively and will not be discussed here. Emphasis will be placed upon the comparative effectiveness of newer steroid esters and upon the long-term effects in patients whose joints have been many times injected.

The comparative effectiveness of prednisolone acetate, prednisolone tertiary-butyl acetate, 6 methyl-prednisolone acetate, triamcinolone di-acetate and triamcinolone acetonide, dexamethasone acetate and dexamethasone tertiary-butyl acetate was evaluated. Seventeen patients with rheumatoid arthritic knees were studied. These patients had all previously received injections of hydrocortisone acetate and were not informed of any change in the type of preparation used. In nearly half the injections no difference between the various preparations was noted, but in the remainder there was a significantly increased duration of effect when any of the t-butyl acetate esters were used. The comparative duration of palliation is summarized in Table 1.

TABLE 1. 17 PATIENTS WITH RHEUMATOID ARTHRITIC KNEES:
COMPARATIVE DURATION OF PALLIATION FROM
INTRA-ARTICULAR STEROIDS

PREPARATION	DOSE INJECTED	DAYS OF RELIEF (AVERAGE)
Hydrocortisone acetate	37.5 mg.	6.0
Hydrocortisone t-butyl acetate	37.5 mg.	12.1
Prednisone acetate	30.0 mg.	2.5
Prednisolone acetate	30.0 mg.	7.8
Prednisolone t-butyl acetate	30.0 mg.	14.5
6-Methyl prednisolone acetate	30.0 mg.	8.2
Triamcinolone di-acetate	30.0 mg.	7.7
Triamcinolone acetonide	30.0 mg.	12.9
Dexamethasone acetate	6.0 mg.	7.6
Dexamethasone t-butyl acetate	6.0 mg.	14.9

The esters of hydrocortisone derivatives all appear to be at least as effective intra-articularly as the parent compound. However, prednisone, a cortisone derivative, showed no objective effect in any instance. The tertiary-butyl acetate esters usually produced prolonged effects, probably because they are hydrolyzed more slowly in the synovial tissues. The effective intra-articular dose of a steroid is not proportional to the effective oral dose. The intra-articular dose required in the knee joint, for example, is more than twice the average daily anti-rheumatic oral dose of the same steroid. None of the newer hydrocortisone derivatives seem to produce a more prolonged local effect than prednisolone TBA. The newer analogues have a definite place in our therapeutic armamentarium, however, since some joints show a decreased response to a given steroid after repeated injection and again show maximal response when another hydrocortisone derivative is substituted.

LONG-TERM RESULTS FROM REPEATED INTRA-ARTICULAR STEROID THERAPY

Although review of our records has not been completed, we have found that more than 200 of our patients have had more than 100 repeated steroid injections into at least one arthritic joint over the past nine years. We have analyzed our data with a view to determining the continued effectiveness of the method and the frequency of major improvement obviating the need for further local therapy, as well as for the incidence of deleterious effects such as increased crippling or instability of the treated joint.

The records of 100 patients with rheumatoid arthritic knees, 62 patients with osteoarthritic hips and 100 patients with osteoarthritic knees were examined (Table 2). All had received at least four intra-articular steroid injections and the majority had received more than 15 injections.

TABLE 2.

NUMBER OF JOINTS	STILL BEING TREATED	REMISSION LOCAL	REMISSION SYSTEMIC	UNSUC-CESSFUL	LOST TO FOLLOW-UP OR DIED	DETERIO-RATED
100 Rheumatoid knees	49 (49%)	27 (27%)	4 (4%)	8 (8%)	12 (12%)	. . . .
62 Osteoarthritic hips	30 (48%)	3 (4.8%)	. .	19 (30%)	. .	10 (17%)
100 Osteoarthritic knees	24 (24%)	59 (59%)	. .	9 (9%)	6 (6%)	7 (7%)

In the group of 100 patients with rheumatoid arthritis of the knees, 49 still received injections of steroid at regular intervals into the joint as needed to relieve symptoms. The average interval between injections was approximately three weeks. In 23 of these patients the steroid employed had been changed to hydrocortisone TBA or prednisolone TBA because of greater duration of effect from the latter compounds. The manifestations of disease did not warrant further local therapy in 31 patients who no longer received injections. Only four of these patients were in remission, however, as 27 of the group still revealed evidence of active rheumatoid arthritis in other joints. In eight patients the relief of pain from the injection was too inadequate to justify further local therapy. Eight more of the group were lost to follow-up, and four of this series had died. One patient of the group had developed a septic infection of the injected joint which necessitated an arthrodesis.

Thirty of the first 62 patients treated intra-articularly for osteoarthritis of the hip continued to benefit from repeated injections. Twenty-six patients of this group, however, received a different steroid than the original hydrocortisone acetate because of decreasing effectiveness of the latter. The injections were abandoned in 19 patients because of inadequate relief. Hip surgery was performed in 10 patients during the observation period. Three patients had a good result from surgery, the results in four were fair, and three had a poor result with no benefit in pain relief or in ability to move the joint. One member of this last group had developed aseptic necrosis of the femoral head after 16 injections (to be discussed below). Of the entire group of 62 patients only three no longer received steroid injections because of sufficient sustained improvement to obviate further need for local therapy.

The results were most satisfactory in the group of 100 patients receiving repeated steroid injections into the knees for osteoarthritis. Local therapy was discontinued in 59 of the group because there were no longer sufficient symptoms in the affected joints to require further therapy. Twenty-four patients continued to receive periodic injections whenever their symptoms warranted it (average, once a month). Seven of the group showed evidence of joint deterioration during the treatment period, either by increased radiographic changes, or because of the need for a hinged knee brace for support of an unstable joint. In nine of the series the injections gave too transient relief to warrant further local treatment, and six patients were lost to follow-up.

Radiographic comparison of treated versus untreated joints over the period of nine years has been only partially carried out. However, control x-ray films and films taken at least four years after the start of intra-articular steroid therapy were obtained in 47 patients. Thirty-eight revealed no perceptible joint deterioration, there was somewhat decreased bony density in nine, and there was some bony absorption and/or increased marginal lipping of bone in three. No joint revealed increased cartilage destruction as evidenced by narrowing of the "joint space." Nearly half of the 52 patients with osteoarthritis of the hip in whom follow-up x-rays were obtained showed definitely more severe degenerative changes, in spite of therapy. In many of these, the opposite hip was also involved but was untreated by steroid in 19 instances. The x-ray comparisons between the left and right hips in these 19 cases showed no difference in the progression of the disease over the years, i.e., the degenerative joint disease seemed to advance not because of the steroid therapy but in spite of it.

Review of 53 comparative sets of x-rays in patients with rheumatoid arthritic joints treated intra-articularly revealed that progression of joint deterioration, mostly osteoporosis, occurred at about the same rate in treated joints as in joints not treated with local steroid. While the maintenance of good joint function was an undeniable result of local steroid therapy in most rheumatoid arthritic joints, it is equally certain that deterioration of the joints was neither hastened nor impeded by therapy as judged by x-ray examination. The disease progressed relentlessly despite the symptomatic improvement and the good functional result. We have been unable to discover any instance of major joint contracture or ankylosis occurring in these steroid-treated joints, with the exception of those in which infection was inadvertently introduced.

The foregoing data are intended to be indicative of trends but represent no more than a sampling of results from long-term intrasynovial therapy. A much more complete review will be presented as a ten-year summary at the next International Rheumatism Congress.

ADVERSE EFFECTS

It is fair to state that it has been impossible to obtain adequate follow-up on many of our patients with regard to beneficial results. However, it has been relatively easy to keep a careful and complete list of all adverse effects from intrasynovial steroid therapy since these are quickly brought to the attention of the physician. Hence, the following figures are probably weighted in favor of adverse effects.

Local inflammatory exacerbations in the injected joint, lasting up to three days, have continued to appear after approximately 2 per cent of all joint injections. The incidence of this "rebound flare" appears to bear no relation to the technique, the type of steroid used or the basic pathologic condition present in the joint. These exacerbations apparently occur at random in a series of treatments of the same joint and are often followed by unusually long periods of symptomatic relief. Synovial fluid aspirated from joints which were the site of this reaction were sterile when cultured. The mechanism of this "flare" is still unknown.

The most common long-term adverse effect has been the occurrence of instability in the oft-injected joint. This complication has been noted with approximately equal frequency in the weight-bearing joints in either rheumatoid arthritis or osteoarthritis. The total occurrence of this untoward effect has been 37 joints in 26 patients from a total of nearly 4000 patients, or an approximate incidence of 0.7 per cent.

So-called "local rebound," occurring several weeks after an intra-articular steroid injection, has not been impressive. Although the symptoms return in most cases to the affected joint, they are rarely more severe than they were prior to the procedure. We do not believe, therefore, that "local rebound" exists as an important clinical phenomenon.

There has been no evidence of loss of sensation or proprioception such as is seen in Charcot's joints, nor have any joints shown the typical x-ray appearance of massive disorganization and bony fragmentation seen with this condition. We therefore differ with the conclusions of Chandler[2, 3] that these are Charcot's joints. Patients with such unstable joints have almost invariably continued activity without major hindrance once proper support has been provided.

Four patients, two with rheumatoid arthritic hips, one with an osteoarthritic hip and one with an osteoarthritic knee, are exceptions to this statement. All four were subjected to surgery, the three diseased hips for removal of a softened femoral head, pathologically diagnosed as "aseptic necrosis." These patients were able to resume ambulation after a prosthetic femoral head had been inserted. The severely unstable osteoarthritic knee was fused.

These patients are still ambulatory and all have quite philosophically accepted the disability and the need to wear the brace.

Although we agree with Chandler that unstable joints may develop coincidentally with intrasynovial steroid therapy, we feel that the risk is so slight that it is not a contraindication to the continued use of this modality of treatment.

Infection of the injected joint was noted in 14 instances in our series of 100,000 injections for an incidence of one in 7000 injections or one in every 286 patients. We do not feel that sterile gown, gloves and drapes are necessary, provided that the skin is carefully prepared and that only autoclaved needles and syringes are used. A detailed description of the clinical course of these patients as well as of others referred to our hospital with joint infections has been reported by our colleagues.[14] Joint infection is always serious, and the degree of difficulty in management is proportional to the delay in time in making the diagnosis and to the nature and antibiotic sensitivities of the infecting organism. The diagnosis of infection was suspected within 48 hours in eight cases, and prompt intra-articular and systemic antibiotic therapy controlled the infection within a relatively few days. The diagnosis of infection was delayed more than four days in six cases, either because the patient did not contact the physician promptly or because the reaction at first appeared as mild as the occasional postinjection flare described above. In these the outcome has been more serious. In spite of prompt surgical drainage, splinting and full doses of appropriate antibiotic therapy, the infection continued for long periods. After months of continuous morbidity, three cases appeared to be effectively suppressed, and the patients were able to resume ambulation although with decreased joint motion and x-ray evidence of increased destruction of cartilage. In two cases fusion of the septic joint was performed and apparently cleared the infectious process. In all cases the organism was *Staphylococcus aureus*. The infection proved much easier to treat if the organism was sensitive to penicillin.

The principles we have learned from experience in managing the adverse effects discussed above are:

1. The patient should be warned of the possibility of a postinjection "flare" and should be told what to do about it if it should occur (ice pack, aspirin and rest of the affected part).
2. If the "flare" occurs later than 24 hours after the injection, or if it persists for longer than 36 hours, the patient should be instructed to contact the physician, who must then take steps to rule out infection.
3. If infection occurs, rapid and massive antibiotic therapy should be employed both systemically and locally into the joint. Adequate drainage must be obtained.
4. An unstable joint should never be injected without correction of the instability, but once this is accomplished there is no contraindication to further local therapy.
5. Activity, particularly weight bearing, should be limited according to the severity of the disease despite symptomatic relief following local steroid therapy.
6. Careful aseptic technique is of utmost importance in this mode of therapy.

SUMMARY

Intra-articular therapy with the esters of hydrocortisone and its derivatives results in temporary, symptomatic suppression of synovial inflammation in a wide variety of rheumatic disorders.

The tertiary-butyl acetate esters of hydrocortisone derivatives have produced the longest consistent results of all preparations assayed thus far.

This mode of therapy is to be considered as an adjunct and must be integrated into an over-all plan of treatment by systemic and other local measures as indicated.

Strict aseptic technique is extremely important, and skill in arthrocentesis must be acquired.

Local steroid therapy is contraindicated in the presence of active or suspected infection. If infections do result, they must be quickly diagnosed and vigorously treated. Infections have occurred in 14 of approximately 4000 patients treated intra-articularly by our group.

Severe deterioration of the injected joint has occurred in less than 1 per cent of our patients. If the painful disability is not severe enough to justify this slight risk, then repeated intra-articular steroid therapy should not be employed.

When viewed in a nine-year perspective, it would appear that intrasynovial steroid therapy has become established as a relatively safe standard adjunct in the local treatment of various rheumatic conditions.

REFERENCES

1. Brown, E. M., Frain, J. B., Udell, L. and Hollander, J. L.: Am. J. Med., 15:656-665, 1953.
2. Chandler, G. N., Jones, D. T., Wright, V. and Hartfall, S. J.: Brit. M. J., 1:952-953, 1959.
3. Chandler, G. N. and Wright, V.: Lancet, 2:661-663, 1958.
4. Duff, I. F., Robinson, W. D. and Smith, E. M.: J. Lab. & Clin. Med., 38:805, 1951.
5. Hollander, J. L.: Bull. Rheum. Dis., 2:21-22, 1951.
6. Hollander, J. L., Brown, E. M., Jessar, R. A. and Brown, C. Y.: J.A.M.A., 147:1629, 1951.
7. Hollander, J. L.: J. Bone & Joint Surg., 35A:983, 1953.
8. Hollander, J. L.: Ann. Int. Med., 39:735, 1953.
9. Hollander, J. L., Brown, E. M., Jessar, R. A., Udell, L., Smukler, N. M. and Bowie, M. A.: Ann. Rheum. Dis., 13:297-300, 1954.
10. Hollander, J. L.: Ann. N. Y. Acad. Sc., 61:511-516, 1955.
11. Murdoch, W. R. and Will, G.: Brit. M. J., 1:1267-1274, 1959.
12. Smyth, C. J. et al.: Twelfth Rheumatism Review. Ann. Int. Med., 50:421, 1959.
13. Stevenson, C. R., Zuckner, J. and Freyberg, R. H.: Ann. Rheum. Dis., 11:112, 1952.
14. Tondreau, R. L., Hodes, P. J. and Schmidt, E. R.: Am. J. Radiol., 82:258-270, 1959.
15. Additional bibliography, in reference 6.

Panel Discussion

JOSEPH J. BUNIM, *Moderator*

DR. BUNIM: To initiate the discussion, I want to ask various members of the panel what the actual indications for institution of steroid therapy in patients with rheumatoid arthritis are. Now, let us assume that a patient is developing rheumatoid arthritis, that he has been put on a strict conservative regimen including comprehensive interest in his individual needs, rest, psychotherapy, removal from a stressful environment, splints and casts as necessary, aspirin, proper supplements in the diet, and physiotherapy and corrective exercises. After three months of this treatment the patient fails to respond and his disease has progressed. First, what would be the next thing one would do, and, second, what would be the indications for steroid therapy?

DR. LOCKIE: I think that steroid therapy occupies a very important place now in the treatment of patients with rheumatoid arthritis. First, it is quite obvious that there are a few patients who need steroid therapy immediately, as exemplified by the patient with far-advanced disease who is in class 3 to 4, who is suffering from severe pain and who has had inadequate care prior to the time he is first seen. I think such a patient should be given steroid therapy for immediate relief, with the hope of salvage and with the hope of relieving symptoms.

Second, there is the patient who has severe systemic rheumatoid disease such as pleurisy, pneumonia or pericarditis and who, in addition, has fever and tachycardia. This patient may die if he is not given steroids in large doses, and in such a patient it may be necessary to continue steroids in some amount forever.

Third, there is the patient who has only a few joints involved, but in whom steroid therapy is indicated to permit the comprehensive physical therapy necessary to rehabilitate him. In this type of patient steroids can be given orally for one week before starting this program, during the two to three weeks of instruction, and then tapered off gradually at the end of three to four weeks.

Fourth, there is the patient who has episodic bouts of rheumatoid arthritis, and this patient can be relieved of a great deal of pain and systemic manifestations by temporary steroid therapy. This is particularly true in children, in whom the episode may last only six to ten weeks followed by recovery even without treatment. If you can relieve these patients with short-term steroid therapy, I think it should be used.

Fifth, there is the patient who has received what I would like to call conservative therapy, including gold salts. If the patient is not doing well at the end of three months, then small amounts of steroids by mouth are indicated.

DR. BUNIM: Dr. Lockie, is there any antagonism between gold and steroids, and is there any reason why one should not give both together?

DR. LOCKIE: If gold salt therapy is part of the program, I do not think corticosteroids should be administered. However, many patients receiving gold salt therapy can be benefited by supplementary intra-articular steroid therapy, and we use it freely under those circumstances, but we do not use large doses of steroids systemically and large doses of gold salts at the same time.

DR. SCHERBEL: If antimalarial drugs are used in these patients, it is obvious that the response will not be at the maximal point for at least three months; in these patients small doses of steroids can be started with the antimalarial drug and tapered off after six to nine months, when the response to the antimalarial drug is maximal.

As far as fulminating disease is concerned, I think the most rapidly effective combination of drugs is ACTH and nitrogen mustard in small doses. We have used these for ten years, and only 2 to 3 mg. per day of the nitrogen mustard and 10 units of ACTH intravenously need to be used. The disease is rapidly suppressed, and the more acute it is the more rapidly it will respond. By this means one can avoid getting into the dilemma of using large doses of steroids, which then eventually will have to be reduced with a possible relapse.

DR. BUNIM: I would be curious to know how many patients coming to an arthritis clinic are getting steroid therapy. Dr. Lockie, would you be willing to estimate how many patients in your care are on steroid therapy?

DR. LOCKIE: The figures are different for our clinic and private patients. In the clinic, 10 per cent of the patients, and in private practice 5 per cent of the patients receive steroids.

DR. BUNIM: Dr. Neustadt, what percentage of your patients are on steroids?

DR. NEUSTADT: I would say our percentage is much, much higher than that. It depends on the type of patient that is presented to you. If most of your patients have early mild rheumatoid arthritis, a large percentage can be controlled without steroids. However, the type of patients that I see are in poor condition when they first arrive and in order to do anything at all, we almost have to rely on steroids. I would estimate that at least 50 per cent of our patients take steroids at some time during the course of their treatment.

DR. BUNIM: Dr. Lockie, of the patients you have seen, how many have never received steroids?

DR. LOCKIE: I would say about 30 per cent.

DR. BUNIM: In other words, about 70 per cent of the patients you have seen received steroids at one time or another—not necessarily under your care but under the care of someone else?

DR. LOCKE: Yes.

DR. BUNIM: I think that is about the right figure. Our percentage is about the same or, if anything, higher than 70 per cent. I might also tell you of a special experience which is fresh in my memory since I have just returned from England, having studied very carefully the results of the Empire Rheumatism Council and the Medical Research Council on the relative value of aspirin versus cortisone in rheumatoid arthritis. I was quite astonished to find that steroid therapy in rheumatoid arthritis is enjoying such widespread use in England.

Are there any additional comments that anyone on the panel would like to make?

DR. McCARTY: There are two comments which I want to make about long-term steroid therapy. First, if one takes into consideration the combined reports of several large clinics, it is evident that marked improvement in functional capacity can not be sustained in more than 50 per cent of patients for longer than two years with continued steroid administration. However, this loss of effect can be frequently restored by empirically switching from one preparation to another.

Second, and I think this is most important, improvement in the patient's functional capacity with steroid therapy is often not associated with the cessation of destructive changes in joints even though the patient may be asymptomatic. Freyberg and Berntsen studied a group of 168 patients with rheumatoid arthritis treated for five years or longer with corticosteroids in doses of 5 to 15 mg. of prednisone or its equivalent per day. However, the vast majority of patients exhibited relentless progressive joint damage and the conclusion is inescapable that long-term hormonal therapy fails to retard the natural progression of the disease. The only exception to this in our experience is the virtual absence of ankylosis in patients treated with these agents.

DR. BUNIM: Are there any contraindications to steroid therapy which should be recognized, Dr. Neustadt?

DR. NEUSTADT: As I mentioned in my paper earlier, there are of course contraindications to the use of steroids; however, I personally think that these contraindications are relative. In other words, I think it depends on how important it is for the patient to have corticosteroid treatment. If you have a patient, a young man perhaps, who has an economic responsibility to support his family, as compared, let us say, with an older person who does not have to do hard work, it is much more important to give steroid treatment to the younger patient. If he has a peptic ulcer or arrested tuberculosis, you might still consider giving steroids, taking certain precautions. That is, if he has an ulcer, you would prescibe an anti-ulcer program along with the steroid and watch the ulcer closely; if he has arrested tuberculosis, it might be well to give isoniazid or one of the other antitubercular drugs.

DR. BUNIM: One of the contraindications which we are very concerned about has received very little mention, and that is a patient who is absolutely bedfast. I think the chances are extremely great that such a patient would develop a compression fracture of the vertebrae due to osteoporosis within a short period of time if he is given a steroid, because of the additive effect resulting from complete bedrest. The question arises as to whether there is any real benefit in treating such patients with large doses of estrogens and androgens. If not, what else can you do for a patient who develops a compression fracture of the vertebrae? Is this an indication for discontinuation of the steroid?

DR. HILL: The mechanism of devolopment of osteoporosis during steroid therapy, as was discussed yesterday in one of the panels, is not well understood, but I think there are at least two factors involved. One is the catabolic effect of steroids, and the other is the effect of the steroids on the parathyroid glands either directly or indirectly as a result of intestinal loss of calcium. Certainly, it would seem logical to try to counteract the catabolic effect of steroids and thus, perhaps, prevent the development of osteoporosis by the use of an anabolic substance, and I think androgens would be indicated. Immobility, which Dr. Bunim has mentioned, also leads to osteoporosis. One of the strongest stimuli to the development of bone matrix is the stress and strain that is applied to a bone, and if this is eliminated through complete bedrest, the effects of the steroid are compounded. Therefore, I also think that a rocking bed or some other mechanism to apply stress and strain on the bones should be added in addition to the androgens in the treatment of this complication. I do not think estrogens are necessarily needed.

DR. BUNIM: I must say that, in our own experience and in the experience of those colleagues with whom I discussed this particular question and who have extensive experience with osteoporosis, the administration of large doses of estrogens and androgens has not really been helpful in patients with compression fractures of vertebrae resulting from the osteoporotic effects of steroids in rheumatoid arthritis. We have, in fact, encountered two patients who had been put on this regimen because of compression fractures and who, while on this regimen, proceeded to fracture more vertebrae despite administration of the gonadal steroids.

DR. HILL: Dr. Bunim, I think we have to take into consideration the diet the patient has been on, too. Sometimes, when the patient with osteoporosis is not responding well, a change in the dietary program, with the addition of certain essential and perhaps sulfur-containing amino acids, as was discussed previously, may lead to an anabolic effect on bone; however, I do not have any confirmatory data on this.

DR. NEUSTADT: Dr. Bunim, in regard to your statement concerning the use of anticatabolic agents—and I assume you are including other substances such as Dianabol and Nilevar—do you mean that these drugs were ineffective after the patient had developed a compression fracture and perhaps had pain, or have you had experience with a group of patients receiving corticosteroid therapy, dividing them into a sex hormone treated group and a control group, and found there is no difference in the frequency of compression fractures?

DR. BUNIM: Unfortunately, we have not been able to get a control group. I simply referred to two patients who had developed compression fractures, who were treated to the best of our ability by palliative therapy, and who were allowed to be up and about with a brace. As they were not relieved of their symptoms, estrogen and androgen therapy was initiated; then several months later they were found to have additional vertebral fractures even though estrogen and androgen therapy had been continued.

Dr. Whedon, at the National Institute of Arthritis and Metabolic Diseases, is conducting a very interesting series of studies on osteoporosis, and perhaps his data can be related to what Dr. Hill said about diet, not only in respect to amino acids, but to the effect of calcium intake on calcium balance of patients who have osteoporosis resulting from steroid administration. He found that calcium intake is very important in the treatment of osteoporosis in patients receiving steroids, and is perhaps more important than estrogens or androgens. He was able to obtain a positive calcium balance in such patients, even though he continued the administration of corticosteroids, by increasing the patient's calcium intake; the critical level of intake appeared to be between 1100 and 1400 mg. of calcium a day. Of course, this required supplementary calcium therapy. The role of the level of calcium in the diet in the pathogenesis of osteoporosis, not only in corticosteroid type but in senile osteoporosis as well, must be re-investigated.

Another controversial question related to the adverse effects of steroids is the incidence of peptic ulcer. There are incidence figures ranging from 25 per cent among patients who have prolonged steroid therapy down to about 8 per cent in a recent publication from the Mayo Clinic. I would like to get the opinion of the panelists on this. It seems to me there are a number of variables that have to be considered. First, do patients with rheumatoid arthritis, even when untreated, have a greater susceptibility to peptic ulcer than patients in the general population? Second, what role does aspirin play in the high incidence of ulcer in rheumatoid arthritis? Third, what role does steroid therapy play in causation of this complication in rheumatoid arthritis? Fourth, does peptic ulcer in steroid-treated patients vary in incidence with the daily dose of the steroid, the duration of steroid therapy and the severity of the rheumatoid arthritis? Fifth, is the combination of aspirin and steroid more likely to produce an ulcer than the administration of the steroid alone? The answers to such questions might be able to solve some of the controversies. Dr. Black, what is your opinion on this matter?

DR. BLACK: I would like to begin by citing some of our experiences with peptic ulcer in these patients. As you pointed out, there is a great divergence in the incidence or prevalence of peptic ulcer in various reported series. In our own experience, 25 per cent of the steroid-treated patients have, at one time or another, had gastric or duodenal ulcers. Although the prevalence of ulcers in patients with rheumatoid arthritis who are not treated with steroids is said to be twice that in the general population, this is considerably under the prevalence of peptic ulcer in steroid-treated patients.

There is also the interesting observation that at least half of the peptic ulcers which occurred in our group of patients treated with steroids were gastric in location. This is certainly quite different from the usual ratio of gastric to duodenal ulcers and introduces the question about the effect of some local agent such as aspirin.

The relationship of peptic ulcer to aspirin administration introduces another question, and one which is difficult to answer on the basis of data available at this time. Certainly, most patients with rheumatoid arthritis receive considerable doses of aspirin. Since we were interested in this question, we divided our group of patients who were receiving dexamethasone into two subgroups—those who were receiving the steroid alone and those who were receiving the steroid plus aspirin. It is interesting to note that almost all of those in the aspirin-treated group had guaiac-positive stools, whereas only one patient in the group treated with dexamethasone alone had guaiac-positive stools. The one ulcer that occurred in this small series was in a patient treated with aspirin and the steroid.

DR. BUNIM: I think there is general agreement by those who have studied this question very carefully that aspirin does cause gastrointestinal bleeding, perhaps in most instances to a small degree, but in others to a large degree. This has been studied by injecting chromium-51 tagged red cells and counting the radioactivity in stools collected over a period of several days, and these results have been published. However, the question arises as to whether you can equate gastrointestinal bleeding with ulcer formation. One does not necessarily follow the other, but I think it is something we will have to evaluate, since almost every patient with rheumatoid arthritis takes very large doses of aspirin all the time, even if he is on steroids.

DR. LOCKIE: I think it is very important to use only tablets of aspirin that dissolve and disintegrate quickly. It has been definitely shown that a hard compressed tablet of aspirin is far more apt to produce ulcer-like symptoms or ulcers than aspirin tablets that disintegrate and dissolve very quickly. It would be interesting to check on the effects of these two kinds of aspirin tablets, using the chromium-51 tagged red cell technique, but the evidence indicates very strongly that we should use a tablet made by a good manufacturer which has the properties I mentioned.

Production and Metabolism of Steroids in Rheumatic Fever*

VINCENT C. KELLEY

University of Washington School of Medicine

After a decade of intensive study, the question concerning the possible role of altered production and metabolism of adrenocorticosteroids in patients with rheumatic fever remains unresolved. Early investigators who concerned themselves with this question were handicapped by inadequate methodology and inadequate understanding of normal steroid biogenesis and catabolism, and to a lesser extent this is true today. With increasing knowledge of these aspects of normal steroid physiology has come an enhanced appreciation of the enormous complexity of the problem involved in definitively evaluating steroid production and metabolism in patients. Even despite the advances in steroid methodology that have been achieved

* The investigations reported in this paper were supported in part by grants from the American Heart Association, New York, N. Y.; the Life Insurance Medical Research Fund, New York, N. Y.; The Upjohn Company, Kalamazoo, Mich.; the Washington Heart Association, Seattle, Wash.; the Boeing Research Fund, Seattle, Wash.; and by Research Grants HG-911 from the National Heart Institute and A-765 from the National Institute of Arthritis and Metabolic Diseases, U. S. Public Health Service, Bethesda, Md.

in recent years, at the present time data that have accumulated can be interpreted only tentatively, pending the availability of more definite methodology and the accomplishment of more detailed and comprehensive studies.

During the past ten years the author and his collaborators, first at the University of Utah and more recently at the University of Washington, have carried out rather extensive studies of steroid metabolism in patients with rheumatic fever; the present discussion will be confined almost exclusively to a summarization of the results of these studies. Most of the data arising from these studies have been published elsewhere previously and will not be presented in detail here.

In evaluating adrenocorticosteroid production by the rheumatic fever patient, it is necessary to include a consideration of both quantitative and qualitative aspects of steroid production. Thus, steroid production might be abnormal by virtue of: (1) generalized over- or underproduction of all steroids normally elaborated by the adrenal cortex with no alteration in the relative amounts of individual steroids produced; (2) over- or underproduction of certain steroids without an equivalent parallel alteration in the production of other steroids, resulting in abnormal steroid ratios; or (3) production of "abnormal" steroids or failure to produce one or more steroids which normally are secreted by the adrenal cortex.

One approach to the evaluation of total steroid production by the adrenal cortex is through measurement of urinary excretion of adrenocorticosteroids or their metabolites. Many such studies have been done in patients with "rheumatic disease"[14, 25] but few of these have been concerned solely with rheumatic fever patients. Although the group of so-called "rheumatic diseases" all seem to have certain similarities, they are by no means identical, and there seems little reason to expect identical changes in steroid production or metabolism in the various disease states usually included as members of this group. The methods used in the earlier studies, including biological assay techniques and chemical determinations of urinary "corticoids" and 17-ketosteroids, were of limited value because they lacked either specificity or sensitivity. However, the results of these studies established one point with reasonable certainty: steroid excretion is not increased in patients with rheumatic disease.

Later, the introduction of techniques for measurement of 17-hydroxycorticosteroids (17-OHCS) based on the Porter-Silber reaction[20] provided an improved means of estimating total adrenocorticosteroid production. These methods measure a group of steroids which include cortisol, the principal adrenocortical hormone in normal man, and therefore might be expected to reflect more reliably the function of the adrenal cortex than did previously available methods.

With one of these techniques,[9] a detailed study of urinary 17-OHCS excretion in children with active rheumatic fever was performed.[8] No significant difference was observed between these patients and a group of normal children with regard to 17-OHCS excretion. These data would seem to indicate that adrenal steroid secretion is neither increased nor decreased in patients with active rheumatic fever. However, it should be remembered that urinary 17-OHCS excretion may be influenced by many other factors (rates of conjugation and "metabolism" of steroids, renal function, etc.). Only a relatively small proportion of administered steroid appears in the urine as 17-OHCS, and rather extreme variations in urinary 17-OHCS excretion may occur in an individual patient on different days while the patient is receiving the same daily dose of steroid.[8] These considerations make it apparent that any conclusions regarding steroid secretion by the adrenal cortex based on urinary 17-OHCS excretion data must be regarded with some skepticism.

Plasma 17-OHCS concentrations also were studied in patients with various phases of rheumatic fever activity.[15] In these studies it was observed that, except during the first few days of an acute rheumatic attack, plasma 17-OHCS concentrations were lower than normal. In patients with "well established" active rheumatic fever (more than two weeks after onset of illness) the mean plasma 17-OHCS concentration (5.9 µg./100 ml.) was significantly lower than in normal children. Similarly, in 87 patients with inactive rheumatic fever and in 27 patients with chorea without other overt rheumatic symptoms the plasma 17-OHCS concentrations were significantly lower than in normal children. During the first few days of rheumatic symptoms plasma 17-OHCS concentrations were somewhat elevated (mean = 23 µg./100 ml.); however, these values were considerably lower than those observed in patients acutely sick with other severe illnesses.[4, 13, 16, 17] Thus, in patients with rheumatic fever, plasma 17-OHCS concentrations are uniformly low except during the first few days of illness, at which time they are somewhat greater than normal but are not elevated to the same extent as in patients with other acute, severe illnesses.

The failure of these patients to maintain "normal" plasma 17-OHCS concentrations might be attributable to either a decreased rate of steroid production or an increased rate of disappearance of free steroid from the circulation (decreased half-life). To investigate this latter possibility, which seemed reasonable, the half-life of exogenous cortisol in rheumatic patients was studied.[6] The results of these studies indicate that in children with active rheumatic fever the half-life of cortisol is prolonged rather than shortened. This would seem to indicate that the low plasma 17-OHCS concentrations in rheumatic patients are attributable to decreased steroid production rather than to an increased rate of its disappearance from the circulation.

Decreased steroid production by the adrenal cortex might be due to either a failure of the anterior pituitary to produce adequate ACTH or a failure of the adrenal cortex to respond to ACTH stimulation which in the normal person would be adequate to evoke normal production of steroids. In an attempt to determine which of these factors might be responsible for the low plasma 17-OHCS concentrations, a study was undertaken[3] in which the concentration of ACTH in the blood of a group of patients with various phases of rheumatic activity was estimated by the Sydnor and Sayers adrenal ascorbic acid depletion technique.[22] It was found that in children with "early acute" rheumatic fever (first week of illness), as in normal children[21] and patients with other acute illnesses,[23] blood ACTH concentrations were not high enough to be detected by this method, but in patients with "well established" active rheumatic fever, inactive rheumatic fever, or chorea these concentrations were elevated. It seems evident from these data that the low plasma 17-OHCS levels in patients with rheumatic fever cannot be attributed to failure of the anterior pituitary to produce adequate ACTH, since in the same groups of patients who have low plasma 17-OHCS levels the blood ACTH levels are higher than normal. Rather, it would seem that, in accordance with the current concept of humoral control of ACTH secretion, the elevated ACTH levels in these patients may be considered secondary to the decreased 17-OHCS levels.

The fact that these patients do not maintain plasma 17-OHCS levels as high as usual "normal" levels despite the stimulation provided by higher than usual circulating ACTH levels would suggest that the adrenal cortex in these patients is less than normally responsive to ACTH. Another suggestion that the adrenals in rheumatic patients are not normally responsive to ACTH stimulation may be gleaned from the observed phenomenon that elevated plasma 17-OHCS concentrations do not occur in response to salicylate intoxication in rheumatic patients, whereas they do in previously normal subjects,[7] and this stimulus is known to exert its effect on plasma steroid concentrations by inducing increased release of ACTH by the pituitary.[5]

However, although the adrenals in rheumatic patients may not be normally sensitive to ACTH stimulation, they are by no means completely unresponsive. This has been demonstrated by the fact that in rheumatic patients the plasma 17-OHCS response to a standard test dose of ACTH (25 I.U., I.M.) is normal.[12] This, of course, is a large ACTH dose which provides nearly maximal stimulation. Unfortunately, no data are available to indicate the adrenal responsiveness of these patients to minimal ACTH stimulation. Recently, studies of "pituitary reserve" using Metopirone (SU-4885) have been undertaken[2] to determine the response to this drug in rheumatic patients. These studies are still preliminary, and there are no adequate studies of normal children at various ages with which to compare them. It is apparent, however, that these patients respond to Metopirone by an increased urinary 17-OHCS excretion of approximately the magnitude that would be anticipated for a normal response. This would suggest that the anterior pituitary is normally responsive and that sufficient ACTH is released to evoke a normal increase in 17-OHCS excretion.

No evidence has been advanced nor has it been postulated that any "abnormal" steroid is produced by the adrenal cortex in rheumatic fever patients or that there is complete absence in these patients of any steroid normally produced by the adrenal cortex. If such abnormalities do exist in rheumatic patients, they remain undetected. On the other hand, there has been considerable speculation concerning whether there may be abnormal "glucocorticoid/mineralocorticoid" ratios in rheumatic fever patients and, if these do exist, whether they might be of significance in the pathogenesis of the disease. These questions remain unanswered primarily because adequate methods to resolve them have not been available. Because many steroids are produced by adrenal steroidogenesis,[10, 18, 19] and in reality there is no clear-cut distinction between "glucocorticoids" and "mineralocorticoids," many steroids having considerable potency of each type, it has been difficult to approach the problem of determining "glucocorticoid/mineralocorticoid" ratios.

There have been clear demonstrations in several disease states of simultaneous overproduction of certain steroids and underproduction of others due to decrease or absence of specific enzymes involved in the biochemical process of adrenal steroidogenesis.[1] As mentioned by Axelrod and Goldzieher,[1] there have been no definitive demonstrations of reduced steroid 17-hydroxylating activity of the adrenal cortex, so the syndromes that might result from this have remained undefined. The author recently has suggested[14] that if 17-hydroxylating activity of the adrenal cortex were absent or reduced but 11-β- and 21-hydroxylating activity remained intact, the major product of adrenal steroidogenesis would be corticosterone, and if in addition 11-β-hydroxylating activity were reduced, the major product of adrenal steroidogenesis would be 11-desoxycorticosterone. In either case the production of 17-OHCS (the potent "glucocorticoids") would be reduced, as would the "glucocorticoid/mineralocorticoid" ratio.

Certain studies have been accomplished and others are in progress to determine whether this might be the situation in rheumatic fever patients. Plasma corticosterone concentrations have been determined in children with rheumatic fever and in normal children[11] and found to be significantly higher in the rheumatic patients; consequently, since rheumatic patients have lower plasma 17-OHCS concentrations than normal children, the 17-OHCS/corticosterone ratios are reduced in the rheumatic patients. In addition, the relatively few data available suggest that the increase in plasma corticosterone concentration in response to ACTH was greater in the children with rheumatic fever than in normal children. These observations would be consistent with the concept that the adrenal cortex of the rheumatic fever patient may have reduced 17-hydroxylating activity with intact 11β- and 21-hydroxylating activity.

Further studies to evaluate the 11β-hydroxylating activity of the adrenal cortex in these patients involving determinations of aldosterone and 11-desoxycortisol[24] are in progress. With regard to these studies it can be said at this time only that the adrenal appears capable of converting 11-desoxycortisol to cortisol (11β-hydroxylation) in rheumatic patients, as evidenced by the fact that only insignificant concentrations of 11-desoxycortisol but considerably greater concentrations of cortisol are found in the plasma of these patients. However, the data also suggest the possibility that there is some reduction in 11β-hydroxylating activity in these patients in that, following the administration of Metopirone (SU-4885), plasma 11-desoxycortisol levels appear to remain elevated for an abnormally long time in patients with rheumatic fever.

This latter observation might be explained if the rate of disappearance of free 11-desoxycortisol from the circulation is abnormally slow (prolonged half-life). No data are available with regard to this point. However, it is known that both cortisol and corticosterone have prolonged half-life values in patients with active rheumatic fever.[6, 11] These values return to normal as the patient improves clinically.

All of these data make it apparent that neither production nor metabolism of steroids is completely normal in patients with rheumatic fever. However, the changes observed are subtle and somewhat difficult to evaluate and interpret. What their significance may be with regard to pathogenesis of the disease remains an enigma. It seems obvious that much further investigation is indicated. Perhaps as new techniques and concepts are developed and explored it will be possible to define more accurately the precise alterations in steroid production and metabolism which exist in rheumatic fever patients and to interpret more confidently their significance.

REFERENCES

1. Axelrod, L. R. and Goldzieher, J. W.: The metabolism of 17α-hydroxyprogesterone and its relation to congenital adrenal hyperplasia. J. Clin. Endocrinol., 20:238, 1960.
2. Blaim, A. and Kelley, V. C.: To be published.

3. Brill, A. B., Ely, R. S., Done, A. K., Ainger, L. E. and Kelley, V. C.: Blood adrenocorticotropin (ACTH) in children with rheumatic fever. J. Clin. Endocrinol., 16:262, 1956.
4. Done, A. K., Ely, R. S. and Kelley, V. C.: Studies of 17-hydroxycorticosteroids. XIV. Plasma 17-hydroxycorticosteroid concentrations at death in human subjects. A.M.A. Am. J. Dis. Child., 96:655, 1958.
5. Done, A. K., Ely, R. S. and Kelley, V. C.: Salicylates and the pituitary-adrenal system. Metabolism, 7:52, 1958.
6. Done, A. K., Ely, R. S., Olsen, L. J. and Kelley, V. C.: The *in vivo* half-life of exogenous hydrocortisone in patients with rheumatic fever. Metabolism, 4:416, 1955.
7. Done, A. K., Ely, R. S., Raile, R. B. and Kelley, V. C.: Studies of 17-hydroxycorticosteroids. XIII. Effects of salicylate intoxication in rheumatic and non-rheumatic subjects. J. Pediat. 47:727, 1955.
8. Ely, R. S., Ainger, L. E., Seely, J. R., Done, A. K. and Kelley, V. C.: Studies of 17-hydroxycorticosteroids. X. Urinary excretion of 17-hydroxycorticosteroids in patients with rheumatic fever. J. Clin. Endocrinol., 15:523, 1955.
9. Glenn, E. M. and Nelson, D. H.: Chemical method for the determination of 17-hydroxycorticosteroids and 17-ketosteroids in urine following hydrolysis with β-glucuronidase. J. Clin. Endocrinol., 13:911, 1953.
10. Hechter, O. and Pincus, G.: Genesis of the adrenocortical secretion. Physiol. Rev., 34:459, 1954.
11. Hughes, E. R., Kelley, V. C. and Ely, R. S.: To be published.
12. Kelley, V. C.: Rationale for hormone therapy in rheumatic fever. Ann. N. Y. Acad. Sc., 61(2):369, 1955.
13. Kelley, V. C.: Studies of pituitary-adrenal hormones in children in health and disease. Pediatrics, 15:1, 1955.
14. Kelley, V. C. and Ely, R. S.: Production and metabolism of adrenocorticosteroids in connective tissue disease. Ann. N. Y. Acad. Sc., 86:1115, 1960.
15. Kelley, V. C., Ely R. S., Done, A. K. and Ainger, L. E.: Studies of 17-hydroxy-corticosteroids. VI. Circulating concentrations in patients with rheumatic fever. Am. J. Med., 18:20, 1955.
16. Klein, R., Papadatos, M. D. and Fortunato, J.: Serum corticoids in children under stress. J. Pediat., 43:385, 1953.
17. Nelson, D. H., Samuels, L. T., Willardson, D. G. and Tyler, F. H.: The levels of 17-hydroxycorticosteroids in peripheral blood of human subjects. J. Clin. Endocrinol., 11:1021, 1951.
18. Pincus, G.: The biosynthesis of adrenal steroids. Progr. Allergy, 4:198, 1954.
19. Pincus, G.: The biosynthesis of adrenal steroids. Ann. N. Y. Acad. Sc., 61(2):283, 1955.
20. Porter, C. C. and Silber, R. H.: A quantitative color reaction for cortisone and related 17, 21-dihydroxy-20-ketosteroids. J. Biol. Chem., 185:201, 1950.
21. Sydnor, K. L., Kelley, V. C., Raile, R. B., Ely, R. S. and Sayers, G.: Blood adrenocorticotrophin in children with congenital adrenal hyperplasia. Proc. Soc. Exper. Biol. & Med., 82:695, 1953.
22. Sydnor, K. L. and Sayers, G.: A technic for determination of adrenocorticotrophin in blood. Proc. Soc. Exper. Biol. & Med., 79:423, 1952.
23. Sydnor, K. L., Sayers, G., Brown, H. and Tyler, F. H.: Preliminary studies on blood ACTH in man. J. Clin. Endocrinol., 13:891, 1953.
24. Waxman, S. H., Tippit, D. F. and Kelley, V. C.: To be published.
25. West, H. F.: Corticosteroid metabolism and rheumatoid arthritis. Ann. Rheumat. Dis., 16:173, 1957.

The Evolution of
Rheumatic Heart Disease in Children

Five-Year Report of a
Cooperative Clinical Trial of
ACTH, Cortisone, and Aspirin *

A joint report by the Rheumatic Fever Working Party of the Medical Research Council of Great Britain and the Subcommittee of Principal Investigators of the American Council on Rheumatic Fever and Congenital Heart Disease, American Heart Association.

Members of the Rheumatic Fever Working Party and United Kingdom participating centers: The late Sir James Spence (Chairman), Royal Victoria Infirmary, Newcastle; Professor A. Bradford Hill, Honorary Director, Statistical Research Unit of the Medical Research Council (Vice-chairman, and Chairman following the death of Sir James Spence); Dr. E. G. L. Bywaters (Secretary), Canadian Red Cross Memorial Hospital, Taplow; Dr. E. Ellis, Royal Victoria Infirmary, Newcastle; Professor Stanley Graham, Royal Hospital for Sick Children, Glasgow; Professor R. S. Illingworth, The Children's Hospital, Sheffield; Dr. B. E. Schlesinger Hospital for Sick Children, Great Ormond Street, London; Professor A. G. Watkins, Llandough Hospital, Cardiff.

Members of the Principal Investigators Subcommittee and United States participating centers: Dr. David D. Rutstein (Chairman), Coordinating Center, American Heart Association, New York; Dr. Albert Dorfman, La Rabida Jackson Park Sanitarium, Chicago; Dr. Edward E. Fischel, College of Physicians and Surgeons, Columbia University, New York; Dr. John D. Keith, Hospital for Sick Children, Toronto (Canada); Dr. John A. Lichty, University of Colorado Medical Center, Denver; Dr. Benedict F. Massell, House of the Good Samaritan, Boston; Dr. Currier McEwen, New York University-Bellevue Medical Center, New York.

Associated investigators at cooperating centers: In the United Kingdom: Drs. O. P. Gray and N. Royston, Cardiff; Dr. Gavin C. Arneil, Glasgow; Drs. D. G. Cottom, J. N. Montgomery, and H. J. Weston, London; Dr. Rendle Short, Shef-

* The National Heart Institute of the United States Public Health Service supported the study with grants to the coordinating center and to the cooperating centers in the United States and by a travel grant to the Medical Research Council of Great Britain. The Medical Research Council provided support for the six centers and for a coordinating registrar in the United Kingdom. The center in Toronto received a grant from the Canadian Arthritis and Rheumatism Society. In the United States, the costs of the medical care of its patients were met by each cooperating center, and in Great Britain by the National Health Service. The American Heart Association provided office space for the American Coordinating Center and a grant for statistical services.

This cooperative clinical trial was first proposed by Dr. John R. Mote, then assistant general manager of the Armour Laboratories. For the planning of the study, funds were provided by Armour Laboratories and Merck and Company, and space and services by the Helen Hay Whitney Foundation.

In the planning and conduct of this trial much is owed to the wise advice and guidance of the late Dr. T. Duckett Jones and the late Sir James Spence.

This report was published simultaneously in the British Medical Journal in the United Kingdom, in Circulation (Volume XXII, Number 4, October 1960) in the United States, and in the Canadian Medical Association Journal in Canada. It is reprinted here through the courtesy of the American Heart Association and the publishers of Circulation. The report was presented at the Hahnemann Symposium by David D. Rutstein, M.D., Harvard Medical School.

581

field; Drs. Barbara Ansell, Alan St. J. Dixon, K. Hallidie Smith, and Gerald Thomas, Taplow. In the United States: Drs. Carrol Butler, Florence Mayer, Raymond J. Walther, and Eliot Young, Boston; Drs. John I. Gross, Andrew Lorincz, Irving Rozenfeld, and Katherine Smull, Chicago; Drs. Matthew L. Gibson and John H. Githens, Denver; Drs. Charles W. Frank and Daniel Larson (Columbia) New York; Drs. Janet Baldwin (deceased), Eugenia F. Doyle, Ann G. Kuttner, Gene H. Stollerman, and Harrison Wood (New York University) New York; Drs. R. D. Rowe and A. D. Barry McKelvey, Toronto (Canada).

Statistical consultation and services were provided by Miss Marjorie T. Bellows, Chief Statistician and Mrs. Elizabeth R. Densen of the American Heart Association and Dr. John Knowelden, London School of Hygiene and Tropical Medicine. Mr. Felix Moore, Professor and Chairman, Department of Public Health Statistics, University of Michigan School of Public Health served as statistical consultant. Dr. A. St. J. Dixon, Taplow, served as Coordinating Registrar for the British centers. Mrs. Ruth E. Rutstein was Coordinator for the centers in the United States.

The United Kingdom and United States cooperative clinical trial was set up in 1951-52 to compare the relative merits of ACTH, cortisone, and aspirin in the treatment of rheumatic fever and the prevention of rheumatic heart disease. Over a period of approximately a year and a half, and under closely defined diagnostic criteria, 497 children under the age of 16 were admitted to the trial in 12 centers in the United Kingdom, the United States, and Canada. These patients were allocated at random to one or another of the three treatments under investigation. They were treated according to a specified plan for 6 weeks and, after a further 3 weeks of detailed observation, were followed up at defined intervals. Full details of the plan of the study have been given in an earlier publication.[1]

The previous report compared the three treatment groups in detail throughout the 6 weeks of treatment, 3 succeeding weeks of observation, and at the end of a further year of follow-up. It was concluded that there was no evidence that any of the three agents resulted in uniform termination of the disease and on all treatments some patients developed fresh manifestations during treatment. Treatment with either of the hormones had resulted in more prompt control of certain acute manifestations but this more rapid disappearance was balanced by a greater tendency for the acute manifestations to reappear for a limited period upon cessation of treatment. Treatment with the hormones was followed by a more rapid disappearance of nodules and soft apical systolic murmurs. At the end of 1 year, however, there was no significant difference between the three treatment groups in the status of the heart.

This second joint report records the state of the patients after a follow-up of 5 years. It is concerned with a comparison of the amount and severity of rheumatic heart disease in each of the three treatment groups at the end of this time period. It also demonstrates that the status of the heart at start of treatment is the major factor determining the condition of the heart at the end of 5 years and that no treatment can be properly evaluated if this factor is not taken closely into account.

THE NUMBERS INVOLVED

Of the 497 cases admitted to the trial (240 U.K. and 257 U.S.) 445 (89.5 per cent) were known to be alive at the end of the 5 years and the status of the heart had been recorded for all but 19 of them. Sixteen (3.2 per cent) were known to have died. Thus 92.7 per cent of 497 cases had been traced at 5 years. Of the remaining 36 untraced cases 9 were known to be alive at the end of 4 years, 9 at the end of 3 years, 8 at the end of 2 years, 1 at the end of 1 year, and 9 were lost before the end of the first year.

The numbers of deaths and the numbers successfully followed up are given in more detail in Table 1, where the cases have been divided into three groups according to the status of the heart on admission to the trial: namely Group A, no or questionable carditis and no pre-existing heart disease; Group B, carditis present but no pre-existing heart disease; and Group C, definite or questionable pre-existing heart disease.*

At the end of 5 years the fact of death or the status of the heart among the survivors had been recorded in 88 per cent in Group A, 90 per cent in Group B and 88 per cent in Group C. Similarly, the figures for the three treatment groups were 91 per cent ACTH, 89 per cent cortisone and 87 per cent aspirin. The corresponding figure was 91 per cent for the U.K. and 87 per cent for the U.S.

It is clear that within these classifications no differential losses, which might obscure comparisons, have taken place.

DEATHS

Of the 497 children under the ages of 16 who were admitted to the study and completed the prescribed course of treatment only 14 had died from rheumatic fever or rheumatic heart disease by the end of the 5 years of follow-up.† One of these deaths occurred shortly after the end of treatment and 4 more within the first year of follow-up. There were no deaths in the second year and only 1 in the third, followed by 4 deaths in the fourth year and 4 in the fifth. In addition there were 2 deaths from unrelated causes, namely one in the ACTH group from acute nephritis and uremia in the fourth year and one in the cortisone group from acute intestinal obstruction in the fourth year.

Division by treatment of the 14 deaths due to rheumatic fever or rheumatic heart disease shows 7 among the 162 ACTH cases (4.3 per cent), 2 among the 167 cortisone cases (1.2 per cent), and 5 among the 168 aspirin cases (3.0 per cent). Division by cardiac status at the start of treatment (Tables 1 and 9) shows no deaths at all in the 117 Group A cases (cases with

* The diagnostic criteria for admission to the study specified carditis as shown by any one of the following:
  (a) Development of an organic apical systolic murmur or an aortic diastolic murmur under acceptable observation.
  (b) Change of heart size of more than 15 per cent on standard x-ray film by any standard method of measurement.
  (c) Pericarditis revealed by a definite friction rub or by pericardial effusion.
  (d) Congestive failure, in a patient under 25 years and in the absence of other causes, and shown by one or more of the following: (1) dyspnea, (2) orthopnea, (3) enlargement of the liver, (4) basal pulmonary rales, (5) increased jugular venous pressure, or (6) edema.

In the assessment of carditis as a criterion for entry to the trial, it was assumed in patients with no known pre-existing rheumatic heart disease or history of an attack of acute rheumatic fever, that previous to the current illness the patient's heart was of normal size and that there were no rheumatic murmurs. In other patients observations of changes in heart size and murmurs were used in determining carditis and recorded.

† One child given cortisone who died 20 hours after the start of treatment is not included in the 497 children or the 14 deaths. With this single exception all the patients survived the course of treatment. The death rates following these courses can therefore be compared without the introduction of any bias due to the incidence of deaths during treatment.

TABLE 1. NUMBER OF CASES TRACED AT FIVE YEARS ACCORDING TO CARDIAC GROUP. U.K., U.S., U.K. AND U.S.

CARDIAC GROUP AT START OF TREATMENT	At start of treatment	NUMBER OF CASES				Per cent untraced
		Died	Alive and heart status known	Alive but heart status unknown	Untraced	
U.K.						
Group A—no or questionable carditis; no pre-existing heart disease	41	0	37	0	4	9.8
Group B—Carditis present; no pre-existing heart disease	123	4*	109	4	6	4.9
Group C—with definite or questionable pre-existing heart disease	76	7†	61	3	5	6.6
All groups	240	11	207	7	15	6.2
U.S.						
Group A—no or questionable carditis; no pre-existing heart disease	76	0	66	4	6	7.9
Group B—Carditis present; no pre-existing heart disease	129	1	112	6	10	7.8
Group C—with definite or questionable pre-existing heart disease	52	4	41	2	5	9.6
All groups	257	5	219	12	21	8.2
U.K. and U.S.						
Group A—no or questionable carditis; no pre-existing heart disease	117	0	103	4	10	8.5
Group B—Carditis present; no pre-existing heart disease	252	5*	221	10	16	6.3
Group C—with definite or questionable pre-existing heart disease	128	11†	102	5	10	7.8
All groups	497	16	426	19	36	7.2

* One death from acute nephritis and uremia.
† One death from acute intestinal obstruction.

no or questionable carditis and without pre-existing heart disease), 4 deaths (1.6 per cent) among the 252 Group B cases (carditis present but no pre-existing heart disease) and 10 (7.8 per cent) among the 128 Group C cases (with pre-existing heart disease). Of the Group B cases 1 death occurred among the 37 cases with failure and/or pericarditis at entry (2.7 per cent) and 3 deaths in the remaining 215 cases (1.4 per cent) where these features were absent. Six of the 10 deaths in Group C occurred in a small group of 31 cases where there was already failure and/or pericarditis at the start of treatment. In other words death occurred in 1 out of every 5 of these cases compared with 1 in 25 in the remainder of Group C.

There were more deaths among females (9 in 238 or 3.8 per cent) than among males (5 in 259 or 1.9 per cent) but the difference might very easily be due to chance. There were also more deaths among those whose disease was 6 weeks or more in duration when treatment was started than among those treated within 6 weeks of onset (8 of 104 or 7.7 per cent compared with 6 of 393 or 1.5 per cent). The difference occurred entirely in the Group C cases where the death rate was 17.5 per cent among late treated cases as compared with 3.4 per cent in early treated cases (7 of 40 and 3 of 88 cases). In Group B the rates for late and early treated cases were 1.9 per cent and 1.5 per cent respectively (1 of 54 and 3 of 198 cases). The death rate was not significantly lower among those treated within 2 weeks of onset (3 of 225 or 1.3 per cent) than among those treated at 2 to 6 weeks (3 of 138 or 2.2 per cent).

One of the most remarkable features of this study is the very low case fatality in comparison with previous reports.[2-5] In addition to the modern treatment of the disease there may, however, be a number of other factors concerned in this striking decrease in the severity of the disease. These factors could include a change in the natural history of rheumatic fever or streptococcal infection, the introduction of penicillin and sulfadiazine prophylaxis and environmental features associated with the higher standard of living. There were also six severely ill patients reported in the U.S. as being kept out of the trial of randomized treatments in addition to the one death after 20 hours of treatment (see footnote, page 583). On the other hand, not included in this study are cases of rheumatic fever too mild to be admitted to the study hospitals, a number of which limit their admissions to rheumatic fever and receive referrals from other hospitals. In other words the case fatality rate could have been biased in either direction by these selective factors.

RECURRENCES

The study plan specified that all cases should receive daily prophylaxis with sulfadiazine, after initial eradication of the streptococcus with a 10-day course of penicillin. In spite of this schedule, recurrences did occur and for analytical purposes were defined as the appearance, after an interval of at least 3 months of freedom from rheumatic activity, of manifestations that would have originally qualified the patient for admission to the trial. An analysis was made of all cases retreated for such a recurrence. There were, in total, 64 such retreated recurrences in the 5 years among 56 different cases of the 497 admitted (11 per cent). In addition there were 16 retreated recurrences among 14 cases in which chorea was the only manifestation in the recurrences.

It is more informative, however, to limit attention to the cardiac groups

A and B, since many cases in Group C had continuous rheumatic activity making recurrence impossible to identify. In Groups A and B there were, excluding recurrences of pure chorea, 42 recurrences in 36 cases (10 per cent of the 369 cases). Further, in these two groups the 42 recurrences and 36 cases in which they occurred were divided almost exactly among the three treatment groups. Thus, there were 16 recurrences in 12 of the 114 ACTH cases, 12 recurrences in 12 of the 128 cortisone cases, and 14 recurrences in 12 of the 127 aspirin cases. It is clear that the frequency of retreated recurrences does not bias the subsequent comparisons of the treatments used in this study.

COMPARISON OF THE TREATMENTS

The dosage schedules of ACTH, cortisone, and aspirin were based on published studies and unpublished reports at that time (1950), the aim being to select a dosage likely to be effective over a period of administration short enough to indicate whether the acute attack had been differentially shortened by any one of the three drugs.

The schedules were as follows:*

ACTH   U.K. cases. A daily dosage in U.S.P. units of 80 for the first 4 days, 60 for the next 3 days, 40 for the second and third weeks, 30 for the fourth and fifth weeks, and 20 for the sixth week.

U.S. cases. 120 U.S.P. units for the first 4 days, 100 for the next 3 days, 80 for the second week, 60 for the third week, 40 for the fourth and fifth weeks, and 20 for the sixth week.

Cortisone   A daily dosage of 300 mg. for the first day, 200 mg. for the next 4 days, 100 mg. for the second and third weeks, 75 mg. for the fourth and fifth weeks, and 50 mg. for the sixth week.

Aspirin   A daily dosage of 60 mg. per pound of body weight or 10 Gm. (whichever was less) for the first 2 days, 40 mg. per pound or 10 Gm. (whichever was less) for the next 5 days, and 30 mg. per pound for the second to sixth weeks.

If retreatment was necessary at any time during the 3 months following the original course of therapy, then a 4-week retreatment scheme was followed using the same drug and dosage as in the first 4 weeks of initial therapy. No patient was retreated unless he demonstrated rheumatic activity sufficient to have brought him into the study initially. If, after 3 months without activity, the patient developed a new attack of rheumatic fever, he was treated as in the original course, i.e., for 6 weeks on the same drug and dosage, followed by a 3-week period of observation.

The results among cases followed for 5 years are analyzed in terms of the cardiac groups already defined.

Looking first at Group A (Table 2), it will be seen that 6 of the 37 ACTH cases had a murmur at the end of 5 years (all grade I apical systolic murmurs), 1 of the 33 cortisone treated cases (a basal diastolic murmur), and 1 of the 33 aspirin treated group (a grade I apical systolic murmur). The small excess in the ACTH group is not statistically significant. The striking fact which emerges from this comparison is the exceedingly small proportion of Group A cases treated at these dosage levels of ACTH, cortisone, and

* Further details of the treatment schedule, including control of auxiliary therapy, can be found in the original report.[1]

TABLE 2. NUMBER OF CASES FOLLOWED-UP FOR FIVE YEARS AND PROPORTION WITH ONE OR MORE MURMURS AT THAT TIME, ACCORDING TO TREATMENT GIVEN AND INITIAL CARDIAC STATUS. U.K. AND U.S.

CARDIAC GROUP AT START OF TREATMENT	ACTH			CORTISONE			ASPIRIN		
	No. of cases	With murmurs at 5 years No.	Per cent	No. of cases	With murmurs at 5 years No.	Per cent	No. of cases	With murmurs at 5 years No.	Per cent
Group A—no or questionable carditis; no pre-existing heart disease	37	6	16	33	1	3	33	1	3
Group B—Carditis present; no pre-existing heart disease									
1) Apical systolic murmur grade I, only	5	0	0	19	3	16	15	4	27
2) Apical systolic murmur grade II or III, only	18	4	22	17	7	41	25	8	32
3) Apical systolic and apical mid-diastolic murmurs	12	9	75	15	6	40	17	8	47
4) Basal diastolic murmur only	3	2	67	5	1	20	3	0	0
5) Basal diastolic and other murmurs	16	9	56	9	4	44	9	5	56
6) With failure and/or pericarditis	13	11	85	13	8	62	7	4	57
Group C—with definite or questionable pre-existing heart disease									
1) Without failure and/or pericarditis	26	17	65	27	21	78	27	18	67
2) With failure and/or pericarditis	10	10	100	7	7	100	5	5	100

aspirin, in which there is evidence of heart disease at the end of 5 years of follow-up. The prognosis in cases without carditis, but otherwise meeting the criteria for the diagnosis of rheumatic fever, is so good that it would be unreasonable to expect that large-dose cortisone therapy could significantly improve it. The well recognized occasional severe toxic manifestations in large-dose cortisone therapy also militate against its use in such cases.[6]

In Group B (Table 2), the cases are divided into 6 sub-groups according to their cardiac status, ranging from the mildest with only a grade I apical systolic murmur* to the most severe with pericarditis and/or failure. Examination of these groups shows no consistent difference in favor of any one treatment but the number of cases in each group is small. Direct comparison of the effects of treatment among the total of cases in Group B is not valid because of the unequal distribution of cases of different degrees of clinical severity among the three treatment groups. For example, there were more severely ill cases in the ACTH group and more of the milder cases in the cortisone group. There were only 5 ACTH in comparison with 19 cortisone cases in the group of mild cases with only a grade I apical systolic murmur. On the other hand, there were 16 cases with a basal diastolic and one or more other murmurs in the ACTH group compared with only 9 in the cortisone group. Also there were only 7 cases with pericarditis and/or failure in the aspirin group in comparison with 13 on ACTH and 13 on cortisone treatment.

It is, however, possible to allow for this unequal distribution of cases of varying degrees of clinical severity among the three treatment groups and thus make a valid evaluation of treatment within the entire Group B. Making the assumption that in each of the cardiac sub-groups the three treatments had no differential effects whatsoever, it is possible to calculate the expected outcome in Group B cases for each of the 3 treatment groups.† The expected figures may then be compared with those which actually occurred. Thus, for ACTH the expected number of cases having murmurs at 5 years was 31 as compared with 35 observed, for cortisone 31 expected versus 29 observed, and for aspirin 30 expected and 29 observed. There is no evidence in this comparison that the prognosis has been affected more by one treatment than by another.

An alternative analysis of this important Group B can also be made by comparing separately all cases with a single murmur at the start of treatment and those with two or more murmurs at that time (Table 3). Among

* In this study, the following grades were adopted for reporting apical systolic murmurs:

Grade O—No murmur, or a murmur considered to be "functional" on the basis of its apparent origin at the pulmonic area or along the left sternal border.

Grade P—Murmur apparently localized to the apical area, but so faint as not to be transmitted to or toward the axilla. The "P" murmurs were not considered indicative of carditis.

Grade   I—Soft apical systolic murmur transmitted to or toward the axilla.

Grade   II—Louder similar murmur.

Grade III—Very loud similar murmur, usually transmitted to the back.

† The proportions with murmurs at 5 years were taken separately for the U.S. and the U.K. for each of 6 sub-groups in Group B *for all three treatments combined*. These proportions were applied to the actual number of patients *on each treatment* and in each of the 6 sub-groups (U.K. and U.S. separately) to see how many in the small sub-groups would have had a murmur at 5 years if they had experienced the total rate of occurrence. The "expected" numbers in each small sub-group were then added to give the total number of Group B cases expected to have murmurs. The numbers expected can then be compared with the observed numbers of cases with murmurs at 5 years.

TABLE 3. *CARDIAC GROUP B (CARDITIS PRESENT; NO PRE-EXISTING HEART DISEASE). NUMBER OF CASES FOLLOWED-UP FOR FIVE YEARS AND PROPORTION WITH ONE OR MORE MURMURS AT THAT TIME, ACCORDING TO TREATMENT GIVEN AND INITIAL CARDIAC STATUS. U.K. AND U.S.*

CARDIAC SUB-GROUP AT START OF TREATMENT	ACTH			CORTISONE			ASPIRIN		
	No. of cases	With murmurs at 5 years No.	Per cent	No. of cases	With murmurs at 5 years No.	Per cent	No. of cases	With murmurs at 5 years No.	Per cent
Group B—carditis present; no pre-existing heart disease									
1) One murmur, any grade	26	6	23	41	11	27	43	12	28
2) Two or more murmurs, any grade	28	18	64	24	10	42	26	13	50
3) With failure and/or pericarditis	13	11	85	13	8	62	7	4	57

cases with a single murmur at start of treatment, 23 per cent of those on ACTH, 27 per cent on cortisone, and 28 per cent on aspirin still had one or more murmurs at 5 years, a negligible difference between the treatments. For those who initially had two or more murmurs, the corresponding proportions were 64 per cent ACTH, 42 per cent cortisone, and 50 per cent aspirin. For cases with failure and/or pericarditis at start of treatment the proportions were 85 per cent for ACTH, 62 per cent for cortisone, and 57 per cent for aspirin. In short, in the Group B cases there is no pattern in these results to indicate any advantage for one or another of the forms of treatment.

Finally, of the Group C cases without failure and/or pericarditis at the start of treatment (Table 2) there were 26 on ACTH, 27 on cortisone, and 27 on aspirin. At 5 years 17 (65 per cent), 21 (78 per cent), and 18 (67 per cent) had murmurs. Of the 22 Group C cases with failure and/or pericarditis 10 were treated with ACTH, 7 with cortisone, and 5 with aspirin. In every one of these cases murmurs were present at 5 years. There is once again no evidence of any significant difference between the three treatment groups.

THE EVOLUTION OF RHEUMATIC HEART DISEASE

Since there is no evidence that the treatments varied in their effectiveness, the three groups can be added together for the study of the evolution of rheumatic heart disease in this particular series of patients. The essential division is the cardiac status when treatment was begun.

Cardiac Group A. Of the 103 cases in this group 12 (12 per cent) had a murmur at 1 year. At 5 years* (Table 4) the figure is 8 or 8 per cent (7 with grade I apical systolic murmur and 1 with a basal diastolic murmur). It appears that the outlook is better for the 71 cases without any murmur than for the 32 with a questionable murmur† at the start of treatment, 96 per cent with no apparent heart disease compared with 84 per cent. The difference is not formally significant but it appears in both countries and is in accordance, as shown later, with the general trend of the results.

The number of retreated recurrences in Group A was 10, but none of the 9 cases followed for 5 years had a murmur at that time.

In summary, the prognosis for the cases without carditis when treatment is started (Group A) is excellent. None of the patients had died and 92 per cent were without apparent heart disease 5 years later.

Cardiac Group B. Of the 252 cases in this category originally admitted to the study 5 had died, 10 were known to be alive although their cardiac status was unknown, and the cardiac status at 5 years had been recorded for

* Murmurs in all cardiac groups both appeared and disappeared in the time interval between 1 and 5 years. Thus in some cases murmurs present at 1 year were absent at 5 years, while in other cases that were without murmurs at 1 year a murmur was present at 5 years.

† The questionable apical systolic murmur (P murmur) was defined differently in the United States than in the United Kingdom. This difference affects the comparison of the results between the countries and the interpretation of the natural history of the disease. In the U.S., each principal investigator was permitted to classify a doubtful apical systolic murmur as a P murmur. In the U.K., however, the Working Party agreed that each investigator make a firm decision as to the presence or absence of an apical systolic murmur at the time of admission of the cases to the study. (A few cases, 7, were called doubtful in the U.K.). In the U.K. some patients with doubtful apical systolic murmurs were unquestionably labelled "no murmur," others were labelled "apical systolic murmur" and included in Group B.

TABLE 4. CARDIAC GROUP A (NO OR QUESTIONABLE CARDITIS; NO PRE-EXISTING HEART DISEASE). NUMBER OF CASES FOLLOWED-UP FOR FIVE YEARS AND PROPORTION WITH ONE OR MORE MURMURS AT THAT TIME. U.K., U.S., U.K. AND U.S.

CARDIAC SUB-GROUP AT START OF TREATMENT	U.K.			U.S.			U.K. AND U.S.		
	No. of cases	With murmurs at 5 years No.	Per cent	No. of cases	With murmurs at 5 years No.	Per cent	No. of cases	With murmurs at 5 years No.	Per cent
Group A—no or questionable carditis; no pre-existing heart disease	37	6	16	66	2	3	103	8	8
No murmur	30	3	10	41	0	0	71	3	4
Questionable murmur*	7	3	43	25	2	8	32	5	16

* A murmur apparently localized to apical area but so faint as not to be transmitted to or toward axilla.

221. The remaining 16 had been lost (Table 1). As has already been shown the group is clinically heterogeneous and for analysis of the 5-year results has been subdivided in table 5 into five sub-groups of murmurs (without failure and/or pericarditis) and one sub-group comprising cases with failure and/or pericarditis. The untraced cases were spread evenly over these sub-groups. Confining attention first of all to the total figures (U.K. and U.S.) the following results may be noted:

(1) CASES WITH A GRADE I APICAL SYSTOLIC MURMUR ALONE. Of the 39 cases with only a grade I apical systolic murmur at the start of treatment 14 or 36 per cent had murmurs at 1 year while at 5 years the number had fallen to 7 or 18 per cent (3 with a grade I apical systolic murmur, 1 with a grade III apical systolic murmur, 1 with apical systolic and mid-diastolic murmurs, 1 with basal diastolic, apical systolic and mid-diastolic murmurs, and 1 with apical systolic and pre-systolic murmurs). Thus 82 per cent of this group had no apparent heart disease at 5 years and none had died.

(2) CASES WITH A GRADE II OR III APICAL SYSTOLIC MURMUR ALONE. Of the 60 cases in this category 32 or 53 per cent had at least one cardiac murmur at 1 year. This figure had decreased considerably at 5 years to 19 or 32 per cent (6 with grade I apical systolic murmurs, 5 with grade II or III apical systolic murmurs, 5 with apical systolic and mid-diastolic murmurs, 1 with basal diastolic and apical systolic murmurs, and 2 with known but unspecified murmurs). Thus among these cases 68 per cent had no apparent heart disease at 5 years. Two additional cases originally in this group had died, both in the first year.

(3) CASES WITH AN APICAL SYSTOLIC MURMUR OF ANY GRADE PLUS AN APICAL MID-DIASTOLIC MURMUR. Of the 44 cases in this category 28 or 64 per cent had at least one murmur at 1 year while at 5 years the number was 23 or 52 per cent (6 with an apical systolic murmur grade I, 6 with an apical systolic murmur grade II or III, 4 with an apical systolic and an apical mid-diastolic murmur, 2 with a basal diastolic murmur and an apical systolic murmur, 3 with a basal diastolic murmur, an apical systolic, and a mid-diastolic murmur, and finally 2 with an apical pre-systolic murmur accompanied by an apical systolic murmur in the first and by an apical systolic and a basal diastolic murmur in the second). Thus, among these cases only about half (48 per cent) had no apparent heart disease at 5 years. In addition one had died during the fourth year but not from rheumatic fever.

(4) CASES WITH A BASAL DIASTOLIC MURMUR ALONE. There were only 11 cases in this category of whom 5 or 45 per cent had at least one murmur at 1 year, decreasing to 3 cases or 27 per cent at 5 years (2 with basal diastolic murmurs alone, 1 with unspecified murmurs). Thus, 73 per cent of this group had no apparent heart disease at 5 years. None had died.

(5) CASES WITH A BASAL DIASTOLIC MURMUR AND AN APICAL SYSTOLIC AND/OR A MID-DIASTOLIC MURMUR. Of the 34 cases in this category at 5 years, 33 were reported at 1 year and of these, 22 or 67 per cent had at least one murmur at that time. The figure decreased to 18 out of 34 cases or 53 per cent at 5 years (4 with a grade II apical systolic murmur, 1 with apical systolic and mid-diastolic murmurs, 1 with an apical mid-diastolic murmur alone, 7 with a basal diastolic murmur alone, and 5 with a basal diastolic murmur and another murmur, 4 of which were apical systolic and 1 a mid-diastolic murmur). Thus, almost one half of this group (47 per cent) had no apparent heart disease at 5 years. In addition one patient had died during the fifth year.

(6) Cases with Failure and/or Pericarditis. Turning finally to the cases in Group B with failure and/or pericarditis at the start of treatment, there were 33 such cases, of which 24 or 73 per cent had at least one murmur at 1 year. At five years 23 or 70 per cent had a murmur (4 with a grade I apical systolic murmur, 8 with a grade II or grade III apical systolic murmur, 3 with apical systolic and mid-diastolic murmurs, 2 with a basal diastolic murmur alone, and 6 with a basal diastolic murmur and other murmurs of which 3 were apical systolic, 2 were apical systolic and mid-diastolic, and 1 was apical pre-systolic and mid-diastolic). In other words, only 30 per cent of this group were without apparent heart disease at 5 years. In addition one patient had died during the fourth year.

Comparison of the U.K. and U.S. experiences in all Group B cases (Table 5) reveals no consistent pattern of advantage or disadvantage. The largest difference, which lies in the group with basal diastolic plus other murmurs, is almost entirely a function of a differing standard of interpretation, since the U.K. figure is derived from one center only. Thirty of the total 31 U.K. cases with a basal diastolic murmur at start of treatment whose status was known at 5 years were reported from this center. The basal diastolic murmurs in cases at this center were soft and 25 of the 30 disappeared.

An analysis was made of other factors which might have prognostic effects. These included sex, age, duration from onset, and presence or absence at start of treatment of polyarthritis, nodules, chorea, and prolonged P-R interval. None of these individually appeared to affect the evolution of rheumatic heart disease as measured by the presence of murmurs at 5 years (Table 6). Cardiac enlargement as measured by a cardiothoracic ratio on the teleroentgenogram of 0.60 or greater was present at start of therapy in 16 Group B cases. In 13 of these at least one murmur was present at 5 years. This serious prognosis is explained by the large number of such cases (11 of 16) that had cardiac failure and/or pericarditis at start of treatment, practically all of which (10 of 11) had at least one murmur at 5 years.

Retreated recurrences occurred in 25 Group B cases. The cardiac status at start of treatment among these cases was, on the average, more severe than in the remainder of Group B cases (Table 7). At 5 years these retreated patients had a larger proportion with murmurs than those without retreated recurrences. However, the relationship between cardiac status at start of therapy and at 5 years still held even though retreated attacks had occurred in the interim. Among Group A cases there were no murmurs at 5 years in 9 cases with retreated recurrences; in Group B cases with a single murmur at start of treatment 3 out of 8 cases had murmurs at 5 years as compared with 9 out of 9 in cases with two or more murmurs and 7 out of 8 cases with failure and/or pericarditis.

Summarizing the cases with carditis but without pre-existing heart disease (Group B), it is clear that prognosis is directly dependent on the amount and severity of cardiac involvement at the start of treatment, the proportion with a murmur at 5 years varying from 18 per cent in those with a grade I apical systolic murmur to 70 per cent among those with pericarditis and/or failure. Excluding the group with basal diastolic murmurs for the reason given above and because of the relatively few cases in this category in the U.S., this trend holds when the figures are examined individually for each country. In addition, the proportion of all Group B cases with murmurs is remarkably similar in the two countries.

Cardiac Group C. There were 102 cases with known cardiac status at

TABLE 5. *CARDIAC GROUP B (CARDITIS PRESENT; NO PRE-EXISTING HEART DISEASE). NUMBER OF CASES FOLLOWED-UP FOR FIVE YEARS AND PROPORTION WITH ONE OR MORE MURMURS AT THAT TIME U.K., U.S., U.K. AND U.S.*

CARDIAC SUB-GROUP AT START OF TREATMENT	U.K.			U.S.			U.K. AND U.S.		
	No. of cases	With murmurs at 5 years No.	Per cent	No. of cases	With murmurs at 5 years No.	Per cent	No. of cases	With murmurs at 5 years No.	Per cent
Without failure and/or pericarditis	97	36	37	91	34	37	188	70	37
1) Apical systolic murmur grade I, only	14	4	29	25	3	12	39	7	18
2) Apical systolic murmur grade II or III, only	28	10	36	32	9	28	60	19	32
3) Apical systolic *and* apical mid-diastolic murmurs	24	11	46	20	12	60	44	23	52
4) Basal diastolic murmur only	6	1	17	5	2	40	11	3	27
5) Basal diastolic *and* other murmurs	25	10	40	9	8	89	34	18	53
With failure and/or pericarditis	12	10	83	21	13	62	33	23	70

TABLE 6. CARDIAC GROUP B (CARDITIS PRESENT; NO PRE-EXISTING HEART DISEASE). NUMBER OF CASES FOLLOWED-UP FOR FIVE YEARS AND NUMBERS EXPECTED* AND OBSERVED TO HAVE MURMURS AT FIVE YEARS ACCORDING TO SEX, AGE, DURATION FROM ONSET, AND PRESENCE OR ABSENCE OF VARIOUS SIGNS OR SYMPTOMS. U.K. AND U.S.

STATUS AT START OF TREATMENT	NUMBER OF CASES	NUMBER WITH MURMURS AT 5 YEARS OBSERVED	EXPECTED*
Males	104	41	44
Females	117	52	49
Under 10 years of age	119	55	54
10-16 years of age	102	38	39
0-14 days from onset	102	38	39
15 + days from onset	119	55	54
P-R .18 +	54	15	20
P-R < .18	167	78	73
With joint involvement	76	26	30
Without joint involvement	145	67	63
With nodules	38	20	17
Without nodules	183	73	76
With chorea	30	8	11
Without chorea	191	85	82

* Expected numbers take account of differences in the severity of cardiac involvement among the groups being compared. They were calculated in the following manner: The proportions of cases with murmurs at 5 years were taken separately for the U.S. and the U.K. for each of the six cardiac sub-groups in Group B. These proportions were applied in the U.S. and U.K. separately to the actual number of patients in each cardiac sub-group of the categories listed above to see how many in the small sub-groups would have had a murmur at 5 years if they had experienced the total rate of occurrence. The "expected" numbers in the sub-groups were added to get the total number expected in each category for the U.S. and U.K. combined.

5 years who had definite or questionable pre-existing heart disease at the start of their treatment (Table 8). Of the 80 without failure and/or pericarditis at start of treatment, 70 per cent had heart disease at 5 years and of the 22 with failure and/or pericarditis, all had heart disease. It may also be recalled that in addition 4 and 6 deaths from rheumatic fever had taken

TABLE 7. CARDIAC GROUP B (CARDITIS PRESENT; NO PRE-EXISTING HEART DISEASE). NUMBER OF CASES WITH AND WITHOUT RETREATED RECURRENCES FOLLOWED-UP FOR FIVE YEARS AND PROPORTION WITH ONE OR MORE MURMURS AT THAT TIME. U.K. AND U.S.

CARDIAC SUB-GROUP AT START OF TREATMENT	WITHOUT RETREATED RECURRENCES No. of cases	With murmurs at 5 years No.	Per cent	WITH RETREATED RECURRENCES No. of cases	With murmurs at 5 years No.	Per cent
Group B—carditis present; no pre-existing heart disease						
1) One murmur, any grade	102	26	25	8	3	38
2) Two or more murmurs, any grade	69	32	46	9	9	100
3) With failure and/or pericarditis	25	16	64	8	7	88

TABLE 8.   CARDIAC GROUP C (DEFINITE OR QUESTIONABLE PRE-EXISTING
HEART DISEASE). NUMBER OF CASES FOLLOWED-UP FOR FIVE YEARS
AND PROPORTION WITH ONE OR MORE MURMURS AT
THAT TIME. U.K., U.S., U.K. AND U.S.

CARDIAC SUB-GROUP AT START OF TREATMENT	U.K.		U.S.		U.K. AND U.S.	
	No. of cases	With murmurs at 5 years No. Per cent	No. of cases	With murmurs at 5 years No. Per cent	No. of cases	With murmurs at 5 years No. Per cent
Without failure and/or pericarditis	45	36 80	35	20 57	80	56 70
With failure and/or pericarditis	16	16 100	6	6 100	22	22 100

place respectively in these two groups and one death from other causes in the group without failure or pericarditis.

*   *   *   *

In Table 9 all of the cases in the study followed for 5 years are listed in the order of increasing severity of heart disease at start of treatment. It is abundantly clear that the range from 96 per cent to 0 per cent with normal hearts at 5 years is much more striking than differences reported here or ascribed elsewhere to the effects of treatment. Thus, in the prevention of rheumatic heart disease no evaluation of therapy of acute rheumatic fever can be valid unless this major factor is taken into account in the design of the study or the analysis of the data. This conclusion is reinforced by the occurrence of most of the deaths from rheumatic fever (10 of 14) among cases with pre-existing heart disease, and the absence of deaths among the cases without heart involvement at start of treatment.

TABLE 9.   PROGNOSIS IN RELATION TO CARDIAC STATUS AT START
OF TREATMENT. U.K. AND U.S.

CARDIAC STATUS AT START OF TREATMENT	NO. OF CASES OBSERVED FOR 5 YEARS	PER CENT WITH NO MURMUR AT 5 YEARS	NO. OF DEATHS IN 5 YEARS
Group A			
No carditis	71	96	0
Questionable carditis	32	84	0
Group B			
Apical systolic murmur grade I, only	39	82	0
Apical systolic murmur grade II or III, only	60	68	2
Apical systolic *and* apical mid-diastolic murmurs	44	48	1†
Basal diastolic with or without other murmurs	45 (15)*	53(27)*	1
Failure and/or pericarditis	33	30	1
Group C			
Pre-existing heart disease without failure and/or pericarditis	80	30	5‡
Pre-existing heart disease with failure and/or pericarditis	22	0	6

* Excluding one U.K. center.
† Death from acute nephritis and uremia.
‡ Includes 1 death from acute intestinal obstruction.

No comparisons have been made with the conflicting reports of results obtained with large-dose hormone therapy[7-11] the most recent of which shows no advantage in a well controlled study.[11] A firm decision on the efficacy of large-dose hormone treatment of rheumatic fever will depend on controlled studies of adequate size in which the status of the heart is taken into account.

SUMMARY

1. A study has been made 5 years after the end of treatment of the 497 children who were admitted to the U.K./U.S. cooperative clinical trial of the relative merits of ACTH, cortisone, and aspirin in the treatment of acute rheumatic fever.

2. Four hundred and forty-five of the cases (89.5 per cent) were followed for the complete 5 years and the status of the heart was known for 426 of them. Only 16 (3.2 per cent) had died, 14 of them from rheumatic heart disease; 36 (7.2 per cent) were untraced. The very low fatality rate is striking.

3. At the end of 5 years, there is no evidence that, on the treatment schedule used in this study, the prognosis has been influenced more by one treatment than another. This confirms the findings reported at 1 year.

4. The major factor in determining the incidence of rheumatic heart disease at the end of 5 years is the status of the heart at the time treatment was begun. For cases without carditis initially the prognosis was excellent, since in 96 per cent there was no residual heart disease. In cases with carditis initially but without pre-existing heart disease the proportion without residual heart disease decreased progressively from 82 per cent for those with only a grade I apical systolic murmur to 30 per cent for those with failure and/or pericarditis. In cases with pre-existing heart disease the prognosis was poor. Only 30 per cent of those without pericarditis or failure and none of those with pericarditis and/or failure were without heart disease at 5 years.

5. Cases with carditis and without pre-existing heart disease which had recurrences demanding retreatment during the follow-up period had on the average a more severe cardiac status at start of treatment than did those without recurrences requiring retreatment. At 5 years a larger proportion of these retreated cases had murmurs.

6. These results make clear that treatment of acute rheumatic fever cannot be properly evaluated unless the status of the heart of the patients at the start of treatment is taken closely into account.

REFERENCES

1. The treatment of acute rheumatic fever in children. A cooperative clinical trial of ACTH, cortisone and aspirin. A joint report by the Rheumatic Fever Working Party of the Medical Research Council of Great Britain and the Subcommittee of Principal Investigators of the American Council on Rheumatic Fever and Congenital Heart Disease, American Heart Association. Circulation, *11*:343, 1955, and Brit. M. J., *1*:555, 1955.
2. Findlay, L.: The Rheumatic Infection in Childhood. London, Edward Arnold & Co., 1931, chap. 12.
3. Ash, R.: The first ten years of rheumatic infection in childhood. Am. Heart J., *36*:89, 1948.
4. Wilson, M. G. and Lubschez, R.: Longevity in rheumatic fever. Based on the experience of 1042 children observed over a period of 30 years. J.A.M.A., *138*:794, 1948.
5. Bland, E. F. and Jones, T. D.: Rheumatic fever and rheumatic heart disease. A twenty year report on 1000 patients followed since childhood. Circulation, *4*:836, 1951.

6. Good, R. A., Vernier, R. L. and Smith, R. T.: Serious untoward reactions to therapy with cortisone and adrenocorticotropin in pediatric practice. I. and II. Pediatrics, 19:95 and 272, 1957.
7. Greenman, L., Weigand, F. A. and Danowski, T. S.: Cortisone therapy in initial attacks of rheumatic carditis. Ann. Rheumat. Dis., 12:342, 1953.
8. Markowitz, M. and Kuttner, A. G.: Effect of intensive and prolonged therapy with cortisone and hydrocortisone in first attacks of rheumatic carditis. Pediatrics, 16:325, 1955.
9. Roy, S. B. and Massell, B. F.: Comparison of large and small doses of hormones in treatment of acute rheumatic carditis. Circulation, 14:44, 1956.
10. Ferencz, C., Markowitz, M. and Bunim, J. J.: Effect of large doses of prednisone on acute rheumatic fever: observations on treatment of seventeen patients with carditis with two year follow-up. A.M.A. J. Dis. Child., 97:561, 1959.
11. Combined Rheumatic Fever Study Group. A comparison of the effect of prednisone and acetylsalicylic acid on the incidence of residual rheumatic heart disease. New Engl. J. Med., 262:895, 1960.

Evaluation of Steroid Therapy in Acute Rheumatic Fever

Results of Treatment Related to Other Factors Influencing Prognosis*

BENEDICT F. MASSELL, GABOR CZONICZER, SHEKAR JHAVERI, ROBERT BARNET, and BURTON J. POLANSKY

Children's Hospital Medical Center and Boston City Hospital, Boston, Massachusetts

In papers presented at meetings of the American Heart Association[4] and the New England Cardiovascular Society[1, 2] in October and November 1959, we pointed out that there are a number of factors, in addition to therapy, which may influence the prognosis of rheumatic fever and which must be given consideration in the evaluation of therapy. The International Cooperative Study,[5] in which the House of the Good Samaritan participated, showed similar conclusions. The various factors reported upon by us in 1959 are the interval between the onset of the rheumatic attack and the beginning of therapy, the development of rheumatic fever recurrences subsequent to treatment, and the status of the heart at the beginning of treatment as indicated by the presence of significant murmurs, the intensity of such murmurs, the type of valve lesion, the size of the heart and the presence of congestive failure or pericarditis. In this paper, which is a progress report of our studies, the results of therapy are related to those factors which define the status of the heart.

* This investigation was supported by a research grant (H-4957) from the National Heart Institute, Public Health Service, and by grants from the Massachusetts Heart Association (369-F), the Barnstable County Chapter of the Massachusetts Heart Association, the Schering Corporation, and Merck Sharp and Dohme Research Laboratories.

CLINICAL MATERIAL

The clinical material utilized for the present report consists of 583 patients observed in their first attack of rheumatic fever. As shown in Table 1, these patients are distributed among five study groups.

The "No Therapy" group is a consecutive series of patients who were admitted to the House of the Good Samaritan between 1941 and 1951 and who were carefully screened (for another study[3]) so as to eliminate all those who may have had a recurrence prior to admission to the study. Also excluded from this group are a small number of patients who more appropriately belong to one of the other four study groups. Patients in the "No Therapy" group received either no antirheumatic drugs whatever or, at the most, relatively small amounts of aspirin.

The "Small Dose Hormone" group is a combined group composed of patients selected for ACTH therapy during 1949 and 1950 and of patients given ACTH or cortisone during 1951 and 1952 in connection with the International Cooperative Study.[5, 6] Very few of these patients received a total of more than 2500 units of ACTH or 4.1 grams of cortisone, and very few were treated longer than six weeks.

The "Post-Coop. Hormone" group includes patients selected for a trial of hormone therapy in large dosage during 1952 and 1953. Most of these patients received a total of 13.0 grams of cortisone over a period of 12 to 16 weeks.

The "N.C.S. (New Comparative Study) Hormone" and the "N.C.S. Aspirin" groups are composed of patients included in a new comparative study of large-dose hormone therapy and of aspirin therapy that has been in progress since 1954. In this last study patients meeting specified criteria for rheumatic fever have been selected at random for treatment with aspirin or hormones. Aspirin has been given in a dose of approximately 40 mg. per pound of body weight per day over a period of 12 weeks. Hormones have been given for 12 weeks in total amounts of approximately 4200 units of ACTH gel, 15.5 grams of cortisone, 3.1 grams of prednisone or 310 mg. of dexamethasone. At present the method of random selection is such that the number of patients treated with aspirin is about the same as the number treated with hormones. However, during the first few years of the N.C.S. study there was approximately only one aspirin-treated patient for every two hormone-treated patients. Therefore, in order to increase the number of aspirin-treated patients available for comparison with hormone-treated patients, a small number of patients given aspirin at the House of the Good Samaritan as part of the International Cooperative Study have been included with the N.C.S. Aspirin group listed in Table 1. It is to be noted that all of the 99 patients in the N.C.S. Aspirin group in Table 1 were chosen for aspirin therapy by a method of random selection.

All of the patients in the first three study groups of Table 1 were observed at the House of the Good Samaritan, Children's Hospital Medical Center. Approximately one-third of the patients in the N.C.S. Hormone and N.C.S. Aspirin groups were admitted to the Pediatric Service of the Boston City Hospital. Some of these were started on treatment there and later transferred to the House of the Good Samaritan, while others were given all of their treatment at the Boston City Hospital. The remaining two-thirds of the patients in the N.C.S. Study groups received their care entirely at the House of the Good Samaritan. Patients treated at the Boston City Hospital were

TABLE 1. 583 FIRST ATTACKS OF RHEUMATIC FEVER: CARDIAC STATUS
AT INITIAL OBSERVATION AND DISTRIBUTION OF
CASES IN 5 STUDY GROUPS

| STUDY GROUP | CARDIAC STATUS | | | | TOTAL CASES |
	Normal Heart (cases)	Borderline ? Normal, ? RHD (cases)	Definite RHD (cases)	(%)	
"No Therapy"	139	19	114	41.9	272
Small Dose Hormone	6	3	38	80.9	47
Post-Coop. Hormone	10	2	36	75.0	48
N.C.S. Hormone	51	10	56	47.9	117
N.C.S. Aspirin	45	11	43	43.4	99
Totals	251	45	287	49.2	583

examined and evaluated periodically by members of the Research Staff of the House of the Good Samaritan as well as by members of the Pediatric Staff of the Boston City Hospital.

Follow-up Observations. All of the 583 patients were classified with regard to their cardiac status when they were first observed in the hospital or when therapy was begun (Table 1) and also when they were discharged from the hospital. Thereafter, as the number of years since discharge increased, the number of patients available for classification decreased for the following reasons: Patients who died were excluded from the tabulations after the time of death. Patients developing rheumatic fever recurrences were excluded from the tabulations after the onset of the recurrences. Patients who failed to return to the clinic were eliminated after their last clinic visit. Patients discharged relatively recently from the hospital have, necessarily, a limited potential period of follow-up.

RESULTS

Patients with Normal or Borderline Cardiac Findings at Initial Observation. Most of the 296 patients in these two categories (Table 1) continued to do well and were classified as having normal hearts by the time of discharge from the hospital or within the next few years. Eleven patients, however, developed significant murmurs during hospitalization and were classified as having definite rheumatic heart disease at time of discharge. All of these 11 patients came from the "No Therapy" and N.C.S. Aspirin groups. None of the hormone-treated patients developed significant murmurs.

Patients with Definite Rheumatic Heart Disease at Initial Observation. In approximately one-fourth of 287 patients who initially had definite rheumatic heart disease (Table 1), significant murmurs completely disappeared or became questionable by the time of discharge from the hospital. Thus, at discharge only 74 per cent of these 287 patients were classified as still having definite rheumatic heart disease (Fig. 1). Thereafter, significant murmurs continued to lessen in intensity, and to disappear in some patients, so that the incidence of definite rheumatic heart disease among observed patients reached a level of about 53 per cent between the sixth and seventh years after discharge from the hospital.

Factors Other than Therapy That Influence the Disappearance of Signs of Rheumatic Heart Disease. The cardiac status at the time of the patient's first observation (or at the beginning of therapy) appears to be an important

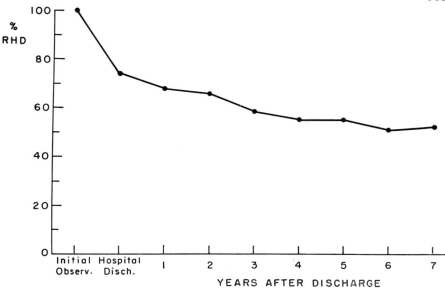

Fig. 1.   Disappearance of signs of rheumatic heart disease: 287 patients with significant murmurs at initial observation.

determinant in the subsequent course of the signs of rheumatic valvular involvement.[1, 4, 5] Some of the factors defining the initial cardiac status and influencing the disappearance of significant murmurs are illustrated in Figures 2, 3 and 4, and in Table 2. Figure 2 demonstrates that patients with enlarged

TABLE 2.   INFLUENCE OF AORTIC REGURGITATION ON DISAPPEARANCE OF SIGNS OF RHEUMATIC HEART DISEASE

	AR II		AR I	
	Observed (cases)	RHD (cases)	Observed (cases)	RHD (cases)
Initial observation	7	7	13	13
Hospital discharge	7	6	13	3
Years after 1	7	6	12	1
discharge 2	5	4	10	1
3	5	4	9	2

Analyses confined to patients with normal size heart and with MR I (mitral regurgitation, Group I), M. INV. I. (mitral involvement, Group I) or no mitral disease.

hearts not caused by pericarditis are less likely to lose all significant murmurs than are patients whose hearts are initially of normal size. Figure 3 shows that the presence of congestive failure (with or without pericarditis) has about the same effect as cardiac enlargement. Figure 3 also suggests that pericarditis without accompanying congestive failure (only 11 cases) is a less unfavorable sign than congestive failure even though most patients with pericarditis also have enlargement of the cardiac silhouette.

Significant apical systolic murmurs were classified according to their intensity in two groups. Group II includes those that were grade 3 or louder (Levine's system of grading). Group I includes significant systolic murmurs of less than grade 3 intensity. Patients with significant systolic murmurs were

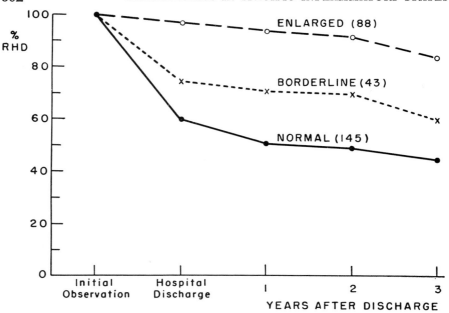

Patients with "pericarditis only" excluded from analysis

Fig. 2. Influence of heart size on disappearance of signs of rheumatic heart disease.

also divided according to whether or not there were accompanying mid-diastolic murmurs. Those patients with a systolic murmur alone were diagnosed as having pure mitral regurgitation (M.R.); those patients with an accompanying mid-diastolic murmur were said to have mitral involvement

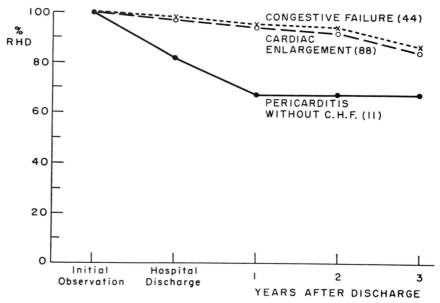

Fig. 3. Comparison of cardiac enlargement, congestive failure and pericarditis without congestive failure in regard to disappearance of signs of heart disease.

(M. Inv.). Figure 4 shows that the intensity of the apical systolic murmur is an important determinant of whether or not signs of valvular disease will disappear, but that the presence of a mid-diastolic murmur (in addition to a systolic murmur) has very little, if any, influence on prognosis.

Aortic diastolic murmurs (definite, long, blowing diastolic murmurs along the left sternal border and/or at the aortic area) were classified in two groups, Group II including those that were of grade 2 intensity or louder, Group I including those that were of less than grade 2 intensity. It is generally believed that signs of aortic regurgitation rarely disappear. The data in Table 2 suggest that this clinical impression is correct for Group II cases but that slight aortic diastolic murmurs (Group I cases) not infrequently disappear completely.

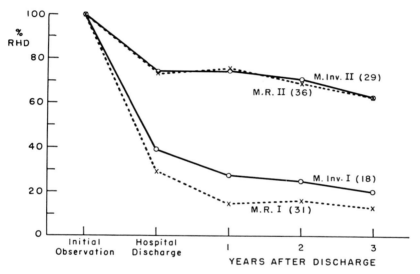

Analysis confined to patients without involvement of the aortic valve and without cardiac enlargement, congestive failure, and pericarditis.

Fig. 4.   Influence of intensity of systolic murmur and presence of a mitral mid-diastolic murmur on disappearance of signs of mitral valve disease.

The cardiac factors influencing the frequency of disappearance of significant murmurs, which have been described in the foregoing paragraphs, are inter-related and can be combined in many different ways. Ten possible combinations are represented by the ten curves shown in Figure 5. The ten groups that correspond to the ten curves can be used for the purpose of classifying the severity of cardiac involvement at the time of initial observation or at the time therapy was begun.

Expected Incidence of Rheumatic Heart Disease for the Five Study Groups. By dividing the 287 cases that initially had definite rheumatic heart disease into the ten groups corresponding to the ten curves in Figure 5, it is possible to calculate the expected incidence of rheumatic heart disease for each of the 287 cases at time of hospital discharge and at one, two and three years after discharge. Furthermore, by recombining the cases according to the five study groups listed in Table 1, it is also possible to calculate the expected incidence of rheumatic heart disease at each interval for each of the study groups.

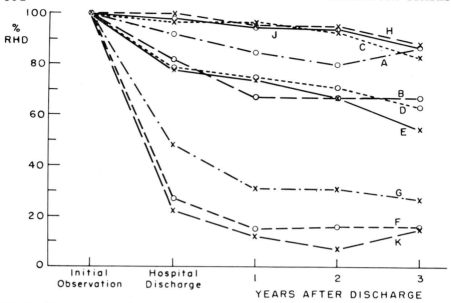

Fig. 5. Disappearance of signs of rheumatic heart disease in groups used for calculating "expected incidence."

The expected incidence data, shown by the five curves in Figure 6, indicate that all of the five study groups were remarkably similar in regard to severity of rheumatic disease—if incidence of residual signs of valvular involvement is used as a measure of severity.

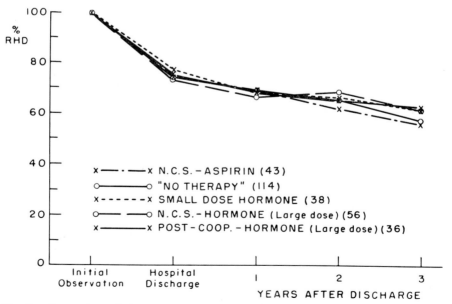

Fig. 6. Comparison of therapy groups in regard to "expected" incidence of rheumatic disease.

Influence of Therapy on Disappearance of Signs of Rheumatic Heart Disease. Because of the close similarity of the five study groups with regard to severity of rheumatic heart disease it is reasonable not only to compare the N.C.S. Aspirin and the N.C.S. Hormone groups (the two groups in which treatment was randomly determined) but also to compare all of the five groups with each other.

Such a comparison is shown in Figure 7, where the actual incidence of rheumatic heart disease at each interval is indicated for each of the study groups. The same data are shown more clearly in Figure 8, in which a somewhat different scale is used and in which the curves indicate the proportion of observed patients in whom all definite signs of rheumatic heart disease have disappeared. From Figures 7 and 8 it is evident that the N.C.S. Hormone

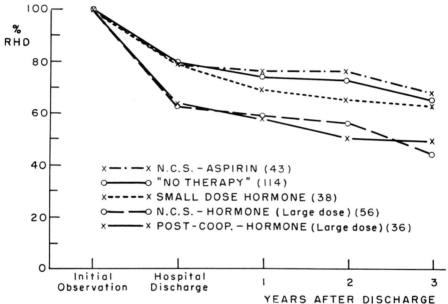

Fig. 7. Comparison of therapy groups in regard to disappearance of signs of rheumatic heart disease.

group of patients fared better than the N.C.S. Aspirin group with regard to disappearance of signs of heart disease. It is also evident that the "No Therapy" group behaved very similarly to the N.C.S. Aspirin group, whereas the course for the Post-Coop. Hormone group was rather similar to that for the N.C.S. Hormone group. The curve for the Small Dose Hormone group falls in between the other curves but somewhat closer to those for the "No Therapy" and N.C.S. Aspirin groups.

These data suggest that treatment with hormones in large amounts increases the frequency with which signs of rheumatic heart disease disappear. Treatment with hormones in relatively small amounts seems to have little if any influence on the disappearance of significant murmurs.

Statistical Analysis of Results and Relation of Results to Severity of Initial Heart Disease. Only preliminary statistical analyses have been completed at this time; at a later date all of the material will be subjected to further statistical review. The results of the preliminary analyses are presented in Tables 3 to 7.

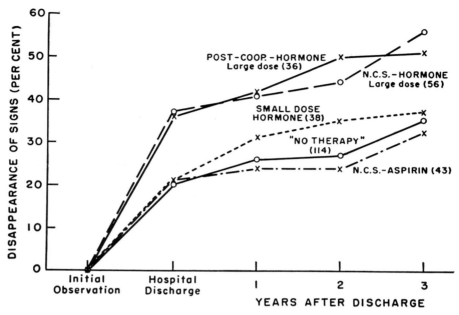

Fig. 8. Comparison of therapy groups in regard to disappearance of signs of rheumatic heart disease.

Table 3 compares the two groups of patients in whom treatment was determined by random selection (N.C.S. Aspirin and N.C.S. Hormone groups). At the time of discharge from the hospital and at one, two and three years after discharge the proportion of patients in whom signs of rheumatic heart disease disappeared was greater for those treated with large amounts of hormones than for those treated with aspirin. However, when the chi square test is applied and the P values are determined, it is found that the observed differences are not statistically significant. This finding, in turn, could be due either to the possibility that there is no real difference in the results or to the possibility that the number of cases observed is still too small to demonstrate that the observed differences are significant. In regard to interpretation of the data, it also is to be noted that the P values for the observed differences at time of hospital discharge (.08) and at one year after discharge (.09) are just slightly above the arbitrary value of .05 that is usually required for "significance."

Because of the foregoing considerations larger numbers of cases were obtained for comparison by combining the data for the two study groups in

TABLE 3. *DISAPPEARANCE OF SIGNS OF RHEUMATIC HEART DISEASE: COMPARISON OF N.C.S. HORMONE AND N.C.S. ASPIRIN GROUPS*

	ASPIRIN Rx			HORMONE Rx			
	Observed (cases)	Loss RHD (cases)	(%)	Observed (cases)	Loss RHD (cases)	(%)	P
Initial observation	43	0		56	0		
Hospital discharge	43	9	21	56	21	38	.08
Years after discharge 1	37	9	24	53	22	42	.09
2	25	6	24	34	15	44	> .10
3	19	6	32	27	15	56	> .10

which large doses of hormones were given (N.C.S. Hormone group and Post-Coop. Hormone group) and by combining the data for the two study groups in which hormone therapy was not used (N.C.S. Aspirin and "No Therapy" groups). The pooling of data in this way seems justified in view of the close similarity of all of the study groups with regard to severity of rheumatic heart disease (Fig. 6).

TABLE 4. *DISAPPEARANCE OF SIGNS OF RHEUMATIC HEART DISEASE: COMPARISON OF N.C.S. HORMONE + POST-COOP. HORMONE GROUPS (COMBINED) WITH N.C.S. ASPIRIN + "NO THERAPY" GROUPS (COMBINED)*

| | ASPIRIN Rx AND "NO THERAPY" | | LARGE DOSE HORMONE | | |
	Observed (cases)	Loss RHD (cases) (%)	Observed (cases)	Loss RHD (cases) (%)	P
Initial observation	157	0	92	0	
Hospital discharge	157	32 20	92	34 37	< .01
Years after discharge 1	126	32 25	89	37 42	< .02
2	106	28 26	68	32 47	< .01
3	88	30 34	60	32 53	.02

When the combined groups are compared (Table 4), it is evident that the data from the patients treated with large doses of hormones and the data from the patients not given hormones are very similar to the corresponding data in Table 3. However, the differences observed with the combined groups in Table 4 are statistically significant since the numbers of cases involved in Table 4 are larger than the numbers of cases in Table 3.

In view of the data in Table 4, which suggest that treatment with large doses of hormones has a favorable influence on the disappearance of signs of rheumatic heart disease, the next and last problem to be considered is whether the differences shown in Table 4 hold for patients with all degrees of cardiac involvement or only for some of these patients.

In order to investigate this problem, patients treated with large doses of hormones and those not given any hormone therapy have been divided into three groups according to the degree of cardiac involvement present when the patients were first observed in the hospital. The expected incidence figures for rheumatic heart disease at various intervals, as shown by the ten curves in Figure 6, have been used as a measure of severity. Thus, the degree of heart disease was considered to be "severe" for patients included in Subgroups A, C, H and J (represented by the top four curves in Figure 6), "moderate" for those in Subgroups B, D, and E (middle three curves), and "slight" for those in Subgroups G, F, and K (lowest three curves).

Table 5 presents a comparison of large dose hormone therapy and no hormone therapy in patients with "severe" rheumatic heart disease. Significant murmurs disappeared in relatively few of these patients, irrespective of therapy given, and there were no significant differences between the two groups being compared. In evaluating these results, especially for purposes of determining the kind of patient for whom hormone therapy should be used, it is important to keep in mind that the data presented here indicate only whether or not signs of valvular involvement persisted. They do not provide any information regarding the severity of residual heart disease among those who continued to have significant murmurs. Furthermore, the

TABLE 5. DISAPPEARANCE OF SIGNS OF RHEUMATIC HEART DISEASE:
ANALYSIS OF "SEVERE" HEART DISEASE CASES IN THE
COMBINED GROUPS

	ASPIRIN Rx AND "NO THERAPY"			LARGE DOSE HORMONE			
	Observed (cases)	Loss RHD (cases)	(%)	Observed (cases)	Loss RHD (cases)	(%)	P
Initial observation	62	0		42	0		
Hospital discharge	62	1	1.6	42	2	4.8	> .30
Years after discharge 1	55	3	5.5	41	2	5.1	> .90
2	43	2	4.7	33	4	12.1	> .20
3	31	3	9.7	28	6	21.4	> .20

present report is not concerned with the problem of whether hormone
therapy may be of value in saving life in critically ill patients, all of whom
would be included in the groups of patients with "severe" rheumatic heart
disease.

An appreciable number of patients with "moderate" heart disease (Table
6) lost their signs of valvular involvement, and the proportion of observed
patients in whom all significant murmurs disappeared was about 100 per cent
to 180 per cent greater among those who were treated with large amounts of
hormones than among those who were treated with aspirin or who received
"no therapy." The chi square test shows that the observed differences are not
quite statistically significant at the time of hospital discharge (P = .09) but
that the differences are significant at all intervals thereafter even though the
number of patients observed at the longer intervals becomes smaller. Although various explanations for the change in "significance" must be considered, one definite possibility is that one or more years are sometimes
required for the complete regression and disappearance of significant murmurs. Hence, the full effect of hormone therapy may not always become
apparent until some time after the completion of treatment.

Table 7 shows that among the patients who initially had "slight" heart
disease the number of those who lost all significant murmurs was relatively
large irrespective of therapy given. However, even in this group the proportion of patients in whom signs of cardiac damage disappeared was on the
average 50 per cent greater among those treated with large doses of hormones than among those who were given aspirin or who received "no therapy." Furthermore the chi square test indicates that the observed differences
are statistically significant.

TABLE 6. DISAPPEARANCE OF SIGNS OF RHEUMATIC HEART DISEASE:
ANALYSIS OF "MODERATE" HEART DISEASE CASES IN
THE COMBINED GROUPS

	ASPIRIN Rx AND "NO THERAPY"			LARGE DOSE HORMONE			
	Observed (cases)	Loss RHD (cases)	(%)	Observed (cases)	Loss RHD (cases)	(%)	P
Initial observation	54	0		23	0		
Hospital discharge	54	9	17	23	8	35	.09
Years after discharge 1	38	7	18	22	10	46	< .03
2	34	7	21	17	10	59	< .01
3	32	10	31	16	11	69	< .02

TABLE 7. DISAPPEARANCE OF SIGNS OF RHEUMATIC HEART DISEASE:
ANALYSIS OF "SLIGHT" HEART DISEASE CASES IN THE
COMBINED GROUPS

	ASPIRIN Rx AND "NO THERAPY"			LARGE DOSE HORMONE			
	Observed (cases)	Loss RHD (cases)	(%)	Observed (cases)	Loss RHD (cases)	(%)	P
Initial observation	41	0		27	0		
Hospital discharge	41	22	54	27	24	89	< .01
Years after discharge 1	33	22	67	26	25	96	< .01
2	29	19	66	18	18	100	< .01
3	25	17	68	16	15	94	.05

SUMMARY AND CONCLUSIONS

1. Among rheumatic fever patients who did not have significant murmurs when they were first observed in the hospital, relatively few subsequently developed signs of rheumatic heart disease. Those instances in which valvular involvement did appear were confined to patients treated with aspirin or given no antirheumatic therapy. None were observed in the groups of patients treated with hormones. Nevertheless, it can be concluded that in the absence, at first observation, of significant murmurs the risk of heart disease developing during the next few years is very slight even in patients who are not given hormone therapy.

2. Among patients who already had significant murmurs when they were first observed, an appreciable number lost their murmurs by the time of discharge from the hospital or during the following few years.

3. The severity of the initial cardiac damage as measured by the size of the heart, the intensity of systolic murmurs and the presence of aortic diastolic murmurs, congestive failure and pericarditis was an important determinant of the subsequent course of the signs of valvular involvement.

4. Therapy also appeared to be a substantial factor influencing the disappearance of significant murmurs. On the whole, patients treated with hormones in large dosage seemed to fare better than did patients treated with aspirin or given no antirheumatic therapy.

5. Since the number of patients in our New Comparative Study, in which therapy is determined by random selection, is still too small to prove statistical significance for the observed differences between aspirin and hormone treatment, and since significant differences could be demonstrated only by pooling data for different study groups, it would seem important that the New Comparative Study be continued until a larger number of patients has been observed.

ACKNOWLEDGMENTS

We are grateful to Drs. David M. Greeley and Sydney S. Gellis for making clinical material from the Boston City Hospital available for this study. We are also indebted to Drs. James Dow, Sujoy Roy, Eliot Young and Raymond Walther and other members of our Clinical and Research Staff for assistance in the evaluation of patients at the House of the Good Samaritan and the Boston City Hospital.

REFERENCES

1. Barnet, R., Czoniczer, G., Jhaveri, S. and Massell, B. F.: Factors affecting the prognosis of first attacks of rheumatic fever and subsequent rheumatic heart disease. II. Role of heart size, valvular lesions, and congestive failure. Proc. New Engl. Cardiovas. Soc., *18*:17, 1959-1960.
2. Jhaveri, S., Czoniczer, G., Barnet, R. and Massell, B. F.: Factors affecting the prognosis of first attacks of rheumatic fever and subsequent rheumatic heart disease. I. Course of the disease during follow-up and role of therapy in the acute phase. Proc. New Engl. Cardiovas. Soc., *18*:15, 1959-1960.
3. Massell, B. F., Fyler, D. C. and Roy, S. B.: The clinical picture of rheumatic fever: diagnosis, immediate prognosis, course, and therapeutic implications. Am. J. Cardiol., *1*:436, 1958.
4. Massell, B. F., Jhaveri, S. and Czoniczer, G.: Therapy and other factors influencing the course of rheumatic heart disease. Proceedings of the 32nd Scientific Sessions of the American Heart Association. Circulation, *20*:737, 1959.
5. The evolution of rheumatic heart disease in children. Five-year report of a cooperative clinical trial of ACTH, cortisone, and aspirin. A joint report by the Rheumatic Fever Working Party of the Medical Research Council of Great Britain and the Subcommittee of Principal Investigators of the American Council on Rheumatic Fever and Congenital Heart Disease, American Heart Association. Circulation, *22*:503, 1960.
6. The treatment of acute rheumatic fever in children. A cooperative clinical trial of ACTH, cortisone and aspirin. A joint report by the Rheumatic Fever Working Party of the Medical Research Council of Great Britain and the Subcommittee of Principal Investigators of the American Council on Rheumatic Fever and Congenital Heart Disease, American Heart Association. Circulation, *11*:343, 1955, and Brit. M. J., *1*:555, 1955.

The Long-Term Effects of
Steroids in Rheumatic Heart Disease

WILLIAM LIKOFF

Hahnemann Medical College and Hospital, Philadelphia

The dramatic effectiveness of steroids in the treatment of rheumatic fever has now been amply confirmed.[3, 4] A review of the long-term benefits must be based upon a consideration of the concepts which prompted their initial use. Therefore, this discussion will include comments concerning the pathogenesis, the natural history and the histopathology of the disease as well as the pharmacodynamics of the steroids, as an antecedent to the comments related to the results which have been obtained.

Although many aspects of its pathogenesis are still poorly understood, rheumatic fever is now generally accepted as a complication of infection with Group A streptococci. This conclusion is based on clinical, epidemiologic, bacteriologic and immunologic observations. However, the nature of the fundamental interaction of the organism and the host which results in the development of rheumatic heart disease in specific patients has not been defined. An explanatory theory of hypersensitivity to the streptococci based on pertinent experimentation with foreign protein sensitization has been formulated.[6]

The streptococcal infections which are presumed to initiate rheumatic fever may be overt and serious or may be so subtle as to go unrecognized by the patient or the physician. The subsequent rheumatic activity likewise may be characterized by classic manifestations or may continue in a protracted subclinical form which defies identification. Unfortunately, the mechanisms which are responsible for the continuing disease and the progressive cardiac damage are unknown. In any case, the disease is characterized by chronicity and recurrent exacerbations.

In many patients the evolutionary patterns of specific valvular deformities are superimposed on the clinical features of rheumatic fever. Because of natural and iatrogenic variables they also are phasic.

As a total result, the natural history of rheumatic fever and rheumatic carditis is predictable only within very gross limits. The major responsible

I. CONCEPTS SUPPORTING TREATMENT

B. NATURAL HISTORY

(DEATH RATE)

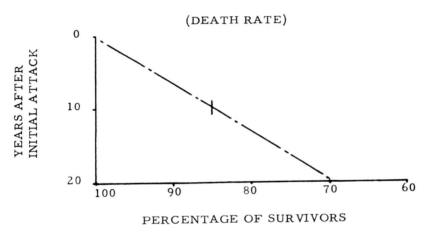

Fig. 1.   Death rate following initial attack of rheumatic activity.

element is the fact that even during the long periods of time when the clinical expressions of the disease are obscure, insidious morphologic tissue changes may continue relentlessly.

In terms of mortality, approximately 15 per cent of the patients succumb within ten years of the initial bout of activity, and 30 per cent within 20 years[10] (Fig. 1). Furthermore, at least 20 per cent of the survivors are disabled within the first decade[9] (Fig. 2).

It is commonly held that the histopathologic lesions are characterized by proliferation and exudative inflammation involving primary collagen tissue or its ground substance. These have a widespread distribution in the endocardium, myocardium, pericardium and conductive system. The histopathologic alterations mature in the valves to produce varying and serious distortions which are responsible for specific interferences in intracardiac blood flow.

Similar distortions obviously do not occur in the myocardium. Nevertheless, significant disturbances in myocardial function are encountered. It has been suggested, therefore, that the histopathology may be myogenic, thereby accounting for the causative relation between rheumatic fever and myocardial failure.[5]

Only two of the clinical effects of the corticosteroids are related to the hypothesis concerning the etiology and the histopathologic expressions of rheumatic fever and rheumatic carditis. Cortisone and related compounds are believed to have important anti-inflammatory and antihypersensitivity actions. At least theoretically, therefore, the foundation for their application to the problem appears secure. If effective, they should bring about both acute and long-term benefits by modifying the early activity and by aborting chronic tissue distortions. When combined with effective antibiotic therapy, they should convert the chronic phasic disease to a more predictable and controlled pattern.

At least the first portion of the total concept, namely, the efficiency of cortisone and its related compounds in the treatment of the acute manifesta-

I. CONCEPTS SUPPORTING TREATMENT

B. NATURAL HISTORY (CONTINUED)

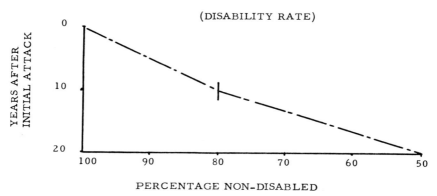

(DISABILITY RATE)

Fig. 2.   Disability rate following initial attack of rheumatic activity.

tions of rheumatic fever, has been confirmed. Whether a true superiority exists over the salicylates is questionable.

An equally serious hesitancy persists regarding the long-term effects or the ability of the steroids to prevent chronic tissue alterations in the heart. Their efficiency in this regard is related to the time of application, the dose system employed and the severity of the initial process.

In patients stricken for the first time, the likelihood of preventing chronic valvular disease decreases as the delay in utilizing the steroids increases (Fig. 3). This is borne out in several comprehensive reviews.[7, 8] Unfortunately, most so-called long-range observations are limited to a year. Thus, in Figure 3, which represents a compilation study, only 2 per cent of the patients are shown to develop a chronic valvulitis when steroid therapy is begun within one week of the onset of activity. This increases to 49 per cent when the drug is given in the second week, to 70 per cent when the delay is extended between the second and fourth week, to 75 per cent when medication is withheld until the fourth to sixth week, and to over 90 per cent when steroids are offered after that time.

The distribution of the valvular lesions which finally occur in the treated

II.   PRACTICAL APPLICATIONS AND RESULTS

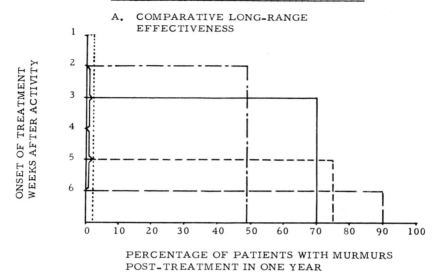

A.   COMPARATIVE LONG-RANGE
EFFECTIVENESS

Fig. 3.   Development of chronic valvular disease as related to the time between the onset of symptoms and initiation of steroid therapy.

and untreated groups is quite similar, mitral deformities being most common. Insufficient time has elapsed to determine whether the natural evolution from mitral insufficiency, the predominant deformity, to stenosis is altered. Nevertheless, it is a firm fact that long-term benefits are not to be expected unless treatment is begun early with the first recognition of the disease.

Studies also suggest that permanent cardiac damage is most likely to be prevented with high dosages of the hormones.[1, 2, 4] To compromise on a minimum daily dose of 60 mg. of prednisolone, for example, is to risk acute and long-term failure. This schedule may be extended two- and threefold if side effects permit. It is maintained until a clinical response is realized and has continued unchanged for at least four weeks. Thereafter a gradual reduc-

II.   PRACTICAL APPLICATIONS AND RESULTS

A.   COMPARATIVE LONG-RANGE
EFFECTIVENESS (CONTINUED)

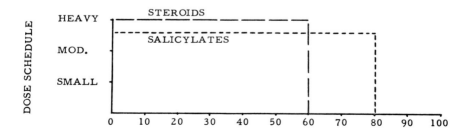

Fig. 4   Development of chronic valvular disease as related to the dose of steroid therapy.

tion over 8 to 12 weeks is warranted, provided that symptoms and signs do
not recur. Figure 4 indicates that the expectation of preventing a persistent
murmur with large doses of steroids is somewhat better than when significant
amounts of salicylates are offered.

The severity of the initial process in many instances is a critical factor in
determining the ultimate long-range effect and may even transcend the
importance of either the time when treatment is offered or the dose sched-
uled. In this matter (Fig. 5) steroids offer more benefit than salicylates.
However, neither agent prevents chronic valvulitis as effectively as when the
activity is only moderate or mild.

The failure to avoid chronic carditis currently can not be explained. A
constant possibility remains that the carditis which does develop in treated

II. PRACTICAL APPLICATIONS AND RESULTS

A. COMPARATIVE LONG-RANGE
EFFECTIVENESS (CONTINUED)

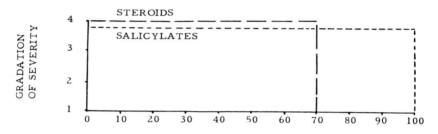

PERCENTAGE OF PATIENTS WITH MURMURS IN ONE YEAR

Fig. 5.   Comparison of steroids and salicylates in the prevention of chronic valvular disease following severe rheumatic activity.

patients may over the years prove more benign than that in untreated persons. The difficulty of assaying the truth of such a premise is self-evident.

The long-range benefits of the steroids, however limited, must be appraised in terms of their noxious toxic and side effects. The preparation of
new potent agents with minimal salt-retaining properties has created a favorable balance in this matter even though the ideal drug is not yet available.

SUMMARY AND CONCLUSIONS

Theoretically, cortisone and related hormones should minimize the acute
expressions of rheumatic activity and the chronic cardiac tissue deformities
which ensue. In respect to the latter, practical experiences indicate that the
best therapeutic response results when these compounds are offered early
in the disease in large doses and are continued for long periods. Side effects
and toxic reactions do not act as serious deterrents to their use. It remains
a matter of current record, however, that treatment failures are common.
There is a growing contention that this stems from delayed and inadequate
application. Whether even under these circumstances the failures are of the
same magnitude as those which occur without therapy is a moot question.

REFERENCES

1. Done, A. K., Ely, R. S., Ainger, L. E., Seely, J. R. and Kelley, V. C.: Pediatrics, *15*:522, 1955.
2. Kropp, I. G.: New York J. Med., *54*:2699, 1954.
3. Massell, B. F.: New Engl. J. Med., *251*:183, 221, 263, 1954.
4. McEwen, C.: Am. J. Med., *17*:794, 1954.
5. Murphy, G. E.: Medicine, *39*:289, 1960.
6. Rich, A. R. and Gregory, J. E.: Bull. Johns Hopkins Hosp., *72*:65, 1943; *73*:239, 1943; *75*:115, 1944.
7. Roy, S. B. and Massell, B. F.: Circulation, *14*:44, 1956.
8. Roy, S. B., Sturgis, G. P. and Massell, B. F.: New Engl. J. Med., *254*:95, 1956.
9. Stroud, W. D., Bromer, A. W. and Gallagher, J. R.: Tr. A. Am. Physicians, *45*:247, 1930.
10. Stroud, W. D. and Twaddle, P. H.: J.A.M.A., *114*:629, 1940.

The Use of Large
Doses of Prednisone
in Acute Rheumatic Fever

CHARLOTTE FERENCZ

University of Buffalo School of Medicine

Ever since the introduction of steroids into the therapy of acute rheumatic fever there has been controversy concerning their effect on the rheumatic process and on the incidence of rheumatic heart disease. A glance back into the salicylate era reveals that many of the questions which plague us today were already debated more than half a century ago. It might, therefore, be of some value to review the historical milestones in the treatment of rheumatic fever and to examine some of the problems which have arisen in connection with salicylate therapy and again with the use of steroids.

In Table 1 are listed the treatment courses of a few selected authors and the results which they reported.

SALICYLATES

Credit is usually given to Stricker[11] of Berlin for recognizing the therapeutic value of salicylic acid in acute rheumatic fever. His was not an unexpected observation since salicylic acid had just become available in powder form and was being tried in various diseases. Stricker reported his initial experience in 1876 and he himself mentioned another worker, Buss, who had found the drug beneficial in rheumatic patients. He further engaged in a lively controversy with Riess, who had apparently also claimed credit for the discovery of this highly effective form of therapy.

The drug, in those early days, was given in a dose of 0.5 to 1.0 gram each hour, except when the patient was asleep, and was continued until signs and

TABLE 1. TREATMENT OF RHEUMATIC FEVER

DRUG	AUTHOR	INITIAL DOSE	DURATION AFTER THERAPY			EFFECT ON HEART
			Fever	Arthritis	ESR	
Salicylates	Stricker (1876)	5-15 gm.	8-10 hrs.	1-2 days		?
	Miller (1914)	10-20 gm.		5 days		−
	Coburn (1943)	10-20 gm. I.V.	<3 days	1-2 days	10 days	+
	Warren (1945)	10-20 gm. I.V.	4 days		54 days (av)	−
		<7 gm.	11 days		58 days (av)	−
Cortisone	Hench (1949)	200 mg.	1-4 days	2-6 days	12-18 days	?
	Co-op study (1955)	200-300 mg.	<7 days	3-8 days	14-35 days	−
	Greenman (1953)	300 mg.		1-2 days*	28 days (av)	+
	Wilson (1953)	300 mg.				+
Prednisone	Ferencz (1959)	75 mg.	5-48 hrs.	1-2 days*	4-20 days	?
	Comb'd study (1960)	60 mg.				−

* In one patient in each series articular effusion lasted 8 or 9 days.

symptoms disappeared. This took "no less than 5 gms. and no more than 15 gms." and thus the medication was usually stopped on the second day. Signs of salicylism, tinnitus and deafness, were then usually present.

As soon as a few cases had been so treated the frequent re-appearance of manifestations after therapy became apparent. The return of fever and joint symptoms occurred rapidly, within two or three days in some patients, or in a delayed fashion, after six to eleven days in others. The course of therapy was therefore modified, and after the initial high dosage, a small daily dose of 1.5 to 2.5 grams was given for a week.

Stricker's initial report is remarkable for the detailed recording of careful observations; little, if anything, can be added to his description of the effect of salicylates in acute rheumatic fever. In addition to the subsidence of fever and arthritis, he noted the beneficial effect of the drug on pericarditis and pericardial effusion. He was certain that pre-existing heart disease was not altered, but he hoped that the favorable effect on acute exudative manifestations would also indicate a favorable effect on endocarditis.

Extensive experience with the use of salicylates accumulated rapidly over the next several years. Miller,[9] in 1914, undertook a review of all the reported cases, which included over 1000 patients treated with salicylates and an approximately equal number of untreated patients. He made the interesting and important observation that recurrence of disease manifestations occurred more frequently in salicylate treated patients (30.3 per cent) than in patients in whom the acute manifestations had subsided spontaneously (6 per cent). Miller noted the difficulty of drawing accurate conclusions in a disease so variable, but it was clear, he said, that heart disease was not prevented by the use of salicylates.

There was renewed interest in the problem of rheumatic fever therapy in 1943, when Coburn[1] asserted that rheumatic heart disease could be prevented if salicylate therapy was sufficiently intense. Coburn gave 10 to 20 grams of sodium salicylate intravenously for two or three days and then continued with high oral doses for a month longer. Thus was initiated the era of "massive salicylate therapy."

It was not long before the literature abounded in controversial opinions. Among the authors of that period were Warren, Higley and Coombs,[12] who reported a controlled study using massive doses of salicylates in one group of patients and conventional doses in the other. They could find no evidence that residual heart disease was prevented by either form of therapy. Thus the pendulum, which had swung from optimism to pessimism and back, now returned to a mid-position and symptomatic treatment was in general use for the next few years.

STEROIDS

With the introduction of steroids we have started on a new but similar cycle, which has not yet been completed. The dramatic anti-inflammatory effects of steroids raised the hope for a permanent, favorable effect on rheumatic lesions of the heart. Although some authors found encouragement in their results, others could not perceive any significant lessening in the incidence of rheumatic heart disease in steroid-treated patients. Inevitably, the dosage and treatment time were increased, and recent courses of steroids have been as high and as long as the patients could tolerate with reasonable safety.

It is not my intention to cast a vote either for or against steroids as a therapeutic agent capable of preventing rheumatic heart disease. The variability of opinion, even among the few authors quoted in Table 1, is evident. I would only point out that over the entire period of time under consideration, there is really no great difference between the results of salicylates and steroid therapy, no matter which parameter is used for comparison. Fever usually subsided in a day or two, arthritis within about one week, and the sedimentation rate returned to normal in approximately one month. If one takes into account that the criteria for improvement are also variable, the differences between the reports become negligible indeed.

The treatment courses quoted in Table 1 are illustrated in Figures 1 and 2.

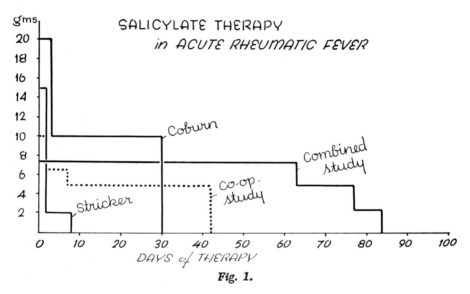

Fig. 1.

Figure 1 shows the courses of salicylate therapy: the short course of Stricker,[11] the "massive" course of Coburn[1] and the recent courses used in the two cooperative studies[2, 15] for comparison with steroids.

In Figure 2 are depicted the early course of cortisone used by Hench,[8] the short intensive courses of Wilson[13, 14] and the slowly tapering course of the International Cooperative Study.[15] Among the high-dose long-term courses is shown the method advocated by Greenman[7] and the slow tapering introduced by Massell and adopted by the Combined Study Group[2] and, finally, the long course which we used at the Harriet Lane Home.[4]

It has already been noted, in connection with Miller's series,[9] that disease manifestations recurred in many patients after salicylate therapy was stopped, whereas only a few failed to remain well if the manifestations subsided without specific therapy. Similarly, in the case of steroid-treated patients, return of abnormalities was frequent; the longer the course of treatment, the later in relation to the initial illness was the return of acute manifestations. Among 17 patients who received the long 99-day course of prednisone shown on the graph, a return of abnormal findings was noted in 14 instances.

Manifestations which had been present during the initial illness and had disappeared during therapy gradually reappeared at the end of the treat-

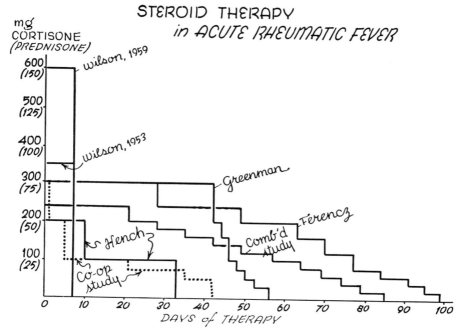

Fig. 2.

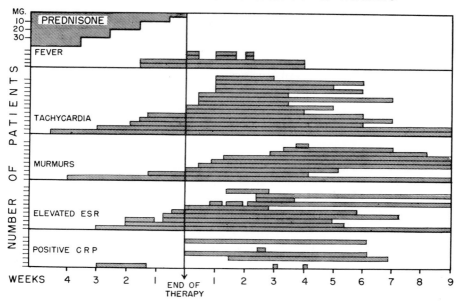

Fig. 3.

ment course. Tachycardia, an elevated sedimentation rate and changing murmurs were the most frequent signs. In some patients these made their appearance during the period of diminishing dosage of steroid; in others, only after the drug was discontinued. The abnormal manifestations usually persisted for a considerable length of time.

There is as yet no satisfactory explanation for this phenomenon. Its relation to the end of therapy, no matter how long the treatment course, suggests a basic alteration in the disease process beyond simple suppression of manifestations.

PATHOLOGY

We turn, naturally, to the pathologists for information about possible alterations in the rheumatic process as a result of suppressive therapy. Valuable information has been published recently by Costero[3] of the National Institute of Cardiology of Mexico. A condensation of his report is presented here with his permission.

TABLE 2.   EFFECT OF STEROIDS ON THE PATHOLOGIC PROCESSES OF ACUTE RHEUMATIC FEVER: 30 FATAL CASES

PATHOLOGIC PROCESS	EFFECT OF STEROIDS	COMMENT
Fibrinous verrucae	No effect on incidence	Favors embolism
	May be larger and more numerous	Less deformity
	Organize more slowly	
Fibrinoid necrosis	Greater incidence	Unfavorable
	More extensive	
	Necrosis of myocardium	
	Less tendency to organization	
Aschoff nodules	Diminished incidence	Favorable even with small doses
	Increase in fibroblasts and collagen	
	Appearance of basophilic cells	
Lymphocytic infiltration	Usual frequency and severity	Unaffected
Cicatrization	Rich in cells	
	Poor in collagen	
	Less retractile	Less deformity
Fibrinous pericarditis	Usual frequency	
	Increased fibrinoid necrosis	More scarring
	Intense fibroblastic reaction	Scar loose
	Less retractile collagen	

Adapted from Costero, I.: Arch. Inst. cardiol. México, 28:155, 294, 427, 1958, by permission.

Costero studied the hearts of 30 patients who had died of acute rheumatic fever and who had been treated with steroids for varying periods of time preceding death.

The findings indicate a complex effect of steroids, favorable on some aspects of the rheumatic process, unfavorable on others.

The three outstanding deviations from the expected pathological findings are: (1) the great tendency to fibrinoid necrosis and even necrosis of the myocardium of an extent never seen before the advent of steroid therapy; (2) the suppression of Aschoff bodies, evident even after relatively small doses of hormone; and (3) the increased fibroblastic activity, but greatly slowed organization resulting in less deformity of affected structures.

These same findings in rheumatic patients have been reported by workers in this country,[5, 6, 10] but since only isolated instances were observed a definite pattern of altered responses was not discerned.

It is of note that these alterations are similar to those observed following steroid administration in experimental inflammatory states, as reported by Drs. Jean and Spain earlier in this symposium.

These findings bring to mind a number of important questions: How is the clinical course of the patient influenced by the altered pathologic processes? How is residual cardiac damage determined? What is the role of Aschoff bodies, or of necrosis in the ultimate outcome of the disease? What is the local biochemical alteration in the heart which produces necrosis of myofibers and calls forth the inflammatory response?

It appears that further studies in rheumatic fever should attempt to bridge the gap between the findings of pathologists and biochemists on the one hand and the observations of clinicians on the clinical course of the disease on the other.

Perhaps this approach could bring about a purposeful method of rheumatic fever therapy and the control of rheumatic heart disease, a goal which clinical trial and error cannot hope to achieve.

REFERENCES

1. Coburn, A. F.: Salicylate therapy in rheumatic fever. Bull. Johns Hopkins Hosp., 73:435, 1943.
2. Combined Rheumatic Fever Study Group: A comparison of the effect of prednisone and acetylsalicylic acid on the incidence of residual rheumatic heart disease. New Engl. J. Med., 262:895, 1960.
3. Costero, I., Barroso-Moguel, R., Chevez, A., Monroy, G. and Contreras, R.: Las lesiones de la fiebre reumatica en los enfermos tratados con cortisona. Arch. Inst. cardiol. México, 28:155, 294, 427, 1958.
4. Ferencz, C., Markowitz, M. and Bunim, J. J.: The effect of large doses of prednisone on acute rheumatic fever, A.M.A. J. Dis. Child., 97:561, 1959.
5. Glaser, R. J. and Smith, D. E.: Rheumatic heart disease with acute rheumatic fever. Clinico-pathologic conference. Am. J. Med., 11:109, 1951.
6. Golden, A. and Hurst, J. W.: Alterations of the lesions of acute rheumatic myocarditis during cortisone therapy. Circulation, 7:218, 1953.
7. Greeman, L., Weigand, F. A., Mateer, F. M. and Danowski, T. S.: Cortisone therapy of initial attacks of rheumatic carditis. A.M.A. J. Dis Child., 89:426, 442, 1955.
8. Hench, P. S., Slocumb, C. H., Barnes, A. R., Smith, H. L., Polley, H. F. and Kendall, E. C.: The effect of the adrenal cortical hormone, 17-hydroxy-11-dehydro-corticosterone (compound E) on the acute phase of rheumatic fever: preliminary report. Proc. Staff Meet., Mayo Clin., 24:277, 1949.
9. Miller, J. L.: The specific action of salicylates in acute articular rheumatism. J.A.M.A., 63:1107, 1914.
10. Spain, D. M. and Roth, D.: Effect of cortisone and ACTH on the histopathology of rheumatic carditis. Am. J. Med., 11:128, 1951.
11. Stricker: Ueber die Resultate der Behandlung der Polyarthritis rheumatica mit salicylsaure. Berl. klin. Wchnschr., 13:1, 14, 99, 1876.
12. Warren, H. A., Higley, C. S. and Coombs, F. S.: Effect of salicylate on the sedimentation rate, fever and occurrence of valvular heart disease in acute rheumatic fever. Proc. Centr. Soc. Clin. Res., 18:30, 1945.
13. Wilson, M. G.: Effect of short term administration of corticotropin in active rheumatic carditis. A.M.A. J. Dis. Child., 86:131, 1953.
14. Wilson, M. G. and Lim, W. N.: Short term hormone therapy: its effect in active rheumatic carditis of varying duration. New Engl. J. Med., 260:802, 1959.
15. United Kingdom and United States Joint Report: Treatment of acute rheumatic fever in children: cooperative clinical trial of ACTH, cortisone and aspirin. Circulation, 11:343, 1955.

Massive Steroid Therapy in Acute Rheumatic Activity and Carditis

DANIEL MASON

Hahnemann Medical College and Hospital, Philadelphia

This report presents the results of a clinical study of 52 children who were diagnosed as having acute rheumatic activity, with concomitant rheumatic carditis in most. The study was conducted during the past two and a half years at the Children's Heart Hospital of Philadelphia. Each patient was given large doses of steroids (usually dexamethasone), and attempts were made to evaluate the effects of these steroids on the acute manifestations of the presenting illness.

There were 24 male and 28 female patients on steroid therapy in this study. Their ages ranged from 3 to 18 years at the time of the initial administration of the steroid drug. The average age was 10.4 years. There were 32 white children, 19 Negro children and one Filipino child. The average hospital stay was five and a half months.

Findings of acute rheumatic activity in this group of patients included fever, migratory polyarthritis, chorea, erythema marginatum, subcutaneous nodules and carditis. Carditis was shown by a significant apical systolic murmur in patients previously known not to have any such murmur, the presence of a basal early blowing diastolic murmur of aortic insufficiency or an apical mid-diastolic murmur in patients without a previous history of rheumatic activity in whom there was reason to believe that there was no pre-existing heart disease, or a significant change in the loudness or quality of any of these murmurs without significant change in heart rate in a patient under observation with a previous history of rheumatic fever or rheumatic heart disease. Other signs of carditis included obvious progressive cardiac enlargement (by x-ray), pericarditis as shown by a pericardial friction rub or by electrocardiographic means (none had a detectable pericardial effusion), or congestive failure in the absence of dynamic valvular disease or other causes. Also included in the congestive failure group were those patients in whom diastolic gallop rhythm developed in the absence of apparent significant valvular disease.

In addition, certain of the patients manifested findings of transient first degree heart block, increased sedimentation rate, increased white blood cell count, positive C-reactive protein reaction, significant changes in antistreptolysin-O titers or a history of positive beta hemolytic streptococcal infection preceding the signs and symptoms of acute rheumatic activity by one week to one month. Two of the patients in this series had a history of scarlet fever preceding acute rheumatic activity.

Other less specific symptoms included fever, recurrent bouts of epistaxis, nausea, vomiting, crampy abdominal pain, pallor, weight loss, anorexia, fatigue and "nervous irritability." One patient had a leukemoid reaction and another had a purpuric rash prior to therapy.

TABLE 1. MANIFESTATIONS OF RHEUMATIC ACTIVITY AND CARDITIS
IN 52 PATIENTS

SIGNS AND SYMPTOMS	NUMBER OF PATIENTS
Migratory polyarthritis	30
Arthralgia	12
Chorea	7
Erythema marginatum	5
Subcutaneous nodules	2

Of the 52 patients, 30 had evidence of migratory polyarthritis or a bona fide history of such prior to steroid therapy, and 12 had arthralgia (Table 1). Chorea was noted in seven patients, erythema marginatum in five and subcutaneous nodules in two. Carditis (Table 2) was manifested by a new apical systolic murmur in one patient, a new mid-diastolic murmur in one patient and changing murmurs in 14 patients. Twenty-six patients had cardiac enlargement, but only eight had changing heart size during the course of therapy. There were two patients with acute pericarditis (both shown by

TABLE 2. MANIFESTATIONS OF RHEUMATIC ACTIVITY AND CARDITIS
IN 52 PATIENTS

SIGNS AND SYMPTOMS	NUMBER OF PATIENTS
Carditis	
Apical systolic murmur (new)	1
Mid-diastolic murmur (new)	1
Basal early diastolic murmur (new)	10
Changing murmurs	14
Cardiac enlargement (x-ray)	26
Pericarditis (pericardial friction rub)	1
(electrocardiogram)	2
Congestive failure	2
Gallop rhythm (diastolic)	3
First degree heart block (transient)	15

electrocardiographic means), and one of these had an associated pericardial friction rub. There were two patients with congestive failure in addition to three patients who developed a diastolic gallop rhythm.

Fifteen patients revealed evidence of transient first degree heart block. An increased sedimentation rate was noted in 39 patients (Table 3) and increased white blood cell count in 16 patients. A positive C-reactive protein reaction was noted in 36 patients, and significant changing ASTO titers were noted in 32 patients.

TABLE 3. MANIFESTATIONS OF RHEUMATIC ACTIVITY AND CARDITIS
IN 52 PATIENTS

SIGNS AND SYMPTOMS	NUMBER OF PATIENTS
Increased sedimentation rate	39
Increased white blood cell count	16
Positive C-reactive protein reaction	36
Changing significant ASTO titers	32
History of preceding beta hemolytic streptococcal infection	
(sore throat)	9
(scarlet fever)	2

TABLE 4. ELECTROCARDIOGRAPHIC FINDINGS

	NUMBER OF PATIENTS
First degree heart block	15
Frequent ventricular premature systoles	1
A-V nodal rhythm	2
Right bundle branch block	1
W-P-W Syndrome	1
Nonspecific T-wave changes	2

There was a history of preceding beta hemolytic streptococcal infection in 11 patients. Nine of these had sore throat and two had scarlet fever.

In addition to the above, it was noted that there was one patient who had transient frequent ventricular premature systoles (Table 4), two patients with transient A-V nodal rhythm, one patient with transient right bundle branch block, one patient with transient Wolfe-Parkinson-White syndrome, and two patients with a myocardial abnormality following no specific pattern, as shown by nonspecific T-wave changes.

Each of the patients in this study was given a course of steroid therapy. This was usually dexamethasone in the dosage of 6 to 10 mg. (depending upon weight and age) for a period of six weeks with gradual decrease in the dosage to zero during the subsequent four weeks. Most of these patients also received concomitant oral penicillin prophylaxis in the dosage of 200,000 units twice daily. All were on complete bed rest during the acute phase of their illness.

Among the 52 patients thus treated, clinical observations revealed the following: In those patients with migratory polyarthritis, all had significant reduction in the joint manifestations. The average duration of joint findings after the institution of steroid therapy was two days.

Of special interest were the results obtained in seven patients with chorea. In four patients with this manifestation, each had a remission of the neurologic signs within 48 to 72 hours; the remaining three patients were greatly improved within one week, although one of these still had choreiform movements of minimal degree for three months. All received concomitant phenobarbital; none had any phenothiazine or other tranquilizing drugs. Several patients with choreiform movements could not walk, speak nor dress prior to steroid therapy; following therapy, they were able to perform these functions within two days.

Erythema marginatum seen in five patients was noted to disappear in all within four days following institution of therapy with steroids.

TABLE 5. CHANGING MURMURS DURING STEROID THERAPY

	NUMBER OF PATIENTS
Apical systolic murmur:	
Disappeared	5
Diminished loudness	4
Mitral insufficiency and mitral stenosis:	
Disappeared	1
Mid-diastolic murmur:	
New	1
Disappeared	1
Diminished loudness	1
Aortic insufficiency:	
Disappeared	2

Subcutaneous nodules seen in two patients were diminished in four days following institution of steroid therapy but did not disappear. These persisted in one patient for one month.

During steroid therapy, it was noted that the apical systolic murmur of mitral insufficiency present initially in 22 cases disappeared in five (Table 5) and diminished in loudness in four. In one patient, the murmurs of mitral insufficiency and mitral stenosis disappeared. The short, blowing, faint apical mid-diastolic murmur disappeared in one patient, became less loud in another and appeared during steroid therapy in one patient. Two patients with aortic insufficiency lost the early basal diastolic murmur during steroid therapy.

Roentgen examination (Table 6) revealed a decrease in heart size in

TABLE 6.   X-RAY FINDINGS

	NUMBER OF PATIENTS
Cardiac enlargement:	
Stationary	18
Smaller	6
Progressive increase	2

six patients; the heart size was not changed in 18 patients. In two patients, the heart size increased while they were on steroid therapy.

Pericarditis, found in two patients, disappeared in one and a half months in one patient (by electrocardiogram). This patient's pericardial friction rub disappeared within one week following institution of therapy. Evidence of pericarditis persisted for three months following the cessation of one course of steroid therapy in the second patient.

Of the five patients with cardiac failure due to acute carditis, there were three patients who responded (without digitalis) to steroid therapy with subsidence of the signs and symptoms of congestive failure within six days. These were the patients who had developed diastolic gallop rhythm as a principal finding of cardiac failure. Two patients also required digitalis and diuretic therapy. The latter two patients had severe dynamic valvular disease, and one had a relapse into congestive failure following the cessation of steroid therapy.

Among the 15 patients with first degree heart block, conversion to normal A-V conduction occurred in 13 in one to four months during the course of steroid therapy. There was no change in one patient, and one patient had a progressive increase in heart block while on steroid therapy. Two patients had A-V nodal rhythm. In one, this arrhythmia persisted for one month; in the other it lasted for four months. One patient with right bundle branch block retained this conduction defect for three months. One patient had a transient W-P-W syndrome for two months while on steroid therapy. One patient had frequent ventricular premature systoles which disappeared on steroid therapy, but with cessation of steroids, the ventricular premature systoles recurred.

The increased sedimentation rate present in 39 of the 52 patients reverted to normal in 31 within one to two weeks. Leukocytosis present in 16 of the patients decreased toward normal within five to seven days in 14 patients but remained persistently elevated in two for two months. In the 30 patients with a positive C-reactive protein reaction, the test became negative in 22 and less positive in four within ten days. In two patients, it increased despite steroid therapy.

Mild anemia (between 9 and 10 grams per cent of hemoglobin) was noted in 38 patients initially. During the course of treatment with steroids, the hemoglobin level had a tendency to rise in most by 2 to 3 grams per cent.

Antistreptolysin-O titers, which were significantly elevated in 32 patients, decreased in all during steroid therapy.

Fever, when present, was almost invariably abolished within 48 hours following institution of steroid therapy. The increased pulse rate decreased to normal with therapy within two days in most patients.

A leukemoid reaction present in one patient disappeared within four days following therapy. In one patient purpura disappeared within one week following therapy.

COMPLICATIONS OF STEROID THERAPY (TABLE 7)

A significant number of the 52 patients developed Cushing-like signs and symptoms. These included nine patients with moon facies, four patients with hyperglycemia and glycosuria, four patients with increased elevation of blood pressure (varying between 146 to 150 millimeters of mercury systolic and 96 to 100 millimeters of mercury diastolic), and five patients with striae on the breasts, abdomen and thighs. In one patient, the blood sugar rose to 305 mg. per cent (fasting, Folin-Wu). In addition, there were six patients who developed acne, one patient who developed adrenal depletion and one patient who developed osteoporosis. Marked weight gain (of more than 20 pounds) was seen in eight patients.

TABLE 7.   COMPLICATIONS ASSOCIATED WITH STEROID THERAPY

	NUMBER OF PATIENTS
Moon facies	9
Hyperglycemia	4
Hypertension	4
Striae	5
Acne	6
Adrenal depletion	1
Osteoporosis	1
Weight gain (> 20 lbs.)	8
Psychosis	2
Paronychia	2
Pneumonitis	3
Appendicitis (atypical)	1

Two patients developed paronychia (due to staphylococcic infection) which appeared to be resistant to antimicrobial agents while they were on steroid therapy. Three patients developed pneumonitis of unknown etiology while on steroid therapy.

One patient developed atypical findings of acute appendicitis while on steroid therapy. The only manifestation of this complication was nausea followed by persistent vomiting during the following day. There was no fever, leukocytosis, abdominal pain, abdominal tenderness or abnormal bowel movements. Two days following the cessation of steroid therapy, the temperature rose above normal and right lower quadrant tenderness became manifest. Operation revealed a highly inflamed appendix. The patient recovered uneventfully following surgery. Two patients developed severe psychoses, and one of these had to be transferred to a psychiatric hospital.

One patient had a gastrointestinal hemorrhage, but roentgen study failed to reveal any point of bleeding.

There were no deaths among these patients while on steroid therapy.

After ten weeks of steroid therapy, 12 patients (19 per cent) redeveloped signs and symptoms of rheumatic activity. These received one or more subsequent courses of steroid therapy. Three patients required almost continuous steroid therapy for more than one year because of persistent rheumatic activity with carditis following cessation of each course of steroid therapy.

Thirty-eight patients with acute rheumatic activity were hospitalized concurrently with the above 52 patients, but these did not receive steroid therapy. All received aspirin and prophylactic therapy as well as complete bed rest.

Among this group, two children lost their apical systolic murmurs, one after one and one half months and one after six months. One patient lost a mid-diastolic murmur in one and one half months, and one patient developed an apical mid-diastolic murmur which later disappeared in two weeks. One child developed a new apical systolic murmur which persisted.

There were two patients with increased A-V conduction. One of these with first degree A-V block had normal A-V conduction within two weeks; another had normal A-V conduction within one month.

One child developed progressive cardiac enlargement. This patient had auscultatory evidence of mitral insufficiency and aortic stenosis.

Joint signs, increased sedimentation rate, increased white blood count and positive C-reactive protein reaction tended to persist longer in this group of patients, although not consistently.

One patient had chorea of mild degree persisting for six months. One patient had a staphylococcic paronychia.

CONCLUSIONS

It is our impression that steroid therapy can affect the acute phase of rheumatic activity by decreasing an elevated temperature, by reducing increased heart rate and by dramatically improving patients with acute severe chorea. Steroid therapy may also be of value in maintaining a more adequate hemoglobin level.

In patients with intractable heart failure due to acute myocarditis, steroid therapy may be life-saving.

Other manifestations of acute rheumatic activity, as noted in this series, however, do not appear to be uniformly controlled by steroids.

No conclusions can be drawn from this study as to the subsequent development of residual valvular damage in patients treated with steroids.

Since the institution of steroid therapy, the average hospital stay of steroid-treated patients at the Children's Heart Hospital has been decreased by one-half, compared with the non-steroid-treated group.

Complications of hypercortisonism occurred frequently. In addition, there were cases of pneumonitis, atypical appendicitis and paronychia in those patients receiving steroid therapy.

It is thought that steroids should be reserved for those patients with acute severe rheumatic myocarditis and possibly for those with severe chorea; but, in general, these drugs should otherwise be withheld in patients with acute rheumatic activity and rheumatic carditis.

Effects of Salicylates on
Adrenal Cortical Function*

VINCENT C. KELLEY

University of Washington School of Medicine

Numerous studies have been done in attempts to evaluate the influence of salicylates on adrenal cortical function. The results of these studies have been summarized in a recent review.[16] Definitive evaluation of the results reported by various investigators has been difficult and still presents some problems, because apparently contradictory data have been obtained with regard to many aspects of this problem. However, as more data are accumulated, it is becoming obvious that many of these differences are more apparent than real. The divergent conclusions expressed by various authors have seldom been based upon inability of one investigator to reproduce the exact experiment of another but have been based rather upon differing interpretations of data from quite dissimilar experiments. It seems apparent that in many instances the differences might be resolved if adequate cognizance were taken of such important factors as: (1) the parameters used for evaluating adrenal function, including the specific methods used for steroid determinations; (2) the dose, route and duration of administration of salicylate; (3) the time relationships between administration of the stimulating dose and measurement of the response; and (4) the species, age, previous state of health and other pertinent factors regarding the experimental subjects.

EFFECTS OF SALICYLATE ON INDIRECT INDICES OF ADRENOCORTICAL FUNCTION

Many investigators have reported that salicylate causes a reduction in adrenal ascorbic acid and cholesterol;[8, 11, 14, 22, 23, 26, 27, 30, 32, 33, 38, 39, 44, 50] this response is eradicated by hypophysectomy[5, 7, 8, 14, 50] or by pretreatment with cortisone.[13, 47] It has also been found repeatedly that large doses of salicylates produce eosinopenia[7, 10, 27,34, 35, 38, 41] and that this effect is abolished by hypophysectomy.[5, 7, 14, 26, 50] In addition, histologic alterations of the adrenals interpreted as indicating hypersecretion have been reported[11, 39, 46] to follow salicylate administration. All these studies were done in animals and employed large doses of salicylates. In man, Roskam and Van Cauwenberge[41] and Kelemen et al.[27] have reported eosinopenia following salicylate administration; Marson[31] failed to confirm this observation, and in our labortories[17] the eosinopenic response was found to be quite unpredictable. The variability of these results in man probably reflects the fact that relatively smaller doses of salicylate have been used.

* The research reported here was supported in part by research grants from the A. H. Robins Co., Richmond, Va., and the Institute for the Study of Analgesic and Sedative Drugs.

EFFECTS OF SALICYLATE ON URINARY
STEROID EXCRETION

Reports concerning the effects of salicylates on urinary steroid excretion have been variable. In guinea pigs, Bertolani et al.[6] found an increase in 17-ketosteroid excretion, and LaBarre and Hans[29] found an increase in the excretion of reducing corticoids following salicylate. In human subjects, several workers have found no consistent increase in the urinary excretion of 17-ketosteroids,[9, 10, 25, 37, 51] 17-ketogenic steroids,[25] reducing corticoids,[9] "cortisone-active material,"[28] "cortisonoids"[12] or 17-hydroxycorticosteroids[37, 45] in response to salicylate administration. However, Van Cauwenberge and Heusghem[51] found an increase in urinary excretion of reducing corticoids, and Roskam,[40] of both reducing corticoids and 17-hydroxycorticosteroids in salicylate-treated adult patients. In salicylate-treated children with rheumatic disease, Pellegrini and Sala[36] found increased excretions of 11-oxycorticosteroids and 17-ketosteroids. In our laboratories, no elevation of urinary 17-ketosteroid or 17-hydroxycorticosteroid excretion following salicylate administration has been found. Rather, in normal adult volunteers given amounts of salicylate within the usual therapeutic dose range[17] and in children with rheumatic fever during salicylate therapy,[20] the urinary excretion of 17-hydroxycorticosteroids was observed to be somewhat decreased, and of 17-ketosteroids, not significantly altered.

EFFECTS OF SALICYLATE ON PLASMA 17-OHCS
CONCENTRATIONS

In Animals. Several studies of the effects of salicylates on plasma 17-OHCS concentrations have been reported. Van Cauwenberge[48] found that rats given sodium salicylate in a dose of 300 mg./kg. developed elevated blood 17-OHCS levels; adrenalectomy abolished this effect.[52] In our laboratories[15, 16, 19, 24] it has been found that large doses of salicylates produce elevated plasma 17-OHCS concentrations in rats, dogs and guinea pigs. It has been demonstrated further[16] that the magnitude of the response in plasma steroid concentration is dependent upon the size of the salicylate dose, that the steroid levels increase following oral, intraperitoneal or intravenous administration of salicylate, and that the steroid response to salicylate is abolished by either hypophysectomy or adrenalectomy.[24] It seems clear from these experiments that in animals of different species salicylates are capable of producing elevated blood 17-OHCS concentrations and that this effect is mediated by activation of the pituitary-adrenal system.

In Man. In man the evidence is more equivocal, and conflicting interpretations have arisen. These may be due in some degree to differences in experimental approach.

IN PREVIOUSLY NORMAL PERSONS. *Toxic doses* of salicylates produce elevations of plasma 17-OHCS concentrations in previously normal children or adults.[18, 19] In those in whom it was possible to determine the amount of salicylate ingested this was found to be roughly comparable, in relation to body weight, to the doses which produced elevated plasma steroid levels in guinea pigs. Also, the plasma salicylate levels in these patients were in the same range as were those in animals that developed elevated 17-OHCS levels.

"Therapeutic" doses, short-term administration. Benard et al.[3, 4] found no increase in circulating concentrations of either free or conjugated 17-

OHCS in normal subjects given a single 4 gram dose of sodium salicylate orally. Peterson et al.[37] studied the effect of a single dose of salicylate (3.6 grams of sodium salicylate orally) on plasma cortisol levels throughout the day. Only two normal subjects were included in this study; one of these had increasing rather than the expected decreasing plasma cortisol levels during the afternoon and the other showed no apparent response.

In our laboratories, with short-term administration (one or more doses on a single day) of amounts of salicylate in the usual therapeutic dose range, no consistent elevation in the plasma 17-OHCS concentration was observed in normal young adults.[17] Rather, striking fluctuations in plasma 17-OHCS concentrations occurred and the response was variable. Analysis of the data obtained indicated that significantly greater increases as well as decreases in plasma 17-OHCS concentrations occurred on the day of salicylate administration than on control days (normal diurnal variation) in the same subjects. Based on these and other findings, it has been postulated[17] that salicylates may cause an increased rate of both production and "metabolism" of steroids.

"Therapeutic" doses, long-term administration. Peterson et al.[37] also studied plasma cortisol concentrations in five normal subjects before and after 3 to 50 days of "therapeutic" doses (3.6 to 6.0 grams/day) of salicylate. No significant differences were observed in the fasting morning plasma steroid concentrations before and after salicylate administration in these subjects. However, Benard et al.[2] report that subjects given 4 grams/day of salicylate for three weeks developed significant elevations in plasma steroid concentrations.

Specificity of salicylate effect. It is apparent from the observations summarized above that stimulation of steroid production by salicylate is dose-dependent. It is clear that in large doses salicylates are capable of increasing the plasma concentrations of steroids both in different species of experimental animals and in normal human subjects. It has been suggested that the elevated steroid levels observed in salicylate-intoxicated persons may represent "an adrenal response to stress of a toxic and non-specific nature." Whereas in a sense this may be true, there is rather extreme variation in the plasma steroid concentrations induced in guinea pigs by equivalent molar doses of various benzoic acid derivatives closely related structurally to salicylates.[15, 16] In these studies it was apparent, as in studies previously published by others,[8, 14, 30, 44, 49] that there is no consistent quantitative correlation between antirheumatic and adrenal-stimulating potencies. On the other hand, the steroid concentrations induced in these animals appeared to bear little if any relationship to the toxicity of the benzoic acid derivative administered.

IN RHEUMATIC SUBJECTS. Increased plasma 17-OHCS concentrations in salicylate-treated rheumatic patients have been reported by some workers[40, 42] but not by others.[1, 37] In studies reported from our laboratory,[21, 43] plasma 17-OHCS concentrations in salicylate-treated rheumatic patients were consistently low throughout the period of salicylate therapy. In addition, even when salicylate intoxication occurred in salicylate-treated rheumatic patients no increases in the circulating 17-OHCS concentrations were found.[18] A similar observation was reported by Peterson et al.[37] in a single rheumatoid arthritis patient (H. G.) with acute salicylate intoxication.

An additional observation that has been made in rheumatic subjects is of some interest but difficult to interpret. Prolonged salicylate therapy appeared to cause decreased responsiveness to ACTH during the immediate post-therapy period,[16] despite the fact that neither urinary nor plasma 17-OHCS concentrations were elevated during the therapy period. This inhibition of adrenal responsiveness was similar in degree to that observed in steroid-treated patients.

It is apparent that in the patient with rheumatic disease the adrenal response to salicylate differs considerably from that in the normal subject. It is also apparent, as pointed out by Bayliss and Steinbeck[1] and re-emphasized by others,[16, 37] that the antirheumatic effects of salicylates are not dependent upon the maintenance of elevated circulating levels of 17-OHCS. However, the suggestion of Kelemen[28] that adrenocortical stimulation may occur but be masked by enhanced "metabolism" of steroids still deserves consideration.

EFFECTS OF SALICYLATE ON RATE OF METABOLISM OF STEROIDS

A few studies have been done in an attempt to determine the effects of salicylates on the rate of steroid "metabolism." As mentioned above, the rapidly fluctuating plasma steroid concentrations observed in normal young adults given "therapeutic" doses of salicylates in acute experiments[17] may afford some evidence that salicylates enhance the "metabolism" of steroids. Studies of the effects of a single dose of salicylate on the half-life of cortisol in normal human subjects, in dogs and in rats have been performed in our laboratories. On repeated occasions a definitely shortened cortisol half-life has been observed following the administration of salicylate, but this has not been a consistent finding; in some instances the cortisol half-life has been unchanged or increased. However, in hypophysectomized rats, administration of salicylate results in a consistent and significant decrease in cortisol half-life.

Peterson et al.[37] have reported an increased cortisol half-life and an unaltered corticosterone half-life in subjects who had received "therapeutic" doses (3.6 to 6.0 grams/day) of salicylates for 6 to 50 days. In this study the cortisol half-life was determined in five subjects (four rheumatoid arthritis patients and one normal subject) and the corticosterone half-life in two subjects (one rheumatoid arthritis patient and one normal subject). In the rheumatoid arthritis patients the half-life of each steroid increased following salicylate administration in each subject studied. However, in the one normal subject the half-life of each steroid decreased after salicylate administration. These data would suggest that the effects of salicylates on steroid "metabolism" in patients with rheumatoid arthritis differ from those in normal subjects.

SUMMARY

Salicylates in large doses are capable of activating the adrenal cortex in different species of animals and in normal human subjects. This response is abolished following hypophysectomy or pretreatment with steroids and may be considered to be mediated through increased ACTH release by the pituitary.

Studies in human subjects with smaller doses of salicylates have yielded apparently conflicting findings regarding the effects on adrenal function.

Data have been cited which support the hypothesis that salicylates not only stimulate the adrenal cortex to produce steroids but also enhance steroid "metabolism." It is suggested that this concept of a dual action of salicylates, although it requires further verification, would explain many of the apparently discrepant results that have been reported.

Patients with rheumatic disease differ from normal persons in their adrenal response to salicylates. The antirheumatic effect of salicylates is not dependent upon maintenance of elevated circulating levels of adrenal hormones. If increased steroid production does occur in rheumatic patients in response to salicylates it is masked by an accelerated "metabolism" of the steroids.

REFERENCES

1. Bayliss, R. I. S. and Steinbeck, A. W.: Salicylates and the plasma level of adrenal steroids. Lancet, 1:1010, 1954.
2. Benard, H., Cruz-Horn, A., Piguet, B. and Seeman, A.: Action d'un traitement salicyle prolongé sur le taux des 17-hydroxycorticosteroides plasmatiques. Compt. rend. Soc. de biol., 150:661, 1956.
3. Benard, H., Cruz-Horn, A., Piguet, B. and Seeman, A.: Influence de l'ingestion d'une dose unique de salicylate de sodium sur le taux plasmatique des 17-hydroxy-corticosteroides conjugués chez l'homme. Compt. rend. Soc. de biol., 150:458, 1956.
4. Benard, H., Cruz-Horn, A., Piguet, B. and Seeman, A.: Action d'une dose unique de salicylate de sodium sur le taux des 17-hydroxycorticosteroides plasmatiques chez l'homme. Compt. rend. Soc. de biol., 150:243, 1956.
5. Bertolani, F., Bonati, B., Lorenzini, R., Bergamini, A. and Mari, E.: Salicylici ipofisi e corticosurrene. Folia endocrinol., 6:61, 1953.
6. Bertolani, F., Lorenzini, R. and Bonati, B.: Letter to editor. Lancet, 1:54, 1951.
7. Betz, H. and Van Cauwenberge, H.: Reactions histologiques a l'injection de salicylate de soude chez le rat. Compt. rend. Soc. de biol., 145:1275, 1951.
8. Blanchard, K. C., Dearborn, E. H., Maren, T. H. and Marshall, E. K.: Stimulation of the anterior pituitary by certain cinchoninic acid derivatives. Bull. Johns Hopkins Hosp., 86:83, 1950.
9. Böe, J. and Stöa, K. F.: The ACTH-like effect of acetylsalicylic acid. Acta endocrinol., 12:20, 1953.
10. Bonati, B., Bertolani, F. and Lorenzini, R.: Action of some hydroxy aromatic acids on the excretion of 17-ketosteroids and on the circulating eosinophils. Farm. sci. e tec., 6:719, 1951.
11. Champy, C. and Demay, M.: Mode of endocrine action of salicylates and gentisates. J.A.M.A., 145:1365, 1951.
12. Coste, F., Bourel, M., Delbarre, F. and Weissenbach, R.: Comment agit le salicylate de sodium. Presse méd., 61:979, 1953.
13. Cronheim, G. and Hyder, N.: Effect of salicylic acid on adrenal-pituitary system. III. Studies on mechanism of this effect. Proc. Soc. Exper. Biol. & Med., 86:409, 1954.
14. Cronheim, G., King, J. S., Jr. and Hyder, N.: Effects of salicylic acid and similar compounds on adrenal-pituitary system. Proc. Soc. Exper. Biol. & Med., 80:51, 1952.
15. Done, A. K., Ely, R. S. and Kelley, V. C.: Influence on circulating 17-hydroxycorticosteroid concentrations of compounds structurally related to salicylate. Proc. Soc. Exper. Biol. & Med., 93:294, 1956.
16. Done, A. K., Ely, R. S. and Kelley, V. C.: Salicylates and the pituitary-adrenal system. Metabolism, 7:52, 1958.
17. Done, A. K., Ely, R. S. and Kelley, V. C.: Response of plasma 17-hydroxycorticosteroids to salicylate administration in normal human subjects. Metabolism, 4:129, 1955.
18. Done, A. K., Ely, R. S., Raile, R. B. and Kelley, V. C.: Studies of 17-hydroxycorticosteroids. XIII. Effects of salicylate intoxication in rheumatic and nonrheumatic subjects. J. Pediat., 47:727, 1955.
19. Done, A. K., Ely, R. S. and Kelley, V. C.: Studies of 17-hydroxycorticosteroids. III. Blood levels in salicylate intoxication. J. Pediat., 44:153, 1954.
20. Ely, R. S., Ainger, L. E., Seely, J. R., Done, A. K. and Kelley, V. C.: Studies of

17-hydroxycorticosteroids. X. Urinary excretion of 17-hydroxycorticosteroids in patients with rheumatic fever. J. Clin. Endocrinol., 15:523, 1955.

21. Ely, R. S., Done, A. K., Seely, J. R., Ainger, L. E. and Kelley, V. C.: Studies of 17-hydroxycorticosteroids. XI. Relation of plasma concentrations to urinary excretion in patients treated for rheumatic fever. J. Pediat., 47:576, 1955.

22. Feeney, G. C., Carlo, P. and Smith, P. K.: Action of salicylates and related compounds on carbohydrate metabolism and on adrenal ascorbic acid and cholesterol concentrations. J. Pharmacol. & Exper. Therap., 114:299, 1955.

23. Forbes, J. C., Board, J. A. and Duncan, G. M.: Adrenal response of rats to salicylamide and sodium salicylate with and without para-aminobenzoic acid. Proc. Soc. Exper. Biol. & Med., 85:37, 1954.

24. Good, T. A., Done, A. K., Ely, R. S. and Kelley, V. C.: Effects of salicylate on plasma 17-hydroxycorticosteroids in hypophysectomized and adrenalectomized guinea pigs. Metabolism, 6:346, 1957.

25. Henly, A. A.: Steroid metabolism in rheumatoid arthritis. Ann. Rep., West London Hosp., 1952, p. 24.

26. Hetzel, B. S. and Hine, D. C.: The effect of salicylates on the pituitary and suprarenal glands. Lancet, 2:94, 1951.

27. Kelemen, E., Majoros, M., Ivanyi, J. and Kovacs, K.: Salicylates, stress and cortisone. Experientia, 6:435, 1950.

28. Kelemen, E., Majoros, M., Soletsz, R. and Tanos, B.: Zum wirkungsmechanismus grosser Salizylätdosen. Deutsche med. wchnschr., 77:1317, 1952.

29. La Barre, J. and Hans, M. J.: Effects comparatifs de differents dérivés salicyles sur l'élimination urinaire des steroïdes reducteurs. Compt. rend. Soc. de biol., 148:723, 1954.

30. Lowenthal, J. and Jaques, L. B.: A comparative study of the effect of a series of aromatic acids on the ascorbic acid content of the adrenal gland. J. Pharmacol. and Exper. Therap., 107:172, 1953.

31. Marson, F. G. W.: Effect of ACTH and salicylate on the urinary uric acid: creatinine ratio and circulating eosinophils in man. Ann. Rheum. Dis., 12:296, 1953.

32. Pasqualini, R. Q.: Corticotrofina y salicilato de sodio en el tratamiento de la fiebre reumatica. Rev. Asoc. med. argent., 64:332, 1950.

33. Pasqualini, R. Q., Dosne de Pasqualini, C. and Garberi, J. C.: Accion del salicilato de sodio sobre el sistema hipofisosuprarenal. Rev. Soc. argent. biol., 26:120, 1950.

34. Pasqualini, R. Q. and Lascalea, M. C.: Tratamiento de la fiebre reumatica con salicilato de sodio y cloruro de amonio. Prense med. argent., 35:1091, 1948.

35. Pasqualini, R. Q., Dosne de Pasqualini, C. and Garberi, J. C.: Action du salicylate de soude sur le système hypophysosurrenal. Compt. rend. Soc. de biol., 145:122, 1951.

36. Pellegrini, U. and Sala, I.: Ricerche sul meccanismo d'azione del Na salicilato nella terapia antireumatica. Pediatria, 61:351, 1953.

37. Peterson, R. E., Black, R. L. and Bunim, J. J.: Salicylates and adrenocortical function in man. Arth. & Rheum., 1:29, 1958.

38. Rivi, E.: Recerca sul meccanismo dell'azione antireumatica del salicilato. Boll. Soc. med.-chir., Modena, 51:253, 1951.

39. Robinson, F. B.: Aspirin and the adrenal cortex. Brit. M. J., 1:300, 1951.

40. Roskam, J.: Un concept nouveau: les médications hormonopoïetiques et ses consequences pratiques. Schweiz. med. Wchnschr., 86:1269, 1956.

41. Roskam, J. and Van Cauwenberge, H.: Effect of sodium salicylate on circulating eosinophils and urinary uric acid: creatinine ratio. Lancet, 2:375, 1951.

42. Roskam, J., Van Cauwenberge, H., Vivario, R. and Vliers, M.: Les modes d'action de la salicylotherapie. Presse méd., 63:1105, 1955.

43. Seely, J. R., Ely, R. S., Done, A. K., Ainger, L. E. and Kelley, V. C.: Studies of 17-hydroxycorticosteroids. VII. Effects of therapy on concentration of 17-hydroxycorticosteroids in the plasma of patients with rheumatic fever. Pediatrics, 15:543, 1955.

44. Smith, M. J. H.: Monohydroxybenzoic acids and ascorbic acid depletion of the adrenal glands of the intact rat. Lancet, 1:991, 1952.

45. Smith, M. J. H., Gray, C. H. and Lunnon, J. B.: Urinary excretion of adrenocortical steroids by patients receiving salicylates. Lancet, 1:1008, 1954.

46. Tronchetti, F. and Nello, P. R.: Salicilato di sodio e ghandiole endocrine. Folia endocrinol., 5:365, 1952.

47. Van Cauwenberge, H.: Contribution a l'étude de la réactivité surrénalienne du rat. Arch. int. pharmacodyn., 106:473, 1956.

48. Van Cauwenberge, H.: Influence de l'ACTH, du salicylate de sodium et de la cysteinamine sur les 17-hydroxycorticosteroïdes sanguins chez le rat. Compt. rend. Soc. de biol., 148:1297, 1954.
49. Van Cauwenberge, H.: Réaction de l'axe hypothalamo-hypophysosurrénalien a quelques derives benzeniques. Compt. rend. Soc. de biol., 147:1118, 1953.
50. Van Cauwenberge, H.: Relation of salicylate action to pituitary gland: observations in rats. Lancet, 2:374, 1951.
51. Van Cauwenberge, H. and Heusghem, C.: Therapeutique par acide acetylsalicylique et excretion urinarie des corticosteroïdes. Acta med. scandinav., 141:265, 1952.
52. Van Cauwenberge, H. and Roskam, J.: Influence du salicylate de soude sur le taux des 17-hydroxycorticosteroïdes sanguins chez le rat surrénalectomisé. Compt. rend. Soc. de biol., 149:1064, 1954.

Salicylate and Steroids
in Rheumatic Fever*

EDWARD E. FISCHEL

The Bronx Hospital, New York City

The relative merits and demerits of various drugs in the management of rheumatic fever may be compared, but it is not necessary to limit oneself to an exclusive choice of one drug alone. Indeed, after appropriate evaluation of the tangible goals of therapy, of the properties possessed by available agents and of the accumulated critical experience in their application, it may well be that a judicious combination of drugs would appear more desirable for certain situations than any one drug alone.

Ideally, a drug should be directed against the cause of a disease, with appropriate concern for its complications as well. The pathogenetic mechanism for the development of rheumatic fever following an initiating streptococcal infection has not been well defined (cf. 4). The prevention or treatment of Group A streptococcal infections with penicillin has been very successful in preventing rheumatic fever.[15, 19] Penicillin therapy, however, has not been satisfactory for the treatment of the acute attack, except perhaps to a degree as described in one report which warrants re-evaluation.[13]

In the absence of any specific agent directed against a known pathogenetic factor, we must rely on criteria for current management which can be considered clinically logical. It appears desirable to stop promptly all manifestations of the disease, cardiac and otherwise. These should be stopped permanently. If acute heart damage has occurred, it should be reversed, preventing the development of heart disease. In addition, an ideal agent should have a lack of hazard associated with its use and with the discontinuance of its use.

It may be that the nature of the disease precludes attaining these goals, but it is also apparent that the drugs presently available are less than ideal. There is little doubt, however, that salicylate and corticosteroids possess to some degree the attributes of good therapeutic agents for rheumatic fever. At varying rates, and to various degrees, both suppress the acute manifesta-

* Supported in part by grant H-2144 from the National Heart Institute, by the Helen Hay Whitney Foundation and by the New York State Chapter, Arthritis and Rheumatism Foundation.

tions of the disease in most instances. The anti-inflammatory action of salicylate was long thought to be merely a masking or falsely suppressive action of the drug. Its use for a short period of time was frequently followed by a recrudescence of signs of active disease. Indeed, the intermittent use of salicylate simply for suppression of fever and joint pains was propounded for many years as a recommended form of management. This probably resulted in an unhappy outcome for the patient and a poor reputation for salicylate, neither of which was justified. The flare-up of activity when salicylate was discontinued was reported by Stricker[17] shortly after Maclagen introduced his classic studies with salicylate. This "rebound" obviously demonstrated that the disease had not been eradicated, and it also demonstrated that a suppression of inflammation *had* occurred during the period of drug administration. The suppressive action could be shown to have occurred in the heart when cardiac signs emerged during the rebound.[5] In retrospect, the drug appeared to have had an effect in the heart. This devious chain of reasoning had to be invoked because the more obvious tests of drug efficacy were difficult to control. Many clinicians were unwilling to accept as cause and effect that the administration of salicylate was related to the subsidence of inflammation. On occasion, subsidence of many or all manifestations of rheumatic fever occurred spontaneously without salicylate therapy, and on other occasions the disease appeared to progress without any noticeable suppressive effect from the drug. Both situations reflect the extreme variability that may be encountered in the clinical course of rheumatic fever. Further reasons for the lack of appreciation of the potential of salicylate derive from difficulties in assessing changes in the cardiac status, particularly after the disease is well established, and from the varying dosage and intermittent regimens that were used. These factors and others gave rise to many conflicting reports about the efficacy of salicylate which have been reviewed elsewhere.[5, 6] Other agents such as amidopyrine and phenacetin were similarly appraised.

With the advent of the clinical use of cortisone and ACTH, there occurred a general appreciation of the anti-inflammatory effect of these drugs. By analogy, other drugs were thought to have similar potential. Early use of the corticosteroids in rheumatic fever was associated with an enthusiasm that was usually well justified. In some reports, however, there was also a condemnation of salicylate therapy which was frequently based on hearsay, on an uncritical experience with casually treated patients in the past, or on a lack of familiarity with the early and acute phase of the disease. In 1950 a cooperative clinical trial was set up at 13 centers in the United States, Canada and Great Britain to compare ACTH, cortisone and aspirin in rheumatic fever. Provision was made for random allocation of cases to treatment groups. In many ways this was a very well controlled and extensive study of this disease. The details of the experience through the first year have been published[1] and the follow-up at the end of five years has been presented by Dr. Rutstein and was recently published.[2] No striking differences were noted in the incidence of heart disease in the three treatment groups.

There have been several reports which also attempted to compare the steroids with salicylate. These have generally been uncontrolled or retrospective, with varying criteria for selection of patients and appraisal of results, and with varying amounts and durations of therapy. Among the controlled studies that should be considered is the experience of Stolzer et al.[16] with young adults selected and treated according to the protocol of the Cooperative Study. In this study, treatment with hormones appeared to result in somewhat less heart disease, principally because there occurred a rather high incidence of aortic lesions in the salicylate group. Long term follow-up was not possible here. The authors concluded that the differences observed "do not allow a definite conclusion as to whether cortisone or corticotropin are superior to acetyl salicylic acid in the prevention of heart damage." In one of Illingworth's reports,[10] salicylate was found to be better than no therapy, even with bias introduced in favor of the group receiving no therapy. A later comparison of the salicylate treated group with groups receiving steroids suggested that the latter were better,[11] although the groups were treated over a nine year period and not concomitantly. More recently, a group of pediatricians with Dr. Anne Kuttner as coordinating director reported[3] on the incidence of residual heart damage in children treated with either prednisone or aspirin for twelve weeks under controlled conditions. Prednisone was not found to be superior to acetylsalicylic acid in preventing residual rheumatic heart disease; indeed, the data suggest that the alternative might have been more likely.

The varying outcomes in the different reported studies may be related to many factors besides differences in therapeutic agents. Some benefit does appear to result from either salicylate or corticoid therapy. Both drugs appear to act independently. This is suggested by the different responses of clinical and laboratory manifestations[1] and by clinical and experimental studies which indicate that salicylate may act when the adrenals are absent[18] or functionally suppressed.[14] Furthermore, the drugs have different metabolic effects.[9, 12] Salicylates and the corticosteroids also differ widely in their manifestations of serious toxicity. The hyperventilation of salicylism may be metabolically and physically taxing for the patient with acute rheumatic fever. The untoward effects of corticosteroids include hypertension, convulsions, lack of resistance to infections, perforated gastrointestinal viscera, severe osteoporosis and psychotic phenomena (cf. 8).

Among the disadvantages of both agents is the hazard associated with discontinuation of therapy. The rebound of rheumatic inflammation which may occur has been mentioned previously to illustrate that a suppressive action had occurred while the drug was being administered. The rebound itself is frequently mild and self-limited, but it may be as serious as any other phase of the disease. Severe inflammatory reactions, progressive disease, congestive heart failure, pericarditis and death have been observed following the cessation of either hormone or salicylate therapy.[1, 5, 7] Under similar conditions of therapy, cessation of ACTH or of cortisone resulted in twice the incidence of rebounds, and these were of greater severity.[1] In a study of the manifestations of the rebound, it appeared that the more frequent and more severe rebounds were directly related to the degree of cardiac involvement on admission and to the occurrence of preceding attacks of rheumatic fever.[7] The latter factors were also related to the condition of the heart at time of follow-up,[2] but no causal relationship could be established between the severity of the rebound and the development of late heart disease.

It appeared logical to attempt to avoid the frequent flare-up of rheumatic inflammation at the end of therapy much as the initial disease activity is suppressed. Accordingly, an uncontrolled exploratory attempt has been made to employ both salicylate and corticosteroids to obtain the advantages of each and to minimize their disadvantages, including their direct toxic effects and the rebound which occurs after either drug is discontinued.[6] Forty-one patients were treated with combined corticosteroid and salicylate therapy to attempt to keep at a minimum the manifestations of inflammation. About half the patients were seen in a first attack of rheumatic fever within 21 days from onset. As might be anticipated, most of these patients appeared to do well. The small number of patients and the large numbers of variables make any over-all summary meaningless. Experience was obtained, however, to indicate that suppression of the anticipated rebound may have been achieved by the continued administration of salicylate while corticosteroids were being discontinued. This was an uncontrolled study, but logically it might be expected that some benefit could be derived from the rapid and sustained suppression of inflammation. Further studies in this direction may permit more definitive conclusions.

REFERENCES

1. The treatment of rheumatic fever in children. A Cooperative Clinical Trial of ACTH, cortisone and aspirin. Circulation, 11:343, 1955; Brit. M. J., 1:555, 1955.
2. The evolution of rheumatic heart disease in children. Five-year report of a Cooperative Clinical Trial of ACTH, cortisone and aspirin. Circulation, 22:503, 1960; Brit. M. J., 2:1033, 1960.
3. Combined Rheumatic Fever Study Group: A comparison of the effect of prednisone and acetylsalicylic acid on the incidence of residual heart disease. New Eng. J. Med., 262:895, 1960.
4. Fischel, E. E.: The role of allergy in the pathogenesis of rheumatic fever. Am. J. Med., 7:772, 1949.
5. Fischel, E. E., Frank, C. W. and Ragan, C.: Observation on treatment of rheumatic fever with salicylate, ACTH and cortisone. I. Medicine, 31:331, 1952.
6. Fischel, E. E., Frank, C. W., Boltax, A. J. and Arcasoy, M.: Observation on treatment of rheumatic fever with salicylate. II. Combined salicylate and corticoid therapy and attempts at rebound suppression. Arth. &. Rheum. 1:351, 1958.
7. Fischel, E. E., Frank, C. W. and Bellows, M.: Manifestations of rheumatic fever following cessation of therapy. Circulation, 18:367, 1958.
8. Good, R. A., Vernier, R. L. and Smith, R. T.: Serious untoward reactions to therapy with cortisone and adrenocorticotropin in pediatric practice. I and II. Pediatrics, 19:95 and 272, 1957.
9. Hailman, H. F.: ACTH and cortisone vs. salicylates. J. Clin. Endocrinol., 12:454, 1952.
10. Illingworth, R. S., Burke, J., Doxiadis, S. A., Lorber, J., Philpott, M. C. and Stone, D. G. H.: Salicylates in rheumatic fever. An attempt to assess their value. Quart. J. Med., 23:177, 1954.
11. Illingworth, R. S., Lorber, J., Holt, K. S., Rendle-Short, J., Jowett, G. H. and Gibson, M. W.: Acute rheumatic fever in children. A comparison of six forms of treatment in 200 cases. Lancet, 2:653, 1957.
12. Ingle, D. J.: The effect of aspirin upon the glycosuria of partially depancreatized rats in the presence and absence of the adrenal glands. Endocrinology, 52:403, 1953.
13. Mortimer, E. A., Jr. et al.: The effects of penicillin on acute rheumatic fever and valvular heart disease. New Eng. J. Med., 260:101, 1959.
14. Petersen, R. E., Black, R. L. and Bunim, J. J.: Salicylates and adrenocortical function in man. Arth. & Rheum., 1:29, 1958.
15. Stollerman, G. H.: The use of antibiotics for the prevention of rheumatic fever. Am. J. Med., 17:757, 1954.
16. Stolzer, B. L., Houser, H. B. and Clark, E. J.: Therapeutic agents in rheumatic carditis. Arch. Int. Med., 95:677, 1955.
17. Stricker: Ueber die Resultate der Behandling der Polyathritis rheumatica mit Salicylsaure. Berl. klin. Wchnschr., 13:15, 1876.
18. Ungar, G., Damgaard, E. and Hummel, F. P.: Action of salicylates and related drugs on inflammation. Am. J. Physiol., 171:545, 1952.
19. Wannamaker, L. et al.: Prophylaxis of acute rheumatic fever. Am. J. Med., 10:673, 1951.

Panel Discussion

WILLIAM LIKOFF, *Moderator*

DR. LIKOFF: I was most interested in the presentation by Dr. Ferencz, and I would like to ask her how she would view the pathologic alterations as created or caused by steroid therapy: in terms of benefit or in terms of detriment?

DR. FERENCZ: You are asking me a question I would very much like to know the answer to, Dr. Likoff. I was very intrigued with the report from the National Institute of Cardiology in Mexico and wanted to quote it at this Symposium but then I learned a great deal in general about the effect of cortisone and steroids on production of both necrosis and inflammation in the course of the last few days from Dr. Spain and Dr. Jean and several other speakers. Apparently there is a depression of the inflammatory process while the noxious agent continues to be present, and it is the noxious agent which produces necrosis—the increase in the amount of the necrosis being due to the fact that the normal inflammatory process is not there to neutralize the noxious agent. In other words, the steroids do not produce as one effect necrosis and as another suppression of inflammatory cells and as another a slowing of fibroblastic activity, but these all go together. The answer we need to know is what this means in terms of those patients we are following in whom there is a murmur. How do steroids affect the long-term course of rheumatic valvular disease?

DR. LIKOFF: Do you or any other member of the panel care to comment on this concept? If the inflammatory reaction leading to necrosis is reduced, will the chronic tissue changes, which supposedly are only postinflammatory, be beneficially affected? For example, if the process of exudation and proliferation in the valvular structures results in the mechanical disease with which we ultimately deal, would it not seem logical that the ability to negate the postinflammatory changes would in all respects be of ultimate benefit?

DR. RUTSTEIN: Dr. Likoff, I think you are asking an impossible question. Nobody has ever followed the course of a rheumatic lesion in the human heart with repeated biopsies and nobody knows whether the necrosis is worse with the inflammation or without it.

DR. MASSELL: Although the lesions may not be identical, the lesions in the heart and in the subcutaneous nodules are certainly very similar, and we have observed over and over again that the nodules respond more rapidly to steroids in large doses than to salicylates. I am not sure just what significance this has, but possibly by observing the nodules which are on the outside of the body, one can get some inference about what is going on in the lesions in the heart.

DR. HILL: Dr. Massell, does your statement also apply to necrosis?

DR. MASSELL: This is a clinical observation, and all I know is that the nodules go away. I have not obtained specimens for histological examination.

DR. FISCHEL: I think it is curious that for many years we have always been taught, and I certainly would not accept it, that rheumatic fever in one area of the body—for example, in the joints or in the pleura—is not comparable to rheumatic fever in the heart. I would agree with Dr. Massell, and I think that the disease is the disease wherever it exists. However, there are many factors involved, depending on the location of the lesions; for example, inflammation in the nodule and in the joints has never resulted in chronic fibrosis, as it does in the heart, and I think there are some differences in the lesions from one area to another although the pathogenesis is probably the same.

DR. BUNIM: I would like to support the statement just made by Dr. Fischel. For documentary evidence I refer you to one of the January issues of the J.A.M.A. in 1955, in which we published photomicrographs of sections of the synovial membrane of one patient with rheumatoid arthritis who was given aspirin in large doses over a long period of time. We obtained a biopsy of the synovia of his knee and then put him on prednisone; 24 days later a second biopsy specimen was obtained from the same knee in exactly the same area. The striking difference between these two sections was the disappearance of the fairly massive deposition of fibrinoid material, and this is exactly the opposite effect from that cited today as occurring in the heart. Once again, we can not predict the effects of steroids on one tissue from the response of another.

DR. LIKOFF: Dr. Rutstein, one of the major points of your paper was that it is difficult to assay the effects of treatment against the variable patterns of rheumatic activity. Would you indicate your general ideas about the so-called evolutionary pattern of rheumatic fever? What can we expect, in general, in regard to the ordinary prognosis of an initially stricken patient, in terms of, not acute disability, but in terms of the chronic progression of the disease?

DR. RUTSTEIN: This is a difficult question, but I will try to answer it briefly. First, I think it is perfectly clear that most of the activity in rheumatic fever, if one accepts the fact that mitral stenosis is a rheumatic lesion, occurs at a subclinical level, because certainly since one-half of the adults develop mitral stenosis without recognizable acute rheumatic fever, many pathological changes occur without any clinical evidence of activity. This raises a lot of questions, because we have two criteria and we mix them up. We talk about activity; at one moment we are talking about a section of the heart muscle with an Aschoff body, and at the next moment we are talking about the sedimentation rate. I do not think there is any evidence at all to indicate that when the sedimentation rate becomes normal the Aschoff body disappears. As a matter of fact, the evidence is opposite to that, because when you do a biopsy at the time of mitral valvulotomy you find that a significant proportion of patients do have lesions. You have to agree that what is going on is going on beneath the surface.

Now, concerning the natural history of this disease, we have seen some changes over the years. In the series reported by Bland and Jones, beginning in the mid 1920's, the patients had a different prognosis than the patients we have today. More patients died, more patients had recurrences and their hospital stays were longer. It seems that many things could be associated with this change. The change in death rates for rheumatic heart disease in the United States started suddenly about 1930 before penicillin was available. Maybe this change had something to do with changes in environment or a lot of things we do not know anything about, such as a change in the streptococcus. Certainly the use of penicillin, when it became available, seemed to add something to this. Changes in standard of living may be another factor. And maybe treatment has done something too—certainly the disease has changed.

Comparing Dr. Massell's results with our results, even if you accept that these were obtained from comparable groups of patients—and I do not know whether they were or not—but if you could, for the sake of the discussion of the moment say they were the comparable groups, we obtained the same results in mild, moderate or severe disease with aspirin that he obtained with large doses of steroids. I do not know why he got such poor results with aspirin, but the reason may be differences in the disease.

In watching the evolution of this disease under treatment, I would agree with Dr. Fischel that we saw major differences between patients getting steroids and patients getting salicylates—so much so that I do not think we can assume that they work in the same way at all, and we did not say that the drugs work in the same way. What we said was that the number of people with heart disease was the same at the end of the study period. The drugs may work quite differently. Now, that is what I say as a scientist. As a clinician, I would say the following. If I had a patient with mild rheumatic fever, in terms of the history of disease, and if he had a good chance of getting better, I think I would use the mildest treatment—that is, aspirin. If the patient were very sick I, as a doctor, would use both drugs since I think the two drugs work differently in this disease, although we do not have any statistical evidence to support this.

Dr. Likoff, I have one final point which I think is very important and that is, in your paper, you compared the results in patients treated early in the disease with the results in patients treated late in the disease. You can not make this comparison and the reason you can not make it is that the sample is so different. You start off, for example, with 100 patients with any chronic disease, not only rheumatic fever, but any chronic disease, in which there is a low death rate initially. In this situation, if treatment is started during the first or second week of disease, there will be many patients in the group who will be well by the fifth or sixth week, so if you subsequently use patients who are still sick in the sixth week, you are not using the same sample of patients; you are picking a residual of patients who are sicker than others. The way to find out whether early treatment is better than late treatment is not to compare early patients with late patients, but to take a group of early patients and randomly distribute them and compare the results of early treatment with the results of late treatment with the same drugs. You can not compare early treatment with late treatment unless you are willing to keep all of the patients in the hospital, and those who are to receive late treatment must be kept in the hospital even if they are well, and treatment must be given even if they are well during the sixth week of disease. In our study, which started in Denver on January 1, 1951, there were three patients who were sick before the beginning of the year, and these patients were retained in the hospital without treatment so they would be available for the study when it started; but when the study was started they were no longer sick, and they did not have enough evidence of activity even to enter the study. You can not compare early with late treatment, unless the criteria which I mentioned are carried out, and this is very important.

In summary, Dr. Likoff, this is a disease of varying prognosis that has changed over the years for the better, at least in this country, although not in Poland or Russia. Recent experiences of mine and of others have shown that there are still many patients with severe rheumatic fever in those countries. The reasons for this are not clear. But in any event, with this change in the United States, patients here now have a better prognosis even without treatment. The only way one can tell about the effect of a therapeutic agent is to control the natural history by having control groups selected on some random basis.

DR. LIKOFF: In defense of the early-late treatment, I would like to say that there was a component correlation in regard to severity and response to severity, which obviously explained, at least in part, the differences involved.

DR. MASSELL: There is one important fact that we must not forget from the practical point of view, which is perhaps the most important thing that has been accomplished in the treatment of rheumatic fever to date, and that is the prevention of recurrences. In our series, patients who had recurrences were removed from the study group, since in many of the patients in whom murmurs disappeared development of a recurrence led to reappearance of the murmur. Some of those who redeveloped murmurs eventually had permanent heart disease. I think that the change in recurrence rates may very well explain the differences in natural history that Dr. Rutstein mentioned. For example, the large series of untreated patients I mentioned in my paper were seen during the period from 1941 to 1951.

The more recent patients do not differ from them if we carefully screen them from the point of view of recurrences.

DR. LIKOFF: What, in effect, has been said thus far is a repetition of the dispute that has occurred in the papers themselves, and I would like to ask Dr. Rutstein one brief question. Did you imply that, despite the statistical evidence against such practice, you condone or advise the use of steroids in the treatment of rheumatic activity?

DR. RUTSTEIN: In serious cases, yes, I would give both. It is a clinical impression, and as I said before, I am talking as a doctor, not as a scientist. In our studies we found no difference. We did not study both drugs together, and I do not know of any statistical evidence supporting their use together. In any disease, if I have a sick patient and there are two possible drugs which might be beneficial and I think that they might act in different ways, I would give the patient both drugs.

DR. LIKOFF: Does anyone have any other comment on this? Would anybody treat a mild case with steroids? If they are effective in severe involvement why are they not effective in mild involvement?

DR. RUTSTEIN: No one said combined treatment was not effective in the mild form of the disease. The point is that you do not have to give steroids to patients with minimal activity, because they get better by themselves.

DR. BUNIM: I feel very strongly about the point Dr. Rutstein made, and I am very happy that he feels this way, because those charged with the responsibility of taking care of a patient during an acute attack are very much concerned about using an effective, dependable anti-inflammatory agent which will produce prompt suppression of the inflammation. Now, provided there is no serious contraindication to, and provided no serious adverse effects are likely to occur from a drug, I think the physician should use the drug he can depend upon for prompt action. Therefore, if a child has serious acute rheumatic carditis, I think it would be good clinical judgment to use a steroid and also to use salicylates. I do not see anything against it, and I think Dr. Rutstein feels the same way. But we are talking about two different things: the treatment of the acute attack, during which in some instances the life of the child may be in danger, and the chronic disease with the possibility of residual damage to the heart three years later. The data, I think, show clearly that there is no difference in the ultimate residual damage whether the patient is treated with salicylates or whether the patient is treated with steroids. This has nothing to do with the indications for steroid therapy during an acute attack of carditis, especially when the child is seriously ill with congestive heart failure and is threatened with death.

DR. RUTSTEIN: I do not wish to be misinterpreted. In our previous report in 1955, we showed that the rate of response as far as pericarditis was concerned and as far as congestive failure was concerned was the same whether the patient received salicylates or small doses of steroids. Now, again, those are the data which we collected. We saw no difference, but I would agree entirely with Dr. Bunim that I would give both drugs to a patient who was very sick. Again, we had no patients who received both, and I do not know of any evidence, of the kind that we tried to get on a control group, that the patient cleared up faster with one drug than with the other.

DR. LIKOFF: Dr. Mason, do you have any comments about this?

DR. MASON: No, but I would like to ask the panel what their feelings are about the use of steroids for chorea. I think the drug is of special benefit in those patients with severe chorea. I know that others will state that certain drugs such as the phenothiazine group may be of value in these patients, but it is our impression that steroids are of greater value in severe cases.

Dr. KELLEY: I certainly agree with what Dr. Mason said. We have treated about 30 really severe cases of chorea. It is difficult to demonstrate a real shortening of the course in mild cases of chorea, but when you treat the really severe ones, there is just no doubt that you can greatly shorten the course of the severe manifestations of the disease, although I doubt that the time required for complete disappearance of the choreiform movements is shortened.

Dr. MASSELL: We do not have any statistical data, but I agree with this. I have the definite impression that we have yet to see a patient with severe chorea who did not respond to steroids. The main problem is that certain patients get better anyway with rest alone, and we have not made any comparative studies. The other problem is that most chorea patients do not have carditis, and the first question is that of weighing the advantages of steroids against the possible risks. The problem is not quite the same as in patients with severe carditis, in whom you are much more concerned about the outcome.

Dr. FERENCZ: We once reviewed a number of patients who had chorea but who did not receive intensive therapy of any kind. There were about 42 patients and the duration of the disease varied from one week to 52 weeks; this makes interpretation of drug response very difficult unless controlled studies are done.

Dr. KELLEY: I think you will agree that it is a very exceptional for an extremely severe chorea patient to convalesce very rapidly, and this is specifically why we chose only the patients with extremely severe involvement.

Dr. RUTSTEIN: Is there anyone here on the panel or in the room who has a controlled experience with the treatment of chorea? When you put these patients into the hospital and put them quietly to bed, they certainly change very fast. Now, does anyone have a controlled study in which he has allocated patients to steroid therapy and to some other therapy to see whether there is any difference? I do not think you can determine the efficacy of therapy just by giving patients steroids without a basis of comparison in a disease as variable as Dr. Ferencz has indicated. Are there such data anywhere?

Dr. KELLEY: We do not have such data.

Dr. LIKOFF: There are very many pertinent unanswered questions in relation to the treatment of rheumatic fever. To turn to another subject, Dr. Massell, what is the mechanism of death in those patients who represented treatment failures with the steroids?

Dr. MASSELL: I think all of the patients who die of rheumatic carditis die from congestive failure, and we assume that congestive failure is due to inflammation of the heart. The question is: Will hormones reverse this? If the steroids are really superior anti-inflammatory drugs, then they should be better than aspirin in congestive failure due to rheumatic carditis; the unfortunate thing is that there are not very many controlled studies in this group of patients because even in the co-operative studies, when the patient was very ill the clinicians who were responsible tended to take them off aspirin and put them on therapy with steroids, or they withheld the patient from the study. In the new studies we are doing, we have great difficulty in getting really sick patients because the clinicians at the Children's Hospital Medical Center would object if they entered a patient in the study and the patient were placed in the aspirin group.

DR. FISCHEL: Dr. Likoff, I think it is fair to say that the data from the coopera-tive study show that there was about the same order of magnitude of switching of the patients, because in those days there were still some men who thought that aspirin was better than cortisone and they took a sick patient and put him in the aspirin group. Actually all of these patients were eliminated from the study, and since it happened in only six out of 497 cases, I do not think this altered the re-sults. Not one of these died. However, it is important to note that the patients who died during the acute phase of the cooperative study were those who had been on cortisone. These patients did not have heart failure before starting cortisone or during the six weeks of therapy, but they developed a rebound phenomenon after cessation of therapy which was of such magnitude that the re-institution of the drug did not stop the progression of the disease. This is one reason why I am extremely reluctant to treat patients with mild disease with cortisone. I have the feeling that the cessation of these drugs constitutes a new introduction to the disease and I do not know how severe it will be or whether it can be controlled if a rebound occurs.

DR. LIKOFF: I think a brief summary is in order at this point. It is very apparent that the effects of the steroids on the basic pathologic process and its devolutionary pattern, speaking in terms of carditis, are not as yet clearly understood. It is also equally apparent that steroids do not have significant benefits over those of the more conservative forms of therapy, at least in the early illness and in patients who are only moderately sick. Some reservations are held by some members of the panel as to whether steroids should be applied under all circumstances; others confine the use of steroids to the more severely ill.

Treatment of Lupus Erythematosus with Steroids*

LOUIS J. SOFFER

Mount Sinai Hospital and State University of New York College of Medicine, New York City

The study presented here extended over a ten-year period and concerned the investigation of 90 patients with disseminated lupus erythematosus. It consisted essentially of two parts, the study and treatment of the disease in general and the investigation of the nature of the renal lesions and their response to therapy. The second aspect of the study is presented in a subse-quent paper in this volume.

Of the 90 patients studied, 11 were males and 79 females; the youngest patient in the group was approximately six years of age and the oldest was 72, but most of the patients were in the age range of 16 to 40.

Table 1 lists the various clinical manifestations in this group of un-treated patients. Almost all patients had arthralgias at some time or another, many had fever, approximately two-thirds had weight loss, and only two-thirds had the typical characteristic skin lesions.

* This study was supported by the National Institutes of Health of the U. S. Public Health Service.

SYMPTOMS	PERCENTAGE OF PATIENTS
Arthralgias	95
Fever	91
Weight loss	65
Rash	62
Arthritis	62
Chest pain	36
Chills or chilliness	31
Abdominal pain	20
Bleeding tendency	11
Convulsions	10

As indicated in Table 1 arthralgias and arthritis are very common manifestations of disseminated lupus erythematosus. Arthralgia frequently occurs for a variable period of time prior to the onset of the more significant manifestations of lupus; in some instances arthralgia was present for a period of years before the patient developed either the rash, fever, renal damage or other symptoms.

Table 2 lists the findings on the physical examination. It is important

TABLE 2. PERCENTAGE INCIDENCE OF PHYSICAL SIGNS IN 90 PATIENTS WITH SYSTEMIC LUPUS ERYTHEMATOSUS

PHYSICAL SIGNS	PERCENTAGE OF PATIENTS
Lymphadenopathy	71
Rash	62
Joint abnormalities	51
Hepatomegaly	47
Cardiac abnormalities (total)	36
Significant murmur (systolic)	11
Gallop rhythm	9
Pericardial friction rub	7
Pericardial effusions	7
Mucous membrane lesions	35
Pulmonary abnormalities (total)	33
Pleural effusion	13
Pleural friction rub	11
Splenomegaly	25
Psychiatric abnormalities	24
Abnormal fundi	21
Edema	20
Petechiae	11
Neurologic abnormalities	9

to emphasize that lymphadenopathy occurs in almost three-quarters of the patients. The lymph nodes are discrete, relatively soft, and as a rule flat; they occur in the anterior and posterior cervical chains, in the axillae and in the inguinal areas. The characteristic rash occurs in perhaps two-thirds of the group. Hepatomegaly, which is a not uncommon physical finding in disseminated lupus erythematosus, occurs in almost half the patients, and splenomegaly is found in perhaps a fourth. There is nothing particularly characteristic about the enlargement of the spleen or of the liver.

Table 3 shows the laboratory data from this group of patients. There are

TABLE 3.   LABORATORY DATA IN 90 PATIENTS WITH SYSTEMIC LUPUS ERYTHEMATOSUS (PER CENT)

Positive L.E. test	100
Elevated sedimentation rate	93
Anemia (Hgb. less than 12.0 grams)	71
Cephalin flocculation test (2 + to 4 +) (of 44 patients)	68
WBC less than 5,000/cu.mm.	64
Urine abnormalities	62
Abnormal EEG (of 30 patients)	50
Azotemia (of 62 patients)	42
Blood creatinine greater than 1.5 mg./100 ml. (of 56 patients)	41
Abnormal chest x-ray	36
C-reactive protein test 1 + or more (of 19 patients)	36
False positive serologic test for syphilis	27
Hyperglobulinemia (of 76 patients)	26
Abnormal ECG	22
Prolonged bleeding time (of 32 patients)	22
Platelets less than 100,000/cu.mm.	16

a number of points of interest. In the first place, a positive L.E. smear was found in all of the patients. It should be emphasized that a positive L.E. smear is not necessarily present the first time a patient is admitted to the hospital. However, careful studies of the slides over a long period of time or repeated examinations for L.E. cells eventually established a positive test in all patients with disseminated lupus erythematosus in our series. An increase in sedimentation rate occurred in almost 100 per cent of the patients, and this is of some interest. The white blood cell count revealed significant leukopenia in two-thirds of the patients; characteristically, an absence of leukocytosis is one of the hallmarks of disseminated lupus erythematosus. A leukocytosis occurs in this illness only in association with some underlying intercurrent infection; leukocytosis without an adequate explanation in a given patient in whom the diagnosis of systemic lupus is suspected usually indicates that the patient does not have this disease. False positive serologic tests for syphilis occurred in about 25 per cent of the group.

Of the 90 patients in our group, 26, or slightly less than 30 per cent, died (Table 4). Of these 26 patients, 22 died of progressive renal failure. The deaths of the other four were avoidable; that is to say, one patient committed suicide, one died from status epilepticus because of insufficient therapy, the third died as a result of inadequate therapy (this was one of an earlier group treated at a time when comparatively small amounts of steroids were available), and the fourth patient died of a disseminated fungus infection. Therefore, it should be emphasized that almost all of the deaths occurred in the presence of significant renal damage.

TABLE 4.   CAUSE OF DEATH IN PATIENTS WITH RENAL DISEASE

CAUSE	NUMBER	PER CENT
Uremia	22	84
Other*		
Status epilepticus	1	4
Disseminated fungus infection	1	4
Suicide	1	4
Inadequate therapy	1	4

* All were azotemic at the time of death.

TABLE 5. EFFECT OF TREATMENT WITH CORTICOTROPIN OR GLUCO-GENIC STEROIDS ON THE CLINICAL MANIFESTATIONS OF SYSTEMIC LUPUS ERYTHEMATOSUS (90 PATIENTS)

CLINICAL MANIFESTATIONS	COMPLETELY IMPROVED (per cent)	PARTIALLY IMPROVED (per cent)	TOTAL IMPROVED (per cent)
Fever	100	0	100
Arthralgias	100	0	100
Pleural friction rub	100	0	100
Pleural effusion	100	0	100
Pericardial friction rub	100	0	100
Pericardial effusion	100	0	100
Rash	41	50	91
Chest pain	55	35	90
Mucous membrane lesions	53	21	74
Abdominal pains	36	36	72
Fundal abnormalities	44	22	66
Weight loss	66	0	66
Psychiatric abnormalities	31	31	62
Gallop rhythm	20	40	60
Edema	25	33	58
Lymphadenopathy	19	36	55
Hepatomegaly	8	12	20
Neurological abnormalities	0	20	20
Splenomegaly	7	7	14
Hypertension	0	0	0
Cardiac murmur	0	0	0

Table 5 presents the results of treatment in our group. In all patients fever responded well to therapy. Arthralgia disappeared very promptly; pleural friction rubs, pleural effusion, pericardial friction rubs and pericardial effusion—when present—vanished, and the rash responded very well in most of the patients. However, splenomegaly, hepatomegaly and hypertension often did not disappear, hepatomegaly subsiding in only a fifth of the group, and splenomegaly in 10 to 15 per cent. Hypertension persisted in all patients in whom it was present.

Table 6 shows the changes in the laboratory findings as a result of therapy. The L.E. test continued to be positive in all instances. Although the frequency with which the typical cell was seen in the smear was perhaps less after treatment or during the course of treatment than it had been during the control period, with careful observation the cell could always be found.

The second point of interest is that hemolysis, when present, disappeared in all instances, although the Coombs' test continued to be positive. Azotemia improved in about a third of the group, and the sedimentation rate improved in two-thirds or perhaps more, of the patients; as a matter of fact, the sedimentation rate is the best criterion to be employed in establishing the maintenance dosage of steroids in patients with lupus. Thrombocytopenia as a rule improved in those patients in whom it was present.

Table 7 lists the glucogenic steroids that were employed at one time or another in the course of the treatment of this group of patients. The figures presented indicate the average initial daily dose—and I must emphasize that this is only the *average* dose, since not infrequently the initial daily dose was very much higher, several patients receiving as much as 1000 mg. a day of cortisone to induce suppression of the disease. Occasionally, the initial dose was lower; but, in general, the majority of patients responded

TABLE 6. EFFECT OF TREATMENT WITH CORTICOTROPIN OR GLUCO-
GENIC STEROIDS ON THE LABORATORY DATA IN SYSTEMIC
LUPUS ERYTHEMATOSUS (90 PATIENTS)

LABORATORY TEST	IMPROVED (per cent)
Positive L.E. test	0
Positive direct Coombs test	0
Abnormal EEG	0
Cephalin flocculation greater than 1 +	14
C-reactive protein test greater than 1 +	25
Urinary abnormalities	
Sediment—occasional to many RBC	32
" " " " WBC	50
" " " " casts	36
Albuminuria 1 + or more	26
Azotemia	35
WBC shift to left (band forms greater than 10 per cent)	41
Abnormal ECG	42
Hyperglobulinemia	46
Hemoglobin less than 10 grams/100 ml.	54
Abnormal chest x-ray	60
Platelets less than 100,000/cu.mm.	63
Elevated sedimentation rate	70
WBC less than 5000/cu.mm.	72
Prolonged bleeding time	75
Hemolysis	100

adequately to the dose level indicated. With cortisone this average initial dose was 200 to 300 mg. a day, and the maintenance dose was 50 to 100 mg. per day; if dexamethasone (which is not included in this table) is used, the patient would require approximately 6 to 10 mg. a day, with a maintenance dosage of 1.5 to 4 mg. a day. The patients responded equally well to all of the adrenal steroids. The incidence of side effects was exactly the same with all steroids except that cortisone and hydrocortisone frequently caused salt retention. Prednisone and most of the other synthetic analogs used did not, as a rule, cause retention of sodium and fluid. This is the major advantage of the analogs, and it is a significant one; however, all the other side effects occurred with an equal degree of frequency with use of the various steroids in the doses I have outlined.

TABLE 7. COMPARATIVE EFFECTIVENESS OF THE ADRENAL STEROIDS AS
ANTI-INFLAMMATORY AGENTS IN MAN

HORMONAL AGENT	ANTI-FLAM-MATORY ACTIVITY	AVERAGE INITIAL DAILY ORAL DOSE (mg.)	AVERAGE DAILY ORAL MAINTENANCE DOSE (mg.)
Cortisone	1	200-300	50-100
Cortisol	1-1.25	200-300	50-100
Prednisone	3-5	40-60	10-25
Prednisolone	3-5	40-60	10-25
6-Methylprednisolone	3-5	32-48	8-24
3-Methylcortisol	4-5	30-50	5-20
Desoxycorticosterone acetate	0	. .	. .
Aldosterone	0-?	. .	. .
9α-Fluorocortisol	10-15	8-12	4-6
9α-Fluoro-16-hydroxyprednisolone	3-5	32-48	8-24

In conclusion, I think that the present day treatment of disseminated lupus erythematosus with steroids represents a very significant advance, and although I do not think it represents a very significant advance in the management of the associated renal disease, the toxic manifestations and all of the other clinical manifestations of lupus respond in very satisfactory manner.

High Dosage Steroid Therapy for Systemic Lupus Erythematosus[*]

EDMUND L. DUBOIS

University of Southern California School of Medicine

The dosage of steroids required in the treatment of systemic lupus erythematosus (S.L.E.) is exceedingly variable. Approximately 3 per cent of our series of 400 cases of this disease required more than the equivalent of 1000 mg. of cortisone daily for periods of weeks in the treatment of acute crises. Ten per cent of the entire group needed 500 to 1000 mg. daily for the control of exacerbations. The aim of this paper is to review indications, techniques and problems associated with high dosage corticoid therapy.

Steroids are not indicated in every case of proved systemic lupus erythematosus; however, approximately two-thirds of our patients eventually require them at some time during the course of their illness. Every effort should be made to avoid their early administration, particularly in the mild cases, since the use of rest, salicylates and antimalarials is a much less hazardous mode of treatment.[2, 3]

INDICATIONS FOR STEROID THERAPY

If salicylates and antimalarials fail to control the disease, if the patient is critically ill, or if there is neurological or renal involvement, steroid therapy should be started. The dosage of corticosteroid required varies directly with the severity of the disease. In the milder cases the estimated amount of hormone is merely added to the therapeutic regimen of the patient. Often this means supplementing a combination of salicylates and antimalarials with small doses of steroids such as 5 mg. of cortisone four times daily. Periods of a week or more are permitted to lapse between dosage changes in the milder cases, and the increments are small, perhaps a 10 to 20 per cent rise at intervals of one or two weeks until symptomatic and laboratory improvement is noted. Similar decrements are utilized in withdrawing steroid therapy. No corticotrophin is employed. Whenever more than 50 mg. per day of cortisone or its equivalent in other steroids is used for longer than

[*] The study was supported by a research grant (A3075) from the National Institute of Arthritis and Metabolic Disease, United States Public Health Service, and by grants from Merck Sharp and Dohme, Lederle Laboratories and The Upjohn Company.

a few weeks, a prophylactic ulcer regimen should be instituted, consisting of six feedings, antacids and anticholinerigic therapy.[4]

TECHNIQUE OF HIGH DOSAGE STEROID THERAPY

If the patient is severely ill, salicylates and antimalarials are not given early in therapy; he is immediately placed on large doses of steroids, such as 400 mg. per day of cortisone. This is done initially with the hope of rapidly reversing the pathological process before irreversible damage occurs. If no response is noted within 24 to 48 hours, the dosage of steroid is increased by 25 to 100 per cent, depending on the clinical situation, until improvement is noted. As much as 2300 mg. per day of cortisone or the equivalent dose of newer steroids has been used successfully in treating acute L.E. crises. It is advisable to continue using high dosages of steroids until all acute abnormal physical findings have subsided.

Early renal involvement is usually benefited by large doses of these hormones. The clinical characteristics of such involvement are the absence of hypertension, presence of proteinuria, hematuria, occasional azotemia, and casts of the red cell, granular and hyaline type. A nephrotic syndrome is often also an early manifestation, and this too may be benefited. If improvement has not occurred after two months of adequate steroid treatment, nitrogen mustard is often helpful.[2] Advanced nephropathy with hypertension and anasarca is usually aggravated by large amounts of corticoids; oliguria, grand mal seizures and death often rapidly ensue following their administration. Nitrogen mustard is occasionally helpful in this terminal stage. Chlorothiazide and related drugs are useful in controlling the edema associated with nephropathy. Many patients develop cutaneous reactions from one of these diuretics, but the lesions do not necessarily recur on changing to another thiazide derivative. Mercurials should be used with caution since severe anaphylactic reactions are more likely to occur in patients with S.L.E. than in others.

Adjunctive therapy is necessary when more than 50 mg. per day of cortisone is used for protracted periods. The necessity for routinely utilizing a prophylactic ulcer regimen has already been mentioned and will be discussed further under side effects. When 100 or more milligrams of cortisone or its equivalent is given daily, sodium usually should be restricted to 2 grams or less per day depending upon the clinical situation. Massive dosages of steroids often lead to sodium retention even when the newer corticoids are used. If the daily equivalent of 200 or more milligrams of cortisone is required, supplementary potassium—preferably in the liquid form—should be given in doses of 8 to 15 grams of potassium salts (such as Elixir Potassium Triplex [Lilly] 15 cc. in juice) after meals or intravenous potassium chloride 6 to 12 grams (80 to 160 mEq.) daily diluted in 3000 cc. of parenteral fluid. The parenteral route should be avoided if possible because of the dangers of a slough if extravasation occurs. Enteric-coated tablets are often not absorbed in critically ill patients. If the patient is unable to swallow and is not vomiting, it is advisable to insert a nasogastric tube and to give food and medication by that means rather than parenterally, since large amounts of steroids and potassium may be required. In critical situations, intravenous hydrocortisone may be used as a continuous drip. The doses required for oral or parenteral use are similar.

Frequent electrolyte determinations as well as urinalyses for glycosuria and acetonuria should be performed. If the patient is receiving several hundred milligrams daily of cortisone or its equivalent for months, chest roentgenograms should be performed every few months and, in addition, lateral views of the thoracic and lumbar spine should be taken every 4 to 6 months in order to detect early osteoporosis. Pulmonary fungus infections such as torulosis are not uncommon in patients on high-dosage corticoid therapy.

GUIDES TO STEROID DOSAGE

The clinical picture and hemoglobin level are used as the major guides to steroid therapy. The temperature curve provides an excellent indicator for dosage adjustment. In general the temperature during crisis approaches normal when the dosage is adequate and the clinical status is improving. If infections are ruled out, the dose of steroid should be adequate to produce a normal temperature within a few days in a moderately ill patient and within one to two weeks in the critically ill patient requiring massive dosages of steroids. Note the temperature responses in the cases discussed below. When steroids are reduced, return of fever may precede clinical relapse. Consequently, if a febrile rebound phenomenon occurs without immediate clinical repercussion, the period between dosage reductions should be lengthened until the temperature curve returns to normal. If significant renal involvement is present, this is followed closely in order to determine when to reduce the dose. The sedimentation rate is never used as the main index to dosage, since it can remain indefinitely elevated in some patients who are in complete clinical remission. The L.E. cell test is helpful in following the over-all picture of the disease but should not be used as a basis to determine therapy, because it requires several weeks for changes to occur. Many patients have had persistently positive L.E. cell tests even though they are in a remission requiring no medication.

Examples of High Dosage Steroid Therapy

Case 1. W. B. is a 21-year-old white plant nurseryman. As a child, he had been in good health until age 9, in August 1948, when he developed a transitory butterfly area blush on his cheeks. In September 1949, after prolonged exposure to the sun, the erythema reappeared, and during the following month, scaly erythema developed on both ears and gradually spread to involve the butterfly area. Soon after this, thrombocytopenia, anemia and polyarthritis appeared. L.E. cells were present. In March 1950, small doses of corticoids were started without much effect. During most of the next two years, the patient received 75 to 100 mg. of cortisone daily. When first seen by the writer in November 1952, the patient was a slightly obese, restless, 13-year-old boy with severe scaling and erythema in the butterfly area of the face. Similar cutaneous changes were present on the ears, the V area of the chest and the lateral surfaces of the arms, thighs and legs. Otherwise, the findings in the physical examination were within normal limits. Laboratory studies revealed a normocytic anemia, with hemoglobin 10.5 grams, a white cell count of 4580 with normal differential, and a slightly reduced number of platelets. The Wintrobe sedimentation rate was 45 mm. per hour, uncorrected. The L.E. cell preparation was negative. The urine was normal. The dose of cortisone was raised to 150 mg. per day, and following this there was gradual improvement in the rash and an increased sense of well-being. In January 1953, arthralgia in the hands recurred, and there were pains in the toes on walking. The dose of cortisone was increased to 350 mg. per day. In March 1953, the tip of the large toe became cyanotic and exceedingly painful. It was believed that an active angiitis of the small blood vessels was present. Pulsation in the larger vessels was normal. The dose of cortisone was raised again to 800 mg. per day with subsequent improvement (see Figure 1). Despite these large doses of cortisone, the white cell count was only 3850, hematocrit 37 and platelet count 54,000. L.E. cells were again found. On April 23, 1953, the patient was slightly Cushingoid and steroids were reduced to 600 mg. per day. A week later the patient was hospitalized because of severe myalgia in the left thigh and bilateral effusion in both knees. On May 2, 1953, his temperature rose to 102°, cortisone was again increased to 800 mg. per day, and the symptoms abated. The patient was given 10 mg. of nitrogen mustard in order to determine whether this would help ameliorate the systemic manifestations. On May 9, 1953, he had normal vital signs and no complications. The hemoglobin was 10.5 grams and white cell count was 3250. Ten hours later he had the first of a series of generalized grand mal seizures. There had been a

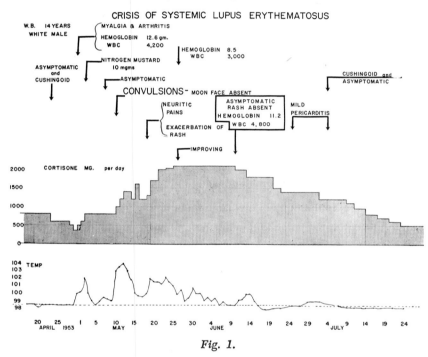

CRISIS OF SYSTEMIC LUPUS ERYTHEMATOSUS

Fig. 1.

vague history of two prior seizures one year before. After the convulsions, the patient complained of pleuritic pain along the dorsal spine from the third to eleventh vertebrae. There was no tenderness. He was now acutely ill and febrile to 103.5° despite taking 800 mg. daily of cortisone. The blood pressure was 130/70; otherwise, there were no significant abnormalities noted on the physical or neurological examinations. The hemoglobin was 11.3 grams and white cell count 6400. Urinalysis now showed a trace of albumin plus a few fine and coarse granular casts. X-rays of the spine revealed advanced osteoporosis and multiple compression fractures throughout the dorsal and lumbar areas (see Figure 2). It was believed that, in view of the persistent fever and recent exacerbation of arthritis and myalgia, the patient had active central nervous system angiitis due to systemic lupus, and cortisone was increased gradually to 1400 mg. per day. In addition, supplementary potassium salts (6 grams daily), an ulcer regimen, prophylactic penicillin, anticonvulsant medication and testosterone (several hundred mg. weekly) were begun. A plaster body cast was made to prevent further collapse of the spine. On May 18 the patient was still febrile and there was persistent pain

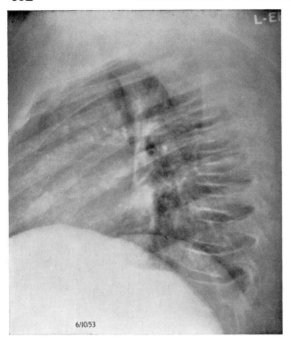

Fig. 2. Case 1, W. B. Steroid-induced osteoporosis with multiple thoracic vertebral compression fractures. June 10, 1953.

in the forearms, fingers and palms for several days, as well as new erythematous papules on the palms and fingers. Greyish ulcers were present on the buccal mucosa and pharynx. Because of these evidences of disease activity, the cortisone dosage was raised from 1300 to 2100 mg. per day. On May 26 the neuritic pains,

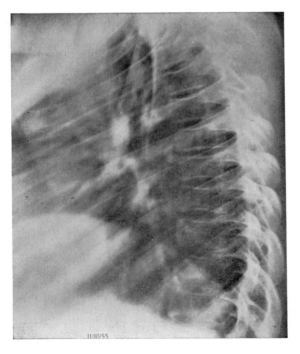

Fig. 3. Case 1, W. B. Healing of the fractures and bone regeneration following reduction in steroid dosage and administration of androgens. November 10, 1955.

back pain and rash began to improve. By June 15 the patient was discharged from the hospital on 1800 mg. per day of cortisone. Because of persistent discomfort in the thoracic and lumbar vertebrae the patient was unable to walk and remained in a wheel chair. During the course of the next few months, steroids were gradually tapered to 300 mg. per day, androgens were continued, and the patient received physiotherapy. By September 1953, he was beginning to walk without assistance. Anticonvulsant medication was gradually discontinued. In November 1953, cortisone had been reduced to 100 mg. daily. During the next two years the patient received between 100 and 200 mg. daily for control of minor exacerbations. X-rays of the spine on November 10, 1955, showed improvement (see Figure 3). By June 1957, the dose had been reduced to 25 mg. daily and the patient has been maintained at that level since. Attempts to reduce the steroid level below this point produced symptoms of adrenal insufficiency. Figure 4 shows a recent roentgenogram of the thoracic spine, illustrating complete recalcification of the vertebrae. Despite advice to the contrary, the patient has been working as a plant nurseryman during the past several years, carrying heavy materials and constantly exposed to desert sun, without a relapse of the rash or other clinical manifestations.

Case Summary. A 21-year-old white male who has had proved systemic lupus erythematosus for 12 years to date developed a severe relapse in the fifth year of his illness, with convulsions, peripheral vasculitis, fever and pancytopenia. In addition he had osteoporosis with compression fractures secondary to steroid therapy and aggravated by the seizures. The exacerbation was controlled by the use of as much as 2100 mg. per day of cortisone for more than two weeks. During the subsequent seven years the patient has entered complete remission, requiring only 25 mg. of cortisone per day during the past three years. The osteoporosis has completely disappeared and the spine has returned to normal.

Case 2. G. H., now a 24-year-old colored female, was admitted to the hospital in August 1951 at the age of 15, complaining of painful joints of one year's duration. The patient had been in good health until the age of 14, when she developed

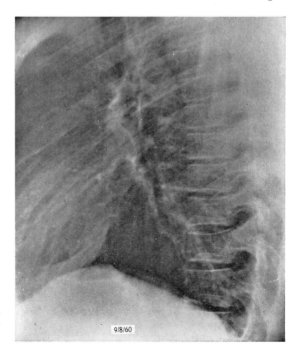

Fig. 4. Case 1, W. B. Normal thoracic spine. September 8, 1960.

9/8/60

migratory polyarthritis involving both the major and minor joints, including the proximal interphalangeal articulations. The following year, when first seen here, she had a relapse of fever and arthritis. Studies revealed evidence of rheumatoid-like arthritis, sero-sanguinous pericarditis, bilateral pleural effusions and a severe normocytic anemia. L.E. cells were present. Cultures for tuberculosis were negative. The patient was initially treated with corticotrophin with excellent results and then was maintained on 50 to 100 mg. per day of cortisone for the next four years. Steroids were completely discontinued during the following two years; in this period the patient gave birth to a normal child. One month post partum, in May 1958, arthralgia recurred and the patient was placed on chloroquine 500 mg. daily in addition to salicylates. In August 1958, dexamethasone 0.75 mg. per day was added to her therapeutic regimen, and this was continued during the next year. In August 1959, arthralgia increased with a relapse of pleuritic pain. The dose of dexamethasone was raised to 2.0 mg. per day with good control. On Sep-

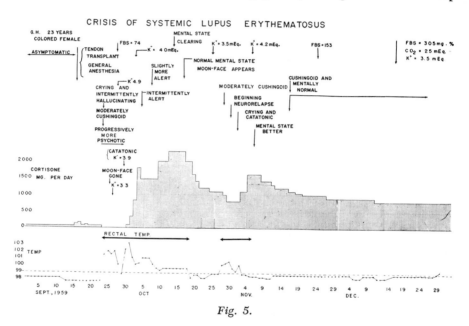

Fig. 5.

tember 15, 1959, the patient was hospitalized for a tendon transplant under general anesthesia because of the flexion contractures of the fourth and fifth digits of both hands. Steroids were increased slightly pre- and postoperatively. In Figure 5, for graphic purposes, all steroids have been converted to cortisone (0.75 mg. of dexamethasone = 25 mg. of cortisone = 20 mg. of hydrocortisone). Several days postoperatively she was again taking 2.0 mg. per day of dexamethasone. On September 23, while the patient was still slightly Cushingoid from the steroids and afebrile, intermittent hallucinations appeared. Serum potassium was 3.3 mEq./L. It was felt that there might be a steroid-induced psychosis; hormones were stopped and supplementary potassium was given. Within 24 hours she became febrile to 102°. Her mental state now began to deteriorate rapidly, with more crying spells, confusion, incontinence and screaming. Repeated serum potassium levels were normal. The fasting blood sugar was 74 mg. per cent. Within the next few days the psychosis became more severe, with alternating screaming and crying. On September 29 she became completely catatonic. At this time her hemoglobin was 13.3 grams and the white cell count was 3400. One competent psychiatrist who saw the patient thought she had a functional psychosis, whereas the other psychiatrist thought it might be an organic one. The results of neurological examination and lumbar puncture were within normal limits. The Cushingoid appearance had disappeared about September 25, 1959. It was now thought, in view of the fever, progressive psychosis despite cessation of steroids and loss of Cushingoid appearance, that this was an organic psychosis due to systemic lupus erythematosus. Since the patient was unable to take oral medication voluntarily, steroids were administered via nasogastric tube and parenterally. Beginning on September 30 with 100 mg. daily of parenteral hydrocortisone, the hormone was rapidly increased to 1440 mg. by October 3. On October 4 the patient was intermittently alert, and during the course of the next few days gradual clearing occurred. On October 9, because of persistent fever, parenteral hydrocortisone was supplemented by triamcinolone 80 mg. daily via the nasogastric tube. For five days, the patient received the equivalent of 2300 mg. per day of cortisone. During this period there was rapid improvement in her mental status, which returned to normal, coincident with the reappearance of a moon-face. On October 28 the patient was quite Cushingoid and mentally clear. Severe leg weakness was noted, and deep tendon reflexes were absent. It was thought that this was due to degenerative changes in the anterior spinal cord secondary to her illness, since both leg strength and tendon reflexes had been intact prior to the neurological episode. The mental state was normal, and triamcinolone was decreased further to 32 mg. four times a day, with discontinuation of parenteral medication. Within 24 hours, fever and intermittent crying spells appeared. By 48 hours, the patient became partially catatonic again. Triamcinolone was increased to 44 mg. four times a day and was supplemented with 400 mg. per day of parenteral hydrocortisone. Two days later she was better and became afebrile again. The fasting blood sugar on November 24 was 153 mg. per cent and on December 17, 305 mg. per cent. CO_2 was 25 mEq./L. and potassium was 3.5 mEq./L. Intermittent glycosuria was noted during the next month but did not require antidiabetic therapy. The dose of steroid was gradually tapered and the patient was discharged on December 14, 1959, taking 128 mg. per day of triamcinolone. Because of persistent muscle weakness which might have been aggravated by triamcinolone, she was changed to methylprednisolone 112 mg. per day. During the next month the patient's medication was reduced to 32 mg. per day without any relapse. By February 17, 1960, her leg strength gradually began to return while she was still receiving 24 mg. per day of methylprednisolone, but deep tendon reflexes were still absent. The following month the patient was fully ambulatory without assistance. On August 10, 1960, methylprednisolone was reduced to 4 mg. daily. Deep tendon reflexes were again present. Her mental state has remained normal.

Case Summary. A 24-year-old colored woman, who had had proved systemic lupus erythematosus since age 14, developed a severe neurological episode with a catatonic schizophrenic state at the age of 23. The equivalent of 2300 mg. of cortisone daily was required to control the exacerbation, and several weeks later reduction of dosage to 800 mg. per day led to an exacerbation of symptoms, but these immediately responded to elevation of the amount of cortisone to 1600 mg. daily. The only complication was glycosuria, which was controlled by diet alone. Ten months after the exacerbation the patient remained asymptomatic on 4 mg. of methylprednisolone daily.

Case 3. A 17-year-old Mexican girl had been in good health until April 1958, when she developed a sore throat, fever, malaise and arthralgia in both the major and the proximal interphalangeal joints. The white cell count and sedimentation rate were elevated. A diagnosis of acute rheumatic fever was made. The patient improved with rest and salicylates.

In September 1958, the patient developed unexplained abdominal pain, left-sided pleurisy, cough productive of bloody sputum, dyspnea and fever. In addition, periorbital edema and weight loss were noted. She was admitted to the Medical Service on November 19, 1958.

Her temperature was 102, pulse 132, respirations 28 and blood pressure 118/72. The patient was an acutely and chronically ill, pale 17-year-old girl with marked periorbital edema. There were signs of pleural effusion at the left base posteriorly, and this was verified radiologically. There were no heart murmurs or evidence of cardiac enlargement.

Laboratory studies showed a white cell count of 9200 with a normal differential. The hemoglobin was 9.5 grams. Urinalysis revealed 2+ albumin with 800 mg. of protein per 24 hours. No abnormal sediment was present. Serum albumin was 2.2 grams per cent and globulin was 4.7 grams per cent. An L.E. cell preparation was strongly positive. Other findings were blood urea nitrogen 12 mg. per cent, thymol

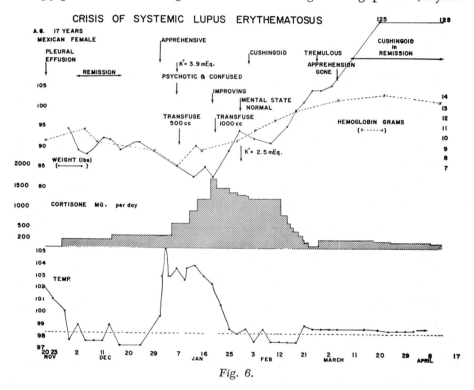

Fig. 6.

turbidity of 9.0 units and cephalin flocculation of 3+. A total of 325 cc. of straw-colored pleural fluid was removed from the left pleural space.

On November 27, 1958, the patient was begun on tetracycline and methyl-prednisolone 32 mg. per day, and there was gradual improvement in her symptoms. (See Figure 6. For charting purposes, steroid doses have been converted to cortisone, using the usual equivalents.) On December 5, methylprednisolone was increased to 48 mg. per day because of generalized weakness and failure to gain weight. At this time her cough was gone and her chest was free of all abnormal signs. The patient was discharged on December 18, 1958, in a good steroid-induced remission on 40 mg. per day of methylprednisolone.

On December 31, 1958, she was readmitted because of nausea, vomiting and fever. The physical examination revealed a febrile, very apprehensive girl with marked intention tremor. Several "cotton wool" exudates were present in the ocular fundi. A grade 2 blowing apical systolic murmur was noted for the first time. The liver was enlarged two fingerbreadths below the costal margin. Hemoglobin was 8.8 grams, and the white cell count was 7000 with a normal differential. The serum potassium was 3.5 mEq./L. On January 6, 1959, the patient became frankly psychotic. At this time the serum potassium was 3.9 mEq./L. and the hemoglobin had fallen to 7 grams. Five hundred cc. of blood was administered. In order to be certain of adequate tissue potassium levels, supplementary liquid potassium was given as Elixir of Potassium Triplex 30 cc. four times daily, containing a total of 360 mEq. of potassium per day. Methylprednisolone was increased to 24 mg. four times daily. Her temperature ranged between 103° and 105°. The psychosis and confusion, which were thought to be due to active central nervous system lupus, persisted. On January 9, methylprednisolone was raised to 36 mg. four times daily. Three days later there was no improvement and the patient began to vomit all oral medication. Steroid therapy was then changed to intramuscular cortisone acetate, 200 mg. every four hours, and this was supplemented by up to 400 mg. of hydrocortisone per day intravenously in her parenteral fluids. At this time the white cell count was 4700 and hemoglobin 8.7 grams. Lumbar puncture revealed a protein of 77 mg. per cent but no other abnormalities. Two days after the equivalent of 1700 mg. per day of cortisone was started the phychosis began to clear. Ten days of high steroid dosage were required before the temperature began to fall. There was no evidence of infection (see **Figure 6**). On January 19, 1959, while the mental state was returning to normal, bilateral transitory ankle clonus was noted. On January 27, the mental state had completely returned to normal. Serum potassium was now 2.5 mEq./L. Elixir of Potassium Triplex was increased to 90 cc. three times daily. By January 30, 1959, after she had received the equivalent of more than 600 mg. per day of cortisone for four weeks, the first signs of Cushing's syndrome appeared. During the following two weeks the patient was mentally improved but very weak. Ankle clonus persisted, with normal reflexes. The serum potassium was 3.3 mEq./L. Cortisone was gradually decreased so that on February 25 she was receiving only 50 mg. per day. Within three days on this dosage increasing anxiety appeared, which cleared promptly after the dose was increased to 200 mg. per day. On April 8, 1959, cortisone was gradually reduced to 100 mg. per day. The patient was continually maintained on approximately this dosage of corticosteroid during the next 18 months and remained in a good steroid-induced remission. Urinalysis in July 1960 showed a persistent albumin of 2+ with several hyaline casts per high power field. The blood urea nitrogen was 16 mg. per cent and serum cholesterol 213 mg. per cent. Despite these massive doses of steroids, there was no evidence at any time that the renal lesion was benefited.

Case Summary. A 17-year-old Mexican girl developed systemic lupus erythematosus at age 15. One month after the initiation of steroid therapy a severe relapse occurred, characterized by psychosis and anemia. The dosage of corticoids was increased, and after 1700 mg. per day of cortisone had been administered for several days the psychosis began to clear. Ten days of this therapy were required before the temperature returned to normal. A minor psychiatric relapse occurred six weeks later when the maintenance dose was lowered to 50 mg. per day; these symptoms promptly cleared when the dose was increased to 200 mg. per day. The patient had a moderate degree of renal involvement which was not benefited by high dosage steroid therapy. During the past eighteen months the steroid-induced remission has been well maintained.

Side Effects of High Dosage Steroid Therapy

Table 1 lists the commonly observed side effects of steroid therapy in S.L.E., based on a series of patients who received an average of 100 mg. per day of cortisone or its equivalent as maintenance therapy. It is noteworthy that, despite the very large doses of steroids utilized in the foregoing cases, Cushingoid appearance was not usually noted until a steroid-

TABLE 1. CORTICOSTEROID SIDE-EFFECTS

NO. OF CASES	DEXA-METHASONE (50)	METHYL-PREDNISOLONE (40)	TRI-AMCINOLONE (29)	PREDNI-STEROIDS (37)
Cushingoid appearance	60%	52%	45%	49%
Hirsutism	28	8	21	3
Acne	10	10	17	16
Striae	4	3	14	3
Ecchymoses	20	27	14	3
Edema	28	5	3	6
Diabetes	4	0	3	6
Dyspepsia	30	17*	37*	33*
Peptic ulcer	22*	22*	18*	19*
Muscle weakness	0	0	19	0
Insomnia	8	0	0	0
Psychosis	2	0	0	0

*Data obtained from a comparable group of patients who had serial upper gastrointestinal tract x-rays while receiving long-term steroid therapy.[2, 3]

induced remission occurred; if present during an exacerbation, it promptly disappeared only to return during a steroid-induced remission. Although this is generally true, exceptions may occur. Apparently during crises of S.L.E. the patient may metabolize sizable amounts of corticoids without developing the Cushingoid effects.

Diabetes is primarily a problem in patients who are receiving high dosage therapy. It occurs in about one-half the patients who are given more than 1000 mg. per day of cortisone or its equivalent over a period of weeks. The appearance of this side effect may be noted without Cushingoid facies and while the basic disease process is yet unregulated. This is especially true in patients who are obese or have a family history of diabetes. These patients will often require large doses of insulin for control of the diabetes while steroids are continued for their anti-inflammatory effect. If ketosis is absent and glycosuria is mild, as often occurs in these cases, diet alone may be sufficient to control the process. Tolbutamide was tried in one patient with severe glycosuria without ketosis but was unsuccessful in controlling the diabetes. Unregulated diabetes leads to severe potassium depletion in the steroid-treated patient. One of our patients received 90 cc. three times daily of Elixir of Potassium Triplex (81 grams of potassium salts daily) for weeks. Normal serum potassium levels appeared only after the diabetes was controlled with 60 to 80 units of insulin daily.

The problem of peptic ulcer induction by the use of steroids in this group of patients has recently been reviewed.[4] The incidence in patients on long-term steroid therapy is approximately the same regardless of the steroid employed. Routine serial gastrointestinal studies in a series of 94 patients have shown a definite correlation between the dose of steroid employed and the incidence of ulcerations. Ulcers are exceedingly rare in patients receiving under 10 mg. per day of prednisone or its equivalent in other steroids; the incidence is 13 per cent in those receiving 10 to 19 mg. per day and rises to 47 per cent in patients taking more than 60 mg. per day for periods of several months. A prophylactic ulcer regimen is of help in reducing these complications.

Osteoporosis is a rare complication which is primarily helped by reduction in steroid dosage and synergistic use of salicylates and antimalarials. Remarkable healing may occur in younger patients, as shown in Case 1.

The dosages and therapeutic value of androgens and estrogens used in conjunction with steroid therapy in the hope of preventing or treating osteoporosis are not known. Calcium and vitamin D therapy have also been used in milder cases with equivocal results.

DISCUSSION

High dosage steroid therapy is required in only a small percentage of cases of systemic lupus erythematosus. Haserick, in 1951, first discussed the successful use of as much as 600 mg. of cortisone daily in treating an acute episode of this disease[6] in a single case. A second patient failed to respond to 2300 mg. per day for one day. Pemphigus and acute leukemia are two other disorders in which this type of therapy may have to be employed.

The typical acute crisis of S.L.E. usually is associated with central nervous system involvement. The psychiatric and neurological disturbances which may occur in this disorder have been well documented. These changes are due to vasculitis in the brain and spinal cord.[1, 5, 7, 8, 9] Unfortunately, many of these episodes occur in patients who are already receiving corticosteroids, and invariably the problem arises as to whether the steroids are inducing these changes. Steroid-induced psychoses in systemic lupus are very rare compared with the large number due to organic disease. This author has seen only two cases of hormonally induced psychiatric difficulties in this large series. If there is doubt as to the etiology of the mental disorder, the cessation of steroids or a sharp decrease in dosage for one or more days will often clarify the picture, as illustrated in the foregoing cases. Supplementary potassium salts in doses of 10 to 15 grams per day should be given in all these cases even if serum levels are normal.

Although this form of therapy is often life-saving in crises of the type described, it is not invariably so. Two patients with clinical pictures similar to those described above have received as much as 4000 mg. per day of cortisone for a week without benefit. Both subsequently died with a persistent psychosis.

SUMMARY AND CONCLUSIONS

During the past ten years 400 patients with systemic lupus erythematosus have been treated with rest, salicylates, antimalarials and corticosteroids. Approximately two-thirds of the patients eventually required some corticoid therapy. Every effort should be made to treat the patient conservatively prior to the use of these hormones. The dosage of steroid used depends entirely on the severity of the illness. Small doses of corticoids should be used as adjunctive therapy in conjunction with salicylates and antimalarials in the patient who has mild symptoms of activity such as active arthritis or anemia. Large doses should be prescribed immediately for patients who have acute exacerbations of the illness which are usually associated with central nervous system manifestations. Three per cent of our patients required more than 1000 mg. per day of cortisone or its equivalent daily for periods of weeks in order to control these exacerbations. Ten per cent needed as much as 500 to 1000 mg. per day for extended periods to control moderately severe flare-ups of their illness. As much as 2300 mg. per day of this steroid has been successfully used to control crises of systemic lupus erythematosus. The importance of a prophylactic ulcer regimen, potassium supplementation and control of steroid-induced diabetes must be stressed when such large doses are used. Almost all psychotic episodes which occur in patients with systemic lupus erythematosus are due to central nervous system vasculitis, regardless of whether the patient has recently been on steroids. These psychoses require massive doses of corticoids which usually are helpful in inducing a remission. High dosage steroid therapy is often a life-saving measure in this disease. Following massive steroid treatment, remissions for as long as seven years have occurred.

REFERENCES

1. Daly, D.: Central nervous system in acute disseminated lupus erythematosus. J. Nerv. & Ment. Dis., 5:461, 1945.
2. Dubois, E. L.: Systemic lupus erythematosus: recent advances in its diagnosis and treatment. Ann. Int. Med., 45:163, 1956.
3. Dubois, E. L.: Current therapy of systemic lupus erythematosus. J.A.M.A., 173:1633, 1960.
4. Dubois, E. L., Bulgrin, J. G. and Jacobson, G.: The corticosteroid-induced peptic ulcer: a serial roentgenological survey of patients receiving high dosages. Am. J. Gastroenterol., 33:435, 1960.
5. Dubois, E. L.: The effect of the L.E. cell test on the clinical picture of systemic lupus erythematosus. Ann. Int. Med., 38:1265, 1953.
6. Haserick, J. R., Corcoran, A. C. and Dustan, H.: ACTH and cortisone in the acute crisis of systemic lupus erythematosus. J.A.M.A., 146:643, 1951.
7. Malamud, N. and Saver, G.: Neuropathologic findings in disseminated lupus erythematosus. Arch. Neurol. & Psychiat., 71:723, 1954.
8. O'Connor, J. F.: Psychoses associated with systemic lupus erythematosus. Ann. Int. Med., 51:526, 1959.
9. Sedgwick, R. P. and Von Hagen, K. O.: The neurological manifestations of lupus erythematosus and periarteritis nodosa. Bull. L. A. Neurol. Soc., 13:129, 1948.

Prognosis in

Systemic Lupus Erythematosus

ROBERT P. MC COMBS

Tufts University School of Medicine

The estimation of prognosis in a disease such as systemic lupus erythematosus is difficult because of the many variations in its severity, the organ systems affected, the time in the course of the disease when the diagnosis is established and variations in treatment. Careful follow-up of many patients over a period of years is essential.

The literature on this subject is scanty. Jessar et al.[3] studied the duration and course of systemic lupus erythematosus in 44 patients over a 15-year period and found that 13 (30 per cent) were alive more than five years after the initial diagnosis; none of these received corticosteroid therapy. Haserick[2] reported upon the course of 83 patients with positive plasma L.E. tests and noted lengthening of life and improvement in morbidity as a result of corticosteroid therapy, but he also noted that some patients, especially those with progressive renal disease, often failed to improve. Objections to statistical methods used by others in recording survival in systemic lupus erythematosus were made by Harvey et al.[1] and elaborated by Merrell and Shulman.[5] These authors believed that in analyzing the influence of various factors upon survival, it was necessary to take as a fixed point the time of diagnosis rather than the estimated time of onset of the disease and, by using the available figures, to construct a life table indicating the percentage of patients surviving each year after diagnosis.

In an earlier paper,[4] we reported our impressions of various factors that seemed to influence the course and prognosis in systemic lupus erythematosus, but we did not subject our data to statistical analysis because of the limited number of cases involved and the relatively short follow-up period in many of the cases. It is now possible to report upon a sufficient number of cases with adequate follow-up data to permit rough statistical comparisons of the effects of various factors upon mortality.

MATERIAL AND METHODS

At the Pratt Clinic–New England Center Hospital the diagnosis of systemic lupus erythematosus has been established beyond reasonable doubt in 104 cases. Only those cases in which there were adequate follow-up data for 36 months after the time of diagnosis (72 cases) were included in this study. In 10 cases follow-up data were inadequate, and in the remaining 22 the diagnosis was established less than 36 months prior to the time of the study. In establishing survival at the 36-month cut-off period, it was important to know only that a patient was living or dead at that point, regardless of what might have been known of his subsequent course. Factors known to have been present prior to or at the time of diagnosis which might have influenced survival were listed and compared in surviving and fatal cases, and mortality rates were subjected to statistical analysis. When significant factors were found, various combinations of these were analyzed by determining the mortality rates in groups where two factors were both present, both absent, or present singly.

The following factors were analyzed: age at time of diagnosis; sex; the course of disease during the first three years after onset; the presence or absence of constitutional, cutaneous, musculoskeletal, serosal, cardiovascular, neurological, renal, hematological and serological manifestations of the disease; and the effects and risks of corticosteroid therapy.

RESULTS

Of the 72 patients included in this study, 36 were dead and 36 were living three years after the time of establishment of the diagnosis, giving a mortality rate in this specially selected group of 50 per cent.

The number of cases, deaths and mortality rates at the 36-month cut-off period, determined by various factors that might affect prognosis, are listed in Table 1.

Age at Time of Diagnosis. Many of the sickest patients seen were in the youngest age group (13 to 21 years). Of 16 patients in this group, 10 were dead within 36 months of the time of diagnosis (mortality rate, 62.5 per cent). With the relatively small number of cases involved, however, this is

TABLE 1. EFFECT OF VARIOUS FACTORS UPON MORTALITY RATE DETERMINED 36 MONTHS AFTER ESTABLISHMENT OF DIAGNOSIS IN 72 CASES OF SYSTEMIC LUPUS ERYTHEMATOSUS

PROGNOSTIC FACTORS	CASES	DEATHS	MORTALITY RATE (%)
Age, time of diagnosis (yrs.)			
13-21	16	10	62.5
22-45	43	20	46.4
46-61	13	6	46.1
Sex			
Male	8	6	75.0
Female	64	30	46.9
Early course of disease			
Nonprogressive	24	3	12.5
Progressive	48	33	68.8*
Manifestations			
A. Constitutional			
Absent	17	2	11.8
Present	55	34	61.8*
B. Cutaneous			
Absent	9	2	22.2
Present	63	34	54.0*
C. Musculoskeletal			
Absent	15	7	46.7
Present	57	29	50.9
D. Serosal			
Absent	37	20	54.0
Present	35	16	45.7
E. Cardiovascular			
Absent	54	26	48.1
Present	18	10	55.5
F. Neurological			
Absent	54	26	48.1
Present	18	10	55.5
G. Renal			
Absent	30	7	23.3
Present	42	29	69.0*
H. Hematological			
Absent	17	3	17.6
Present	55	33	60.0*
I. Serological			
Absent	26	10	38.5
Present	34	16	47.1
(Not tested)	(12)	..	..
Corticosteroid therapy			
Not used	20	17	85.0
	(5)	(0)	(0.0)
Used	47	19	40.4*

* Difference in mortality rate significant ($p < .01$).

not significantly greater than the mortality rates in the middle (46.4 per cent) and older age (46.1 per cent) groups. The risk of death from other causes normally would cause the death rate in the 46 to 61 year age group to be considerably higher than the others. Perhaps the fact that it is not, in this small series, reflects the relative mildness of the disease in the older age group.

Sex. Six of eight males in this series were dead within 36 months of the time of diagnosis; this fact suggests that the disease is more serious in men than in women. However, because of the small number of cases involved, the difference in mortality rate (75 per cent in males and 46.9 per cent in females) was not statistically significant.

Early Course of the Disease. Estimates of the course of such a disease as systemic lupus erythematosus by retrospective analysis of the history are subject to errors because the time of onset is not known. It was helpful in estimating prognosis, however, to judge the early course of the disease by taking as the estimated time of onset the time when *symptoms* characteristically present in this disease first appeared and judging the severity of the early course by the degree of disability and necessity for hospitalization or other medical care, on the basis of the patient's recollection of these events. Using these criteria, cases were listed according to whether the early course was nonprogressive or progressive during the first three years of symptoms irrespective of when the diagnosis was made; then mortality rates were determined in these two groups 36 months *after diagnosis.* Of 24 patients with a nonprogressive early course only three were dead 36 months after establishment of diagnosis, whereas of 48 patients with an early progressive course 33 were dead within 36 months of the time of diagnosis. As a matter of fact, in 25 of these 33 cases death occurred within 36 months of the apparent *onset* of the disease.

Constitutional Manifestations. (FEVER AND/OR WEIGHT LOSS.) In those patients who had fever at the time of diagnosis or a history of recent febrile episodes or weight loss, the 36-month mortality rate was significantly higher than in those patients in whom these findings were lacking (61.8 per cent vs. 11.8 per cent). Obviously, constitutional manifestations reflect involvement of various body systems, but the presence of fever and weight loss, was of greater prognostic significance than any single visceral manifestation, since, as shown in Table 1, the presence or absence of involvement of certain viscera did not prove to be of prognostic importance.

Cutaneous Manifestations. (ERYTHEMATOUS RASH, VASCULAR PURPURA, URTICARIA, DRUG AND SUN SENSITIVITIES, ALOPECIA AND RAYNAUD'S PHENOMENON.) It is well known that, in themselves, cutaneous lesions in this disease are not particularly harmful. Patients with the most extensive skin involvement often exhibited the least systemic involvement. Like constitutional manifestations, cutaneous manifestations were almost invariably evident when the more serious visceral changes that influenced mortality were present. There were only nine patients in whom no cutaneous changes were present, and only two of these died within 36 months of the time of diagnosis, whereas in the 63 cases with cutaneous involvement the mortality rate was 54 per cent. The difference was statistically significant.

Musculoskeletal Manifestations. (ARTHRALGIAS, MYALGIAS, ARTHRITIS AND MYOSITIS.) These were among the most common of the manifestations of the disease, but their presence or absence did not significantly influence the 36-month mortality rates (50.9 per cent vs. 46.7 per cent).

Serosal Manifestations. (PLEURISY, PERICARDITIS, PERITONITIS.) These are among the most dramatic manifestations during the "toxic" phase of systemic lupus erythematosus. Yet in the over-all statistical study the slight difference between mortality rates of those with and those without this manifestation was not statistically significant (45.7 per cent vs. 54.0 per cent). The reason for this apparent inconsistency became evident when the effect of corticosteroid therapy upon various manifestations was calculated.

Cardiovascular Manifestations. (ENDOCARDITIS, MYOCARDITIS.) There was an insignificant difference in mortality rates between those with and those without these manifestations (55.5 per cent vs. 48.1 per cent). The lack of statistical difference was partly due to the small number of cases involved and partly due to effects of treatment.

Neurological Manifestations. (PSYCHOSES, CONVULSIONS, NEUROPATHIES.) At times it was difficult to determine whether psychosis was a manifestation of the disease (encephalitis) or was induced by corticosteroid therapy. In other cases encephalopathies accompanied uremia and were therefore attributed to this rather than to brain involvement by the disease. Recognizing these difficulties in diagnosis, we thought that 15 of our 72 patients had important involvement of the central nervous system; only five of these were dead 36 months after time of diagnosis. The mortality rate (33.3 per cent) in this group was less than in the group without these manifestations (54.4 per cent) but the difference was not statistically significant. The small number of cases involved makes it difficult to draw inferences from these figures.

Renal Manifestations. (ALBUMINURIA, HEMATURIA, DECREASED RENAL FUNCTION, HEMATURIA.) The affected and nonaffected groups were nearly equal in size, but the number of deaths in the affected group was more than four times as large as in the nonaffected group, and the difference in mortality rate (69.0 per cent vs. 23.3 per cent) was statistically significant. The way in which renal involvement affected the statistics in other categories is discussed later.

Hematological Manifestations. (ANEMIA, LEUKOPENIA, THROMBOCYTOPENIA.) In cases exhibiting hematologic abnormalities there was a significant increase in the mortality rate (60 per cent vs. 17.6 per cent). This increase occurred chiefly in cases with anemia; when mortality rates for patients with leukopenia were analyzed separately no significant difference was evident in positive or negative groups, and the number of cases with thrombocytopenia was too small to analyze. The fact that most of the deaths in this group occurred in cases with renal involvement is discussed later.

Immunological Abnormalities. (REVERSAL OF ALBUMIN-GLOBULIN RATIO, BIOLOGICALLY FALSELY POSITIVE SEROLOGICAL TESTS.) It has been postulated that systemic lupus erythematosus may be caused by some disturbance in the immunological mechanisms because abnormal antibodies and hypergammaglobulinemia are often encountered. In the 60 cases of this series in which both the albumin-globulin ratio and the serology were determined, abnormalities were encountered in 34. The death rate in this group (47.1 per cent) was not significantly greater than it was in the group in which these tests were normal (38.5 per cent).

Corticosteroid Therapy. Eighteen patients were seen before the advent of corticosteroid therapy and 15 of these were dead within 36 months of the time of diagnosis. Two others received corticosteroids only briefly because of the development of psychoses shortly after treatment was initiated; these patients both died shortly after withdrawal of corticosteroids. Thus, the mortality rate in the "untreated" group was 85 per cent. There were an additional five patients in whom corticosteroids were not used because of the mildness of the disease and the lack of any serious systemic manifestations; these were all living at the end of 36 months. The remaining 47 patients all received corticosteroids for varying periods of time in varying dosage,

TABLE 2. EFFECT OF RENAL INVOLVEMENT UPON MORTALITY RATE ATTRIBUTED TO OTHER FACTORS

PROGNOSTIC FACTOR	MORTALITY (%)	RENAL DISEASE ABSENT			RENAL DISEASE PRESENT		
	(All cases)	Cases	Deaths	Mort. (%)	Cases	Deaths	Mort. (%)
Age, time of diagnosis							
13-21	62.5	6	2	33.3	10	8	80.0
22-45	46.4	18	5	27.8	25	15	60.0
46-61	46.1	6	0	0*	7	6	85.6
Early course							
Nonprogressive	12.5	19	0	0*	5	3	60.0
Progressive	68.8	11	7	63.6	37	26	70.3
Constitutional manifestations							
Absent	11.8	10	0	0	7	2	28.6
Present	61.8	20	7	35.0*	35	27	77.1
Hematological manifestations							
Absent	17.6	11	0	0	7	3	42.9
Present	60.0	19	7	36.8	35	26	74.3*
Corticosteroid therapy							
Not used	68.0	7	3	42.9	18	14	77.8
Used	40.4	23	4	17.4*	24	15	62.5

* Difference in mortality rate significant (p < .01).

and the mortality rate in this group was 40.4 per cent. The difference between the treated and the untreated group was statistically significant.

Analysis of the effect of corticosteroid therapy upon various prognostic factors could not be done effectively because of the relatively small number of untreated cases. Certain observations were of interest, however. For example: No deaths occurred among 16 treated patients in whom the early course was benign; only three of 21 treated patients with serosal manifestations and only one of nine treated patients with neurological manifestations died; only four treated patients without renal manifestations died, whereas of 24 treated patients with renal disease, 15 died (Table 2).

Effect of Renal Manifestations upon Mortality Rate Attributed to Other Factors (Table 2). No deaths occurred among six patients over the age of 45 with no renal disease.

No deaths occurred among 19 patients who had a benign early course and who did not have renal involvement at time of diagnosis.

No deaths occurred among ten patients without constitutional manifestations or renal disease. Most of the deaths in the group with constitutional manifestations occurred when renal disease was present.

Most of the deaths occurring in the group with hematologic abnormalities occurred among those who also had renal disease, suggesting that, in most cases, anemia (the most significant hematological abnormality) was due to uremic bone marrow suppression.

Twenty-four patients with renal disease were treated with corticosteroids, and there were 15 deaths (mortality rate, 62.5 per cent). Twenty-three patients with no renal disease were treated with corticosteroids and there were only four deaths (mortality rate, 17.4 per cent); two of these deaths were attributable to the therapy.

Causes of Death. Of the 72 patients comprising this series, 36 were known to have died within three years of the time of diagnosis. Seven patients known to have been living three years after diagnosis are known to have died subsequently; three of these were in the "untreated" group and four in the corticosteroid-treated group. It is of interest to compare the causes of death in these two groups (Table 3).

There was a distinct difference between corticosteroid-treated and "untreated" groups. Death occurred most commonly in the untreated group during the "toxic" phase of the disease, which was characterized by high fever, polyserositis and carditis, the exact mechanism of death being difficult

TABLE 3.   CAUSES OF DEATH IN SYSTEMIC LUPUS ERYTHEMATOSUS*

	"UNTREATED"	TREATED WITH CORTICOSTEROIDS
Renal failure	2	11
Cardiac failure	5	2
"Toxic"	8	0
Infection	3	5†
Other	0	2‡
Unknown	2	3
	20	23

* This list includes 3 cases in the untreated group and 4 cases in the treated group in which death occurred more than 36 months after establishment of diagnosis.

† Pancreatitis, tuberculosis (2 cases), pneumococcal meningitis, staphylococcal endocarditis.

‡ Gastrointestinal bleeding, diabetes (vascular accident).

to ascertain even at autopsy because of the multiple systems involved. On the other hand, death did not occur in a single case in the "toxic" stage in the treated group. Infection was a more common cause of death in the treated than in the untreated patients; these infections were either difficult to recognize or of an overwhelming type resistant to antibiotics. They are logically considered as complications of treatment. Two other patients died as a result of complications of treatment, one with an uncontrollable gastro-intestinal hemorrhage from a peptic ulcer and the other with corticosteroid-induced diabetes and severe vascular disease from an apparent cerebral-vascular accident.

SUMMARY

In a series of 104 cases of systemic lupus erythematosus seen at the Pratt Clinic–New England Center Hospital sufficient follow-up data were available to permit a study of survival three years following establishment of diagnosis in 72 cases. Various factors thought to influence mortality were subjected to statistical analysis.

The data indicated that there was a favorable prognosis when the severity of the disease did not progress during the first three years after onset, and when constitutional manifestations, cutaneous manifestations, renal involvement or hematological abnormalities were not present at the time of diagnosis. Adequate doses of corticosteroids aided in prolonging life to 36 months from the time of diagnosis in nearly all cases except those with renal involvement, and even in cases with renal involvement chances of survival to 36 months were more likely with corticosteroids. The prolonged use of corticosteroids in this disease carried with it some risks, as evidenced by the fact that complications of therapy constituted the second most common cause of death in the treated group. The evidence cited suggests that in all but mild cases these risks were justified.

REFERENCES

1. Harvey, A. M., Shulman, L. E., Tumulty, P. A., Conley, C. L. and Schoenrich, E. H.: Systemic lupus erythematosus: review of literature and clinical analysis of 138 cases. Medicine, *33*:29, 1954.
2. Haserick, J. R.: Effect of cortisone and corticotropin on prognosis of systemic lupus erythematosus: Survey of eighty-three patients with positive plasma L.E. tests. Arch. Dermat. & Syph., *68*:714, 1953.
3. Jessar, R. A., Lamont-Havers, R. W. and Ragan, C.: Natural history of lupus erythematosus disseminatus. Ann. Int. Med., *38*:717, 1953.
4. McCombs, R. P. and Patterson, J. F.: Factors influencing the course and prognosis of systemic lupus erythematosus. New Engl. J. Med., *260*:1195, 1959.
5. Merrell, M. and Shulman, L. E.: Determination of prognosis in chronic disease, illustrated by systemic lupus erythematosus. J. Chron. Dis., *1*:12, 1955.

Panel Discussion

THOMAS M. DURANT, *Moderator*

DR. DURANT: First, I think it would be fair to say that a great many patients with disseminated lupus need steroid therapy at one time or another during the course of their disease. If that is agreed to by the panel, the main problem relating to it is to decide which patients should and which patients should not get steroids. Apparently, steroids in some way alter the abnormalities in the antibody response of the body that occur in this disease, which Dr. Harvey has referred to as the epilepsy of the immune mechanism. In regard to the indications for steroid therapy, there is one question I would like to ask now because I think it drives home a very important point, and that is, would the patient with systemic lupus erythematosus who has no symptoms and only a positive LE preparation require any therapy at all? In other words, are we going to treat a laboratory test? Dr. Dubois, would you give us your opinion about that?

DR. DUBOIS: I do not think it is necessary to treat the patient who has no symptoms just because of a positive laboratory test. Those patients who are completely asymptomatic with a positive LE test are extremely rare; possibly a few of us may have seen one patient. One also has to consider that before the advent of steroids 40 per cent of the patients who had systemic lupus erythematosus had spontaneous remissions; so there is a very good possibility that a spontaneous remission will occur in these patients on one or more occasions if you wait long enough and just prescribe aspirin and rest.

DR. DURANT: That is a very important point. This is a disease that fluctuates, and spontaneous exacerbations and remissions occur, which make it difficult to evaluate the effects of therapy.

DR. ZARAFONETIS: I would like to discuss one point, and that is what you tell the patient who is in a clinical remission and who is not presently being treated but who has a positive LE prep or some of the other stigmata of the disease, such as protein abnormalities. I tell them to avoid ultraviolet light and sulfonamide and penicillin therapy because these have been precipitating factors in some cases. Since other members of the panel may have another approach to this problem, I would like to hear their ideas.

DR. DUBOIS: We tell our asymptomatic patients about the same thing, but eventually, after some months of being asymptomatic, they often begin to increase their activity, even including water skiing and being out in the sun. A moderate number can tolerate this without getting a recurrence of disease even though in the past some may have been sun-sensitive. Although we warn them. some patients still do what they want, often without difficulty, but at times severe reactions occur.

DR. DURANT: What would you tell a young woman who comes for a routine premarital examination and has a positive serology, proved to be biologically false, if she is healthy and has no other protein abnormalities? Should she be told anything? Should she be told not to marry? Should she be told not to have children?

DR. ZARAFONETIS: I would tell her the same thing I tell patients with lupus—to avoid sunlight, sulfonamides and so forth.

668

Dr. Pollak: In this connection, one just needs to repeat the facts which Dr. Harvey presented. In his eight-year follow-up of 184 patients with biologic false positive tests for syphilis, 12 now have definite SLE, and 38 have features suggestive of a connective tissue disease. Although these patients are asymptomatic, they have a high chance of getting a connective tissue disease and probably SLE in the future.

Dr. Rose: I think many of the manifestations of SLE will declare themselves readily enough to the patient, and no harm will be done by delaying therapy until that happens. There is an exception, though, in case of renal involvement, and regular urine examination should be carried out in people who potentially may develop lupus erythematosus.

Dr. McCombs: That point should be re-emphasized. Of the patients given steroids in our series, none developed renal disease during the period that they were on steroids, whereas some who did not take steroids, even though they were in remission, did develop renal involvement; this has an ominous prognostic significance. Now, I am not advocating that one should use steroids prophylactically, but the patient should be followed very closely so that the earliest signs of renal involvement may be detected.

Dr. Soffer: In the days before the advent of steroids and ACTH, exposure to sun was almost invariably associated with a recrudescence of the rash, fever and illness; however, in patients who are treated with steroids, exposure to the sun is apparently a harmless episode and a recrudescence apparently does not occur under such circumstances. Therefore, the type of treatment the patient is getting determines whether or not it is important to emphasize the hazards associated with exposure to the sun.

The question has also arisen about the prophylactic effects of steroids in relation to the development of renal disease. In our experience, the development of renal disease occurred independently of whether or not the patient received steroid therapy. I cannot emphasize this point too much. It seemed to us that either the patient had renal disease at the time of the first hospital admission or he never developed it.

Whether you treat a patient who has a positive LE smear but who has no symptoms is dependent on how one conceives of lupus erythematosus. Is the presence of a positive LE smear in itself an adequate indication for the existence of disseminated lupus, or is it not? I must hasten to add that I am not quite sure how to answer this question. If you study patients in clinics which deal exclusively with rheumatoid arthritis, about 10 per cent of them will have positive LE smears. As far as one can tell, these 10 per cent are no different from other patients with rheumatoid arthritis in the clinic. We had occasion to observe a group of these patients over a period of five years; a few of the 10 per cent have developed the typical picture of disseminated lupus erythematosus, but the majority have not. Whether the latter are still patients with disseminated lupus erythematosus is hard to say. It would be easier for us in an effort to assay the value of the steroids in lupus if we bore in mind that the disease is a serious one, a significant one, an important one and, in a sense, a characteristic one. Therefore, in our clinic the diagnosis of lupus is established only in patients who have more than just a positive LE smear; the majority of those in whom we make this diagnosis have had fever at some time in the course of the illness or have had involvement of the pleura or pericardium, and a significant number have had involvement of the kidneys. The point, in effect, which I want to make is that I do not quite think it is fair to say that the patient has lupus in the absence of other clinical manifestations, solely on the basis of a positive LE smear.

DR. ZARAFONETIS: I would agree with that. I would not make a diagnosis of lupus on this basis necessarily, but I certainly think that it is only fair to the patient to give advice which may prevent precipitation of the disease.

DR. DUBOIS: The entity we are talking about—an asymptomatic patient with LE cells—must be exceedingly rare. I have yet to find the first; I know that they exist, and a few of us have talked about them, but there must be a reason why an LE smear is done in these people; they must have had some symptoms. Another fact, pointing up the rarity of this, is that in the thousands of control LE preps we have done as an investigative study, we have yet to obtain one positive smear from a blood bank donor.

DR. DURANT: How about the families of patients who have had proved lupus? Have you checked many of those people?

DR. DUBOIS: We have done LE preps on some of the families of patients with proved lupus, and although we have not done this routinely in the relatives of our patients, we did not obtain a positive smear from any of about 30 or 40 relatives whom we did study; however, other people have found one or two positives in their studies.

DR. SOFFER: All of the family members of our patients have been investigated for the possible existence of a positive LE smear. In each of two families there were two siblings who had the illness, a brother and sister in one instance and two sisters in another. In no instance was either the father or mother involved in the disease in terms either of clinical manifestations or of a positive LE smear.

DR. DURANT: Dr. Dubois, will you tell us when a patient with systemic lupus should have steroids?

DR. DUBOIS: Steroids should be used when the patient is seriously ill and has not responded to therapy with rest, salicylates and antimalarial compounds. In other words, we would start steroids immediately if the patient has a significant degree of anemia with a hemoglobin of 8 grams or less, if he has proteinuria or very definite proteinuria and casts, if he has central nervous system involvement of lupus, if he has extensive pleuritis with effusion or if he has severe carditis. In other words, steroids should be used in patients with severe extensive inflammation due to the disease, which we have found will not respond to more conservative therapy.

DR. DURANT: Is the panel in essential agreement on these indications? Dr. Rose, as far as the dosage is concerned, should we use steroid therapy to obtain complete suppression of disease activity or merely palliation?

DR. ROSE: In those patients whose lives are threatened, and that means those with renal involvement and those with central nervous system involvement, a dose of steroids sufficient to abolish all evidence of active disease, including maintenance of a more or less normal sedimentation rate, should be used. In patients in whom the disease is only a nuisance and not a general danger, including those with skin eruptions, joint pains, pleurisy, and so forth, the least dose needed to keep the patient tolerably comfortable and leading a fairly reasonable life should be used.

DR. POLLAK: I would agree essentially with Dr. Rose, but I would like to differ with him and with Dr. Soffer about the sedimentation rate. I think it is a very poor criterion for judging activity in lupus. We have recently completed a study on the correlation of the titer of antinuclear factors with the activity of the disease. This shows a good correlation So, too, is there a good correlation of activity with serum albumin levels, with serum gamma globulin levels, with the hematocrit, and with the leukocyte count, but there is no correlation in these data whatever of the level of the sedimentation rate with activity, and in virtually none of the patients did the sedimentation rate come down to normal. This has always been our experience, and I think it is an unreliable indication of normality.

DR. SOFFER: A disturbance in the globulin component occurred in only about half of our patients and in the serum albumin component in a few less than this, so that many patients with characteristic clinical signs and symptoms of disseminated lupus erythematosus had no alterations in the protein components of their blood. Therefore, I do not think that this is a very useful index to indicate the presence or absence of active disease. In addition, anemia in lupus is one thing which is very difficult to correct. It takes a great deal of treatment for a long period of time before a significant increase in the hemoglobin and red blood cell count appears, and if renal disease is present, it practically never improves. In about half of the patients there is definite leukopenia, and in the remainder there is a normal white blood cell count, but it is true that as improvement in the disease occurs, either with therapy or during a spontaneous remission, the white blood cell count returns to normal in those patients with leukopenia. In our experience, the sedimentation rate constitutes the most significant indication of the adequacy of therapy, and elevation of sedimentation rate often precedes a relapse of the disease a few days before the relapse is evident clinically, either by a recrudescence of the joint pains, or by the development of fever or rash. So, I think that the sedimentation rate is a very good indication of the efficacy of therapy. In almost all patients who are treated vigorously and actively for a long enough period of time, the sedimentation rate will tend to return to normal as the acute manifestations of the disease subside. It may not return entirely to normal, but it increases appreciably with relapses and therefore can be used as an indication of the adequacy of steroid therapy.

DR. DUBOIS: Our experience has been very similar to that of Dr. Pollak. The sedimentation rate, although usually quite elevated, comes down somewhat but does not return to normal, and in our experience it is a poor guide to therapy. It will often persist in women at a level of 30 to 40 by the Wintrobe method even during periods when the patient is in a good clinical remission. One can reduce the sedimentation rate to normal in most of these patients by giving very large doses of steroids, but we found that the sedimentation rate very often remained high with or without steroids in asymptomatic patients. The LE cells will also decrease in numbers with high doses of steroid after four to six weeks, and in about half of the patients these cells completely disappear. Admittedly, if one searches the LE preparation for half an hour to an hour, one may find a few LE cells; however, since before treatment there may be literally thousands of these cells, for practical purposes one can say they just about disappear completely. This again is not a guide to therapy, although it is an interesting way to follow the patient.

DR. MILLS: Many patients with lupus can have a clinical remission from a subjective and also to a great extent from an objective standpoint, and still have an elevated sedimentation rate. Some of these patients with so-called clinical remissions have evidence of continued activity in terms of an abnormal urinary sediment, and this indicates active renal disease. By raising the dose of the steroid somewhat in these patients who *feel* well, one can often diminish the sedimentation rate and abolish the urinary findings, particularly hematuria, although albuminuria, if high, tends to persist for a long time. I wonder if it is not better for the patient to try to abolish all of these manifestations. Now, obviously, when you try to do this, you often have to use doses of steroids which are quite high, and of course, you increase the risk of possible toxicity from the steroids. However, from the standpoint of the effects of steroids on the progression of the patient's disease, and for the sake of discussion leaving aside the problem of toxicity, I wonder what the opinion of some of the panel members would be regarding the possible beneficial effects of long-term, high dose therapy?

DR. DUBOIS: We have found that although some of the manifestations can be suppressed with very high doses of steroids, such as 500 mg. a day of cortisone, one does have to consider the risks of such chronic maintenance therapy. For example, in one patient we had, severe demineralization of the spine occurred as a result of these doses of cortisone, even though the patient was ambulatory. This is really the limiting problem. If we had a steroid that we could safely administer for years, it would certainly be very useful, but one must keep in mind that lupus is a disease with remissions and exacerbations going on over a period of many years and that it is very risky to keep the patient on hundreds of milligrams of cortisone a day for many years based on a theoretical assumption that maybe the patient will be benefited. In addition, we do not have any very good evidence that large doses of steroids will increase his life span as compared to more conservative therapy with smaller doses.

DR. POLLAK: I would agree that the risk of side effects is increased in lupus patients who are given high doses of steroids for long periods of time. In our group of 16 patients who received large doses of prednisone, 15 developed full-blown Cushingoid features, and the other patient probably would have too, but she died shortly after being placed on therapy. However, subsequently, after the initial six-month period of treatment with high doses, most of these manifestations disappeared when the dose was gradually reduced to the maintenance level. In addition, in this group of 16 patients there were four who developed infections, and although these were not serious in three of the patients, one patient developed severe herpes zoster, which resulted in loss of vision due to corneal scarring. This patient had been previously exposed to chicken pox, and it is difficult to say whether or not the course would have been different had she not been on steroids. One patient in the series had developed a tuberculous lesion while on low dose therapy prior to this study, but was still given high dose therapy; at the time of her death, which was due to another cause, there was no evidence of active tuberculosis. One patient in the series developed a peptic ulcer, which perforated on one occasion, but this healed with conservative management and gastric suction, and without surgery, in spite of the fact that steroids were continued. On another occasion this same patient had hematemesis and melena, which also responded to conservative therapy. Five of the 16 patients developed diabetes. One patient developed severe osteoporosis, and one other had mild osteoporosis. Troublesome mental agitation and depression occurred in two patients. One patient had a severe Addisonian-like crisis, when she suddenly, of her own volition, stopped all steroid therapy. However, in spite of these complications, I have the general impression, although we have not yet statistically analyzed our data in the low dose and high groups, that the incidence of serious side effects was not much greater in the group receiving high dosage than it was in the group receiving low dosage. However, I am sure the risk is at least somewhat greater, and it must be taken into consideration and these patients should be followed carefully.

DR. DURANT: So far, although we disagree somewhat on what the best criteria of therapeutic efficacy are, we agree that sufficient amounts of steroids should be given to suppress adequately the dangerous manifestations of the disease, and that a smaller dose should be given only when the less serious manifestations are present and other therapy is ineffective. When steroids are used, the dangers of the therapy must always be kept in mind, and that suggests a question which I think is a very interesting one. Dr. Pollak, do you think peptic ulcer is as common a complication of steroid therapy in patients with SLE as it is in patients with rheumatoid arthritis?

DR. POLLAK: We have not made a thorough study of this problem. In our own institution, we discuss this about once a year at grand rounds, and it seems apparent from these discussions and from our own experience that the incidence of peptic ulceration in patients with rheumatoid arthritis who are treated with steroids is comparatively high. In our own series of patients with lupus, we have seen one or two patients out of 100 or more who have developed clinical evidence of a peptic ulcer. We have not studied this radiologically, but clinical evidence of peptic ulcer has occurred only in 1 or 2 per cent. Among Dr. Kushner's patients with ulcerative colitis, the incidence is of the same order, and certainly in hematological disorders in which large doses of steroids are used—for example, in leukemia and other diseases of this nature—the incidence also appears to be very low.

DR. DUBOIS: We have had quite a problem with peptic ulcers. However, on the basis of clinical symptoms, out of a few hundred patients who have received steroids, we have had only one definitely perforated ulcer and only two or three others with severe ulcer symptoms and bleeding; but when these patients were surveyed before, during and after steroid therapy with routine gastrointestinal x-rays, the incidence of peptic ulcer was found to rise in direct proportion to the dose of steroid given, up to a maximum of 47 per cent in patients receiving more than 50 mg. a day of prednisone or its equivalent when other steroids were used. The patients on these larger doses of prednisone were not given salicylates, but patients who received smaller doses of prednisone in the range of 20 to 30 mg. a day did get salicylates. In the latter, the incidence of peptic ulcer was in the range of about 20 to 25 per cent. The results are very comparable to the experience of people who studied patients with rheumatoid arthritis on steroid therapy by radiological methods. I do not think there is any difference in incidence of ulcer in the patients with lupus and rheumatoid arthritis.

DR. KUSHNER: Our experience in a much smaller group of patients with lupus nephritis is much more consistent with the data of Dr. Dubois than with those of Dr. Pollak, and I wonder whether there is a population difference, since our patients are obtained in large part from a malnourished population which is in large part also alcoholic. Such patients may be more prone to develop peptic ulcers than the type of patients in the hospital of the University of Illinois.

DR. DURANT: Do you think that is possible, Dr. Pollak?

DR. POLLAK: I think there are certain differences between the Cook County Hospital population and ours, but they are not very great. I think we must look for other factors, and we must determine what the incidence of peptic ulcer is in these diseases when the patients are not treated with steroids.

DR. DUBOIS: We have some data on that. The incidence of ulcer in about 50 patients with lupus treated before steroids were available was about 5 per cent, so the incidence is not particularly high.

DR. SOFFER: In our group of 90 patients, seven patients developed peptic ulcer during steroid therapy, with clinical and x-ray evidence of the ulcer. In the period before the advent of steroids, we had a large number of lupus patients in the hospital and the incidence of ulcer was almost nil; there is a definite relationship between the treatment and the presence of peptic ulcer. One of the interesting things observed in our studies was that when steroid therapy was reinstituted because of recrudescence of the disease, after having been stopped because of peptic ulceration, the ulcer responded to ordinary, orthodox treatment with antacids and a Sippy diet, as if the patient had not been on steroid therapy.

DR. DURANT: Then you had no reason to regret such a course in any case?

DR. SOFFER: No.

DR. POLLAK: There is one thing which must be kept in mind when we discuss the complications of steroid therapy in lupus patients. It certainly has been our impression that a number of complications are very much more likely to occur during the phase of the illness when the patient is on steroids and the disease is not adequately controlled. In this circumstance the patient is still sick, often has a poor appetite, and as a result is malnourished; we have seen complications particularly under these circumstances. Our general impression is that when patients are adequately treated and not allowed to have definite systemic symptoms, there are fewer complications than if they are somewhat inadequately treated.

DR. McCOMBS: I think the problem of peptic ulcer is dependent upon how well the patient will follow the prescribed anti-ulcer therapy. However, to me this is a small problem compared to the more serious problem of infection in patients on continuous steroid therapy. As I indicated, we had two patients who died of tuberculosis, both of whom were followed carefully. The diagnosis was not made clinically, but only at autopsy. In two others, there were overwhelming infections that could not be controlled by the available antibiotics, even though the diagnosis was made antemortem. I am sure that others who prescribe steroids must have had similar experiences.

DR. DURANT: Another complication of steroid therapy that should be mentioned here is suicide. Practically everyone's series of patients includes such a patient. On the other hand, osteoporosis is a complication that is not as likely to be as serious in this disease as it is in rheumatoid arthritis because lupus patients are sufficiently active, in contrast to those with rheumatoid arthritis, to keep the stimulus to bone formation active.

Dr. Hurley, in some patients with lupus, the skin rash persists in spite of therapy with steroids. How would you treat patients of this type as far as the skin rash is concerned?

DR. HURLEY: I think that many times it is possible to improve the eruption to some extent by avoidance of factors which are known to flare or produce exacerbations of the disease and the cutaneous changes. For instance, exposure to sunlight is an important precipitating factor, and occasionally the use of topical steroids will reduce the local inflammation; the concurrent use of "sun screen" preparations is also helpful.

I have not had a great deal of experience with the use of chloroquin in patients with lupus, but I know it has been used extensively by Dr. Dubois. Since patients with lupus have a great tendency to develop drug hypersensitivity, I wonder whether the use of chloroquin should be avoided in these patients? There have been some reports in the literature of peculiar reactions to chloroquin—precipitation of porphyria, for example—and I am curious to know whether Dr. Dubois has noted any reactions in terms of exacerbation of systemic lupus erythematosus from the use of chloroquin.

DR. DUBOIS: We have had very successful results with the use of chloroquin. In one patient, seen in 1953, the skin lesions persisted despite extremely large doses of cortisone. Atabrine was available then and large doses of this drug were the only thing that would control the rash. Such compounds definitely seem to be of value in any lupus patient who has a skin lesion, regardless of the stage of the disease. The main problem with the use of antimalarial drugs is, as Dr. Scherbel has mentioned, that these compounds do not work as dramatically as the steroids. A number of weeks are required before a sufficient level of the drug is obtained in the body, and increasing the dose to obtain a high level initially will result in nausea and vomiting. Therefore, it may take several weeks to obtain an effect on the skin lesions. In addition, since lupus is an illness with remissions and exacerbations, an exacerbation occurring a few days after beginning chloroquin is not necessarily due to the drug. Chloroquin and hydroxychloroquin are both exceptionally safe drugs and lupus patients have an amazing tolerance to them; the most severe reaction is the development of skin lesions which occur in possibly 10 to 15 per cent of patients, and changing from one antimalarial to another often controls this.

DR. DURANT: Dr. Zarafonetis, do you think potassium para-aminobenzoate is of value in the therapy of lupus?

DR. ZARAFONETIS: We tried this compound in the treatment of discoid lupus and in some of the less severe forms of systemic lupus years ago, before cortisone was available, and noted some beneficial effects. However, the efficacy was not great enough to justify the recommendation of this therapy for these disorders. After the advent of cortisone, we thought this drug might be useful in patients who required 200 to 300 mg. a day of cortisone and who, in spite of this, still had symptoms. We treated a number of such patients, adding 12 grams of potassium para-aminobenzoate per day to their regimen. In many instances we were able to reduce gradually the cortisone requirements to 12.5 mg. every eight hours. Some patients have been on this regimen for eight years or more without any signs of hypercortisonism and with much better control of their illness than they had before. Periodically, we withdrew all medication to make sure they were not in a natural remission or that they were not taking therapy unnecessarily. I think there is a place for combined therapy in order to try to minimize the side effects of long-term administration of the higher doses of corticosteroids, and we have found this regimen to be satisfactory in many instances.

Part VIII | TREATMENT OF
OTHER DISEASES

The Modification
of Polyarteritis
Nodosa by Steroid Therapy

GEOFFREY A. ROSE

St. Mary's Hospital, London, England

In its natural course, as in all its characteristics, polyarteritis nodosa is tremendously variable. At one extreme one may see a man fit and well one week and dead the next. At the other extreme is the patient who still has active disease after 10 years or more. Between these limits are the few in whom active disease remits, but in the majority recurrent crops of new lesions are still appearing when the patient dies. This means that any therapeutic trial faces formidable difficulties, for where the natural course of a disease is variable, *ipso facto*, large numbers are needed to demonstrate significant effects—and here one is dealing with an uncommon condition. Furthermore, it means that one can scarcely hope to answer the question: does treatment shorten the duration of active disease? For since without treatment most patients still had active disease when they died, it is clearly impossible to predict how long activity would have lasted had they survived. The most that can therefore be expected is to discover whether treatment obviously prolongs life or mitigates suffering.

THE MEDICAL RESEARCH COUNCIL TRIAL

Table 1 illustrates the situation with which physicians treating this disease were faced when cortisone was first introduced. It lists the various treatments that had been given to a total of 104 patients with proven polyarteritis nodosa in a British Medical Research Council survey.[5] In one patient

TABLE 1. TREATMENTS GIVEN TO 104 PATIENTS WITH PROVEN POLYARTERITIS NODOSA, AND THEIR APPARENT EFFECTS

TREATMENT	NUMBER OF PATIENTS	APPARENT EFFECTS
Sulphonamides	24	Transient urticaria in 1
Antibiotics		
Penicillin	50	None
Tetracyclines	9	,,
Chloramphenicol	9	,,
Salicylates, high dosage	13	Arthritis (? rheumatic) improved in 1
Antihistamines	6	None
Blood transfusion	12	,,
Anticoagulants	2	,,
Iodides	3	,,
Oestrogens	2	,,
Chloroquine, calciferol, gold, urethane	1 each	,,

sulphonamides caused transient urticaria but no change in the polyarteritis; a second course had no effect at all. In another patient, who very probably had rheumatic fever as well as polyarteritis nodosa, salicylate therapy relieved the arthritis, but again the polyarteritis seemed to be unchanged. Allowing for natural variations in disease activity, in no other instance did it appear that treatment had any effect at all.

In 1950 came the discovery of the dramatic effects of cortisone in this disease.[4, 7] In most patients the response was such that no clinical trial was needed to prove its reality. Faced with such a situation, and recalling the serious prognosis of the disease and the total failure of all other therapies, the Collagen Diseases Panel of the Medical Research Council decided that a controlled trial of steroids would be ethically wrong. This being so, it may be that we were foolish to attempt any sort of trial at all. But it would clearly have been wrong to assume too readily that a drug with a good immediate effect would necessarily prove to confer long-term benefit in a chronic disease, especially since the drug itself had very real drawbacks and dangers. It was therefore decided to undertake a trial, but using retrospective instead of concurrent controls.[2, 3]

Because suitable patients were few, the trial was undertaken on a cooperative basis jointly by ten hospitals. The essential criterion for admission was biopsy evidence of necrotising arteritis in a clinically suggestive case. We tried to minimise the limitations of retrospective control by collecting consecutive cases from the period immediately before the introduction of cortisone, the series being drawn mainly from the same hospitals as the treated series. The same criterion of biopsy proof was applied, and sections from both series were reviewed by the same pathologists.

In all, 19 "control" and 21 treated cases were obtained, the period of follow-up being a minimum of three years from biopsy diagnosis. Careful comparison of the two series showed that at the time of diagnosis they were similar in most respects, including age distribution, duration of disease, sex ratio, frequency of involvement of the various major organs and the incidence of renal failure. Unfortunately, in one major respect they differed: Hypertension, well known to carry a bad prognosis in this disease,[6] was present in eight untreated patients but in only one of the treated series. We have been unable to explain this difference, but its presence means that the effects of treatment upon survival can be assessed fairly only when patients with initial hypertension have first been excluded.

Treatment was started with cortisone, 200 mg. per day, with weekly adjustments thereafter according to the patient's progress. Individual physicians varied a good deal in the rigour of their management. Some aimed at achieving complete suppression of active disease, including the maintenance of a normal blood sedimentation rate. It has been the impression of this group of physicians that active disease can always be controlled completely in this way, although it may sometimes need as much as 400 to 500 mg. of cortisone (or its equivalent) daily, and occasionally as much as 1 gram. Such levels may prove intolerable, especially over a long period. For this reason other physicians followed the principle that is often adopted in managing a case of rheumatoid arthritis, namely, to give the least dose which makes life tolerable. They were prepared to permit, for example, a raised blood sedimentation rate or microscopic haematuria, provided that the patient felt reasonably well.

All the patients showed an early, and often a dramatic, response. Their

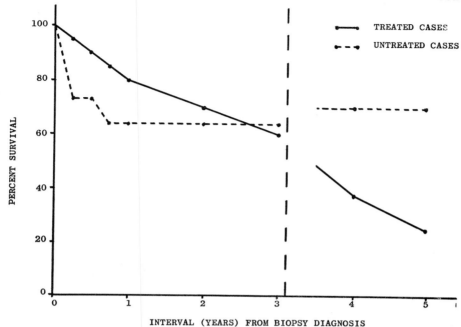

Fig. 1. Percentage survival rates in treated and untreated groups, excluding cases with initial hypertension.

subsequent experience is summarised in Figure 1, and shown more fully in Table 2. Among the untreated there was a heavy early mortality. If we consider, as we should, only those patients who were initially free of hypertension, then 36 per cent of the "control" series failed to survive nine months from diagnosis; by contrast, nine-month mortality in the treated series totalled only 14 per cent. In comfort, too, the treated patients generally fared better; they had less fever and less pain, and more of them were able to return to work. Beyond nine months, however, the picture gradually changes. There were no more deaths among the "control" patients, but among those receiving steroids there was a small but continuing mortality

TABLE 2. COMPARISON OF THE TREATED AND UNTREATED GROUPS AT VARIOUS INTERVALS AFTER BIOPSY

INTERVAL FROM BIOPSY DIAGNOSIS	NO. ALIVE		% ALIVE	
	Treated	Untreated	Treated	Untreated
0 months	21(20)	19(11)	100(100)	100(100)
3 "	20(19)	11 (8)	95 (95)	58 (73)
6 "	19(18)	9 (8)	90 (90)	47 (73)
9 "	18(17)	7 (7)	86 (85)	37 (64)
12 "	15(16)	7 (7)	71 (80)	37 (64)
2 years	15(14)	7 (7)	71 (70)	37 (64)
3 "	13(12)	7 (7)	62 (60)	37 (64)
4 "	6/14(5/13)	7/18(7/10)	43 (38)	39 (70)
5 "	2/5 (1/4)	7/18(7/10)	40 (25)	39 (70)

The numbers in parentheses refer to those patients in whom there was no initial hypertension.

throughout the whole period of observation. By three years, the survival rates in the two groups are very much the same. Follow-up beyond three years is based on incomplete numbers; but in the fourth and fifth years death among the treated patients numbered three, against none in the untreated. This gives a slight advantage to the untreated group.

Summarising the conclusions from this trial, one might say that its structure and size prevent really valid deductions. The results suggest that steroid therapy may prolong life in this disease; nevertheless, they provide no evidence that, in the dosage given, it improves the ultimate chance of survival.

OUTSTANDING QUESTIONS

Several other questions of great practical importance remain to be answered. These include (a) Which type of treatment is better: rigorous suppression or mere palliation? (b) Does treatment cause any aggravation of the underlying disease process? (c) What practical guidance can be given on the best treatment for different types of patients? Unfortunately, the answers to these questions must at present be founded more on guesswork than on factual observations.

Suppression v. Palliation. In the Medical Research Council trial the results were better at those centres where fully suppressive treatment was the aim. Numbers are too small for proper comparison. One does, however, know that in untreated or partially treated patients disastrous complications of the disease may occur without warning. Coronary or cerebral polyarteritis may prove suddenly fatal. Renal destruction may first be recognised by the appearance of irreversible uraemia or hypertension. For this reason, and because such evidence as we have suggests that the benefits may outweigh the dangers, I personally in most cases favour an attempt at rigorous suppression.

The Effect of Steroids on the Underlying Disease. Many physicians believe that if a patient with rheumatoid arthritis is treated for a time with steroids, stopping the treatment may leave the patient with worse disease than if steroids had never been given. Furthermore, there is good evidence[1] that steroid treatment of rheumatoid arthritis predisposes to a form of arteritis which may or may not be the same as polyarteritis nodosa. The normal pattern of polyarteritis nodosa is so unpredictable that it is difficult to make any direct assessment. But I have seen two patients in whom over a fairly long period without treatment the disease had run a mild course confined to skin and joints. Within a short time of starting steroid therapy each had an attack of asymmetrical peripheral neuropathy. Furthermore, I have several times had the impression, when side effects necessitated a reduced dosage, that the disease flared up with much greater severity than it had shown in the earlier untreated stage. Clearly the whole question is still very open, but these small pointers to a possible danger do exist.

A Practical Scheme. In the practice of medicine one is compelled to develop a practical scheme of action, even though this may often have to be based on guesses. In the light of our present limited knowledge, the following plan is suggested:

1. Never start treatment unless the diagnosis is certain, or unless it is almost certain and the patient's life is threatened.

2. If the disease seems to be confined to the skin or to the skin and joints,

and if it is not disabling, withhold treatment but watch with very great care and at short intervals. Although such patients may at any time, even after years, develop generalised disease, the risk of this is possibly outweighed by the dangers and discomforts of prolonged high-dosage steroid therapy.

3. In cases where it is clear that the battle is already lost, and *possibly* also in some cases where the disease is already very chronic, give the minimum dose that will keep the patient reasonably comfortable.

4. In all other cases one should aim at full suppression of all clinical manifestations of active disease and the maintenance of a normal blood sedimentation rate. A reasonable initial dose might be prednisone, 40 mg. daily. Sometimes this may have to be considerably increased, the only limitation being a threat of dangerous side effects. Such rigorous treatment, although it may make life very unpleasant for a few patients, will improve the comfort and perhaps prolong the lives of the majority. There may even be a few whose lives are saved.

ACKNOWLEDGMENT

I am indebted to the Medical Research Council for permission to quote their data.

REFERENCES

1. Kemper, J. W., Baggenstoss, A. H. and Slocumb, C. H.: The relationship of therapy with cortisone to the incidence of vascular lesions in rheumatoid arthritis. Ann. Int. Med., *46*:831, 1957.
2. Medical Research Council: Treatment of polyarteritis nodosa with cortisone: results after one year. Brit. M. J., *1*:608, 1957.
3. Medical Research Council: Treatment of polyarteritis nodosa with cortisone: results after three years. Brit. M. J., *1*:1399, 1960.
4. Rose, B., Pare, J. A. P., Pump, K. and Stanford, R. L.: Preliminary report on adreno-corticotrophic hormone in asthma. Canad. M. A. J., *62*:6, 1950.
5. Rose, G. A.: The natural history of polyarteritis nodosa: a report to the Collagen Diseases and Hypersensitivity Panel of the Medical Research Council. (Unpublished.)
6. Rose, G. A. and Spencer, H.: Polyarteritis nodosa. Quart. J. Med., n.s., *26*:43, 1957.
7. Shick, R. M., Baggenstoss, A. H., Fuller, B. F. and Polley, H. F.: Effects of cortisone and ACTH on periarteritis nodosa. Minn. Med., *34*:852, 1951.

Treatment of Dermatomyositis

HARRY J. HURLEY

Hahnemann Medical College and Hospital, Philadelphia

The treatment of dermatomyositis, like that of most other diseases of unknown etiology, is still far from satisfactory. However, with the introduction of the corticosteroid drugs the therapy of this disease was greatly facilitated. Prior to the availability of these compounds, neither the course of dermatomyositis nor its symptoms could be predictably altered to a significant degree. Improvement in some patients had been noted after the use of testosterone, para-aminobenzoic acid and other empirical therapy. Moreover, physical therapy and orthopedic management to minimize or prevent contractures was helpful. However, it was only with the advent of the corticosteroids that consistent improvement of the general well-being of these patients and some extension of their life expectancy could be anticipated. These compounds, therefore, are the basis for a more rational, if not an ideal, approach to the treatment of dermatomyositis.

The interesting association of an internal malignant condition with dermatomyositis is, in the opinion of most observers, more than coincidental, for it occurs in 10 to 20 per cent of patients with this connective tissue disease.[1, 2, 3, 7, 11] Ovarian, mammary and gastric carcinoma have been described most frequently, but pulmonary, adrenal, rectal and testicular cancer, osteosarcoma, lymphoma and leukemia have also been observed. In many cases the cancer has clearly preceded the onset of dermatomyositis by months to several years; in others the dermatomyositis apparently developed prior to any detectable sign of the tumor. The etiologic relationship between the neoplastic process and dermatomyositis has not yet been decisively demonstrated. Hypothetically, the pathologic dynamics responsible have been variously presented as auto-immune in origin, due to release of toxic or allergic substances by the tumor, or due to the effects of other chemicals produced by the cancer. Removal or destruction of the associated cancer has resulted in resolution or arrest of dermatomyositis in a significant number of instances.[3] Thus, the detection and treatment of a possible associated neoplasm should be a primary consideration in the management of all patients with dermatomyositis. It should be mentioned that the presence of an underlying cancer with dermatomyositis is much less likely in children than in adults with the disease.

Dermatomyositis may present an acute fulminant picture or it may follow a subacute to chronic course, undulating in severity, with remissions of variable duration, generally not exceeding several months.[12] Spontaneous recovery after a prolonged and difficult course has been described but this outcome is exceptional. The diagnosis of dermatomyositis depends upon a consideration of the clinical features, biopsy of involved muscle and electromyography. Determination of serum glutamic oxalacetic acid transaminase (aminopherase) is also of diagnostic importance and may be utilized to follow the course of the disease.

CORTICOSTEROID THERAPY

The administration of corticosteroids is generally indicated in all cases of dermatomyositis. Even in those patients in whom an underlying or associated malignancy is being treated, the use of corticosteroids to reduce inflammation and minimize parenchymal damage is desirable. The principal effect of these drugs in dermatomyositis is apparently anti-inflammatory, although the concept that they may interfere with an antigen-antibody reaction of possible etiologic importance should also be borne in mind. Because they diminish muscle inflammation and degeneration, the corticosteroids tend also to reduce the nitrogen loss seen in this disease.

The dosage of corticosteroid to be employed varies according to the acuteness of the dermatomyositis. In the severely ill patient, 60 to 100 mg. of prednisone or its equivalent of another steroid (hydrocortisone, methylprednisolone, triamcinolone, dexamethasone or fluprednisolone) should be given daily. Prednisone and methylprednisolone would seem preferable to the other steroids mentioned because of a lower incidence of side effects.[4] Because of the muscle-wasting sometimes seen with triamcinolone, it would seem judicious to avoid this drug in dermatomyositis. The dosage of any of the corticosteroids employed should be increased to to the requisite level which produces clinical improvement. This dosage level is to be maintained until subsidence of the acute phase is apparent. Parenteral administration of the steroids, either intramuscularly or through the use of an intravenous infusion, may be the most satisfactory method during the acute period. As the patient shows evidence of clinical improvement, a reduction of the dosage of the corticosteroids may be carried out gradually until a maintenance level is determined. This may be as little as 5 to 10 mg. of prednisone daily. At times it may be possible to stop the corticosteroids altogether, although they should be promptly restarted with any indication of an exacerbation. The usual considerations in the prolonged administration of corticosteroids in any patient should apply in the management of dermatomyositis also. Thus, a low salt diet, administration of potassium chloride and the use of antacids are recommended.[9] The possibility that these patients may in time develop other evidence of steroid toxicity, such as osteoporosis, should also be anticipated.

GENERAL SUPPORTIVE CARE

A high protein diet is desirable for all patients with dermatomyositis in an effort to counteract the catabolic effect of muscle degeneration. Proper maintenance of fluid and electrolyte balance is also to be observed. Occasionally certain patients with dermatomyositis present involvement of the muscles of deglutition or of respiration. The use of suction to insure a free airway and the importance of a respirator in such patients should be stressed. In acutely ill patients, changes of position to prevent the development of hypostatic pneumonia are recommended. When necessary, antibiotic therapy should be employed to control a secondary infection complicating the dermatomyositis.

ANABOLIC AGENTS

The loss of tissue protein incident to the degeneration of muscle is a matter for serious concern in most cases of dermatomyositis. Moreover, the intrinsic catabolic effect of the corticosteroids would seem to compound this tendency toward a negative nitrogen balance. However, because the corticosteroids produce a decrease in tissue inflammation and thus retard or arrest the muscle damage in dermatomyositis, a relative anabolic effect may be achieved with these compounds.

A direct or positive anabolic effect may be achieved through the use of testosterone or one of the newer "nonandrogenic" tissue-building agents. Testosterone propionate, in a weekly intramuscular dosage of 75 to 100 mg., has been used in dermatomyositis for this effect for years. It is cheaper than the newer anabolic drugs, but produces undersirable androgenic stimulation. Newer anabolic agents such as norethandrolone (Nilevar), nandrolone phenpropionate (Durabolin) and 17-methyl-17-β-hydroxyondroste-1, 4-dien-3-one (Dianabol) all possess reduced androgenic potential. Of this group, Dianabol, which is relatively inexpensive and may be given orally, seems promising. A dosage of 5 mg. two to four times daily is recommended. If therapy is to be carried beyond six to eight weeks, a rest period of two to four weeks before continuing the drug is advised. The drug is contraindicated in the presence of prostatic carcinoma or severe liver damage.

PHYSICAL THERAPY

The use of physical therapy is important in the management of patients with dermatomyositis, since it minimizes or prevents severe contractural sequelae. It is sometimes difficult to determine the optimal time to begin physical therapy. If it is started too late, some contractures may have already developed. On the other hand, it would seem judicious to defer such therapy until signs of the acute inflammation have subsided. Initially, passive exercise and heat and, later, active exercise should be instituted and regulated as the patient improves and is maintained on other therapy. Once contractures have developed, some improvement may be obtained by the use of diathermy and stretching, although the most extreme contractures may not be helped by these measures. In recent years the use of ultrasonic therapy has been advocated for such patients and may be of value. Heavy muscular work should always be avoided by these patients even during what appears to be a long remission.

ANTIMALARIAL COMPOUNDS

The apparent efficacy of antimalarial compounds in many cases of chronic discoid and disseminated lupus erythematosus led to the use of these drugs in other inflammatory connective tissue disorders, including derma-tomyositis.[6, 13] The precise mechanism of action of these compounds in such diseases is still obscure. A reduction in tissue inflammation is achieved, apparently not as a result of stimulation of the pituitary-adrenal system.[5]

There are no clear indications as to which patients should be given the antimalarial compounds. They have been used in acute dermatomyositis in conjunction with the corticosteroids. However, it may be more appropriate to consider their use during the period in which the corticosteroid compounds are being reduced, since it may be possible to maintain some patients on the antimalarial drug alone. Chloroquine in a dosage of 250 mg. twice daily or hydroxychloroquine in a dosage of 200 mg. three or four times a day are the most commonly used antimalarial compounds. An effort should be made to reduce the dosage of these drugs whenever possible or to discontinue them completely, if the patient's remission permits. Ophthalmalogic exami-nation for evidence of corneal opacification or retinopathy that may be produced by these drugs should be performed periodically.

PARA-AMINOBENZOIC ACID (PABA)

The para-aminobenzoates have been employed in the therapy of sclero-derma and dermatomyositis for more than ten years. Many observers have been unenthusiastic in their appraisal of the efficacy of these compounds in these conditions; others, notably Zarafonetis et al.,[10, 15] have found them useful. The mechanism of action of PABA is not entirely clear. Improvement in dermatomyositis is presumed to be mediated through an anti-inflammatory effect and possibly through an anabolic action. It has been suggested that combination of PABA with corticosteroids might enhance the beneficial effect of each compound.

Although the evidence clearly indicates the secondary importance of PABA in the management of dermatomyositis, a description of its administration is included here. The potassium salt is generally preferred since it has no water-retaining effect and induces fewer gastrointestinal symptoms than does the sodium salt. A daily dosage of 8 to 10 grams is desirable. It is generally given in four to five doses, each consisting of 20 cc. of a 10 per cent solution. Side effects are uncommon, but drug fever, a drug eruption or spontaneous hypoglycemia may occur when large doses are used (10 to 20 grams/day).

CHELATION

The use of Na_2EDTA (disodium ethylenediaminetetracetate) has been advocated in scleroderma and in sclerodermatomyositis as well. This compound was originally employed to mobilize calcium from areas of calcinosis in scleroderma.[8] It was subsequently found to be of value in patients without overt clinical evidence of calcinosis.[10] In dermatomyositis its use is best considered in those patients with calcinosis, although it might also find occasional application in therapy-resistant patients without this complication. The drug is administered in an intravenous infusion (3 grams of Na_2EDTA in 500 cc. of 5 per cent glucose in water), given at a rate of 30 to 40 drops a minute over a four to six hour period. These infusions are given daily in three series of five days each with a two-day rest between series. The concurrent administration of pyridoxine, 100 mg. daily, has been advocated by some observers. Daily urinalyses should be performed to detect the development of any nephrotoxicity. In addition, a complete blood count and platelet determination every four to six days is desirable, although a reduction of various blood elements in patients on this medication is an uncommon complication. Hypocalcemia is not a concern if the infusion is not given too rapidly. Occasionally, some increase in reflex activity and muscle cramps, notably in the muscles of the abdomen, may be observed. Some local thrombophlebitis may also be seen in the area of the injection. It is recommended that the course of chelation should not be repeated for at least two to three months.

SUMMARY

Corticosteroid therapy remains the primary approach to the management of all patients with dermatomyositis. The acute phase of the disease demands the use of these drugs in any dosage which will produce clinical improvement. Reduction of corticosteroids to the appropriate maintenance dosage is carried out after the acute phase has subsided. In some patients, remissions may allow the cessation of corticosteroid therapy. The importance of general supportive care, anabolic medication and physical therapy in the management of these patients is also emphasized.

The administration of other drugs which have been employed in dermatomyositis, such as the antimalarials, para-aminobenzoic acid and disodium EDTA, is also considered in detail.

Special emphasis is placed upon the diagnosis and treatment of an associated or underlying neoplasm which may be seen in patients with dermatomyositis.

REFERENCES

1. Bezecny, R.: Dermatomyositis. Arch. Dermat. u. Syph., 171:242, 1935.
2. Brunner, M. J. and Lobraico, R. V., Jr.: Dermatomyositis as an index of malignant neoplasm. Ann. Int. Med., 34:1269, 1951.
3. Curtis, A. C., Blaylock, H. C. and Harrell, E. R., Jr.: Malignant lesions associated with dermatomyositis. J.A.M.A., 150:844, 1952.
4. Dubois, E.: Methylprednisolone (Medrol) in the treatment of systemic lupus erythematosus. J.A.M.A., 170:1537, 1959.
5. Epstein, J., Forsham, P. H. and Friedman, E.: Effect of chloroquin on adrenal corticoid metabolism. J. Invest. Dermat., 32:109, 1959.
6. Everett, M. A.: Dermatomyositis. In Conn, H. F. (ed.): Current Therapy. Philadelphia, W. B. Saunders Co., 1959.
7. Lansbury, J.: Collagen disease complicating malignancy. Ann. Rheum. Dis., 12:301, 1953.
8. Mendelson, C. G.: The use of disodium EDTA in dermatology, with particular reference to scleroderma. In Seven, M. J. (ed.): Metal Binding in Medicine. Philadelphia, J. B. Lippincott Co., 1960, p. 187.
9. Richards, J. W. and Staley, C. J.: Acute perforation of gastric carcinoma during steroid therapy for dermatomyositis. A.M.A. Arch. Surg., 80:167, 1960.
10. Rukavina, J. G., Mendelson, C., Price, J. M., Brown, R. R. and Johnson, S. A. M.: Scleroderma (acrosclerosis). I. Treatment of three cases of the non-calcific variety by chelation (EDTA). J. Invest. Dermat., 29:273, 1957.
11. Sheard, C., Jr.: Dermatomyositis. Arch. Int. Med., 88:640, 1951.
12. Talbott, J. H. and Moleres Ferrandis, R.: Collagen Diseases. New York, Grune & Stratton, 1956.
13. Ward, R. W.: Antimalarials in the treatment of dermatomyositis. J. M. Soc. N. J., 57:317, 1960.
14. Zarafonetis, C. J. D.: Treatment of scleroderma. Ann. Int. Med., 50:343, 1959.
15. Zarafonetis, C. J. D., Curtis, A. C. and Gulick, A. E.: Use of para-aminobenzoic acid in dermatomyositis and scleroderma. Arch. Int. Med., 85:27, 1950.

The Treatment of Scleroderma: Results of Potassium Para-aminobenzoate Therapy in 104 Cases

CHRIS J. D. ZARAFONETIS

Simpson Memorial Institute for Medical Research, University of Michigan

This report is concerned with the treatment of scleroderma. It is based on personal experience accumulated over the past 12 years during the direct management of 104 patients with this disorder. There was no selection of subjects, each being placed on the treatment regimen employed regardless of the severity of the disease. Many of these patients had been previously treated unsuccessfully elsewhere with corticosteroids, adrenocorticotrophin, Releasin, Bistrimate, androgens and various antimalarials. Six had been subjected to one or more courses of chelation with EDTA, and several had undergone cervical sympathectomy. Eighty-three females and 21 males constitute the series, with a range in age of from 3¼ to 75 years at the time of admission to the treatment program followed in this clinic.

TREATMENT PROGRAM

This program has been previously recorded[8, 9, 11, 12] and need not be described in detail here. Briefly, it consists of (1) systemic antifibrosis therapy through the long-term administration of potassium para-amino-benzoate (Potaba), (2) physiotherapy, including deep breathing exercises and dynamic traction splints where applicable, and (3) Urecholine for the relief of dysphagia.

Potaba Therapy. It should be emphasized that adults with scleroderma require 12 grams of Potaba daily, in divided doses, in order to achieve the optimal therapeutic result. Most patients prefer to take the medication in capsules or as a 10 per cent chilled aqueous solution. Individual doses of 2.0 grams, 2.5 grams or 3.0 grams each are taken six times, five times or four times daily, respectively. The exact schedule depends on individual factors, including convenience at work or schedules for shopping or other activities. The first dose of each day is taken at breakfast, however, and the last at bed-time in order to obtain the widest temporal range of drug action. All patients are instructed to interrupt therapy in the event anorexia or nausea occurs. This permits the prompt subsidence of symptoms and prevents the possible development of hypoglycemia, which may occur if the administration of the drug is continued through a period of inadequate food intake. As soon as the patient is eating normally, treatment is resumed.

Aside from an adequate dosage schedule, the most important requirement of Potaba therapy is that of long-term administration. After a few weeks of treatment, some patients show improvement which may be striking at times. In others, it is only by careful checking of the involved skin over the clavicles or wrists, or about the mouth and forehead, that it is possible to note that softening of the skin has begun. This is evident from the illustrative cases shown in Figures 1, 2 and 3, and from the over-all results

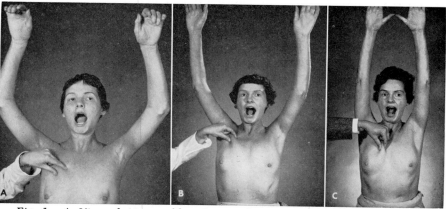

Fig. 1. A, View of 44-year-old patient on June 18, 1958. Note tightness of skin, limitation of joint range of shoulders, elbows, mouth and hands. Onset in May 1957, with progression despite relaxin and stilbestrol therapy. Placed on Potaba; other medications stopped.

B, View showing improvement achieved in this patient by September 14, 1959.

C, Latest view taken October 3, 1960, showing further improvement. Potaba therapy sustained throughout and is continuing.

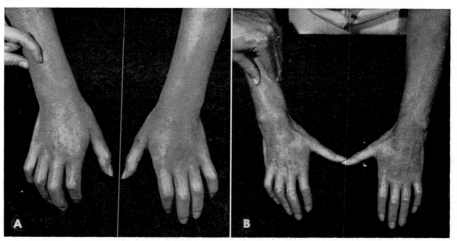

Fig. 2. A, View of hands of patient shown in Figure 1, taken June 18, 1958. Maximum extension of fingers and abduction of thumbs depicted, along with tightly bound, nonwrinkling involvement of skin of forearms.

B, Improved extension of fingers and thumbs as of October 3, 1960; skin of forearms now movable and can be wrinkled. Dynamic traction extension splints were added to regimen in August 1958.

presented in Table 1. Moderate to considerable cutaneous improvement was observed in 97 of the 104 patients. Five of seven who had slight to no improvement were on treatment for less than three months (Table 1 A). It should be noted that all 32 patients treated since 1958 experienced significant skin improvement. Moreover, a number of subjects who had experienced only moderate improvement at the time of their evaluation in 1958 (Table 1 A)[11] have since shown continued benefit which would permit their re-classification into the "considerable improvement" category.

Patients are usually kept on Potaba until it is judged that no further benefit is to be expected. Some patients have reached essentially complete clinical remissions on this program and therapy has been discontinued. The longest post-treatment follow-up period without relapse is now 8½ years. Most subjects, however, show some signs of residual activity or change. In such cases, treatment is continued indefinitely. Two men, for example, who were iron mill workers and exhibited pronounced pulmonary fibrosis, have remained on therapy for more than 9 years. Both have had excellent clinical results[11] insofar as the overt aspects of scleroderma are concerned, but it is believed that the presence of pulmonary fibrosis, though of probably mixed etiology, warrants the continued administration of Potaba.

Physiotherapy, Deep Breathing Exercises and Dynamic Traction Splints. One of the main difficulties in the management of scleroderma is that of overcoming the consequences of pericapsular and other fibrous tissue shortening. In many patients, there may be marked improvement in skin pliability without concomitant improvement in the range of motion of the underlying joint. For this reason, physiotherapeutic measures are instituted as early as possible. Active and passive physiotherapy and range-of-motion exercises of all joints should be regular features of the patient's program. Deep breathing exercises should be included, for relative rigidity of the thoracic cage is not an uncommon feature of diffuse systemic sclerosis. Dynamic traction splints[8, 9, 11, 12] have been of aid in overcoming limitation of either flexion or extension of the fingers (Fig. 2). The value of such splints, of course, is directly proportional to the regularity of use and total time they are employed each day.

Dysphagia. Esophageal symptoms are relatively common in scleroderma. Indeed, one or more symptoms related to the esophagus were present in 35 (74 per cent) of 47 patients in whom special studies were performed by Lorber and Zarafonetis.[3] Dysphagia and pyrosis were the most common complaints. Transport studies disclosed absence or nonprogression of a

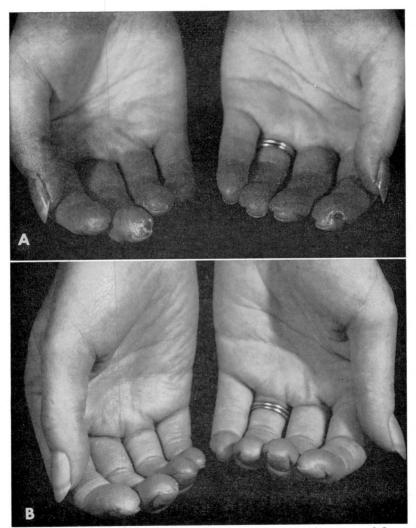

Fig. 3. *A,* Sclerodermatous changes with chronic necrotic ulcerations of finger tips of hands of 31-year-old woman with 3-year history of disease activity. Progressive changes despite hydrocortisone therapy for 3 years. No relief of Raynaud's phenomena following right cervical sympathectomy. Photograph of February 2, 1960, at time of start of Potaba therapy, 12 grams daily, orally. Other medications discontinued.

B, Photograph of March 29, 1960, showing rapid healing of ulcerations as part of general improvement on Potaba program.

peristaltic wave in 68 per cent of the patients, and dilatation of a mild degree was exhibited by half of them. Evidence of retention was observed during the basal examination in 28, or 60 per cent, of the patients, and in 27 of these the administration of 5 mg. of Urecholine subcutaneously lessened or completely abolished the finding within 15 minutes. An injection of Dibuline, on the other hand, increased the degree of retention present in 23 of the patients. Some degree of improvement in esophageal emptying was noted

TABLE 1. A. DURATION OF THERAPY WITH POTASSIUM PARA-AMINOBENZOATE RELATED TO SKIN IMPROVEMENT AT TIME OF EVALUATION OF 72 CASES OF SCLERODERMA (OLD SERIES)

| SKIN IMPROVEMENT | PERIOD OF TREATMENT | | TOTAL |
	Less than 3 months	More than 3 months	
None to slight	5*	2**	7
Moderate	5	34***	39
Considerable	2	24	26
Total	12	60†	72††

* One patient died of acute cardiac insufficiency early in course of treatment.

** In one subject, weight loss continued while on Potaba therapy; treatment was changed to cortisone without benefit, and he later succumbed.

*** Addition of Meticorten, 5 mg. every eight hours, to therapeutic program of one patient was followed by development of hypertension, cardiac failure, "scleroderma kidney" and death.

† Four patients died of cancer while under treatment.

†† Personal communications dealing with 10 additional cases of scleroderma treated with Potaba indicate moderate to considerable improvement in nine, and no noticeable improvement in one subject who received medication for only three months.

(From Ann. Int. Med., 50:343, 1959.[11])

B. DURATION OF THERAPY WITH POTASSIUM PARA-AMINOBENZOATE RELATED TO SKIN IMPROVEMENT AT TIME OF EVALUATION OF 32 CASES OF SCLERODERMA (NEW SERIES)

| SKIN IMPROVEMENT | PERIOD OF TREATMENT | | TOTAL |
	Less than 3 months	More than 3 months	
None to slight	0	0	0
Moderate	3	17*	20
Considerable	0	12	12
Total	3	29	32

* One patient died of cardiac arrhythmia complicating cor pulmonale; another died with fulminating hypertension, cardiac failure and acute renal necrosis.

C. SUMMARY OF 104 CONSECUTIVE CASES TREATED WITH POTASSIUM PARA-AMINOBENZOATE

| POTABA-TREATED CASES | SKIN IMPROVEMENT | | | TOTALS |
	None to Slight	Moderate	Considerable	
Old-series, 1948-58	7	39*	26	72
New series, 1958-60	0	20	12	32
Totals	7	59	38	104

* A number of subjects in this group have continued therapy and changed to "considerable improvement" category.

after administration of Dibuline to 11 subjects, but in only one was this greater than that which followed the administration of Urecholine.

In view of these observations, Urecholine has been prescribed for those scleroderma patients who complain of dysphagia. One or two 5 mg. tablets, crushed and swallowed about one-half hour before each meal, usually suffice to control this difficulty.

Pyrosis is another problem often encountered in these patients. The nature of the esophageal involvement in scleroderma favors reflux, and pyrosis may be more troublesome when the patient is recumbent. It is treated with milk, antacids and postural measures—not always with complete success.

DISCUSSION

It is believed that the cumulative experience gained in the management of this series of 104 patients clearly demonstrates that the long-term administration of Potaba in adequate dosage will produce moderate to considerable improvement in the great majority of patients with scleroderma. It should be recognized, however, that Potaba is not a complete treatment for this disorder. In a minority of patients who exhibit a highly active, rapidly progressive form of the disease, the process may be only retarded by this medication. Moreover, the contractive features of the disease must be actively combated by physiotherapeutic measures, as described above. Similarly, esophageal symptoms require supplemental therapeutic attention, as already discussed. With regard to the Raynaud's phenomena which are commonly present in scleroderma, little of therapeutic value has been observed from the use of various medications with the patients of this series. In those patients who had undergone cervical sympathectomy, none experienced more than transitory relief at best. We generally advise the avoidance of sharp temperature changes and of emotional stresses, but this is not always feasible. Reserpine and triiodothyronine have recently been reported by Peacock to be of value in the control of Raynaud's phenomena.[5] His regimen deserves trial, particularly for those subjects who experience these neurovascular manifestations to an almost disabling degree.

It is to be emphasized that the program of management outlined herein is necessarily empirical, since scleroderma is a disease of unknown etiology. The original reason for employing Potaba in this disorder stemmed from observations made more than a decade ago. At that time large doses of the drug were administered to a patient with clinical features of both dermatomyositis and scleroderma.[12] The compound was used for the dermatomyositis, but striking improvement also occurred in the areas of sclerodermatous involvement. This experience naturally led to the further use of Potaba in scleroderma[8, 9, 11, 12] and in other conditions associated with excessive fibrosis.[10, 13]

The mechanism by which Potaba exerts antifibrotic and other effects remains obscure. Nevertheless, a number of observations have been made in recent years which are of interest in this connection. First, a patient was observed who had features of scleroderma in association with a functioning carcinoid syndrome.[17] The conjunction of these findings was interpreted as a potential clue to the pathogenesis of the fibrotic changes of scleroderma and other fibrotic states as well as those of the carcinoid syndrome.[11, 17] It was postulated that "fibrosis might result from a deranged interaction of serotonin-mono-amine oxidase mechanisms at the tissue level. Fibrosis was believed to occur whenever an excess serotonin effect was sustained over a sufficient interval of time. This could result from too much serotonin or too little mono-amine oxidase activity."[11] Subsequent studies in the author's laboratory and elsewhere lend support to this general thesis, but with an extension to embrace other mechanisms which function to decrease the tissue level of serotonin in addition to the mono-amine oxidase system.[14] This concept is presented schematically in Figure 4. It should be noted that aside

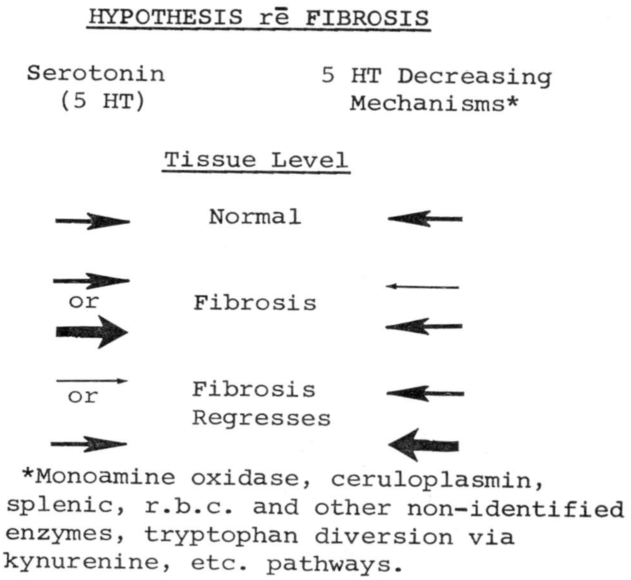

HYPOTHESIS r̄e FIBROSIS

```
     Serotonin              5 HT Decreasing
      (5 HT)                 Mechanisms*

              Tissue Level

      ────>        Normal        <────

      ──>
        or         Fibrosis        ───
      ═══>                        <────

      ──┐
        or         Fibrosis      <────
      ──>          Regresses     <════
```

*Monoamine oxidase, ceruloplasmin, splenic, r.b.c. and other non-identified enzymes, tryptophan diversion via kynurenine, etc. pathways.

Fig. 4. Schematic presentation of an hypothesis regarding the interrelation of serotonin mechanisms and the pathogenesis of fibrosis. This same concept may be extended to explain certain aspects of rheumatoid arthritis, Raynaud's phenomena, pain of glomus tumors and the pain and necrosis of envenomation wounds. (See text).

from the clinical observations regarding fibrosis in the carcinoid syndrome, fibrosis has been induced experimentally in rats by repeated injection with serotonin.[4] Of importance also in this regard is the finding of Scherbel and Harrison that patients with scleroderma are hyper-reactive to local injections of serotonin.[7] Further evidence that tryptophan metabolism is deranged in scleroderma has been provided by the careful studies of Price et al.[6] These workers detected increased excretion of kynurenine and other metabolites of this pathway of tryptophan metabolism. Whether this is a primary defect or a compensatory diversion of tryptophan to nonserotonin metabolites, or both, is not yet clear. Of added interest was the demonstration of an accompanying depletion of pyridoxine in scleroderma. It will be of future interest to determine whether the administration of supplements of vitamin B_6 will produce improvement in the over-all results obtained with the therapeutic regimen described herein.

In any event, there appears to be increasing support for the thesis that serotonin is causally related not only to the fibrotic element but also to certain other features of scleroderma. It may be that an interplay of serotonin and certain catechol amines is responsible, for example, for the occurrence of Raynaud's phenomenon, as suggested by Halpern et al.[2] Moreover, on the basis of histochemical studies of glomus tumors, it appears that serotonin contributes significantly to the pain which is characteristic of these lesions.[16] In the scleroderma patient, it seems likely that glomus-serotonin, probably acting with catechol amines, gives rise to the painful, necrotic ulcerations of the finger tips such as those shown in Figure 3 A. Attention has recently been drawn to the relationship of serotonin and catechol amines to the production of pain and necrosis in envenomation wounds.[15] Serotonin has also been implicated in rheumatoid arthritis and in other clinical areas which are beyond the scope of this discussion. It is believed, however, that enough evidence has been cited to warrant consideration of serotonin mechanisms as operative in the production, directly or indirectly, of certain manifestations of scleroderma and related disorders.

Finally, mono-amine oxidase and several other enzymes which participate in tryptophan-serotonin metabolism are oxygen-dependent. Potaba increases oxygen uptake at the tissue level.[1] Thus, its beneficial effects in scleroderma and other fibrotic states may be mediated through these pathways.

SUMMARY

Program for the safe, long-term management of patients with scleroderma has been described. It consists of (1) systemic antifibrosis therapy through the prolonged administration of 12 grams daily of Potaba, (2) physiotherapy, deep breathing exercises and dynamic traction splints where applicable, and (3) Urecholine for the relief of troublesome dysphagia.

Of 104 consecutive, unselected patients so far treated with Potaba, 97 showed moderate to considerable improvement of the involved skin. Five of the seven subjects who failed to show significant improvement had received the drug for less than three months.

Although scleroderma remains a disease of unknown etiology, a hypothesis is presented which assigns a major role to serotonin in the pathogenesis of fibrosis and of certain other manifestations in scleroderma and related disorders.

REFERENCES

1. Greiff, D.: Biology of the *Rickettsiae*. In The Rickettsial Diseases of Man. Washington, D. C., American Association for the Advancement of Science, pp. 51-53.
2. Halpern, A. et al.: Raynaud's disease, Raynaud's phenomenon, and serotonin. Angiology, 11:151, 1960.
3. Lorber, S. H. and Zarafonetis, C. J. D.: Esophageal transport studies in patients with scleroderma. To be published.
4. MacDonald, R. A., Robbins, S. L. and Mallory, G. K.: Dermal fibrosis following subcutaneous injections of serotonin creatinine sulfate. Proc. Soc. Exper. Biol. & Med., 97:334, 1958.
5. Peacock, J. H.: The treatment of primary Raynaud's disease of the upper limb. Lancet, 2:65, 1960.
6. Price, J. M., Brown, R. R., Rukavina, J. G., Mendelson, C. and Johnson, S. A. M.: Scleroderma (acrosclerosis). II. Tryptophan metabolism before and during treatment by chelation (EDTA). J. Invest. Derm., 29:289, 1957.
7. Scherbel, A. L. and Harrison, J. W.: Response to serotonin and its antagonists in patients with rheumatoid arthritis and related diseases. Angiology, 10:29, 1959.
8. Zarafonetis, C. J. D.: Therapeutic possibilities of para-aminobenzoic acid. Ann. Int. Med., 30:1188, 1949.
9. Zarafonetis, C. J. D.: Clinical use of para-aminobenzoic acid. Texas State J. Med., 49:666, 1953.

10. Zarafonetis, C. J. D.: Para-aminobenzoic acid in the treatment of scleroderma and other disorders associated with excessive fibrosis. J. Mich. State M. Soc., 53:782, 1954.
11. Zarafonetis, C. J. D.: Treatment of scleroderma. Ann. Int. Med., 50:343, 1959.
12. Zarafonetis, C. J. D., Curtis, A. C. and Gulick, A. E.: Use of para-aminobenzoic acid in dermatomyositis and scleroderma. A.M.A. Arch. Int. Med., 85:27, 1950.
13. Zarafonetis, C. J. D. and Horrax, T. M.: Treatment of Peyronie's disease with potassium para-aminobenzoate (Potaba). J. Urol., 81:770, 1959.
14. Zarafonetis, C. J. D. and Kalas, J. P.: Serotonin degradation by ceruloplasmin and its inhibition by isoniazid and iproniazid. Am. J. M. Sc., 239:203, 1960.
15. Zarafonetis, C. J. D. and Kalas, J. P.: Serotonin, catechol amines, and amine oxidase activity in the venoms of certain reptiles. Am. J. M. Sc., 240:764, 1960.
16. Zarafonetis, C. J. D., Kalas, J. P. and Watts, H. M.: To be published.
17. Zarafonetis, C. J. D., Lorber, S. H. and Hanson, S. M.: Association of functioning carcinoid syndrome and scleroderma. I. Case report. Am. J. M. Sc., 236:1, 1958.

Systemic and Topical Steroids in the Treatment of Dermatoses

NORMAN B. KANOF

New York University Post-Graduate Medical School

The applicability of adrenocortical steroids to the treatment of a wide range of dermatologic disorders, systemically, topically and intralesionally, undoubtedly makes this group of compounds the most important addition to dermatologic therapy in recent times.

Steroids enable the dermatologist to prolong, perhaps even save, the lives of patients with previously rapidly fatal dermatoses, to make life dignified and productive—"worth living"—for patients with certain chronic, disabling, humiliating dermatoses, and to shorten the course of the disease and lessen the discomfort of patients with many an acute dermatitis. With full awareness of the facts that these drugs do not cure and that they are no substitute for accurate diagnosis and elimination of etiologic agents, the judicious and skillful use of steroid therapy is essential to dermatologic practice today.

TOPICAL THERAPY

A variety of steroids are available for topical use. Triamcinolone acetonide 0.1 per cent and dexamethasone 0.1 per cent are most effective topically, and hydrocortisone 0.5 to 1.0 per cent, prednisone/prednisolone 0.25 to 0.5 per cent and methyl prednisolone 0.25 to 1.0 per cent are all very satisfactory. Lower concentrations tend to be less consistently effective though they are economically compelling. Higher concentrations are rarely necessary and are very expensive. These active agents are now available as sprays and foams and in an adherent base for application to mucosal surfaces in addition to the ointment, cream and lotion vehicles. Antibiotics are frequently used topically in combination with steroids. Neomycin is most often employed for this purpose, but preparations with bacitracin, gramicidin, polymyxin and the tetracyclines are also available. Such combinations are very effective in primary and secondary pyodermas, but I feel that their routine prophylactic use in grossly uninfected dermatoses has been overemphasized. Topical steroids are also available with nystatin for those inflammatory dermatoses attributable to *Candida albicans* and with various tars and halogenated hydroxyquinolines for a variety of dermatoses.

The most effective topical therapeutic agents for atopic dermatitis in all its phases (infantile eczema, localized and generalized neurodermatitis) are the steroids, either by themselves or combined with an antibiotic, a tar or one of the halogenated hydroxyquinolines. Allergic eczematous contact dermatitis also responds very well to topical steroid therapy. Lesions of seborrheic dermatitis involving the face, the ears, the scalp margins, the folds of the axillae and groins are also indications for topical steroids. Some cases of rosacea and acne will improve with topical steroids. Anogenital pruritus in most instances responds dramatically to topical steroids, and external otitis does also. Vesicular, pustular eczematous dermatoses of the hands and nummular eczema anywhere on the body also are benefited by these preparations. Psoriasis of the glabrous skin rarely clears with the topical steroid therapy available today, but lesions in the intertriginous folds and the anogenital region sometimes respond, particularly to triamcinolone.

Topical steroids are among the safest agents in dermatologic therapy. Allergic sensitivity to them has not been reported (though it does occur to the antibiotics and other compounds with which the steroid may be combined), and systemic side effects from absorption have not been observed even when tremendous amounts of hydrocortisone have been applied over large body areas for long periods of time.

SYSTEMIC THERAPY

In the topical use of steroids, the physician's question can be a simple one: "Will it work or won't it?" When we turn to systemic steroid therapy in dermatology, our question is no longer so simple. Because of the troublesome side effects associated with systemic steroid administration, we must answer for each condition, for each patient, not only "Will it work?" but "Though it will work, should I use it?"

None will deny the necessity for steroid therapy in those dermatoses in which life is threatened and alternate therapy offers little. In pemphigus, systemic lupus erythematosus, dermatomyositis, widespread scleroderma, sclerema neonatorum, exfoliative erythrodermas and some cutaneous lymphomas, the indication is clear.

Few will interdict the use of systemic steroids in those dermatoses with a (relatively) predictable and limited course which are incapacitating and painful. Severe contact dermatitis, severe urticaria due to drugs and other drug eruptions, erythema multiforme and intense sunburn, respond very well to short courses of systemic steroid therapy.

It is a group of dermatoses that do not fall into either of these categories in which systemic therapy with steroids presents both a problem and a challenge to the dermatologist. These dermatoses are chronic and recurrent. They are not a threat to life, but they are uncomfortable, unpleasant and incapacitating physically, economically and psychologically. They are controlled by systemic steroids but recur when the steroid is withdrawn or its dose is reduced below a maintenance level. In this group are atopic dermatitis, psoriasis, widespread nummular dermatitis, disseminated discoid lupus erythematosus, chronic contact dermatitis (frequently occupational), chronic urticaria (cause undertermined) and alopecia areata totalis. Psoriasis responds well to systemic therapy with triamcinolone but poorly to the other steroids currently available. The other conditions respond well to all the steroids now in use.

The decision for or against systemic steroid therapy must rest on the physician's evaluation of the individual patient. The risks inherent with systemic steroids must be weighed against the benefits which may be expected. These will depend on the severity of the condition and its response to other forms of therapy. Relative contraindications such as diabetes, hypertension or peptic ulcer need concomitant active or prophylactic therapy. Each patient should be aware of the type of therapy being used and of the possibility of side effects and complications. The necessity for regular examinations to reveal and minimize these difficulties must be stressed.

The dose of steroid will depend on the particular drug used and the severity of the dermatosis. The initial dose should be high enough to suppress the condition quickly. After this has been accomplished, the dose is gradually reduced to the least amount which will control the clinical signs and symptoms. These need not remain completely abolished. Some slight activity at a low maintenance steroid dosage is often to be preferred to complete clearing which requires a much higher dose. Concomitant therapy with other modalities will help to hold down the steroid requirements and to deal with the inevitable exacerbations. The steroid dose level may need to be increased to cope with episodes of increased severity of the condition, but the constant aim of the physician should be to probe for a lower and lower maintenance dose and the eventual discontinuance of steroids altogether.

Several special points deserve mention. Since systemic steroid therapy in the young growing child interferes with proper skeletal growth and maturation, the use of this form of treatment in childhood atopic dermatitis should be sharply limited, even though the results are most gratifying. This limitation applies even more stringently to alopecia areata totalis occurring before puberty. The problem of continuing steroid therapy during pregnancy also arises. In my experience such therapy, even though continued through the entire period of gestation, has not affected the pregnancy, the delivery or the newborn child. A third problem arises from the very ease and efficacy of systemic steroid therapy itself. It seems so easy and safe to the patient that the temptation to self-medication and lapse of proper follow-up is great. An awareness by the patient of the possible side effects and complications of steroid therapy will discourage such unsupervised therapy.

INTRALESIONAL THERAPY

The local injection of relatively insoluble suspensions of corticosteroids into (or in many instances beneath) dermatologic lesions has received increasing attention. Localized neurodermatitis (lichen simplex chronicus), hypertrophic lichen planus, alopecia areata and psoriasis respond well to such intralesional therapy. Psoriasis responds best to triamcinolone; the other conditions respond equally to any of the steroid suspensions. The clearing which results from this form of steroid therapy will usually last for one to six months. Intralesional steroid therapy is also of value in pustular and cystic acne and in the treatment of small sebaceous cysts. It is occasionally beneficial in necrobiosis lipoidica but has been disappointing in keloids, scleroderma and the cutaneous lymphomas. The local injection of insoluble steroid suspensions is sometimes followed by atrophy which may persist for many months. Occasionally superficial ulceration occurs at the site of such injections. If large amounts of steroids are used for intralesional therapy, systemic effects may sometimes occur.

SUMMARY

The corticosteroids occupy a pre-eminent position in dermatologic therapy today. Skillfully employed topically, systemically and intralesionally, they relieve the itching and discomfort of many an acute dermatitis, suppress the distress and disability of certain chronic and recurrent dermatoses and prolong or save the lives of some patients with otherwise fatal dermatoses.

Treatment of Ocular Inflammations

DAN M. GORDON

Cornell University Medical College

Ocular inflammation has many possible causes. Since redness and swelling are often the only visible manifestations, a thorough examination of the eye and adnexa is essential in making an accurate diagnosis and in prescribing effective treatment.

FOREIGN BODIES

Conjunctival and corneal foreign bodies, a frequent source of eye trauma, may lead to serious loss of vision. They may carry bacteria into the cornea or may cause corneal abrasions resulting in ulcers. Eversion of the upper eyelid to rule out the presence of foreign bodies is the first step in the examination of an irritated eye. If a foreign body is found, a moistened toothpick applicator will usually serve to lift it from the lid.

Corneal foreign bodies and minute lesions are often difficult to see. The use of 1 or 2 per cent fluorescein (preferably as fluorescein strips) will stain the denuded area of the corneal epithelium green and thus highlight the foreign body or lesion. Foreign bodies of the cornea can frequently be irrigated off with a squeeze bottle containing sterile saline or water after the eye has been subjected to topical anesthesia, or may be lifted off the anesthetized surface with the point of a sterile hypodermic needle. Attempts to wipe the object off with a moistened applicator may damage the cornea.

After foreign bodies have been removed from the eyelid, no further treatment is required. However, corneal foreign bodies cause varying degrees of epithelial loss and discomfort. For that reason it is wise to apply an eye patch for several hours. If a sterile instrument has been used for removal of the irritant and if the eye does not appear to be infected, simple irrigation with any bland, sterile solution suffices; medication is unnecessary.

LESIONS OF THE EYELIDS AND CONJUNCTIVA

Inflammation of the eyelids arising from an internal sty (meibomitis) or an external sty (hordeolum) is always associated with tender swelling of the involved lid.

Inflammatory lesions of the conjunctiva produce engorgement of the conjunctival vessels, visible as an injection of the mucosal covering of the eye (bulbar conjunctiva) if that portion is affected. At times the injection (conjunctivitis) is confined to the palpebral conjunctiva which lines the lids. The inner eyelid surface may be red, with or without discharge. When the bulbar conjunctiva is involved, the eye may appear almost malignantly inflamed. The conjunctival vessels are irregular in their course and emanate from the lid areas. By contrast, the ciliary vessels are straight and fan out from the limbus. Differentiation between a conjunctival injection and the ciliary injection occurring in involvement of the iris or ciliary body and in acute or chronic congestive glaucoma presents an important diagnostic problem. If the physician presses the patient's lower lid firmly against the limbus with his thumb and, while maintaining that pressure, slowly draws the lower lid downward, an area of paleness will appear at the site of pressure. If the injection is conjunctival, the area of pallor will persist as the lower lid is drawn down under pressure. This indicates that the disease is superficial. If the area pales momentarily, only to redden again immediately as the lower lid is pulled down under pressure, one can deduce that ciliary injection is present and that the causative lesion probably lies within the eye itself.

All forms of conjunctivitis tend to cause discomfort rather than pain, accompanied by a sandy or scratchy sensation. If the conjunctiva is injected, with or without discharge, one may assume that he is dealing with inflammation, possibly with infection. Steroid-antimicrobial combinations are indicated and are usually gratifyingly effective. If the palpebral conjunctiva appears pale and watery, the inflammation is probably allergic and calls for a topical steroid preparation.

EPISCLERITIS AND SCLERITIS

In episcleritis, an inflammation of the episcleral tissues, the red area characteristically is localized, although it may sometimes be widespread. Contrasted with conjunctivitis, there is a red or mildly purplish area, exquisitely tender when palpated through the overlying lid. Episcleritis usually responds to topical steroids frequently applied. Occasionally, however, episcleritis precedes iridocyclitis.

Inflammation of the sclera (scleritis) is a grave condition which should be treated by an ophthalmologist. Often associated with rheumatoid arthritis and perhaps progressing to nodular involvement or actual ulceration, scleritis produces a deep purplish discoloration of the white of the eye, with overlying conjunctival injection. It demands intensive systemic and topical steroid therapy.

KERATITIS AND OTHER CORNEAL LESIONS

Inflammation of the cornea (keratitis), usually accompanied by pain and localized or generalized ciliary injection, conjunctival injection, or both, is always serious. Part or all of the normally mirror-like surface of the cornea appears irregular or glazed and the light reflexes from it are roughened or irregular. It is important to rule out herpes simplex (dendritic keratitis), which characteristically consists of a single lesion or multiple branching lesions with a round, knoblike excrescence at the terminus of each branch. Normally the cornea is sensitive to touch when tested with a tightly wound wisp of cotton. Dendritic keratitis, commonly unilateral, produces corneal hypesthesia or anesthesia. One should test the unanesthetized eye to determine whether it is anesthetic. Sensation in the uninvolved eye should also be tested for comparison. If the affected eye is anesthetic, dendritic keratitis is to be suspected until the condition is proved otherwise. Topical steroids are contraindicated in herpes simplex keratitis as well as in the rarer fungal keratitis. In localities where pathogenic fungi are endemic, the possibility of fungal keratitis should be kept in mind. Appropriate culture techniques are necessary for accurate diagnosis. Fluorescein staining facilitates diagnosis when corneal epithelium has been destroyed. If a dendritic (branching-type) lesion is evident, the physician is very likely dealing with herpes simplex keratitis. Since all keratitides are true emergencies, they should be treated by an ophthalmologist.

Catarrhal (limbal) ulcers appear as staining infiltrated areas at one margin of the corneal limbus with a contiguous area of conjunctival injection. These lesions respond well to topical steroid-antimicrobial combinations, applied frequently (four to eight times daily).

True corneal ulcers usually occur away from the limbus and cause a definite loss of epithelium. Often an associated iritis or actual pus (hypopyon) is seen in the anterior chamber. Ulcers frequently follow trauma, and identification of the offending organism by culture facilitates treatment. During the interval before the laboratory report is received, the patient may be treated with systemic as well as with topically applied broad-spectrum antimicrobials. Concomitant topical and occasionally systemic steroids benefit the patient, provided that herpes simplex or fungal involvement is absent. All these medicaments should be given frequently and in large doses. Any patient with a corneal ulcer should be referred to an ophthalmologist at once.

HEMORRHAGIC OR PURULENT CONDITIONS

Hyphema, i.e., blood in the anterior chamber, indicates damage to the inner eye and is usually traceable to trauma or intra-ocular neoplasm. An associated secondary rise in intraocular pressure frequently occurs. A fixed or distorted pupil, a tremulous iris, a shallow anterior chamber or a serious disturbance in the red pupillary reflex as seen with the ophthalmoscope indicates intraocular damage, especially when preceded by trauma. Pus in the anterior chamber (hypopyon) may be associated with serpiginous ulcer of the cornea, uveitis or intraocular infection.

INTRAOCULAR INFLAMMATION

Inflammation of the inner eye may cause external redness and, although it is rarely as obvious as conjunctivitis, it is of much more serious import. It usually produces blurring or loss of vision. The most common internal cause of external redness is iritis (iridocyclitis), which produces ciliary injection. Mild edema as well as deposits on the endothelial (posterior) surface of the cornea may be evident. The iris markings exhibit varying degrees of obscuration. The pupil may be smaller than normal and sluggish in its responses. Grayish fibrin in the anterior chamber may tend to obliterate the normal black appearance of the pupil. Since iritis may be a sign of disease of the posterior eye, e.g., choroiditis, generalized uveitis or optic neuritis, injection of the external eye demands inspection and ophthalmoscopic examination of the inner eye. All inflammations and diseases of the inner eye should be treated by an ophthalmologist.

Acute choroiditis (inflammation of the choroid) may involve the retina as well. Ophthalmoscopically, it appears as a raised yellow area, poorly delineated and often associated with vitreous opacities. Inflammation of the optic nerve (optic neuritis) may sometimes be accompanied by uveitis or external ocular inflammation. Optic neuritis and uveitis demand immediate treatment.

GLAUCOMA

When full-blown, acute glaucoma is an excruciatingly painful condition. Attacks vary in severity. The consistency of the eye may range from hard to rock-hard. The greater and more rapid the rise in pressure, the more sudden and intense the visual loss. The cornea becomes edematous and glazed, losing its normal mirror-like appearance. Iris markings are muddy and the pupil is dilated and fixed. To get an idea of intraocular pressure, the globe should be palpated through the upper lid. While the physician holds the eye firm with one index finger, he uses the other to make gentle

TABLE 1.   DIFFERENTIAL DIAGNOSIS OF THREE FREQUENTLY
ENCOUNTERED OCULAR ABNORMALITIES

SYMPTOM OR SIGN	ACUTE CONJUNCTIVITIS	ACUTE IRITIS	ACUTE GLAUCOMA
Injection	Conjunctival (superficial)	Ciliary (deep)	Intense conjunctival and cilary
Pain	Sandy sensation	Moderate	Severe
Vision	Normal	Impaired	Severely impaired
Pupil	Normal	Small	Dilated
Discharge	Watery to purulent	None	None
Anterior chamber	Normal	Normal	Shallow
Media	Clear	Corneal deposits Hazy aqueous	Steamy cornea
Iris	Normal	Muddy markings	Congested
Intraocular pressure	Normal	Usually normal	Elevated

pressure against the globe. This procedure will serve to reveal whether the pressure is significantly elevated, especially in comparison with findings in the other eye if the latter is not involved. Tonometry is more accurate.

Although iridocyclitis is not as painful as glaucoma and rarely causes rapid, intense visual loss, it may be confused with acute glaucoma. Table 1, comparing the signs and symptoms typically encountered in acute conjunctivitis, acute iritis and acute glaucoma, respectively, presents helpful differential points. Since the treatments for these eye diseases are diametrically different, one must not prescribe the wrong therapy if serious harm is to be avoided. If the physician is not sure of the diagnosis, he should use neither miotics nor mydriatics, for their improper use can be dangerous. Acute iritis responds to steroids administered topically and systemically in adequate doses. Many doctors prescribe atropine routinely in the treatment of iritis. Acute glaucoma, however, demands intensive miotic therapy in addition to the use of carbonic anhydrase inhibitors, such as dichlorphenamide. When an ophthalmologist is not available and the physician cannot differentiate between acute iridocyclitis and an acute glaucoma, a double to quadruple dose of a carbonic anhydrase inhibitor may be given without ill effects. However, one should not risk the error of using a miotic when a mydriatic is indicated, or the reverse. Topical steroids are beneficial in acute iritis and to a degree in acute glaucoma in preventing formation of anterior synechiae. When acute iridocyclitis goes untreated, posterior synechiae often develop between iris and lens. If these adhesions completely bind the pupil down to the lens, seclusion of the pupil results, thus preventing the aqueous behind the iris from coming forward into the anterior chamber. The aqueous pushes the iris anteriorly, creating a ballooning appearance (iris bombé) with secondary glaucoma, which must be treated.

SOME GUIDING PRINCIPLES OF THERAPY

In the management of the inflamed eye, the maxim that all therapy should have a rational basis and not be given simply for the sake of doing something is particularly applicable.

The introduction of steroids has revolutionized the treatment of many ocular diseases, especially inflammations and allergies. It is a *sine qua non* of steroid administration as well as of most other ocular therapy that the lesion be saturated with the medication. To that end, it is usually essential to apply steroid or antimicrobial topical preparations every hour, or oftener, during the acute phase of the disease. If the eye has good vision, one should order drops rather than ointments for daytime use, since ointments blur vision. Ointments are usually reserved for use at night, for drops have less duration of contact and activity than ointments and must be applied more frequently. If vision is severely decreased, or if the situation is serious, ointments can be used continuously.

It is important that medication be administered by the proper route to reach the site of disease. As a rule, if the lesion can be seen with the naked eye, frequent topical applications of drops or ointments will arrest progress in most lesions of the lids, conjunctiva, episclera, sclera (in some cases), cornea and iris (in many cases). When the lesion is posterior, affecting the choroid, retina, optic nerve or orbit, full systemic medication by oral or parenteral route is mandatory. Inflammation or allergic involvement which normally should respond to topical medication demands systemic treatment if the condition fails to improve or if it becomes worse after a day or two of topical therapy. The physician must also decide whether failure results from the fact that the therapy employed has been given by an inappropriate or contraindicated route, or from incorrect diagnosis.

Herpes simplex keratitis is a contraindication to steroid therapy. It is treated by broad removal of the diseased and surrounding corneal epithelium. Fungal keratitis, in which steroid therapy is also contraindicated, is difficult to treat but may respond to antifungal agents such as amphotericin B, systemically and topically, or nystatin.

To patch or not to patch is a question raised frequently. If purulent discharge is present, one should not patch, if it can be avoided, for the retained pus will macerate and infect the cornea.

In the presence of infection, antimicrobials are indicated. Their action is often enhanced by the simultaneous use of steroids. The tendency is to employ topically those antimicrobials which are not commonly used systemically. For that reason, neomycin sulfate, which possesses a rather broad range of action (including Morax-Axenfeld diplobacillus, staphylococcus, pneumococcus, Koch-Weeks bacillus, *Proteus vulgaris* and streptococcus), is a favorite.

Some patients with episcleritis and most of those with scleritis do not respond to topical steroids alone, but require additional steroids systemically for good results. This is also true of many patients with iridocyclitis.

The organisms causing true corneal ulcers should be identified by means of cultures. In the interim, broad-spectrum antibiotics plus either polymyxin B sulfate or colistin should be applied topically, with penicillin and broad-spectrum antibiotics given systemically. *Pseudomonas aeruginosa,* most refractory of all ocular infective agents, can prove highly resistant to treatment. Accordingly, polymyxin B sulfate or colistin, or both, should be added to the regimen while a specific diagnosis is being made.

It is wise to use systemic steroids in adequate doses (3.0 to 4.5 mg. or more of dexamethasone or the equivalent in other steroids, or 80 to 120 units of corticotropin) in iritis, choroiditis and optic neuritis, adding topical steroids in iritis. Mydriatics are indicated in iritis if adhesions between the iris and the lens are present or forming. Development of synechiae usually is inhibited by or dissipated during steroid therapy.

Acute glaucoma should be treated immediately by 200 mg. of dichlorphenamide or the equivalent of other carbonic anhydrase inhibitors. If this has not adequately reduced the intraocular pressure within approximately ninety minutes, an intravenous injection of acetazolamide (500 mg.) or urea (1 gram per kg. of body weight) should be given. One should explain to the patient that he may expect subsequent attacks, which can probably be prevented by peripheral iridectomy following the first attack.

Treatment of
Allergic Diseases and Asthma

WILLIAM B. SHERMAN

Columbia University College of Physicians and Surgeons

In discussing the allergic diseases, it is essential to distinguish between the immediate type of allergic reaction in which the phenomena of hypersensitivity are manifested within a few minutes after contact with the antigen and the delayed type which becomes apparent only after many hours. In general, the immediate type of hypersensitivity is accompanied by the presence of circulating antibodies in the plasma and is manifested by reactions of blood vessels, smooth muscles and mucus glands stimulated by histamine or other intermediate substances released as a result of antigen-antibody union. Delayed hypersensitivity, on the other hand, is essentially a cellular reaction. No free antibodies are demonstrable in the plasma or serum, but the hypersensitivity reaction may be transferred in most cases by lymphoid or mononuclear cells. Likewise, the reaction which occurs on exposure to the antigen involves individual cells rather than tissues or organs. There is no clear evidence that release of histamine or other intermediate substances plays a determining role in the delayed reaction.

This discussion is concerned primarily with the immediate type of allergy. Clinically, this type is usually subdivided into anaphylactic sensitization which may be induced in essentially all individuals of susceptible species by a sufficiently heavy, usually parenteral, exposure to antigen, and atopic sensitization which develops in certain individuals predisposed by heredity after normal contacts with antigens in the environment. The former represents the natural response of a normal immune mechanism to an unusual exposure, the latter an unusual response of an abnormal immune mechanism to normal contacts. Many manifestations of the two types of immediate hypersensitivity are similar, and the difference is perhaps one of degree rather than kind.

In clinical medicine, the anaphylactic type of sensitization is exemplified by serum sickness following therapeutic use of heterologous antisera, the atopic form by hay fever and asthma due to extrinsic antigens. In both instances, the specific sensitization is readily demonstrable by an immediate urticarial response to skin tests with the antigen, and the plasma contains reagins which transfer the reaction to normal skin. However, in regard to bronchial asthma, it should be noted that a large proportion of typical cases, including many in which atopic susceptibility is suggested by the family history or the record of previous illnesses, do not show specific reactions to environmental antigens. There is considerable evidence, which cannot be reviewed here in detail, that such "intrinsic" asthma is due in most cases to respiratory infection.[3, 4]

Once the susceptibility to asthma has developed, either through sensitization to a specific antigen or through respiratory infection, attacks may be produced by a variety of specific and nonspecific causes. Thus, the symptoms may be produced by exposure to the specific antigen or by an exacerbation of respiratory infection. Attacks may occur during acute respiratory infections in patients whose asthma is due primarily to specific antigens, or they may be precipitated by exposure to nonspecific irritants such as chemical fumes, smoke or even cold damp air, regardless of the basic cause of susceptibility. Exertion and emotional stress may also act as nonspecific factors precipitating attacks.[7]

The basic principle of allergic treatment of asthma is to identify the basic causes producing the susceptibility in the individual case and to correct them either by avoidance of contact or by immunization with the specific agent. If this can be accomplished, the effects of secondary nonspecific factors usually become insignificant. In asthma due to extrinsic antigens, the percentage of success is high. The specific antigens can usually be identified by skin tests, and a considerable proportion can be avoided by due care. In the cases of allergy to house dust, atmospheric pollens and mold spores, which cannot easily be avoided, the results of suitable immunizations are generally good, with 85 per cent success in asthma due to a single pollen such as ragweed.

In asthma due to respiratory infection, on the contrary, specific causative organisms can only occasionally be proved, avoidance is difficult, and satisfactory immunization rarely is possible. Antibiotics are particularly useful during acute exacerbations of infection, but continuous control of symptoms by antibiotics alone rarely is practical. In contrast to the prophylaxis of rheumatic fever, which involves a single susceptible organism, the respiratory infection in asthma is usually due to a mixed and changing flora, often including resistant organisms. Thus, the results of allergic methods in these cases are often discouraging and the physician is more dependent upon nonspecific therapy.

For the nonspecific symptomatic relief of asthma, three main groups of drugs are available, the adrenergic drugs, the theophylline derivatives and the steroids. The antihistamine drugs, which are useful in most other allergic diseases, are relatively ineffective, since the bronchospasm of asthma results from the release not only of histamine but also of the slow-reacting substance SRS-A, against which the antihistamine drugs have no effect.[2]

The action of steroids in asthma is apparently related to their anti-inflammatory effects, but details of the mode of action have not been completely defined. In general, asthmatic patients have normal adrenal cortical function, and treatment depends upon providing a mild excess of hormone activity rather than correcting a deficiency. Doses adequate to control symptoms do not inhibit the reaction of the skin to tests with the specific antigen or with histamine. Short-term treatment does not change the amount of sensitizing antibody in the plasma or the acceptance by the skin of passive sensitization by the sera of other allergic patients.[5] The therapeutic effects of steroids are similar in asthma due to specific antigens and that due to respiratory infection.

In general, the same effects in the treatment of asthma can be produced by the use of any of the commonly available steroid drugs. In numerous instances of shifting patients with asthma from one steroid to another, we have found 25 mg. of cortisone equivalent to 20 mg. of hydrocortisone, 5 mg. of prednisone or prednisolone, 4 mg. of triamcinolone or methyl prednisolone and 0.75 mg. of dexamethasone. Prednisone and prednisolone are preferred for reasons of economy. The same effects may be produced by injections of corticotrophin. Usually, its effects are somewhat more rapid than those of the oral steroids, but prednisone or prednisolone is substituted as soon as the initial effect is obtained to avoid the salt and water retaining effects of corticotrophin.

The use of steroids in asthma has been cautious. Since the fatality rate of asthma is low and the course usually chronic, fear of the long-term side effects of the steroids has caused most physicians to use them in asthma only as a last resort when other drugs fail. As a result of remarks by physicians and articles in popular magazines, many patients with asthma have developed such exaggerated fear of steroids that they are reluctant to use them at all. Actually, the steroids are among the most effective drugs for the treatment of asthma, giving more comfortable continuous relief with fewer immediate side effects than any other drugs for the purpose. The doses required for asthma are usually relatively small and the incidence of serious side effects is low when they are used with care.

For prompt relief of acute attacks of asthma, epinephrine is faster than the steroids and generally is preferable. Mild attacks are better controlled by self-administration of aerosols of epinephrine and related compounds or by oral use of compounds of ephedrine and theophylline than by spasmodic doses of the steroids.

The use of steroids for asthma may be divided into three categories: (1) short-term use during status asthmaticus, (2) intermittent use in chronic asthma and (3) long-term continuous use in intractible asthma.

The clearest indication for the use of steroids is in status asthmaticus, severe persistent asthma in which epinephrine and aminophylline are ineffective or produce such transitory relief that they are not suitable for continuous control. In cases in which epinephrine and aminophylline are ineffective, the most prompt relief may be attained with an infusion containing soluble hydrocortisone or corticotrophin. In less urgent cases, treatment may be initiated with an intramuscular injection of corticotrophin gel. In either case, oral preparations of steroids are started simultaneously and parenteral injections discontinued as soon as relief is obtained. Initial doses are usually 20 to 30 mg. of prednisone or prednisolone per day. Occasionally, this may be increased to 40 mg. a day before relief is effective, but rarely higher. When the asthma is well controlled, the dosage is reduced by 5 mg. every day or two.

If the asthma has been precipitated by respiratory infection, or if the sputum is purulent, an antibiotic is given concurrently with the steroid. Since this type of severe persistent asthma most often results from respiratory infection, antibiotics are used in a large proportion of such cases. Usually tetracycline is started with doses of 250 mg. every six hours, and sputum cultures with sensitivity tests are made as soon as convenient. Often the infection has been controlled before these tests are reported, but if necessary, appropriate changes of antibiotic can be made on the basis of the results. If the severe asthma has been precipitated by respiratory infection, and the use of antibiotics is successful, it is anticipated that the use of steroids may be discontinued in a week or ten days, and the dose is gradually tapered off with this intention.

In chronic asthma, which recurs frequently despite allergic treatment, an attempt is made to control exacerbations by the use of adrenergic and theophylline drugs in preference to steroids. When these other medications must be used frequently and produce only partial relief, the use of steroids for periods of a week or so is safe and usually satisfactory in securing results. In such cases, doses of 10 to 15 mg. of prednisone a day are often adequate and the risk of side effects is negligible. One should remember that most such exacerbations occurring in patients under careful allergic management are due to respiratory infections, and one should consider the advisability of concurrent use of an antibiotic. In seasonal asthma due to pollens, steroids may be given for a week or two at the peek of the season without hesitation.

The third and most difficult category is that of severe chronic asthma in which really complete relief can never be maintained by adrenergic and theophylline drugs. These patients are severely limited in their activities and tend to develop emphysema with progressive respiratory disability. In such cases, the prolonged use of steroid drugs often makes the difference between chronic invalidism and a relatively comfortable, useful life. On the other hand, the possibility of discontinuing the drug is small and the chances of significant side effects greater. In balancing the advantages against the risks, much depends on the dosage of steroids needed for relief. In many cases, a decided improvement may be produced by the use of 10 mg. or less of prednisone per day. Most adults who are free of other diseases can tolerate such doses for indefinite periods without a serious incidence of side effects. In children, however, even smaller doses may cause suppression of growth.[8] The use of 15 or more milligrams a day by adults causes a higher incidence of undesirable effects. In general, if 10 mg. per day of prednisone enable the adult patient to keep ambulatory and to control residual symptoms with adrenergic or theophylline drugs, this dosage is preferable to the larger amounts that may be needed to completely suppress the asthma by steroids alone. If higher doses are needed for this practical degree of control, the possibility of side effects must be weighed against the certainty of respiratory distress and the patient must be watched carefully. Two patients in this category who incurred collapse of vertebral bodies insisted that they continue prednisone rather than suffer from asthma.

In the other allergic diseases, the need for steroids is less frequent than in asthma since the diseases are less disabling and the antihistamines are more often effective. One hesitates to use steroids for relatively mild conditions of prolonged or indefinite duration, but they may be used more freely in allergies in which the duration of symptoms is limited for various reasons. In hay fever, the disability is not great and the antihistamines are usually effective, so that the need for steroids is relatively infrequent. However, patients who are acutely uncomfortable at the peak of the pollen season may be given prednisone for a period of a week or two with the knowledge that the need will soon be over. Usually doses of 10 to 15 mg. a day are adequate. On the other hand, one hesitates to start steroids in chronic perennial rhinitis, in which the symptoms may be expected to persist indefinitely. The same reasoning applies to the use of steroids in urticaria; they may be used freely for the treatment of severe acute attacks, but one should consider carefully before starting their use in chronic urticaria.

One of the definitely self-limited allergic diseases in which steroids are particularly useful is serum sickness due to prophylactic or therapeutic use of heterologous antiserum. No other single drug will control the varied symptoms of skin rashes, edema, arthralgia and fever; combinations of aspirin, codeine and antihistamine drugs are often only partially successful in affording relief. Since the duration of serum sickness depends chiefly on the number of different heterologous antigens included in the serum injection, attacks produced by modern preparations of highly concentrated therapeutic antisera rarely last more than a week. Prednisone or other steroid drugs may be used freely in doses up to 30 or 40 mg. per day until the symptoms are controlled; then the doses are rapidly tapered off in the course of five or six days. The results are usually most gratifying, and the chances of recurrence after the steroid is discontinued are small.

In the similar reactions due to injection of penicillin, the therapeutic effects are equally good while the steroid is given, but the possibility of recurrence is greater. Some such reactions persist for many weeks or even months without further use of penicillin, and the advisability of continuing the steroid for such a period is doubtful. In general, the steroids may be given for a week or ten days initially. If the symptoms recur after the steroid is discontinued, treatment with penicillinase is instituted.[1, 6] The steroids are used first because they are less apt to produce unfavorable reactions than the presently available preparations of penicillinase.

Unlike most other drugs, the steroids are effective in suppressing both the immediate and delayed types of allergic reactions. For severe poison ivy dermatitis, they are the most effective treatment. For this purpose, prednisone 15 to 30 mg. per day may be given orally, and creams or lotions containing prednisone or hydrocortisone may be applied locally.

In the most severe immediate allergic reactions of the anaphylactic type, such as sudden collapse after a bee sting, an injection of penicillin or other exposure to an antigen, the action of steroid drugs is not sufficiently rapid to permit their use as the only medication. Epinephrine should be given first and as promptly as possible. If epinephrine alone does not control the reaction, it may be followed by intravenous hydrocortisone, antihistamines and, if necessary, Levophed.

In summary, it may be noted that the steroid drugs are among the most effective, although not the most rapid, drugs for the relief of a variety of allergic diseases of both the immediate and delayed types. They are not curative and do not replace the allergic method of diagnosis and treatment. They are most often used during acute exacerbations of chronic allergic diseases and in allergic reactions of short duration. In chronic disabling asthma, continuous use over prolonged periods of time may produce relief that far outweighs the possibility of undesirable side reactions.

REFERENCES

1. Becker, R. M.: Effect of penicillinase on circulating penicillin. New Engl. J. Med., *254*:952, 1956.
2. Brocklehurst, W. E.: A slow reacting substance in anaphylaxis "SRS-A." In Ciba Symposium on Histamine. Boston, Little, Brown & Co, 1956, p. 175.
3. Cooke, R. A.: Infective asthma: indication of its allergic nature. Am. J. M. Sc., *183*:309, 1932.
4. Cooke, R. A.: Allergy in Theory and Practice. Philadelphia, London, W. B. Saunders Co., 1947, p. 130.
5. Cooke, R. A. et al.: ACTH and cortisone in allergic disease. J. Allergy, 22:211, 1951.
6. Minno, A. M. and Davis, G. M.: Penicillinase in the treatment of penicillin reactions. J.A.M.A., *165*:222, 1957.
7. Sherman, W. B.: The allergic reaction. Med. Clin. North America, *39*:751, 1955.
8. Van Metre, T. E., Jr. and Pinkerton, H. L., Jr.: Growth suppression in asthmatic children receiving prolonged therapy with prednisone and methyl prednisolone. J. Allergy, *30*:103, 1959.

Panel Discussion

Hobart A. Reimann, *Moderator*

Dr. Reimann: I have been dissatisfied with the name "periarteritis nodosa" because nodes are not common and I have never seen them myself. The disease is much more than just periarteritis; "polyarteritis" or even "polyvasculitis" would be better terms. Dr. Rose, will you comment on the selection of a better term for this entity?

Dr. Rose: I certainly agree with you about the undesirability of the term "periarteritis nodosa." I think it was about the turn of the century that the Italian Ferari suggested that the term "periarteritis" should be used for the vascular lesions seen in a whole range of conditions in which there is inflammation of arterial walls but no necrosis and that "polyarteritis" should be used for the disease with arterial necrosis. I would also quite agree that the nodes are rare; on the other hand, it is perhaps not unjustifiable to transfer the term "nodosa," as they used it, to the type of disease which we usually see, in which there is a focal reaction rather than a diffuse one, a segment of the arterial wall or small artery usually being affected. It is, in a microscopic sense, still nodular in that there is a segmental or nodular distribution of the lesions. I would speak of the human disease as "polyarteritis nodosa" and use the term "polyarteritis" alone to describe the other types of necrotizing arteritis that one sees in association with other diseases in man or in animals and which are not necessarily the same as the classic disease.

DR. REIMANN: I am a little concerned that there has not been more argument about the therapy of these diseases, because it seems that everyone who has spoken is in favor of the use of corticosteroids. Dr. Kushner, do you have any reservations about the use of steroids in any of these conditions?

DR. KUSHNER: I have been concerned about the influence of steroids, especially in scleroderma and perhaps also in polyarteritis, in regard to the possible acceleration of renal lesions, when they are present, with the rapid production of renal insufficiency. This stems from observations we made in 1950 and 1951 of rapidly accelerating renal insufficiency in the first two patients, one with scleroderma and one with polyarteritis, that we treated with steroids, and a similar experience was reported in that same year by the Mayo Clinic. I wonder whether this was a chance observation or whether this has been observed by the other panelists? If it is a real phenomenon, one should obtain histological information on the type of renal lesion present in patients with scleroderma before steroids are started and then follow this carefully during therapy.

DR. ROSE: In trying to treat the patient with polyarteritis nodosa who already has renal failure, almost certain death awaits the patient if you do not treat him; whereas, there is a real risk of acute progression of renal failure when steroids are given. I do not know what the pathological explanation for this is, but I think it is a real risk. It does not always happen and there is an exceptional patient in whom there is an improvement in renal function during treatment. Therefore, personally I would give steroids cautiously, but if there is rapid rise in blood urea nitrogen then obviously one must reduce or stop treatment.

DR. POLLAK: Investigators in our laboratory have recently completed a study of the serial biopsy and autopsy findings in about 25 patients with scleroderma. One or two rather intriguing things have emerged from this study in relation to the renal lesion. Like others, we were initially impressed by the acute renal lesion which appears in scleroderma in association with the rapid development of severe hypertension and death from renal failure; but this lesion, in fact, has been present only in a minority of these patients and in our material is present in those patients who have had an acute clinical course in other ways. This lesion has occurred in five of our patients, and in all five it occurred within two years after the onset of scleroderma. On reviewing the literature, this impression was confirmed, because in the 27 cases found with this type of renal lesion, 20 of the patients had developed the lesion within two years of the onset of scleroderma and all 27 within four years of the onset. In our five patients who had this renal lesion, two did not have steroid therapy at any stage of their illness and in these two the lesion was obviously not associated with or precipitated by steroid therapy. One of the striking things about the study was the demonstration by renal biopsy of very gross changes in the renal interlobular and smaller interlobular arteries in patients who by all clinical methods appeared to have normal renal function and had normal urinalyses; some of these patients had had scleroderma for as long as 20 years. The histological findings are somewhat different in character from those that are found in the acute lesions that

I mentioned first, and are very impressive histologically in the sense that the vessels appear to have virtually no lumen at all, and the vessel wall contains very large amounts of elastic tissue. These abnormalities do not appear to be associated with any clinical evidence of renal disease or hypertension. This has certainly been very surprising in view of the histological appearance.

DR. ZARAFONETIS: With regard to the renal lesion in scleroderma, we had one patient who developed this lesion during the administration of steroids. Steroids were prescribed reluctantly only after another physician, the patient and the patient's family insisted that treatment with cortisone be given. I pointed out the possible risk of hypertension and of a severe renal exacerbation, but the family still insisted on this type of therapy. The patient was then given 5 milligrams of prednisolone every eight hours and in two weeks she felt well; however, after two more weeks of therapy she was hypertensive and we stopped the steroid, but in spite of this the patient developed acute congestive heart failure and had severe necrotizing disease of the kidneys. To me this is more than coincidental. This is not to say that the data Dr. Pollak described are incorrect, but nevertheless, there are occasions when we may produce this particular phenomenon by steroid therapy. Therefore, I do not treat patients with scleroderma with cortisone; the only time we use it is when scleroderma is associated with active lupus erythematosus.

DR. POLLAK: In this connection, it should be pointed out that the type of patient who is liable to be treated with cortisone is the type of person who does get this acute renal lesion; these patients have acute scleroderma, and physically often have features of lupus or dermatomyositis or other connective tissues diseases as well.

DR. DUBOIS: We have had the same experience—severe exacerbations of scleroderma following the use of steroids—and I think part of the problem is that one can not predict the severity of the renal disease at the time therapy with steroids is initiated; because of this we do not use steroids in most patients with scleroderma.

In addition, in our experience with about eight patients with scleroderma, we were unable to note any improvement after several months of therapy with potassium para-aminobenzoate.

DR. REIMANN: Not long ago, Dr. Smyth presented a series of remarkable slides showing the production of polyarteritis by the prolonged use of steroids. This has been a subject of controversy. Dr. Daeschner, would you discuss this?

DR. DAESCHNER: I have not seen this happen, but I have seen Dr. Smyth's slides, and they are very impressive. It appears to be related to the steroid withdrawal syndrome, which I believe someone will discuss in a later panel.

DR. REIMANN: If steroids are used to cure the disease, is it not surprising that steroids could also cause the lesions? Dr. Dubois, can you clarify this problem?

DR. DUBOIS: Part of the problem has been that the doses of steroids in the experimental studies have been fantastically large and not comparable to the human doses. Such reactions have also occurred when steroids have been given in combination with large amounts of salt and DOCA. The circumstances are just not the same as in patients.

DR. REIMANN: A few days ago Dr. Rose discussed the natural history of pan-arteritis or polyarteritis. Several years ago, I observed two patients who had trichinosis and in whom there was unquestioned polyvasculitis; both patients recovered from the trichinosis, and evidence of vasculitis disappeared histologically in biopsy specimens. Chronic nephritis persisted in both patients. One survived for two years or longer and the other died. At postmortem, there were no traces of polyvasculitis. I would like to ask Dr. Rose if he believes that polyarteritis does disappear in some patients? Perhaps this occurs in many more patients than we realize, if the cause of the condition is corrected or if there is a spontaneous remission.

DR. ROSE: This is one of the features of the pathology of polyarteritis that are not generally appreciated. One tends to assume that a scar in the arterial wall and destruction of the internal elastic lamina must be permanent features once they have occurred. However, I have seen a number of patients who in life had quite undoubted evidence of extensive disease in particular organs and who at necropsy have shown no lesions at all in the arteries of those organs. One man, in particular, had fulminating polyarteritis nodosa affecting clinically most of his viscera and peripheral nerves, and he had a positive muscle biopsy. The disease remitted spontaneously, and he died of another cause 18 months later. In about 50 sections from most of the organs of the body, I could not find a trace of active arteritis or of healed arteritis anywhere, and I think, quite apart from therapy, that this is part of the natural course of healing.

DR. REIMANN: Do you think there are some patients who have polyarteritis in which the lesions disappear and the disease is never diagnosed?

DR. ROSE: One can only guess in answer to that. One other patient whom I saw about the same time had rheumatoid arthritis and had an episode of ulnar neuropathy quite unexplained. Subsequently this cleared up and she remained well for the next eight years; a muscle biopsy done originally was negative and at that time there was never any real proof that she had polyarteritis at all. She then developed generalized polyarteritis nodosa and died. If it had not been for the final episode, the disease would never have been identified. It may be that there are many such cases. I just do not know. If we did biopsies more extensively, we might get some better idea of this.

DR. McCOMBS: I thought for some time that there was an error in nomenclature here. Polyarteritis is the condition Dr. Rose described in his paper. However, there is a group of patients in whom the vascular disease is much less severe and often self-limited; serum sickness in which there is a definite etiologic agent is a prototype of this; trichinosis is another. Vasculitis also occurs in schistosomiasis, which again is due to a definite etiologic factor. This lesion may be present in patients who have certain types of drug reactions. We have chosen to call it "allergic vasculitis"; others have used other terms. I think that this type of vasculitis should be differentiated from polyarteritis nodosa, because the clinical course is apt to be much different, the response to steroids is often dramatic and complete, and remissions are likely to be permanent. There are a group of patients, however, in whom there is no apparent etiologic factor and who follow a course similar to that seen in systemic lupus erythematosus. I believe Dr. Harvey would call this "probable lupus," but we have not done so because it is more apt to occur in men, there is no skin rash, and antinuclear antibodies and LE cells do not appear. This process seems to be a clinical entity with low grade, chronic vasculitis, and it never involves the larger muscular arteries which are affected in polyarteritis nodosa.

DR. REIMANN: Dr. McCombs, what is the frequency of polyarteritis, scleroderma and dermatomyositis as compared to systemic lupus erythematosus and other collagen diseases?

DR. McCOMBS: In our clinic during a specific time interval we have had over 100 patients with systemic lupus erythematosus, about 30 with scleroderma, about 15 with periarteritis or polyarteritis nodosa and about 50 or 60 with allergic vasculitis.

Dr. Dubois: What is the incidence of dermatomyositis in your clinic? The incidence of this disease seems to vary considerably from one institution to another.

Dr. McCombs: We have had only about 15 patients with dermatomyositis.

Dr. Dubois: This is about the same incidence we have found. There are great differences in the frequency with which this diagnosis is made. This is apparently not a result of geographic factors, because in our own city the incidence varies greatly in two hospitals from which I have data. We consider it to be a very rare disease, but in other areas it is apparently seen much more frequently. I think this is possibly due to different interpretations of clinical pictures of dermatomyositis, which often overlaps lupus. Most of the patients I see who have been said to have dermatomyositis elsewhere usually develop other manifestations sooner or later, and eventually LE cells are demonstrated, so I think most of them have a clinical picture more compatible with lupus or with other of the collagen diseases. The diagnostic criteria must vary greatly from one medical center to another.

Dr. Reimann: Are circumstances about the same in England, Dr. Rose?

Dr. Rose: I can give figures only in regard to systemic lupus and polyarteritis. During the Medical Research Council therapeutic trials, patients were obtained from many hospitals during the same time period, and the proportion of lupus to polyarteritis was about 5 to 1. The dermatologists in England treat most of the patients with scleroderma and dermatomyositis, and the general physicians do not have a very good idea of the frequency of these diseases. I suspect that scleroderma is more common than polyarteritis, but less common than lupus, and that dermatomyositis is very rare; I have seen only three cases.

Dr. Reimann: Dr. Sherman, what is the mechanism of the effect of steroids in bronchial asthma? You mentioned this briefly in your paper. Would you elaborate on it further?

Dr. Sherman: There is little information on this subject, but I can say, in general, that the reaction to skin tests with a specific allergen are not appreciably changed during effective treatment with steroids. There is also no appreciable change in the level of sensitizing antibodies in the plasma of those patients with asthma due to extrinsic allergens, and in whom these are present before therapy. The reaction of the skin to histamine is not changed, and the ability of the skin of the treated patient to accept passive sensitization to the serum of another patient who has sensitizing antibodies is not changed. All of the information that we have so far is negative. The benefit of steroids in this process is generally considered to be related to the anti-inflammatory effect of the drug, but we do not have a really clear idea of what the mechanism is.

Part IX | EFFECTS OF STEROIDS
ON SPECIFIC NEPHROPATHIES

Effect of Steroid Therapy on Acute Lupus Nephropathy*

LOUIS J. SOFFER

Mount Sinai Hospital and State University of New York
College of Medicine, New York City

The results to be presented are part of a study instituted approximately a decade ago. Over the course of this period, 90 patients with systemic lupus erythematosus have been admitted to the wards of the hospital on my service and have been followed over the ten-year period by the same group of investigators, headed by me. Upon discharge from the hospital they have been sent to the lupus clinic, where they have been followed by the same group of investigators. I make these administrative points to emphasize the controlled nature of this study in the light of the conclusions to be presented.

Of the 90 patients with disseminated lupus erythematosus, approximately 56 had renal disease. In our experience, the single most important prognostic sign in disseminated lupus erythematosus is the presence or absence of renal disease. I must emphasize that in our experience no form of therapy currently available has served to alter permanently the development of renal disease once it is present. It pursues an inexorable course, eventually resulting in the death of the patient. The administration of nitrogen mustards, massive amounts of steroids, antibiotic agents and antimalarials sometimes has resulted in a temporary remission of the renal process in the nephrotic syndrome or in what has appeared to be acute nephritis, but in every instance, despite continuation of the therapy, the renal disease has eventually manifested itself again and has eventually resulted in a fatal outcome. However, there is one type of involvement of the kidney in which the results are somewhat different. A patient with disseminated lupus erythematosus may be admitted to the hospital acutely ill with considerable elevation of the temperature. At that stage it is not unusual to find red cells, casts and albumin in the urine and an elevation of the blood urea nitrogen. These findings are not necessarily characteristic of renal disease of disseminated lupus erythematosus. Renal biopsies, of which we have a fairly sizeable number, distinguish this group from those with actual lupus nephropathy, in the sense that the kidneys of the former patients show cloudy swelling with a moderate amount of débris in the tubules; they do not, however, show the renal histological findings suggestive of disseminated lupus erythematosus. In the former group, after the acute manifestations of the disease are suppressed or brought under control, the renal abnormalities frequently disappear.

To summarize our results, we find that the renal disease in disseminated lupus erythematosus is progressive, and the currently available therapeutic measures, in our experience, have exerted no permanent effect in terms of alteration of the renal findings.

* Supported by the National Institutes of Health of the U. S. Public Health Service.

717

TABLE 1. SEX AND RACE DISTRIBUTION

	WITH RENAL DISEASE	WITHOUT RENAL DISEASE	TOTAL
Sex			
Male	6	5	11
Female	50	29	79
Race			
White	47	29	76
Negro	6	2	8
Puerto Rican	3	3	6
Total patients	56	34	90

Table 1 lists the incidence of renal disease in our 90 patients, of whom 56 had such involvement. At some time in the course of the illness more than half of the patients with disseminated lupus erythematosus developed impairment of renal function. As McCombs (see p. 660) points out, renal disease is more apt to occur in the younger age group than in the older.

One very interesting observation in our studies was that of the 56 patients with lupus nephropathy 53 showed evidence of renal disease upon first admission to the hospital ward service (Table 2). In two of the other three

TABLE 2. ONSET OF RENAL DISEASE IN RELATION TO TIME OF FIRST HOSPITAL ADMISSION

	NUMBER	PER CENT
Present on first hospital admission	53	94
Absent on first hospital admission but present within one year of that admission	2	4
Absent until more than one year after first hospital admission	1	2
Total	56	100

patients, involvement of the kidneys occurred within the course of the subsequent year, and in the other patient it occurred just after one year from the initial hospital admission. We found that by the time a patient was seen in our study group either renal disease was present or it was not likely to occur. It is important to bear in mind, however, that it is difficult to determine how long this group had had lupus erythematosus prior to the hospital admission.

Table 3 lists the clinical manifestations in the patients with renal disease. The three parameters which concerned us most were the blood pressure, the presence or absence of edema and the ocular fundi. Approximately half of the patients with disseminated lupus erythematosus who have renal

TABLE 3. CLINICAL MANIFESTATIONS

MANIFESTATIONS	WITH RENAL DISEASE		WITHOUT RENAL DISEASE	
	Number*	Per cent (of those with renal disease)	Number*	Per cent (of those without renal disease)
Blood pressure above 140/90	24 (55)	44	2 (34)	6
Edema present	18 (52)	35	0 (34)	0
Abnormal fundi	16 (53)	30	3 (34)	9

* Number in parentheses is the number of patients in whom the presence or absence of the manifestation is known.

disease have hypertension. However, I think the most significant way to state it is that half of the patients with renal disease and lupus do not have hypertension; hence, the absence of hypertension does not indicate the absence of renal disease. However, the presence of hypertension almost invariably indicates the presence of renal involvement. Edema occurred in about one-third of the patients, and the abnormal ocular fundi, showing hemorrhages, exudates, A-V nicking or other abnormalities, similarly occurred in one-third of the group. The presence of hypertension was not a contraindication to treatment with steroids, particularly since, with the advent of the synthetic analogues, salt and fluid retention are so much less likely to occur.

The urinary findings are those one would expect in a patient with renal disease (Table 4); from the examination of the urine, differentiation of lupus nephropathy cannot be made from chronic diffuse glomerulonephritis or from the nephrotic syndrome. All patients with lupus and renal disease in our series had albuminuria, which varied from a trace to very considerable amounts; almost all had hematuria and the majority had casts; several had pyuria.

Extensive renal function studies were performed in this group of patients (Table 5). In addition to renal biopsies, which were obtained in 20 patients, the tests most commonly done were the PSP excretion in 15 minutes and in two hours, the creatinine clearance test, the urine concentration test and the blood urea nitrogen. Of these, the PSP excretion in 15 minutes proved to be the simplest and perhaps the most satisfactory test. The results obtained with the creatinine clearance test were equally satisfactory, but the procedure is more complicated. The PSP excretion in 15 minutes yielded more significant information than did the total PSP excretion over a two-hour period. In the majority of the patients with renal disease, less than 25 per cent of the PSP was excreted in 15 minutes. The urine concentration test proved to be inadequate. Impairment of urine concentration almost always occurred only in the presence of far-advanced renal disease and did not help to pick out the patient with early renal damage. The blood urea nitrogen was elevated in a considerable number of patients, but only late in the course of the illness.

Sixteen, or 30 per cent, of the 56 patients with renal disease had the clinical picture of the nephrotic syndrome, characterized by edema, albuminuria and hypoalbuminemia (Table 6). The course in these 16 patients, both with and without hypercholesterolemia, was disturbing, since ten died within a period of eight months after the onset of the nephrotic syndrome. This occurred despite the fact that several had a satisfactory remission of the other general clinical manifestations of lupus with the administration of either large amounts of steroids or nitrogen mustards. Therefore, the development of nephrosis in the patient with disseminated lupus erythema-

TABLE 4. URINARY FINDINGS IN PATIENTS WITH RENAL DISEASE

MANIFESTATION	NUMBER IN WHICH PRESENT*	PER CENT IN WHICH PRESENT
Albuminuria	56 (56)	100 per cent
Hematuria	49 (55)	88 "
Pyuria	34 (55)	63 "
Casts	38 (55)	70 "

* Number in parentheses is the number of patients in whom the test was done.

TABLE 5. KIDNEY FUNCTION TESTS

TEST	NUMBER OF PATIENTS STUDIED	MEAN	MAXIMUM	MINIMUM	NUMBER OF PATIENTS IN WHOM VALUES WERE ABNORMAL	
					Number	Per cent
Phenolsulphonphthalein excretion in 15 min.* With R.D.	21	16	35	0	13	62
Without R.D.	14	36	65	10	1	7
Phenolsulphonphthalein excretion in 2 hrs.** With R.D.	26	56	90	20	9	35
Without R.D.	19	73	100	40	3	16
Creatinine clearance cc./min.*** With R.D.	9	45	85	12	8	89
Without R.D.	3	86	99	54.5	1	33
Urinary Concentration Test† With R.D.	18	1.017	1.040	1.006	5	28
Without R.D.	14	1.024	1.032	1.016	1	7
Blood urea nitrogen‡ With R.D.	38	70	266	8	26	68
Without R.D.	24	14	20	9	0	0

* Normal, > 25 per cent
** Normal, > 50 per cent
*** Normal, > 80 cc./min.
† Normal, > 1.022
‡ Normal, < 22 mg. per cent
R.D. = Renal disease

TABLE 6.   THE DURATION OF SURVIVAL IN NEPHROSIS IN RELATION
TO THE PRESENCE OR ABSENCE OF HYPERCHOLESTEROLEMIA

MODE OF PRESENTATION	NUMBER OF PATIENTS	NUMBER DIED	MEAN SURVIVAL AFTER ONSET OF NEPHROTIC SYNDROME
Nephrotic syndrome with hypercholesterolemia	10*	8	8 months
Nephrotic syndrome without hypercholesterolemia	6**	2	1 month

* 2 lost to follow-up.
** 1 lost to follow-up.

tosus should be viewed with concern. Remissions of the nephrotic syndrome generally occur with steroid therapy; however, such remissions are temporary.

Table 7 summarizes the course of events in the group with renal disease. Of the 56 patients there have been adequate follow-up data for 51. Of these, 26 have died, and 25 are living. Most of those who died did so within a period of three years, although some lived for as long as seven years. The reneal disease continued to progress, despite remissions occurring either spontaneously or as a result of treatment, with an eventual fatal outcome.

TABLE 7.   SURVIVAL PERIOD OF PATIENTS WITH RENAL DISEASE*

YEARS	DIED	STILL LIVING
Less than 3	22	13
4 to 7	4	12
More than 7	0	0

* Of 26 patients without renal disease in whom the follow-up has been adequate, none have died up to this writing. The period of observation thus far varies from 6 months to 10 years.

Of the 26 deaths in our group of patients, 22 occurred in association with progressive renal failure; in the remaining four patients, death was due to other causes and could have been avoided with the use of present day therapeutic measures.

The Use of Steroids
and Diuretics in the
Treatment of Lupus Nephropathy

LEWIS C. MILLS, GEORGINA FALUDI and
JOHN H. MOYER
Hahnemann Medical College and Hospital, Philadelphia

The kidney is frequently involved in systemic lupus erythematosus. In reported series in the literature proteinuria is present in 50 to 75 per cent of patients.[1] When the incidence is studied by renal biopsy, lesions are found in an even greater number of patients,[5] and in one postmortem series the incidence was found to be 100 per cent,[3] although only 82 per cent of the latter patients had clinical or laboratory evidence of renal disease during life. These figures are not merely of academic interest; in many patients, clinical manifestations of the nephrotic syndrome, lupus nephritis or renal insufficiency are present. The latter has been an important cause of death from this disease in the past and was directly responsible for the patients' deaths in 41 per cent of the cases in the series of Harvey et al.[4]

It is therefore of considerable importance to develop adequate therapeutic approaches to this aspect of systemic lupus erythematosus. There is no doubt about the fact that steroid therapy leads to dramatic clinical improvement in the majority of patients with acute systemic manifestations of the disease, definite benefit often occurring within 48 hours. In many, remission can be maintained with lower doses of steroids and/or administration of antimalarial compounds. In spite of this, there is a divergence of opinion as to the therapeutic efficacy of steroids in the renal disease, both from a clinical and laboratory viewpoint, some authors stating that there is little or no effect[1, 7] and others reporting definite improvement.[1, 2, 6] In addition to this problem of control of the renal lesions, there is also the problem of management of the edema which occurs, either associated with the nephrotic syndrome or as a result of steroid therapy. The following report summarizes the experience in this hospital in the management of and the results obtained in the treatment of lupus nephropathy.

METHODS

The records of all of the patients with a diagnosis of lupus erythematosus admitted to the Hahnemann Hospital in the last ten years were analyzed. From these, 35 patients were found in whom a definite diagnosis was established. In many, treatment had been carried out by other physicians and no attempt had been made to determine the effects of "adequate suppressive doses" as opposed to "minimal suppressive doses" of anti-inflammatory steroids or ACTH. However, in some of the more recently treated patients this method of approach was used and, in addition, there was a tendency to give higher doses over a longer period of time.

RESULTS

Of the 35 patients, 21 had clinical or laboratory evidence of renal disease. In the latter, adequate follow-up information and urinalyses were not available in nine, leaving a total of 12 patients in whom the data were adequate for presentation (Table 1). Five of these patients had clinical and laboratory evidence of the nephrotic syndrome at some time during the observation period; seven had some degree of renal insufficiency, the blood urea nitrogen being over 20 mg. per cent. In 10 of the 12 patients, the acute inflammatory process in the kidney responded to steroids, as judged by complete or almost complete disappearance of red blood cells from the urine. Proteinuria was more resistant to therapy, clearing in only five of the 12 patients; however, it was reduced to minimal levels in two others, bringing the total number responding to seven. In evaluating the total effect of therapy on the kidney as judged by the blood urea nitrogen and urinalysis, the results were considered to be good in six, fair in three and poor in three.

In one of the patients having a poor result (Patient 10, Table 1), red

TABLE 1. EFFECT OF STEROID THERAPY ON LUPUS NEPHROPATHY

| | BLOOD STUDIES | | | | | | URINALYSES | | | | | | THERAPY AND COMMENTS |
| | ESR | | LE cells | | BUN | | Protein | | RBC | | Casts | | |
	Initial	During treatment	Initial	During treatment	Initial	During treatment	Initial	During treatment	Initial	During treatment	Initial	During treatment	
1. L.E. nephritis	32	..	+	..	12	..	2+	0	TNTC	0-1	2-3	0	Rapid disappearance of urinary abnormalities with cortisone in 12 days. Initial dose, 200 mg./day; discharge dose, 60 mg./day.
2. L.E. nephritis	35	15	+	0	38	20	4+	1+	6-8	0-1	10-12	0	Dramatic response to therapy over 29 days. BUN fell to upper limit of normal. Cortisone, 300 mg./day; then methylprednisolone, 80 mg./day. Steroids discontinued after several months. Remission maintained on antimalarial therapy.
3. L.E. nephritis	40	21	0	0	17	9	2+	0	4-6	0	0	0	Urine cleared after 18 days on triamcinolone. 300 mg./day. Discharged on 75 mg./day.
4. L.E. nephritis	37	34	+	..	13	20	2+	tr	TNTC	0	2-4	0	Urine cleared after 18 days on triamcinolone. Initial dose, 64 mg./day; final dose, 12 mg./day.
5. Nephrotic syndrome-renal insufficiency	32	20	+	0	170	38	4+	0	TNTC	0	TNTC	0	Good response to cortisone during 1 year of therapy. Initial dose, 300 mg./day; maintained on 100 mg./day. Some residual but inactive renal disease over next 3 years on prednisone in average dose of 30 mg./day.
6. L.E. nephritis, 1954	43	..	+	..	10	..	1+	..	2-5	..	0	0	Followed for 6 years. No evidence of progression of renal disease; one acute episode during 5th admission controlled by increasing steroid dosage. Controlled during early years with cortisone, 50 to 100 mg./day and later with triamcinolone, 10 mg./day and chloroquine.
2nd admission, 1955		34	..	..	..	..	..	0	..	0	0	0	
3rd admission, 1956		43	..	..	..	..	..	tr	..	0	0	0	
4th admission, 1957		37	..	..	..	8	tr	0	50	2-3	1-2	0	
5th admission, 1958		46	..	0	..	13	..	tr	..	0	0	0	
6th admission, 1959		53	..	..	..	14	..	0	..	0	0	0	
7th admission, 1960		..	..	..	..	..	..	..	..	..	..	..	
7. L.E. nephritis	34	25	+	..	8	..	1+	0	2-4	0-2	0-1	0	Triamcinolone, 32 mg./day gradually reduced to 2 mg./day after 39 days. Partial control of SLE, but high sedimentation rate persisted. During 2nd admission 1 year later for mild clinical recurrence, there was further evidence of renal involvement. Urine cleared on prednisone, 10 mg./day.
2nd admission, L.E. nephritis	..	20	..	..	..	15	2+	0	5-6	0-1	15-20	0-1	
8. Nephrotic syndrome-renal insufficiency	47	13	+	0	255	68	4+	4+	TNTC	2-6	10-12	1-3	Prednisone, 50 mg.; maintenance dose, 25 to 50 mg. Peritoneal dialysis done, but BUN stable at lower level with control of SLE by the 14th week of therapy.

TABLE 1. EFFECT OF STEROID THERAPY ON LUPUS NEPHROPATHY—(Continued)

| | BLOOD STUDIES | | | | | | URINALYSES | | | | | | |
| | ESR | | LE cells | | BUN | | Protein | | RBC | | Casts | | THERAPY AND COMMENTS |
	Initial	During treatment	Initial	During treatment	Initial	During treatment	Initial	During treatment	Initial	During treatment	Initial	During treatment	
9. Nephrotic syndrome-renal insufficiency	23	..	+	..	47	78	4+	4+	TNTC	0	3-4	2-3	Hematuria cleared after 18 days of therapy with ACTH, 20 units every 6 hours. No effect on proteinuria or azotemia. Advanced renal disease.
10. L.E. nephritis	54	54	+	..	14	..	4+	4+	8-10	0	28-30	0	Initial Rx with I.V. ACTH; then prednisone, 15 mg./day. RBC and casts disappeared from urine, but proteinuria and high sedimentation rate persisted. Rapid progression of renal disease at this dose level over 8-month period.
2nd admission, L.E. nephritis	28	..	..	..	..	..	4+	..	1-2	..	10-12	..	
3rd admission, neph. syndrome	..	..	..	..	50	40	4+	..	35-40	..	6-8	..	
11. L.E. nephritis	36	40	+	+	..	..	4+	2+	4-6	TNTC	7-10	0	Moderately good clinical response to cortisone, 300 mg./day. Later received prednisone, 30 mg./day. However, had persistent low grade fever, urinary abnormalities and high sedimentation rate on this dose, and continued to have exacerbations of her disease during 2 years up to 2nd admission. Died with pulmonary edema.
2nd admission, L.E. nephritis	..	..	..	..	90	90	4+	3+	0	20-25	0-2	2-4	
12. Nephrotic syndrome-renal insufficiency	..	..	0	0	52	300	4+	4+	16-18	1-2	12-16	0-1	Died of renal failure. SLE of 7 years duration. On prednisone, 2.5 mg./day prior to this admission. Maximal dose of prednisone, 30 mg./day.

ESR: Erythrocyte sedimentation rate.
I: Values obtained when patient first seen.
DT: Values obtained during therapy.

cells and casts cleared from the urine during the first hospital admission, but proteinuria was unaffected and erythrocyte sedimentation rates remained high on a maintenance dose of prednisone of 15 mg. per day. A few months later proteinuria was still present, with casts and a few red cells in the urine. The sedimentation rate was still elevated at this time. At the time of the third admission, eight months after the patient had first been seen, the blood urea nitrogen was 50 mg. per cent and continued hematuria and cylindruria were present. It seems likely, as judged from other patients treated and evidence of inadequate suppression of the disease from a laboratory standpoint, that steroid therapy in this patient was suboptimal.

In the second patient with a poor response (Patient 11, Table 1), larger doses of anti-inflammatory steroids were used; however, the sedimentation rate remained high, and during the two-year interval between the first and second admissions, the patient had many episodes in which mild to moderate clinical symptoms of lupus erythematosus were present, indicating continued activity of the disease. In this patient, since the dose of prednisone was already in the range in which toxicity is common, higher dosage, at least as a therapeutic trial, should have been given, since the risk of additional toxicity would probably have been minimal.

The third patient (Patient 12, Table 1) having a poor result with corticosteroid therapy had SLE of seven years' duration before admission to Hahnemann Hospital. Renal insufficiency and a nephrotic syndrome were present on admission. He had been taking only insignificant amounts of prednisone (2.5 mg./day) prior to this time. The maximum daily dose of prednisone used during hospitalization was 30 mg. Although it seems likely that he had considerable permanent renal damage at the time of admission, the fact that hematuria almost cleared with steroid therapy indicates that there was some element of acute inflammation in the kidney. Here, again, higher dosage may have been indicated as a therapeutic trial.

TABLE 2. EFFECT OF STEROID DOSAGE ON LUPUS NEPHROPATHY
(PATIENT 8, TABLE 1)

WEEKS	ESR	LE CELLS	BUN	PROTEIN	RBC	CASTS	STEROID	DOSE*
0	47	+	255	4 +	TNTC	10-12	0	..
2	18		180	4 +	TNTC	15-20	Prednisone	50
6			58	4 +	TNTC	0-2	Prednisone	5
10			51				Prednisone	25
14	13	0	68	4 +	2-6	1-3	Prednisone	35
20	12		62	4 +	0-2	0-1	Prednisone	25
24	18		60	4 +	6-8	15-20	Prednisone	25
25	34			4 +	15-20	0-5	Prednisone	25
26	40		76	4 +	TNTC	0-2	Prednisone	25
27				4 +	10-15	0	Prednisone	50
28	32			4 +	5-7	0-1	Prednisone	50
29	30		41	4 +	0	0	Prednisone	50
30				4 +	20-30	0	Prednisone	37.5
31	28		108	4 +	40-50	30-40	Prednisone	25
32	21		122	2 +	5-7	2-7	Prednisone	50
33	12		80	2 +	2-4	3-5	Prednisone	50
34			76	4 +	25-30	30-40	Prednisone	37.5
35				4 +	TNTC	20-30	Prednisone	37.5
36	15			2 +	15-20	0	Prednisone	50
37			51	2 +	10-15	0	Prednisone	50
41				2 +	2-3	0	Prednisone	50
42	32			4 +	12-16	2-4	Prednisone	37.5

* Indicates dose at time of examination. Patient started on next dose listed below immediately after each examination.

The effects of varying the dose of anti-inflammatory steroids on the sedimentation rate, blood urea nitrogen and urinalyses of one of the patients (Patient 8, Table 1) are shown in Table 2. This patient had been treated for systemic lupus erythematosus for a period of three years before she was referred for consultation. Cortisone had been given intermittently on the basis of clinical symptoms. On admission she was severely uremic and had all of the manifestations of the nephrotic syndrome. Following peritoneal dialysis and institution of prednisone therapy, 50 mg. per day, she improved. Subsequently, the dose of prednisone was reduced on three occasions. On

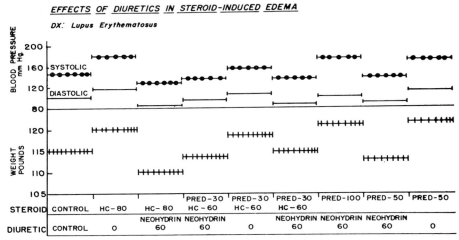

Fig. 1. Note increase in edema and (as judged by increase in patient's weight) blood pressure when hydrocortisone was given; however, this was readily controlled by administration of Neohydrin, 6 tablets daily. When prednisone was added to the regimen, even though the dose of hydrocortisone was reduced slightly, edema increased, and was further intensified when Neohydrin was stopped. The edema responded partially when Neohydrin was again administered, but increased when the dose of prednisone was at the level of 100 mg. per day. When this dose was lowered to 50 mg./day, weight and blood pressure decreased, but again increased when Neohydrin was stopped.

each occasion there was a gradual increase in the number of red blood cells in the urine, indicative of activation of the renal lesions. The process could be controlled by again raising the dose of prednisone, but it appeared to be more difficult to resolve after each period of activation. This illustrates the importance of maintaining adequate suppression of the disease process.

Treatment of the edema associated with nephrotic syndrome may also require intensive therapeutic measures. Of the five patients in this series with nephrosis, edema cleared with continued steroid and diuretic therapy in two, although proteinuria was unchanged in one of these patients. In two other cases edema persisted, although with intensive diuretic therapy it diminished. The fifth patient with nephrosis also had renal insufficiency (Patient 12, Table 1) and died of uremia with persistent edema.

In the treatment of the nephrotic syndrome large doses of anti-inflammatory steroids are of great importance during the initial three or four weeks of therapy. In the patient who had the best response (Patient 5, Table 1), 300 milligrams of cortisone was given per day for several days until adequate control of the basic disease process was obtained. Thereafter, the dose was gradually reduced to 100 milligrams per day and this dosage was maintained during the next 12 months. Because of the salt-retaining properties of this compound, concurrent diuretic therapy was required; Neohydrin, 6 tablets per day, was given. With this regimen the patient became edema-free and protein disappeared from the urine. In the subsequent year, prednisone became available and the patient was transferred to this drug, as initially the sodium-retaining properties of this compound were thought to be minimal. However, diuretic therapy was still required for control of hypertension and mild edema. This is depicted in Figure 1, which shows the effects of altering the dose of both the steroid and Neohydrin.

Occasionally, when the edema of the nephrotic syndrome fails to respond to high-dose steroid therapy given for an adequate period of time, it may be helpful to lower the dose to minimal levels, as sometimes a diuretic phase will occur when this is done. Such was the situation of one of the patients responding in this series (Patient 8, Table 1). This patient initially required peritoneal dialysis because of uremia and fluid retention. Following dialysis and administration of prednisone, 50 mg. per day, some edema persisted even with diuretic therapy. When prednisone was reduced to 5 mg. per day with careful observation, a rapid diuresis occurred and edema disappeared. Subsequently it was possible to control the edema with the previous diuretic therapy even though the dose of prednisone was raised to 50 mg. per day. Sudden reduction of the dose of the steroid carries a considerable degree of risk and should be undertaken with great caution in this group of patients as opposed to those with nephrosis associated with glomerulonephritis, because of the likelihood of an acute exacerbation of the basic disease process in those with lupus. However, in this particular patient, no untoward complications occurred.

DISCUSSION

The data presented indicate that it is possible to control the acute inflammatory involvement in the kidney resulting from the basic abnormality in lupus erythematosus. Patients treated early in the course of the renal lesions with *adequate* suppressive doses of anti-inflammatory steroids will have a satisfactory response, and the renal lesions can often be held static. When the nephrotic syndrome has occurred, or if renal insufficiency is present, therapy is less effective and not always predictable. However, even patients with severe renal insufficiency may occasionally respond when adequate therapy is given, if active disease is present as manifested by clinical symptoms of lupus erythematosus, elevation of the sedimentation rate and hematuria. Although these results are contrary to those obtained by some investigators,[1, 7] others[1, 2, 6] have found that the dosage schedule of steroid therapy has an extremely important bearing on the course of lupus nephropathy.

Ideally, for control, sufficient amounts of anti-inflammatory steroids should be given to suppress all clinical and laboratory evidences of active inflammation to or near normal. When this occurs, the dose should be reduced gradually, following the above indices of activity closely. Adjuvant therapy with antimalarial compounds should be given concurrently, although at the present time there are insufficient data on the effects of the latter drugs on the renal lesion to determine their final therapeutic role in stabilizing the renal process. Unfortunately, the amount of steroids necessary for adequate suppression of the disease process is often in the toxic range, and infection or other well known complications of steroid therapy may occur. Because of this, it may not always be practical to follow the above regimen for a long period of time. However, it is of great importance to try to achieve an initial remission of the disease; once this has occurred, the dose can often be decreased to a level lower than that required for only partial control before a remission has been induced. Although such vigorous therapy may not be indicated in a chronic, non-life-threatening disorder such as rheumatoid arthritis, the course of systemic lupus erythematosus is often short and fatal once clinical manifestations of renal involvement occur. In this situation, higher dosage of steroids seems indicated and necessary if the process is to be controlled; however, extremely careful and frequent follow-up visits are required if side effects of steroid therapy are to be avoided, and prophylactic measures such as administration of antacids and restriction of sodium in the diet should be carried out.

Use of newer improved anti-inflammatory steroids such as triamcinolone or methyl prednisolone should simplify therapy in patients with the nephrotic syndrome, as these two compounds exhibit little, if any, sodium-retaining effect; in fact, there is some evidence to suggest that these drugs may increase sodium and water excretion (Table 3). In addition, newer, more potent

TABLE 3. EFFECT OF TRIAMCINOLONE ON WATER AND
ELECTROLYTE BALANCE

COMPARISON	NUMBER OF PATIENTS	DIETARY SODIUM	URINE VOLUME (ml./24 hours)		URINE SODIUM (mEq./24 hours)		URINE POTASSIUM (mEq./24 hours)	
			1	2	1	2	1	2
C vs. C	19	27	1086	1060	33	26	30	31
C vs. TCL	23	34	1477	1872	37	53	42	53

C: Control period.
TCL: Triamcinolone.
1: Average of 3-day period.
2: Average of next 3-day period.

diuretics are available for prolonged oral administration, such as chlorothiazide or its derivatives. Hospitalization is usually desirable initially so that intensive therapy can be given. Parenteral mercurial diuretics are still probably the most potent compounds available. Once diuresis has been obtained, control can often be maintained with a less potent oral drug. At times in refractory cases the combination of two diuretics, such as a mercurial and a thiazide derivative, is of value. Close attention should also be given to the patient's serum electrolyte concentrations and adequate replacement therapy given as indicated. With such a regimen, it should be possible to control the nephrotic syndrome in most patients.

REFERENCES

1. Cross, R. J., Larson, D., Holman, H., Snyder, A. and Kabat, E.: Combined staff clinic: Systemic lupus erythematosus. Am. J. Med., 28:416, 1960.
2. Dubois, E. L.: Methylprednisolone (Medrol) in the treatment of systemic lupus erythematosus. J.A.M.A., 170:1537, 1959.
3. Griffith, G. C. and Vural, I. L.: Acute and subacute disseminated lupus erythematosus. Circulation, 3:492, 1951.
4. Harvey, A. M., Shulman, L. E., Tummulty, P. A., Conley, C. L. and Shoenrich, E. H.: Systemic lupus erythematosus: review of literature and clinical analysis of 138 cases. Medicine, 33:291, 1954.

5. Muehrcke, R. C., Kark, R. M., Pirani, C. L. and Pollak, V. E.: Lupus nephritis: a clinical and pathologic study on renal biopsies. Medicine, 36:1, 1957.
6. Pollak, V. E.: The effect of large doses of prednisone on the clinical and histological progression of lupus glomerulonephritis. In Mills, L. C. and Moyer, J. H. (eds.): Inflammation and Diseases of Connective Tissues. Philadelphia, W. B. Saunders Co., 1961, p. 729.
7. Soffer, L. F.: Effect of steroid therapy on acute lupus nephropathy. In Mills, L. C. and Moyer, J. H. (eds.): Inflammation and Diseases of Connective Tissues. Philadelphia, W. B. Saunders Co., 1961, p. 717.

The Effect of Large Doses of Prednisone on the Clinical and Histological Progression of Lupus Glomerulonephritis*

VICTOR E. POLLAK

University of Illinois College of Medicine

In 1957 a detailed study of the natural history of renal involvement in systemic lupus erythematosus (SLE) was reported from this laboratory.[3] Serial clinical studies and serial tests of renal function and percutaneous renal biopsies from 31 patients ill with SLE were discussed in detail. On the basis of the histology in the initial renal biopsy, the patients were divided into three groups:

1. Those in whom the initial renal biopsy was *normal.*

2. Those in whom *lupus glomerulitis* was diagnosed in the initial renal biopsy. The term "glomerulitis" was used to indicate proliferative and/or membranous lesions of the glomerular tufts in the absence of any tubular damage or changes in the interstitial tissue.

3. Those in whom *lupus glomerulonephritis* was diagnosed in the initial renal biopsy. The term "glomerulonephritis" was used to indicate a proliferative and/or membranous lesion of the glomeruli associated with tubular and interstitial tissue changes. The glomerular lesions were invariably mild in lupus glomerulitis and were very much more severe in lupus glomerulonephritis.[3]

These patients were first studied in 1953 to 1955, and were treated with only sufficient cortisone or hydrocortisone to control their clinical symptoms. They received, on the average, 50 mg. of cortisone daily.

Eleven of these patients had *normal* renal biopsies at the time of the initial study. Seven are still living an average of five and a half years after the initial renal biopsy and none has severe renal disease. Three have died

* This study was supported by Grant H-2253(c) from the National Institutes of Health, U. S. Public Health Service, and Contract DA-49-007-MD-637 from the Surgeon General's Office, U. S. Army.

and one has been lost to follow-up. Of the three patients who died, none died of renal failure but two had histologic evidence post mortem of renal involvement by SLE.

Lupus glomerulitis was diagnosed in the initial renal biopsy of ten patients. Five are living an average of five and a half years later and do not have significant decompensation of renal function. The other five died. One patient died of accidental carbon monoxide poisoning six years after the initial renal biopsy; there was no evidence of progressive renal disease three months before his death. The other four patients with lupus glomerulitis have died in renal failure an average of 40 months after the initial renal biopsy.

Lupus glomerulonephritis was diagnosed in the initial renal biopsy of ten patients. All of these patients died an average of 13.8 months after the initial renal biopsy. Eight died of renal failure and two died when severely azotemic with acute exacerbations of SLE. From these studies it was apparent that the prognosis of lupus glomerulonephritis was very grave and that cortisone in the dosage used (an average of 50 mg. daily) did not significantly affect the course of lupus glomerulonephritis.

When these results became available to us, we decided to treat a second series of patients with lupus glomerulonephritis, using large doses of prednisone for a minimum period of six months. This decision was made because of a chance observation on one patient diagnosed as having lupus glomerulonephritis. Her systemic illness was so severe that for more than six months 150 to 300 mg. of cortisone each day was required to control her symptoms. Serial studies indicated no significant deterioration of renal function nor of renal histology during this time. In all other patients with lupus glomerulonephritis studied, there had been definite clinical, functional and histologic evidence of progression of the renal lesions while the patients were treated with small doses of cortisone. In addition, we believed on theoretical grounds that it was possible that the prolonged administration of large doses of cortisone might influence the renal lesions favorably by suppressing effectively the antibody-producing mechanism.

From 1956 to 1958 every patient in whom a diagnosis of lupus glomerulonephritis was made in the first renal biopsy was treated deliberately for a period of approximately six months with large doses of prednisone, irrespective of the clinical symptoms. No patient received less than 40 mg. of prednisone daily, and the average dose was 47.5 mg. daily. At the end of the six-month period, a second renal biopsy was done and the dosage of prednisone was lowered gradually to between 15 and 25 mg. daily. The sole criterion for admission of patients to this series was the histological diagnosis of lupus glomerulonephritis in the first renal biopsy.

The first series of patients with lupus glomerulonephritis, studied initially from 1953 to 1955 and treated with an average of 50 mg. of cortisone daily, is referred to hereafter as *the low steroid group.* The second series of patients with lupus glomerulonephritis, studied initially from 1956 to 1958, is referred to hereafter as *the high steroid group.* Except for the dose of cortisone or prednisone, the treatment of the two groups of patients was the same. It should be pointed out that our first experiences with the use of large doses of prednisone in the treatment of lupus glomerulonephritis were so gratifying that we considered it to be unjustifiable ethically to treat patients by random allocation to two series, one receiving small and the other large doses of prednisone. For this reason, we considered that it was particularly important to demonstrate that the two series of patients with lupus glomerulonephritis were comparable when the first renal biopsy was done and before treatment was started.

It was shown that the duration of SLE, the known duration of renal involvement, and the initial blood pressure readings were similar at the outset in the two series of patients.[4] It was also shown that the renal function at the time of the initial biopsy was comparable in the two groups save for the fact that the serum urea nitrogen level was greater than 30 mg./100 ml. in five of the ten patients in the low steroid group and in five of 16 patients in the high steroid group.[4] A detailed analysis of the histologic findings showed that they were comparable in the initial renal biopsies in the two series of patients.[4] The methods of detailed semiquantitative analysis used to score the histologic changes have been described previously.[3, 4]

RESULTS

The effect of treatment on survival is shown in Table 1 and Figure 1. The initial serum urea nitrogen level was greater than 30 mg./100 ml. in five patients in the low steroid group. All died, on the average 15.0 months after the initial renal biopsy. The initial serum urea nitrogen level was less than 30 mg./100 ml. in the other five patients in the low steroid group. They survived, on the average, 12.8 months.

TABLE 1. SURVIVAL TIME IN LUPUS GLOMERULONEPHRITIS IN RELATION TO RENAL FUNCTION AT TIME TREATMENT WAS STARTED

RENAL FUNCTION WHEN TREATMENT WAS STARTED	LOW STEROID*			HIGH STEROID†		
	Number of patients	Number alive	Average survival time (months)	Number of patients	Number alive	Average survival time (months)
Serum urea nitrogen ≦ 30 mg./100 ml. or Serum nonprotein nitrogen ≦ 45 mg./100 ml.	5	0	12.8	11	9	33.8‡
Serum urea nitrogen > 30 mg./100 ml. or Serum nonprotein nitrogen > 45 mg./100 ml.	5	0	15.0	5	0	6.5

* Patients studied initially 1953-1955.[3]
† Patients studied initially 1956-1958.[4]
‡ Survival time of 2 patients; duration of follow-up on 9.
(From Pollak, V. E. et al.[4]: J. Lab. & Clin. Med., 57:495-511, 1961, by permission of The C. V. Mosby Company, publishers.)

In the high steroid group the initial serum urea nitrogen level was higher than 30 mg./100 ml. in five patients. All five died in uremia, three within one month, one five months and one 26 months after treatment began. The initial serum urea nitrogen level was less than 30 mg./100 ml. in 11 patients in the high steroid group. Only two have died, 22 months and 41 months, respectively, after starting treatment with large doses of prednisone. The exact cause of death could not be determined clinically or by postmortem examination. There was no evidence of deterioration of renal function three months and one week, respectively, before death. The other nine patients are living, on the average, 33.8 months after treatment with large doses of prednisone was started. In none is there evidence of progressive deterioration of renal function.

The effect of treatment on the survival and renal histologic findings is shown in Figure 1 (A and B). In all, 25 serial renal histologic studies were made on 8 patients in the low steroid group, and 37 serial studies were made

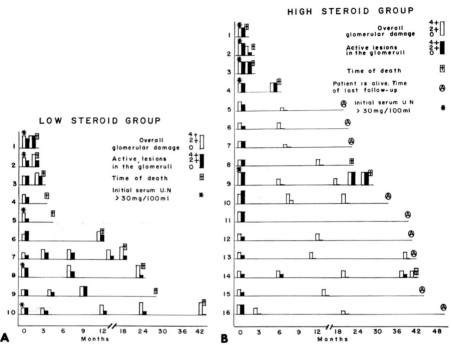

Fig. 1.　Summary of the over-all glomerular damage and of the activity of the glomerular lesions in two groups of patients with lupus glomerulonephritis: (A) those treated symptomatically with small doses of cortisone, (B) those treated with large doses of prednisone for six months. In the low steroid group the over-all glomerular damage increased with the passage of time, and histologic activity persisted. In the high steroid group the over-all glomerular damage did not increase, and histologic activity decreased or disappeared in most patients. (Reproduced by permission of The C. V. Mosby Company from Pollak, V. E. et al.[4]: J. Lab. & Clin. Med., 57:495-511, 1961.)

on 14 patients in the high steroid group. The degree of over-all glomerular damage and of activity of the lesions in the glomeruli of each biopsy and autopsy specimen are plotted for each patient in Figure 1 on a scale from 0 to 4+. In the low steroid group (Figure 1A), over-all glomerular damage increased with the passage of time; histologic evidence of activity persisted throughout the period of study except in Patient 10, who died with "end stage kidneys." In the high steroid group (Figure 1B), the over-all glomerular damage was unchanged or decreased with the passage of time (Patients 9 and 16). Histologic evidence of activity persisted in Patients 2, 3 and 4; histologic evidence of activity decreased in Patient 10, and it disappeared completely in the other ten patients. In the glomeruli of these patients, thickening of the capillary basement membrane, a few wire loop lesions and adhesions between the glomerular tuft and Bowman's capsule persisted.

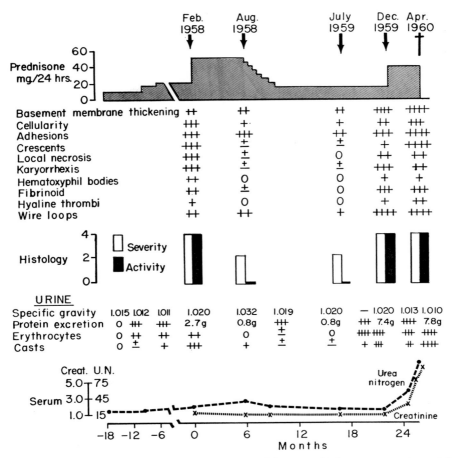

					Feb. 1958	Aug. 1958		July 1959	Dec. 1959	Apr. 1960

Prednisone mg./24 hrs. 60 40 20 0

Basement membrane thickening					++	++		++	+++	++++
Cellularity					+++	+·		+	++	+++
Adhesions					+++	+++		±	+++	++++
Crescents					+++	±		±	+	++++
Local necrosis					+++	±		0	++	++
Karyorrhexis					+++	±		±	+++	++
Hematoxyphil bodies					++	0		0	+	+
Fibrinoid					++	±		0	+++	+++
Hyaline thrombi					+	0		0	+	++
Wire loops					++	++		+	++++	++++

Histology 4 2 0   □ Severity ■ Activity

URINE

Specific gravity	1.015	1.012	1.011	1.020		1.032	1.019	1.020	— 1.020	1.013 1.010
Protein excretion	0	+++	+++	2.7g		0.8g	+++	0.8g	+++ 7.4g	+++ 7.8g
Erythrocytes	0	++	++	++		0	±	0	+++ +++	+++ +++
Casts	0	±	+	+++		+	±	±	+ +++	++ +++

Creat. U.N. 5.0 ┬ 75 Serum 3.0 ┼ 45 1.0 ┴ 15

Urea nitrogen

Creatinine

-18 -12 -6 0 6 12 18 24

Months

Fig. 2. Summary of the serial histologic and laboratory findings in a patient with lupus glomerulonephritis. Systemic lupus erythematosus was first diagnosed in this patient 20 months before the initial renal biopsy. A severe acute exacerbation of SLE was treated successfully with 25 to 50 mg. of prednisone daily and she was discharged from the hospital and followed in the outpatient clinic. At this time she was treated with prednisone 10 mg. daily. Evidence of renal involvement appeared *first* while the patient was receiving 10 mg. of prednisone daily, and abnormal urinalyses persisted thenceforth. When the first renal biopsy was done the lesions were extremely severe and very active. Treatment with large doses of prednisone for six months, from February to August 1958, resulted in a decrease in severity of the lesions and a remarkable decrease in the activity. Note particularly the disappearance of fibroepithelial crescents, local necrosis, karyorrhexis, hematoxyphil bodies, fibrinoid and hyaline thrombi. The dosage of prednisone was subsequently lowered gradually to a level of 15 mg. daily. In the third biopsy, in July 1959, note that the histologic improvement was maintained. Subsequently, however, while the patient was still receiving prednisone, 15 mg. daily, a second episode of severe renal involvement occurred and this failed to respond to prednisone 40 mg. daily. Note the reappearance of the histologic signs of activity in the biopsy taken in December 1959. Note, also, the fact that the initial successful treatment with large doses of prednisone resulted not in a normal glomerulus, but in a glomerulus in which diffuse capillary basement membrane thickening was the predominant change. These observations are typical of those in the patients who were treated successfully for active lupus glomerulonephritis with large doses of prednisone.

In summary, severe active lupus glomerulonephritis appeared for the first time and progressed while the patient was on small doses of prednisone; the progression of the renal lesions was halted by the use of large doses of prednisone; active lupus glomerulonephritis subsequently recurred while the patient was again receiving small doses of prednisone. (Reproduced by permission of The C. V. Mosby Company from Pollak, V. E. et al.[4]: J. Lab. & Clin. Med., 57:495-511, 1961.)

Fibrinoid, local necrosis, karyorrhexis, hematoxyphil bodies and hyaline thrombi disappeared. One patient (No. 9) had a second recrudescence of active lesions 11 months after the dosage of prednisone was reduced to 15 mg. daily.

A typical example of the effects of small and large doses of prednisone in the individual patient is shown in Figure 2.

DISCUSSION

The two groups of patients with lupus glomerulonephritis were comparable when they were first studied. From the data presented it is clear that treatment with large doses of prednisone for six months increased the life span of the patients, delayed the onset of renal failure and led to the disappearance of the active renal lesions.

The histologic data presented in Figures 1 and 2 are summarized in terms of severity and activity of the renal lesions. The activity of the renal lesions was graded in terms of the presence and severity of local necrosis, karyorrhexis, hematoxyphil bodies, fibrinoid and hyaline thrombi. The evidence that these histologic parameters were signs of active and rapidly progressive renal lesions has been presented elsewhere.[3, 4]

When the study of the effects of large doses of prednisone on lupus glomerulonephritis was initiated, it was thought that this treatment might decrease or suppress completely those histologic features indicative of activity. The data in Figure 1B indicate clearly that this objective was attained in 10 of the 16 patients studied serially and treated with large doses of prednisone.

Three patients, however, who had severe azotemia and very severely damaged glomeruli, died after less than one month of treatment with large doses of prednisone. Serial histologic studies in two (Figure 1B, Patients 2 and 3) suggested that, if the patients had survived, a longer period of treatment would have been necessary to achieve suppression of the active lesions. The striking decrease in the activity of the renal lesions in two other patients with less severe azotemia (Figure 1B, Patients 9 and 10) indicated that adequate treatment was effective if started early enough, even when the kidneys were very severely involved.

It is common practice for the dosage of prednisone used to control the *systemic* manifestations of SLE to be regulated by the clinical response to treatment, but, in point of fact, treatment should be adequate to suppress effectively *all* disease activity.[6] Relatively small amounts of the drug suffice in many patients, but occasionally as much as 100 mg. of prednisone daily, or more, is necessary. Unfortunately, we had no satisfactory clinical or biochemical criteria to assess whether or not effective suppression of active renal lesions had been achieved. The dose of 40 to 60 mg. of prednisone daily was chosen because we thought that this dose of the drug would suppress the active renal lesions effectively in most patients. In one instance, however, the activity of the renal lesions was not affected by treatment with prednisone, 55 mg. daily, for five months (Figure 1B, Patient 4). In another (Patient 9), the active renal lesions were suppressed completely by treatment with 50 mg. of prednisone daily, but a later exacerbation was unaffected by treatment with 40 mg. of prednisone daily. That complete suppression of histologic activity was not achieved in every patient is not surprising, as the dosage used was chosen arbitrarily and its effects on the kidney could not be assessed adequately by clinical observations.

When this study was planned, it was decided to treat the patients for six months before reducing the dosage of prednisone below 40 mg. daily. Except in one patient, this empirically chosen period was adhered to rigidly because of the lack of valid and reliable clinical and biochemical criteria of activity of the renal lesions. Clearly, in view of the complications of this treatment, it is probably desirable to use such large doses of prednisone only until adequate and complete suppression of the activity of the renal lesions has been attained. For these reasons we have studied recently the relationship between the titer of antinuclear factors in the serum on the one hand, and the clinical activity of SLE and histologic activity of the renal lesions on the other.[2] A relationship was found between clinical activity of SLE and the titer of antinuclear factors. Most patients with active renal lesions had high titers of antinuclear factors in the serum, but enough serial studies have not yet been done to make this a reliable test in determining the duration of therapy in lupus glomerulonephritis.

Thickening of the glomerular basement membrane, with or without fibrinoid, has been observed as a constant feature of the histology of lupus nephritis.[3] In other diseases affecting the kidney, e.g., membranous glomerulonephritis, our observations and those of others indicate that significant thickening of the glomerular basement membrane is a permanent change and that it is not affected by treatment with cortisone, prednisone or other drugs.[1, 5] In lupus nephritis, likewise, simple thickening of the glomerular basement membrane, without fibrinoid, was not influenced significantly by treatment with low or high doses of prednisone. Adhesions between the glomerular tuft and Bowman's capsule also persisted. However, the use of large doses of prednisone resulted in the disappearance or decrease of the histologic signs of activity. Complete suppression of active lesions with little or no residual chronic damage occurred only in the less severely involved cases. When the active lesions had been suppressed in the more severely involved glomeruli, permanent changes such as local fibrosis, glomerular adhesions and diffuse capillary basement membrane thickening were invariable residua. The majority of the glomerular capillaries remained patent, and rapidly progressive destruction of functioning glomeruli was halted. Unless fresh active lesions develop in the future, it is probable that progressive changes in these glomeruli will occur slowly and that renal failure will be delayed for a long period of time.

ACKNOWLEDGMENTS

The prednisone used throughout this study was kindly supplied as Meticorten through the courtesy of Dr. C. J. Szmal, the Schering Corporation, Bloomfield, New Jersey.

We wish to thank the Editor, Dr. William D. Robinson, and the publishers of the Journal of Laboratory and Clinical Medicine, The C. V. Mosby Company, for permission to quote from and reproduce figures from the data originally presented in that journal (Pollak, V. E., Pirani, C. L. and Kark, R. M.: The effect of large doses of prednisone on the renal lesions and life span of patients with lupus glomerulonephritis. J. Lab. & Clin. Med., 57: 495-511, 1961).

REFERENCES

1. Blainey, J. D., Brewer, D. B., Hardwicke, J. and Soothill, J. F.: The nephrotic syndrome. Diagnosis by renal biopsy and immunological analyses related to the response to steroid therapy. Quart. J. Med., 29:235, 1960.
2. Mandema, E., Pollak, V. E., Kark, R. M. and Rezaian, J.: Quantitative observations on antinuclear factors in systemic lupus erythematosus. J. Lab. & Clin. Med. To be published (September 1961).
3. Muehrcke, R. C., Kark, R. M., Pirani, C. L. and Pollak, V. E.: Lupus nephritis: a clinical and pathologic study based on renal biopsies. Medicine, 36:1, 1957.
4. Pollak, V. E., Pirani, C. L. and Kark, R. M.: The effect of large doses of prednisone on the renal lesions and life span of patients with lupus glomerulonephritis. J. Lab. & Clin. Med., 57:495-511, 1961.
5. Pollak, V. E., Pirani, C. L. and Kark, R. M.: Unpublished observations.
6. Soffer, L. J.: The therapy of systemic lupus erythematosus. J. Mount Sinai Hosp., 26:297, 1959.

Effect of Steroids in Nephrosis

C. W. DAESCHNER, JR. and WARREN F. DODGE

University of Texas Medical Branch, Galveston

In earlier portions of this volume detailed accounts are given concerning the possible mechanisms operable in the development of hypersensitivity states generally and the nephrotic state specifically. In addition, the manner in which adrenal glucocorticoids may modify these events has been described. Others have discussed the more complex problem of nephrosis in relation to systemic lupus erythematosus, chronic glomerulonephritis and diabetes mellitus. A consideration of the effects of steroid therapy on the nephrotic syndrome may, therefore, reasonably be limited to answering the question: How effective have the steroids been in modifying the clinical course of patients with the nephrotic syndrome?

Although the nephrotic syndrome is generally thought of as an entity, it is in fact a symptom complex representing a wide variety of etiologic circumstances and a variable spectrum of renal histologic changes. This has led to some disparity among reports concerning the clinical effectiveness of steroid therapy in nephrosis. For this reason, any consideration of the treatment of nephrosis must begin by defining not only the clinical circumstances, but also the type and degree of renal histologic change.

In this paper, only patients with the idiopathic or "pure" nephrotic syndrome, sometimes called lipoid nephrosis, will be considered. This is the form of the disease usually seen in childhood and in most instances characterized histologically by mild to moderate diffuse thickening of the glomerular basement membrane. Some adults (especially young adults) manifesting clinical evidence of the nephrotic syndrome demonstrate this same renal lesion, but more often the adult subject is found to have long-standing, destructive renal disease and reduced renal function. The latter patients are usually not improved by steroid therapy and, if given steroids, they may show progressive edema, hypertension and azotemia.[1]

THE IDIOPATHIC NEPHROTIC SYNDROME OF SHORT DURATION

The influence of steroid therapy on the course of the idiopathic form of the nephrotic syndrome may be divided conveniently into two areas: (1) the immediate clinical response and (2) the long-term prognosis. At this time sufficient experience has not accumulated to state the latter with certainty. However, the clinical results of the last ten years clearly support the effectiveness of steroids in the control of the patient's signs and symptoms.

Influence of Steroids on the Clinical Course. In the typical patient with the nephrotic syndrome there is the insidious onset of massive edema, marked proteinuria, hypoproteinemia (principally hypoalbuminemia) and hyperlipemia. Though uncommon, the presence of a mild degree of hypertension, hematuria and/or azotemia is compatible with the diagnosis. Such patients demonstrate nearly normal renal histology when renal tissue is examined by standard H & E stains, and only mild, diffuse glomerular basement membrane thickening by PAS staining technique. Electron microscopy of the glomerulus usually demonstrates moderate basement membrane thickening and loss of the foot processes from the glomerular tuft epithelial cells.[3] Uncertainty exists as to whether the first change occurs in the glomerular basement membrane or in the epithelial cell foot processes, but most workers favor the former as the site of the primary event. In any case these changes parallel the appearance of proteinuria, which is the cardinal finding in this disease.

Patients with proteinuria of short duration are the best candidates for steroid therapy, and good results may be anticipated if an adequate dosage is utilized and treatment is begun promptly. Delay in the institution of steroid therapy beyond four months after the appearance of symptoms not only decreases the chances of successful therapy but may delay the complete clearing of proteinuria in those who do respond.

An adequate dosage is usually considered to be in the range of 40 to 50 mg. per square meter of body surface area per day of a delta-1 steroid (e.g., prednisone) or its equivalent* given in divided doses every six hours. This daily dose stated in terms of body weight is approximately 1 mg. per pound in infancy, 0.75 mg. per pound in the preschool child, 0.67 mg. per pound in the older child and 0.5 mg. per pound in adolescent and adult patients. The details of steroid therapy have been described previously.[2]

Treatment must usually be continued for 10 to 14 days and occasionally for as long as 28 days before proteinuria ceases. It is important that, whenever possible, the *total absence* of proteinuria be taken as the end point for treatment rather than *diuresis*, since the latter often precedes complete clearing of protein from the urine. If treatment is discontinued prematurely, recurrent proteinuria is likely. As the proteinuria and edema clear, the total serum protein value returns to normal and the various protein moieties achieve a normal distribution more gradually. Usually the last item to return to normal is the elevated serum lipids. At this point the patient has no clinical or chemical evidence of the nephrotic syndrome. His resistance to infections is normal, as are his appetite and general physical vigor. In many patients a period of prophylactic steroid therapy† introduced at this point and con-

---

* Equivalent therapeutic daily doses per square meter of body surface area are approximately as follows: cortisone 250 mg., hydrocortisone 200 mg., prednisone 50 mg., methylprednisone 50 mg., prednisolone 40 mg., triamcinolone 40 mg., and dexamethasone 7.5 mg.

† Prophylactic steroids (e.g., prednisone) are given three consecutive days each week in a dose of 30 mg. per square meter per day divided into three equal doses.

tinued for six months to a year may minimize the tendency to recurrence. In certain patients in whom proteinuria fails to clear completely during the period of intensive steroid therapy, it may do so during prolonged prophylactic steroid administration. In either case, daily examination of the urine at home for proteinuria is an essential feature of management if the earliest recurrences of proteinuria are to be detected and re-treated promptly (i.e., within one to two days and prior to the return of edema). Such an approach to treatment will not only minimize proteinuria, but will also prevent recurrences of edema. In these respects, then, the control of the clinical signs and symptoms with steroids can be said to improve the immediate outlook for these patients and significantly prolong their lives. These patients are to all appearances well at this point, though experience tells us that they still retain a propensity to new episodes of proteinuria following a variety of antigenic challenges (e.g., acute infections, immunizations, insect bites, etc.).

Steroids and the Renal Lesion. The central problem in establishing the long-term prognosis in patients with the idiopathic nephrotic syndrome lies in the evaluation of the influence of successful clinical therapy on the underlying glomerular lesion. It is well established that in untreated nephrosis the mild membranous thickening of the glomerular tuft will by successive stages go on to the sclerotic, hyalinized, nonfunctioning glomerulus of terminal renal insufficiency. The *basic objective* of steroid therapy is to prevent the latter course of events and to preserve kidney function. Several workers have shown that the disappearance of proteinuria parallels the return of the epithelial cell foot processes, and these cells appear to return to complete normalcy. Changes in the basement membrane are less predictably influenced. Serial renal biopsy studies have been helpful in evaluating this point. Our own experience and that of others suggests that a few patients with very minimal basement membrane changes prior to treatment may appear to have entirely normal glomeruli following steroid-induced remission of proteinuria. Similar studies in other patients suggest that although the basement membrane changes present before steroid therapy are not abolished, they do not progress during periods when the patient is free of proteinuria. However, certain patients have been followed in whom some degree of progressive glomerular scarring was demonstrated during periods in which there was no detectable proteinuria. These patients have been in a minority in our experience, but they constitute an important group prognostically. Whether this represents new and progressive renal disease or merely the influence of aging on the histologic appearance of the original basement membrane changes is often difficult to decide. If progressive glomerular scarring is occurring in patients in clinical remission, it would appear that at least the rate of change is slower than would be expected for the untreated nephrotic. The question then becomes whether successful steroid therapy prevents glomerular scarring entirely or merely slows the succession of events. Only much more clinical experience coupled with careful light and electron microscopic evaluation of serial renal biopsy specimens can settle this question with certainty. In any event, present evidence would encourage us to use steroid therapy as the cornerstone of treatment in patients with the nephrotic syndrome.

THE IDIOPATHIC NEPHROTIC SYNDROME OF LONG DURATION

The patient who has experienced many months of nephrotic proteinuria has a more complex therapeutic problem and a more guarded prognosis.

The Clinical Signs and Symptoms. These patients usually show evidence of chronic illness and long-standing massive protein loss. There is often a tendency for edema to be less apparent in their thin extremities, but ascites is very noticeable. The degree of hypoalbuminemia and hyperlipemia is extreme. Although a therapeutic program similar to that described earlier should be tried initially, the failure rate is high and some patients show no evidence of a therapeutic response. In others, gradually decreasing proteinuria encourages the physician to continue, and, in a few, complete cessation of proteinuria ensues. The quantitative determination of urine protein excretion is often helpful in the evaluation of the course of these patients, particularly when improvement is so gradual as to be discouraging to both the physician and his patient. A progressive fall in the quantity of urine protein may provide the only interim index of therapeutic response.

Renal Histology. Examination of the renal biopsy specimens from patients with long-standing proteinuria usually reveals more definite morphologic changes. These vary from glomerular basement membrane thickening and a tendency to tuft lobulation to glomerular sclerosis. In many of these patients the biopsy specimen reveals a spectrum of disease, sometimes of such severity as to make it difficult to differentiate on a histologic basis late idiopathic nephrosis from other forms of chronic nephritis. These glomerular scars are not likely to regress in response to steroid therapy, and one can only hope that they will remain static. It has been suspected that in some patients the reduction in proteinuuria may be due to progressive glomerular sclerosis and ischemia rather than to a decrease in glomerular membrane permeability. Our experience would suggest that in patients who tolerate steroid therapy well (i.e., show no evidence of progressive hypertension, edema or azotemia during treatment) the reduction in proteinuria is due to decreased glomerular membrane permeability and not to progressive glomerular sclerosis.

Although steroid therapy is not as consistently effective in these patients as in those first discussed, it offers the most likely means of preserving their remaining renal function if well tolerated. In some of these patients steroids may be as effective as they are in nephrosis of short duration.

REFERENCES

1. Daeschner, C. W. and Dodge, W. F.: Specific and supportive therapy of patients with the nephrotic syndrome. In Moyer, J. H. and Fuchs, M.: Edema: Mechanisms and Management. Philadelphia, W. B. Saunders Co., 1960, p. 553.
2. Daeschner, C. W., Dodge, W. F. and Hill, L. L.: Management of the nephrotic syndrome, with particular reference to the use of triamcinolone. J. Pediat., 56:48, 1960.
3. Farquhar, M. G., Vernier, R. L. and Good, R. A.: An electron microscope study of the glomerulus in nephrosis, glomerulonephritis and lupus erythematosus. J. Exper. Med., 106:649, 1957.

Effect of Steroid Therapy on the Rate of Progress of Glomerular Changes of Chronic Glomerulonephritis as Studied by Serial Renal Biopsy*

DANIEL S. KUSHNER, S. HOWARD ARMSTRONG, JR., PAUL B. SZANTO, EUGENE SCHUPAK and MICHAEL GLYNN

Hektoen Institute for Medical Research of the Cook County Hospital, Northwestern University Medical School, University of Illinois College of Medicine and Chicago Medical School

A full understanding of the natural history of the nephrotic syndrome in the adult requires: (1) knowledge of the prognosis—variables and limits for each etiologic entity in the untreated state; (2) critical evaluation of responsiveness to therapy at various stages of impaired function and altered structure; and, perhaps most important, (3) an assessment of the histogenesis of the renal lesion and its modification by therapy.

Existing studies have suggested variously that minimal membranous glomerulonephritis is the most commonly encountered lesion in the nephrotic state,[1, 12] that in its presence a therapeutic response to steroids is more likely to be anticipated,[1, 21] to the contrary, that membranous glomerulonephritis accounts for only 20 per cent of nephrotics,[3, 4, 9, 10, 16, 20] and that patients with membranous lesions are unlikely to respond.[4] Limited studies reported to date of histologic alterations during steroid therapy have suggested reversal to normal of minimal foot process changes demonstrable only by electron microscopy in otherwise normal-appearing renal biopsies,[18] a change recently ascribed to proteinuria as a secondary phenomenon. Few have observed in serial renal biopsy either the regressive or progressive histopathologic changes in association with improvement or resistance to steroid therapy specifically in the nephrotic states of glomerulonephritis, as compared with the untreated state.[4, 5, 6, 8, 11, 19, 22, 23]

The present study of Cook County Hospital adult nephrotics excluded patients with nephrosclerosis, S.L.E., amyloidosis, renal vein thrombosis and diabetes mellitus. Thirty patients remained, with histologic diagnoses of a variant of diffuse glomerulonephritis. Follow-up periods ranged from 2 to 84 months. Our experience with three initial therapeutic failures, following the administration of intermittent corticotropin therapy (80 mg. ACTH gel for 10-day periods), which appeared either to precipitate or accelerate renal insufficiency, discouraged for several years further attempts by us to alter the course of the nephrotic stage of glomerulonephritis, thus providing for analysis the course of 16 untreated patients.

* This work has been made possible by Grants A927 and A1300 from the National Institutes of Health of the United States Public Health Service.

In view of the appalling mortality rate in our nephrotic-nephritic population, exceeding 60 per cent at two years and approaching 90 per cent at four years,[2] we embarked upon an attempt to evaluate the efficacy of intensive-dosage long-term continuous steroid therapy, with serial biopsy evaluations of renal structural alterations in correlation with clinical, functional and biochemical response.[7, 13, 14, 15, 17]

Therapy consisted of prednisolone in an initial dosage of 125 mg./day maintained either until maximum response was obtained or until reduction in level was forced by a complication; maintenance dosage averaged about 37.5 mg./day. Treatment was discontinued only if after six months no amelioration in any aspect of the nephrotic state had been achieved. Renal biopsies, obtained whenever possible, were performed at intervals ranging

TABLE 1. RACE IN SURVIVAL OF NEPHROTIC GLOMERULONEPHRITICS

	NEGRO	SURVIVAL IN MONTHS, MEAN (RANGE)	CAUCASIAN	SURVIVAL IN MONTHS, MEAN (RANGE)
Alive	7*	29 (5-63)	8	37 (10-84)
Dead	14	19 (2-43)	1	33
Total	21	22	9	36

* One patient (G. Ba.) lost to follow-up in the 28th month.

from 1 to 40 months after the onset of edema, a total of 18 biopsies being performed in 8 intensively treated patients.

Fifteen of the entire series of 30 patients have survived. Consideration of race as a possible variable in survival rates (Table 1) reveals a 70 per cent predominance of Negroes in our material, with a mortality rate of 66 per cent and a mean duration of only 19 months to death. Among the 9 Caucasians, only one died at 33 months, and 8 were surviving at a mean duration of disease of 37 months. The over-all mean survival was only 22 months in the Negro, as contrasted with 36 months in the Caucasian.

TABLE 2. STEROID TREATMENT IN SURVIVAL OF NEPHROTIC
GLOMERULONEPHRITICS

	LIVING	MEAN DURATION OF FOLLOW-UP	DEAD	DURATION FROM ONSET
No steroids	5*	40 (28-63)	11	20 (2-43)
Minimal steroids	3	40 (16-84)	3	24 (14-40)
Intensive steroids	7	25 (5-45)	1	10
Total	15	33 (5-84)	15	20 (2-43)

* One patient (G. Ba.) lost to follow-up in the 28th month.

TABLE 3. INTERACTION OF RACE AND INTENSITY OF STEROID
THERAPY IN SURVIVAL

	UNTREATED (OR MINIMAL)			INTENSIVE STEROIDS			Grand Total
	Dead	Alive	Subtotal	Dead	Alive	Subtotal	
Negro	13	3	16	1	4	5	21
White	1	5	6	0	3	3	9
Total	14	8	22	1	7	8	30

Steroid treatment had been offered to 10 of the 15 who survived and to only 4 of the 15 who died (Table 2). Although the numbers in each category are small, it would appear that minimal steroids offer little or no advantage over none. Half of those surviving have been treated intensively, but only one of the 15 dead had been so treated.

TABLE 4. INITIAL HISTOLOGIC CLASSIFICATION IN SURVIVAL OF NEPHROTIC GLOMERULONEPHRITICS

DIAGNOSIS	LIVING	MEAN DURATION FOLLOW-UP	DEAD	DURATION FROM ONSET (MONTHS)	TOTAL
Proliferative	3	37 (28-47)*	2	21 (9-32)	5
Membranous	5	47 (16-84)	2	(2-7)**	7
Lobular	6	20 (5-45)	10	23 (10-43)	16
Sclerosing	1	31	1	18	2
Totals	15		15		30

* Patient (G. Ba.) lost to follow-up in the 28th month.
** Patient (R. J.) died of asthma in 2nd month unrelated to nephrosis.

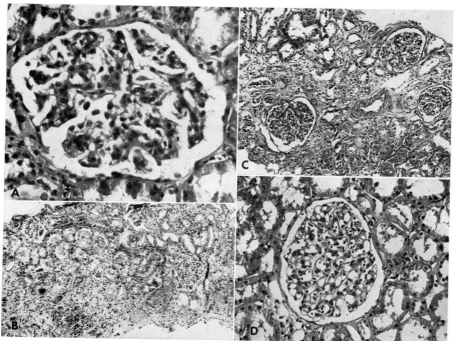

Fig. 1.   *A,* The first biopsy (in patient Ev. Sm.), performed during initial evaluation 12 months after onset of edema, shows moderate thickening of basement membranes of glomerular capillary loops (280 ×).

B, The second biopsy, one month later, shows in addition focal interstitial leukocytic infiltration (55 ×).

C, The third biopsy, 28 months after onset and after 12 months of intensive steroid therapy, shows thickened glomerular capillary basement membranes, focal interstitial fibrosis and inflammatory reaction, and atrophic tubules (100 ×).

D, The fifth biopsy, 40 months after onset and after 24 months of "successful" intensive steroid therapy, shows a nearly normal glomerulus. Not shown are indistinct thickening of basement membranes in other glomeruli, two fibrosed glomeruli, and focal tubular atrophy (280 ×).

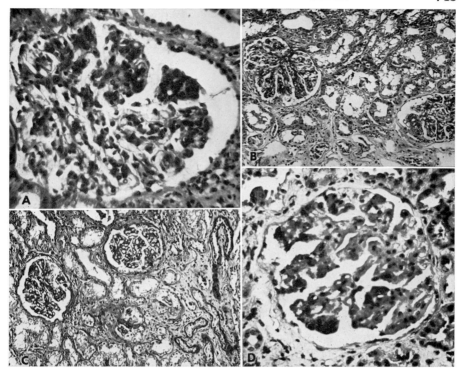

Fig. 2.   A, The first biopsy (in patient Ho. Ja.), performed during initial evaluation 2 months after onset of edema, shows moderate thickening of the basement membranes of the glomerular capillary loops (280 ×).

B, The second biopsy, 3 months later, shows a finger-like matting together of glomeular capillary loops (lobularity), and an adjacent area of tubular atrophy (80 ×).

C, The third biopsy, 19 months after onset. Intensive steroid therapy was given during the 10th-13th months of observation after which the patient was lost to follow-up. Two glomeruli show matting of thickened capillary loops, with intervening areas of tubular atrophy and interstitial fibrosis (80 ×).

D, The fourth biopsy, 30 months after onset (no steroid therapy for 17 months), shows definite progression of capillary basement membrane thickening, matting of loops tending toward lobularity, and periglomerular fibrosis. Not shown are several fibrosed glomeruli and interstitial fibrosis (280 ×).

The interaction of race and intensity of steroid therapy suggests that such treatment of the Negro is mandatory in that 13 of the 16 untreated have died, while 4 of the 5 Negroes intensively treated have a mean survival to date of 20 months (Table 3).

The initial histologic classification makes clear the poor prognosis in the untreated state of the predominating lobular and membranous forms (Table 4). Consideration of the interaction of histologic classification and intensive steroid therapy suggests responsiveness of the lobular group to such therapy (Table 5).

The serial renal biopsies in two intensively treated patients with membranous glomerulonephritis are contrasted in Figures 1 and 2.

The first patient, a 41-year-old Caucasian housewife on continuous therapy over a 24-month period, has achieved complete clinical and biochemical remission of the nephrotic state, with no deterioration in renal function. Basement membrane thickening has diminished; on the other hand, a few

TABLE 5. INTERACTION OF HISTOLOGIC CLASSIFICATION AND INTENSITY
OF STEROID THERAPY IN SURVIVAL

	UNTREATED (OR MINIMAL)			INTENSIVE STEROIDS			Grand total
	Dead	Alive	Subtotal	Dead	Alive	Subtotal	
Proliferative	2	2	4	0	1	1	5
Membranous	2	3	5	0	2	2	7
Lobular	9	2	11	1	4*	5	16
Sclerosing	1	1	2	0	0	0	2
Total	14	8	22	1	7	8	30

* Mean follow-up in living treated patients in lobular group is 17 months to date compared with mean of 25 months in the 9 who died without treatment.

glomeruli have fibrosed and an active chronic interstitial nephritis has developed.

The second patient, a 34-year-old Negro man, was given intensive steroid therapy for only four months before he rebelled and was temporarily lost to follow-up. No clinical response was obtained. When again seen 17 months later, he was still nephrotic but renal function had not deteriorated. However, the glomerular changes had undergone considerable progression, with increased basement membrane thickening.

A third intensively treated patient expired with tuberculosis and uremia after 10 months of observation and only 4 of therapy. Five others are living, with total follow-ups ranging from 5 to 45 months. Histologic progression was documented in 11 of the 12 untreated patients with serial comparative histopathology, and regression with therapy was observed in only one of four with serial biopsies (Table 6).

TABLE 6. COMPARATIVE HISTOPATHOLOGY

	SUBSEQUENT HISTOLOGY			
INITIAL BIOPSY	Untreated	No.	Treated	No.
Proliferative	Lobular	1	Progression	1
Membranous	Membranous	1	Progression	1
	Sclerosing	1	Regression	1
Lobular	Progression	2	Sclerosing	1
	Sclerosing	6		
Sclerosing	Progression	1		
Totals		12		4

It seems clear that (1) the rate of progress of the nephrotic phase of chronic glomerulonephritis is particularly rapid in the Negro, in whom the high mortality rate justifies heroic therapy; (2) orthodox, minimal corticotropin or steroid therapy probably offers little to alter this course; (3) initial presentation with membranous or lobular forms of glomerulonephritis in this patient population carries grave prognostic implication; (4) intensive steroid therapy may well diminish the high mortality rate even in the lobular form and perhaps also in membranous glomerulonephritis; (5) the histologic variants of chronic glomerulonephritis appear to be simply temporally related stages of a common process with an order of progression from proliferative or membranous to lobular to sclerosing stages; (6) little correlation appears to exist between steroid suppression of proteinuria and, thereby, of the nephrotic syndrome, and the rate of progress of the glomerular lesion.

ACKNOWLEDGMENTS

The authors are grateful to Warden Fred A. Hertwig of the Cook County Hospital and to President Daniel Ryan and the Board of Commissioners for provision of basic laboratory facilities.

The authors are grateful to Doctors B. P. Maduros, J. M. Levine, G. L. River, T. N. Gynn, J. P. Pendras, J. Greenwald and G. Buckman, and to A. Poulos, H. A. Dyniewicz, E. Hackett, R. Nelson, A. Costos and J. Cremin for their several contributions to this work.

REFERENCES

1. Allen, A. C.: The clinico-pathologic meaning of the nephrotic syndrome. Am. J. Med., *18*:277, 1955.
2. Armstrong, S. H., Jr. and Kushner, D. S.: Current status of steroid therapy in chronic adult glomerulonephritis; the unnatural history of Bright's disease. Am. J. Med., *29*:377, 1960.
3. Berman, L. B. and Schreiner, G. E.: Clinical and histologic spectrum of the nephrotic syndrome. Am. J. Med., *24*:249, 1958.
4. Blainey, J. D., Brewer, D. B., Hardwicke, J. and Soothill, J. F.: The nephrotic syndrome. Quart. J. Med., *29*:235, 1960.
5. Chasis, H.: Glomerulonephritis and pyelonephritis. Bull. New York Acad. Med., *36*:664, 1960.
6. Daeschner, C. W. and Dodge, W. F.: Specific and supportive therapy of patients with the nephrotic syndrome. In Moyer, J. H. and Fuchs, M. (eds.): Edema, Mechanisms and Management. Philadelphia, W. B. Saunders Co., 1960, p. 553.
7. Goodman, H. C. and Baxter, J. H.: The nephrotic syndrome; clinical observations and therapy with prednisolone and other steroids. J.A.M.A., *165*:1798, 1957.
8. Howe, J. S.: Renal Biopsies in Renal Diseases. In Metcoff, J. (ed.): Proc. 7th Ann. Conf. on Nephrotic Syndrome. New York, The National Nephrosis Foundation, 1955, p. 167.
9. Joekes, A. M., Heptinstall, R. H. and Porter, K. A.: The nephrotic syndrome: a study of renal biopsies in twenty adult patients. Quart. J. Med., *27*:495, 1958.
10. Johnson, J. R. and Reader, R.: Prognosis in the nephrotic syndrome: a study with particular reference to the adult and older child. Australasian Ann. Med., *8*:200, 1959.
11. Kark, R. M.: Observations on various types of clinical nephrotic syndrome. In Metcoff, J. (ed.): Proc. 7th Ann. Conf. on Nephrotic Syndrome. New York, The National Nephrosis Foundation, 1955, p. 141.
12. Kark, R. M., Pirani, C. L., Pollak, V. E., Muehrcke, R. C. and Blainey, J. D.: The nephrotic syndrome in adults; a common disorder with many causes. Ann. Int. Med., *49*:751, 1958.
13. Lange, K.: In Metcoff, J. (ed.): Proc. 7th Ann. Conf. on Nephrotic Syndrome. New York, The National Nephrosis Foundation, 1955, p. 203.
14. Lange, K., Strang, R., Slobody, L. D. and Wink, E. J.: The treatment of the nephrotic syndrome with steroids in children and adults. A.M.A. Arch. Int. Med., *99*:760, 1957.
15. Lange, K.: In Metcoff, J. (ed.): Proc. 10th Ann. Conf. on Nephrotic Syndrome. New York, The National Kidney Disease Foundation, 1958, p. 244.
16. Parrish, A. E., Watt, M. F. and Howe, J. S.: Membranous glomerulonephritis. A.M.A. Arch. Int. Med., *100*:620, 1957.
17. Pollak, V. E., Kark, R. M., Pirani, C. L., Soothill, J. F. and Muehrcke, R. C.: The significance and potential value of renal biopsy in Bright's disease. J. Chron. Dis., *5*:67, 1957.
18. Pollak, V. E., Folli, G., Pirani, C. L., Reid, R. T. W. and Muehrcke, R. C.: On the electronmicroscopic recognition and clinical cure of lipoid nephrosis in adults. J. Clin. Invest., *37*:922, 1958.
19. Post, R.: Results of steroid therapy of the nephrotic syndrome in adults. In Metcoff, J. (ed.): Proc. 10th Ann. Conf. on Nephrotic Syndrome. New York, The National Kidney Disease Foundation, 1958, p. 236.
20. Schreiner, G. E.: Glomerulonephritis and pyelonephritis. Bull. New York Acad. Med., *36*:666, 1960.

21. Sharpe, A. R., Jr. and Unger, A. M.: The nephrotic syndrome. A.M.A. Arch. Int. Med., *104*:684, 1959.
22. Vernier, R.: In Metcoff, J. (ed.): Proc. 10th Ann. Conf. on Nephrotic Syndrome. New York, The National Kidney Disease Foundation, 1958, p. 243.
23. Vernier, R. L.: Kidney biopsy in the study of renal disease. Pediat. Clin. North America, 7:353, 1960.

Panel Discussion

John H. Moyer, *Moderator*

Dr. Moyer: Since there seems to be some difference of opinion relative to the effectiveness of steroids in lupus nephropathy, I thought we might begin the discussion on this point. Dr. Pollak, could you postulate why your results are different from those of Dr. Soffer? There is probably some specific reason, perhaps referable to dosage or other factors.

Dr. Pollak: I can not answer this question without knowing what dose of steroids Dr. Soffer gave his patients and, particularly, how long the steroids were given. All I can say is that we designed our study using an empirically chosen dose and an empirically chosen duration. There were some reasons for doing this, but essentially both the dose and time chosen were somewhat empirical, and we wished to determine whether steroids given in high doses and for a long time would in fact alter the findings. I think it is quite clear from the serial histological studies we have collected that the disappearance of active lesions which we have been able to demonstrate at six months does not occur within weeks, and possibly not within several months, but instead this is a gradual process. This may well be a very important factor involved in the difference between our results and those of Dr. Soffer.

Dr. Moyer: Would you review the exact dosage schedule used in your patients?

Dr. Pollak: We gave 40 to 60 milligrams of prednisone a day, and the average dose which our patients received was 47 milligrams per day. The minimum period of treatment was six months.

Dr. Moyer: Do you think the type of steroid used could lead to differences in results?

Dr. Pollak: I do not really know. We have always been satisfied with prednisone as compared with any of the newer analogues and we prefer it to cortisone; comparative investigation has not been carried out in our clinic. Certainly, in other diseases involving the kidney I have not been impressed by any particular difference between one steroid and another.

There is one point which I would like to emphasize, and it may be a point about which there is some confusion. Although I do not recall the exact figures, there were approximately equal numbers of nephrotic patients in both the low and high dose steroid-treated groups. Although the larger doses of prednisone, in general, prevented the appearance and progression of renal failure and prevented the deterioration of the over-all renal histologic picture, the glomeruli did not return to normal and the diffuse basement membrane thickening in the glomeruli persists when severe basement membrane thickening is present initially. Proteinuria also persists. In other words, what I am saying is that while renal excretory function does not deteriorate in the group treated with high doses of steroids, there is little or no effect in measurable time on the proteinuria, and it persists.

DR. MOYER: Dr. McCombs, what is your experience relative to the dose and duration of therapy, since these seem to be important factors in determining the type of results obtained with steroid therapy?

DR. McCOMBS: There are two aspects to this question. The use of steroid therapy for patients with existing evidence of renal involvement in our series has not been very successful. We used the higher doses of steroids, perhaps not continuing the doses for six months at the level Dr. Pollak does, but using large doses at least for a period of two or three months. We have had only two patients out of about 28 treated who have shown improvement in renal function and disappearance of renal findings or hematuria. In both of these patients, the treatment was instituted quite early in the course of the disease—in one, within a week or two of the apparent onset.

One other aspect of the disease that I have wondered about, and the question is again raised by Dr. Soffer's data, is: How many of the patients who did not get renal disease were being treated with steroids? In our series of 28 patients who did not get treatment with steroids, four developed renal disease some time after the diagnosis was established; whereas, of 30 patients who were treated with steroids for other aspects of the disease and who did not have renal disease at the time the diagnosis was made, only one subsequently had renal involvement. We have the distinct impression that the use of steroids before renal involvement occurs may prevent the subsequent development of the renal lesions. Do any of the other panelists have this impression?

DR. POLLAK: I can not give a definite answer to that question at the present time, but like Dr. Soffer, I have been impressed by the fact that many patients who have normal renal biopsies initially do not subsequently develop renal disease; however, there are some who do, whether they are on steroid therapy or not. From a practical point of view, I would say that it is unjustified, on the basis of our present knowledge, to give steroid therapy either in high doses or low doses specifically in order to prevent the occurrence of renal disease.

DR. McCOMBS: I would agree with this in principle, but as I said yesterday, patients with lupus who do not have renal disease should be followed very closely, and if they develop albuminuria or hematuria, high dosage therapy should be initiated immediately in the hope that it will have some suppressive effect.

DR. POLLAK: I would agree entirely with that. I think our major mistake in the past, even though we had been trying to follow our patients closely, was the failure to obtain frequent urinalyses. We now have a policy which requires every patient in our clinic to have a urinalysis at least every two months, even if they are clinically well and visiting us infrequently.

DR. DUBOIS: Actually, I think there is a reasonable amount of agreement about the renal problem. Most of us would agree that the early acute toxic nephropathy with hyaline casts, red cells and albuminuria in association with high fever and other manifestations of lupus which Dr. Soffer described will almost invariably respond to steroids. Most of us have also seen patients with the moderately advanced renal problem which Dr. Pollak described, and the renal lesions in these patients will respond to large doses of steroids. I also think that there is agreement that high dosage steroid therapy often causes problems in the patient who comes in with hypertension, a BUN over 30 mg. per cent, a high cholesterol and the nephrotic syndrome, but in whom the temperature is normal and in whom there is not a lot of catabolism going on. These patients have advanced nephritis. In our experience, nitrogen mustards often produce a fairly good remission in this group. The course of lupus nephrosis and lupus nephropathy, in general, is a very variable thing, and some of our patients have lived as long as nine years after repeated courses of mustards and intermittent dosages of the adrenal steroids.

DR. MOYER: Dr. Zarafonetis, would you comment on the effectiveness of nitrogen mustards in lupus nephropathy?

DR. ZARAFONETIS: I have had some experience with the use of nitrogen mustards in lupus nephritis, but in the particular patients we treated, the results were not particularly good.

DR. MILLS: In regard to the statements of Dr. Dubois about the prognosis in patients with lupus who have severe azotemia and nephrotic syndrome, I would agree in general that these patients have a poor prognosis. However, there are certainly patients in that situation who do respond to steroid therapy. We had one patient with a BUN which was over 300 initially, who had severe anemia with only 5 grams of hemoglobin and who responded to steroid therapy and stabilized at a BUN level of about 50; the hematuria disappeared, and although she had persistent albuminuria, there was no clinical evidence of progression of the renal disease during a period of one and a half years that we followed her. I know of another patient with the same clinical syndrome who had an even better result from therapy. In fact, this particular patient had been given an injection of hydro-cortisone into one renal artery at another institution in the hope that high dose local steroid therapy would have a beneficial effect on the renal lesion, but it did not; in fact, it almost destroyed the kidney on the injected side. She had a severe nephrotic syndrome at that time, but with subsequent steroid therapy the nephrotic syndrome cleared up and her renal status remained stable after that for a period of about four years. At the time of her death, which unfortunately was the result of a steroid complication, her renal lesion was stable and there was no evidence of active lupus nephritis at postmortem examination.

DR. MOYER: In regard to the dose of steroids, we observed a few patients in whom we could titrate the dose of the steroid very exactly by examination of the urine. In one patient, for example, if the dose of prednisone was reduced below 50 milligrams, many red cells would begin to appear in the urine, but just by the addition of another 10 mg. of prednisone the hematuria would clear up very dramatically, and changes in the urinary findings could be produced at will. It took about a week or so after reduction of dosage for the exacerbation of the hematuria to occur and a week or two for hematuria to disappear again after reinstitution of larger doses of the steroids. I also want to emphasize that there were no subjective or objective changes in the patient aside from the changes in the urinalysis and sedimentation rate when the dose of the steroid was changed. It seems to me, then, that one important aspect of this problem is that the dose of the steroid is not actually adjusted to each individual patient. All too often the patients either receive a standard dose, just because this dose is said in the literature to be the usual dose required, or they receive a dose just sufficient to relieve most of their subjective complaints even though there is objective or laboratory evidence of persistent activity.

DR. POLLAK: I think this is essentially true, Dr. Moyer, and this has been our experience. However, we set up our study for a specific purpose, and the dose and duration of therapy were somewhat empirical, as I have indicated. The renal lesions in one patient in this study, as determined by serial biopsies, did not change at all during a period of steroid therapy which should have been long enough to obtain a response. Clearly, in retrospect, this patient should have been given larger doses of the steroid. I think there are many examples of this. However, there are as yet insufficient data available from which to draw final conclusions as to correct dosage and length of therapy. I would not say that the dosages we used in this study were necessarily ideal.

DR. ROSE: In regard to Dr. Mills' point, I think it is important to remember what we have heard this morning about the usual progress of lupus in patients with azotemia, but I agree that we should not have the attitude that the prognosis is hopeless in these patients. For example, five and a half years ago I observed a patient who had severe classic systemic lupus, with a diastolic blood pressure of 145, papilledema, proteinuria, total blood urea nitrogen of 92 and edema with a low plasma albumin. Steroids were given for a period of two years, using prednisone in an initial dose of about 50 milligrams a day, with a gradual reduction in dose thereafter. Steroid therapy was stopped three and a half years ago, and the patient is now back at work, has no proteinuria, has an almost normal blood urea nitrogen, and her blood pressure has been entirely normal for two years, although for three years previously it had been elevated.

DR. KUSHNER: I have two comments with respect to Dr. Soffer's data. First, he told me that he has done about 22 renal biopsies in patients with lupus and that eight of these were normal histologically. This is in striking contrast to our own experience; in an approximately equivalent number of biopsies, none of the biopsies were normal, all showing diffuse glomerular involvement. This, I think, suggests that we are studying somewhat different populations. Secondly, I think the dosage level of steroids is critical, because in following the lead of Dr. Pollak's group during the past two years we have treated all of our patients with active lupus nephritis with 125 milligrams of prednisone per day, as we have done in chronic nephritis, and I do not remember a single patient in whom steroids in this dose failed to suppress the manifestations of renal activity. This includes patients with the nephrotic syndrome as well as other lesions.

DR. DUBOIS: In our experience, large doses of steroids have caused gradually rising hypertension and gradual elevation of the BUN and creatinine in the group of patients who have had renal disease for several years and who have had an advanced nephrotic syndrome. This is the group that we have had a great many problems with. It is true that the acute symptoms that occur with sudden exacerbations of the disease will often respond to steroids, but, in our experience, hypertension does not improve and often becomes worse in the patient who has progressive disease and who has approached the end of his advancing renal problem. We have tried steroids in large doses, but in addition to increased hypertension, convulsive seizures often occur. We have had to cease doing this. As Dr. Larson mentioned, his experience at Columbia was similar. I think most of the discrepancies in our results are due to the fact that each panelist is talking about a little different type or stage of renal disease, and good evidence for this has just been pointed out by Dr. Kushner. There is certainly no question that patients with advanced renal disease and other manifestations of disease activity, such as rash, pleuritis, anemia, and so forth, should have a trial with steroids, but steroids should be used very cautiously in those patients with advanced renal disease.

DR. MOYER: Dr. Kushner, would you discuss the origin of hypertension in lupus?

DR. KUSHNER: In response, I can only ask what is the mechanism or etiology of hypertension in primary vascular disease of the kidneys—that is, benign or malignant nephrosclerosis?

DR. MOYER: May I state the question in another way? In a patient who has chronic glomerulonephritis, significant hypertension is not usually a problem. There is only relatively mild diastolic hypertension. Severe hypertension in chronic glomerulonephritis is usually a terminal event, and therefore I would think that this has a direct bearing on the question that was raised here as to the effect of the steroids on the hypertension associated with lupus nephritis, and that is, if the hypertension is a terminal event, one is less likely to see a beneficial effect from steroid therapy. Would you care to comment on that, Dr. Rose?

DR. ROSE: First, I would like to make an analogy with polyarteritis nodosa. In polyarteritis nodosa with acute glomerulonephritis one does not usually see any elevation of the blood pressure; in fact, there may even be a fall, and the development of hypertension which occurs later in this disease seems to be associated with renal scarring subsequent to the initial involvement. I wonder whether the same is true in lupus glomerulonephritis. In the stage of acute activity is the blood pressure likely to be normal, and have those who have done renal biopsies found this to be so?

DR. POLLAK: In our patients with lupus nephritis who died rapidly, we usually found large "white kidneys" or large, somewhat hemorrhagic kidneys, but not contracted kidneys. Most of these patients, while they may have had some mild hypertension, did not have any really significant elevation of blood pressure, although there were occasional exceptions to this. In patients who have been treated with large doses of steroids, there is a much higher incidence of significant hypertension. It is difficult to say how much of this is due to the steroids and how much of it is associated with the fact that the renal lesion is not progressing as rapidly and that some interstitial fibrosis is occurring at this time and that you therefore have a more chronic type of renal lesion. In those patients with hypertension in whom the dose of the steroids has subsequently been reduced to the range of about 15 milligrams per day, the blood pressure often decreases somewhat, but the diastolic pressure often persists at about 100 mm.

DR. BREST: Hypertension is not infrequently absent in patients with lupus erythematosus. When it is present, it is often mild. When it does occur in the course of lupus, one should be sure that it is not steroid-induced. One should also be alert to the possibility that some patients with lupus may have malignant hypertension. Finally, there is the possibility that the hypertension is due to renal ischemia and the liberation of renin and the subsequent production of angiotensin.

DR. DUBOIS: Generally, in our experience, the untreated lupus patient has a normal or low blood pressure, and one of the best single clinical guides relating to prognosis is the blood pressure of the untreated lupus patient. If blood pressure is higher than 140/90 in the non-steroid-treated patient, the outlook is generally not quite as good, and the higher the pressure, the worse the prognosis is. I think this reflects the degree of vasculitis in the kidney of the untreated patient. However, it is true that in acute exacerbations of the disease there may be an arteritis in the kidney and this patient will respond to steroids, but this applies to the very acute hypertension and not to the chronic progressive hypertension seen in the advancing renal disease of chronic lupus nephritis.

DR. ZARAFONETIS: In regard to hypertension in lupus, I want to emphasize what Dr. Comens said earlier, and that is that some people with essential hypertension treated with Apresoline will develop an LE syndrome. Once some of these interesting observations are elucidated, I am sure we will have information about some of the basic mechanisms which we are quite naive about at present.

DR. MOYER: Dr. Hurley, from a dermatological point of view, is there any correlation between the response to steroids of the skin lesions and the response of the systemic manifestations of lupus, particularly those related to the kidney? Does activity in these two areas correlate?

DR. HURLEY: I think this varies somewhat. In general, exacerbation of the skin lesions is an indication of the exacerbation of the underlying disease and therefore is a rough guide to other inflammatory activity. From the practical standpoint, I am not sure what type of regimen should be instituted in those patients who do have very active disease, whether manifested by skin lesions, anemia or other lesions. Should very large doses of steroids be used to obtain complete suppression in an effort to prevent or minimize the development of kidney disease, or should smaller doses, just sufficient to control the other symptomatic phases of the disease, be used?

DR. KUSHNER: The ideal method would be to obtain a renal biopsy before making this decision. If the patients are similar to those of Dr. Soffer, the group will include several patients beyond the first year who do not have renal involvement, and these patients should do well with symptomatic suppressive therapy. If the group is similar to ours, a significant number of patients will be found to have lupus nephritis whether or not it is clinically manifested, and then I think it becomes imperative to use intensive steroid therapy.

DR. BREST: Have serial renal biopsies been done in untreated lupus patients, and if so, do the glomerular lesions of lupus show evidence of healing at one time and evidence of activity at another? If so, this might be an important factor in judging the response to the different therapeutic regimens.

DR. KUSHNER: All of our patients with lupus have been quite ill and all have required treatment, so I have no data on that.

DR. MOYER: Has anyone on the panel obtained serial renal biopsies from untreated lupus patients?

DR. POLLAK: We have single biopsies from untreated patients, but as Dr. Kushner stated, most of the patients require treatment and we have had very few opportunities to do serial biopsies in this group.

DR. MOYER: Would you comment on the findings in the few you have done?

DR. POLLAK: The findings are similar to those in the patients receiving low dose steroid therapy, but the number is too small to draw any definite conclusions.

DR. MOYER: Dr. Daeschner, is the response to lupus erythematosus particularly different in a child as compared to the adult phase of the disease?

DR. DAESCHNER: In general, the disease is more severe, and I have seen only one child who did not have renal disease at the time he was first seen. The majority have rather severe glomerulosclerosis or vascular changes. Most of our patients have had hypertension, and, in general, if the hypertension can be controlled by reserpine we go ahead with steroid therapy; if hypertension can not be controlled, we give only that amount of steroids which will not significantly increase the hypertension.

DR. ZARAFONETIS: In regard to the disease in children and to the age at which the greatest activity of systemic lupus occurs, it is my impression that before the age of puberty there are just as many males as females with systemic disease; similarly after the climacterium, the same situation exists. In the five adults we have seen whose lupus began after the age of 60, four were men. During the reproductive period in women, the systemic form of the illness occurs about 8 to 10 times more commonly in women than in men; however, if we include all of the men who have discoid LE and subacute LE in the figures, we find that there is a far greater incidence in men than we have suspected. In 100 patients with all types of LE that I investigated before 1950, 40 were men; to be sure, most of them had discoid LE, but I think that the sex differences relate to the expression of the disease rather than to the incidence. I hope some of the other panel members will comment on this.

DR. McComBS: The incidence in men is much higher, if one includes patients with illnesses that we call allergic vasculitis in the lupus group, but they do not have a rash. In our experience, discoid lupus occurs in both men and women, and I do not think it is more frequent in men than it is in women.

DR. HURLEY: As I recall, discoid lupus occurs in about equal frequency in both sexes.

DR. POLLAK: There is one point that Dr. Zarafonetis raised which is quite important. I am impressed, as he is, that the sex incidence may not be very different after the age of the menopause in women. I also wonder whether the clinical manifestations of the disease are not somewhat different, and particularly whether it is not a considerably milder disease. Perhaps some of these patients may not be diagnosed because of the somewhat different clinical spectrum, but this is just speculation.

DR. ROSE: Systemic lupus is a disease which, more than almost any other in medicine, has a remarakble sex predilection. It is a disease which has its maximum incidence in women during the reproductive age of life and its most severe manifestations often occur at that age. The patient that I referred to earlier, who had a complete remission after two years of steroid therapy, appears in some respects to be a unique case in that her condition improved at the time of the menopause. Should one consider oophorectomy in these otherwise almost hopeless cases?

DR. DUBOIS: I have also noticed that there is a slight shift in the sex incidence in the younger and the older age groups. The incidence is generally about 12 per cent in males in an over-all series, but in small groups of patients under the age of 10 and over the age of 60, the proportion of males may be 20 to 30 per cent. This certainly seems to be a valid observation, as does the observation that the disease is apparently more malignant in the younger patient and more benign in the older patient.

Part X | STEROIDS AND INFECTION

Development of Intercurrent Infections in Patients Receiving Steroids

EDWIN M. ORY, HANNA ABU-NASSAR and ELLARD M. YOW

Ben Taub Infectious Disease Research Laboratory, Jefferson Davis Hospital, and Baylor University College of Medicine

The possible adverse effect of the administration of exogenous adrenocortical steroids on infections was appreciated very early in accumulated experience with these agents. By the time that they had been released for general use, this danger was emphasized in the medical literature and in the package literature furnished by the pharmaceutical industry. These warnings stemmed as much from experimental observations that inflammatory reactions and immune mechanisms were inhibited by steroids as from actual clinical observations.

With the perspective of more than a decade of experience with these agents, we may now assess the relative danger of intercurrent infections against the possible beneficial effects of steroids. It is difficult to set up a controlled study utilizing comparable patients treated with and without steroids. In reviewing our own results, it is evident that patients who have received steroid therapy have been those with the most serious and life-threatening illnesses. Many have had prolonged debilitating illnesses which in themselves are often associated with lowered resistance to infection and altered clinical manifestations. This paper will therefore not be a statistical review of the side effects of steroid therapy, but rather a résumé of certain principles and generalities derived from a review of the literature and from our own experience. Observations concerning altered susceptibility to infection during steroid therapy come from both experimental and clinical sources.

EXPERIMENTAL

The phenomenon of decreased resistance to infections induced by steroids has been observed in mice, rats, guinea pigs, rabbits, monkeys and other animals. Among the infections studied have been those due to bacteria, viruses, fungi, protozoa and helminthes. The reported effects of steroid administration on resistance to infection in experimental animals have varied with the species, age of the animal, the pathogen, dose of ACTH or cortisone, pretreatment with the hormone, duration of therapy, and whether antibiotics were given before, simultaneously or after challenge with the pathogenic organism. The dosage of steroid has often been far in excess of that employed therapeutically in humans.

Several conclusions concerning the influence of cortisone on infectious processes now seem justified:

1. Cortisone has no direct antimicrobial effect upon the infectious agents.

2. Steroids have a "detoxifying effect" and an antipyretic effect which may alter the manifestations of infection.
3. Steroids inhibit the ability of the host to localize infection. This most important effect of steroids on the development of intercurrent infections is enhanced by the following mechanisms:
   a. Suppression of inflammation
      (1) Decreased cellular, fluid and protein exudation.
      (2) Reduced reflex vasomotor reactions, leading to reduced capillary permeability and vascular tone.
   b. Depression of reticuloendothelial function
      Apparently there is no interference with phagocytosis by either polymorphonuclear leukocytes or reticuloendothelial cells, but the latter system is unable to dispose of bacteria and particulate matter. It becomes blocked and infection may become disseminated after residing in the phagocyte for variable periods of time.
4. ACTH and cortisone do not interfere with the actual union of antigen and antibody in hypersensitivity reactions. They do not interfere with cutaneous reactions that are associated with release of histamine-like substances.
5. Steroids do interfere with delayed hypersensitivity reactions such as those seen with tuberculin, Frei and streptococcal products.
6. Although cortisone diminishes antibody production in very high dosage, it does not interfere with the development of antibody titers in the usual clinical dosage.

A few specific experimental reports may be cited to illustrate the above generalizations.

Mogabgab et al.[14] showed that Group A hemolytic streptococcal infections in mice were intensified by cortisone, but immunized rabbits were resistant to a dose that was lethal for nonimmunized rabbits even when treated with cortisone. Increasing the size of the inoculum overwhelmed the immunity in both groups. The production of antibodies was not prevented. Penicillin was effective in large doses when given within three days after infection. Cortisone given alone without streptococcal challenge resulted in spontaneous bacterial infections, but the animals displayed little evidence of illness despite severe bacteremia.

Denny and Thomas[3] demonstrated that cortisone-treated rabbits infected with Group A hemolytic streptococci develop septicemia and die without localizing manifestations. They observed that the administration of cortisone as late as 104 days after an acute infection can result in a recrudescence and lethal outcome.

LeMaistre[11] reported similar findings in mice and rats with experimental tuberculosis in which cortisone converted a chronic smoldering infection into an acute progressive process. Morgan et al.[15] demonstrated that the infection-intensifying effect of cortisone on experimentally induced tuberculosis in rabbits was greater in nonsensitized rabbits.

In their observations on experimental pneumococcal and influenza virus infections in mice, Kass et al.[10] found that steroids decreased the capacity of the host to survive a given concentration of virus in the lungs and diminished the survival time of mice infected with the pneumococcus.

Cortisone administered shortly before and after infection with *Candida albicans* was shown by Seligman[19] to produce a generalized fatal infection.

Selye reported the frequent occurrence of pulmonary abscess formation or generalized septicemia in animals treated with steroids in large doses. The organisms included a variety of species ordinarily considered nonpathogenic.

Robinson et al.[18] demonstrated that adrenalectomized animals, when infected with pneumococci, were rapidly overwhelmed, but that when small doses of cortisone were added their resistance was restored to normal; on increasing the dose the resistance of these animals to infection again disappeared.

CLINICAL

It is interesting to note that in hyperadrenalism (Cushing's syndrome) infection is the leading cause of death, and the incidence of infection as a cause of death has not decreased significantly since the advent of chemotherapy. Patients with Addison's disease are also more susceptible to infection. These observations suggest that there is an optimal level of steroid activity for maximum resistance to infection.

The hazard attributable to intercurrent infections during corticosteroid therapy is greatest in chronic diseases such as disseminated lupus erythematosus, sarcoidosis, rheumatoid arthritis, etc. In such cases there is also a greater susceptibility to infection, with or without steroid therapy. In acute self-limiting infections characterized by prolonged convalescence such as rheumatic fever, when debility is not prominent, the hazard is less. During severe illnesses of brief duration, such as pneumonia, gram-negative septicemia, infectious mononucleosis, etc., the danger is minimal, especially if steroid therapy is given for a brief period.

Not all of the reported cases represent activation or appearance of new infection. In many instances patients with fever of unknown origin were treated for collagen disease, although the diagnosis of tuberculosis or mycotic infection had not been excluded.

In a series of 510 patients of rheumatoid arthritis receiving prolonged steroid therapy, Hench reported that eight exhibited lowered resistance to infection. Benedek and Montgomery[1] analyzed 900 patient-months of hormone therapy and did not demonstrate significant differences from untreated controls. Phillips et al.[16] reported one case of staphylococcal septicemia and endocarditis secondary to cortisone-treated exfoliative dermatitis due to penicillin and cited three other cases. We have observed a similar case that has not been reported.

Only two patients, one with disseminated histoplasmosis and one with reactivation of latent tuberculosis, were encountered by Spink[21] among 81 selected patients treated for short periods of time and with large doses of steroids.

Lepper and Spies[12] reported 12 cases of serious bacteremia during a clinical study of steroid treatment in 84 seriously ill patients with infection. The frequency of infection was attributed to the severity of the illness and an available portal of entry.

Six intercurrent infections occurring during steroid therapy (four staphylococcal, one monilial and one histoplasmosis) were seen by Smith and Cleve[20] during one year.

Gelfand[5] cited five infections associated with steroid therapy. These included two cases of nonspecific pericarditis, two of cellulitis, and one of pneumonia.

Levy and Cohen[13] presented a case of generalized fungus infection following three months of corticotropin therapy. The same authors, mentioning the experience of others, cited three fatal cases of systemic moniliasis and aspergillosis complicating steroid therapy. Thirteen cases of fungus infections associated with antibiotic and/or steroid therapy were reviewed by Torack.[24] In the patients who received steroid therapy, lesions were invasive into tissue; in those who received antibiotics alone, the fungi remained limited to the mucous membranes by surface proliferation only. Most of these infections were moniliasis, aspergillosis and mucormycosis.

We have observed one case of sporotrichosis that became disseminated during prolonged steroid therapy; the patient later developed staphylococcal septicemia and died during steroid therapy.

The hazard of intercurrent viral infection is dramatized by a report of 12 fatal cases of varicella in children receiving steroids. These cases were collected after a poll of 65 physicians from various medical centers representing a large experience, as pointed out by Kass and Finland.

Two cases of unusually severe herpes zoster in children who received hormone therapy are cited by Good et al.

The following is a summary of our own experience:

1. Development of disseminated tuberculosis in a patient with congenital heart disease while on steroid therapy.

2. Development of tuberculous pleural effusion in a patient with intractable asthma treated with steroids.

3. Dissemination of sporotrichosis in a patient treated with steroids for arthritis; patient died of staphylococcal septicemia.

4. Septic staphylococcal arthritis following intra-articular injection of hydrocortisone.

5. Development of staphylococcal septicemia in a patient during steroid therapy for exfoliative dermatitis.

6. Severe varicella causing death of an adult patient with Cushing's disease.

7. Development of active pulmonary tuberculosis in a patient with asthma treated for three years with prednisone.

8. Development of extensive staphylococcal abscess of leg in a patient with disseminated lupus erythematosus; destruction of gastrocnemius muscle; minimal clinical signs.

Corticosteroid therapy suppresses fever, inflammation and the constitutional symptoms of many infections. It particularly suppresses those manifestations that are attributed to hypersensitivity to the infectious agent or its products. Finland and Kass demonstrated the persistence of pneumococcal bacteremia in pneumococcal pneumonia despite the decrease in most other clinical manifestations of pneumonia. This effect tends to make infections acquired during the course of hormone therapy more difficult to recognize. Such infections are often occult and advanced before either the patient or the physician becomes aware of them. We have seen septic joints in which complete destruction of the joint occurred before the development of sepsis was recognized. This has been especially true following intra-articular injection of hydrocortisone or its analogs into joint spaces.

We have observed parenchymal pulmonary lesions due to tuberculosis progress in two patients while there was amelioration of the clinical symptoms. Another patient developed a tuberculous pleural effusion while under long-term steroid therapy for intractable asthma.

To place this problem in its true perspective, it should be pointed out that in the majority of patients who are on steroid therapy intercurrent infection does produce signs and symptoms of infection. These are recognizable by the usual clinical manifestations in most cases, but in debilitated patients they may be less severe and may go unrecognized for a longer period of time than usual.

SUMMARY AND CONCLUSIONS

Intercurrent infection constitutes a small but definite hazard during steroid therapy. The danger is greatest in patients who are under long-term therapy for a chronic debilitating illness which in itself constitutes a hazard. There is minimal risk in patients with relatively brief illnesses. Proper evaluation of such patients prior to institution of therapy and close vigilance during therapy permit earlier recognition and therapy.

Prevention may be difficult. Chemoprophylaxis is ineffective and leads to antibiotic-resistant infections.

Steroids inhibit inflammation and may alter the manifestations of infection. The most important effect is interference with mechanisms that localize infection, so that dissemination of infection constitutes the chief hazard.

REFERENCES

1. Benedek, T. G. and Montgomery, M. M.: The influence of ACTH and cortisone on the incidence of infections. J. Lab. & Clin. Med., 44:766, 1954.
2. Bloch, R. G., Vennesland, K. and Gurney, C.: The effect of cortisone on tuberculosis in the guinea pig. J. Lab. & Clin. Med., 38:133, 1951.
3. Denny, F. W., Jr. and Thomas, L.: Persistence of Group A streptococci in tissues of rabbits after infection. Proc. Soc. Exper. Biol. & Med., 38:260, 1955.
4. Frenkel, J. K.: Evaluation of infection-enhancing activity of modified corticoids. Proc. Soc. Exper. Biol. & Med., 103:552, 1960.
5. Gelfand, M. L.: Infections associated with steroid therapy. New York J. Med., 58:3461, 1958.
6. Haggerty, R. J. and Elcy, R. C.: Varicella and cortisone (letter to editor). Pediatrics, 18:160, 1956.
7. Kass, E. H. and Finland, M.: Adrenocortical hormones and the management of infection. Ann. Rev. Med., 8:1, 1957.
8. Kass, E. H. and Finland, M.: Corticosteroids and infections. Adv. Int. Med., 9:45, 1958.
9. Kass, E. H. and Finland, M.: Adrenocortical hormones in infections and immunity. Ann. Rev. Microbiol., 7:361, 1953.
10. Kass, E. H., Lundgren, M. and Finland, M.: Observations on the effect of corticosteroids and growth hormone on resistance to experimental pneumococcal and influenza virus infections. Ann. N. Y. Acad. Sc., 56:765, 1953.
11. LeMaistre, C. et al.: The effects of corticosteroids upon tuberculosis and pseudotuberculosis. Ann. N. Y. Acad. Sc., 56:772, 1953.
12. Lepper, M. and Spies, H.: A clinical study of the use of cortisone, hydrocortisone, and corticotropin in the treatment of seriously ill patients with infection. Antibiotics Ann., 57:447, 1956.
13. Levy, E. S. and Cohen, D. B.: Systemic moniliasis and aspergillosis complicating corticotropin therapy. Arch. Int. Med., 95:118, 1955.
14. Mogabgab, W. J. and Thomas, L.: The effects of cortisone on bacterial infection. J. Lab. & Clin. Med., 39:271, 1952.
15. Morgan, T. E., Wanzer, S. H. and Smith, D. T.: Effect of cortisone and streptomycin on experimentally induced pulmonary tuberculosis in rabbits. J. Bact., 67:257, 1954.
16. Phillips, L. V., Romansky, M. J. and Nasou, J. P.: Staphylococcal septicemia and endocarditis secondary to cortisone-treated exfoliative dermatitis due to penicillin. Antibiotics Ann., 5:68, 1954.

17. Robinson, H. J.: Adrenal cortical hormones and infection. Pediatrics, 17:770, 1956.
18. Robinson, H. and Smith, A. L.: The effect of adrenal cortical hormones on experimental infection. Ann. N. Y. Acad. Sc., 56:757, 1953.
19. Seligman, E.: Virulence enhancement of *Candida albicans* by antibiotics and cortisone. Proc. Soc. Exper. Biol. & Med., 83:778, 1953.
20. Smith, F. and Cleve, E. A.: Infections complicating cortisone therapy. New Engl. J. Med., 256:104, 1957.
21. Spink, W. W.: Adrenocortical steroids in the management of selected patients with infectious diseases. Ann. Int. Med., 53:1, 1960.
22. Thomas, L.: Cortisone, ACTH and infection. Bull. N. Y. Acad. Med., 31:485, 1955.
23. Thomas, L.: Infectious diseases; effects of cortisone and adrenocorticotropic hormone on infection. Ann. Rev. Med., 3:1, 1952.
24. Torack, R. M.: Fungus infections associated with antibiotic and steroid therapy. Am. J. Med., 22:872, 1957.
25. Wanzer, S. H., Morgan, T. E. and Smith, D. T.: Effect of corticotropin (ACTH) and streptomycin on experimentally induced pulmonary tuberculosis in rabbits. J. Bact., 67:264, 1954.

Effects of Steroids on the Natural Course of Infection

MONROE J. ROMANSKY

The George Washington University School of Medicine

Adrenal cortical steroids alter manifestations of a variety of clinical disorders, including infectious diseases. Finland and Kass[5, 15] demonstrated this when adrenal cortical steroids were given to carefully selected patients with lobar and viral pneumonias. Their observations clearly showed that the steroids could induce, in patients with pneumonia, striking defervescence and symptomatic relief, with a decrease or disappearance of not only the subjective signs but also the objective findings. These remarkable changes occurred despite the persistence of pneumococci in the sputum, the presence of bacteremia and, in one instance, the spread of pneumonia to other lobes with subsequent development of empyema. Subsequently, many clinical and laboratory data[14, 26] have been accumulated in an attempt to clarify the meaning of some of these observations. There are broad questions which as yet have not been answered: Are steroids really valuable in infectious diseases or useful in any particular area of infectious diseases? Since these agents may not be helpful but may be harmful, can one be specific in their use, so that advantages may be obtained without serious consequences?

The simultaneous administration of penicillin and cortisone to patients with pneumococcal pneumonia produced defervescence and symptomatic improvement more promptly than in those given penicillin alone. This was a controlled study.[28] No adverse bacteriologic results occurred, but renal insufficiency and prolonged hypothermia occurred in one patient treated with cortisone. Hypothermia has been reported by others[12] as a complication of cortisone therapy.

In a controlled blind study[17] we have compared the effects of tetracycline alone with those of tetracycline and 6-methyl prednisolone in 42 patients with pneumococcal pneumonia. Figure 1 illustrates the effect on fever. Thirteen patients (72.2 per cent) of the 21 in the tetracycline-steroid group were afebrile in 24 hours and seven (33.3 per cent) of the 21 in the tetracycline group were afebrile in 24 hours. One patient in each group had a pleural effusion; this was minimal in the tetracycline-treated patient. However, the patient who received the tetracycline-steroid combination had a 300 cc. effusion removed, which was sterile, and in addition slow resolution of his right lower lobe pneumonic process occurred. He was discharged asymptomatic but returned eight weeks later with a right lower lobe pneumonia and died 24 hours after admission despite vigorous penicillin therapy. A cautious approach should be employed in the administration of steroids

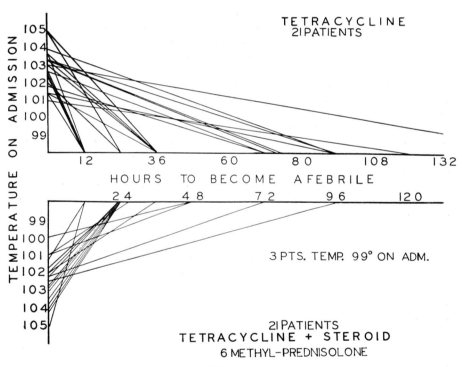

A CONTROLLED BLIND STUDY OF PNEUMOCOCCAL PNEUMONIA

Fig. 1.

with chemotherapy until additional data are available, and steroids should not be used in uncomplicated pneumococcal pneumonia.

Steroids[10, 13] without antibiotics have been used in a variety of infections, such as tuberculosis, typhoid fever, bacterial pneumonia and bacterial endocarditis. Steroids in these patients with acute febrile illnesses brought about rapid remission and reversal of the distressing clinical evidences of the illness. When the etiologic agent could be demonstrated, as in bacterial pneumonia, typhoid fever and subacute bacterial endocarditis, there was frequently evidence of increased multiplication and spread of the micro-organism despite the remission of the clinical syndrome.

It is difficult to detect the depression of immunity. However, in certain areas, controlled studies have been helpful. For example, in infectious hepatitis, the use of steroids leads to rapid symptomatic improvement and a rapid fall in level of serum bilirubin. However, it has been shown[4] that relapses occurred in 20 per cent of the treated patients and did not appear in controls. The hormone should not be employed in the average case but only for patients who are very ill, especially those with severe anorexia.[21]

The effects of steroids have been observed in a controlled study on the course of poliomyelitis,[2] as well as in acute streptococcal disease;[9] no particular effect on the acute disease nor on the sequelae was noted.

The effects of steroids in mumps orchitis are controversial; controlled studies[18] have indicated no difference in response to corticotropin or placebo. However, in these control studies the doses were not very large.

The degree of hazard of infection in patients receiving corticosteroids is not easy to evaluate. These agents may so camouflage the appearance of septicemia that the infection may be noted only at autopsy. Intercurrent infection is more likely to develop in patients with a debilitating type of illness who receive steroids than in those with a milder illness or with a chronic illness such as rheumatic fever, in which debilitation is not a prominent factor.

Examples of the hazard of infection in patients receiving steroids are the 12 fatal cases of varicella in children collected by Hagerty and Eley.[8] The children were receiving steroids at the time of exposure to the disease.

Experimentally it has been demonstrated that large doses of steroids definitely depress resistance to infections. This has been documented by experimental studies[13] with bacteria, viruses, fungi, protozoa and even helminthic agents.

One would anticipate from the foregoing that the chemotherapeutic agents would counteract the adverse effect of the steroids. However, as has been shown in experimental animals, increasing the dose of steroids may overcome the effect of a given dose of a specific protective chemotherapeutic agent.

A careful attitude was assumed early in the use of steroids in the management of patients with active tuberculosis. It has been demonstrated experimentally that steroids suppress inflammation in the tissues, but that tubercle bacilli multiply more rapidly. Therefore, it is interesting that so few patients have been reported with spread of the disease while receiving steroids.

It is well to bear in mind, however, that numbers of controlled observations are few and that considerable improvement in the management of tuberculosis in recent years makes it necessary to evaluate carefully whether the steroids have really contributed to the ultimate outcome.

Substantial symptomatic relief will usually occur when steroids are used with effective antibiotics. However, many infections, particularly those due to staphylococci and certain gram-negative bacteria, are difficult to manage with available agents. It is conceivable that the steroids in these situations may produce more pronounced adverse effects because the antibiotic agents are not as effective.

Difficulties in evaluation of the use of steroids in infectious diseases have been noted by Lepper and Spies,[19] who studied these agents over a six-year period in more than 1000 patients. Although the effects were difficult to evaluate, they could not ascribe any marked benefits.

Figure 2[23] illustrates the hospital course of a young man with severe staphylococcal pneumonia following the Asian influenza syndrome. The severity of his illness is demonstrated in the figure, and one notes the improvement at the time both ristocetin and hydrocortisone were initiated. This patient made an excellent recovery. One might attribute the reversal of the toxic symptoms and recovery to the steroids.

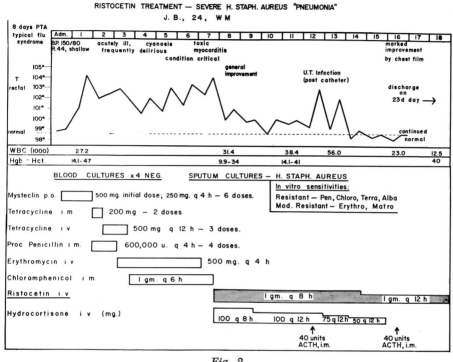

Fig. 2.

However, Figure 3[23] demonstrates an almost identical situation: a patient with staphylococcal pneumonia secondary to Asian influenza in whom the same excellent response occurred after the administration of only ristocetin.

Figure 4[23] demonstrates a different problem in evaluation of the effect of steroid therapy. This 26-year-old woman with puerperal endometritis and staphylococcal septicemia did not have a negative blood culture despite various antibiotics until ristocetin was administered. As one notes from the figure, however, the febrile pattern continued until steroids were given. Actually the administration of the steroids camouflaged the picture since, as soon as the steroids were decreased, the temperature again spiked despite treatment with chloromycetin and erythromycin. The reversal of this serious situation did not occur until the removal of the necrotic uterus was accomplished. Although this may have been a difficult undertaking, nevertheless it was the proper procedure, illustrating the urgent need for surgical removal of the necrotic focus. Although the steroid seemingly was helpful in this patient, it was the removal of the focus of infection which led to the clinical improvement. We might add that the continuation of antibiotics would also

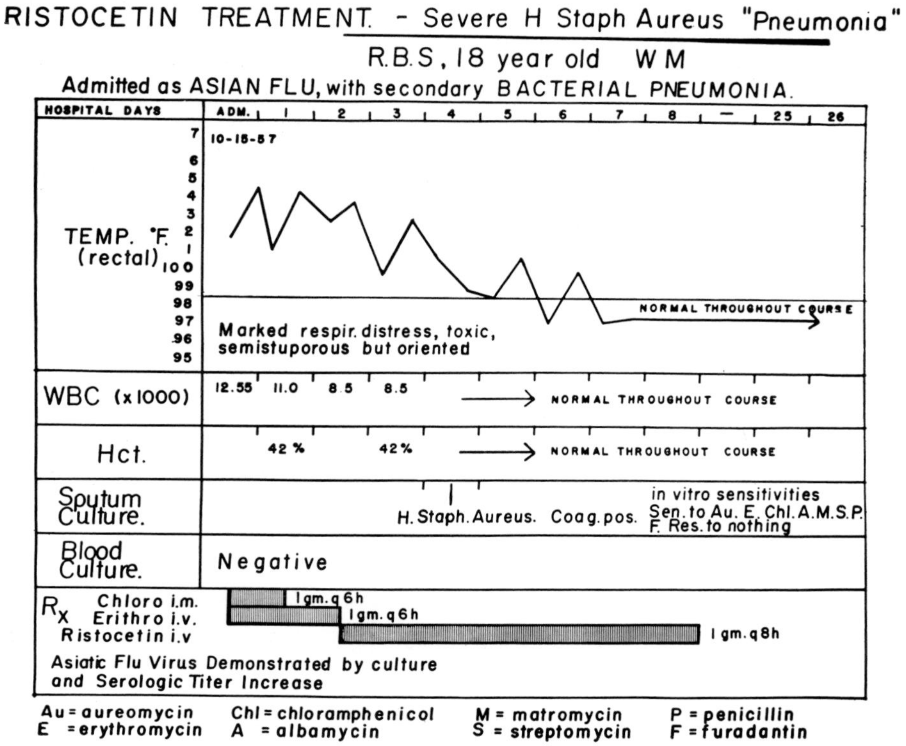

RISTOCETIN TREATMENT. – Severe H Staph Aureus "Pneumonia"

R.B.S., 18 year old   W M

Admitted as ASIAN FLU, with secondary BACTERIAL PNEUMONIA.

HOSPITAL DAYS	ADM.	1	2	3	4	5	6	7	8	—	25	26

TEMP. °F. (rectal)

Marked respir. distress, toxic, semistuporous but oriented

NORMAL THROUGHOUT COURSE

WBC (x1000)   12.55   11.0   8.5   8.5   → NORMAL THROUGHOUT COURSE

Hct.   42%   42%   → NORMAL THROUGHOUT COURSE

Sputum Culture.   H. Staph. Aureus. Coag. pos.   in vitro sensitivities   Sen. to Au. E. Chl. A.M.S.P.   F. Res. to nothing

Blood Culture.   Negative

Rx   Chloro i.m.   1 gm. q 6h
    Erithro i.v.   1 gm. q 6h
    Ristocetin i.v   1 gm. q 8h

Asiatic Flu Virus Demonstrated by culture and Serologic Titer Increase

Au = aureomycin   Chl = chloramphenicol   M = matromycin   P = penicillin
E = erythromycin   A = albamycin   S = streptomycin   F = furadantin

Fig. 3.

PUERPERAL ENDOMETRITIS AND SEPTICEMIA
(H. Staph. Aureus, coag. pos.)

L.G., 26, C.F.

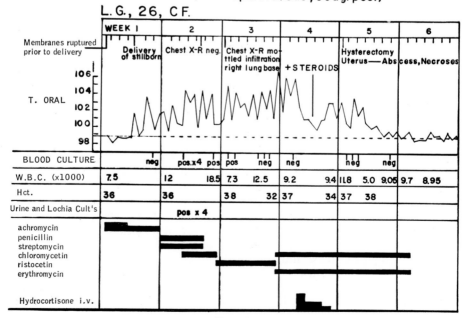

Fig. 4.

have been to no avail without the surgical procedure. This emphasizes the extreme importance of removal of infected foci when antibiotics are administered. Antibiotics alone under circumstances of this type are of limited value.

Antibacterial agents have been used as a prophylactic measure in patients receiving steroids. This is indeed a complex problem. Chemoprophylaxis generally has been effective when it has been used to eliminate susceptible microorganisms such as Group A beta hemolytic streptococci or the meningococci, but it has not been particularly so with staphylococci or with gram-negative bacteria, particularly those which readily become drug-resistant. Prophylactic regimens can hardly be expected to confer adequate protection.

With the common antibiotic-resistant organisms, the feeling of security that the clinician may have in supposedly protecting the patient by chemoprophylaxis is hardly justified. It is particularly important, when prophylactic chemotherapy is used, that the dose of the agent be an adequate therapeutic one.

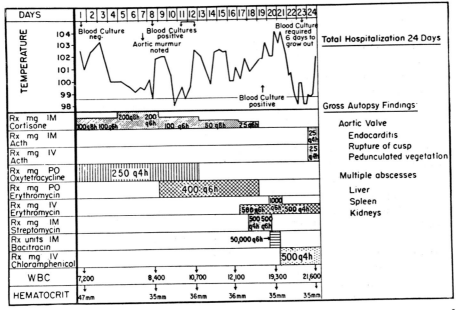

Fig. 5. Staphylococcal septicemia and endocarditis secondary to cortisone-treated exfoliative dermatitis due to penicillin (40-year-old colored woman).

Figure 5[22] shows vividly the complex problem of steroid therapy of allergy to penicillin and the complications which ensued. The patient was a 40-year-old woman who received an injection of penicillin for a small ulcer on the leg. This history was not obtained and later she received a second injection of penicillin. She was subsequently admitted to our hospital with a severe exfoliative dermatitis. We obtained a history of allergy to penicillin over the previous two years. As noted in the figure, not only did her exfoliative dermatitis improve with the administration of steroids but there was a subsidence of her fever. Despite improvement with the steroid and the administration of oxytetracycline for control of her cystitis, present because of a catheter, a staphylococcal endocarditis of the aortic valve developed. Her subsequent course was adverse and she ultimately died. The various postmortem findings are shown. Delipidization of the adrenal cortex was found on histological examination. This case illustrates many problems but in particular the development of a staphylococcal sepsis during steroid therapy and the inability of small doses of an antibiotic to prevent the progression of infection.

The evidence is questionable that adrenal insufficiency occurs as a consequence of severe sepsis in the absence of pre-existing adrenal cortical hypofunction (Addison's disease). It has been shown[24] that endotoxins from gram-negative bacteria inhibit steroidogenesis in the perfused adrenal gland. Large amounts of endotoxin were used in this experiment—that is, large by *in vivo* standards. The possibility of direct damage to the adrenal as a cause of adrenal insufficiency cannot be discounted despite the fact that the circulating corticosteroid levels in the animals given lethal doses of endotoxin are generally above the normal range.[20] Recent studies[27] suggest that large doses of steroids may have a definite value in patients with shock and sepsis.

Of the clinical syndromes considered to be associated with adrenal insufficiency, none is more likely than meningococcal toxemia with collapse, in which the use of corticosteroids and related compounds is generally recommended as part of therapy.

Failures have occurred in spite of the use of steroids,[19] and the collapse in this infection has been successfully corrected by treatment with levarterenol (norepinephrine) without corticosteroids.[25] Some authors[7, 11] emphasize the need for a pressor agent such as levarterenol to be administered along with adrenal hormones and chemotherapy. It is quite apparent that more information is needed concerning the value of the corticosteroids in the management of meningococcal infection with shock.

All of us are aware that adrenal insufficiency may occur if infection appears in patients in whom exogenous steroids have suppressed steroidogenesis. Under such circumstances, there is justification for increasing the dose of steroids. Relatively little objective support exists for the concept that adrenal insufficiency is common in severe infections and that the use of steroids is justified on that basis.

It has already been noted that the steroid levels are usually elevated in patients during severe infections. It is possible that under certain circumstances small doses of exogenous hormone might conceivably cause more steroid to enter tissue cells.

Adrenal corticosteroids are effective in diminishing the inflammatory response regardless of the stimulus. In general, the effects of steroids on inflammation and repair can be explained[3] on the basis of their effect on vascular tone and permeability. The effects of corticosteroids on hypersensitivity reactions and similar tissue responses to immunologically active stimuli probably reflect the general anti-inflammatory effect of these steroids rather than a specific effect on purely immunologic mechanisms.

At present, it is generally agreed that steroids depress antibody production but do not alter the degradation rate of the pre-formed antibodies.[1, 6, 16] The mechanism by which this happens is not quite clear.

In conclusion, it is obvious that the exact status of steroids in the collateral management of infections is still not definitive and requires much in the way of further cautious controlled clinical study.

REFERENCES

1. Bjørneboe, M., Fischel, E. E. and Stoerk, H. C.: Effect of cortisone and adreno-corticotrophic hormone on concentration of circulating antibody. J. Exper. Med., 93:37, 1951.
2. Coriell, L. L., Siegal, A. C., Cook, C. D., Murphy, L. and Stokes, J., Jr.: Use of pituitary adrenocorticotropic hormone (ACTH) in poliomyelitis. J.A.M.A., 142:1279, 1950.
3. Dougherty, T. F. and Schneebeli, G. C.: Use of steroids as anti-inflammatory agents. Ann. N. Y. Acad. Sc., 61:328, 1955.
4. Evans, A. S., Sprinz, H. and Nelson, R. S.: Adrenal hormone therapy in viral hepatitis: effect of ACTH in acute disease. Ann. Int. Med., 38:1115, 1953.
5. Finland, M., Kass, E. H. and Ingbar, S. H.: Effects of ACTH in primary atypical (viral) pneumonia and in pneumococcal pneumonia. Proc. 1st Clin. ACTH Conf. Philadelphia, Blakiston Co., 1950, pp. 529-534.
6. Fischel, E. E., Stoerk, H. and Bjørneboe, M.: Failure of cortisone to affect rate of disappearance of antibody protein. Proc. Soc. Exper. Biol. & Med., 77:111, 1951.
7. Griffin, J. W. and Daeschner, C. W.: Meningococcal infections with particular reference to fulminating meningococcemia (Waterhouse-Friderichsen syndrome) treated with cortisone and norepinephrine. J. Pediat., 45:264, 1954.
8. Haggerty, R. J. and Eley, R. C.: Varicella and cortisone. Pediatrics, 18:160, 1956.
9. Hahn, E. O., Houser, H. B., Rammelkamp, C. H., Jr., Denny, F. W. and Wannamaker, L. W.: Effect of cortisone on acute streptococcal infections and post-streptococcal complications. J. Clin. Invest., 30:274, 1951.
10. Johnson, J. R. and Davey, W. N.: Cortisone, corticotropin and antimicrobial therapy in tuberculosis in animals and man; a review. Am. Rev. Tuberc., 70:623, 1954.
11. Kanter, D. M., Mauriello, D. A. and Learner, N.: Acute meningococcemia with vascular collapse: analysis of 10 recently treated cases. Am. J. M. Sc., 232:674, 1956.
12. Kass, G. H.: Hypothermia following cortisone administration. Am. J. Med., 18:146, 1955.
13. Kass, E. H. and Finland, M.: Adrenocortical hormones and management of infections. Ann. Rev. Med., 8:1, 1957.
14. Kass, E. H. and Finland, M.: Corticosteroids and infections. Adv. Int. Med., 9:45, 1958.
15. Kass, E. H., Ingbar, S. H. and Finland, M.: Effects of adrenocorticotropic hormone in pneumonia: clinical, bacteriological and serological studies. Ann. Int. Med., 33:1081, 1950.
16. Kass, E. H., Kendrick, M. I. and Finland, M.: Effects of corticosterone, hydrocortisone and corticotropin on production of antibodies in rabbits. J. Exper. Med., 102:767, 1955.
17. Kirby, J. C., Jr., Polis, G. and Romansky, M. J.: A controlled blind study of pneumococcal pneumonia treated with tetracycline and tetracycline plus 6-methyl prednisolone. Am. J. M. Sc., 240:30, 1960.
18. Klemola, E. and Somer, P.: Treatment of mumps orchitis with cortisone and corticotropin. Nord. Med., 56:1128, 1956.
19. Lepper, M. H. and Spies, H. W.: Clinical study of the use of cortisone, hydrocortisone and corticotropin in the treatment of seriously ill patients with infections. Antibiot. Ann., 447-454, 1956-1957.
20. Melby, J. C. and Spink, W. W.: Production and catabolism of cortisol in experimental endotoxin shock. J. Clin. Invest., 37:1791, 1958.
21. Nelson, R. S.: Present indications for cortisone therapy in acute viral hepatitis. Ann. Int. Med., 46:685, 1957.
22. Phillips, L. V., Romansky, M. J. and Nasou, J. P.: Staphylococcal septicemia and endocarditis secondary to cortisone-treated exfoliative dermatitis due to penicillin. Antibiot. Ann., 68, 1954-1955.
23. Romansky, M. J.: Ristocetin, an effective antibiotic in staphylococcal infections and short-term therapy of endocarditis. Med. Hyg., Sept. 11, 1959.
24. Rosenfeld, G.: In vitro influence of bacterial pyrogens in adrenocortical function of perfused calf adrenals. Am. J. Physiol., 182:57, 1955.
25. Sokoloff, L., King, B. D. and Wechsler, R. L.: Role of l-norepinephrine in treatment of shock. Med. Clin. North America, 38:499, 1954.
26. Spink, W. W.: ACTH and adrenocorticosteroids as therapeutic adjuncts in infectious diseases. New Engl. J. Med., 257:979, 1031, 1957.

27. Spink, W. W.: The pathogenesis and management of shock due to infection. Arch.
    Int. Med., *106*:433, 1960.
28. Wagner, N. H., Bennett, I. L., Lasagna, L., Cluff, L. E., Rosenthal, M. B. and
    Mirick, G. S.: Effect of hydrocortisone upon course of pneumococcal pneumonia
    treated with penicillin. Bull. Johns Hopkins Hosp., *98*:197, 1956.

The Effect of Steroids
on Shock Due to Endotoxin*

MAX H. WEIL and KENNETH S. ALLEN

School of Medicine, University of Southern California

There is an increasing number of reports that a favorable clinical response
is obtained with large doses of steroids in cases of shock caused by bacterial
infection.[4, 11] The potential value is in the use of corticosteroids as drugs
rather than as replacement therapy. Because of the precarious and complex
clinical picture presented by the patients, these impressions can be only
partly supported by controlled, quantitative measurements at the bedside.
Case history data are impressive, but a variety of therapeutic procedures in
addition to the administration of corticosteroids are usually involved. It is
possible that the very fact that these patients are closely observed results
in therapeutic advantages. Such close observation, with careful attention to
maintenance of a clear airway, the administration of oxygen at a critical
time, or special alertness to fluid and electrolyte balance, may account for
the observed differences in mortality.

At present, insufficient objective data are available to evaluate the therapeutic indications or the value of corticosteroids for the treatment of shock
due to infection. Animal investigations provide the basis for much of the
basic information. However, if tentative therapeutic implications on the
effects of corticosteroids in the human patient are to be derived from animal
experimentation, additional insight may be obtained by studying several
species under controlled conditions. This has been accomplished in shock
produced by endotoxins, which we use as an experimental model for study
of shock due to infection. The findings demonstrate the therapeutic effects of
corticosteroids.

THE RELATIONSHIP BETWEEN PRETREATMENT AND TREATMENT

Pretreatment with corticosteroid hormones has been shown to be remarkably effective in preventing the lethal course of endotoxin shock in the
mouse,[1, 2, 12] the rat[14] and the dog.[7] This is graphically illustrated in Figure 1.
However, the relationship between prophylactic and therapeutic effects is
controversial. In the mouse, Geller, Merrill and Jawetz[2] reported that intraperitoneal injection of a corticosteroid one hour following injection of

* Supported by Grant H-5570, National Heart Institute, National Institutes of Health,
United States Public Health Service, and by grants-in-aid from The American Heart
Association and The Los Angeles County Heart Association.

endotoxin provided only minimal protection. In view of incidental observations in our own laboratory that treatment did promote survival, the comparative effectiveness of pretreatment and treatment was studied again in male Swiss Webster mice weighing between 20 and 25 grams. The mice were injected intraperitoneally with purified endotoxin (lipo-polysaccharide) derived from *Escherichia coli.** Amounts of endotoxin were injected which previously proved lethal for 90 per cent of the animals. Prednisolone phosphate in amounts of 60 mg./kg. was administered intraperitoneally at intervals up to 12 hours before and 12 hours following endotoxin. The result of these experiments, expressed on the basis of survival after 24 hours, is illustrated in Figure 2. With employment of the soluble prednisolone preparation, both prophylactic and therapeutic effects were demonstrated, confirming original observations by Spink and Anderson.[12] The prophylactic effect was greatest with pretreatment given in the period between one-half and two hours prior to injection; however, an even greater therapeutic effect occurred when the steroid was given at the same time or up to four hours

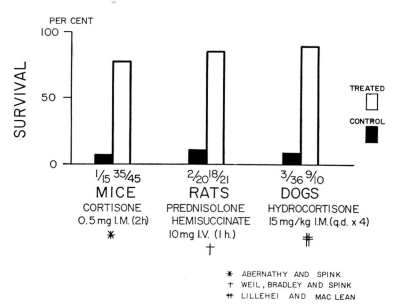

Fig. 1.   Increased survival of mice, rats and dogs shocked with endotoxin after pretreatment with corticosteroid.

after injection of the endotoxin. A corroborative study in which two injections of prednisolone were employed is summarized in Table 1. When one of the injections was given one or four hours prior to the endotoxin, the results were not better than when the two injections were both given following the injection of endotoxin. It is concluded that the early administration of the steroid following intraperitoneal injection of endotoxin provides therapeutic effect equal to or exceeding the effectiveness of pretreatment with a similar amount of corticosteroid.

Protective and therapeutic actions of prednisolone phosphate were also

* Obtained from Difco Laboratories, Detroit, Michigan (Lot #0127:B8).

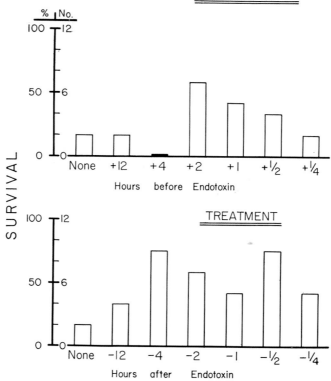

Fig. 2. Duration of protection in endotoxic shock in mice after pretreatment or treatment
with corticosteroid.

studied in the rat. Crude endotoxin (*E. coli* cells) prepared according to
methods previously described[15] was injected intravenously into the tail vein
of male rats, Wistar strain, weighing between 90 and 120 grams. Amounts
were used which were previously found to be lethal for 90 per cent of the
animals. Prednisolone phosphate was injected in amounts of 40 mg./kg.

TABLE 1. *EFFECT OF TIME OF ADMINISTRATION OF TWO INJECTIONS OF
PREDNISOLONE ON THE SURVIVAL OF MICE SHOCKED
WITH ENDOTOXIN*

	NO. OF MICE	PREDNISOLONE INJECTION		SURVIVAL	
		1st	2nd	No.	%
I	12	+ 4	− 4	10	83
II	12	+ 1	− 4	9	75
III	12	− ¼	− 4	10	83
Control	12	0	0	2	17

+ = hours prior to endotoxin.
− = hours following endotoxin.

Male Swiss Webster mice weighing 20 to 25 grams were given intraperitoneal injections of *E. coli* endotoxin.

Prednisolone phosphate, in amounts of 30 mg./kg., was administered intraperitoneally
at times indicated.

intravenously at intervals preceding and following injection of endotoxin. The results of these experiments are graphically demonstrated in Figure 3. Under the circumstances of these studies, the therapeutic action of corticosteroid during the first hour following injection of endotoxin was less impressive. Beneficial effects that followed administration of steroid between two hours before and 15 minutes following endotoxin are highly significant (p < .001). Quantitative differences between the effectiveness of treatment and pretreatment in the mouse and rat are believed to be related largely to the route of administration of the endotoxin. It is likely that endotoxin is absorbed at a much slower rate from the intraperitonal site, allowing the corticosteroid to be therapeutically active for a more prolonged period.

Lillehei and MacLean[8] demonstrated that pretreatment of the dog with hydrocortisone sodium succinate (15 mg./kg. intramuscularly daily for four

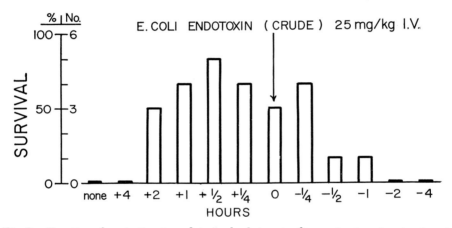

Fig. 3.   Duration of protection in endotoxic shock in rats after pretreatment or treatment with corticosteroid.

days) protects the dog against the lethal effects of crude endotoxin (7.5 mg./kg. intravenously). Under the circumstances of their experiments, only three of 36 untreated control animals survived, whereas nine out of ten dogs pretreated with hydrocortisone recovered. Recent studies in which prednisolone phosphate in amounts of 20 mg./kg. was injected intravenously 15 minutes after crude endotoxin (6.6 mg./kg.) are summarized in Table 2.

The therapeutic effect was much less striking than that observed following pretreatment by Lillehei and MacLean. However, the therapeutic employment of corticosteroid, when used following endotoxin, clearly improved the duration of survival (p < .02).

TABLE 2.   EFFECT OF PREDNISOLONE ON FATALITY TIME AND SURVIVAL FOLLOWING PRODUCTION OF SHOCK WITH ENDOTOXIN IN DOGS

THERAPY	NO. OF DOGS	FATALITY TIME (hours)	NO. OF SURVIVORS
Prednisolone	9	13.0 ± 3.8	3
		p < .02	
Control	9	6.6 ± 1.6	2

Endotoxin (6.6 mg./kg.) was administered intravenously and prednisolone phosphate (20 mg./kg.) was also administered intravenously 15 minutes later.

DOSE OF CORTICOSTEROID

Initial experience in the treatment of endotoxin shock with corticosteroids was not impressive because replacement rather than pharmacological doses were used.[15] The adrenalectomized mouse is sustained by 10 μg. of cortisone

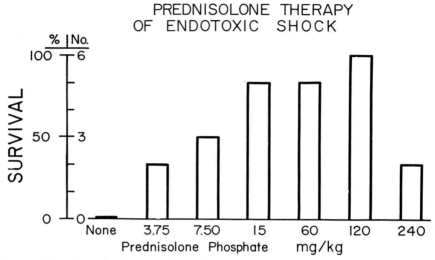

Fig. 4.   The relationship between dose of corticosteroid and survival in therapy of endotoxic shock.

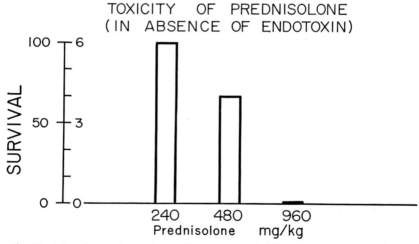

Fig. 5.   Toxicity of very large doses of corticosteroid following intraperitoneal injection into mice.

and requires a maximum of 100 μg. during stress. However, these amounts of corticosteroids provide negligible benefit following injection of endotoxin. The quantities of cortisone that are required to obtain maximum survival are approximately 200 times greater. Relationship of the therapeutic dose to 24-hour survival in experiments with mice is demonstrated in Figure 4. Maximum benefit followed treatment with two injections, each containing prednisolone in a quantity of 120 mg./kg. This remarkably large dose of prednisolone injected into a single 20-gram mouse would be equivalent to the dose that would provide optimal replacement for one day for a human adult with complete adrenal ablation. The increased mortality at higher doses is related to the toxicity of prednisolone itself, a feature which is demonstrated in Figure 5. Thus, the protective effect of the steroid increases up to the point where its beneficial action is compromised by the toxic effect of the drug itself.

MECHANISM OF CORTICOSTEROID PROTECTION

The mode of action of corticosteroids has been studied with the view of elucidating the mechanism by which they protect against lethal effects of endotoxin. Ribble and co-workers[10] found that the rate of removal of radioactive *E. coli* endotoxin and its distribution in organs was unaltered by cortisone. Levitin, Kendrick and Kass,[6] who measured blood levels of cortisol, demonstrated a close relationship between the concentration of the steroid and therapeutic effectiveness. Observations on dosage and duration of effectiveness in the course of studies detailed above led to some similar conclusions. The evidence favors the postulation that the steroids, by their physical presence, protect the tissues against the damaging effects of endotoxin or a secondary product that results from the interaction of endotoxin and blood.[3]

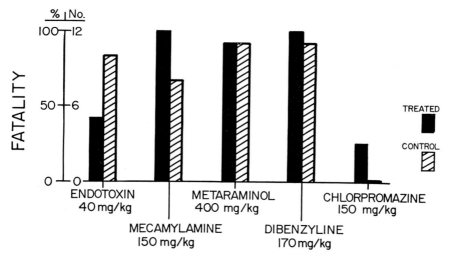

Fig. 6. The effect of corticosteroid treatment on lethal response to ganglionic blocking drugs, adrenergic blocking agents, and sympathomimetic amines in comparison to its action against lethal response to endotoxin.

The suppression of increased serum transaminase by hydrocortisone noted by Melby and Spink[9] probably reflects this protection against tissue injury.

Steroids are sometimes assumed to protect in a "nonspecific manner" against insults that produce hypotension. An exploratory experiment summarized in Figure 6 gives no support to this assumption. Treatment with prednisolone phosphate (60 mg./kg.) intraperitoneally, which protects against the lethal effects of endotoxin, is not effective in protecting against lethal amounts of ganglionic blocking agents (mecamylamine, chlorpromazine), adrenergic blocking drugs (dibenzyline) or sympathomimetic amines (metaraminol). On the contrary, treatment with corticosteroid is associated with a significant increase in fatality in animals injected with mecamylamine and chlorpromazine (p <.01).

Lillehei and MacLean[8] proposed that the beneficial effect of corticosteroids was related to their ability to counter a selective vasospastic effect produced by endotoxin. This conclusion was based on experiments in dogs

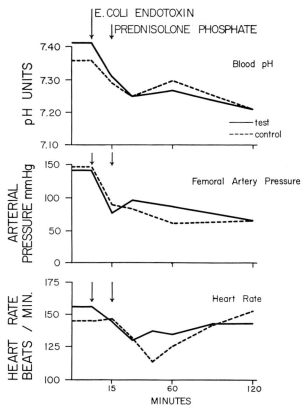

Fig. 7. The effect of corticosteroid therapy on heart rate, arterial pressure, and blood pH of dogs during the first two hours following production of shock with endotoxin.

in which vasopressor amines, especially metaraminol, in large amounts, were administered simultaneously with the endotoxin. The vasopressor agent was found to potentiate shock when used in this fashion. Since hydrocortisone also protected against fatal epinephrine shock, an adrenergic blocking action was ascribed to the steroid. Subsequent studies in dogs, in which metaraminol was administered after endotoxin to maintain arterial pressure at physiological levels, did not show potentiation of shock.[13] Experiments in mice (Fig. 6) did not indicate that corticosteroid protected against lethal effects of metaraminol. Additional experiments in mice in which metaraminol was administered with and without corticosteroid are summarized in Table 3. No beneficial or detrimental effects were observed after the administration of relatively large amounts of the vasopressor drug.

The effectiveness of a vasopressor agent has been shown to be augmented following administration of corticosteroids.[5] Spink[11] has reported that in dogs with endotoxin shock, large doses of hydrocortisone greatly reduced the requirement of metaraminol to sustain arterial pressure at physiological levels. The relationship between therapeutic effects of vasopressor agents and corticosteroid, and their effect on the progression of endotoxin shock, require additional study. However, on the basis of data presently available, it may be concluded that the beneficial action of corticosteroid is not related to an adrenolytic effect.

The hemodynamic and pH changes produced in dogs by endotoxin have been intensively studied. Detailed measurements have been made in an attempt to define the hemodynamic alterations that immediately follow administration of corticosteroid for treatment of shock. No immediate effect on arterial pressure, heart rate, or blood pH was observed in the two hours

TABLE 3. COMPARISON OF THERAPEUTIC RESPONSIVENESS TO METARAMINOL AND CORTICOSTEROID SEPARATELY AND IN COMBINATION FOLLOWING ENDOTOXIN

	SURVIVORS/TOTAL	SURVIVORS (%)
Metaraminol	2/18	11
Prednisolone	10/18	56
Metaraminol and prednisolone	10/18	56
Control (no therapy)	2/18	11

Male Swiss Webster mice weighing 20 to 25 grams were given *E. coli* endotoxin (35 mg./kg.) intraperitoneally. Metaraminol bitartrate (10 mg./kg.) and prednisolone phosphate (60 mg./kg.) were administered intraperitoneally at one-fourth and at four hours following injection of endotoxin.

following the administration of prednisolone phosphate. In Figure 7, these variables are compared in dogs treated with prednisolone and in untreated control animals. No definite alterations were observed during the first two hours in animals treated with the corticosteroid.

CORTICOSTEROID PREPARATIONS

A formulation of hydrocortisone or of one of its analogues that is soluble in blood is required for the emergency treatment of patients in shock. When an indication for such a corticosteroid drug exists, the agent may be injected intravenously to provide almost instantaneous increase in the effective blood concentration of the steroid. Table 4 shows a comparison of the response of mice with endotoxin shock to treatment with four preparations in common use. Doses were adjusted to provide amounts which were approximately equal in therapeutic value. Except for the lesser effectiveness of methyl prednisolone, the response to each of the formulations was approximately the same. Improvement which followed doubling of the dose indicates that the decreased protection obtained during the initial trial with methyl prednisolone was probably related to initial underestimation of the equivalent dose. Clinical and laboratory observations have to date not demonstrated therapeutic superiority for the analogues of hydrocortisone. It is possible that when hypotension is complicated by congestive heart failure, prednisolone may have a practical advantage because of the lessened renal retention of sodium.

TABLE 4. COMPARISON OF THERAPEUTIC RESPONSIVENESS TO COMPARABLE AMOUNTS OF CORTISOL AND ITS ANALOGUES

	DOSE (mg./kg.)	SURVIVORS/ TOTAL	SURVIVORS (%)	TOTAL DOSE	SURVIVORS/ TOTAL	SURVIVORS (%)
Hydrocortisone sodium succinate (Solu-Cortef)	165	16/24	67	330	8/12	67
Prednisolone phosphate (Hydeltrasol)	30	16/24	67	30	12/12	100
Methyl prednisolone sodium succinate (Solu-Medrol)	21	9/24	38	42	10/12	83
Dexamethasone phosphate (Decadron)	4.4	16/24	67	8.8	12/12	100
Untreated	..	3/24	13	..	2/12	17

Male Swiss Webster mice weighing 20 to 25 grams were given intraperitoneal injections of *E. coli* endotoxin (31 mg./kg.). Corticosteroid was administered intraperitoneally at 15 minutes and again at 4 hours after endotoxin.

COMMENT

The present studies in experimental animals have demonstrated the effectiveness of corticosteroids as therapeutic agents in endotoxin shock. The method by which shock has been produced in the experimental animal deserves comment. In each case, purified endotoxin or non-viable bacterial cells were used. In the human patient, bacterial toxin is released in the presence of active infection. The ability of adrenocortical hormones to promote bacterial multiplication and remove natural barriers in the face of spreading infection is recognized. However, clinical and laboratory observations indicate that the concurrent use and judicious choice of antibiotics in patients treated with corticosteroid make this a relatively small hazard.

SUMMARY AND CONCLUSIONS

Previous observations on the effectiveness of pretreatment with corticosteroids in preventing fatal reactions to endotoxin were confirmed. Experiments in mice, rats and dogs also demonstrated their therapeutic value when administered during the four hours that followed injection of endotoxin. Increments in dosage of steroid resulted in corresponding improvement in survival until a point was reached where beneficial effect was limited by toxicity of the drug itself. The value of the corticosteroids is attributed to a pharmacological rather than a physiological action of the hormone.

Studies were made to elucidate mechanisms of corticosteroid protection. The hormone failed to protect against "nonspecific" reactions produced by hypotensive agents. On the contrary, treatment resulted in a significant increase in fatalities in animals injected with mecamylamine and chlorpromazine. No sympatholytic action was demonstrated. Measurements in dogs with endotoxin shock failed to demonstrate major changes in arterial pressure, pulse rate, or blood pH in the early period following prednisolone therapy, in spite of significant improvement in survival of the treated animals. The reason for the protective action of the hormone against the lethal injury produced by endotoxin is not clear. Physical presence of the steroid hormone in extremely large amounts is associated with therapeutic effectiveness. Equivalent doses of soluble preparations of hydrocortisone or one of its newer analogues demonstrated quantitatively similar results.

REFERENCES

1. Abernathy, R. S. and Spink, W. W.: Resistance to endotoxin after protection against initial lethal challenge with adrenocorticoids or chlorpromazine. Proc. Soc. Exper. Biol. & Med., 95:580, 1957.
2. Geller, P., Merrill, E. R. and Jawetz, E.: Effects of cortisone and antibiotics on lethal action of endotoxin in mice. Proc. Soc. Exper. Biol. & Med., 86:716, 1954.
3. Hinshaw, L. B., Bradley, G. M. and Carlson, C. H.: Effect of endotoxin on renal function in the dog. Am. J. Physiol., 196:112, 1959.
4. Kinsell, L. W.: Nutritional and metabolic aspects of infection. Ann. N. Y. Acad. Sc., 63:240, 1955.
5. Kurland, G. S. and Freedberg, A. S.: The potentiating effect of ACTH and of cortisone on pressor response to intravenous infusion of l-norepinephrine. Proc. Soc. Exper. Biol. & Med., 78:28, 1951.
6. Levitin, H., Kendrick, M. I. and Kass, E. H.: Effect of route of administration on protective action of corticosterone and cortisol against endotoxin. Proc. Soc. Exper. Biol. & Med., 93:306, 1956.
7. Lillehei, R. C. and MacLean, L. D.: The intestinal factor in irreversible endotoxin shock. Ann. Surg., 148:513, 1958.

8. Lillehei, R. C. and MacLean, L. D.: Physiological approach to successful treatment of endotoxin shock in the experimental animal. A.M.A. Arch. Surg., 78:464, 1959.
9. Melby, J. C., Bossenmaier, I. C., Egdahl, R. H. and Spink, W. W.: Suppression by cortisol of increased serum transaminase induced by endotoxin. Lancet, 1:441, 1959.
10. Ribble, J. C., Zalesky, M. and Braude, A. I.: Endotoxin and cortisone in mice. Bull. Johns Hopkins Hosp., 105:272, 1959.
11. Spink, W. W.: The pathogenesis and management of shock due to infection. Arch. Int. Med., 106:433, 1960.
12. Spink, W. W. and Anderson, D.: Experimental studies on the significance of endotoxin in the pathogenesis of brucellosis. J. Clin. Invest., 33:540, 1954.
13. Weil, Max H.: Experimental studies on the therapy of circulatory failure produced by endotoxin. J. Lab. & Clin. Med. (in press).
14. Weil, M. H., Bradley, G. M. and Spink, W. W.: Unpublished observations.
15. Weil, M. H. and Spink, W. W.: A comparison of shock due to endotoxin with anaphylactic shock. J. Lab. & Clin. Med., 50:501, 1957.

Steroid Therapy in Bacterial Endocarditis

ALFRED VOGL and BENNET P. LUSTGARTEN

New York University College of Medicine

Until now little use has been made of steroid treatment in bacterial endocarditis, and yet the steroids appear likely to aid in managing the particular problems with which we are presented in this disease—the serious local and the life-threatening systemic manifestations of an inflammatory process. Locally, the disease tends to destroy the valvular structures of the heart and, at the same time, tends to protect the invading organisms by granulomatous tissue proliferation against antibacterial agents carried in the blood stream. Systemically, it often threatens the patient's life directly with overwhelming toxemia. All these are biologic phenomena which are known to be modified and ameliorated by the action of corticosteroids.

Objections to their use are based upon well documented observations of a breakdown of immunologic body defenses in other infectious diseases and upon animal experiments in which there is heightened virulence and subsequent spread of the infection while the outward manifestations of these events are being masked by the steroid effect. The only available answer to this aspect of the problem lies in the simultaneous use of adequate doses of antibiotics with a view to containing the infectious organisms during this period.

Other side effects of the steroids usually associated with their prolonged use may also give rise to concern but are, of course, of much less practical importance in a disease of limited duration.

It is therefore understandable that there has been, and still is, great hesitation to use the steroids in bacterial endocarditis primarily for their presumable beneficial effect on the local disease process, and one is likely to defer their use unless one's hand is forced by severe systemic manifestation of the infection with toxemia of such a degree that it as such becomes an immediate threat to the patient's life.

Such a situation prevailed in the case which we reported in 1959, of a patient who is still under our observation. An abstract of his case history follows:[5]

The patient was 53 in 1958, when he became acutely ill. He had suffered from bronchial asthma since childhood and had had rheumatic fever at the age of 32. During 1957, he had experienced increasing exertional dyspnea. He presented the signs of chronic asthmatic bronchitis and of rheumatic heart disease with mitral insufficiency and aortic stenosis and insufficiency. The symptoms and findings indicated the presence of moderate congestive failure and renal involvement at that time. Within a three-day period, he developed in rapid succession chills, fever up to 103° F. (39.4° C.) (Fig. 1), anterior chest pain, pleuritic type pain in his left chest, moist rales at the bases of both lungs, hematuria, pyuria and electrocardiographic changes including Wenckebach periods, inversion of T waves in leads 1, 2 and V_6,

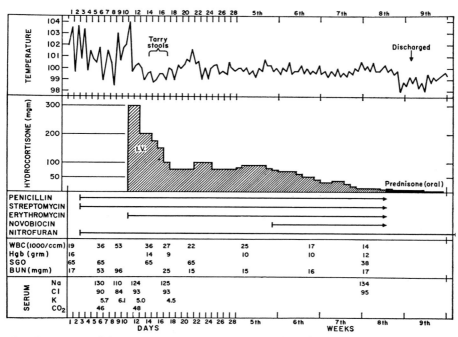

Fig. 1. Course of disease in patient with bacterial endocarditis. (From Lustgarten, B. P. and Vogl, A.: J.A.M.A., *170*:800, 1959.)

and appearance of a Q wave in aVF. These findings appeared indicative of *bacterial endocarditis* superimposed upon *rheumatic heart disease*.

Five specimens of blood were drawn on the first hospital day, and treatment with 3,600,000 units of penicillin and 1 gram of streptomycin a day was started thereafter.

On the second day, the patient developed symptoms of mesenteric embolism consisting of severe abdominal pain, distention and constipation, progressive clinical and radiologic signs of intestinal obstruction and, a week later, passage of tarry stools.

During the first 10 days of hospitalization the fever was septic in type, and dyspnea and chest rales increased. The patient coughed up fresh and clotted blood. He was frequently confused and had several episodes of pulmonary edema and shock. Subsequently he developed uremia with intractable singultus and generalized convulsions. Repeatedly he appeared moribund. On the sixth hospital day the murmurs over the aortic area suddenly became much louder and the diastolic pressure dropped to zero while the systolic remained at 160 mm. (suggesting rupture of an aortic cusp.)

Blood urea nitrogen rose to 53 and later to 96 mg. per cent and the blood developed a leukemoid picture with 50,000 white cells.

This syndrome of septicemia, in a patient with rheumatic valvular heart disease and evidence of multiple embolism (mesenteric and renal) and changing cardiac murmurs, appeared to corroborate the diagnosis of bacterial endocarditis. The blood cultures showed no growth; the causative organism thus remained obscure. Because of the septic complications, the penicillin dosage was increased to 40 million units daily. But despite the antibiotic and supportive therapy the patient's condition was rapidly becoming desperate: he was in stupor most of the time; spiking temperatures and congestive failure with repeated pulmonary edema and severe cyanosis continued, and striking muscular wasting and prostration developed rapidly.

In this critical situation, which was dominated by severe septicemia, it was decided on the 11th hospital day to try vigorous steroid treatment. A single intravenous injection of 100 mg. of hydrocortisone was given and another 200 mg. were added to the infusions of penicillin in 5 per cent dextrose solution in the course of the first day. By midnight the temperature had dropped from 104° F. to 99.8° F. and remained from then on generally about 100° F. for the rest of the hospitalization. The lowering of the temperature was associated with a striking improvement in the patient's symptoms, general appearance and physical findings. Convulsions ceased, cyanosis subsided, congestive failure became easier to manage, the mental status improved markedly and the patient developed a voracious appetite.

The persistence of a severe infection and/or stress despite the obvious clinical improvement was, however, apparent from the leukocyte count of 43,000 per cubic millimeter with a marked shift to the left, the persistence of hematuria and pyuria and a high serum transaminase level which suggested continued tissue destruction, possibly of the kidney.

The hydrocortisone dosage of 200 mg. was reduced to 170 mg. a day after two days, when melena occurred and lasted three days, apparently as the result of a mesenteric infarction (see above). The hydrocortisone dosage was gradually reduced further in the course of the next eight weeks while antibiotics (penicillin, streptomycin, erythromycin and novobiocin) and treatment for congestive failure were continued. During these weeks there was progressive improvement except for a brief breakthrough of fever on the 20th and 21st hospital day which was promptly controlled with a temporary increase in hydrocortisone dosage (from 75 to 100 mg. a day). The blood urea nitrogen fell from 96 mg. per cent before steroid treatment to 25 mg. per cent 10 days later. Leukocytosis, pyuria and albuminuria persisted for seven weeks. The hemoglobin, which was 9 grams after the melena, rose to 12 grams before discharge from the hospital. At that time all antibacterial drugs were stopped. Nitrofurantoin only was continued for another month.

The patient remained afebrile and asymptomatic for 6 months except for extreme fatigability. When presented at the hospital staff conference four months after discharge, he looked and felt well and denied symptoms of congestive heart failure. Six months after discharge he was readmitted for acute rheumatic fever. He responded well to several weeks of salicylate medication. The patient has since been able to perform light manual work despite symptoms of chronic asthmatic bronchitis and mild congestive heart failure. Pyuria recurred but there has been no more azotemia.

In summary, this was the case of a middle-aged man with rheumatic valvular heart disease and bacterial endocarditis manifested clinically by septicemia, rapidly developing left heart failure and signs of mesenteric embolism and focal-embolic glomerulonephritis with uremia. Blood cultures remained negative. The rapidly progressive deterioration to the point of apparently imminent death was dramatically reversed by steroid therapy together with continued massive antibiotic treatment. The subsequent course of the illness was favorable and the patient is now, 2½ years later, able to perform light manual work.

At the time of our report a therapeutic conference took place at the Hôpital Necker in Paris on the treatment of subacute bacterial endocarditis with negative blood culture.[2] Dr. Bertrand-Fontaine discussed the possible role of steroids in these circumstances. She thought it justified to employ steroids together with antibiotics in resistant cases and enumerated the advantages: rapid and spectacular improvement of the general condition with a fall in temperature and a sense of well-being, improvement of the inflammatory signs, improvement of the glomerulonephritis and disappearance of Osler's nodes, improvement of the biologic signs and reduction of the gamma globulin. Dr. Bertrand-Fontaine stressed in the discussion that she regarded the steroids as a weapon not to be used immediately but only in those cases of bacterial endocarditis that prove resistant to antibiotic treatment. She added, however, that no valid criteria for this indication and no controls are as yet available.

In the recent American literature (since the publication of our report) we could find only one reference to the therapeutic use of steroids in bacterial endocarditis. Spink[6] mentioned one patient who was treated with penicillin for bacterial endocarditis and, at the same time, with cortisone because of his penicillin sensitivity. The result was "most favorable." The author refers briefly to sporadic case reports on the use of steroids in subacute bacterial endocarditis along with antibiotics.

Other recent reviews on the treatment of this disease[3, 4, 7] consider steroids only for the purpose of control of drug sensitivity or of facilitating the recovery of positive blood cultures. The latter use is, however, not recommended by Dormer because of the risk of dissemination of the infection.

All the articles mentioned above agree that the present standard methods of therapy of subacute bacterial endocarditis are, in spite of all the progress made, still far from perfect considering the persistent high rate of morbidity and mortality. It may therefore be wise to consider more often the addition of steroids to the routine measures in view of their ability to suppress the local and systemic reactions to the infectious process, as well as the frequently coexistent active rheumatic carditis. The possible drawbacks and dangers of steroid treatment will, no doubt, tend to limit its use to severe and refractory cases. Among these are cases with persistently negative blood cultures or those caused by resistant organisms. An unquestionable indication for the use of steroids in massive doses exists, in our opinion, in cases with severe fulminant toxemia which threatens to overwhelm the patient before there is time to control the infection with antibacterial agents. Only much wider experience will permit a considered opinion with regard to the use of steroids in *early* cases of subacute bacterial endocarditis. Theoretically, it appears conceivable that the unfavorable tissue reaction of the cardiac valves could be blocked in the early course of the disease, and that a more favorable course could be thus produced.

In summary, from our experience and the scanty reports in the literature, it appears that steroids deserve a definite place in the treatment of cases of subacute bacterial endocarditis with overwhelming toxemia.

Whether the use of steroids can improve the results of treatment in less severe cases of bacterial endocarditis over those obtained with present standard treatments, only future experience will show. On theoretical grounds it is conceivable that the entire course of the disease may be favorably influenced if steroid therapy is instituted early in the disease before extensive fibrin deposition or necrotizing lesions have developed.

REFERENCES

1. Barritt, D. W. and Gillespie, W. A.: Subacute bacterial endocarditis. Brit. M. J., 1:1235, 1960.
2. Bertrand-Fontaine, et al.: Le traitement des endocardites à hémoculture négative, Presse méd., 66:941, 1958.
3. Dormer, A. E.: Treatment of bacterial endocarditis. Brit. M. J., 1:1235, 1960.
4. Jawetz, E.: The tough cases of bacterial endocarditis. Circulation, 20:430, 1959.
5. Lustgarten, B. P. and Vogl, A.: Steroid therapy in severe bacterial endocarditis. J.A.M.A., 170:800, 1959.
6. Spink, W. W.: Adrenocortical steroids in the management of selected patients with infectious diseases. Ann. Int. Med., 53:1, 1960.
7. Swenson, D. B. and Borg, J. F.: Diagnosis and treatment of subacute bacterial endocarditis. Lancet, 79:512, 1959.

Effect of Steroids on the Therapeutic Efficacy of Antibiotics

HANNA ABU-NASSAR and ELLARD M. YOW

Baylor University College of Medicine

Since the addition of steroids to the physician's armamentarium during the last decade, very few human diseases have escaped their trial. Their use in infectious diseases has been no exception.

In the wake of such unprecedented enthusiasm, the problem of steroids and their general infection-augmenting properties has received much attention.[6, 18] The effect of steroids on the therapeutic efficacy of antimicrobial agents in infectious diseases has been studied experimentally *in vitro* and in artificially produced infections in animals, but very few controlled human studies have been reported.

EXPERIMENTAL STUDIES

Except for a few isolated reports, most investigators are essentially in agreement that the effects of steroids appear to be solely upon the host and that there is no apparent alteration in the rate of growth, virulence or morphology of the bacterial cells or in the antibacterial activity of antibiotics *in vitro*.[5, 6, 9, 18] This view is not shared by Kull,[7] who demonstrated that a number of aminosteroids had definite antimicrobial activity against a number of fungi and bacteria *in vitro*. Seneca,[13] however, reported that certain oxysteroids did not inhibit bacterial growth, but did interfere significantly with the inhibitory action of penicillin and streptomycin alone or combined and less so with the action of polymyxin B. No such interference was observed on the inhibitory action of neomycin, carbomycin, penicillin plus oxytetracycline, and the tetracycline group on bacteria. On the other hand, the inhibitory effect of neomycin was found by Wilkins[21] to be enhanced in the presence of certain steroids, but only against strains of Micrococci and Streptococci. The antibiotic activities of penicillin, chloramphenicol, chlortetracycline and erythromycin, however, were not affected by steroids.[21]

In experimental infections in cortisone-treated mice, Jawetz[5] demonstrated that steroids in optimal doses interfered significantly with the therapeutic efficacy of penicillin, streptomycin and chlortetracycline in lethal infections induced with *Klebsiella pneumoniae* and Streptococci. It was found that steroids interfered much more with the therapeutic effectiveness of a predominantly bacteriostatic agent (chlortetracycline) than with that of predominantly bactericidal agents (penicillin, streptomycin). The depressant effect of steroids was no longer significant when the antibiotic was administered in doses greatly in excess of the minimum curative dose or when synergism between streptomycin and penicillin, each in subcurative doses alone, achieved a bactericidal curative effect.

In streptococcal infections, Ilavsky[4] observed that steroids had little or no effect on the protective action of penicillin when the penicillin was administered in doses which regularly protected non-cortisone-treated mice. Streptomycin, chlortetracycline and oxytetracycline, even in excessive dosage, failed to protect mice treated with large doses of cortisone but did protect mice treated with small doses of cortisone. The adverse effect of steroids on infections caused by various gram-negative bacteria (*Klebsiella pneumoniae, Salmonella pullorum, Pasteurella multocida, Brucella abortus*) were not reversed by streptomycin, chlortetracycline, oxytetracycline, neomycin, polymyxin B and chloramphenicol given in doses which were sufficient to protect non-cortisone-treated controls.

Steroids in doses equivalent to those used therapeutically in human beings were given early to rabbits with experimental tuberculosis; the infection progressed more rapidly than in controls in spite of the action of streptomycin.[11] In guinea pigs the efficacy of streptomycin was also decreased in cortisone-treated animals as contrasted with animals treated with streptomycin alone.[1] However, when combined treatment was begun 24 days after inoculation, the animals had somewhat less disease than the corresponding streptomycin-treated group and less than controls. This suggests that cortisone treatment after the development of hypersensitivity did not seem to impair the effect of streptomycin.

When some degree of immunity could be induced by passive or active immunization in mice, the therapeutic effect of chlortetracycline and oxytetracycline was found not to be depressed by cortisone in group A streptococcal infections in contrast to the effect in nonimmunized mice.[2] Penicillin, however, was effective in cortisone-treated nonimmunized mice.

Several biologic substances have been used experimentally to reverse the depressive effect of cortisone on antibiotic efficacy, but the results are not conclusive. Among the substances used were vitamin B_{12}, choline, growth hormone, aldosterone and lymphoid extracts from splenic and thymic tissues.

The limitations inherent in an experimental approach stem from the fact that these infections are acute and primarily induced and that often large doses of steroids are used as compared to those used in human studies. In addition, variable factors enter into the nature of the experimental design itself. However, most of the information derived from experimental studies indicates that steroids do depress the therapeutic efficacy of antibiotics.

CLINICAL STUDIES

It is generally known that the only specific indication for steroid therapy is replacement in adrenal insufficiency and that its use in other conditions is nonspecific. There are now many reports suggesting an effect of the addition of steroids to the usual methods of treatment in the course of certain infectious processes. The nature of such interaction in human studies, however, is more difficult to define because such studies cannot be as rigidly controlled as animal studies. Therefore, conclusions about specific effects of steroids on antibiotic efficacy are hard to arrive at because of insufficient data and because such effects are the result of the causative agent-host-antibiotic-cortisone interrelationships. Besides, the dose of an antibiotic used in human studies is almost always greater than the minimum effective dose.

Clinical studies undertaken by various authors on the use of steroids in seriously ill patients have revealed conflicting results.[3, 8, 10, 12, 14, 15, 17, 19, 20] In one study, the administration of large doses of steroids to seriously ill patients for a brief period of time is reported to have been beneficial in selected cases of tuberculosis, brucellosis, infectious mononucleosis and the complications of mumps (including orchitis, purpura and encephalomeningitis); in acute rheumatic fever, hepatitis, trichinosis and severe drug reactions; and in infection and peripheral vascular collapse due to gram-negative organisms.[17] In other reports, beneficial effects were also noted from the use of steroids as an adjunctive measure in the therapy of pneumonia, generalized peritonitis, typhoid fever and meningococcemia,[10] and in the therapy of pneumococcal meningitis along with penicillin.[12] Similar favorable results were observed in the acute exudative forms of tuberculosis (miliary, meningeal, pneumonic and lymphatic) when steroids were accompanied by adequate doses of antimicrobial drugs to which the patient's tubercle bacilli were sensitive.[14, 20] Steroids were also found to have a place in the drug-allergic patient but were contraindicated in chronic, fibrotic, nodular tuberculosis. Equally convincing, however, were reports of unfavorable or equivocal results.[3, 8, 15, 19] In spite of dramatic symptomatic improvement observed in most of these cases no amelioration of the disease process itself was noted, nor was there any difference in the incidence occurrence of bacteremia, relapse or complications. When beneficial effects of steroids were observed, the effect was postulated to be due to their general anti-inflammatory effect regardless of the stimulus, to their protection against endotoxin, to their correction of adrenal insufficiency, and to the potentiating action on vasopressor drugs, often required in the treatment of associated shock.

SUMMARY AND CONCLUSIONS

1. Most *in vitro* studies reveal that steroids exert no direct effect on the activity of antibiotics or on the morphology, growth and virulence of bacteria.

2. In experimental infections steroids reduce the effectiveness of antibiotics. Interference is greater when bacteriostatic drugs are used than when bactericidal agents are used. The adverse effects of steroids may be overcome

by increasing the dose of the effective antibiotic, more successfully in hosts with great natural resistance and in those in whom active or passive immunity has been induced.

3. In human studies the paucity of controlled experiments and the multitude of variable factors involved make reported results inconclusive, but it seems likely that whatever beneficial or harmful effect is produced is the result of the effect of cortisone on the host rather than on the action of the antibiotic. It is recommended that antibiotics be used in larger doses than those usually employed to control infectious diseases in cortisone-treated patients, and bactericidal drugs or synergistic drug combinations should be used whenever possible. Harmful effects may result from prolonged use of steroids in seriously ill patients, particularly when effective antibiotics are not available or when dosage is inadequate.

REFERENCES

1. Bloch, R. G., Vennesland, K. and Gurney, C.: The effect of cortisone on tuberculosis in the guinea-pig. J. Lab. & Clin. Med., 38:133, 1951.
2. Foley, E. J.: Therapeutic effect of chlortetracycline and oxytetracycline in immunized mice treated with cortisone. Antibiotics & Chemother., 5:1, 1955.
3. Hahn, E. O., Houser, H. B., Rammelkamp, C. H., Jr., Denny, W. F. and Wannamaker, L. W.: Effect of cortisone on acute streptococcal infections and post-streptococcal complications. J. Clin. Invest., 30:274, 1951.
4. Ilavsky, J. and Foley, E. J.: Observations on antibiotic treatment of bacterial infections of cortisone-treated mice. Proc. Soc. Exper. Biol. & Med., 84:211, 1953.
5. Jawetz, E.: Effect of cortisone on the therapeutic efficacy of antibiotics in experimental infections. A.M.A. Arch. Int. Med., 93:850, 1954.
6. Kass, E. H., Finland, M.: Adrenocortical hormones and the management of infection. Ann. Rev. Med., 8:1, 1957.
7. Kull, F. C., Castellano, G. A. and Mayer, R. L.: The in vitro antimicrobial activities of certain amino steroids. J. Invest. Dermat., 21:227, 1953.
8. Lepper, M. H. and Spies, H. W.: A clinical study of the use of cortisone, hydrocortisone, and corticotropin in the treatment of seriously ill patients with infection. Antibiot. Ann., 447, 1956-1957. (Medical Encyclopedia Inc., New York.)
9. Lepri, G.: Studies on cortisone in ophthalmology. Am. J. Ophth., 35:935, 1952.
10. Magill, G. B., Killough, J. H. and Said, S. I.: Cortisone and combined antibiotic therapy of acute brucellosis melitensis. Am. J. Med., 16:810, 1954.
11. Morgan, T. E., Wanzer, S. H. and Smith, D. T.: The effect of cortisone and streptomycin on experimentally induced pulmonary tuberculosis in rabbits. J. Bact., 67:257, 1954.
12. Ribble, J. C. and Braude, A. I.: ACTH and adrenal steroids in treatment of pneumococcal meningitis in adults. Am. J. Med., 24:68, 1958.
13. Seneca, H. and Bergendahl, E.: Effect of oxysteroids on the inhibitory action of antibiotics on cultures of bacteria and Endamoeba histolytica. Antibiotics & Chemother, 6:41, 1956.
14. Shane, S. J. and Riley, C.: Tuberculous meningitis—combined therapy with cortisone and antimicrobial agents. New Engl. J. Med., 249:829, 1953.
15. Smadel, J. E., Levy, H. L., Jr. and Diercks, F. H.: Treatment of typhoid fever. I. Combined therapy with cortisone and chloramphenicol. Ann. Int. Med., 34:1, 1951.
16. Speirs, R. S.: Effect of oxytetracycline upon cortisone-induced pseudotuberculosis in mice. Antibiotics & Chemother., 6:395, 1956.
17. Spink, W. W.: Adreno-cortical steroids in the management of selected patients with infectious diseases. Ann. Int. Med., 53: No. 1, July, 1960.
18. Thomas, L.: Cortisone, ACTH and infection. Bull. New York Acad. Med., 31:485, 1955.
19. Wagner, H. N., Jr., Bennett, I. L., Jr., Lasagna, L., Cluff, L. E., Rosenthal, M. B. and Mirick, G. S.: The effect of hydrocortisone upon the course of pneumococcal pneumonia treated with penicillin. Bull. Johns Hopkins Hosp., 98:197, 1956.
20. Weinstein, H. J. and Koler, J. J.: Adreno-corticosteroids in the treatment of tuberculosis. New Engl. J. Med., 260:412, 1959.
21. Wilkins, J. R.: In vitro studies on increased antibacterial activity of neomycin in the presence of certain steroids. Antibiotics & Chemother., 9:464, 1959.

Steroids and Tuberculosis

WINTHROP N. DAVEY

The University of Michigan Medical Center

The use of chemicals in an attempt to control tuberculous disease has assumed ever-increasing importance during the past 15 years. Indeed, the use of specific antituberculosis drugs has become the foundation of treatment, and the observed remarkable declines in the mortality from this disease have been most gratifying. Tuberculosis, however, remains a serious infectious disease for the individual patient, and the more severe and acute forms do not respond uniformly, promptly or without important sequelae to even the best of the antimicrobial regimens. This has prompted interest in and a search for adjuvant forms of treatment in an effort to better the prognosis, shorten the morbidity and reduce the residua of tuberculosis of all types.

Following the initial reports of the effects of cortisone and corticotropin on rheumatic fever and rheumatoid arthritis by Hench and associates,[25, 26] there were observations of the effect of these substances upon infectious disease in experimental animals[45, 47] and in human subjects.[34, 35] When administered to patients with infection, they usually produced reduction in fever and other manifestations of toxicity, and increase in the patients' sense of well-being, even while the underlying disease process followed its expected course.[34] The principal action of the glucocorticoids leading to these manifestations of symptomatic improvement appeared to be a suppression of the usual inflammatory response of the host to the invading microorganisms, with impairment of granulation tissue formation, macrophage activity and fibroblastic repair.[15, 47]

In experimental tuberculous infections in animals, cortisone affects in a fundamental fashion all the essential mechanisms involved in the pathogenesis of the disease.[15, 40, 47] It increases the accumulation of tubercle bacilli within macrophages and suppresses nonspecific and allergic inflammation as a result of the protective effect exerted by the hormone against many agents that increase capillary permeability. Such tuberculous disease in animals may react in a variety of ways when corticosteroids are employed, depending apparently on the species of the animal and the experimental condition; of these the drug employed, the dosage and the animals' native susceptibility and prior experience with tuberculous infection[36] appear most important. These observations have been reviewed previously.[31]

The deleterious effects of the corticoids on human tuberculosis are well documented.[1, 16, 22, 31] Such therapy may cause serious exacerbation of apparently inactive tuberculosis, and though this is not an inevitable consequence, no criteria exist to determine which patients will do poorly. The obscuration of the signs and symptoms of progressive and toxic tuberculosis by these substances further increases the hazard to the patient. The greatest problem has been observed in the treatment of patients with apparently inactive tuberculosis for debilitating diseases such as lymphoma or disseminated lupus erythematosus.[27, 31] In such instances, if there is no indication for treatment of the tuberculosis, careful and thorough examination of the patient must be made and frequent serial chest x-rays and sputum examinations should be done during and following such hormonal therapy.

On the other hand, there are numerous observations indicating that combined corticoid-antimicrobial drug therapy can be administered for as long as several weeks with considerable immediate safety to patients with active tuberculosis of any organ or system of organs. Early, these observations, by and large, were made on patients with tuberculosis who had apparent indications for treatment with corticoids for a nontuberculous condition (e.g., lupus erythematosus,[32] drug hypersensitivity,[28] or sarcoidosis[29]) or for control of acute tuberculous disease, most often with meningeal involvement.[30]

In recent years, combined therapy has been employed by many groups in the management of all forms of tuberculosis, and a considerable mass of published data has accumulated.[2, 17, 19, 43, 49] Many of the observations have been reported from European countries,[4] particularly France[5, 12, 20, 46, 51, 53] and Great Britain.[6, 11, 40, 44, 55] The striking feature of these data is that when patients harboring drug-susceptible tubercle bacilli are given corticoids with concurrent administration of antituberculosis antimicrobials, in accepted dosages, there are no reports of significant deleterious effects upon the tuberculous disease. According to some of the reports, there are no significant deleterious effects when low-dosage corticoids are given even to patients with drug-resistant infections.[55]

There has been great interest in the use of hormones in the management of tuberculous meningitis, and there is increasing evidence[2, 10, 33, 54] that many patients so treated have definitely shown more rapid clinical and laboratory evidence of improvement than would otherwise have been expected. Significant neurologic sequelae are common, and the problem of internal hydrocephalus is great.[21] It has appeared reasonable to expect that the patient with tuberculous meningitis treated with combined therapy might manifest fewer such sequelae.[2, 30, 33] Controlled studies, however, are lacking, and there is some evidence that the problem of internal hydrocephalus is not lessened,[2] at least in children. It has become widely accepted, however, that the meningitic who is seriously ill, who has evidence of cerebrospinal block or who is not responding to the usually effective chemotherapeutic agents is a candidate for such combined therapy.

Indications for the use of combined corticoid-antimicrobial therapy in other forms of tuberculosis are less clearly evident. European authors describe the most beneficial effects in patients with acute pleuritis, with or without effusion, [4, 12, 17, 19, 20, 43, 46, 51, 53] and the least benefit in cases of chronic fibroid pulmonary tuberculosis.[4, 12, 19, 43] Its use in the severely ill with acute pulmonary disease[11, 18] or diffuse exudative disease[23] and in terminal illness[38] has been described repeatedly. Treatment of chronic tuberculous lymphadenitis and tuberculous pericarditis[7, 17, 43] has been attempted. Opinion is uniform that no significant incidence of exacerbation of the tuberculosis has occurred,[50] but differences exist as to the correlation between clinical improvement and x-ray evidence of improvement in pulmonary tuberculosis.[6, 19, 23, 24] Most observations indicate that very gratifying radiologic evidence of improvement appears in patients with acute disease and that this is maintained after corticoid therapy is discontinued.[18, 52, 53]

Explanations for the observed beneficial effects of combined corticoid-antimicrobial therapy of many forms of tuberculosis are not immediately available.[48] Alteration in adrenocortical function in patients with tuberculosis has been considered,[8, 9] but detailed anabolic and catabolic studies of adrenal hormones in tuberculous patients are wanting. As outlined by Spink,[48, 49, 50] it has been established that the inflammatory reaction elicited by noxious agents, including the products of infecting organisms, can be suppressed or averted by the corticoids, but the basic mechanism of this hormonal activity is not understood. There may be an effect at the cellular level by preservation or stabilization of the cell membrane.[13, 14, 39] There are suppression of inflammation, reduction in capillary permeability and increase in phagocytosis, but there is also increase of the rapidity of multiplication of the tubercle bacilli.[15, 40]

This latter effect may be of the greatest importance in the observed beneficial effects of combined corticoid-antimicrobial therapy of acute tuberculosis. The suppression of inflammation by corticoids may be of obvious immediate value to patients and has led to the establishment of broad indications for their use in many medical problems. In infectious disease the increased rapidity of multiplication of the invading microorganisms has often resulted in deleterious effects upon the patient because of his inability to maintain local control of the disease. With the concurrent administration of appropriate antimicrobials, however, it is apparently possible not only to maintain satisfactory control of the infecting organisms, while local and general host factors are mustered, but to enhance the bacteriocidal action of the antimicrobials on these rapidly multiplying organisms,[37, 41, 42, 56] resulting in a net benefit to the host which is qualitatively and quantitatively superior to that obtained by the use of antimicrobials alone.

The chronicity of tuberculosis and the relatively slow and sometimes wavering host-responses to invading tubercle bacilli render a decision for the adjuvant use of corticoids difficult to reach. Discounting the usual contraindications and complications of the use of these hormones, however, it appears that their administration for tuberculous disease is justified in an attempt to enhance the patient's initial improvement, when he is acutely ill and toxic, or to reduce the undesirable and disabling sequelae of tuberculous infection when meningitis, pleuritis with effusion or pericarditis is present. However, such patients should be harboring drug-susceptible tubercle bacilli, and the possible deleterious effects of such management must always be balanced against the apparent need and benefits to be gained.

REFERENCES

1. American Trudeau Society: The effect of cortisone and/or corticotropin on tuberculous infection in man: A statement prepared by the Committee on Therapy. Am. Rev. Tuberc., 66:254, 1952.
2. American Trudeau Society: Indications for adjuvant corticotropin and corticosteroid therapy in tuberculosis: A statement of the Committee on Therapy. Am. Rev. Tuberc., 76:708, 1957.
3. Aspin, J. and O'Hara, H.: Steroid-treated tuberculous pleural effusions, Brit. J. Tuberc., 52:81, 1958.
4. Bergsmann, O. and Karlhuber, F.: Erfahrungen mit Cortison bei der Behandlung der Lungentuberkulose. Wien. med. Wchnschr., 106:554, 1956.
5. Bethoux, L. and Merle, M.: La delta-cortisone en phtisiologie (à propos de 19 cas). Rev. Tuberc., 21:289, 1957.
6. Bland, C. Y.: Corticosteroid and tuberculosis. Brit. J. Tuberc., 51:379, 1957.
7. Bouvrain, Y., Thibier, R. and Abivers, M.: Le traitement de la pericardite tuberculeuse et de la pericardite cryptogenetique par l'ACTH et la cortisone. Press med., 63:1544, 1955.

8. Campbell, G. D., Biggs, R. H. and Boswell, H.: Adrenocortical function in pulmonary tuberculosis. Am. Rev. Tuberc., 66:364, 1952.

9. Clark, E. R., Jr., Zahn, D. W. and Holmes, T. H.: The relationship of stress, adrenocortical function and tuberculosis. Am. Rev. Tuberc., 69:351, 1954.

10. Cocchi, G.: Cortisone and corticotropin in the treatment of tuberculosis in infancy and childhood. Am. Rev. Tuberc., 74(Suppl.):209, 1956.

11. Cochran, J. B., Hislop, J. A. and Clayson, C.: Cortisone and chemotherapy in pulmonary tuberculosis. Brit. J. Tuberc., 50:269, 1956.

12. Despierres, G., Phelip, H. and Hollard, D.: Cortisone et tuberculose pulmonaire. Rev. Tuberc., 19:1329, 1955.

13. Dougherty, T. F.: Some observations on mechanisms of corticosteroid action on inflammation and immunologic processes. Ann. New York Acad. Sc., 56:748, 1953.

14. Dougherty, T. F. and Schneebeli, G. L.: Use of steroids as anti-inflammatory agents. Ann. New York Acad. Sc., 61:328, 1955.

15. Ebert, R. H.: In vivo observations on the effect of cortisone on experimental tuberculosis using the rabbit ear chamber technique. Am. Rev. Tuberc., 65:64, 1952.

16. Editorial: Cortisone, ACTH and infection. New Engl. J. Med., 254:41, 1956.

17. Editorial: ACTH, cortison en tuberculose. Hormoon (Oss), 20:57, 1956.

18. Elsbach, P. and Edsall, J. R.: ACTH and cortisone as adjuncts in the treatment of advanced pulmonary tuberculosis. Ann. Int. Med., 46:332, 1957.

19. Even, R., Sors, C., Delaude, A., Roujeau, J., Trocme, Y. and Commare, G.: La place des hormones hypophyso-surrenales dans le traitment de la tuberculose. Etude clinique, anatomo-pathologique et experimentale. Rev. Tuberc., 19:1249, 1955.

20. Favez, G. and Aguet, F.: Les indications de l'hydrocortisone et de la prednisone dans le traitment de la tuberculose pulmonaire evolutive. Schweiz. med. Wchnschr., 30:1, 1956.

21. Foltz, E. L. and Sheehy, T. F., Jr.: Pneumoencephalography in tuberculous meningitis. Am. Rev. Tuberc., 74:835, 1956.

22. Golding, I. M., Lester, W., Jr. and Berg, G. S.: Adrenocortical steroids and tuberculosis: A reminder. New Engl. J. Med., 254:1026, 1956.

23. Handley, A. E.: The use of corticosteroids in combination with isonicotinic acid hydrazide in the treatment of advanced bilateral progressive pulmonary tuberculosis. South African M. J., 30:605, 1956.

24. Harris, J.: Cortisone-antimicrobial therapy in tuberculosis. Brit. J. Tuberc., 51:98, 1957.

25. Hench, P. S., Kendall, E. C., Slocumb, C. H. and Polley, H. F.: The effect of a hormone of the adrenal cortex (17-hydroxy-11-dehydrocorticosterone: compound E) and of the pituitary adrenocorticotropic hormone on rheumatoid arthritis. Proc. Staff Meet., Mayo Clin., 24:181, 1949.

26. Hench, P. S., Slocumb, C. H., Barnes, A. R., Smith, H. L. and Poelly, H. F.: The effects of the adrenal cortical hormone 17-hydroxy-11-dehydrocorticosterone (compound E) on the acute phase of rheumatic fever: preliminary report. Proc. Staff Meet., Mayo Clin., 24:277, 1949.

27. Hill, H. J. and Kirshbaum, J. D.: Miliary tuberculosis developing during prolonged cortisone therapy of systemic lupus erythematosus. Ann. Int. Med., 44:781, 1956.

28. Houghton, L. E.: Combined corticotropin therapy and chemotherapy in pulmonary tuberculosis. Lancet, 1:595, 1954.

29. Hoyle, C., Dawson, J. and Mather, G.: Treatment of pulmonary sarcoidosis with streptomycin and cortisone. Lancet, 1:638, 1955.

30. Johnson, J. R.: Tuberculous meningitis; use of corticotropin as an adjunct to chemotherapy. Case report and review of literature. Am. Rev. Tuberc., 72:825, 1955.

31. Johnson, J. R. and Davey, W. N.: Cortisone, corticotropin and antimicrobial therapy in tuberculosis in animals and man: a review. Am. Rev. Tuberc., 70:623, 1954.

32. Johnson, J. R. and Davey, W. N.: Treatment of a patient with lupus erythematosus and pulmonary tuberculosis with ACTH, streptomycin and para-aminosalicylic acid. Ann. Int. Med., 42:1109, 1955.

33. Johnson, J. R., Furstenberg, N., Patterson, R., Schoch, H. K. and Davey, W. N.: Corticotropin and adrenal steroids as adjuncts to treatment of tuberculous meningitis. Ann. Int. Med., 46:316, 1957.

34. Kass, E. H., Ingbar, S. H. and Finland, M.: Effects of adrenocorticotropic hormone in pneumonia. Ann. Int. Med., 33:1081, 1950.

35. Kass, E. H. and Finland, M.: The role of adrenal steroids in infection and immunity. New Engl. J. Med., 244:464, 1951.

36. Kass, E. H., Hechter, O., Mou, T. W. and Lurie, M. B.: Effects of adrenal steroids on resistance to infection. Arch. Int. Med., 96:397, 1955.
37. Kass, I., Russell, W. F., Jr., Heaton, A., Miyamoto, T., Middlebrook, G. and Dressler, S. H.: Changing concepts in the treatment of pulmonary tuberculosis. Ann. Int. Med., 47:744, 1957.
38. Katz, S. et al.: Use of hydrocortisone in pre-terminal tuberculosis. Tr. Fourteenth Veterans Administration-Army-Navy Conference on the Chemotherapy of Tuberculosis, 1955, p. 299.
39. Kinsell, L. W.: The clinical application of pituitary adrenocorticotropic hormones. Ann. Int. Med., 35:615, 1951.
40. Lurie, M. B., Zappasodi, P., Dannenberg, A. M., Jr. and Cardona-Lynch, E.: The effect of cortisone and ACTH on the pathogenesis of tuberculosis. Ann. New York Acad. Sc., 56:779, 1953.
41. Middlebrook, G.: Sterilization of tubercle bacilli by isonicotinic acid hydrazide and the incidence of variants resistant to the drug in vitro. Am. Rev. Tuberc., 65:765, 1952.
42. Middlebrook, G. and Yegian, D.: Certain effects of streptomycin on mycobacteria in vitro. Am. Rev. Tuberc., 54:553, 1946.
43. Moreau, L.: ACTH, cortisone et tuberculose. Concours med., 78:1813, 1956.
44. Prednisolone in treatment of pulmonary tuberculosis. A controlled trial. Preliminary report by the research committee of the Tuberculosis Society of Scotland. Brit. M. J., 2:1131, 1957.
45. Robinson, H. J. and Smith, A. L.: The effect of adrenal cortical hormones on experimental infection. Ann. New York Acad. Sc., 56:757, 1953.
46. Sors, C. and Troccme, Y.: Le traitement des pleuresies sero-fibrineuses tuberculeuses par l'ACTH. Rev. de la tuberc., 18:167, 1954.
47. Spain, D. M. and Molomut, N.: Effects of cortisone on the development of tuberculous lesions in guinea pigs and on their modification by streptomycin therapy. Am. Rev. Tuberc., 62:337, 1950.
48. Spink, W. W.: Adrenocorticotropic hormone and adrenal steroids in management of infectious diseases. Ann. Int. Med., 43:685, 1955.
49. Spink, W. W.: ACTH and adrenocorticosteroids as therapeutic adjuncts in infectious diseases. New Engl. J. Med., 257:979, 1031, 1957.
50. Spink, W. W.: Adrenocortical steroids in the management of selected patients with infectious disease. Ann. Int. Med., 53:1, 1960.
51. Turiaf, J., Marland, P. and Blanchon, P.: Association en cures prolongées des antibiotiques du bacille de Koch et des hormones hypophyso-surrenalionnes dans le traitement de l'infection tuberculeuse. Poumon, 12:89, 1956.
52. United States Public Health Service Tuberculosis Therapy Trials: Preliminary observations from a controlled trial of prednisolone in the treatment of pulmonary tuberculosis. Am. Rev. Resp. Dis., 81:598, 1960.
53. Verrator, R. and Chenebault, J.: Hormones hypophyso-surrenales et tuberculose. Rev. Tuberc., 21:1008, 1957.
54. Voljavec, B. F. and Corpe, R. F.: The influence of corticosteroid hormones in the treatment of tuberculous meningitis in Negroes. Am. Rev. Resp. Dis., 81:539, 1960.
55. Warembourg, H. and Gernez-Rieux, C.: Essais de corticotherapie en tuberculose. Acta tuberc. Belg., 47:94, 1956.
56. Youmans, G. P., Raleigh, G. W. and Youmans, A. S.: The tuberculostatic action of para-aminosalicylic acid. J. Bact., 54:409, 1947.

Panel Discussion

ROBERT I. WISE, *Moderator*

DR. WISE: In the preceding series of papers the relation of steroids and infection was discussed. Of particular interest is the fact that steroids may be detrimental in some types of infection and may have a beneficial effect in others. In this regard, 1 would like to ask Dr. Davey to comment about an unusual situation that I observed in a 21-year-old patient who had been treated with steroids by her local physician for a rheumatic condition, perhaps rheumatic fever, for a period of two months. At the end of that time she developed tuberculous meningitis, and she was so critically ill that we thought she would expire in a matter of a few hours. She was given correct antimicrobial therapy, but did not improve. Steroids were given then, and an amazing thing happened. She improved neurologically, the Babinski test became normal, the nuchal rigidity disappeared, she became responsive, she began to eat, and the protein in the spinal fluid decreased. However, as we decreased the dose of the steroid while maintaining antimicrobial therapy in the same dosage, all of these signs and symptoms reappeared. When we increased the dose of the steroid, the same beneficial effect as she had initially occurred and this sequence of events was observed on four different occasions after changes in steroid dosage. Did she or did she not have adrenal insufficiency? What is the mechanism of response?

DR. DAVEY: I am sure I can not answer specifically as to what was occurring; however, this response has been observed not infrequently in the management of tuberculous meningitis with combination therapy, using corticoids and antituberculous drugs. I think it is related completely to the duration of the corticoid therapy. Several of the patients whom we treated initially had a return of all their symptoms and signs, including cerebrospinal fluid block, when corticoid dosage was decreased after a short period of three to four weeks. I think the only solution is to give corticoids for a longer period of time; of course, this increases the risk, for the longer that corticoids are used even with good antituberculous drugs in the treatment of tuberculosis, the greater the risk is. There is no reason to suppose that she had adrenal cortical insufficiency, on the basis of what you have told me.

DR. WISE: Since we were having difficulty in maintaining electrolyte balance, we measured aldosterone production and found it to be zero.

DR. DAVEY: Certainly, patients with tuberculous meningitis, as do those with chronic respiratory disease, have changes in metabolism of that type resulting in sodium depletion upon occasion. We talk about the "salt-losing" meningitic patient frequently. I believe this is another indication for the use of corticoids.

DR. DI RAIMONDO: I also would agree that this patient did not have adrenal insufficiency and that the response to the steroid was due to its effect on the infection. However, the use of large doses of steroids in tuberculosis may lead to miliary disease. On the other hand, some experiments done at the University of Kansas suggest that local levels of hydrocortisone play a role in the disposition and the growth of organisms locally, and suppression of the adrenals by the steroid may prevent localization of the organisms in this tissue and thereby prevent its possible destruction.

DR. ROMANSKY: Dr. Wise, did you do sensitivity tests during the exacerbations?

DR. WISE: No, we did not, Dr. Romansky, and we do not know the sensitivity of the organisms; however, the patient had an excellent recovery and is now back in college.

DR. ROMANSKY: I was thinking about the possibility of increasing resistance of the organisms during the relapse phases; since relapses occurred when the steroid was decreased, the effectiveness of the antibiotics would be lessened if the mechanism we have been talking about was operative.

DR. WISE: Certainly, corticosteroids in combination with adequate antimicrobial drugs seem to be of great benefit in many patients with tuberculous meningitis, and I believe the panel is in essential agreement on this point.

To start the discussion on another aspect of steroids and infection, I will ask Dr. Weil to comment on another case that was most interesting to us. A 24-year-old girl developed retinitis of some type and was treated with steroids for one month. Three weeks after the steroids were stopped she went to another physician to have the retinitis treated. He gave her an injection of typhoid vaccine which produced a severe shock reaction. In spite of administration of steroids and vasopressor drugs in high doses, she died with continuing shock three days later.

DR. WEIL: I did not see the patient, so it is difficult to be sure of the exact mechanism involved in her demise, but I can make some conjectures. The injection of the typhoid vaccine, which contains killed typhoid cells, is, for all practical purposes, an injection of endotoxin. Both the lipopolysaccharide and the protein moieties are present. If the patient was not receiving steroids at the time she received the typhoid vaccine, then the insult that was provided by the typhoid vaccine and that was associated with the development of shock involved the patient at a time when possibly adrenal function was decreased because of prior administration of steroids. One would have to know more about the dose of the steroid used and the duration of the previous treatment before one could really settle this point. However, if adrenal suppression was present and the patient did not receive the steroid very promptly and in very large doses after the onset of the reaction, the damage could have been done and the shock state could not have been controlled. I have found that it is extremely important to administer steroids in very, very large doses and very, very early in the course of the disease because the time available for reversal of this process is extremly short.

DR. WISE: Would you comment on the relative value of steroids in comparison with vasopressor agents in shock caused by gram-negative bacteria? What is the value of the steroids? It has been my impression that the important drug is the vasopressor agent, and I have been teaching that the steroids are less important, although they may be helpful. I gather from your remarks that you think steroids definitely enhance the vasopressor action.

DR. WEIL: On the basis of data that I did not present today, I do not believe that the steroid effect and the vasopressor effect are directly related. I think that the protective pharmacologic effect of the steroids which I reviewed today represents an anti-endotoxin effect in that the steroids protect tissue which is being injured in some way by the endotoxin. The value of the early clinical use of high doses of steroids appears to result from protection of the tissues against the damaging effects of endotoxin. The use of vasopressor agents rests on two concepts. First, the majority of patients who develop shock related to gram-negative bacteria are most frequently in an older age group and are seen most frequently on the urological service following transurethral resections or lower urinary tract infections, but it also occurs not infrequently in patients on the surgical service who have malignancies and infections within the peritoneal cavity. In a large series of patients that we reported from Minnesota, the average age of the patients was about 62, and none were under the age of 35. Most of these patients have vascular disease, particularly coronary artery disease. If there is a reduction in blood flow related to the shock stage, cardiac function is not maintained very long, and in these circumstances, it would seem to me, on the basis of the evidence presently available, very wise to use a drug that will maintain blood flow through the coronary arteries. Secondly, there is the possibility that the vasopressor agent will reverse the presumed pooling that occurs in consequence of the reaction to endotoxin. However, this has been demonstrated only in experimental animals and not as yet in the human patient, and it is therefore a much more tenuous thing. For these reasons, I do not think that the effects of the two drugs are closely related. If I had to choose between the two, I think I would choose the steroid first and the vasopressor agent second. In younger patients not having vascular disease I would withhold final judgment as to the effectiveness of the vasopressor agents until further evidence of their value can be obtained.

Dr. Di Raimondo: In regard to the problem of adrenal insufficiency in your patient, how much drug did she receive during the month of therapy?

Dr. Wise: I do not know the exact amount given, because she was treated elsewhere.

Dr. Di Raimondo: It is very unusual for a patient to have shock three weeks after discontinuing steroid therapy when steroids have been given in the usual suppressive doses for only one month. This would be the exception rather than the rule, and while it is possible to have such a situation occur, it is unlikely. We have studied several patients who have been on steroids for approximately a month; within one week they have a good clinical response to stress in terms of hydrocortisone secretion, and particularly if they are young people and are not too sick.

Dr. Wise: Dr. Yow, are steroids really helpful in the treatment of patients with acute infectious diseases?

Dr. Yow: Several indications were mentioned in the preceding papers for the use of steroids in infectious diseases, but most of the speakers also said that there was much disagreement about this and that no definite conclusions regarding the value of steroids could be arrived at. This may have engendered some doubt in the minds of the audience about the value of steroids in acute infectious diseases. However, most people who have been working in this area have the feeling that there are specific circumstances in infectious diseases in which administration of steroids may be life-saving. It is impossible, in my opinion, to list specific types of infectious diseases in which steroids can be expected to be beneficial or in which steroids should be used routinely. It is the specific circumstance or type of organ involvement that is important rather than the etiologic agent. For example, if a patient has an infectious process or an inflammatory process that is threatening the function of some vital organ, very often the anti-inflammatory effect of cortisone or related steroids can make the difference between life and death. Some very striking examples of this are seen in patients with severe viral encephalitis in whom swelling of the brain in itself can be fatal, in patients with severe viral pneumonia and severe bronchiolitis or bronchopneumonia in whom oxygenation of blood or gas exchange is so strikingly altered that the patient's life is threatened, and in many other patients in whom swelling itself or inflammation itself is threatening the patient's life. In addition, the situation in the patients with endocarditis discussed by Dr. Vogl represents another type of specific indication for the use of the steroids in infections; that is when fever and the hemodynamic changes resulting from fever and infection are great and they threaten the patient's life. In this situation the so-called detoxifying and antipyretic effects of steroids may give the physician time to administer an effective antibiotic and may allow sufficient time for the antibiotic to have an antibacterial effect and in turn have an anti-inflammatory effect. I think it is the circumstance resulting from the infection and not the specific disease which is important, and I am convinced that some patients with acute infections who were treated with steroids had their lives saved as a result of this therapy.

DR. WISE: Dr. Romansky, would you comment on this? Are steroids really help-ful in the treatment of infectious diseases?

DR. ROMANSKY: I think Dr. Yow has expressed this very succinctly. There is no specific infectious disease in which steroids should always be used, but situations have already been mentioned, such as gram-negative endotoxic shock, in which these drugs are of value. In the patients Dr. Vogl mentioned, it is not necessarily the effect on the bacteria, but on the complications of the disease for which the steroids were effective.

DR. WISE: My opinion about and objection to the use of steroids in the manage-ment of patients with infections is that sometimes the physician resorts to the use of steroids without thinking of better methods of diagnosis or better methods for specific treatment of the patient. When steroids are contemplated, I would make a plea that there be a great deal of thought about the possibility of misdiagnosis and about other methods of therapy.

DR. YOW: Short-term intensive steroid therapy does not often create any serious problems except for one thing, and that is distortion of the clinical picture which is normally a part of a specific infectious disease. This makes evaluation of therapy difficult. For example, fever is one of the most valuable things that a physician can observe for evaluation of the effect of antibiotic therapy. One of the greatest objections I would have to using steroids in the treatment of endocarditis is the abolishment of fever, which is extremely important in judging whether or not the patient is doing well. Ultimately the blood cultures become negative and then you know how effective the therapy has been, but in the meantime it is difficult to determine this if the patient's fever has been abolished by steroids and the patient is feeling well.

In regard to the use of steroids in the treatment of shock, many physicians, at least in our part of the country, and I suspect in many other parts of the country, are using steroids routinely. Anesthesiologists also tend to give steroids every time a patient has a drop in blood pressure, and the same is true of surgeons and in-ternists. Many of the patients whom I have seen who had been given steroids for so-called bacteremic shock did not really have this type of shock. They had hypo-tension of the type that is associated with fever or the hypotension that is associ-ated with a severe illness, but not true circulatory collapse. I believe that many of the patients who have been treated for shock with steroids by surgeons and anes-thesiologists would have responded just as well to fluid replacement, blood trans-fusion, vasopressor drugs and other means. The use of such other agents would obviate the problem of distortion of the clinical picture that steroid therapy pro-duces when it is given for any length of time.

DR. GRAY: I also want to comment on the masking of symptoms by steroids. Not only do they prevent the febrile response, but they may completely mask acute peritonitis or an acute surgical abdomen. The abdomen often remains soft and there may be no pain, fever or leukocytosis, and yet the patient may have an acute abdominal condition with an acute perforation or a fulminant peritonitis. This has to be kept in mind in the evaluation of surgical conditions in patients who are on steroid therapy.

DR. WISE: Dr. Dubois, in the treatment of sarcoidosis with steroids, should one use prophylactic measures? In other words, are there instances in which one would give steroids and would want to use prophylactic antibiotics to prevent infections, particularly, for example, to prevent the possibility of tuberculosis?

Dr. Dubois: I think I would proceed with the steroid alone and follow the patient carefully if the tuberculin test was negative and if there was no evidence of coexisting tuberculosis, since statistics indicate that the incidence of tuberculosis in patients with sarcoidosis is low. Of course, the toxicity of INH is minimal, and if one is concerned about this possibility it would be reasonably safe to give INH at the same time.

Dr. Good: I want to comment about the presence or absence of leukocytosis when corticosteroids are used in infection. When adequate amounts of adrenal cortical steroids are present, the patient usually has a definite leukocytosis with the appearance of an intercurrent infection, but when the patient has relative adrenal insufficiency due to relative or absolute deficiencies in secretion from his own adrenal glands or due to insufficient dosage of exogenous steroids there is a normal white count or a leukopenia. The appearance of leukopenia in a patient on steroids is serious and should be so regarded, because it is a paradoxical response to most severe infections.

Dr. Weil: Some years ago, Dr. Spink and I studied the relationship of endotoxic shock to anaphylactic shock. With gram-negative bacteremias, perhaps most notably in typhoid fever, leukopenia may be a part of the clinical picture, and I would be very reticent to use leukopenia as a reflection of the steroid level in the patient. In addition, I would be strongly disinclined to emphasize relative adrenal insufficiency except in those very few patients who do have Addison's disease or iatrogenic adrenal insufficiency following treatment with steroids. I think our colleagues in surgery and anesthesiology have overused this therapy to the detriment of the patient, and, furthermore, they use relatively small doses of steroids. When steroids are required, and this is not often, large doses are needed, not merely replacement doses.

Dr. Dubois: Infection in patients receiving long-term steroid therapy for disseminated lupus has been a problem. In addition to the common infections that often occur, we have had two cases of disseminated torulosis. When one observes psychotic symptoms in a lupus patient receiving long-term steroid therapy, it is important to do repeated examinations of spinal fluid to detect bizarre infections as well as the common ones discussed previously.

Part XI | UNDESIRABLE EFFECTS
OF STEROIDS

Undesirable Effects of Steroids: General Comments, Development of Cushing's Syndrome, the Hypercortisone Syndrome

LEWIS C. MILLS

Hahnemann Medical College and Hospital, Philadelphia

As in many other forms of drug therapy, undesirable effects may occur when anti-inflammatory steroids are used in the treatment of disease states. At times these effects appear to be intimately related to the desired therapeutic action of the steroid and to result from it. An example is the well known tendency for infection to become disseminated when these drugs are used to reduce the inflammatory reaction and systemic toxicity in a patient with a serious infectious disease. In contrast, certain side effects, such as sodium retention and elevation of blood pressure, are not related to the desired therapeutic action of the steroids, except when they are used in the treatment of adrenal insufficiency. By appropriate chemical modification it has been possible to eliminate these properties in certain of the newer anti-inflammatory steroids, while still retaining or even potentiating their anti-inflammatory and desired therapeutic action.

GENERAL COMMENTS

Since the possible side effects of steroid therapy are many and varied, and since many of the following papers deal at length with these effects, it is important at the outset to have a proper perspective of them in their relationship to the therapeutic use of steroids. Even aspirin, which is one of the most innocuous and most frequently used drugs, may cause severe toxic reactions and death and therefore should not be used indiscriminately; however, when it is used intelligently, side effects are very uncommon. Considerably more perspicacity is necessary during administration of steroid therapy, but undesirable effects may be minimized, if not completely prevented, by a thorough knowledge of the disease state being treated, by an appreciation of the potential hazards of steroid therapy, and by the intelligent use of prophylactic and adjuvant therapeutic measures.

The first and most important procedure relating to successful steroid therapy is to determine whether or not there is an actual indication for the administration of steroids. In those conditions in which topical therapy is to be used, there is relatively little cause for concern, since undesirable reactions with this form of therapy are almost nonexistent and therapeutic trials may be done with relative impunity, although it should be remembered that certain dermatologic and ophthalmologic conditions may be worsened by topical steroid therapy. Administration of steroids systemically, on the other hand, requires that many factors be considered. Some of these are:

(1) the severity and probable responsiveness of the disease state to be treated; (2) the dosage and length of therapy likely to be required; (3) the therapeutic, pharmacologic and metabolic properties of the steroid to be used; (4) the presence of a concomitant disease state which might be adversely affected by therapy; (5) complications or peculiarities of the primary disease state which increase the likelihood that certain undesirable effects will occur from therapy; (6) the use of adjuvant therapeutic measures; and (7) the use of prophylactic measures.

1. Although there are many disease states which respond favorably to administration of anti-inflammatory steroids, a large number of them respond satisfactorily to or are significantly ameliorated by other drugs. It is indeed unfortunate that a steroid and another drug, such as aspirin or a vitamin combination, have sometimes been combined into a single tablet or capsule and marketed under a trade name which may suggest antirheumatic or anti-inflammatory activity, often without indicating the steroid content. All too often neither physician nor patient has been aware of presence of a steroid. Such combinations are frequently used in the treatment of minor rheumatic and arthritic conditions, the daily dosage often being regulated primarily by the patient on the basis of the intensity of his symptoms, and numerous instances of preventable side effects or of post-therapy hypo-adrenalism have been observed.

Some of the many disease states for which steroid therapy is actually indicated are discussed in the preceding papers in this volume, and the indications for therapy, the doses used and the responses obtained are adequately considered. The risk of producing undesirable side effects is entirely justified when steroids are used in the treatment of a serious, often life-threatening, disease such as lupus erythematosus, but more consideration must be given to the development of undersirable side effects in a disease such as rheumatoid arthritis, which, although often severe and disabling, is rarely life-threatening. In this situation the possibility that a side effect more serious than the primary disease could develop must be weighed against the benefits to be gained, and steroids should be given only in specific phases of the disease to accomplish certain well defined objectives.

2. The dosage and length of therapy likely to be required are also important factors in the development of side effects, high dosage and long periods of therapy almost always being associated with unwanted effects. Conversely, patients are often maintained on exogenous steroids in a dose which has less anti-inflammatory potency than that of the normal daily amount of hydrocortisone secreted by their own adrenal glands. Most of these patients should be treated with other nonsteroidal anti-inflammatory drugs and the steroid stopped entirely. Finally, in regard to dosage, there is the problem of the ideal amount of steroid which should be prescribed for a given condition, since there is little unanimity as to whether it is better to try to suppress completely all indices of activity of a given disease state and accept the risk of increased undesirable side effects, or to give minimal suppressive doses of steroids with a resulting lessening or abolition of side effects. There is little evidence at present to indicate that "minimally suppressive" doses do much to alter the progression of rheumatoid arthritis, rheumatic valvular disease or lupus nephropathy; in contrast, there are increasing numbers of isolated but probably nevertheless valid reports that large doses of steroids are effective in halting the progression of certain of these disease processes. Unfortunately, this problem is not yet solved and

must await further confirmatory studies, the synthesis of a new, less toxic steroid, or the development of new types of anti-inflammatory compounds.

3. It is also important to be familiar with the therapeutic, pharmacologic and metabolic properties of the steroid to be used. For example, administration of hydrocortisone, cortisone or ACTH in therapeutic doses often leads to sodium and water rentention and edema. Although this is more frequent in patients with cardiovascular or renal disease, it also occurs in some others in whom these systems are functioning normally. For these patients, it is now possible to select a steroid, such as dexamethasone, methyl prednisolone or triamcinolone, which has minimal, if any, sodium-retaining effect; in fact, these compounds may cause diuresis of sodium and water in certain circumstances. Likewise, the other characteristics of the steroid to be used, such as the effect on appetite, protein metabolism and other aspects of metabolism, should be considered in relation to the clinical condition of the patient. Selection of a steroid on this basis will lead to the use of the one with the greatest anti-inflammatory effect and the least toxic effect for the particular patient.

4. In deciding whether to prescribe steroid therapy, the presence or absence of concomitant disease must also be taken into consideration. Patients with inactive tuberculosis or other subclinical infections may develop active infection; patients with prior, although healed, peptic ulcers are more likely to have a recurrence; those with latent diabetes are likely to develop clinical diabetes, and those with overt diabetes require more insulin. These examples, far from complete, indicate that the physician must consider all of the patient's medical history in the development of a satisfactory therapeutic program with the anti-inflammatory steroids.

5. Peculiarities or complications of the patient's primary disease must also be considered. It is known, for example, that peptic ulcer occurs more frequently in association with certain collagen diseases, especially when steroids are used in therapy. Patients with nephrosis and lupus erythematosus are more susceptible to infection; if steroids, which in themselves alter the tissue reaction to infection, are to be used, this complication must be watched for carefully.

6. The use of adjuvants is particularly indicated in steroid therapy. Adjuvant therapy may be in the form of physiotherapy, bed rest, diet or the use of other drugs such as aspirin and nonsteroidal anti-inflammatory agents, depending on the nature of the disease state to be treated. With such a program it is often possible to reduce the dose of the steroid or to discontinue it, thereby lessening or preventing the development of steroid toxicity. Unfortunately, because of the great amount of literature concerning the benefits of steroid therapy, and indeed, the often dramatic subjective clinical response in the patient, there has been a definite tendency to treat a disease such as rheumatoid arthritis with steroids alone, when in actuality a better result could have been obtained with other forms of therapy. This should not be taken to imply that steroids are not the most effective treatment for certain of these diseases, but rather, as with any disease process for which there is no specific cure, that a multifaceted approach designed to give the patient the best therapeutic result with a minimum of therapeutic risk should be used.

7. Finally, after the above factors have been considered and the therapeutic regimen has been decided on, prophylactic measures should be instituted as indicated by the likelihood that a given undersirable side effect

from the steroid might occur. For example, for the patient with a history of peptic ulcer, a dietary and antacid regimen should be instituted if more than moderate doses of steroids are to be given or if they are to be given for more than a two- to three-week period. Similarly, antimycobacterial antibiotics should probably be given in this circumstance to patients with inactive tuberculosis. Other examples could also be given, but these problems are discussed at length in subsequent papers.

CUSHING'S SYNDROME

Cushing's syndrome or a Cushingoid appearance occurs frequently, if not always, in patients receiving large doses of anti-inflammatory steroids for any significant length of time or in patients receiving moderate doses for long periods of time. It is pointless to attempt to state that any specific percentage of patients will develop the clinical manifestations of this syndrome since it is so dependent on a time-dosage relationship, but it is of some interest to compare the incidence of various clinical features of this syndrome in patients with the naturally occurring disease and in those with the exogenously induced disease. As with the over-all incidence, the figures in Table 1 are dependent on dose-time relationships; however, since the averages were obtained from various reported clinical series, the percentages are representative of the incidence which might be expcted in the average patient receiving *cortisone* or *ACTH* at the indicated dose levels. If one of the newer steroids is used, the percentage of certain clinical features, such as hypertension and edema or others, depending on the steroid used, will

TABLE 1. *COMPARISON OF THE MANIFESTATIONS OF CUSHING'S SYNDROME WITH THE SIDE EFFECTS OF EXOGENOUS CORTISONE AND ACTH THERAPY**

SYMPTOM OR SIGN	CUSHING'S SYNDROME	LONG-TERM ACTH AND CORTISONE THERAPY**	HIGH-DOSE ACTH AND CORTISONE THERAPY***
	222 Patients	69 Patients	100 Patients
	Per cent	Per cent	Per cent
Edema	35	45	46
Infection	33	32	39
Mental symptoms	40	36	35
Obesity	97	85	84
Weakness	58	36	44
Hirsutism	70	40	39
Acne	37	15	13
Plethora	60	23	23
Purpura	30	7	10
Hypertension	85	24	25
Menstrual disturbances	75	20	19
Headache	39	8	7
Glycosuria	27	6	3
Polydipsia	28	4	6
Striae	68	3	3
Exophthalmos	7	0	0
Virilism	6	0	0

* Collected cases from the literature.
** Average duration 14.8 months.
*** 75 mg. or more of cortisone per day or 30 units or more of ACTH per day.

be altered. In the collected series listed in Table 1, the incidence of edema was more common in the steroid-treated patients than in those with the natural Cushing's syndrome; the incidence of obesity, mental symptoms and infection was about the same in the two groups. Hirsutism and weakness occurred less frequently, and other symptoms and signs were much less frequent in the steroid-treated patients. Although the frequency of occurrence of these manifestations is high and although they are often a source of concern to the patient, many of these abnormalities are well tolerated or can be adequately treated by appropriate therapeutic measures. However, certain side effects such as mental abnormalities, infection, osteoporosis with compression fractures and peptic ulcer are more serious and require intensive therapy or reduction in steroid dosage. These will be discussed in subsequent papers.

THE HYPERCORTISONE SYNDROME

The hypercortisone syndrome,[1, 2, 3] in addition to having the usual features of Cushing's syndrome described previously, is characterized by an increase in fatigability, cyclic and significant emotional instability and generalized aching in the muscles, bones and joints. Although perhaps more likely to occur in patients with rheumatoid arthritis to whom steroids have been administered in large doses or for long periods of time, it also occurs in other patients receiving "pharmacologic" doses of steroids. Various other terms such as "chronic hypercortisonism" and "steroid pseudorheumatism" have also been applied to this syndrome. In an occasional patient the reaction may proceed into a phase with a diffuse mesenchymal reaction resembling systemic lupus erythematosus or polyarteritis nodosa which may be fatal unless appropriate modifications of the steroid regimen are instituted. The management of such a patient should include very gradual reduction in the total steroid dosage, more evenly spaced and frequent doses, addition of other anti-inflammatory drugs, and extra rest; however, therapy is difficult, if not unsuccessful, when the process has passed into the phase in which there is a diffuse mesenchymal reaction.

In conclusion, it should be emphasized that successful therapy with steroids depends on the thoughtful consideration of the many factors relating both to the clinical condition of the patient and to the steroid to be used. If this is done, the patient will be significantly benefited, and the undesirable effects of therapy will be few.

REFERENCES

1. Good, R. A., Vernier, R. L. and Smith, R. T.: Serious untoward reaction to therapy with cortisone and adrenocorticotropin in pediatric practice (Part I). Pediatrics, *19*:95, 1957.
2. Rotstein, J. and Good, R. A.: Steroid pseudo-rheumatism. Arch. Int. Med., *99*:545, 1957.
3. Slocumb, C. H., Polley, H. F., Ward, L. E. and Hench, P. S.: Diagnosis, treatment and prevention of chronic hypercortisonism in patients with rheumatoid arthritis. Ann. Int. Med., *46*:86, 1957.

Steroid Withdrawal Syndrome

THOMAS A. GOOD

University of Maryland Medical School

Sudden cessation of corticosteroid therapy sometimes produces reactions which may be frightening and confusing. The reactions may be grouped under the following general headings: (1) rebound of disease,[7] (2) addisonian-like crisis,[2] (3) panmesenchymal-panangiitic reaction of Slocumb.[10, 11]

REBOUND OF DISEASE

The rebound of disease symptoms and signs during discontinuation of corticosteroids is frequently seen and is often used as a clinical guide to determine the lowest effective dosage of a steroid which may be used to suppress symptoms of a disease, particularly a chronic disorder such as rheumatoid arthritis. However, in certain instances, especially in acute diseases, rebound may exceed the initial manifestations of disease and may actually be devastating. The following case, previously reported in detail,[5] illustrates this problem.

Case 1. A three-year-old boy was admitted to the Salt Lake County Hospital with a generalized bullous erythema multiforme. He was critically ill, febrile and irrational. Intravenous hydrocortisone was started after initial evaluation. The course of his demise is illustrated graphically in Figure 1. Until the time when his hydrocortisone dosage was lowered he showed progressive improvement.

Within 24 hours following lowering of intravenous hydrocortisone dosage by 60 mg. per day, the patient began showing increased temperature as the first manifestation of disease rebound. His oral intake was good, so he was changed abruptly to oral delta-1-hydrocortisone, 50 mg. per day in four equally spaced doses. In the ensuing 24 hours he showed progressive symptoms of collapse with the appearance of diarrhea, restlessness, polydipsia, abdominal distention, vomiting, peripheral vascular collapse, subnormal temperature and severe leukopenia. Autopsy showed hypertrophy of lymphatic tissue of the ileum, eosinophilia of the spleen sinusoids, fresh massive hemorrhage of the right adrenal gland and decrease in the sudanophilic staining material of the left adrenal cortex.

Certainly a skin disease such as this in which toxicity is a major problem would warn against abrupt changes in the kind, amounts and route of administration of suppressive corticosteroids.

ADDISONIAN-LIKE CRISIS

The withdrawal of steroids during long-term maintenance corticosteroid therapy may result not only in the recurrence of disease symptoms but in the manifestation of an addisonian-like crisis (if withdrawal is abrupt)

* This study was aided in part by a grant from The Upjohn Co., Kalamazoo, Michigan.

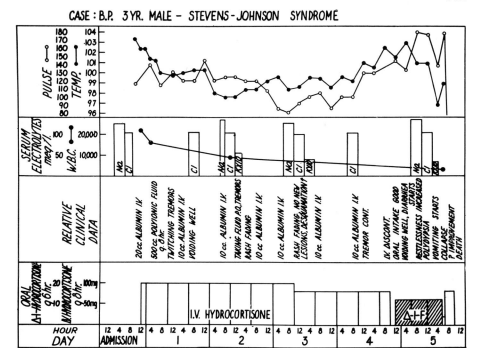

Fig. 1. A child with severe bullous erythema multiforme developed fatal toxic collapse similar to that seen in the Waterhouse-Friderichsen syndrome following abrupt change in steroid therapy. Note the low white blood cell count shortly before death.

and in symptoms which appear to be related to arteritis, as suggested by Slocumb,[10, 11] and Rotstein and Good.[9] The following two cases illustrate these clinical phenomena.

Case 2. A six-year-old boy who had had juvenile rheumatoid arthritis for more than four years had been maintained on corticosteroid dosage sufficient to keep him relatively free of joint pain. For the preceding six months he had been receiving delta-1-hydrocortisone 5 mg. b.i.d. Four days previous to his admission he became withdrawn and anorexic, began to refuse all solid foods, and 60 hours before admission began to vomit so that he received no more steroids until hospital therapy was initiated. On admission he was very uncooperative, withdrawn and whining from discomfort. Any movement of his extremities produced pain and he had severe limitation of movement of all his major joints including his spine. Palpation of his abdomen and over the intercostal areas elicited sharp pain, and it appeared that he was generally quite tender to touch everywhere.

The interesting aspects of this child's hospital course are recorded in Figure 2. Emergency determination of electrolytes showed only slightly low chloride and CO_2 combining power, and he was started on a regimen of half-strength saline and intravenous hydrocortisone. On this therapy the electrocardiogram, which initially had shown low T waves and supraventricular tachycardia, showed intensification of abnormalities in conduction and repolarization compatible with a severe electrolyte disturbance. Serum sodium and serum potassium were then found to be greatly reduced. With intensification of electrolyte therapy which included potassium, and con-

CASE D.A. 6 YR. MALE R.A.

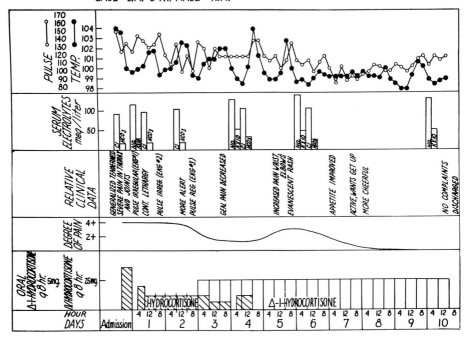

Fig. 2. A child with rheumatoid arthritis who had had cessation of steroids suddenly at home suffered an addisonian-like crisis and symptoms of "pseudorheumatism." Control of symptoms was achieved by resumption of corticosteroid therapy and intensive fluid and electrolyte loads.

tinuous intravenous corticosteroid therapy, the child's symptoms abated and and he was gradually changed to oral delta-1-hydrocortisone and continued to require low-dose maintenance therapy for the suppression of his rheumatoid arthritis.

PANMESENCHYMAL-PANANGIITIC REACTION

The clinical evidence of a panmesenchymal-panangiitic reaction (pseudorheumatism) is manifested by psychic deficits, visceral involvement and skin disorders or rashes.

Case 3. On February 3, 1959, a 58-year-old woman was admitted to the University of Maryland Hospital Psychiatric Service because of chronic rheumatoid arthritis of one year's duration and concomitant personality problems with increasing invalidism for the preceding four months. The diagnosis of rheumatoid arthritis was based upon chronic bilateral symmetrical involvement of the joints, a strongly positive latex agglutination test and negative L.E. tests. X-rays showed moderate hypertrophic arthritis of the spine and wrists. She had developed hoarseness at the onset of her arthritis. Her chest x-ray had been normal 10 days before admission and she had had no known visceral involvement during her illness. The patient had sustained a fracture of T-12 in a fall four months previously and x-rays had shown osteoporosis of the spine. She had been receiving various corticosteroid preparations in fluctuating amounts for the preceding year. Since her response to steroid therapy had not been satisfactory, in the preceding two weeks her private physician had been decreasing the steroid dosage. Concomitant deterioration of personality had resulted in referral to the psychiatric service.

When the patient was admitted she was emotionally labile and was depressed at intervals, particularly in the morning. She was rapidly weaned from the remaining dexamethasone therapy with the resulting events shown in Figure 3. Dexamethasone dosage was cut from 1.5 mg. per day to 0.75 mg. on February 4. On February 8 the last dose was given. On February 9 she suffered increased pain and swelling of the wrists, had puffy edema of the dorsum of the feet, became very depressed, talked hesitantly, and could not

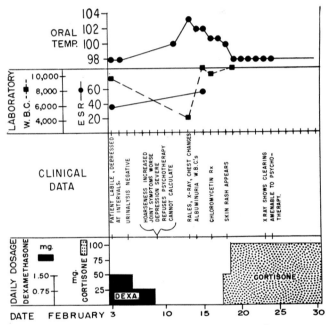

Fig. 3. A "panangiitic-panmesenchymal" reaction developed in a 58-year-old woman following cessation of steroids. The clinical pathology involved the brain, lungs, kidneys and skin. Note the low white count during the height of the reaction.

subtract sevens serially. By February 10 she had become more hoarse and on the 13th she developed fever, generalized diffuse rales and a positive chest x-ray (Fig. 4). Her urine, which previously had been negative, showed 25 to 35 W.B.C. per high power field and 1+ albuminuria. Her peripheral W.B.C. was 4100.

Chloromycetin was started on February 16 because nasal pharyngeal cultures were positive for *D. pneumoniae* and beta hemolytic staphylococci. On February 18 the patient developed a macular annular rash which was felt to be nonspecific. At this time she was started on cortisone 25 mg. every six hours. On the following day she felt better but was still hoarse and had a nonproductive cough. The rales in her chest had disappeared, but there was no change in her x-ray picture. The skin rash was less prominent and her W.B.C. was 11,000. She continued to improve clinically; by February 23 there was clearing of her chest x-ray picture, and on the next day it was

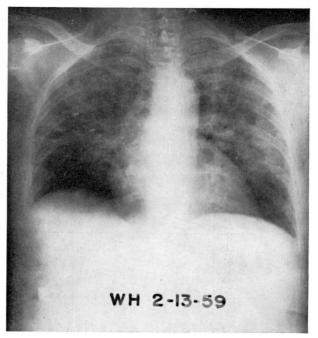

Fig. 4.   The x-ray demonstrates the widespread involvement of the lung. These changes
are similar to those seen in lupus erythematosus and periarteritis nodosa.

possible to resume psychiatric interviews. With steroid therapy, psychotherapy and physical therapy the patient became ambulatory and was discharged
by May 2, 1959.

DISCUSSION

These cases illustrate some of the clinical phenomena of corticosteroid
withdrawal. Certainly in many situations the rapid decrement of steroid
dosage may not be associated with any disturbing reactions. This appears to
be the situation in patients with the nephrotic syndrome. However, withdrawal reactions, particularly disease rebound, are frequent and severe
enough to warn against sudden large decreases of exogenous steroid dosage.

Especially prone to withdrawal reactions are patients requiring prolonged
steroid therapy for rheumatoid arthritis, particularly those in whom low
dosages are not sufficient to maintain suppression of the disease.[9-11]

We have seen transient rheumatic-like symptoms in normal human volunteers following a single large dose of corticosteroid preparations.[5]

Case 2 illustrates the addisonian-like crisis as well as some of the "pseudorheumatism"[9] features of a withdrawal reaction.

The electrolyte imbalance may include hypopotassemia, especially in the
early phase of re-institution of steroid therapy. The rheumatic symptoms
illustrated by both Case 2 and Case 3 involve the joints, muscles, skin and
internal organs. The psychic manifestations are chiefly severe depression, but
the inability to calculate even simple problems is striking.[9-11] Whether the
convulsions reported as side effects of corticosteroid therapy[4] are the result
of withdrawal of steroid is uncertain at the present time.

Case 3 illustrates the postmenopausal female, who appears to have a greater degree of intolerance to steroid therapy and is more prone to develop the relative hypocortisonism syndrome of Slocumb.[10, 11] Such patients in whom this syndrome (or "pseudorheumatism") develops may be devastated by sudden cessation of steroid therapy and may require very slow and gradual decrements of steroid dosage. It should be reiterated that all of the serious implications of acute fulminating lupus erythematosus or periarteritis nodosa apply to the "panangiitic-panmesenchymal" reaction which may result in these patients upon lowering the dosage, by even moderate decrements such as 5 mg. per day of delta-1-hydrocortisone, and weaning decrements should be small (1 mg. or less) and spaced at intervals of approximately 4 to 10 days.

The major underlying pathological lesion which is aggravated by steroid decrement appears to be a nonspecific inflammatory arteritis.[9-11] The pathogenesis of this lesion is probably related to rheumatoid disease,[1, 3, 8] but the development of arteritis in experimental animals has been aggravated by the administration of cortisone.[12] The authors of a recent paper concerning the development of vascular lesions in patients with rheumatoid arthritis have noted that the patients in whom these lesions were prominent had received fluctuating steroid dosage.[6]

Speculatively, one wonders whether the development of dependency of the connective tissue on amounts of corticosteroid has any similarity to the dependency of the highly developed endometrial tissue in the secretory phase of the menstrual cycle on estrogen and progesterone.

REFERENCES

1. Bevans, M., Nadell, J., Demartini, F. and Ragan, C.: The systemic lesions of malignant rheumatoid arthritis. Am. J. Med., *16*:197, 1954.
2. Calkins, E., Engel, L. L., Mitchell, D. M., Carter, P. and Bauer, W.: Clinical, metabolic and endocrinologic effects of abrupt cessation of maintenance cortisone acetate therapy in rheumatoid arthritis. Arth. & Rheum., *3*:204, 1960.
3. Cruicksank, B.: The arteritis of rheumatoid arthritis. Ann. Rheum. Dis., *13*:136, 1954.
4. Good, R. A., Vernier, R. L. and Smith, R. T.: Serious untoward reactions to therapy with cortisone and ACTH in pediatric practice. Pediatrics, *19*:95, 1957.
5. Good, T. A., Benton, J. M. and Kelley, V. C.: Symptomatology resulting from withdrawal of steroid hormone therapy. Arth. & Rheum., *2*:299, 1959.
6. Johnson, R. L., Smyth, C. J., Holt, G. W., Lubchenco, A. and Valentine, E.: Steroid therapy and vascular lesions in rheumatoid arthritis. Arth. & Rheum., *2*:224, 1959.
7. Kelley, V. C., Adams, F. A. and Good, R. A.: Serum mucoproteins in patients with rheumatic fever. Pediatrics, *12*:607, 1953.
8. Kemper, J. W., Baggenstoss, A. H. and Slocumb, C. H.: The relationship of therapy with cortisone to the incidence of vascular lesions in rheumatoid arthritis. Ann. Int. Med., *46*:831, 1957.
9. Rotstein, J. and Good, R. A.: Steroid pseudorheumatism. A.M.A. Arch. Int. Med., *99*:545, 1957.
10. Slocumb, C. H.: Relative cortisone deficiency simulating exacerbation of arthritis. Bull. Rheumat. Dis., *3*:39, 1952.
11. Slocumb, C. H.: Symposium on certain problems arising from clinical use of cortisone: Rheumatic complaints during chronic hypercortisonism and syndromes during withdrawal of cortisone in rheumatic diseases. Proc. Staff Meet., Mayo Clin., *28*:265, 1953.
12. Thomas, L. and Good, R. A.: The effect of cortisone on the Shwartzman reaction. The production of lesions resembling the dermal and generalized Shwartzman reactions by a single injection of bacterial toxin in cortisone-treated rabbits. J. Exper. Med., *95*:409, 1952.

Steroid Diabetes

VINCENT C. DI RAIMONDO

University of California Medical Center, San Francisco

Although the incidence of diabetes mellitus is high in Cushing's syndrome due to an adrenocortical tumor or hyperplasia,[6] the development of steroid diabetes is a rare complication of glucocorticoid therapy.[1] The clinical manifestations as well as the therapy for steroid diabetes are dependent upon available endogenous insulin reserves. With rare exceptions the decreased tolerance for glucose is reversible with resumption of normal glucocorticoid levels.

PATHOGENESIS

Following the administration of excessive quantities of glucocorticoids to animals one observes increases in blood sugar, hepatic glycogen and urinary excretion of nitrogen. Long, Katzin and Fry[3] twenty years ago suggested that the glucocorticoids increased the synthesis of glucose and liver glycogen from endogenous sources of protein. Since then, considerable evidence has accumulated in support of their theory. The subject has been reviewed recently by Renold and Ashmore.[4] There is very little evidence to support any significant peripheral antagonism of the action of insulin by the glucocorticoids. The currently accepted sequence of events following excessive glucocorticoid therapy is as follows: (1) increased breakdown of protein with an increase in amino acid production, (2) increased hepatic trapping, transamination and deamination of amino acids, (3) a probable increased synthesis of p-enolpyruvate from pyruvate via maleate and oxaloacetate, (4) increased hepatic glucose via fructose-1,6-diphosphate, fructose-6-phosphate and glucose-6-phosphate. Associated with these changes one observes an alteration in serum pyruvate and lactate levels. With the increase in glucose production a rise in insulin maintains normal blood sugar levels. In the presence of inadequate quantities of insulin the metabolism of glucose is not sufficiently accelerated, and an elevation of blood sugar results. Although glucocorticoids protect the animal against ketosis,[2, 5] the "brittle" diabetic who has no endogenous insulin can develop ketosis and coma if inadequately treated with insulin. His coma will be complicated by an exaggerated breakdown of proteins. The diabetogenic effects of currently available glucocorticoids, i.e., cortisone, cortisol, prednisone, prednisolone, 6-methylprednisolone, 16-hydroxy,9-alpha fluoroprednisolone, 16-methyl,9-alpha fluoroprednisolone and 9-alpha fluorocortisol, are proportional to their anti-inflammatory potencies.

CLINICAL MANIFESTATIONS

Whether or not a patient develops steroid diabetes is determined by the dose of glucocorticoid used as well as by his endogenous insulin reserve. Since patients with normal adrenocortical function normally secrete approximately 15 mg. of hydrocortisone per square meter of surface area per day,

810

they must receive more than this amount of hydrocortisone or its equivalent before any increased tendency for diabetes occurs. Urinary nitrogen excretion can increase with as little as 30 mg. of hydrocortisone or its equivalent per square meter per day. A maximum nitrogen excretion is usually achieved in normal subjects by administration of approximately 150 mg. of hydrocortisone or its equivalent per square meter per day. Any increase in blood sugar depends upon the insulin reserves of the patient. The rise in blood sugar for a given dose of glucocorticoid is proportional to the insulin reserves. The brittle diabetic frequently notes an increase in the intensity of his diabetes, and the stable diabetic has variable, usually mild, changes in his diabetic state. Another factor contributing to the changes in the diabetic state is the increased food intake associated with the appetite-stimulating effect of the steroids. While on glucocorticoids, patients are resistant to the hypoglycemic effects of insulin. An occasional patient shows resistance to insulin. A decrease in the renal threshold for glucose has been reported. With rare exceptions, steroid diabetes is reversible with the cessation of glucocorticoid therapy.

TREATMENT

Insulin. Brittle diabetics, those without endogenous insulin, usually require increased doses of insulin during glucocorticoid therapy. Stable diabetics who are being treated with insulin usually require more insulin. The increase in the requirement is proportional to the dose of glucocorticoids used.

Oral Hypoglycemic Agents.[7] The sulfonylureas are of no value in patients with no endogenous insulin or in patients who, prior to glucocorticoid treatment, are being managed on maximal doses of these agents. They can be used in patients with mild diabetes who are on small doses of glucocorticoids. Since many patients develop nausea and vomiting with doses of DBI in excess of 150 mg., this drug is of limited value except in patients who have minimal changes in glucose tolerance while on the corticoids.

Diet. While on glucocorticoids, many patients eat more. Because of the protein-wasting effects of the glucocorticoids, it may be unwise to restrict dietary intake severely. High protein intakes and administration of anabolic agents may be wise measures. Dietary intake should maintain body weight. After glucocorticoid therapy has been completed, patients with steroid diabetes should be treated as prediabetics even though their tolerance to glucose returns to normal. They should be encouraged to maintain ideal weight and to increase physical activities. One might use the oral hypoglycemic agents prophylactically.

REFERENCES

1. Bookman, J. J., Drachman, S. R., Schaefer, L. E. and Adlersberg, D.: Steroid diabetes in man. The development of diabetes during treatment with cortisone and corticotropin. Diabetes, 2:100, 1953.
2. Engel, M. G. and Engel, F. L.: Fasting ketosis in the adrenalectomized and cortisone treated rat. Endocrinology, 55:593, 1954.
3. Long, C. N. H., Katzin, B. and Fry, E. G.: The adrenal cortex and carbohydrate metabolism. Endocrinology, 26:309, 1940.
4. Renold, A. E. and Ashmore, J.: Metabolic effects of adrenal corticosteroids. In Williams, R. H. (ed.): Diabetes. New York, Paul B. Hoeber, Inc., 1960, p. 194.

5. Scow, R. O., Chernick, S. S. and Guarco, B. A.: Ketogenic action of pituitary and adrenal hormones in pancreatectomized rats. Diabetes, 8:132, 1959.
6. Thorn, G. W., Renold, A. E. and Cahill, G. F., Jr.: The adrenal and diabetes; some interactions and interrelations. Diabetes, 8:337, 1959.
7. Williams, R. H.: Oral drugs in diabetes. In Williams, R. H. (ed.): Diabetes. New York, Paul B. Hoeber, Inc., 1960, p. 481.

Impairment of Fat Metabolism by Prolonged Administration of Steroids

DONALD BERKOWITZ

Hahnemann Medical College and Hospital, Philadelphia

Since 1949 when steroids were first introduced for the treatment of rheumatoid arthritis, more and more indications are being recognized for their use. Thus, an increasing number of patients are receiving this form of therapy for prolonged or even indefinite periods of time.

During these years an extensive literature has accumulated concerning the effects of the administration of steroids on carbohydrate, protein and mineral metabolism. Much less is known, however, about their effects on lipid metabolism.

The purpose of this presentation is to report three cases which give suggestive evidence that prolonged administration of cortisone or its derivatives may unfavorably affect fat metabolism, specifically leading to hypercholesterolemia, hypertriglyceridemia and impaired radioactive fat tolerance.

CASE REPORTS

Case 1. (Fig. 1). A. W., a 36-year-old male, was first studied by us in March 1958. At that time he was in excellent health with a negative medical

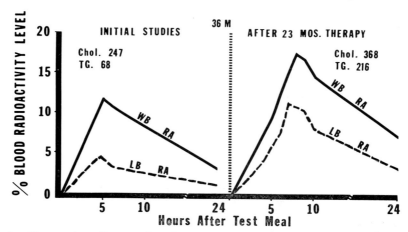

Fig. 1. Changes in radioactive fat tolerance test in a 36-year-old male after 23 months' treatment with steroids (WB = whole blood, LB = lipid blood, RA = radioactivity).

history and normal laboratory findings. The cholesterol was 247 and the triglycerides 68 mg. per cent. A radioactive fat tolerance test showed a normal response. Approximately two years later we were able to restudy this patient. In the interim he had developed pains in both knees for which steroids had been prescribed continuously for more than 18 months. The serum cholesterol was now 368, the triglycerides 216 mg. per cent, and the radioactive fat tolerance curve was markedly abnormal.

Case 2. (Fig. 2). G. H., a 41-year-old female, was first studied in April 1959. At that time, except for a history of migratory arthralgias, she offered no complaints. Physical examination was entirely normal, as were all the laboratory tests including the fat tolerance. The cholesterol was 258 and the triglycerides 86 mg. per cent. Approximately 16 months later a repeat study was done. In the interim the patient had been receiving hydrocortisone for more than a year for her joint pains, which had become more severe. Otherwise she felt perfectly well. The cholesterol was now 322, the triglycerides 186 mg. per cent and the fat tolerance curve abnormal.

Case 3. (Fig. 3). M. W., a 36-year-old female, was first examined in May 1959, during hospitalization because of severe neck pain. A complete laboratory survey was within normal limits. The cholesterol was 236 and the triglycerides 78 mg. per cent. X-rays showed evidence of advanced degenerative joint disease involving the cervical spine, and steroid therapy was instituted. Another opportunity to study this patient presented itself during August of 1960 when she was admitted to the hospital for a minor gynecological procedure. During the 15-month interval she had continued to take the steroids with good relief of her complaints. The serum lipids were now grossly elevated with visible turbidity of the fasting blood serum (cholesterol 372 and triglycerides 314 mg. per cent), and the radioactive fat tolerance test was markedly abnormal.

DISCUSSION

The relationship of the adrenal steroids to fat metabolism and the blood lipids has not been fully clarified. The short-term use of corticotropin has been found to result in a decrease of the blood cholesterol.[2] Administration

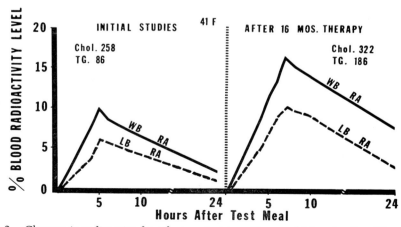

Fig. 2.   Changes in radioactive fat tolerance test in a 41-year-old female after 16 months' treatment with hydrocortisone.

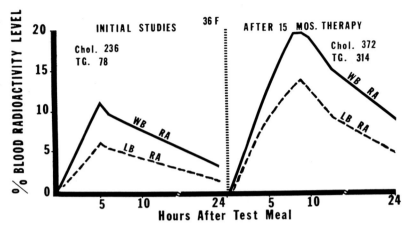

Fig. 3.   Changes in radioactive fat tolerance test in a 36-year-old female after 15 months'
treatment with steroids.

of cortisone or ACTH over longer periods of time may lead to hypercholesterolemia.[1, 5]

More recent evidence for a direct relationship between the adrenals and
lipid metabolism has been suggested by data showing changes in the serum
cholesterol and blood clotting time in men subjected to cyclic occupational
stress.[3] Another report has indicated that the mobilization of free fatty acids
and lipoproteins by epinephrine is dependent upon intact adrenal function
and particularly on the simultaneous availability of cortisone or cortisone-
like steroids.[4]

In the cases presented in this report, marked changes occurred in the
serum lipids and fat tolerance over a long term period during which steroids
were being taken. Other side effects such as weight gain, acne, striae, edema
or hyperglycemia were not present. Although a definite cause-and-effect
relationship has not been established, the data certainly suggest that chronic
administration of cortisone and/or its derivatives may effect unfavorable
changes in lipid metabolism. Furthermore, in line with current thinking concerning the role of hyperlipemia and impaired fat tolerance in the genesis of
atherosclerosis, the steroids may possibly be considered as potentially athero-
genic. Further studies on this problem are in progress in our laboratory.

SUMMARY

Three cases are reported in which an elevation of the serum cholesterol
and triglycerides, together with impairment of radioactive fat tolerance,
developed after long-term steroid therapy.

The possibility is suggested that chronic administration of cortisone or
related steroids produces unfavorable lipid metabolic changes in some
patients which may be a factor in the development of atherosclerosis.

REFERENCES

1. Adlersberg, D., Schaefer, L. E. and Drachman, S. R.: Development of hyper-
    cholesterolemia during cortisone and ACTH therapy. J.A.M.A., *144*:909, 1950.
2. Conn, J. W., Vogel, W. C., Louis, L. H. and Fajans, S. S.: Serum cholesterol: probable
    precursors of adrenal cortical hormones. J. Lab. & Clin. Med., *35*:504, 1950.

3. Friedman, M., Rosenman, R. H. and Carroll, V.: Changes in the serum cholesterol
   and blood clotting times in men subjected to cyclic variations of occupational stress.
   Circulation, 17:852, 1958.
4. Shafrir, E. and Steinberg, D.: The essential role of the adrenal cortex in the response
   of plasma free fatty acids, cholesterol, and phospholipids to epinephrine injection.
   J. Clin. Invest., 39:310, 1960.
5. Stamler, J., Pick, R. and Katz, L. N.: Effect of cortisone, hydrocortisone, and
   corticotropin on lipemia, glycemia, and atherogenesis in cholesterol-fed chicks.
   Circulation, 10:237, 1954.

Effects of Steroids on Wound Healing

DEMETRIOS TZIROS and JOHN M. HOWARD

Hahnemann Medical College, Philadelphia

Evidence at present indicates that cortisone in large doses affects wound healing in a deleterious manner. Studies have been almost entirely experimental. No clinical series is known to the authors, but the clinical impression is widely held that wound healing is impaired in patients receiving cortisone therapy. The impediment to wound healing in animals is due to or associated with a delay or decrease in wound exudation, a delay in capillary formation and a definite decrease in subsequent contracture.

Wound healing, primarily described by histologic studies, has been classically characterized as developing in three stages: (1) the initial or exudative phase, (2) granulation and fibroplasia, and (3) contraction. The initial or exudative phase appears to be preparing the wound for fibroplasia. During the initial stage, exudative fluid brings leukocytes, histiocytes and macrophages into the wound. These cells, aided by proteolytic enzymes, assist in the removal or dissolution of dead tissue. A fibrin clot forms about the second or third day; capillaries and fibroblasts appear in the wound and increase rapidly. By the fourth or fifth day any necrotic tissue is clinically apparent and within another day or two granulation tissue is evident by macroscopic examination. After the sixth day, fibroplasia becomes extensive, forming a scar which later contracts with a resultant decrease in the capillaries and in the interstitial fluid. Epithelization begins early, extending into the depth of the wound and progressing rapidly unless necrotic tissue is present. Capillaries probably develop only by branching from pre-existing capillaries. The degree and possibly the quality of the wound exudate appear to exert a profound influence on the vascular growth. Normally, the vascularity of the wound is reduced by the 24th day.

As stated above, fibroplasia parallels the early proliferation of capillaries. Algire described fibroblasts as arising by proliferation of local cells, by metaplasia from specialized wandering cells in the blood stream, or by proliferation from the vessel walls themselves.[11] Algire credits Carrell with demonstrating that leukocytes stimulate the growth of fibroblasts.

In recent years, Gould[7, 8] Schilling,[12] Dunphy[5] and their colleagues have developed interesting techniques of collecting wound fluid through the implantation of small sponges or wire mesh cylinders into the depths of closed wounds. These studies indicate that during the first few days there is deposited in the wound an amorphous ground material having the staining properties of acid mucopolysaccharide. It is water-soluble and has been studied fairly extensively by chemical analysis. It has been found to contain mucopolysaccharides of several types. The mucopolysaccharides contain hexosamine, an amine containing carbohydrate. The serial changes in hexosamine levels have been interpreted as representing the serial changes in concentration of the ground substances.

The concentration of hexosamine in the wound parallels somewhat the deposition of the amorphous ground material as described histologically. Evidence points toward the plasma glycoproteins as a major source of the hexosamine.[6] Dunphy[11] found that mucopolysaccharides (as hexosamine) increased rapidly in the wound, appearing as early as six hours after injury. A peak concentration was reached by about 48 hours. By the eighth or ninth day, the hexosamine levels had fallen to levels approximating those seen in normal connective tissue.

By the fourth day fibroblasts largely replace inflammatory cells. Edwards, Pernokas and Dunphy[6] demonstrated fibroblasts throughout a wound-embedded sponge at this stage, the fibroblasts being intermingled with the amorphous ground substance.

About the sixth day, wound-implanted sponges contain delicate collagen fibers, which become more abundant by the eighth day.[6] By the twelfth day the sponges contain less of the amorphous ground material but a maximal number of collagen fibers. Jackson[10] found the increase in collagen concentration, which occurred very rapidly between the fifth and fourteenth day, to be paralleled by an increase in tensile strength of the wound and believes that the fibroblasts probably begin synthesizing a collagen precursor as early as the third day. The precursor is deposited in the extracellular space where it aggregates into a fibrous structure.

Several excellent studies of wound healing having been based on the observation that the amino acid, hydroxyproline, exists in the wound in significant quantities only in collagen and therefore its concentration has been accepted as an index of the production of collagen. In review, Dunphy[11] pointed out that all observers agree that there is little or no hydroxyproline present early in the postwounding period. It can first be found in the wound between the fourth and sixth day and its concentration rises rapidly from the sixth day to the twelfth day, after which it declines slightly. *Again, it is the collagen which accounts principally for the restoration of tensile strength.*

How does cortisone effect the process of wound healing? First, it is the impression of W. Cole and his co-workers[3] that when used in characteristic therapeutic doses, neither cortisone nor ACTH affects clinical wound healing. Similarly, in a small group of experiments with dogs, J. Cole and associates[4] gave cortisone subcutaneously in daily doses of 2 mg. per kilogram. The drug was begun one day prior to operation and was continued for 20 days after operation. Two incisions each 11 cm. long were made over the chest wall. The wounds were closed by suture. In this small group of experiments no difference was noted in wound healing as determined histologically between the control animals and those receiving cortisone.

Experimental data points, however, to a retardation of wound healing when cortisone is given in larger doses. Howes and associates[9] gave cortisone to rats and rabbits in doses of 2 to 10 mg. per kilogram of body weight, the drug being given subcutaneously. Open wounds were found to lack exudation and at the end of eight days a wound looked almost the same as it had originally. These investigators found that the mucopolysaccharide content of the wound was decreased. If less cortisone was given, wound healing was better than with the larger doses of cortisone. Small tissue hemorrhages seemed to be absorbed more slowly. In other experiments gastric incisions were made in rats after which the gastric wounds were sutured. Measured on the sixth day after operation, the tensile strength was decreased to the greatest extent in those animals which had received the most cortisone. A decrease in tensile strength associated with cortisone therapy was also noted when the wound consisted of incision of muscle or skin, the wounds having been sutured at the end of the operation.

Sobel[14] gave cortisone subcutaneously in large doses to uninjured rats. Although the animals were not wounded, the hexosamine (mucopolysaccharides) decreased in concentration in both soft tissues and in bones.

Asboe-Hansen[1] gave cortisone and ACTH to humans and demonstrated that the mast cells in the skin became degranulated. At the same time, the hyaluronic acid content of the ground substance disappeared. He believed that the hyaluronic acid was produced by the mast cells and that this accounted for the mechanism by which the connective tissue ground substance was depleted following therapy.

Siuko[13] gave hydrocortisone acetate intramuscularly (10 to 25 mg. per day for 22 days) to guinea pigs. The animals were not wounded, but he found that the alkali-soluble collagens decreased in the skin. He also quoted the work of Roberts and associates, which indicates that adrenocortical hormones diminished the synthesis of hydroxyproline. Sobel[14] has demonstrated that preformed collagen remains essentially unchanged after the administration of cortisone.

In one of the best studies reported to date, Billingham and Russell[2] excised a full thickness of skin in rabbits, allowing the wound to heal by contracture and re-epithelization. The time for the wound to heal was measured. That time required for the surface of the wound to heal by 50 per cent was called the "half-life" of the wound. The wounds consisted of an excision of 34 to 50 square centimeters of skin; they required approximately 50 days to heal. The "half-life" of the wound was nine to ten days. When 10 mg. of cortisone acetate was given daily subcutaneously to the rabbits, granulation tissue was slow to develop. It remained sparse, pale and dry. The granulation tissue did not fill the wound until the 25th day in the animals so treated. Cortisone in the doses administered reduced the rate of contracture by about one half, doubling the "half-life" to 18.7 days. When cortisone was not started until the 16th day after the excision, the wound was already filled by granulation tissue but the rate of contraction slowed immediately after the cortisone was begun. If cortisone was given to the animals as in the original experiment, but was stopped during the later phases of healing, a normal rate of contracture developed thereafter.

SUMMARY

In experimental animals cortisone appears to diminish wound exudation, to delay the development of granulation tissue, to depress proliferation of capillaries and to retard the contraction of wounds. With small doses this depressing effect is not always clinically noted.

REFERENCES

1. Asboe-Hansen, G.: The mast cell. Cortisone action on connective tissue. Proc. Soc. Exper. Biol. & Med., *80*:677, 1952.
2. Billingham, R. E., and Russell, P. S.: Studies on wound healing with special reference to the phenomenon of contracture in experimental wounds in rabbits' skin. Ann. Surg., *144*:961, 1956.
3. Cole, W., Grove, W. and Montgomery, M.: Use of ACTH and cortisone in surgery. Ann. Surg., *137*:718, 1953.
4. Cole, J., Orbison, L., Holden, W., Hancock, T. and Lindsay, J.: A histological study of the effect of cortisone on wounds healing per prima. Surg. Gynec. & Obst., *93*:321, 1951.
5. Dunphy, J. E.: Repair of tissue after injury. Ann. New York Acad. Sc., *73*:426, 1958.
6. Edwards, L. C., Pernokas, L. N. and Dunphy, J. E.: The use of a plastic sponge to sample regenerating tissue in healing wounds. Surg. Gynec. & Obst., *105*:303, 1957.
7. Gould, B. S.: The biosynthesis of collagen. III. The direct action of ascorbic acid on hydroxyproline and collagen formation in subcutaneous polyvinyl sponge implants in guinea pigs. J. Biol. Chem., *232*:637, 1958.
8. Gould, B. S. and Woessner, J. F.: Biosynthesis of collagen. The influence of ascorbic acid on the proline, hydroxyproline, glycine and collagen content of regenerating guinea pig skin. J. Biol. Chem., *226*:289, 1957.
9. Howes, E., Plotz, C., Blunt, J. and Ragan, C.: Retardation of wound healing by cortisone. Surgery, *28*:177, 1950.
10. Jackson, D. S.: Some biochemical aspects of fibrogenesis and wound healing. New Engl. J. Med., *259*:814, 1958.
11. Patterson, W. B. (ed.): Wound Healing and Tissue Repair (Symposium). Chicago, University of Chicago Press, 1959. Includes discussion quoted by Algire, G. H., Dunphy, J. E., Gluckman, A., Gross, J., Levenson, S. M. and Urist, M. R.
12. Schilling, J. A., Milch, L. E. and Cardiovascular Research Group: Fractional analysis of experimental wound fluid. Proc. Soc. Exper. Biol. & Med., *89*:189, 1955.
13. Siuko, H., Savela, J. and Kulonen, E.: Effects of hydrocortisone on the formation of collagen in guinea pig skin. Acta endocrinol., *31*:113, 1959.
14. Sobel, H., Gabay, S. and Johnson, C.: Effect of cortisone on connective tissue of the rat. Proc. Soc. Exper. Biol. & Med., *99*:297, 1958.

Steroid Myopathy

GEORGINA FALUDI, LEWIS C. MILLS and ZEV W. CHAYES

Hahnemann Medical College, Philadelphia

Muscle weakness is a common finding in Cushing's syndrome. Many of these patients have weakness as their only complaint initially. Although the patient becomes stout, heavier and moonfaced, the extremities and especially the thighs remain remarkably thin. Cushing himself described muscle weakness in about half of his cases[3] and it has been recorded repeatedly since then;[15] however, detailed systematic investigation of the underlying pathological process of muscular weakness in Cushing's syndrome was not carried out until very recently.

In patients with Cushing's syndrome the weakness involves the proximal muscles of the lower limbs to the greatest extent, resulting in difficulty in climbing stairs or in rising from a squatting position. Only a few patients have weakness of the shoulder girdle. Abdominal, cervical and facial muscles are not affected. Although patients may have severe weakness in the involved muscles, atrophy or muscular fasciculation has not been reported.[3, 15] Reflexes are usually normal and sensory changes do not occur.

Microscopic examination of muscle fibers from these patients may reveal slight to moderate degeneration,[15] which is much less pronounced than would be expected on the basis of the clinical findings. The muscle fibers are often somewhat thinner than normal and may be partly replaced by connective tissue or fat. Occasionally, a few degenerated, hyalinized fibers with obscured striations are found between normal muscle fibers. The sarcolemmal nuclei usually retain their shape and hypolemmal position. No inflammatory changes are seen. The vessels and nerves are normal. There is no evidence of regeneration of muscle fibers. In general, all of these changes are rather minimal.

In view of the muscular abnormalities in patients with Cushing's syndrome, it is not surprising that muscle weakness may occur in patients given high doses of glucocorticoids. Widespread degeneration of skeletal muscle following the administration of massive doses of cortisone to rabbits has been noted repeatedly.[5, 6, 8, 9]

Ellis investigated the development of muscular lesions in cortisone-treated rabbits in 1955;[6] the earliest histological change was swelling of large segments of muscle fibers to three or four times their normal size. The protoplasm of the swollen fibers then became necrotic and was partly phagocytized. Before phagocytosis was complete, however, regeneration began; this finding is in contrast to reports on patients with Cushing's syndrome. After 21 days, 40 to 80 per cent of the muscle fibers showed various phases of degeneration and regeneration, and interstitial edema and mononuclear cells were usually present. After injections of cortisone were discontinued, complete healing occurred.

Dubois and Freyberg in 1958 were the first to report progressive loss of weight accompanied by muscle wasting as a result of steroid therapy in humans.[4, 7] In one group of patients with lupus erythematosus given large doses of triamcinolone, muscle wasting developed in two patients after three weeks of therapy.[4] In these two patients the flexor and extensor muscles of the hip and the quadriceps muscles were extremely weak, but function in the muscles below the knee was normal.

Moderate or severe muscle weakness as a result of steroid therapy is most likely to occur in patients receiving triamcinolone (9α fluorohydroxyprednisolone)[4, 7, 14, 17, 23] and occurs only rarely in patients treated with other steroid compounds.[10, 22] According to Dubois,[4] absolute correlation between the magnitude of the dose of triamcinolone and the development of muscle weakness does not exist; however, muscular weakness is most likely to occur in patients treated with large doses for periods longer than three weeks. Aside from these clinical observations, specific comparative studies have not been done to determine which of the anti-inflammatory steroids is most likely to produce myopathy or to determine the necessary time-dose relationships. Although some authors think that only the halogenated steroids produce pronounced muscle changes and that it is the fluorine atom in the 9α position which is responsible for these effects,[14] changes in muscular function also may occur in Cushing's syndrome and when nonfluorinated antiinflammatory steroids are given. Therefore, it seems likely that this property resides in the basic chemical configuration of this entire group of compounds, but perhaps particularly potentiated by 9α fluorination.

Strausz believes that myopathy may be produced by ACTH therapy,[22] but his case reports are not conclusive since the patients were on intermittent prednisone and ACTH therapy.

There is no report in the literature of a comparative study concerning the effects of the newer anti-inflammatory steroids on muscle tissue from this point of view. For this reason an experimental study to investigate the development of myopathy induced by various anti-inflammatory steroids was done.

METHODS

Twenty-four mongrel dogs each weighing 30 to 40 pounds were divided into six groups, each group except the control animals receiving daily intramuscular injections of one of the steroids listed in Table 1.* The doses

TABLE 1. DOSAGE SCHEDULE OF STEROIDS

DOG GROUP NO.		DAILY DOSE
I	Hydrocortisone	100 mg.
II	Prednisolone	25 mg.
III	Methylprednisolone	20 mg.
IV	Dexamethasone	4 mg.
V	Triamcinolone	20 mg.
VI	Control group	

selected were equivalent to those that might be used in intensive therapy of human disease states and were of approximately equal anti-inflammatory potency, except for the dose of dexamethasone, which was about 60 per cent greater, depending on which estimate of equivalency is used. The injections were given daily in the morning in the anterior extremities for five weeks. All dogs were on a standard diet without supplementation. Initially and thereafter at weekly intervals, each dog was weighed and the circumference of the muscles of the posterior extremities was measured. At the same time blood samples were taken for determination of sodium, potassium and hematocrit. Each animal had a baseline electromyographic examination using skin leads and also using the coaxial needle technique. This test was repeated when muscle weakness or wasting was noticeable or after three weeks and thereafter at weekly intervals until steroid administration was stopped; a final electromyogram was obtained three weeks later. All dogs had a biopsy of the quadriceps femoris and gluteal muscles at the completion of five weeks of steroid administration. Subsequently the steroids were gradually discontinued, but the dogs were observed until their weight and muscle measurements had returned to the initial normal level.

RESULTS

Clinical Signs and Symptoms. All dogs except the control group lost weight during the period of steroid administration; however, there was a

---

* The drugs used in these studies were supplied as follows: triamcinolone (Aristocort), by Lederle Laboratories, Pearl River, N. Y.; dexamethasone (Decadron) and prednisolone (Hydeltrasol), by Merck Sharp and Dohme, Philadelphia, Pa.; hydrocortisone (Solu-Cortef) and methylprednisolone (Solu-Medrol), by The Upjohn Company, Kalamazoo, Mich.

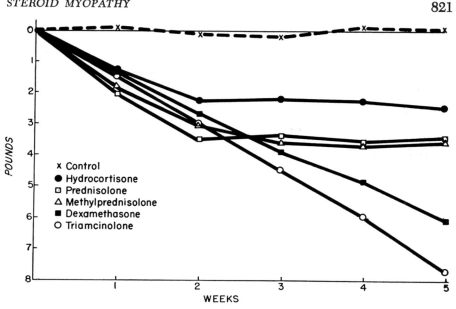

Fig. 1. Average loss of weight in steroid-treated dogs.

notable difference in the amount of weight loss from one group to another (Fig. 1). The dogs receiving hydrocortisone lost an average of 1¼ lbs. during the first week and 1 lb. in the second week, but maintained their weight thereafter. The weight loss in the dogs given prednisolone and methylprednisolone was similar but greater, amounting to about 3½ lbs. in the five-week period. In contrast, the dogs receiving dexamethasone and triamcinolone had a steady weight loss, the average being 6 lbs. for the former group and 7¾ lbs. for the triamcinolone-treated group. In the latter, fatigue and weakness were very pronounced and the dogs had to be forced to move; these animals had definite signs of muscle wasting after 2½ weeks, and it increased thereafter.

The change in weight was associated with a decrease in the circumference of the hind limbs (Table 2 and Fig. 2), indicating a reduction in tissue mass. The quadriceps, gluteal and lower back muscles showed the most involvement, and the dogs had difficulty in walking and were unable to go

TABLE 2. MEASUREMENTS OF THIGHS (IN CM.) OF
STEROID-TREATED DOGS

		UPPER THIGH		MID THIGH		ABOVE KNEE	
Control	Before treatment	36	0	27.5	+ 0.5	23.5	0
	After treatment	36		28		23.5	
Hydrocortisone	Before treatment	34.5	− 0.5	26.5	− 0.5	22	0
	After treatment	34		26		22	
Dexamethasone	Before treatment	33.5	− 0.5	26	− 1.0	21.5	− 0.5
	After treatment	33		25		21	
Prednisolone	Before treatment	31.5	− 0.5	25.5	− 1.5	20.5	− 1.0
	After treatment	31		24		19.5	
Methylprednisolone	Before treatment	31	− 0.5	25	− 1.0	21.5	− 1.5
	After treatment	30.5		24		20	
Triamcinolone	Before treatment	35	− 1.0	25.5	− 2.0	21.5	− 2.0
	After treatment	34		23.5		19.5	

upstairs. As time went on and treatment was continued, the symptoms became more severe and the weakness of the muscles more pronounced; at the end of the fourth week of triamcinolone injection, the dogs had to be carried, as they were unable to walk at all or to stand for any prolonged period of time. Similar changes but of a much lesser degree were noted after three weeks in the dexamethasone group. In the dogs receiving methyl-prednisolone the effects, although noticeable, were less pronouncd. The dogs receiving prednisolone and hydrocortisone did not show any localized muscle wasting even after five weeks and maintained their full strength.

Electromyography. The electromyographic findings tended to support the clinical observations and were similar to those previously reported.[10, 14, 22] The voltage of the motor unit was somewhat decreased for all dogs after

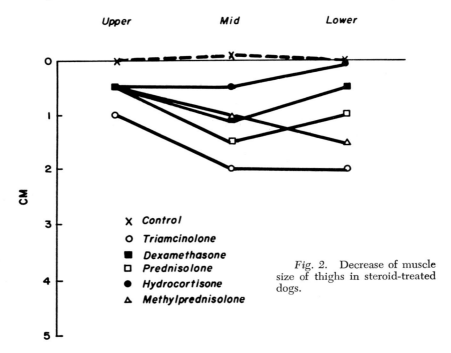

Fig. 2.   Decrease of muscle size of thighs in steroid-treated dogs.

three weeks of treatment; otherwise the findings were similar to those from normal dogs. Fibrillation potentials were not detected in any of the record-ings. The nerve conduction velocity was within normal limits in all animals, a finding which would exclude neurological abnormalities as the cause of the muscle changes.

Electrolytes. The serum electrolytes were within normal limits through-out the experiment, suggesting that abnormalities in electrolyte concentration were not important in the development of the observed muscular changes; however, the possibility of depletion of intracellular or total body potassium was not studied. There was no significant change in the hematocrit during the experiment.

Pathology. Microscopic examination of the muscle obtained by biopsy from each group of dogs revealed notable differences in the size of the muscle fibers from one group to another. As compared with the control group, there was no definite change in the size of the muscle fibers in the

TABLE 3.   FIBER THICKNESS OF QUADRICEPS MUSCLE
IN STEROID-TREATED DOGS

Normal control	25 μ
Methylprednisolone	24.2 μ
Dexamethasone	21.5 μ
Prednisolone	20 μ
Hydrocortisone	19.2 μ
Triamcinolone	14.5 μ

Average measurements; biopsy done after 5 weeks' treatment.

methylprednisolone-treated group; a moderate decrease in the fiber size was found in the dexamethasone-treated group. The fibers were even smaller in the group treated with hydrocortisone and prednisolone, and there was a great reduction in size in the triamcinolone-treated group. The average diameters of the muscle fibers in each group are summarized in Table 3.

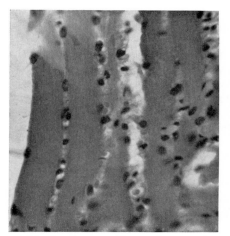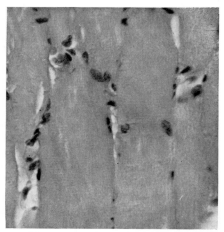

Fig. 3.   Section of biopsy from quadriceps muscle. $\times$ 500. Left: Triamcinolone-treated dog. Right: Normal control.

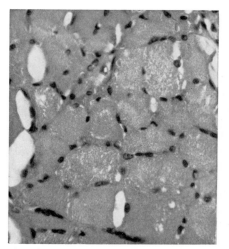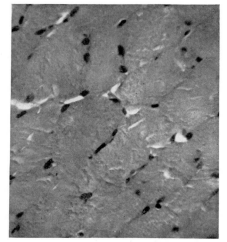

Fig. 4.   Cross section of biopsy from quadriceps muscle. $\times$ 500. Left: Triamcinolone-treated dog. Right: Normal control.

Aside from the changes in fiber thickness, the muscle fibers appeared to be normal, and no evidence of degenerative changes was present (Figs. 3 and 4). No other pathological changes were noted; the vessels and nerves appeared to be normal, and there was no evidence of inflammatory or toxic changes.

Reversibility of Myopathy. After cessation of steroid therapy all dogs regained their weight and strength rapidly; 3½ weeks later all of the animals had returned to their pretreatment state.

DISCUSSION

It is obvious that all of the steroids used had a definite effect on the muscles studied; however, the actual mechanism by which steroid myopathy is produced is still unknown. Kilbourne and Horsfall[12] considered the possibility that a latent viral infection activated by steroids caused the myopathy. Other experiments indicate that this possibility is very unlikely, since homogenates obtained from muscles of rabbits showing cortisone-induced myopathy were found to be nonpathogenic for suckling mice and rabbits, and repeated blood cultures from the rabbits were sterile.[5]

The numerous biochemical studies relating to changes in intermediary metabolism during steriod therapy have so far failed to elucidate this problem definitely; however, there are observations of increased blood creatine levels accompanied by creatinuria[16, 21, 22] and of increased SGOT levels[22] during steroid therapy. These are often higher when the underlying disorder—the reason for steroid therapy—is already in remission.[16] Zierler ascribed creatinuria in patients receiving cortisone due to decreased tubular reabsorption,[24] but this mechanism is unlikely in patients with elevated serum creatine levels.[16] Whether creatinuria and increased creatine levels are due to increased creatine synthesis or to increased breakdown of protein containing creatine is still uncertain; perhaps both are responsible for the occasional really massive serum creatine elevation and creatinuria.[16] However, all these laboratory findings are nonspecific and support only the well known catabolic effect of steroids and their interference with normal protein metabolism, which is at present our only explanation for the muscle wasting.

Bajusz and Strausz[1, 22] claim that inactivity is a major factor in the development of muscle wasting. This was not confirmed in the present study since muscle changes occurred in spite of the fact that all dogs were normally active until severe myopathy occurred.

It is also evident that there is a definite spectrum of activity of each of the steroids studied at least insofar as the posterior limb and quadriceps muscles of the dog are concerned. In equivalent anti-inflammatory doses, hydrocortisone had the least over-all deleterious effect, and triamcinolone had the greatest effect; the other steroids had intermediate effects. The dogs treated with triamcinolone and dexamethasone had the most impressive clinical symptoms of lethargy, muscle weakness and weight loss. However, in the interpretation of these results, it should be noted that the dose of dexamethasone was somewhat greater than that of the other steroids in terms of reported equivalency derived from human and other animal studies. In addition, when dexamethasone is given to humans there is usually a gain in body weight, rather than a loss as observed in these studies.

From the data obtained it appears that the mechanism of the muscle effect is a complex one and that it is probably slightly different for each steroid since changes in the thickness of muscle fibers, circumference of the posterior limb and the amount of body weight lost did not occur in a completely parallel fashion in each group. For example, in the dexamethasone group the changes in muscle fiber thickness and circumference of the hind limb were minimal in comparison to the amount of total body weight lost and clinical findings, particularly when compared with corresponding findings in the group of dogs receiving triamcinolone. Although the hydrocortisone-treated group had only slight weakness and localized muscle wasting, the fiber thickness of the quadriceps muscle decreased more than in any other group except those receiving triamcinolone. Further studies to elucidate these differences in mechanism of action are indicated.

Clinical Diagnosis. Classic steroid myopathy caused by therapeutic administration of large doses of steroids is manifested first by muscle weakness only, first noticeable and most pronounced in the muscles of the lower extremities, mainly in the extensors of the hip and especially in the quadriceps femoris. It is characterized by difficulty in walking, inability to get up from the squatting position or difficulty in going up stairs. Then, a few days or weeks later, there may be visible wasting of the muscles associated with a further reduction in muscle power. In the upper extremities there are few if any signs of weakness. Weakness and wasting of the deep muscles of the back occur only rarely.

It is characteristic that the entire process is reversible; if steroid therapy is discontinued, all symptoms rapidly disappear (usually within three weeks), and the muscle returns to its normal size and shape.[4]

The evaluation and diagnosis of myopathy in the human are often very difficult during the early stages since slight changes may be undetected until there is interference with the activity of the patient; this may occur rather late since patients receiving large doses of steroids are often bedridden and do not use these muscles sufficiently to detect the weakness. In addition, the underlying disease may cause such severe weakness itself that the evaluation of muscle wasting due to steroids is difficult or even impossible. In such patients the use of electromyography and examination of specimens of muscle obtained by biopsy may be of value.

Electromyography. In all kinds of myopathies in which the lesion is located in the muscle tissue itself the electromyogram reveals the duration and voltage of the motor unit to be decreased.[2, 5] The interference pattern shows no diminution in the number of units. With minimal activity there are narrow, low-voltage, normal-appearing motor units with a good interference pattern although it is of lower voltage than usual.

Pathology. The reported histological pattern of steroid myopathy is inconsistent, some authors describing the muscle as normal except for reduction in muscle fiber size and moderate increase in size of subsarcolemmal nuclei,[14] and others describing diffuse uneven atrophy of muscle fibers with clumping and string formation of nuclei, degeneration and necrosis with mononuclear cells in the fiber.[23] Vacuolization, similar to that found in thyrotoxic myopathy, has also been reported.[16] The findings in our study suggest that the typical pathologic change is the decrease in the size of the individual muscle fibers without any additional abnormal findings.

Differential Diagnosis. Many other processes affecting muscles may resemble steroid myopathy, e.g., neurological diseases, potassium deficiency, etc. Measurement of nerve conduction velocity, using the electromyographic apparatus in conjunction with a stimulator, may be of value in the distinction between neuropathic and myopathic involvement. The normal nerve conduction speed is about 50 meters per second. This speed does not change in myopathic involvement, whereas in neurogenic diseases such as amyotrophic lateral sclerosis and progressive muscular dystrophy it may be considerably slowed.

Myopathies induced by potassium deficiency can be differentiated from steroid myopathy by determination of serial serum potassium levels. Morphologically, cortisone-induced myopathy in the skeletal muscle of rabbits resembles that induced by potassium-deficient diets; however, although cortisone-treated rabbits do not exhibit pathological changes in the myocardium, rabbits on potassium-deficient diets do so regularly.[5, 20] The cortisone-treated rabbits have normal serum potassium levels, and the muscular changes occurring in them are not prevented by large doses of potassium, though oral potassium prevents the development of muscle changes in potassium-deficient animals.[20]

SUMMARY

Muscle weakness is a frequent finding in Cushing's syndrome. It also occurs in artificially produced hyperadrenocorticism and is associated with muscle atrophy. It was first described in patients treated with triamcinolone.

Animal experiments were carried out in an attempt to induce myopathy with large doses of anti-inflammatory steroids. Weight loss and signs of muscle wasting could be observed in all groups except the control group; they were most pronounced in the triamcinolone-treated dogs.

Clinical, electromyographic and histologic changes are discussed. No explanation is presently available to account for the differences in the ability of various steroids to induce myopathy and for the peculiar localization of the lesion.

ACKNOWLEDGMENTS

We wish to thank Shinazo Irie, M.D., for his help in the preparation of electromyograms and Maryanne Girardo for her valuable technical assistance.

REFERENCES

1. Bajusz, E.: Disuse atrophy of skeletal muscle in the rat, aggravated by cortisol and various stress conditions. Canad. J. Biochem. & Physiol., 36:825, 1958.
2. Blodgett, W. H.: Clinical application of electromyography. Grace Hosp. Bull., 38:3, 1960.
3. Cushing, H.: The basophil adenomas of the pituitary body and their clinical manifestations. Bull. Johns Hopkins Hosp., 50:137, 1932.
4. Dubois, E. L.: Triamcinolone in the treatment of systemic lupus erythematosus. J.A.M.A., 167:1590, 1958.
5. Ellis, J. T.: Necrosis and regeneration of skeletal muscles in cortisone-treated rabbits. Am. J. Path., 32:993, 1956.
6. Ellis, J. T.: Degeneration and regeneration in the muscles of cortisone-treated rabbits. Am. J. Phys. Med., 34:240, 1955.
7. Freyberg, R. H., Berntsen, C. A., Jr. and Hellman, L.: Further experiences with triamcinolone in treatment of patients with rheumatoid arthritis. Arth. & Rheum., 1:215, 1958.
8. Germuth, F. G., Jr., Nedzel, G. A., Ottinger, B. and Oyama, J.: Anatomic and histologic changes in rabbits with experimental hypersensitivity treated with compound E and ACTH. Proc. Soc. Exper. Biol. & Med., 76:177, 1951.
9. Glaser, G. H. and Stark, L.: Excitability in experimental myopathy. Neurology, 8:640, 1958.

10. Golding, D. N.: Dexamethasone myopathy. Brit. M. J., 2:1129, 1960.
11. Harman, J. B.: Muscular wasting and corticosteroid therapy (Letter to the Editor). Lancet, 1:887, 1959.
12. Kilbourne, E. D. and Horsfall, F. L., Jr.: Lethal infection with Coxsackie virus of adult mice given cortisone. Proc. Soc. Exper. Biol. & Med., 77:135, 1951.
13. Lehoczky, T.: Triamcinolone myopathy (Letter to the Editor). Lancet, 1:994, 1959.
14. MacLean, K. and Shurt, P. H.: Reversible amyotrophy complicating treatment with fludrocortisone. Lancet, 1:701, 1959.
15. Muller, R. and Kugelberg, E.: Myopathy in Cushing's syndrome. J. Neurol., Neurosurg. & Psychiat., 22:314, 1959.
16. Perkoff, G. T., Silber, R., Tyler, F. H., Cartwright, G. E. and Wintrobe, M. M.: Studies in disorders of muscle. XII. Myopathy due to the administration of therapeutic amounts of 17-hydroxycorticosteroids. Am. J. Med., 26:891, 1959.
17. Robinson, C. E. and Robinson, H. S.: Triamcinolone in rheumatoid arthritis. Canad. M. A. J., 80:245, 1959.
18. Rogoff, J. B.: Clinical electromyography. Usefulness in differentiating myopathies from neuropathies. New York J. Med., 60:512, 1960.
19. Smith, M., Burke, H. A., Coppage, W. S. and Liddle, G. W.: The newer steroids. Practitioner, 183:519, 1959.
20. Smith, S. G., Black-Schaffer, B. and Lasater, T. E.: Potassium deficiency syndrome in the rat and the dog. Arch. Path., 49:185, 1950.
21. Sprague, R. G. et al.: Observations on the physiologic effects of cortisone and ACTH in man. A.M.A. Arch. Int. Med., 85:199, 1950.
22. Strausz, I. and Janikovszky, B.: Corticosteroid-myopathia. Orv. Hetil., 101:946, 1960.
23. Williams, R. S.: Triamcinolone myopathy. Lancet, 1:698, 1959.
24. Zierler, L. L., Folk, B. P., Magladary, T. W. and Lilienthal, F. L., Jr.: On creatinuria in men. Role of renal tubule and muscle mass. Bull. Johns Hopkins Hosp., 85:370, 1949.

Effects of Steroids on Mental Processes and Their Treatment

SELWYN BRODY

Children's Village, Dobbs Ferry, N. Y.

The dramatic effect of cortisone and ACTH was heralded as the beginning of a new era in medicine, which would provide not only a panacea for all diseases, but also the key to the understanding of the fundamental processes of disease and health.

The hormones were originally used in the treatment of a vast panorama of diseases and were more spectacular than other "miracle drugs," since they were employed with apparent benefit in some malignant diseases and some severe neurologic and psychiatric disorders.

However, the deluge of sensational reports soon became counterbalanced by increasing evidence of unfavorable side effects. It was primarily the so-called "collagen" and related connective tissue diseases which aroused our interest at the introduction of steroid therapy. As a psychiatrist, I was drawn to the victims of these diseases because of an apparent remarkable connection between the physical symptoms and the emotional disturbances observed during the administration of cortisone and ACTH.[1, 2, 3]

Approximately 80 patients with collagen and related diseases, receiving hormone treatment, were therapeutically studied, the majority through bedside interviews. Because of the dominance of the medical symptoms, only a few of the patients were observed and treated more extensively, but I have had the opportunity to treat several such cases in private practice, one of whom has been under psychoanalytic treatment three times weekly for the past four years.

The most casual observer has acknowledged that profound psychic effects accompany this type of organic disorder. Some nonpsychiatric physicians have conceded that "they are all mental cases." Severe depressions, often psychotic in degree, as well as other neuropsychiatric manifestations, were noted before, during and after hormone therapy in many of these patients. A survey of the literature reveals comments that in the early days of the use of the steroid drugs psychoses occurred more frequently and were considered among its major hazards. Such reactions were attributed to the wide and indiscriminate use of the steroids. Recently, more careful selection of patients and the growing awareness of the effects of the steroids have reduced the number and severity of emotional disorders.[8] According to some studies, the adverse reactions are not related to dosage.

Table 1 lists the diagnoses for the 82 patients observed and treated by

TABLE 1.   DIAGNOSIS IN 82 PATIENTS OBSERVED OR TREATED
FOR PSYCHIATRIC MANIFESTATIONS

Systemic lupus erythematosus	44 (of whom 38 were treated with hormones)
Diffuse vascular disease	7
Rheumatoid arthritis	4
Rheumatoid arthritis and gout	1
Rheumatoid arthritis and chronic lymphatic leukemia	1
Rheumatic fever and rheumatic heart disease	5
Pemphigus	3
Pemphigus, lymphoblastoma and asthma	1
Scleroderma	3
Hyperthyroidism and psoriasis	2
Lymphatic leukemia	1
Lymphosarcoma and lymphoblastoma	1
Chronic lymphatic leukemia and follicular lymphoblastoma	1
Myelogenous leukemia and bronchial asthma	1
Thrombocytopenic purpura	1
Dermatomyositis	2
Uveitis and glaucoma	2
Ulcerative colitis	1
Carcinoma of prostate	1
Total	82

the author. The patients with lupus erythematosus were studied more intensively, and the incidence and course of psychotic manifestations in this group is presented in Table 2. These patients also had several nonpsychotic neuropsychiatric reactions, and these are listed in Table 3.

The incidence of psychotic and neuropsychiatric reactions in the 38 patients with diseases other than lupus erythematosus is presented in Table 4. Of those who had psychotic reactions, two had diffuse vascular disease, two had pemphigus, one had scleroderma, and one had carcinoma of the prostate.

TABLE 2. INCIDENCE OF PSYCHOTIC MANIFESTATIONS IN
PATIENTS WITH LUPUS ERYTHEMATOSUS

	NO.	PER CENT
Total patients (Note: 2 additional patients were added after this study had been made.)	42	100
Total patients with psychotic manifestations	22	52
Psychotic manifestations before therapy	12	29
Improvement during therapy	5	12
Unchanged or provoked during therapy	13	31
Associated with remission or improvement of physical symptoms	15	36
Symptoms on discontinuation of therapy	2	5
Relief of symptoms on discontinuation of therapy	3	7
Psychosis associated with death	7	17
Estimated average duration of psychosis: Patients who survived, 30 days Patients who succumbed, 6 days		

TABLE 3. INCIDENCE OF OTHER NEUROPSYCHIATRIC REACTIONS
IN 42 PATIENTS WITH LUPUS ERYTHEMATOSUS

NONPSYCHOTIC MANIFESTATIONS	NO.	PER CENT
Convulsions	9	21
Convulsions associated with death	6	14
Convulsions, but subsequent improvement	3	7
Depressive reactions (before and during therapy)	10	24
Persistent euphoria during therapy	1	2
Overcompliance	9	21

TABLE 4. PSYCHOTIC OR NEUROPSYCHIATRIC REACTIONS
IN 38 NON-LUPUS PATIENTS

	NO.	PER CENT
Psychotic reactions	6	16
Depressions, severe to moderate, including 1 suicide*	12	32
Euphorias (transient)	19	50
Euphorias (persistent)	4	11
Ambivalence	4	11
Sexual changes	1	2-3
Overcompliance, with underlying hostility and anxiety	11	30
Convulsions	1	2-3

* In a personal communication in 1956, Mark D. Altschule, M.D., of Harvard Medical School, reported collecting "eight instances of suicide in medical patients previously non-psychotic who received ACTH . . . 50 to 100 mg. daily for several weeks."

In order to obtain further statistics on the incidence of mental reactions resulting from steroid therapy, ten representative papers published from 1953-1960 were examined (Table 5). A total of 1057 cases were found. In these, 138, or 13 per cent, had mental, personality or sexual changes.

It is of interest that there has been a tapering off of reports of mental reactions to steroids, and most recent medical articles minimize adverse psychiatric reactions. This can be ascribed to better selection of patients, improved administration of the drugs and the refinement of the newer steroid derivatives. Yet there are investigators who find the picture inconsistent,

TABLE 5. INCIDENCE OF MENTAL SYMPTOMS DUE TO STEROID THERAPY: SURVEY OF LITERATURE

	TOTAL NO. OF CASES	NO. OF REACTIONS	PER CENT
Levin, M. H. et al.: Prolonged treatment of rheumatoid arthritis with cortisone and corticotrophin. Am. J. Med., *14*: 265, 1953.	50		
Mental or CNS side effects		5	10
Personality changes		29	58
Sexual changes		11	22
Ragan, C.: Steroids in clinical medicine. Bull. N. Y. Acad. Med., 29:355, 1953.	100		
High dosage	69		
Mental side effects		25	36
Low dosage	31		
Mental side effects		12	41
Bunim, J. J. et al.: Evaluation of prolonged cortisone therapy in rheumatoid arthritis. Am. J. Med., *18*:27, 1955.	59		
Mental side effects		4	7
Toone, E. C. and Irby, R.: Effects of cortisone in the long-term therapy of rheumatoid arthritis. Am. J. Med., *18*:41, 1955.	35		
Mental side effects		3	9
McMahon, F. G. and Gordon, E. G.: Side effects noted in treatment with medrol. J.A.M.A., *368*:1208, 1958.	67		
Mental side effects including convulsions		10	14
Kendall, P. H. and Hart, H. F.: Side effects following triamcinolone. Brit. M. J., *1*:682, 1959.	47		
Mental side effects		4	9
Nordin, B. E. C.: Side effects of systemic adrenal steroid therapy. Brit. J. Dermat., *72*:40, 1960	450		
Mental side effects		18	4
Thompson, W. T., Jr. and Kelly, J. J., III: Hazards of adrenocortical therapy. Virginia M. Month., *87*:80, 1960.	70		
Mental side effects		3	4
Sherwood, H. and Epstein, J. I.: Long-term evaluation of triamcinolone in allergic diseases. J. Allergy, *31*:12, 1960.	24		
Mental side effects		4	17
Dubois, E. L.: Current treatment of S. L. E., J.A.M.A., *173*:1633, 1960.	155		
Mental side effects		2	1.3
Insomnia		8	5
Total	1057		
Reactions mentioned in the literature		138	13

confused and far from convincing. One author goes so far as to say, "Physicians vary in the care with which they look for side effects and in the way in which they report those that they do observe. . . . Only a small proportion of observed side effects is ever published. . . . The picture one can glean from the literature is at best very imperfect."

Brief summaries of illustrative cases are presented in Table 6.

Electro-encephalographic changes were found to have no relationship to the neuropsychiatric reactions, as positive EEG changes were present in some patients without any observable psychic symptoms and negative EEG's were sometimes present during violent episodes.[6] Epileptiform seizures are not uncommon in L.E., with or without hormone treatment.[9] In one case, relief of symptoms following such a seizure was described as, "She gave herself her own shock treatment."

An extraordinary observation in the lupus patients was that death never occurred in this often fatal disease when a sustained overt psychosis supervened, particularly during hormone treatment. It appeared that the psychosis had a therapeutic effect, a survival function, so to speak, and one which could prevent a fatal outcome. This contrasts with the more usual, conventional attitude that a psychosis is the ultimate in adverse reactions.[3] The issue of correlation of psychosis and organic disease continues to hold interest.[4, 5, 11]

I hesitate to recommend agents for provoking psychoses to save lives, but could this be considered more egregious than injecting malarial parasites to kill the spirochetal parasites of a syphilitic?

In one report, psychosis was not found to be a contraindication to use of the steroid drugs.[12] It would be indeed satisfactory to be able to report with pinpoint precision all of the reactions quantitatively correlating dosage and other important variables (including the objectivity of the researcher), but to my knowledge this has not yet been done.[10]

SUMMARY AND CONCLUSIONS

Extended studies of cortisone-treated patients confirmed the impression that many of these patients were literally destroying themselves with their often fatal diseases. It was observed that: (1) the hormone stimulated personality as well as metabolic functions; (2) metabolic changes induced by hormone therapy affected personality; (3) emotional and personality reactions influenced metabolic processes.

The stimulating action of cortisone as well as its withdrawal induces an abrupt change in severe physical symptoms deeply incorporated in the patient's way of life. Although euphoria was usually evoked initially, it persisted in only a few of the patients, giving way to various mental reactions in keeping with the individual personality structure. "It is possible that since cortisone produces a feeling of elation, addiction may be a serious problem in emotionally predisposed people. Therefore, withdrawal of the drug may precipitate a crisis with possible suicide or psychosis as consequences."[7]

The data suggest the importance of intense investigative psychotherapy in conjunction with the steroid therapy to accomplish the following objectives: (1) to help these patients to organize methods for the healthy discharge of destructive impulses; (2) to help them to acquire healthy, protective insulating barriers against hypersensitive responses to stimuli; (3) to reduce hypersensitive stressful reactions; (4) to restore and improve homeo-

(Text continues p. 840)

TABLE 6. ILLUSTRATIVE CASES

CASE	AGE	SEX	CLINICAL DIAGNOSIS	DURATION OF ILLNESS	ONSET FACTORS	PERSONALITY	THERAPY	PHYSICAL REACTIONS	PSYCHOLOGICAL REACTIONS
1. F. W.	13	M.	Lupus	1 yr.	Death of father; sexual and emotional conflicts of puberty.	Compliant, evasive, "nice boy", on superficial level; distorted ideas of sexuality and masturbation; denies interest or curiosity.	Cortisone 150 mg./day (9 admissions).	Oscillation between recurrences of symptoms on lowered dosage; renal failure and death.	Suppression of anxiety and hostility beneath superficial cooperation; "Appearances are deceiving."; had nightmares of being attacked by doctors with needles; listless and lethargic; terminal psychosis exposed primitive sexual impulses; only at the point of irreversibility would he let himself go and express his real feelings.
2. M. F.	36	F.	Lupus	2 yrs.	Deserted by husband; illness of father; sole support of self and child; "no one to turn to."	Unstable, moody, depressive; need for conformity; no sexual life since husband deserted 15 yrs. ago.	150 mg./day cortisone for 17 days. 200 mg./day cortisone.	Restive to moderate dosage, but remarkable response to 200 mg. per day; oscillation with improvement maintained on therapy; discharged after six months.	Hypomanic-euphoric; agitated; paranoid during improved physical phase; delusions of cancer; "I want to join God. I want to die"; psychosis subsides with reduced dosage, but still depressed: "I think I'd be better off dead."
3. E. L.	35	M.	Lupus	4 mos.	Hypertension; sympathectomy (1940 and 1944) rheumatic fever (1933).	Compliant, apprehensive; tries to conceal anxiety and hostility.	2 admissions. ACTH, then cortisone 10 days 200-250 mg./day.	Fever down, elevation of B.P.; improvement superficial; moon-faced; readmitted for recurrence of symptoms; improvement with therapy; discharged.	Delusional psychosis alternating with euphoria subsided when therapy discontinued; lethargic during cortisone administration.
4. I. S.	26	F.	Lupus	6 mos.	Severe personality disturbance; schizophrenia.	Seclusive; rejects heterosexuality; visual hallucinations; schizoid.	Cortisone, then ACTH.	Definite improvement in 3 days with both, so that brother-in-law who had accompanied her from N. Mex. was permitted to leave for home. 5 wks. after admission, relapse, death in convulsive state.	Psychosis; catatonia, delirium, delusions and hallucinations on admission; showed superficial clearing; suspicious, refused to participate in interviews when brother-in-law left; sullen; acutely agitated; "I want to die; I think I'm going crazy"; states her main trouble is that brother-in-law has gone; "made up her mind" to go crazy, to die.

Case	Sex	Disease	Duration	Precipitating factor	Personality	Treatment	Physical result	Mental effects
5. R. C. 53	F.	Lupus	5 yrs.	Illness of husband; forced to live in mother's home; constant quarreling.	Reactive depressions on death of children and mother; suspicious; unfriendly; pessimistic; "Hard life and nerves brought on my sickness."	Cortisone by mouth for 3 wks., 40 mg. for 5 mos.; increased dosage of ACTH; 3 admissions.	Fever controlled on reduced dosage; returned home to full duties for 3-4 mos.; then recurrence and new symptoms; hypertension with increased dosage; death.	Overt psychosis; **cleared** during hormone therapy; no spontaneous complaints, but uncheerful and uncommunicative; lethargy; incontinence; hostile on readmission; defiant; refuses interviews, **saying, "You know everything on my mind", death.**
6. W. E. 50	M.	Lupus	11 yrs.	Illness of child; forced to move south.	Idealistic; "superior morally"; identified with pious father; effort to control hostility and sexuality.	Cortisone, ACTH. Repeated courses during 9 mos. (2 admissions).	Dramatic improvement; recurring symptoms; diabetes; increased sexual energy on ACTH.	Euphoric: "it's a miracle"; insisted on being optimistic and patient; covered up resentment and anxiety.
7. E. W. 15	F.	Lupus	6 mos.	Regents exams.; puberty; serious friction of parents (mixed marriage).	Perfectionist in performance and behavior; pseudo-mature; fantasies of death of parents and of self.	ACTH, cortisone. 2 admissions in 8 mos.	Physical symptoms checked, but delusions more severe; discharged 5 mos. after admission, physically improved, but psychotic.	Psychosis preceding hormone therapy; increased in severity during therapy; psychosis cleared at home after father's suicide and mother's commitment to mental institution.
8. E. M. 39	F.	Lupus	1 yr.	Loss of job.	Schizoid-schizophrenic; evasive; seclusive; brief psychotic outbursts.	ACTH.	Improvement.	Uncommunicative; evasive: "nothing to say"; unmanageable and terrified when injections given.
9. R. B. 34	M.	Lupus	5 yrs.	Army desert training; readjustment to civilian status and marriage.	"Naturally pessimistic"; likes to "drive self bats"; "Can't let myself go"; infantile; oversensitive; nightmares of crying for help; concerned about masturbation: "ugly."	Cortisone, ACTH.	Immediate improvement in chronic joint pains, retained during 3½ mos. of therapy.	Transient euphoria soon gave way to pessimism: "I could go into a relapse. I think scientifically"; exacerbation of depression after self-revealing interview.
10. E. M. 39	F.	Lupus	1 yr.	Loss of job.	Schizoid; evasive; inappropriate emotionally; affect flat; psychotic during acute phase of the lupus.	ACTH.	Improvement, then death.	Unspontaneous; uncommunicative, evasive, but with weeping, cringing; shrieks when hormone is injected, but insists at interview. "Nothing bothers me."
11. R. V. 20	F.	Lupus		Severe mental stress; social anxiety.	Schizoid; immature; low I.Q. (82); timid; afraid of hostile impulses.	ACTH 5 mos.	Dramatic improvement initially; then stormy course; convulsive seizures; jaundice; then improvement.	Depressed before therapy; then marked improvement on ACTH; lethargy; apathy.

TABLE 6.   ILLUSTRATIVE CASES (Continued)

CASE	AGE	SEX	CLINICAL DIAGNOSIS	DURATION OF ILLNESS	ONSET FACTORS	PERSONALITY	THERAPY	PHYSICAL REACTIONS	PSYCHOLOGICAL REACTIONS
12. M. B.	20	M.	Lupus	17 mos.	Stress of "making grade", as college freshman; obesity; cryptorchidism.	Superficial compliance; covertly apprehensive.	ACTH 100 mg. for 4 days; cortisone 150 mg. for 21 days.	Prompt response in alleviation of joint pains, but low grade fever persisted; improvement for 2 mos. after discharge.	Jolly attitude obviously covering up apprehension; never complains.
13. W. G.	28	F.	Lupus	1 yr.	Severe emotional conflict.	Psychotic-paranoid; completely coherent with intact sensorium when she "felt understood"; homosexual and aggressive impulses; refused to permit doctors to examine her; personality changes following encephalitis with convulsions 6 yrs. prior to admission.	Cortisone 150-300 mg./day, discontinued after 30 days.	Symptoms resistant to ordinary dosage; better response of fever and joint pains to high dosage, but with cerebral disturbances, which gradually improved during cessation of treatment; convulsive seizure transferred to chronic hosp. unimproved after 3 mos. (acute neural defect with paralysis of extraocular movement).	Fluctuation of psychosis; paranoid outbursts at first diminished, only to become intensified as neurological complication with marked depression; "They (drs. and nurses) are making me worse. They are trying to kill me, I am peculiar, nuts. Wish I could die. The drs. gave me drugs to get well, but I am going to be sick the rest of my life. I am . . . I'll die a virgin."
14. A. D.	16	F.	Lupus	4-6 mos.	Severe economic and emotional deprivation; Puerto Rican orphan; change of culture.	Immature; extreme anxiety, allayed whenever she felt accepted by staff; intellectually slow.	ACTH.	Improvement.	Anxiety lessened, except when home situation and discharge discussed.
15. C. B.	34	F.	Lupus	19 mos.	Birth of child; financial stress.	Anxious; psychotic-paranoid; concerned about "dirt."	ACTH 100 mg./day for 2½ mos.	Prompt improvement in symptoms; recurrence on reduced dosage; hirsute after 3 wks. of therapy; free of symptoms 1 yr.	Initial increase in psychotic outbursts with hallucinations and delusions; gradual subsidence of overt psychosis; euphoric alternately with apprehensiveness.
16. S. L.	17	F.	Lupus	4 mos.	Acute pressure by mother to get dates before illness and during improvement at home; severe mental stress; social pressures exerted by mother.	Depressed; complete refusal to discuss personal feelings and family situation; attitude hostile although superficially cooperative; "snippy" and sarcastic; struggling with anxiety; spoiled only child.	Cortisone, ACTH; 3 admissions.	Moderate improvement; discharged after 8 mos. therapy; received cortisone at home; relapse and readmission; hypertension; Cushing's; renal failure and death.	No spontaneity; preoccupied; hostile to efforts to talk with her; became acutely depressed at home; pressure of mother, but could not discuss their quarreling; readmission and death.
17. C. S.	27	F.	Lupus	1½ yrs.	Pregnancy and birth of child.	Compliant; attempt to conceal anxiety; only child.	Cortisone 900 mg., ACTH 800 mg., 3 wks.	Marked fading of lesions; discharged improved.	Jittery; shaky.

No.	Name	Age	Sex	Diagnosis	Duration		Personality	Drug/Dosage	Result	Notes
18.	J. D.	13	F.	Lupus	18 mos.		Agitated and depressed; attempts to be cheerful.	ACTH 8 days. Dosage: 1st day: 25 mg. 2nd–5th: 100 mg. 6th day: 75 mg. 7th day: 70 mg. 8th day: 70 mg.	Dramatic improvement in 2 days, until 8th day, then headaches on 7th and 8th days; generalized convulsion on 9th day; drug discontinued; status epilepticus; pulmonary edema on 11th day and death (2 days after discontinuance). (EEG 2 days after discontinuance showed "possible convulsive disorder.")	At first, cheerful, then irritable and depressed, crying for mother on 6th day; on 7th day, cheerful despite "no visitors" and wants to go home; states resolutely. "It's good to do things for yourself." Then increased depression; wants mother and to go home; status epilepticus; death.
19.	N. M.	30	F.	Lupus	2 mos.	Discharged from job.	Infantile; moody, sensitive; "took things too hard"; must be near mother; psychotic; visual hallucinations.	Cortisone.	Marked improvement.	Psychotic on entry; gradual clearing of hallucinations, but showing poor emotional control; deficient insight; cries easily; unstable.
20.	B. P.	32	F.	Lupus	8 yrs.		Discouraged; depressed after 8 yrs. of temporary remissions and relapses after various therapies; emotionally immature.	ACTH, 2 courses, 100 mg. Cortisone, 2 courses, 3 mos.	Symptoms subsided; symptoms recurred after 3 mos. of therapy. Discharge note: "Clinical picture shows remarkable remission. Cushing's syndrome during cortisone promptly cleared when drug was discontinued; discharged improved."	Org. delusions and hallucinations; delusions subsided; psychotic during relapse; gradually improved during therapy, then showed oscillation of cheerfulness and alertness with depression and lethargy until therapy was discontinued; then apprehension; essentially cheerful on the last course of ACTH prior to discharge.
21.	H. C.	60	M.	Diff. vasc. Periarteritis nodosa.		Lifelong struggle with sexual feelings.	Obsessive; schizoid; depressed; withdrawn.	ACTH, cortisone (Cushing's).	Dramatic improvement initially; downhill course.	Temporary euphoria.
22.	L. P.	38	F.	Rh. arthritis.	19 yrs.		Unhappy; discouraged after many remissions and relapses.	Cortisone 2000 mg. in 2 courses.	Marked reduction of joint pains; increased menstrual flow.	Despite initial pleasure at relief of pain, frequently restless; refused injections; was dissatisfied; required constant enemas; passed flatus, said, "Cortisone may have affected my bowels"; other hypochondriacal complaints; disagreeable.
23.	D. A.	58	F.	Rh. arthritis.	3 yrs.			Cortisone 2000 mg. in 5 wks.	Moderate improvement in joint mobility and pains.	Marked subjective improvement.

TABLE 6. ILLUSTRATIVE CASES (Continued)

CASE	AGE	SEX	CLINICAL DIAGNOSIS	DURATION OF ILLNESS	ONSET FACTORS	PERSONALITY	THERAPY	PHYSICAL REACTIONS	PSYCHOLOGICAL REACTIONS
24. E. M.	60	M.	Rh. arthritis.	20 yrs.	Current exacerbation wife's desertion.	Meek, docile, appeasing; tries to rationalize his financial and marital losses; "can't lose temper."	Cortisone.	Questionable improvement in joint symptoms.	Externally agreeable and optimistic; submissive: "I hope this drug is good. You have to have faith."
25. S. D.	45	F.	Rh. arthritis.	10 yrs.	After marriage and birth of child; rejected by family.	Denial; ambivalent attachment to parents.	Cortisone 200 mg.	Marked improvement; severe headaches; rectal bleeding; elevated blood pressure.	Cheerful, but labile and depressed on discharge.
26. I. G.	56	F.	Rh. arthritis and gout.	15 yrs.	Mother's death; marital failure; husband killed.	Superficial appearance of "sweet," kindly disposition; actually hostile, stubborn begrudging.	ACTH 1000 mg. in 3 wks.	Dramatic improvement until discontinuance of drugs; reappearance of symptoms.	Guarded responses; "Isn't this all research and experimental?" Refused to discuss personal matters; defiant; "You can read my mind anyway. I know I'm not cooperative."
27. C. C.	39	M.	Rh. heart dis.; essential hypertension; polyarthritis; diffuse vascular allergy (?)			Easy-going, dull, uncomplaining, undemanding; insensitive.	Cortisone.	Complete subsidence of symptoms; blood pressure unaltered; sedimentation rate remained elevated.	During therapy, drowsy, submissive; offered few complaints; rarely ventured to admit physical pain; "Every place I lie I feel pain; otherwise I wouldn't know I was sick." Tried to appear cheerful and comfortable, even when he had constant joint pains, which recurred upon cessation of the hormone treatment.
28. J. V.	43	F.	Vascular allergy; periarteritis nodosa.	8 mos.	Enucleation of mother's eye and then her death.	Spinster; tied to mother; pessimistic; gloomy; childishly sulky; super-self-critical; "I brought this on myself."	Cortisone and ACTH.	Unsatisfactory; partially beneficial effects.	Begrudges any improvement; defiant; negativistic and uncooperative; occasional dry cheerfulness, counterbalanced by weeping, depressed mood; hostile.
29. R. M.	14	M.	Rh. heart disease.		Father's desertion; mother living with another man.	Unspontaneous; lonely; likes to be talked to; complains of dreams in which he can't see his own face.	Cortisone 1½ mos.	Gradual improvement.	No affective reaction; no improvement; compulsive; hostile.

No. / Initials	Age	Sex	Diagnosis	Duration	Personality / History	Treatment	Physical response	Mental response
30. A. A.		F.	Acute rh. fever.		**Agreeable, quite, conforming submissive.**		Subsidence of physical symptoms.	No complaints; no spontaneous remarks; complaint and conforming; submissive; no apparent anxiety or apprehension.
31. M. S.	32	M.	Acute rh. fever.	3 wks.	Tied to mother; enuresis until 20; depressed since loss of mother. Broken home since mother's death.	Cortisone 9 days.	"Remarkable response."	Lacking in spontaneity, no display of well-being; despite physical response; no enthusiasm: "I'm the quiet type."
32. M. L.	50	F.	Pemphigus.	8 mos.	"Psychoneurotic"; extremely infantile, rages, tantrums, difficult and intractable according to her family. Dependent tie to son; excessive fear of breaking tie.	Cortisone 3.6 gm. ACTH 2 gm.	Dramatic improvement; gradual recurrence of skin lesions.	Negativistic, hostile, psychotic outbursts; screams; "Don't believe those doctors. I'm getting worse and worse." Agitated, uncooperative; death wishes.
33. J. G.	45	M.	Pemphigus.	5 mos.				Alternately depressed and euphoric.
34. C. G.		M.	Pemphigus; lymphoblastoma.			ACTH.	Dramatic disappearance of skin lesions at 200 mg., but on reducing dosage, lesions reappeared.	Acute psychosis "organic type"; depressed; paranoid.
35. V. Z.	20	F.	Scleroderma.	1½ yrs.	Insists it is "all emotional," due to her reaction to brother's marriage; disease started in rt. arm, subject to undue stress on industrial job (sister has same disease).	ACTH in another hospital; cortisone 150 mg./day, 5 days; 100 mg./day, 15 days; total, 2.35 gm. ACTH, 800 mg. in 18 days.	In 1 wk. improved, skin softer. Improved, but hirsutism of face; recurrence of induration.	Generalized and sexual excitement; was euphoric before cortisone, now more so: "It's like going to a party." Underlying anxiety: "What will happen when it's through? I can't be excited all the time."
36. S. S.	35	F.	Scleroderma; uveitis.	7 yrs.	Serious emotional struggle with family; mixed marriage; psychotic sister. Blind from age 21 (chemical injury); history of "nervous breakdowns."	10 days after discontinuance 6 mos. later, cortisone 300 mg./wk. ACTH and cortisone as high as 400 mg./day.	Doubtful improvement.	Still superficially cheerful, euphoric, optimistic. Paranoid psychosis; cleared after therapy stopped.

TABLE 6.   ILLUSTRATIVE CASES (Continued)

CASE	AGE	SEX	CLINICAL DIAGNOSIS	DURATION OF ILLNESS	ONSET FACTORS	PERSONALITY	THERAPY	PHYSICAL REACTIONS	PSYCHOLOGICAL REACTIONS
37. M. H.	28	F.	Grave's dis.; hyperthyroidism.	8 yrs.	Death of father, and mother's subsequent alcoholic break-down (8 yrs. prior to admission); recurrence after automobile accident (2 yrs. prior to admission).	Compulsive need to be agreeable no matter how provoked; extremely ambivalent tie to mother.	Cortisone 7 days.	No decrease in exophthalmos.	No decrease in tremulousness; deep apprehension and guilt as to effects of her illness upon mother.
38. P. M.	38	F.	Grave's dis.; enlarged thymus; Psoriasis; colitis; fissure in ano.	10 yrs.	Family wiped out in Warsaw in 1939.	Superficially agreeable; easily hurt; weeps easily; can't stand hostile or critical feelings.	Cortisone.	Questionable; no effect on thymos.	Expresses happiness and optimism "whenever I feel someone is helping me" concerning the therapy; no change visible in behavior and anxiety.
39. R. J.	46	F.	Periarteritis nodosa; asthma.	2½ yrs.	Crisis regarding disposition of mentally defective son.	Emotionally unstable; disintegrating from generalized agitation.	ACTH 80-100 mg./day for 5 wks. then cortisone 200 mg./day.	Asthma cleared, but painful nodules persisted; new symptoms whenever discharge was imminent.	Initially depressed, hostile, but seeking sympathy; expressed despair even at the point of greatest physical improvement; "When will it all end?"
40. L. H.	47	M.	Asthma; periarteritis nodosa.	3½ yrs.	Death of father-in-law.	Obsessive-compulsive; paranoid schiz.; passive homosexual.	ACTH, cortisone.	Marked relief, then recurrence.	Euphoric; constant erections.
41. R. S.	17	F.	Periarteritis nodosa.	1 yr.	Rejection and defeat in love affair.	Hysterical, obsessive, masochistic, self-pity; stirs herself up to excitement temperatures; transparent Oedipal conflict, marked ambivalence.	1700 mg. cortisone in 25 days.	Striking improvement after 4th day; symptoms returned on discontinuance.	Euphoric but ambivalent; rejected cortisone: "All my trouble is emotional." Then rejected psychotherapy: "Cortisone will cure me." "Whenever I improve, I want to keep myself sick."
42. S. M.	50	F.	Polyarteritis.	2 yrs.	Psychotic breakdown of sister who was "pillar of the family."	Labile, required previous psychotherapy for depression, before organic breakdown; disturbed family background; traces depressive trends to mother; dependent needs, was psychotic on admission, talking to self, incontinent; history of allergic rhinitis.	Cortisone 150 mg. in 7 days. ACTH total 2.05 gm. Tapered off.	Improvement. Improvement. Recurrence, shock and death.	Improvement in psychosis, although frequent depressed moods; recurrence of psychosis with ACTH; attributes depression to doctors' losing interest; wants to die: "Don't let me wake up."

	Age	Sex	Diagnosis	Duration	History	Drug	Physical effect	Mental effect
43. A. L.	60	M.	Chronic leukemia.	2 yrs.		Cortisone 10 days.	Questionable improvement in blood picture; splenectomy; death.	Feels stronger physically; confusion: "All mixed up in my feelings"; "Should I feel hopeful or not?"
44. L. Z.	58	M.	Chronic myelogenous leukemia; asthma, bronchitis.	2½ yrs.	Followed T & A. Optimistic; cheerful; known in neighborhood for good-natured disposition; "I'm never jealous of anyone."	Cortisone.	No appreciable effect on blood picture; asthmatic attacks during therapy.	Optimistic; "Thanks to the doctors, I'll pull through. I'm fighting the sickness easy; the boys are helping me and I'm with them." Readmitted, apprehensive.
45. F. B.	28	M.	Asthma; bronchiectasis; eczema; puritus anl.	21 yrs.	Father's loss of job; family's poverty during the depression. Bitter; hostile; antagonistic; blames society and hospital for treating "only the rich or racketeers"; demands ACTH; "I'd get rid of my sickness if I didn't have to worry about money."	ACTH.	Dramatic relief of asthma and eczema; immediate relapse on discontinuance of drug.	Despite remarkable relief of physical symptoms, displayed no enthusiasm or cheerfulness; during relapse, requested psychotherapy, which he had previously spurned.
46. M. B.	63	M.	CA of the prostate.			Cortisone.	Death; post mortem: no gross cerebral findings.	Acute organic psychosis with organic features; paranoid; death.

static adrenal-cortical-endocrine behavior; and finally, (5) to moderate, relieve and possibly cure the patients of their intensely painful symptom complexes.

REFERENCES

1. Brody, S.: Phychiatric observations in patients treated with cortisone and ACTH. Psych. Med., *14*:94, 1952.
2. Brody, S.: Psychological factors associated with disseminated lupus erythematosus and effects of cortisone and ACTH. Psych. Quart., *30*:44, 1956.
3. Brody, S.: Psychophysiological factors in the collagen diseases. Psychoanalysis, 5:71, 1957.
4. Cleghorn, R. A.: Recent Developments in Phychosomatic Medicine. Philadelphia, J. B. Lippincott Co., 1956, p. 157.
5. Editorial: Some medical aspects of freedom. J.A.M.A., *162*:1161, 1956.
6. Hoefer, P. F. A. and Glaser, G. H.: Electroencephalographic and Neuropsychiatric Changes in Patients Treated with Adrenocorticotropic Hormone (ACTH). Philadelphia, The Blakiston Co., 1950, p. 536.
7. Hollender, M. H.: Psychological reactions to cortisone. Psych. Med., *14*:306, 1952.
8. O'Connor, J. F.: Psychoses associated with systemic lupus erythematosus. Ann. Int. Med., *51*:526, 1959.
9. Russell P. W., Haserick, J. R. and Zucker, E. M.: Epilepsy in systemic lupus erythematosus: effect of cortisone and ACTH. A.M.A. Arch. Int. Med., *88*:78, 1951.
10. Sherman, L. J.: The significant variables in psychopharmaceutic research. Am. J. Psych., *116*:208, 1959.
11. Sperling, M.: Psychosis and psychosomatic illness. Internat. J. Psychoanal., *36*:320, 1955.
12. Stern, M. and Robbins, E. S.: Psychoses in systemic L. E. Arch. Gen. Psych., 3:205, 1960.

Effect of Various Steroids
upon Gastric Secretion
and Uropepsin Excretion*

SEYMOUR J. GRAY

Peter Bent Brigham Hospital, Boston

Corticotropin or the adrenal steroids may produce peptic ulcer *de novo* with hemorrhage or perforation or may reactivate a previously healed ulcer. The incidence varies considerably depending upon the dose administered, duration of treatment and disease treated.

There are probably several factors involved in the production of the steroid ulcer. Although gastric acid and pepsin and urinary uropepsin are increased in susceptible individuals after steroid administration, hypersecretion is not invariably found in patients with the steroid-induced ulcer, and

* This work was supported in part by grants from the United States Public Health Service, The Miles-Ames Laboratories and Gastrointestinal Fund of the Peter Bent Brigham Hospital.

achlorhydria has been reported in some instances. It is not to be anticipated that every patient will respond with increased gastric secretion or that an ulcer will develop in every patient receiving adrenal glucocorticoids.

THE GASTRIC RESPONSE TO ADRENAL STEROIDS IN THE HUMAN GASTRIC ACID AND PEPSIN

It is generally agreed that the adrenal steroids may increase gastric acid and pepsin secretion in some instances, but the response varies considerably depending upon individual susceptibility and the dose and duration of hormone administered. There is no evidence that one glucocorticoid evokes a greater response than another, although comparisons are difficult because experimental conditions vary considerably.

The daily intramuscular or intravenous administration of corticotropin to normal subjects for three or four weeks may induce in some a significant increase in the basal and nocturnal gastric secretion of acid and pepsin, approximating 150 per cent.[11, 12] Gastric secretion may increase during hormone administration to levels observed in patients with active duodenal ulcer. Epigastric ulcer-like pain has been reproduced in some instances during the maximal gastric secretory response. Vagotomy or antrectomy does not alter the effect.

The adrenal steroids, however, must be administered in large doses for considerable periods of time (three to four weeks or longer) to produce a significant gastric response. In the original studies, 100 to 160 mg. of corticotropin were administered intramuscularly daily, or 20 mg. were given daily intravenously in 5 per cent glucose and water over an eight-hour period. An identical gastric response was elicited by the intramuscular administration of 40 mg. of corticotropin gel twice daily for three weeks. Others have failed to observe a gastric response after cortisone (100 mg. intramuscularly daily for 31 days)[7] or prednisone (15 to 20 mg. daily for 24 days).[1]

Short-term administration of corticotropin or the adrenal glucocorticoids increases gastric secretion in only a small percentage of patients. Intramuscular corticotropin (40 to 80 units of the gel daily) or cortisone (100 to 150 mg. daily) for periods of three to ten days increased the acid and pepsin secretion in only 4 of 17 subjects in our experience.[11] Carbone and Liebowitz[2] noted a significant rise in gastric acidity in 8 of 14 students given 40 mg. of prednisone daily for three to seven days. Similarly, Farmer[9] administered 200 mg. of cortisone daily for ten days and demonstrated an increase in gastric acidity in only three of ten patients. Failure to demonstrate a significant increase in gastric secretion has been reported by others following the administration of (1) corticotropin gel, 50 units daily for six days,[15] (2) corticotropin (25 to 45 mg.), hydrocortisone (25 to 85 mg.) or prednisolone (50 mg.) over a six-hour period,[6] and (3) prednisone (30 mg. daily) for seven days.[1] Reactivation of a duodenal ulcer has been observed, however, after the administration of corticotropin gel for four days, accompanied by an increase in acid and pepsin on the third day of adrenal stimulation.

Crean[4] has reported that the cortisone (100 to 200 mg. daily) administered over a prolonged period (19 to 99 days) significantly increases the gastric secretory response to *maximal histamine stimulation* in humans and attributed the response to increased metabolic activity or to an increase in the number of parietal cells. One might speculate whether the differences among individuals may be predicated upon genetically determined differences in the number and responsiveness of the parietal and peptic cells or variations in the potential parietal cell mass, but this remains to be determined.

It has been suggested that the reaction of the gastric mucosa to high local drug concentrations achieved during oral administration of adrenal steroids may be of significance.[19] The local action on the gastric mucosa, however, has not been definitely established, although animal experiments suggest that cortisone given orally may induce a greater response than that following stimulation by parenteral corticotropin. Oral steroids should be administered with food and antacids as a prophylactic measure.

Decrease in Mucus Protective Barrier. A decrease in gastric juice viscosity has been observed following adrenal steroid administration, suggesting an alteration in the mucus protective barrier. Quantitation of the mucus fractions has not as yet been reported, although recent studies indicate that cortisone inhibits the incorporation of radioactive sulfur into mucin and presumably into the mucus protective moieties.[5]

Interference with Tissue Repair. Delayed healing of experimental ulcers in dogs during cortisone administration has been reported by Janowitz et al.[18] Interference with normal healing of ulcers has also been observed in rats.

Vascular Effects. The adrenal steroids may significantly alter the gastric circulation. An increase in the blood content of the mucosa of the rat's stomach following corticotropin administration and a marked decrease after adrenalectomy have been observed. This is of interest since agents which stimulate glandular activity usually increase the mucosal vascularity.

EFFECT OF CORTICOTROPIN UPON GASTRIC SECRETION OF ACID, PEPSIN AND ELECTROLYTES IN ANIMALS

An increase in acid, pepsin and chloride has been demonstrated in the gastric juice of intact, vagally denervated and antrectomized dogs following the intramuscular injection of 40 international units of crystalline corticotropin. A significant fall in gastric juice, sodium and potassium accompanied the increase in acid, pepsin and chloride. The basal hourly secretion of acid from the intact stomach increased more than 200 per cent during corticotropin stimulation in the intact animals. The concentration of acid rose from 12 to 63 mEq./L. in the Heidenhain-pouch and vagotomized dogs. An increase in gastric acid production following corticotropin (30 mg. intravenously) has also been demonstrated in vagotomized dogs.[27] Porter et al.[20] demonstrated an increase in gastric acidity in monkeys unaltered by vagotomy after a single corticotropin stimulus (10 units per kilogram). In a further study French et al.[10] observed a maximal acid response three to four hours after the subcutaneous administration of corticotropin (5 units per kilogram) or cortisone (5 mg. per kilogram) before and after vagotomy.

An increase in gastric secretion has also been noted by others in animals after prolonged corticotropin stimulation (75 units daily for 10 to 12 days) with or without vagotomy, and after cortisone (100 mg. daily for 14 to 30 days).[28] Shay demonstrated that 100 mg. of hydrocortisone caused a significant decrease in pH and an increase in total acid and pepsin output in each of three trials in Heidenhain-pouch dogs.[23] On the other hand, several observers have failed to demonstrate an increase in gastric secretion with (1) 25 mg. of cortisone daily for one month in either innervated or denervated pouch dogs,[7] (2) corticotropin (40 to 80 units intramuscularly), cortisone (200 mg. intramuscularly) or hydrocortisone (50 mg. intravenously).[21]

The oral route of administration appears to accentuate the gastric response. Plainos reported a 300 to 400 per cent increase in gastric acid and pepsin following the administration of 60 mg. of prednisone daily for ten days directly into the stomachs of dogs.

Of considerable interest is the possibility that there is a synergistic effect upon gastric secretion between the adrenal corticoids and the vagus nerve. The gastric acid output in Heidenhain-pouch dogs after combined hydrocortisone (100 mg.) and methacholine stimulation is considerably greater than with either stimulus alone as noted by Sun and Shay.[25] Recently Clarke, Neill and Welbourn[3] demonstrated that corticotropin gel (25 units), cortisone (50 mg. intramuscularly twice daily) or prednisolone (4 mg. by mouth three times daily) consistently and significantly increased the basal secretion of acid in dogs with denervated gastric pouches and also augmented its secretion in response to histamine and antral stimulation. Three to five days of stimulation were required. The concentration of sodium was reduced considerably, and potassium to a lesser extent. Cortisone, moreover, increased the *maximal* secretory response to histamine as well. The number of parietal cells was increased by about 50 per cent after steroid administration. It was concluded that the adrenal steroids increased parietal cell mass and stimulated the parietal cells to secrete as well.

UROPEPSIN AND PLASMA PEPSINOGEN RESPONSE TO CORTICOTROPIC HORMONE AND ADRENAL STEROID ADMINISTRATION

The urinary uropepsin excretion is derived from the secretion of pepsinogen directly into the blood stream, where it can be measured as plasma pepsinogen. Pepsinogen is then transported to the kidneys and is excreted in the urine as uropepsin. The uropepsin levels may not always reflect gastric pepsin secretion since the adrenal steroids may increase the renal clearance of pepsinogen.

Corticotropin or the adrenal steroids increase uropepsin excretion within 24 to 72 hours to levels ordinarily seen in active duodenal ulcer. This response is not altered by vagectomy or antrectomy and has been verified by numerous observers with almost no disagreement.

Although an increase in uropepsin excretion is accompanied by an increase in gastric pepsin secretion after prolonged adrenal stimulation, an increase in uropepsin excretion is often observed within the first day of hormone administration without an associated demonstrable increase in gastric pepsin. This initial rise in uropepsin excretion may be attributed either to a temporary alteration of renal threshold or to an increased endocrine secretion of pepsinogen relative to its exocrine output into the gastric lumen. The latter appears more likely since an increase in plasma pepsinogen has been observed in humans two to four hours after the administration of 40 to 50 units of corticotropin gel.[26] A similar increase in plasma pepsinogen has been demonstrated in the gastric-venous blood of dogs within four to six hours after an intravenous corticotropin infusion.[16] Finally, corticotropin increases the gastric tissue pepsinogen in the rat, and adrenalectomy significantly reduces gastric pepsinogen.

In summary, the adrenal steroids appear to (1) increase gastric acid and pepsin in some humans and in animals, (2) increase the pepsinogen content in the gastric tissue, plasma and urine, (3) decrease the mucus protective barrier, (4) interfere with tissue repair, (5) alter the blood content of the gastric mucosa, (6) increase parietal cell mass, and (7) sensitize the stomach to a number of stimuli.

As far as can be determined, the only steroids which influence acid peptic activity are the adrenal glucocorticoids. No consistent effect has been demonstrable after the administration of deoxycorticosterone, testicular and adrenal androgens, progesterone and potent estrogen preparations. The only pituitary hormone which induces a gastric response is corticotropic hormone. Present evidence indicates that growth hormone, thyrotropic and gonadotropic hormone are without effect.

"PERMISSIVE" AND "CONDITIONED" ACTIONS OF ADRENAL STEROIDS UPON THE STOMACH

The adrenal cortex may have a dual role in the gastric responses to stress, according to the "permissive" concept of Ingle[17] and the "conditioned" theory of hormonal activity proposed by Selye.[22] The adrenal may function as an agent which "permits" a gastric response to occur which could not occur in its absence. Under normal conditions of daily existence the stomach acts semi-autonomously relative to the adrenal cortex, requiring normal adrenal cortical function for variable acid-peptic activity.

The second role casts the adrenal in a more directive relationship between the levels of adrenal cortical hormone attained and the extent of the gastric response, allowing a more direct and integrated control of gastric secretion in time of severe stress. Excess adrenal hormone such as that resulting from stress may sensitize the stomach to respond more readily to a number of outside ulcerogenic influences. The adrenal glucocorticoids, for example, augment the gastric acid response to histamine, antral or vagal stimulation. Secondly, stress itself may "condition" or sensitize the stomach to a constant level of adrenal hormone without necessarily increasing adrenal secretion.

There are numerous examples of the "permissive" influence of the adrenal steroids upon gastric secretion and peptic ulceration. When adrenal cortical function is diminished, gastric secretion is decreased or absent. Addison's disease in man is often associated with achlorhydria, an observation which has been confirmed repeatedly by many investigators.[13] The gastric mucosa of these patients demonstrates atrophy and replacement of the glandular cells by mucoid chief cells with almost complete disappearance of the parietal cells. Similarly, in animals bilateral adrenalectomy produces involution of gastric zymogen and mucoid chief cells and markedly reduces the volume and acidity of gastric juice. The administration of amphenone, which presumably inhibits the production of adrenal glucocorticoids, reduces gastric secretion to the low levels observed after bilateral adrenalectomy.[13]

The "permissive" effect of the adrenal gland on gastric secretion was demonstrated by Stempien and Dagradi,[24] who elicited a positive acid response in a patient with untreated Addison's disease and histamine anacidity, following the administration of cortisone, deoxycorticosterone (DOCA) and salt. In the dog the response of the stomach to histamine after adrenalectomy varies directly with dose of cortisone administered.

The gastric mucosa in Addison's disease appears to be unusually sensitive to the adrenal glucocorticoids since a secretory response is demonstrable with small daily doses of cortisone (12.5 to 25 mg.) which do not affect the gastric response in normal subjects.[13] The development of chronic duodenal or gastric ulcers in a number of patients with Addison's disease after two to three years of maintenance cortisone therapy in minimal doses of 12.5 to 50 mg. daily has been reported.[13] This is particularly pertinent since chronic peptic ulcer is extremely rare in Addison's disease and was found in only three instances in a collected series of 363 patients.

Engel[8] has described a patient with known Addison's disease of four years' duration who developed a small prepyloric ulcer while on cortisone (25 mg. daily) over a two and one-half year period. Although histamine anacidity had been demonstrated two and one-half years previously, before cortisone therapy was instituted, a repeated gastric analysis at the time the ulcer was diagnosed revealed free acid after histamine stimulation. Cortisone replacement therapy in physiological quantities to the Addisonian or bilaterally adrenalectomized patient may produce gastric hypersecretion and peptic ulcer as a manifestation of the "permissive" action of the hormone.

Increased gastric activity to ulcer levels may be attained by the administration of large doses of cortisone to patients with Addison's disease. Such an occurrence has also been reported by Griep and Buchholz[14] in an Addison's disease patient whose history of chronic duodenal ulcer antedated the onset of adrenal insufficiency. On receiving large doses of cortisone (3900 mg. over a 12-day period) to correct an episode of adrenal crisis, the patient developed an acute perforation of a duodenal ulcer 12 days after intensive therapy was begun.

REFERENCES

1. Beck, I. T., Fletcher, H. W., McKenna, R. D. and Griff, H.: Effect of small and massive doses of prednisone on gastric secretory activity. Gastroenterology, *38*:740, 1960.
2. Carbone, J. V. and Liebowitz, D.: Effect of adrenal corticoids on gastric secretion and suppression of corticoid-induced hypersecretion by anticholinergics. Metabolism, *7*:70, 1958.
3. Clarke, D. S., Neill, D. W. and Welbourne, R. B.: The effects of corticotrophin and corticoids on secretion from denervated gastric pouches in dogs. Gut, *1*:36, 1960.
4. Crean, G. P.: The effects of ACTH and corticosteroids on gastric secretion in humans. Gut, *1*:82, 1960.
5. Denko, C. W.: Effect of hydrocortisone and cortisone on fixation of S[35] in stomach. J. Lab. & Clin. Med., *51*:174, 1958.
6. Dreiling, D. A. and Janowitz, H. D.: Effects of ACTH and adrenal steroid hormones on gastric secretion. Clin. Res. Proc., *5*:110, 1957.
7. Drye, J. C. and Schoen, A. M.: Studies on mechanisms of activation of peptic ulcer after nonspecific trauma: effect of cortisone on gastric secretion. Ann. Surg., *147*:738, 1958.
8. Engel, F. L.: Addison's disease and peptic ulcer. J. Clin. Endocrinol., *15*:1300, 1955.
9. Farmer, D. A., Burke, P. M. and Smithwick, R. H.: Surg. Forum, *4*:316, 1954.
10. French, J. D., Longmire, R. L., Porter, R. W. and Movius, H. J.: Extravagal influences on gastric hydrochloric acid secretion induced by stress stimuli. Surgery, *34*:621, 1953.
11. Gray, S. J.: Present status of endocrine influences upon the stomach and their relationship to peptic ulcer disease. Proc. World Congress of Gastroenterology, Washington, D. C. Baltimore, Williams & Wilkins Co., 1958.
12. Gray, S. J. and Ramsey, C. G.: Adrenal influences upon the stomach and the gastric responses to stress. Rec. Progr. Hormone Res., *13*:583, 1957.

13. Gray, S. J., Ramsey, C. G. and Thorn, G. W.: Adrenal influences on the stomach; peptic ulcer in Addison's disease during adrenal steroid therapy. Ann. Int. Med., 45:73, 1956.
14. Griep, A. H. and Buchholz, R. R.: Perforation of chronic duodenal ulcer during cortisone therapy for Addison's disease. Am. J. Surg., 85:703, 1953.
15. Hirschowitz, B. I., Streeten, D. H. P., Pollard, H. M. and Boldt, H. A., Jr.: Role of gastric secretions in activation of peptic ulcers by corticotropin (ACTH). J.A.M.A., 158:27, 1955.
16. Hoar, C. S., Jr. and Browning, J. R.: Plasma pepsinogen in peptic ulcer disease and other gastric disorders. New Engl. J. Med., 255:153, 1956.
17. Ingle, D. J.: Permissive action of hormones. J. Clin. Endocrinol., 14:1272, 1954.
18. Janowitz, H., Weinstein, V., Shaer, R., Cereghinini, J. and Hollander, F.: Effect of cortisone and corticotropin on healing of gastric ulcer: experimental study. Gastroenterology, 34:11, 1958.
19. Morton, E. V. B.: Discussion on the complications of steroid therapy. Proc. Roy. Soc. Med., 51:317, 1958.
20. Porter, R. W., Movius, H. J. and French, J. D.: Hypothalamic influences on hydrochloric acid secretion of the stomach. Surgery, 33:875, 1958.
21. Ragins, H., Dragstedt, L. R., II, Landor, J. H., Lyon, E. S. and Dragstedt, L. R.: Duodenal ulcer and hypophysis-adrenal stress mechanism. Surgery, 40:886, 1956.
22. Selye, H.: "Conditioning" versus "permissive" actions of hormones. J. Clin. Endocrinol., 14:122, 1954.
23. Shay, H.: Emotional stress and parietal cell mass: their role in etiology of peptic ulcer. Am. J. Digest. Dis., 4:846, 1959.
24. Stempien, S. J. and Dagradi, A.: The histamine response of the gastric mucosa in a patient with adrenal insufficiency: effect of cortisone administration. Gastroenterology, 27:358, 1954.
25. Sun, D. C. H. and Shay, H.: Potentiation of mecholyl or histamine-stimulated gastric secretion by hydrocortisone in Heidenhain-pouch dogs. Physiologist, 1:77, 1958.
26. Varro, V., Faredin, I. and Novaszel, F.: Plasma pepsinogen concentration and adrenocortical activity. Acta med. scandinav., 153:211, 1956.
27. Villarreal, R., Ganong, W. F. and Gray, S. J.: Effect of adrenocorticotrophic hormone upon gastric secretion of hydrochloric acid, pepsin and electrolytes in the dog. Am. J. Physiol., 183:485, 1955.
28. Zubiran, J. M., Kark, A. E. and Dragstedt, L. R.: Effect of ACTH on gastric secretion in experimental animals. Gastroenterology, 21:276, 1952.

The Corticosteroid-Induced Peptic Ulcer:

A Serial Roentgenological Survey of Patients Receiving High Dosages*

EDMUND L. DUBOIS, JAMES G. BULGRIN and
GEORGE JACOBSON

University of Southern California School of Medicine

During a period of three years, 92 patients who were candidates for or were receiving steroid therapy, were observed for peptic ulcer. Most of them were examined roentgenologically at three-month intervals. This made it possible to correlate ulcer incidence with dose, duration of therapy and effect of individual drugs, as well as to add to the very sparse information upon behavior of ulcers during continuous steroid administration. Almost all of the patients had systemic lupus erythematosus and required large amounts of steroids. The incidence of peptic ulcer in this treated group was compared with the incidence in a similar group of patients not receiving these hormones. Since there are relatively few reports of roentgenological surveys of patients treated with steroids, and none with such extensive serial studies on patients receiving high dosage, it was thought that presentation of our findings and comparison with previous data would be of interest.

Up to 1954, Sandweiss[20] and Wollaeger[24] were able to collect from the literature only 50 to 55 instances of peptic ulcer occurring during steroid therapy. Since then the reported incidence has varied from 0 to 31 per cent. The more widely quoted reports and all roentgenological surveys have been tabulated in Tables 1 and 2. Table 1 comprises those reporting a relatively low and Table 2 those reporting a relatively high incidence of ulcer. It was thought that such a division might emphasize variations in dosage, length of treatment or effect of individual drugs if such exist.

In Table 1, ulcer incidence varies from 0 to 7.8 per cent. It is noted that in most reports patients were receiving cortisone and that, using generally accepted dosage equivalents, the amounts of drug were far less than is the case in Table 2. There seems to be some dose-ulcer incidence correlation in the report of the American Rheumatism Commission[8] which shows that the incidence of ulcer in patients receiving more than 50 mg. of cortisone was nearly double that in those receiving less than this amount. Bunim et al.[5] comment that all three of the patients in their group of 64 receiving more than 100 mg. of cortisone developed an ulcer. No conclusions can be drawn regarding length of therapy and its relation to ulcer incidence from Table 1.

In Table 2, the reported ulcer incidence varies between 12.5 and 31.0 per cent. Kern, Clark and Lukens[16] and Kammerer et al.[9, 15] both show a rather

* This study was supported by grants from Lederle Laboratories and the Upjohn Company and research grant A 3075 from the National Institute of Arthritis and Metabolic Diseases, United States Public Health Service.

TABLE 1. SUMMARY OF LITERATURE SHOWING RELATIVELY LOW INCIDENCE OF PEPTIC ULCER DURING STEROID THERAPY

AUTHORS AND DATES OF REPORTS	NO. OF PATIENTS	PER CENT INCIDENCE OF ULCER	REMARKS
Arbesman and Richard,[1] 1954	75	0	Asthmatics on cortisone. Dosage sometimes intermittent. Average maintenance dose from 50 to 75 mg. per day.
Henderson,[11] 1955	1440	5.3	No dosage correlation. Figures based on survey of literature.
American Rheumatism Assn.	564	6.6	Figures from questionnaires. On doses of 50 mg. or less of cortisone per day, incidence of ulcer was 4.4 per cent; on doses of more than this it was 8.3 per cent.
Bunim, Ziffe and McEwen,[5] 1955	64	7.8	While the over-all incidence of ulcer was low, the only 3 patients to receive more than 100 mg. cortisone daily all developed ulcer, 2 of which perforated.
Boland,[3] 1956	141	4.9	Gastric complaints in 26 patients. G.I. series on these showed 7 ulcers. Dose 8 to 14 mg. prednisone or prednisolone. Adverse reactions of all kinds increased with dose increase.
Kirsner, Sklar and Palmer,[17] 1957	180	0	Cases of chronic ulcerative colitis. Initial large, but smaller maintenance doses cortisone. Long treatment time.
Meltzer et al.,[19] 1958	115	Under 3.6	All examined roentgenologically. Average dose 13.8 to 14.2 mg. prednisone.

TABLE 2. SUMMARY OF LITERATURE SHOWING RELATIVELY HIGH INCIDENCE OF PEPTIC ULCER DURING STEROID THERAPY

AUTHORS AND DATES OF REPORTS	NO. OF PATIENTS	PER CENT INCIDENCE OF ULCER	REMARKS
Bollet, Black and Bunim,[4] 1955	18	16	Serial G.I. studies on all patients. Two of the 3 ulcer patients had negative pretreatment studies. All ulcers asymptomatic and occurred on doses of 25 to 30 mg. daily prednisone or prednisolone.
Howell and Ragan,[13] 1956	75	26	No precise dose-incidence relationship. Doses generally 43 to 75 mg. cortisone or 10 to 25 mg. prednisone or its equivalent daily. Often only slight epigastric distress with objective ulcer.
Kern, Clark and Lukens,[16] 1957	169	12.5	Ulcers occurred 5 to 30 months after initiation of therapy. Three of 14 patients developed ulcers on 20 mg. or more prednisone daily. No ulcers in 54 patients with dose of 15 mg. or less. No definite relationship between length of therapy and development of ulcer. Statistical analysis indicates a 20- to 60-fold increase over normal expectation of ulcer development.
Black, Yielding and Bunim,[2] 1957	39	16	Doses of prednisone over 20 mg. per day.
Hilbish and Black,[12] 1958	49	24	This data is from review of all steroid-treated patients at National Institutes of Health. Atypical ulcer symptoms. Time-dose relationship to ulcer variable, but most patients received over 15 mg. prednisone daily. Two fatal hemorrhages from steroid-associated ulcers.
Evans,[7] 1958	23	26	All patients studied roentgenologically. One-third asymptomatic. Average dose 20 mg. prednisone daily.
Gedda and Moritz,[10] 1958	69	19	All patients studied roentgenologically. Doses of 5 to 15 mg. prednisone daily for at least 6 months. Length of treatment increased ulcer risk. Often slight symptoms. Control group of autopsied rheumatoid arthritis, 31 in number, 10 per cent ulcer.
Kammerer, Freiberger and Rivelis,[9, 15] 1958	117	31	All patients treated 6 months or more. 40% asymptomatic. Dose and relation to ulcer incidence (prednisone equivalent, mg./day): 2.5 to 7.5 mg. = 4.7 per cent ulcer (21 patients). 10 to 15 mg. = 45.0 per cent ulcer (61 patients). over 15 mg. = 40.0 per cent ulcer (6 patients). Control group of 33 patients = 9 per cent ulcer. Single roentgenologic study of each patient.

clear-cut increase in ulcer incidence with increasing steroid dosage. The data of the latter workers is especially striking both as to total ulcer incidence and dosage correlation. They report an over-all incidence of 31 per cent. When a dosage of 10 mg. of prednisone or its equivalent was given, there was an almost tenfold increase in ulcer incidence over those given lesser amounts. All of their patients had received steroids for six months or more, and a single roentgenologic study was made of each patient. Prolongation of therapy beyond six months did not affect ulcer incidence. Gedda and Moritz[10] found an increased risk of peptic ulcer with increasing length of treatment. Others failed to make such a correlation.

Since we employed roentgenological methods of diagnosis, we were particularly interested in studies using similar diagnostic criteria. Bollet, Black and Bunim,[4] Evans,[7] Gedda and Moritz[10] and Kammerer et al.[9, 15] reported ulcer incidences of from 16 to 31 per cent. In each of the studies, the authors remarked upon the frequency with which the patients were asymptomatic or had symptoms atypical for ulcer in the face of an objectively demonstrated lesion. The only radiologic survey showing an extremely low incidence of ulcer is that of Meltzer et al.[19] In this study there was no obvious variation in dose, duration of treatment or individual drug to explain this.

MATERIALS AND METHODS

Ninety-two patients from the Collagen Disease Clinic of the Los Angeles County General Hospital were studied. Seventy-eight of them received steroid therapy. All but two were ambulatory outpatients. Eighty-one per cent were female. Aside from three cases of rheumatoid arthritis and four of other collagen diseases, they were diagnosed as having systemic lupus erythematosus. An attempt was made to examine all patients roentgenologically prior to instituting steroid therapy, but, since many were on such treatment when the study began and others required therapy immediately, this was achieved in only 52. Once steroid therapy had begun, serial roentgen studies were performed at intervals of approximately three months. The program was carried on for three years, and the 92 patients received a total of 279 examinations (Table 3). Only two of the 14 patients who did not receive steroids were examined more than once. Although a patient receiving over 10 mg. per day of prednisone or its equivalent in our Clinic normally is placed on a prophylactic ulcer regimen, such prophylaxis was given in only seven of the 92 patients in this series. One of the seven had a

TABLE 3.   FREQUENCY OF SERIAL GASTROINTESTINAL STUDIES

NUMBER PER PATIENT	NUMBERS OF PATIENTS
1	28
2	25
3	10
4	9
5	4
6	8
7	4
8	1
9 or more	3

Total number of gastrointestinal studies = 279.

TABLE 4. COMPARATIVE THERAPY IN ULCER AND NON-ULCER PATIENTS: RESULTS OF ROENTGENOLOGIC STUDIES CORRELATED WITH DRUG, DOSAGE AND DURATION OF OBSERVATION

STEROID	No. of patients receiving drug	Median duration steroid therapy, months to last x-ray	Total patient months x-ray observation	PATIENTS WITH ULCER					PATIENTS WITH NO ULCER SHOWN			
				Patients	Per cent	Dose range 4 to 8 weeks prior to demonstration active ulcer (mg./day)	Median dose (mg./day)	Average period x-ray observation (months)	No. of patients	Dose range during x-ray observation	Median dose (mg./day)	Average period x-ray observation (months)
Prednisone and prednisolone	27	10	98	5	18.5	12.5-100	40	4.8	22	10-50	30	3.2
Methylprednisolone	18	12.5	94	4	22.0	36-144	60	3.7	14	8-48	20	5.6
Triamcinolone	23	21.5	169	4	17.4	12-96	40	13.7	18	8-100	28	6.3
Dexamethasone	27	13	154	6	22.2	1-20	10.7	5.4	21	0.5-16	2.0	5.8
Total	95*		505	19					75			

* A number of patients received more than one steroid.

TABLE 5. PEPTIC ULCERS OCCURRING DURING STEROID THERAPY

PATIENT	NORMAL BASE LINE STUDY	STEROID ADMINISTERED AND DOSE (MG./DAY) DURING THE 4 TO 8 WEEK PERIOD PRIOR TO DEMONSTRATION OF THE ULCER	DURATION STEROID THERAPY BEFORE ULCER (MONTHS)	DESCRIPTION AND LOCATION OF NICHE	HEALING AND/OR BEHAVIOR OF ULCER	REMARKS	PROPHYLACTIC REGIMEN	SYMPTOMS	THERAPEUTIC REGIMEN
Z.K.	Yes	Prednisone 60	18	Initial ulcer on greater curvature fundus	Initial ulcer showed variable behavior, finally healing in 7 months.	Reduction in steroid dosage after appearance of each ulcer. Change of drug to hydrocortisone 70 mg. after initial lesion, hence second ulcer developed while on this therapy.	0	+	+
Z.K.		Hydrocortisone 70	23	Second ulcer-antral on lesser curvature	Second ulcer healed in 11 months.		+	+	+
T.F.	Yes	MK 117 20	3	Moderate size prepyloric	Healing in 5½ months.	16-alpha-hydroxy-hydrocortisone 20 mg./day during healing.	0	+	+
S.R.	Yes	Prednisone 20	18	Duodenal	Fully healed in 4 months.	8 gastrointestinal studies before appearance of crater. Mucosal change preceded niche.	0	+	+
J.G.	Yes	Methylprednisolone 64	6	Duodenal	Healing in 5 weeks.	Reduced dose and change of steroid after ulcer. Melena at time of diagnosis.	+	+	+
O.J.	Yes	Triamcinolone 48	10	Small, prepyloric	Healing in 5 months.	Mucosal changes preceded niche. Dose of steroid unchanged during healing.	0	0	0
M.P.	Yes	Methylprednisolone 36	7	Moderate size, antral lesser curvature	Fully healed in 3 months.	Psychosis, no symptoms.	0	?	+
R.M.	Yes	Methylprednisolone 144	2	Lesser curvature, mid fundus	Healing in 2 months.	Psychosis, no symptoms. Reduced dose of steroid during healing.	+	?	+
D.M.	Yes	Dexamethasone 3.5	16	No crater. Normal bulb, then deformity 6 months later.	Repeated examinations merely confirmed deformity.	The only roentgenologic diagnosis made without demonstrating crater.	0	+	+
M.F.	Yes	Dexamethasone 1.5	2½	Pyloric canal	Healed in 3 months.	Symptom appeared 5 weeks after start of therapy.	0	+	+
G.L.	Yes	Dexamethasone 15.0	2.0	Antral	Not observed.		0	0	+

L.J.	No	Methylpred-nisolone 56	2½	Small, prepyloric, lesser curvature	Healing in 5 months.	Healing on 10 mg. dexamethasone.	0	0	0
A.C.	No	Prednisone 12.5	9	Small, prepyloric, lesser curvature	No healing over a 10-month period.	Steroid changed to 8 mg. methylprednisolone.	0	+	0
E.M.	No	Cortisone 100	6	Lesser curvature, antral	Healing in 7 months.	Reduced steroid dose during healing.	0	+	+
E.M.	No	Dexametha-sone 1.0	11	Recurrence at same site	Healing in 4 months.	Healing on 1.0 mg. dexamethasone.	0	+	+
P.B.	No	Cortisone 75	72	Duodenal	Not observed.		0	+	+
E.B.	No	Prednisone 15	36	Duodenal	Healed in 2 months.	Parenteral cortisone during healing.	0	+	+
B.B.	No	Triamcino-lone 32	9	Small, pyloric	Healing within 1 year.	Reduced steroid dose during healing.	0	0	0
J.W.	No	Triamcino-lone 12	4	Initial ulcer pyloric. Second pyloric ulcer 4 months after healing of 1st.	Initial ulcer healed in 2½ months.	Known previous ulcer and deformed bulb at start of steroid therapy. Reduced steroid dose during healing.	+	+	+
B.T.	No	Dexametha-sone 2.25	16	Lesser curvature pylorus	Symptoms appeared 6 months after start of therapy.	Initial x-ray taken after 16 months of dexamethasone therapy.	0	+	+
R.B.	Yes	Triamcino-lone 32	4	Normal roentgenologic study. Died 2 months later.	Autopsy proved perforated duodenal ulcer.	Prednisone 100 mg./day given latter part of 4-month period of observation.	+	+	+
S.S.	Yes	Dexametha-sone 18	4	Two normal roentgenologic studies	2 episodes of massive hematemesis.	Ulcer regimen. Hematemesis subsided, as did symptoms.	0	+	+

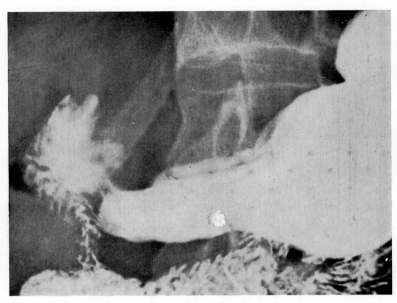

Fig. 1.   Base line normal study (T. F.).

pre-existing peptic ulcer. Four were on unusually high dosage of steroids. Another had gastrointestinal symptoms prior to our study, and the final patient had been on a prophylactic ulcer regimen elsewhere.

RESULTS

Base Line Studies or Control Group.   In the 52 patients examined prior to institution of steroid therapy, only two (approximately 4 per cent) showed

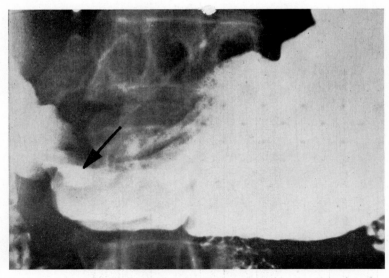

Fig. 2.   After 3 months of steroid therapy, development of a moderate sized, shallow preplyloric ulcer (T. F.).

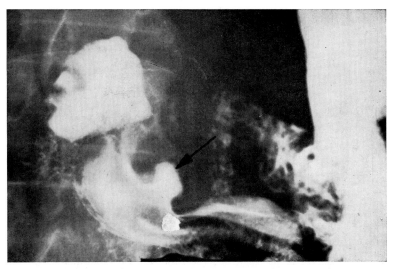

Fig. 3. Large lesser curvature, antral ulcer (E. M.).

any roentgenological abnormality. In each case this consisted of deformity of the duodenal bulb. One of these patients showed no change during steroid therapy while the other developed active ulceration. Fourteen of this group of 52 patients did not receive steroids while the others were so treated subsequent to their base line examination.

Steroid-treated Patients Examined Roentgenologically. Of the 78 patients receiving steroid therapy, 59 showed no evidence of active peptic ulceration. The comparative therapeutic data in this group and in those with positive

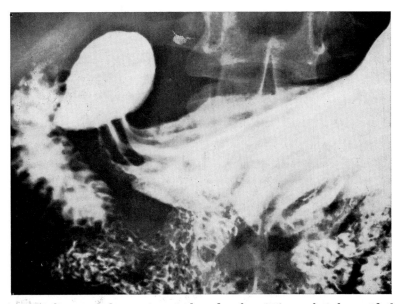

Fig. 4. Base line normal gastrointestinal study after 16½ months of steroid therapy (Z. K.). (Prednisone 15 mg./day.)

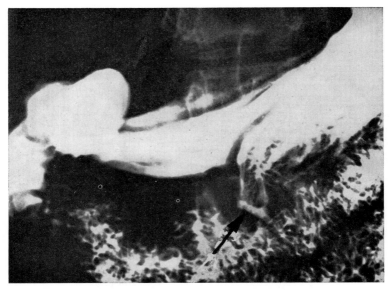

Fig. 5.   Within 6 weeks of increased dosage of steroid therapy, development of a penetrating greater curvature ulcer (Z. K.). (Prednisone 60 mg./day.)

evidence of ulcer is presented in Table 4. Drug dosage was higher and duration of therapy longer in the group developing ulcer.

Twenty-one active peptic ulcers were demonstrated roentgenographically in 19 patients. In addition, two patients with normal radiographic findings were diagnosed as having peptic ulcer for a total incidence of 27 per cent. One was diagnosed on the basis of a perforated duodenal ulcer proved at

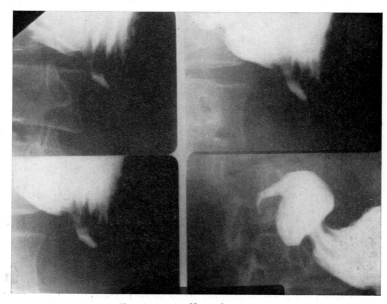

Fig. 6.   Spot films of Figure 5.

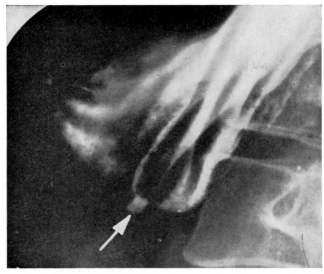

Fig. 7. Two months after appearance of greater curvature ulcer, reduction in its size (Z. K.).

autopsy, the other on the basis of repeated episodes of massive hematemesis. The data on all patients developing ulcer is presented in Table 5.

LOCATION AND RADIOLOGIC APPEARANCE OF ULCERS. Sixteen ulcers were gastric and six duodenal. Fourteen of the gastric ulcers were in the distal

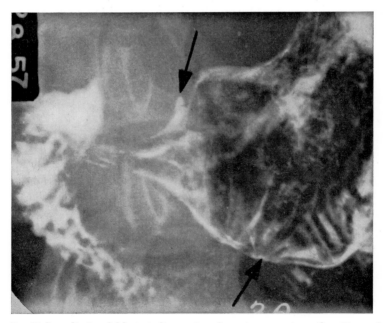

Fig. 8. Only radiating folds to indicate site of greater curvature ulcer 7 months after the initial ulcer. Note development of entirely new, small lesser curvature antral ulcer. Coincident with appearance of second ulcer, observe change in contour of distal stomach compared with previous studies (Z. K.).

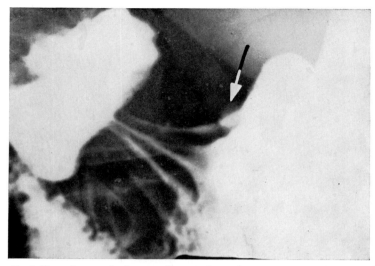

Fig. 9. Spot film of second ulcer-small, antral, on lesser curvature two months later (Z. K.).

stomach and only two in its mid portion (see Figs. 1-3). One was located on the greater curvature (see Figs. 4-9). In one-half of the cases, the ulcers were shallow and surrounded by mucosal edema, as emphasized by other workers.[9, 15] In the others, however, the appearance was not different from the usual gastric ulcer. In a few cases in which many examinations were performed, mucosal changes, presumably based upon edema, preceded appearance of the niche. This was also demonstrated in one case of duodenal ulcer (see Figs. 10-11). The other four duodenal ulcers were not unusual in appearance or location. Only one diagnosis of ulcer was made without demonstration of a niche. In this case a normal gastrointestinal study was followed by observation of a deformed duodenal bulb.

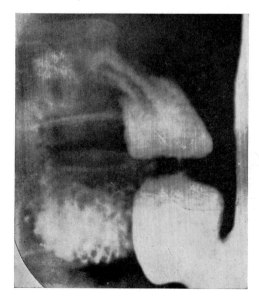

Fig. 10. Base line normal. Note mucosa of duodenal cap (S. R.).

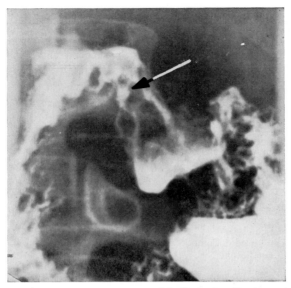

Fig. 11. Crater on lesser curvature aspect of bulb in its distal portion with marked mucosal edema after 18 months of steroid therapy (compare with base line) (S. R.).

SEX INCIDENCE OF PEPTIC ULCER IN STEROID-TREATED PATIENTS. Of 13 males, five (39 per cent) developed ulcer; of 65 females, 16 (25 per cent) were shown to have peptic ulcer.

CORRELATION OF ULCER INCIDENCE WITH LENGTH OF TREATMENT. The duration of steroid therapy in patients showing peptic ulcer is given in Table 5 and the duration of such therapy in patients developing ulcer as compared with those who did not in Table 4. In all but eight instances, steroid therapy had been administered for more than six months before peptic ulcer was diagnosed. The minimum time for the roentgenographic appearance of an ulcer was two months in two instances. It is noteworthy that in these exceptional cases a dose of 144 mg. of methyl prednisolone was administered daily to one patient and 15.0 mg. per day of dexamethasone to another.

CORRELATION OF ULCER INCIDENCE WITH DOSE. The specific dosage data for each patient developing ulcer are given in Table 5. The considerably higher median dose and the dose ranges in the patients with ulcer compared to those not developing ulcer is demonstrated in Table 4. Table 6, however, presents the most striking correlation of steroid dosage with ulcer incidence. Since there was no difference in occurrence of peptic ulcer on various drugs, dosage is expressed in milligrams of prednisone equivalent by use of conversion factors appended to Table 6. Ulcer incidence of 25 per cent with dosages of 40 to 49 mg./day and of 47 per cent with dosages over 60 mg./day furnishes a striking correlation. The minimum dose of individual drugs (mg./day) associated with occurrence of peptic ulceration is: prednisone and prednisolone 12.5; triamcinolone 32.0; methyl prednisolone 36.0; dexamethasone 1.0. The patient who developed the ulcer on 1.0 mg. of dexamethasone had had a prior ulcer at the same site 18 months before. The minimum dose for induction of a new ulcer in patients treated with this steroid was 1.5 mg. per day.

BEHAVIOR OF ULCERS. In the single patient who showed a deformed bulb

TABLE 6.   CORRELATION OF STEROID DOSAGE AND ULCER INCIDENCE

DOSAGE IN MG./DAY EXPRESSED AS PREDNISONE EQUIVALENT	TOTAL NUMBER OF PATIENTS	NUMBER OF PATIENTS DEVELOPING ULCER	PERCENTAGE OF PATIENTS DEVELOPING ULCER
Under 10	10	1*	10*
10-19	29	5	17
20-39	26	1	4
40-59	12	3	25
Over 60	19	9	47

* Recurrent antral ulcer at prior site while receiving 1.0 mg. per day of dexamethasone for 11 months without a strict ulcer regimen.

CONVERSION DATA FOR INDIVIDUAL STEROIDS

STEROID	EQUIVALENT UNITS
Prednisone and prednisolone	5
Triamcinolone	4
Methyl prednisolone	4
Dexamethasone	0.75
Cortisone	25
Hydrocortisone	20

following a normal gastrointestinal study, repeated examinations showed only persistence of the deformity. Three patients were lost to observation following demonstration of a single active ulcer. Another showed a persistent niche for ten months. Thirteen patients who were followed by serial roentgenological studies after the appearance of an active ulcer showed healing, and this observation of behavior is one of the unique features of

TABLE 7.   OBSERVATIONS ON HEALING OF ULCERS ASSOCIATED WITH STEROID THERAPY

CASE	TIME REQUIRED FOR HEALING	MANAGEMENT DURING HEALING PERIOD
O.J.	5 months	Dose of steroid unchanged. No ulcer regimen.
L.J.	5 months	Change of drug, but equivalent dosage. No ulcer regimen.
B.B.	12 months	Reduced dose of steroid. No ulcer regimen.
J.G.	5 weeks	Change of drug with reduced dosage and ulcer regimen.
R.M.	2 months	Reduced dose of steroid. This patient was on prophylatic ulcer regimen because of the enormous dose of steroid administered.
E.B.	2 months	Change of drug (parenteral cortisone).
T.F.	5½ months	Change of steroid. Ulcer regimen.
E.M.	7 months	Reduced steroid dosage and ulcer regimen.
	4 months	Almost healed. Strict ulcer regimen. Same steroid dose.
Z.K.	7 to 11 months	Recurrent ulcer. Reduced steroid dosage and ulcer regimen.
J.W.	2½ to 6 months	Recurrent ulcers with healing under reduced steroid therapy. This patient had an ulcer history before steroid therapy and a deformed bulb at the start of treatment. She was on continuous prophylactic ulcer regimen.
M.P.	3 months	Reduced dose of steroid and ulcer regimen.
S.R.	4 months	Dose of steroid unchanged. Ulcer regimen.
M.F.	3 months	Ulcer regimen and steroid reduction.

this study. The healing time and management during healing in these patients are given in Table 7. Among the 13 patients, perhaps the most unusual phenomenon is that in two instances (O.J. and L.J.) healing occurred at the end of five months without either an ulcer regimen or reduction in steroid dosage, and both were asymptomatic. The ulcers in the other 11 patients healed with reduced steroid dosage and/or administration of an ulcer regimen. Healing time was variable and in the majority was between five and 12 months. While healing was observed, it must be remembered that there were two patients who had recurrence of ulcer and that ulcer behavior was most unfavorable in two additional patients with one instance of repeated hematemesis and one fatal perforation.

ASSOCIATION OF ULCERS WITH SYMPTOMS. Two patients with peptic ulceration were asymptomatic. Two others were psychotic. In the rest of the group (80 per cent) subjective manifestations varied from classic post-prandial pain relieved by food to heartburn and vague upper abdominal distress. When gastrointestinal complaints in the non-ulcer as well as the ulcer groups were tabulated it was found that, of a total of 78 patients treated with steroids, 31 had gastrointestinal symptoms. Sixteen of these had peptic ulcer and 15 did not. There was no variation in incidence of subjective distress when one steroid was compared with any other. Generally, the occurrence of symptoms coincided with positive roentgen findings but, in one case, symptoms preceded demonstration of an ulcer by seven months.

INFLUENCE OF A PROPHYLACTIC ULCER REGIMEN. Four of the patients developing peptic ulcer had received a prophylactic ulcer regimen for some time prior to the demonstration of the lesion. One of these had a known gastric ulcer two years before steroid therapy and a deformed bulb when therapy was initiated. The others were the patients receiving the highest dosages of steroids in the entire group—prednisone 100 mg., triamcinolone 96 mg. and methyl prednisolone 144 mg. per day, respectively. Only three patients in the non-ulcer group received prophylaxis.

COMMENT

Early reports of a low incidence of steroid-associated peptic ulcer (up to 7.8 per cent), largely on low dosages of cortisone, have not been confirmed by more recent investigations where higher doses of newer steroids have been employed (up to 31 per cent). Using prednisone equivalents in mg./day, Kern et al.[16] found an ulcer incidence of approximately 20 per cent when 20 mg. or more was administered and 0 per cent with 15 mg. or less, while Kammerer et al.[9, 15] cited an almost tenfold increase in incidence when doses of more than 10 mg. were compared with amounts less than this. Roentgenologic surveys especially have, with one exception, shown incidences of from 16 to 31 per cent. Correlation of ulcer occurrence with length of treatment is not so clear, although in the series with the highest rate of ulceration, all patients were treated for more than six months.

In our series of 92 patients undergoing numerous roentgenologic examinations over a long period of time, there was no unusual incidence of ulcer in a control group and an incidence of approximately 25 per cent during steroid therapy. One-half of the gastric ulcers varied in appearance from the ordinary type in that ulcerations were shallow and mucosal changes unusual. In a few cases with multiple examinations, mucosal changes were almost evolutionary, preceding and almost predicting appearance of a niche. Variability from the usual in location was evidenced by occurrence of one greater curvature ulcer and appearance of 88 per cent in the distal stomach. The frequency of gastric compared to duodenal ulcers was notable —2.7:1 as compared to the normal expectation of 1:10. Most ulcers appeared after six months of treatment. Dose-incidence correlation was very significant, rising to 47 per cent with 60 mg./day or more of prednisone or its equivalent. Behavior of ulcers with continued steroid administration was interesting in that healing was usual, although five months or more were required in more than 60 per cent of instances. Laitinen et al.[18] observed fairly prompt healing under the same conditions in seven patients. No other large series of observations upon ulcer behavior with continued steroid administration are known to us. Healing with continued therapy did not imply benignity or preclude recurrence. There were three recurrent ulcers and one fatal perforation. One instance of severe melena occurred at the time of demonstration of a crater, and in another patient severe hematemesis appeared in the face of negative roentgen studies. Sex incidence, higher in the male, correspond to the usual experience with peptic ulcer. Although the frequency of an asymptomatic state commented upon by other roentgenologists surveying steroid-treated patients was not confirmed, there were two patients with objective ulcer and no symptoms in this series. Eighty per cent of our patients with x-ray-demonstrated ulcers were symptomatic. Only half of those with symptoms had ulcer objectively. While this study does not allow conclusions regarding the effectiveness of the usual ulcer regimen, either prophylactically or therapeutically, such a regimen is to be recommended for both purposes, especially when higher doses of steroids are employed (over 10 mg./day of prednisone or its equivalent).

The significance of the steroid-induced ulcer problem can best be realized if one attempts to compare the increase in incidence of peptic ulceration during the short period of steroid therapy with the normally expected occurrence of ulceration in these patients or in a closely allied disease, rheumatoid arthritis. In a careful study in England, it was determined that the expectation rate of developing a new peptic ulcer in men between the ages of 35 and 64 was 0.327 per cent per year.[6] Since the incidence in males in our series during their treatment period of approximately one year was 39 per cent, or about 32 per cent more than the average expected incidence of 7.5 per cent for males with nonsteroid-treated rheumatoid arthritis, the rise in risk during their year of steroid treatment is about 100-fold more than if no hormones were given.[22] Utilizing half this occurrence rate for women, or 0.163 per cent per year, there were 25 per cent ulcers versus the average expected incidence in this group of about 3.8 per cent, and therefore the rise in risk is about 130-fold.

The etiology of the higher incidence of peptic ulceration in the steroid-treated patient is still an unsettled problem. Studies have shown no consistent differences in secretion of hydrochloric acid, uropepsin and gastric mucus in patients before and during steroid hormone therapy. The best evidence to date is that these hormones act by inhibition of local healing of normal ulcerations via two mechanisms. The first in the case of oral corticosteroids is the high local concentration of the hormone, particularly in the stomach. This may account for the much higher incidence of steroid-induced gastric ulcers compared to the spontaneous form (72 per cent in our series compared to about 10 to 12 per cent normally). The low incidence of peptic ulceration in patients receiving corticotrophin intramuscularly also suggests the importance of these local factors. Savage and West reported a total of 115 cases of rheumatoid arthritis patients treated as long as two and one-half years with daily injections of this hormone.[21, 23] No routine roentgenological studies were made of the gastrointestinal tract, but only two patients developed symptomatic ulcers. Clinically we have observed several steroid-treated patients with intractable ulcers which healed after transfer from oral to parenteral cortisone. In order to avoid the prolonged local concentrations of corticosteroids, it may be advisable to give these hormones immediately before meals, so that the material leaves the stomach as soon as possible rather than to employ the usual practice of administration after meals or with a small amount of food. The second mechanism is due to inhibition of healing by circulating hormones, as shown by Janowitz and his group in dogs with gastric explants who received both cortisone and ACTH intramuscularly; both inhibited healing of experimentally induced ulcers.[14]

CONCLUSION

Sixty-four patients, most of whom had systemic lupus erythematosus requiring large doses of corticosteroids, had serial upper gastrointestinal x-rays performed at intervals of three months. An additional 28 patients had one examination. The incidence of peptic ulcer in 41 of these who were treated with salicylates and antimalarials was 5 per cent. Twenty patients, or 27 per cent of the steroid-treated group, developed peptic ulcers. Five of the 13 treated males in the series, or 39 per cent, showed these changes, and 25 per cent of the female patients.

In 21 cases in which definite ulcer craters were found, 15 were gastric in location and six duodenal. The occurrence of ulceration was directly proportional to the dosage of corticosteroid employed. There was no statistically significant difference in incidence of ulceration between prednisone, prednisolone, methyl prednisolone, triamcinolone or dexamethasone. Converting the dosage of steroids utilized to prednisone equivalents, the incidence ranges from the occurrence of one recurrent peptic ulcer below 10 mg. per day, 4 to 25 per cent from 10 to 59 mg. per day, and 47 per cent when the dosage was over 60 mg. per day for two months or more. Four patients who developed ulcers had been on a prophylactic ulcer regimen. One of them had a deformed duodenal bulb and ulcer symptoms at the start of the therapy, and the other three received the highest doses of the steroids, namely, 100 mg. per day of prednisone, 96 mg. per day of triamcinolone and 144 mg. per day of methyl prednisolone.

Ulcer symptoms were present in 16 of the 21 patients with lesions. Two others were psychotic. Two additional patients had their ulcer craters appear and fully heal without symptoms, change in steroid therapy or ulcer regimen. One ulcer healed with only reduction in steroid dosage.

A total of 31 patients, of 78 given corticosteroids, had ulcer symptoms while taking the newer hormones and 16 of the symptomatic cases developed proved peptic ulcers. Consequently, complaints of dyspepsia during steroid therapy should be given serious consideration and a full ulcer regimen should be begun.

During the period in which the patient receives steroid therapy, the chances of developing peptic ulcer are 100 to 130 times greater than for the nonsteroid-treated patient. The only preventive method is the use of prophylactic ulcer regimens with antacids and anticholinergic therapy in patients receiving 10 mg. per day of a prednisteroid or its equivalent. All patients with an ulcer history or those who develop dyspepsia on steroids should be placed on a regular ulcer schedule regardless of steroid or dose employed.

REFERENCES

1. Arbesman, C. E. and Richard, N. B.: Prolonged cortisone and hydrocortisone therapy. J. Allergy, 25:306, 1954.
2. Black, R. L., Yielding, K. L. and Bunim, J. J.: Observations on new synthetic antirheumatic steroids and critical evaluation of prednisone therapy in rheumatoid arthritis. J. Chron. Dis., 5:751-769, 1957.
3. Boland, E. W.: Prednisone and prednisolone therapy in rheumatoid arthritis. J.A.M.A., 160:613-621, 1956.
4. Bollet, A. J., Black, R. and Bunim, J. J.: Major undesirable side-effects resulting from prednisolone and prednisone. J.A.M.A., 158:459, 1955.
5. Bunim, J. J., Ziff, M. and McEwen, C.: Evaluation of prolonged cortisone therapy in rheumatoid arthritis. Am. J. Med., 18:27, 1955.
6. Doll, R. and Jones, F. A.: Occupational Factors in the Etiology of Gastric and Duodenal Ulcers. Med. Res. Council Special Report Series 276, 1951.
7. Evans, K. T.: Peptic ulceration associated with prednisolone therapy. Brit. J. Radiol. 31:307, 1958.
8. Experience with cortisone in the management of rheumatoid arthritis; report of a co-operative study conducted by a committee of the American Rheumatism Association, Dr. Culver McEwen, Chairman. Ann. Rheum. Dis., 14:325-336, 1955.
9. Freiberger, R. H., Kammerer, W. H. and Rivelis, A. L.: Peptic ulcers in rheumatoid patients receiving corticosteroid therapy. Radiology, 71:543, 1958.
10. Gedda, P. O. and Moritz, U.: Peptic ulcer during treatment of rheumatoid arthritis with cortisone derivatives. Acta rheum. scandinav., 4:249, 1958.
11. Henderson, E.: New developments in steroid therapy of rheumatic diseases. J. M. Soc. New Jersey, 52:609-615, 1954.
12. Hilbish, T. F. and Black, R. L.: X-ray manifestations of peptic ulceration during corticosteroid therapy of rheumatoid arthritis. A.M.A. Arch. Int. Med., 101:932, 1958.
13. Howell, D. S. and Ragan, C.: The course of rheumatoid arthritis during four years of induced hyperadrenalism. Medicine, 35:83-119, 1956.
14. Janowitz, H. D. et al.: Effect of cortisone and corticotropin on healing of gastric ulcer: experimental study. Gastroenterology, 34:11-20, 1958.
15. Kammerer, W. H., Freiberger, R. H. and Rivelis, A. L.: Peptic ulcer in rheumatoid patients on corticosteroid therapy; clinical, experimental and radiologic study. Arth. & Rheum., 1:122-141, 1958.
16. Kern, F., Jr., Clark, G. M. and Lukens, J. G.: Peptic ulceration occurring during therapy for rheumatoid arthritis. Gastroenterology, 33:25-33, 1957.
17. Kirsner, J. B., Sklar, M. and Palmer, W. L.: The effect of ACTH and adrenal steroids in the management of ulcerative colitis. Observations on 180 patients. Am. J. Med., 22:264, 1957.
18. Laitinen, H., Meurman, K. and Virkunen, M.: Roentgenological appearance of corticosteroid produced peptic ulcers. Acta rheum. scandinav., 4:205, 1958.
19. Meltzer, L. E., Bockman, A. A., Kanenson, W. and Cohen, A.: The incidence of peptic ulcer among patients on long-term prednisone therapy. Gastroenterology, 35:351, 1958.
20. Sandweiss, D. J.: Effect of adrenocorticotrophic hormone (ACTH) and of cortisone on peptic ulcer; clinical review. Gastroenterology, 27:604, 1954.
21. Savage, O. et al.: The clinical course and corticosteroid excretion of patients with rheumatoid arthritis during long-term treatment with corticotrophin. Brit. M. J., 2:1257, 1957.
22. Short, C. L., Bauer, W. and Reynolds, W. E.: Rheumatoid Arthritis. Cambridge, Mass., Harvard University Press, 1957.
23. West, H. F.: Effects of prolonged adrenocortical stimulation on patients with rheumatoid arthritis. Ann. Rheum. Dis., 16:322, 1957.
24. Wollaeger, E. E.: Untoward effects of cortisone and corticotropin on the gastrointestinal tract. Minnesota Med., 37:626, 1954.

Comparative Effects of Steroids on Water and Electrolyte Balance

LEWIS C. MILLS, ZEV CHAYES and BENJAMIN NEWMAN

Hahnemann Medical College and Hospital, Philadelphia

Edema due to sodium and water retention is one of the frequent side effects resulting from administration of therapeutic doses of cortisone or hydrocortisone. It occurs in almost half of the patients receiving more than 75 mg. of cortisone per day for any significant length of time. Although edema is usually self-limited in patients not having cardiovascular or renal disease, the development of cardiac failure or severe edema in those with these disorders often presents a difficult therapeutic problem. Fortunately, many of the newer synthetic anti-inflammatory steroids have little, if any, sodium- and water-retaining activity. Since the choice of a steroid to be used for a given disease condition should be based on its metabolic and pharmacologic properties in relation to the patient's disease, knowledge of the relative sodium-retaining potency of the commonly used anti-inflammatory steroids is of value in making this selection. Several comparative studies are reported elsewhere in this volume and these data will not be reiterated here.

TABLE 1. EFFECTS OF CORTICOSTEROIDS ON GLOMERULAR FILTRATION RATE AND URINARY EXCRETION OF SODIUM AND POTASSIUM*

DRUG	DOSE mg./day	Na mEq./day	K mEq./day	GFR ml./min.
Hydrocortisone	100	− 34	+ 2	+ 12
Prednisolone	25	− 11	+ 2	+ 19
Methyl prednisolone	16	0	− 4	+ 22
Triamcinolone	16	+ 39	− 2	+ 37
Hydrocortisone	200	− 55	+ 23	+ 14
Prednisolone	50	− 22	+ 7	+ 5
Methyl prednisolone	32	− 2	− 2	+ 30
Triamcinolone	32	+ 66	+ 3	+ 54

* McMahon et al., Metabolism, 9:511, 1960.

In one of the best comparative studies reported elsewhere[1] the renal and electrolyte effects of hydrocortisone, prednisolone, triamcinolone and methyl prednisolone were compared in normal subjects receiving a constant diet containing 230 mEq. of sodium and 122 mEq. of potassium per day (Table 1). In these studies all steroids were given at two dose levels approximately equivalent in anti-inflammatory potency to 100 and 200 mg. of hydrocortisone, respectively. Administration of hydrocortisone and prednisolone at both dose levels led to retention of sodium, although it was considerably less with prednisolone than with hydrocortisone. Methyl prednisolone had no effect on sodium excretion, and a noticeable increase occurred when triamcinolone was given. None of the steroids significantly increased potassium excretion except for hydrocortisone at the higher dose level.

865

Glomerular filtration rate increased during administration of each steroid and was particularly elevated by triamcinolone.

Since the experiments noted above and most of the other reported studies have been carried out in normal subjects, it seemed important to reassay these compounds in patients with various disease conditions. To accomplish this, 55 patients with various illnesses such as cardiac failure, cirrhosis of the liver, asthma and leukemia were placed on a constant low

TABLE 2.   EFFECTS OF ANTI-INFLAMMATORY STEROIDS ON
WATER AND ELECTROLYTE EXCRETION

COMPARISON		DOSE		UV Δ ml./24 hrs.	P	UR Na Δ mEq./24 hrs.	P	UR K Δ mEq./24 hrs.	P
1	vs 2	1	2						
C	C	0	0	− 26	NS	− 7	< .05	+ 1	NS
CV	TCL	0	30	+ 395	< .001	+ 16	< .10	+ 11	< .01
TCL	C	16	0	− 504	< .05	− 21	< .01	− 1	NS
TCL	TCL	22	22	− 12	NS	− 5	NS	− 2	< .10
TCL	MP	34	34	− 96	NS	+ 6	NS	− 2	NS
MP	TCL	34	34	− 21	NS	− 2	NS	+ 6	NS
MP	MP	51	47	+ 176	NS	− 6	NS	+ 5	NS
MP	Pred	46	50	− 45	NS	− 7	NS	+ 8	NS

Key:
UV—Urine volume. Ur Na—Urine sodium. Ur K—Urine potassium.
Δ—Change from first period to second period. (Each period is the average of a 3-day urine collection period.)
C—Control. TCL—Triamcinolone. MP—Methyl prednisolone. Pred—Prednisone. P—p Value.

sodium diet. After sufficient time for stabilization, consecutive 24-hour urines were collected during a three-day control period, after which the steroid to be studied was administered orally. The effects on urine volume and urine sodium and potassium excretion were determined. These results are summarized in Table 2 and are reported elsewhere in greater detail.[2] The differences shown in the table represent the change from the first period to the second, each period being the average value for three consecutive days of urine collection. A minus value indicates that the average urine excretion decreased by the indicated amount and a plus value indicates an increase in excretion. The results again show that triamcinolone has a diuretic effect on water, sodium and potassium excretion. In these studies little difference could be shown between triamcinolone, methyl prednisolone and prednisone.

In a subsequent experiment, 10 patients with various diseases were again placed on a constant sodium diet. This experiment was similar to the above study, except that each patient, after an initial control period, received each of five steroids for a three-day period. The steroids used were hydrocortisone, prednisone, methyl prednisolone, triamcinolone and dexamethasone. Approximately equal anti-inflammatory doses were used in a given patient in the ratio of 20:5:4:4:1 mg., respectively, the usual dose being equivalent to 80 mg. of hydrocortisone. The drugs were also given in random order to avoid bias on the basis of the possibility that the initial effects of a given steroid might be different from those occurring from the same steroid several days later. The data were then averaged for each three-day period. The changes in relation to the control period are presented in Table 3.

In these studies there was no significant change in urine volume or in potassium excretion, with the possible exception of increased potassium

TABLE 3. EFFECTS OF FIVE COMMONLY USED ANTI-INFLAMMATORY
STEROIDS ON WATER AND ELECTROLYTE EXCRETION

DRUG	UV Δ ml./24 hrs.	UR Na Δ mEq./24 hrs.	UR K Δ mEq./24 hrs.
Hydrocortisone	+ 31	+ 2	+ 3
Prednisone	+ 189	+ 26	+ 4
Dexamethasone	+ 243	+ 28	+ 12
Methyl prednisolone	+ 137	+ 38	0
Triamcinolone	− 154	+ 38	− 3

For key to abbreviations see Table 2.

excretion with dexamethasone. Sodium excretion increased with all but hydrocortisone, but more with triamcinolone and methyl prednisolone than with prednisone and dexamethasone.

The results presented here and elsewhere in this volume are in essential agreement and indicate that hydrocortisone and cortisone have the most sodium-retaining effect and therefore are the most likely to induce edema and to contribute to the development of cardiac failure in patients with heart disease. Although the results vary somewhat, prednisolone and prednisone are the drugs next most likely to produce sodium retention. Dexamethasone and methyl prednisolone appear to have about the same effect on sodium excretion, either producing little change or increasing its excretion, and triamcinolone usually has a diuretic effect.

The results reported by McMahon et al.[1] again serve to emphasize that the effects of these steroids on sodium excretion reflect the balance between the increase in renal glomerular filtration rate and the increase in tubular reabsorption of sodium. If glomerular filtration rate is only slightly increased, as with hydrocortisone, reabsorption of sodium by the tubules exceeds the increase in filtered sodium so that there is a net retention. Conversely, if the filtration rate is greatly increased as with triamcinolone, the increase in filtered sodium exceeds the increased amount reabsorbed, so that a net sodium loss or diuresis occurs. Undoubtedly, there are also other factors, as yet incompletely explored, such as the effect of these compounds on cellular electrolyte transport other than in the kidney, which may be important in explaining their effects on electrolyte balance. The significance of these other factors must await further investigation.

In addition, it should be remembered that edema may occur during administration of any of the anti-inflammatory steroids; in patients with severe renal disease, in whom glomerular filtration rate can not increase or increases very little, the tubular effects predominate and sodium retention and edema can occur. Contrariwise, all of the commonly used anti-inflammatory steroids may, on occasion, lead to diuresis, as, for example, in nephrosis, or diuresis may occur when the steroid is combined with a diuretic agent when neither produces diuresis alone, as, for example, in ascites due to cirrhosis of the liver.

REFERENCES

1. McMahon, F. G., Gordon, E. S., Kenoyer, W. C. and Keil, P.: Renal and pituitary inhibiting effect of exogenous corticosteroids in normal subjects. Metabolism, 9:511, 1960.
2. Mills, L. C., Pontidas, E. and Faludi, G.: Comparative salt-retaining effects of common steroids in clinical use. In Moyer, J. H. and Fuchs, M.: Edema, Mechanisms and Management. Philadelphia, W. B. Saunders Co., 1960, p. 356.

Hypertension and Edema
Due to the Therapeutic
Administration of Steroids*

JOHN H. MOYER and ALBERT N. BREST

Hahnemann Medical College and Hospital, Philadelphia

Hypertension and edema due to the therapeutic administration of steroids occur frequently, but fortunately the occurrence of these side effects is usually not serious, being reversible when the steroids are discontinued. Even when the continued administration of steroids is mandatory, these side effects can be treated effectively, i.e., by the administration of diuretic agents in the case of edema and by a combination of diuretics and anti-hypertensive agents which depress the sympathetic nervous system in the case of blood pressure elevation.

HYPERTENSION

Blood pressure elevation is seen frequently in certain naturally occurring endocrinopathies, e.g., primary aldosteronism and Cushing's syndrome (Table 1). This finding raises the questions of whether essential hypertension is due to abnormal adrenal cortical steroid metabolism and whether the therapeutic administration of steroids triggers off the stimulus that is responsible for blood pressure elevation in patients with essential hypertension. At this time, there is no definite evidence that the latter consideration is valid or that abnormal adrenal cortical function is of etiological significance in essential hypertension. Instead, it is more likely that blood pressure elevation associated with abnormal adrenal function is merely one specific type of hypertension. Although Laragh et al.[3, 4] have found that patients with malignant hypertension have increased excretion rates of aldosterone, their data suggest that a well defined biochemical difference exists between the group of patients with benign essential hypertension (which iatrogenic hypertension resembles) and those who manifest the clinical picture of malignant hypertensive disease. These investigators found increases in the secretion rate of aldosterone in all but one of 15 patients with malignant hypertension. In contrast, all of their patients with primary benign essential hypertension secreted normal amounts of aldosterone. It is noteworthy that patients rarely develop malignant hypertension as a result of the therapeutic administration of steroids. The latter finding suggests that the increased secretion of aldosterone in patients with malignant hypertension is probably a secondary phenomenon.

There is further evidence to indicate that the therapeutic administration of steroids, whether these are naturally occurring adrenal cortical steroids

* Supported in part by grants from the Eastern Pennsylvania Heart Association, The Mary Bailey Foundation and the National Institutes of Health of the United States Public Health Service.

868

or synthetic anti-inflammatory steroids, produces an increase in blood pressure by enhancing the vasopressor response to norepinephrine at the neuroeffector site of the sympathetic nervous system as well as by a secondary phenomenon of renal salt and water retention. The severity of the increase in blood pressure is dependent on the steroid, the dose and the length of administration; the larger the dose and the longer the period of drug administration, the more likely is the development of diastolic hypertension (Tables 1 and 2). The protracted course may explain the high incidence of hypertension in naturally occurring syndromes associated with increased aldosterone secretion[1,2] (Table 1).

TABLE 1. INCIDENCE OF PERIPHERAL EDEMA AND HYPERTENSION EXPRESSED IN PER CENT OF THE NUMBER OF PATIENTS OBSERVED

	PRIMARY ALDOSTERONISM*	CUSHING'S SYNDROME	LONG-TERM[†] THERAPY WITH HYDROCORTISONE	LARGE DOSES OF HYDRO-CORTISONE ($>$ 60mg./day)
Number of patients	50	40	50	100
Hypertension (%)[‡]	80	82	22	26
Edema (%)	$<$ 10	30	42	48

* Conn.[1]

† Patient received steroid daily for 36 weeks or more.

‡ Increase in mean arterial blood pressure of more than 10 mm.Hg.

It seems likely that a significant part of the mechanism of iatrogenic hypertension following steroid administration is due to a direct central nervous system stimulatory effect. Most of the patients have associated anxiety manifestations and they may become severely agitated and/or depressed. Sodium retention is also a significant factor, but the association of hypertension with peripheral edema is erratic, the latter occurring in only about half of the patients with blood pressure elevation.

TABLE 2. THE INCIDENCE OF HYPERTENSION RESULTING FROM THE THERAPEUTIC ADMINISTRATION OF HYDROCORTISONE AND PREDNISONE

	INCIDENCE OF HYPERTENSION (PER CENT)
PREDNISONE	
5 to 20 mg.	5
20 to 40 mg.	18
40 to 80 mg.	36
More than 80 mg.	54
HYDROCORTISONE	
20 to 50 mg.	4
50 to 100 mg.	22
100 to 200 mg.	38

The incidence of hypertension associated with prednisone and hydrocortisone administration is given in Table 2. It is evident that there is a significant relationship between incidence and the size of the dose.

Treatment of Hypertension due to the Therapeutic Administration of Steroids.   It is obvious that the best treatment is to discontinue the steroid. When this course is not feasible, however, the blood pressure elevation can be controlled by the same measures ordinarily used in the treatment of

COMPARISON OF THE EFFECT OF A PARENTERALLY ADMINISTERED MERCURIAL
DIURETIC (MERCUHYDRIN) ON SODIUM AND WATER EXCRETION IN A PATIENT
WHO HAS SODIUM AND WATER RETENTION DUE TO PREDNISONE AND
ONE WHO HAS RETENTION DUE TO CARDIAC FAILURE

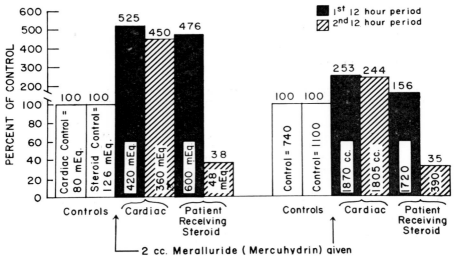

Fig. 1. The open bar graphs on the left represent the sodium excretion (mEq./L)
for a 12-hour control period prior to drug administration; those on the right indicate the
rate of water excretion (cc.) during the same period. Following drug administration, the
increase in sodium excretion is about the same in the patient with heart failure as compared with the patient with edema due to steroid administration. However, during the
subsequent 12-hour period, the patient with edema due to heart failure continues to have
a natriuretic response, whereas the patient with edema due to steroid administration retains sodium.

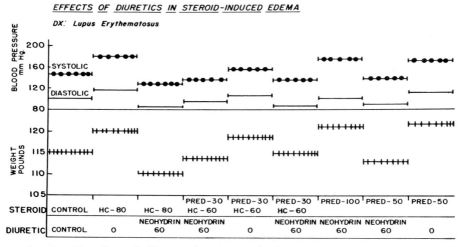

Fig. 2. The effect of chlormerodrin (Neohydrin) in a patient with moderate blood
pressure elevation and edema due to the therapeutic administration of prednisone or
hydrocortisone. When the mercurial (chlormerodrin) was given, the blood pressure decreased. The accompanying diuresis is reflected in the weight loss.

essential hypertension. Only when the pressure elevation is significant and progressive should specific antihypertensive therapy be instituted. Probably a fixed diastolic pressure above 115 mm.Hg is adequate indication for drug management.

When treatment is indicated, a thiazide derivative (e.g., chlorothiazide in a dose of 500 to 1000 mg. twice a day) is usually effective. Mercurials are also useful but are less easy to administer. When mercurials are given parenterally they must be administered with adequate frequency, usually every 24 hours (Fig. 1). About half of the patients will respond adequately to diuretic therapy so that additional drugs are not required (Fig. 2). However, the blood pressure will return to normotensive levels in only a very few patients despite a significant concomitant reduction of total body sodium. The latter finding suggests that salt and water retention is not the only mechanism involved in the blood pressure elevation.

When the response to chlorothiazide is inadequate, an additional drug

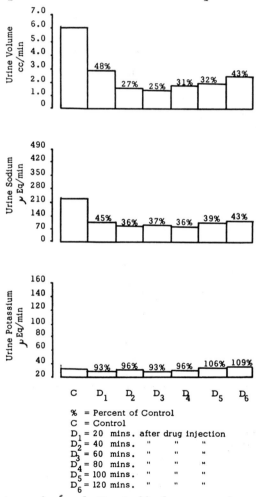

% = Percent of Control
C = Control
D₁ = 20 mins. after drug injection
D₂ = 40 mins.   "   "   "
D₃ = 60 mins.   "   "   "
D₄ = 80 mins.   "   "   "
D₅ = 100 mins.   "   "   "
D₆ = 120 mins.   "   "   "

Fig. 3. Following a sharp reduction in blood pressure when guanethidine is administered parenterally, there is a significant decrease in the excretion rate of water and sodium.

which depresses the transmission of neurogenic impulses is indicated. Guanethidine, a drug which inhibits the release of norepinephrine from the postganglionic sympathetic fibers, seems to be the most effective agent for this purpose. Rauwolfia is not indicated since it has limited potency and it may seriously aggravate any accompanying central nervous system effects of the steroids. When guanethidine is used (concurrently with chlorothiazide) the initial recommended dose is 10 mg. per day. Thereafter the dosage can be increased by 10 mg. increments at five- to ten-day intervals until the desired reduction in blood pressure (standing) is obtained. A reduction in pressure to approximately 150/90 is usually considered adequate.

Excessive reduction in blood pressure should be avoided, otherwise increased retention of salt and water may ensue. This phenomenon is especially likely to occur with the acute reduction in blood pressure following the parenteral administration of a potent sympathetic depressant drug such as guanethidine (Fig. 3). Although these patients do respond to the latter drug, the response obtained is not as good as that achieved in the patient with essential or simple neurogenic hypertension.

PERIPHERAL EDEMA

The major mechanism responsible for the development of edema in patients receiving steroids seems quite obvious, i.e., renal retention of sodium and water. Although peripheral edema is usually associated with this phenomenon, localized edema may also occur secondary to a simple redistribution of body fluids without a demonstrable retention of salt and water or a significant increase in total body sodium and water. Presumably the steroids affect the body distribution of electrolytes and water by their effects on cell membrane permeability.

Treatment of Peripheral Edema. The treatment of steroid-induced edema is detailed in the next paper, but the following principles are worthy of emphasis. When edema is due to the renal retention of salt and water, it can usually be treated effectively by the use of diuretic agents. However, diuretics of adequate potency must be used, and they must be administered frequently enough so that the secondary sodium retention which occurs after the diuretic effect is spent does not negate the primary therapeutic response. For example, in Figure 1, the response to a mercurial diuretic is presented. It is obvious that if this compound were given every 12 hours, it would be effective in controlling the sodium and water retention associated with the administration of the steroid. On the other hand, if it were given every 48 hours, it would not be adequately effective. This is different from the situation encountered in the patient with congestive heart failure, and it is important that the therapist recognize this fact.

Because of their ease of administration, chlorothiazide and its derivatives seem to be the most useful agents for the treatment of iatrogenic steroid edema. A dose of 500 to 1000 mg. given twice daily (or its equivalent when other thiazide compounds are employed) is usually adequate. Although the dose varies with the different thiazide derivatives, their natriuretic effects are quantitatively similar (Fig. 4). Switching to another thiazide compound is frequently effective when the continued use of any one has ceased to be adequate. In addition, the co-administration of mercurials with a thiazide derivative will produce a further natriuretic and diuretic response (Fig. 5).

When thiazide derivatives are used concurrently with steroids in therapy,

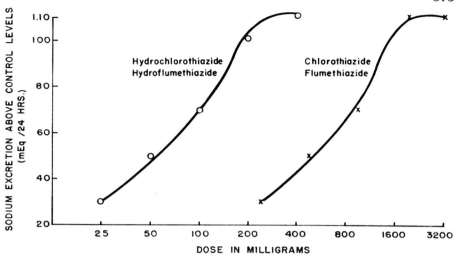

Fig. 4. Dose response (comparing sodium excretion as the significant modality) to 4 thiazide derivatives. There was no difference between chlorothiazide and flumethiazide and no difference between hydrochlorothiazide and hydroflumethiazide. Although the hydrogenated compounds (hydrochlorothiazide and hydroflumethiazide) require a lesser dosage, the maximum natriuretic response is the same.

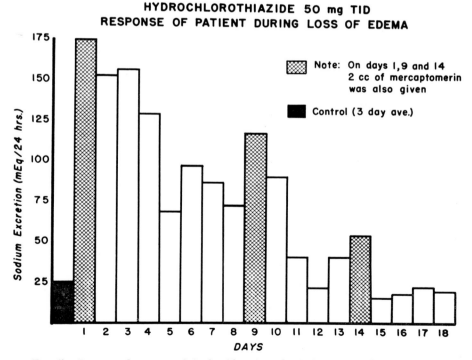

Fig. 5. Patient who received hydrochlorothiazide daily. When the mercurial was given, there was an additional natriuretic response. As the patient approached dry weight, the natriuresis resulting from the chlorothiazide decreased and the added response to the mercurial was less significant.

potassium supplements should be given if there is a tendency to hypokalemia. The potassium salts may be given in liquid solution (potassium triplex) with meals in a dose of 30 to 45 milliequivalents. It is noteworthy that there is very little difference in the kaluretic effect produced by various thiazide derivatives (Fig. 6).

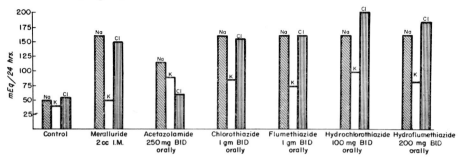

Fig. 6. Electrolyte excretion pattern of various diuretics as compared with the excretion rates during the control periods. All of the thiazide derivatives showed a significant, but similar, kaluretic response.

REFERENCES

1. Conn, J. W.: Adrenal factors in hypertension. Circulation, *17*:743, 1958.
2. Flynn, P.: Adrenal cortical tumors with fulminating hypertension. J. Irish M. A., *39*:77, 1956.
3. Holten, C. and Peterson, V. P.: Malignant hypertension with increased secretion of aldosterone and depletion of potassium. Lancet, 2:918, 1956.
4. Laragh, J. H., Ulick, S., Januszewicz, V., Deming, Q. B., Kelly, W. G. and Lieberman, S.: Aldosterone secretion and primary and malignant hypertension. J. Clin. Invest., *39*:1091, 1960.

Therapy of Steroid Edema

MORTON FUCHS

Hahnemann Medical College and Hospital, Philadelphia

The use of adrenal steroids has become a cornerstone in the therapy of many pathologic syndromes. As with any potent therapeutic agent, the incidence of side effects with the steroids demands an understanding of the pharmacologic activity and requisite indications and contraindications for the use of these drugs.

By their inherent structure and activity on the renal tubule, most available steroids are capable of producing sodium retention and are therefore capable of producing edema. When the adrenal steroids are used as replacement therapy for adrenal insufficiency, the presence of edema would indicate an excessive dose beyond the physiologic requirements of the patient. Reduction in dosage of the drug usually is adequate for controlling the excess sodium and water retention. On the other hand, when the adrenal steroids are used primarily for their anti-inflammatory effects, out of therapeutic necessity the dose may far exceed the routine physiologic range of the drug and may produce positive sodium and fluid balance with resultant edema. To reduce the dose of the drug under these circumstances may reduce the fluid retention, but the objectives of the steroid therapy may be negated. In order to retain the desired therapeutic influence of the steroid and still keep the patient free of edema, other measures are frequently necessary to maintain a physiologic sodium balance.

The steroid that is administered will have significant influence on the degree of sodium retention by the kidney. The goal in development of the newer adrenal steroid preparations is the separation of the various actions of these hormones. The discrete separation of the glucocorticoid (anti-inflammatory) action from the mineralocorticoid (sodium-retaining) action of the adrenal steroids would be ideal in those conditions in which a large dose of the drug is necessary for anti-inflammatory activity. The development of steroids with increased anti-inflammatory activity and markedly decreased sodium-retaining effect has been realized with such drugs as prednisone, prednisolone, methyl prednisolone, triamcinolone and dexamethasone. The incidence of edema with these agents has varied but is usually less than 8 per cent. The action of these steroids on the renal mechanisms is not completely understood, but there is much evidence to indicate that these drugs may produce increased sodium excretion.

The approach to the therapy of the patient with edema of exogenous steroid origin is one primarily of using those steroids with the least sodium-retaining effects. If edema is still a problem, sodium retention must be reduced by restricting sodium intake and if necessary by increasing sodium excretion.

SODIUM RESTRICTION

The edema associated with chronic steroid administration may be in part due to the shift of fluid into the extracellular compartment in the absence of significant sodium retention.[6] This is most probably due to the effects of the steroid on the cell membranes. However, for the most part, the edema of steroid origin is based on the effects of excess sodium retention by the kidney.

Sodium restriction in the diet has the net effect of reducing the total quantity of sodium available for retention by the renal tubular mechanisms. With adequate sodium restriction and the use of those steroids that have negligible effects on sodium retention the majority of patients do quite well. In addition to the advantage of decreased fluid retention with the use of a low sodium diet, there is a definite sparing effect on potassium excretion in the presence of steroid administration.[5] Figure 1 demonstrates the effects of a 1-gram (50 mEq.) sodium diet on the 24-hour urine sodium and potassium excretion in a patient given 60 mg. of prednisone daily. This patient was a 32-year-old white woman with idiopathic thrombocytopenic purpura. When the patient received the diet alone, the 24-hour urinary sodium excretion remained relatively constant and the patient evidenced no significant weight gain or edema. The potassium content of the diet was approximately 50 mEq. per day. The 24-hour urinary potassium excretion also remained relatively constant, but there was a tendency toward a negative potassium balance. During this phase of the study the patient was free of complaints representing potassium deficiency and hypokalemia. Upon the addition of

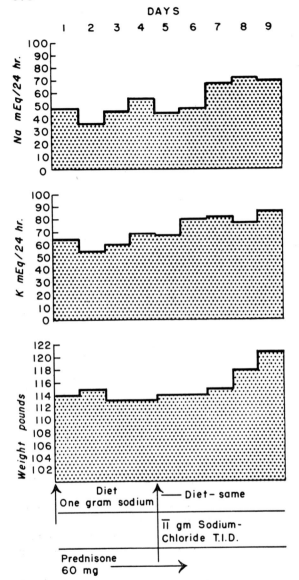

Fig. 1. A patient with idiopathic thrombocytopenic purpura receiving 60 mg. of prednisone daily and a 1 gram (50 mEq.) sodium diet. Twenty-four hour urinary sodium and potasssium excretion remain relatively constant. With the addition of 2 grams of sodium chloride three times daily there is an increase in sodium and potassium excretion and a significant weight gain.

2 grams of sodium chloride three times daily to the above diet, there was increased sodium excretion. However, the net result was a positive sodium balance, and the patient's weight increased significantly from 114 pounds to 121 pounds. At the end of this phase of the study the patient manifested peripheral edema with noticeable pitting edema in the lower extremities and generalized puffiness about the face. At this time she also complained of headaches and generalized weakness. The potassium excretion was also increased during the administration of the additional sodium chloride, denoting an increased negative potassium balance. This experiment bears out the previously established evidence that sodium restriction has a sparing effect on the urinary excretion of potassium. The quantity of sodium allowed

in the diet of this patient (50 mEq.) could have been reduced further, had it been necessary, in order to prevent the accumulation of edema fluid. However, in this particular patient restriction of sodium to 50 mEq. per day was sufficient to prevent significant weight gain and edema over a period of several weeks. When 1 gram of potassium chloride was given four times daily to this patient while she was still on the 1-gram sodium (50 mEq. sodium) diet, the 24-hour urine sodium excretion remained relatively constant, as did the potassium excretion. However, in this phase of the study there appeared to be a positive potassium balance (Fig. 2). The patient had no significant complaints on this regimen, and edema and weight gain were not evident.

The over-all effect of adequate sodium restriction in the patient requiring large doses of steroid drugs is to reduce the net retention of the sodium ion

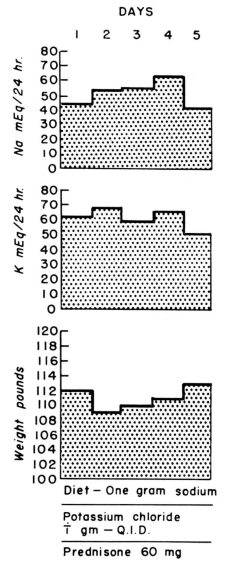

Fig. 2. The addition of supplementary potassium chloride to the diet did not influence urinary sodium or potassium excretion in this patient.

Diet — One gram sodium

Potassium chloride
1 gm — Q.I.D.

Prednisone 60 mg

and thereby to prevent excess fluid retention. In addition, the restriction of sodium chloride in the diet conserves the body potassium and therefore allows for a more physiologic response to the effects of steroids on the renal tubule. The degree of sodium restriction that must be maintained will vary with the individual patient, and when a 1-gram sodium (50 mEq. sodium) diet is not adequate restriction, further reduction in the sodium ion content of the diet can be prescribed. The degree of restriction will be governed by the socio-economic status of the patient as well as by his willingness to cooperate. Palatability of the low sodium diet can be improved by adequate addition of condiments, oils, flavorings, etc. When sodium restriction is severe the supplemental use of potassium salts may be indicated, since gradual insidious deficiency of body potassium may occur. In addition, by possibly augmenting the cation exchange mechanism of the renal tubule, the addition of potassium salts to the diet may reduce the intensity of sodium retention.[4]

DIURETICS

When sodium restriction is not sufficient for maintenance of the edema-free state or when the patient is unable to maintain sodium restriction adequately, the use of those agents that will increase sodium excretion is indicated. Numerous diuretics are available for the therapy of steroid edema, but the most practical compounds for use today are the potent orally administered drugs. The parenteral mercurials still remain the most active diuretic agents available. The necessity for continuous diuretic activity frequently becomes mandatory with steroid edema, and therefore the necessity for frequent mercurial injections becomes a problem. Occasionally in a case of severe steroid edema, which is unusual with the more recent steroid derivatives, the necessity for maintenance of saluretic activity may require a mercurial injection twice daily.

The carbonic anhydrase inhibitors such as acetazolamide (Diamox) or ethoxzolamide (Cardrase) have only moderate natriuretic activity and have a high potential for potassium and bicarbonate excretion. Since excess potassium excretion is frequently a problem in the patient with edema due to steroid effects on the renal tubule, the use of the carbonic anhydrase inhibitors does not appear indicated. In addition, these drugs lose their effectiveness after two to four days of continuous administration and cannot be used when persistent natriuretic activity is required.

The more recent benzothiadiazine derivatives have served efficiently in the therapy of steroid edema since they can be administered orally and as frequently as necessary to maintain sodium excretion at efficient levels. There is no apparent refractoriness to these drugs as is found with the carbonic anhydrase inhibitors. Their toxicity is negligible, and tolerance over prolonged periods of continuous therapy is rarely a problem. Chlorothiazide (Diuril) and flumethiazide (Ademol) have an effective dose range of 200 to 200 mg. daily. Hydrochlorothiazide (Hydrodiuril, Esidrix, Oretic), hydro-flumethiazide (Saluron) and 3-benzylthiomethyl chlorothiazide (Naclex) have a dose range of 25 to 200 mg. Benzhydroflumethiazide (Naturetin), trichlormethiazide (Naqua) and methylchlorothiazide (Enduron) have a dose range of 1 to 10 mg. It should be noted that although these drugs differ in their milligram potency the effective sodium excretion with the maximum effective dose of all the thiazides available to date is approximately the same.

Therefore, these drugs can be used interchangeably when equivalently effective doses are prescribed.[1, 2]

Another recent addition to the diuretic armamentarium is phthalimidine (Hygroton). This drug is a potent saluretic agent and has the ability to effect significant sodium excretion for as long as 48 hours or more after a single dose.[3]

The administration of diuretics to the patient with steroid-induced edema presents the problem of negative potassium balance. The steroid alone is prone to produce potassium deficiency, and the additive effect of the prolonged administration of diuretics may produce severe potassium deficiency. In Figure 3 the 24-hour urine sodium and potassium excretion with the administration of 100 mg. of hydrochlorothiazide daily to the previously

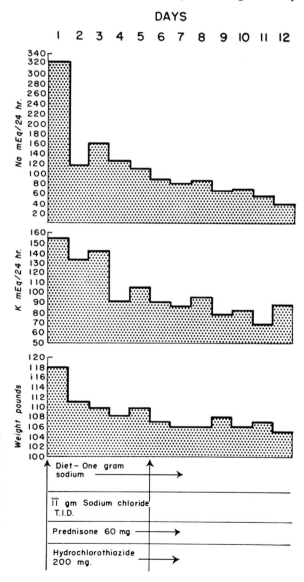

Fig. 3. The use of 100 mg. of hydrochlorothiazide with supplementary sodium chloride produces extremely high sodium and potassium excretion with a significant weight loss. When supplementary sodium is stopped and only a 1-gram sodium diet is used, potassium excretion remains elevated with the continued use of the diuretic.

described patient are demonstrated. The patient was maintained on a 1-gram sodium (50 mEq. sodium) diet and 60 mg. of prednisone daily. An additional 6 grams of sodium chloride were administered daily. The sodium excretion reached extremely high levels and the patient lost all evidence of edema; there was a significant weight loss of nine pounds. Potassium excretion increased, however, although not as much as sodium excretion. During this period the patient's clinical manifestations of edema improved but she developed rather noticeable weakness. This also demonstrates the wide range of salt tolerance the patient may accept with diuretic therapy. When the supplementary sodium was stopped on the sixth day of the study and diuretic therapy was continued, sodium excretion progressively fell toward the previous levels seen with the use of the 1-gram sodium diet alone. This most probably indicated a depletion of excess sodium stores at this time. However, the potassium excretion remained at elevated levels while the diuretic was continued, indicating a persistence of the negative potassium balance. The necessity for supplementary potassium salts in the patient receiving diuretics for steroid edema even though sodium restriction is maintained is demonstrated.

The use of anti-aldosterone agents such as the spironolactone (Aldactone) is usually not required since the diuretic agents available are extremely potent drugs. The effectiveness of Aldactone in edema due to exogenous steroid therapy has been unpredictable in our hands.

In summary, the prescribed approach to the edema of exogenous steroid origin is one in which we attempt to prevent edema by using those steroids that have the least sodium retaining potential and sodium restriction in the diet. If edema still occurs or if sodium restriction is impossible or adherence to a low sodium diet by the patient is impractical, the use of diuretics is indicated. The smallest dose of the diuretic necessary to maintain the edema-free state should be used. The addition of supplementary potassium salts is indicated when diuretics are used.

REFERENCES

1. Beyer, K. H. and Baer, J. H.: The pharmacology of chlorothiazide and its analogues. Int. Rec. Med., 172:413, 1959.
2. Fuchs, M. and Mallin, S. R.: Clinical pharmacology of thiazide derivatives. In Moyer, J. H. and Fuchs, M.: Edema: Mechanisms and Management. Philadelphia, W. B. Saunders Co., 1960, p. 276.
3. Fuchs, M., Moyer, J. H. and Newman, B. E.: Human clinical pharmacology of the newer diuretics: benzothiadiazine and phthalimidine. Ann. N. Y. Acad. Sc., 88:795, 1960.
4. Liddle, S. W., Bennett, L. L. and Forsham, P. H.: The prevention of ACTH-induced sodium retention by the use of potassium salts. J. Clin. Invest., 32:1197, 1953.
5. Seldin, D. W., Welt, L. G. and Cort, J.: Effect of pituitary and adrenal hormones on metabolism and excretion of potassium. J. Clin. Invest., 30:673, 1951.
6. Soffer, L. J.: The adrenal gland and its effect on electrolyte and fluid distribution. In Moyer, J. H. and Fuchs, M.: Edema: Mechanisms and Management. Philadelphia, W. B. Saunders Co., 1960, p. 107.

Panel Discussion

CHARLES M. THOMPSON, *Moderator*

DR. THOMPSON: Many of the undesirable effects of steroid therapy have been discussed by the various speakers, but no one has mentioned any detrimental effect of steroids on the liver. I wonder whether long-term steroid therapy does have any effect on liver function or histology, since, as we all know, steroids have a profound effect on metabolism, and the liver is certainly involved in this process in many ways. Dr. Gray, would you comment on this?

DR. GRAY: I do not think that the steroids have any detrimental effect on the liver. Steroids may cause a decrease in serum bilirubin, but that is thought to be due to a change in the synthesis of bilirubin and not to a choleretic effect. As a matter of fact, steroids may be beneficial in some types of liver disease, and they are used in massive doses in some cases of acute fulminating hepatitis. This was started in Chile, where they have epidemics of it, and this therapy has been reported to be life-saving in certain instances of acute fulminating hepatitis.

DR. THOMPSON: Dr. Mills, have you seen diabetic steatorrhea as a result of diabetic neuropathy, and, if you have, are steroids beneficial in this process? Or would steroids be contraindicated in this situation because of their hyperglycemic effect?

DR. MILLS: I can not give a definite answer to that question from personal experience. Steatorrhea on that basis is very infrequent, and I do not remember seeing a single patient in the last three years who has had this particular difficulty. We have had two or three patients with minor difficulties in bowel function, but not with steatorrhea. I do not know what the effect of steroids would be on the steatorrhea.

DR. GRAY: I believe steroids would make the diabetes worse and would not help the steatorrhea. Steatorrhea is thought to be on a neurogenic basis in the diabetic patient.

DR. THOMPSON: Then there is apparently no evidence of villous atrophy?

DR. GRAY: That is correct. It is not a primary malabsorption syndrome.

DR. THOMPSON: I think recent work has shown that the steatorrhea in diabetics may be associated with a secondary infectious process, a situation similar to that in many patients with the malabsorption syndrome. Some people are treating these patients with neomycin.
  Dr. Berkowitz, could the abnormalities in fat metabolism which you mentioned in your paper be a nonspecific effect of steroids? Could they be simply due to increased absorption?

DR. BERKOWITZ: I can not answer that definitely. I was rather impressed that the changes observed were more specific, because they were associated with not only elevated lipid levels but also a more fundamental process, an abnormality in the fat tolerance test, and I thought this was more than just a nonspecific effect. I think it is due to an abnormality in metabolism of fat after it is absorbed.

DR. MOYER: Since we are talking about comparative effects of various steroids,

I would like to ask Dr. Gray if he has noticed in his studies any difference relative to the ulcerogenic effect of the various steroids, particularly of the synthetic steroids as opposed to the natural steroids.

DR. GRAY: It is difficult to be sure unless gastrointestinal x-ray examinations are done routinely, but as far as I can determine, there is no specific difference in the incidence of ulcer when equivalent anti-inflammatory doses of the various steroids are used; however, there has been insufficient time for proper evaluation of the newer steroids.

DR. MOYER: Is this also true in the studies you have done on the effects of these drugs on gastric secretion?

DR. GRAY: Yes, the effects are about the same.

DR. THOMPSON: Dr. Gray, I think you referred to the fact that peptic ulcer is very rare in patients with Addison's disease. Certainly today we see many ulcers in patients with Addison's disease, especially in Negro patients in charity hospitals. What do you think the actual incidence of peptic ulcers in Addisonian patients is? I think it is high.

DR. GRAY: Do you see it in patients who are not on steroids?

DR. THOMPSON: No, the patients I referred to were all on steroids .

DR. GRAY: That is an exciting fact relating to the whole problem of the pathogenesis of ulcers. Prior to the availability of steroids, patients with Addison's disease practically never had peptic ulcers unless they were in an adrenal crisis or shock, and that is a different situation. Chronic peptic ulcer disease is extremely rare in patients with untreated Addison's disease, but when the Addisonian patient is given steroids, secretion of gastric acid and pepsin is often above normal, and ulcer production is not at all uncommon. This is also seen with replacement steroid therapy after bilateral adrenalectomy. In those patients steroids should be given only with food and with antacids. Our concept is that the adrenal steroids potentiate the histamine, antral and vagal processes related to gastric secretion. For example, in a patient with Addison's disease and histamine anacidity, histamine causes decided hyperacidity after only small doses of cortisone.

DR. THOMPSON: That has been our experience. In other words, there seems to be increased susceptibility to ulcer disease in patients with Addison's disease who are treated with steroids.

DR. HOWARD: Dr. Thompson, the British have reported acute pancreatitis as a complication of steroid therapy on several occasions. Have you or has anyone on the panel seen this?

DR. THOMPSON: No, I have not. Has anyone else here seen it? Apparently not.
   Dr. Brody, I was interested in your discussion about the psychological effects of steroid therapy. What is the first sign of a serious emotional disturbance in people who are receiving steroids? What are the early manifestations preceding severe mental symptoms or psychoses?

DR. BRODY: There is general agreement that the minor psychological reactions —that is, euphoria, restlessness and insomnia—may be the forerunners of major psychiatric reactions. However, I would like to point out an interesting phenomenon. A colleague of mine is treating a patient who had ulcerative colitis. The colitis cleared up completely after a year and a half of steroid therapy, but then the patient developed a classic paranoid psychosis. There seems to be a peculiar reciprocal relationship between psychoses and certain organic syndromes, and although there are many who scoff at the whole idea of such a relationship, there are others who have observed such a relationship in patients with asthma, rheumatoid arthritis and various other organic diseases.

DR. MOYER: Dr. Brody, in the first case you presented in your paper I was somewhat confused about the relationship of steroid therapy to the mental reaction. You stated that the patient had a definite psychiatric background going back to childhood, and then said the patient had a mental reaction as a result of steroid therapy. How did you differentiate between the already existing psychopathology and that due to the steroid?

DR. BRODY: This is a very important question. Many of the psychiatric articles stress the difficulty in trying to distinguish which factor started the process. In fact, some psychiatrists do not believe that the premorbid personality or prediseased personality is as important as the biochemical, physiological and pharmacological effects of the hormones on the central nervous system. There are others, however, including myself, who think that the premorbid personality is very important. In the patient that you are referring to, there is no question but that he had had life-long personality difficulties and a difficult family situation.

DR. MOYER: Then you are saying that you think the steroids act to trigger off a mechanism which is just waiting to be triggered?

DR. BRODY: I think that is a very good point, but it is likely that steroid treatment, plus the disease itself, plus all the other things that are going on in and about the patient play a vital role.

DR. GRAY: We observed a very similar situation in a patient with ulcerative colitis who was given steroids and became psychotic. He sued the hospital, but we found out that he had been a patient at Boston Psychopathic Hospital several years before, and that he had had an established psychosis which was not recognized at the time steroids were started. Administration of steroids just precipitated a new episode. I think that the most important premonitory sign is insomnia. Patients will often state that thoughts race through their minds so that they can not control them; this keeps them up all night and they become very excited and agitated. It is similar to the situation all of us have encountered from time to time when we are overly tired; it is difficult to go to sleep and all sorts of thoughts keep going through our minds. This is exactly the sort of thing that the patient first experiences, and whenever this occurs, I immediately reduce the dose of the steroids.

DR. MOYER: This is an interesting point; it is almost typical of the mental effects of Rauwolfia. Patients develop early morning insomnia and agitation which then may go on to a classic depression if Rauwolfia is not stopped.

DR. THOMPSON: In regard to the situation in ulcerative colitis, Dr. Brody's comments were quite interesting. I am sure both of us have seen patients who seem to be almost normal emotionally develop an acute psychotic reaction after colectomy. This reaction may become very serious, although it varies from a mild depression to a catatonic stupor.

DR. FUCHS: Dr. Brody, did you mean that the patient who develops a psychosis with steroid therapy has a personality which is possibly psychopathic to begin with, or would the theoretically normal person who is given steroids develop a psychosis? Must he have a neuropsychiatric disorder to begin with? In other words, does the person with ulcerative colitis get a psychosis because he was already abnormal to start with, or do perfectly normal, well-balanced people ever become psychotic as a result of steroid therapy?

DR. BRODY: The factors are complicated. Ulcerative colitis patients are rather familiar patients in psychiatrists' offices, and even internists tell me that all of these patients have mental difficulty. This also applies to severely ill patients with collagen diseases. It is often quite difficult to determine whether a given patient has a mental disorder, and even trained psychiatrists occasionally have difficulty.

DR. GRAY: Perhaps steroids could be used in a diagnostic fashion to make this tendency more obvious, as is done in patients with latent diabetes.

DR. THOMPSON: Dr. Howard, what preoperative preparation must be made in patients presently being treated with steroids and in those who have been treated with steroids in the recent past? For example, in patients with ulcerative colitis who have been treated with steroids for one to two years and who now require a colectomy, do you see a hazard in wound healing, and is there a need for any particular precaution in preparation?

DR. HOWARD: I think two problems may arise. One is the possibility of wound infection, and the other is difficulty in wound healing. I would anticipate these in many patients because of the nature of ulcerative colitis and the often associated malnutrition.

DR. TZIROS: I would agree with Dr. Howard. In many instances there is some evidence of delayed wound healing, and stay sutures should probably be used, but of course, this depends on the exact situation present.

DR. GRAY: Many of our patients with ulcerative colitis who have been on steroids for periods of two to four years have been operated on, and we have noticed a remarkable lack of wound healing problems; the wounds in these patients heal up very well. Most of the surgeons around Boston have remarked on this as being the difference between the theoretical and practical effect. However, we have had some infections due to accidental spillage of intestinal contents during surgery, since the bowel in these patients is very friable. I think the most important thing to do in patients having surgery after prolonged steroid therapy, or after any form of steroid therapy, is to give hydrocortisone intravenously during the operation—in the operating room. If you do not, sudden death may occur as in the instance quoted in the last panel discussion in a steroid-treated patient following injection of typhoid vaccine.

DR. THOMPSON: I would like to add to what Dr. Gray said. It always surprises me that in such a morbid process as ulcerative colitis we do not see more side effects from steroid therapy. In fact, I rarely see steroid ulcers in patients with ulcerative colitis, but I know the incidence is high in these patients, as has been brought out here. I have not encountered trouble with wound healing in ulcerative colitis, and, even when pyoderma is present, I have not seen spreading infections. Patients with ulcerative colitis seem almost immune to the side effects of steroid therapy.

DR. GRAY: We have done skin grafts in some patients with pyoderma gangrenosum, and although they have been on large doses of steroids for two or three weeks prior to surgery, the skin grafts have taken very well and have healed up completely.

DR. THOMPSON: Dr. Faludi, what methods do you use to make the diagnosis of steroid myopathy?

DR. FALUDI: In some patients, especially in the early stages, it may be very difficult to make the diagnosis. Many of the patients who receive high doses of steroids have a severe underlying condition and are bedridden. Neither the patient nor the physician may notice muscle weakness in this circumstance, or the patient may have a disease which in itself causes muscle weakness. Biopsies and electro-myographic examinations may be of help in some patients. However, if the patient has the classic symptoms and signs—weakness in the lower extremities, difficulty in walking, difficulty in getting up from sitting or squatting positions, evidence of muscle atrophy in the thigh and gluteal muscles—and particularly if the patient is taking triamcinolone, the diagnosis is not difficult.

DR. MILLS: Unfortunately, Dr. Dubois is not present on this panel, but he told me about a patient with steroid myopathy whom he had seen recently, the myopathy developing during triamcinolone therapy. In this patient, the total body potassium pool was normal. Because of the myopathy the dose of triamcinolone was reduced gradually to 8 milligrams per day; however, even on this relatively low dose, the myopathy persisted. Triamcinolone was then discontinued and cortisone was substituted in an equivalent anti-inflammatory dose of 50 milligrams per day. In spite of cortisone therapy, the myopathy disappeared and the muscles returned to normal. Since the myopathy disappeared in this circumstance, it appears that there was something specific about the triamcinolone structure which led to the development of the myopathy and that it was not due to potassium loss or due to the general protein catabolic or anti-anabolic properties that characterize this group of steroids.

INDEX

887